Understanding Your Health

Eleventh Edition

Wayne A. Payne, Ed.D.

Dale B. Hahn, Ph.D.

Ellen B. Lucas, Ph.D.

All of Ball State University
Muncie, Indiana

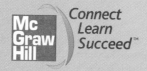

Mc Graw Hill

Connect
Learn
Succeed™

*To all our students, with the hope that the
decisions they make will be healthy ones.*

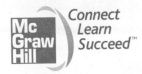

Published by McGraw-Hill, an imprint of The McGraw-Hill Companies, Inc., 1221 Avenue of the
Americas, New York, NY 10020. Copyright © 2011, 2009, 2007, 2005, 2002, 2000, 1998, 1995, 1992,
1989, 1986. All rights reserved. No part of this publication may be reproduced or distributed in any
form or by any means, or stored in a database or retrieval system, without the prior written consent
of The McGraw-Hill Companies, Inc., including, but not limited to, in any network or other
electronic storage or transmission, or broadcast for distance learning.

This book is printed on acid-free paper.

1 2 3 4 5 6 7 8 9 0 RMN/RMN 1 0

ISBN: 978-0-07-338088-9
MHID: 0-07-338088-1

Vice President, Editorial: *Michael Ryan*
Director, Editorial: *William R. Glass*
Executive Editor: *Christopher Johnson*
Marketing Manager: *William Minick*
Director of Development: *Kathleen Engelberg*
Development Editor: *Sarah Hill*
Editorial Coordinator: *Lydia Kim*
Production Editor: *Rachel J. Castillo*
Production Service: *Melanie Field, Strawberry Field Publishing*
Manuscript Editor: *Robin Gold*
Design Manager: *Ashley Bedell*
Photo Researcher: *Poyee Oster*
Production Supervisor: *Louis Swaim*
Media Project Manager: *Jennifer Barrick*
Composition: *10.5/12 Minion by Laserwords Private Limited*
Printing: *45# New Era Matte Plus, R.R. Donnelley & Sons*

Cover: © *Tay Rees/The Image Bank/Getty Images*

Photo credits: The photo credits section for this book begins on page 583 and is considered an
extension of the copyright page.

Library of Congress Cataloging-in-Publication Data

Payne, Wayne A.
    Understanding your health/Wayne Payne, Dale Hahn, Ellen Lucas.—11th ed.
      p. cm.
    ISBN-13: 978-0-07-338088-9 (alk. paper)
    ISBN-10: 0-07-338088-1 (alk. paper)
    1. Health. 2. College students—Health and hygiene. I. Hahn, Dale B. II. Mauer, Ellen. III. Title.

RA777.3.P39 2011
613—dc22

                            2009047281

The Internet addresses listed in the text were accurate at the time of publication. The inclusion of
a Web site does not indicate an endorsement by the authors or McGraw-Hill, and McGraw-Hill does
not guarantee the accuracy of the information presented at these sites.

www.mhhe.com

Brief Contents

Contents

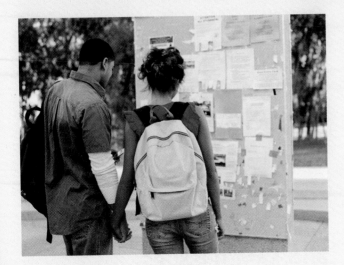

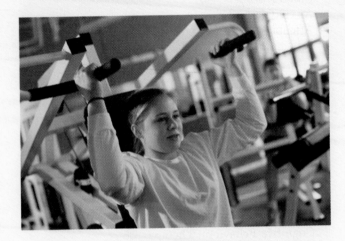

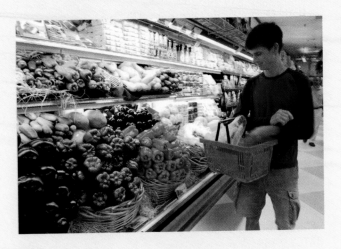

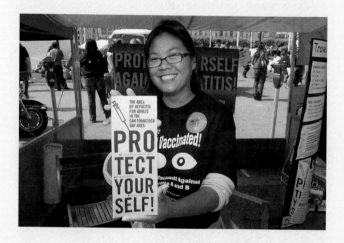

Part Five: Sexuality and Reproduction   386

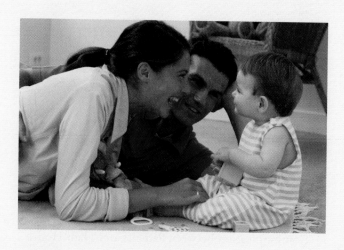

Boxes in Text

Building Media Literacy Skills

Changing for the Better

Learning from Our Diversity

Discovering Your Spirituality

Considering Complementary Care

Star

Preface

As a health educator, you already know that personal health is one of the most exciting courses a college student will take. Today's media-oriented college students are aware of the critical health issues of the new millennium. They hear about environmental issues, substance abuse, sexually transmitted diseases, fitness, and nutrition virtually every day. The value of the personal health course is its potential to expand students' knowledge of these and other health topics. Students will then be able to examine their attitudes toward health issues and modify their behavior to improve their health and perhaps even prevent or delay the onset of certain health conditions.

Understanding Your Health accomplishes this task with a carefully composed, well-documented text that addresses the health issues most important to both instructors and students. As health educators, we understand the teaching issues you face daily in the classroom and have written this text with your concerns in mind.

Hallmarks of the Text

Several unique themes and features set *Understanding Your Health* apart from other personal health texts. These successful features continue to define *Understanding Your Health* in its eleventh edition.

A Text for All Students

This book is written for college students in a wide variety of settings, from community colleges to large four-year universities. The content is carefully constructed to be meaningful to students of all ages. We have paid special attention to the increasing numbers of nontraditional-age students (those over age 25) who have decided to pursue a college education. *Understanding Your Health* continues to encourage students of all ages and backgrounds to achieve their goals.

Two Central Themes

Throughout the text, two central themes—the multiple dimensions of health and the developmental tasks—offer students a foundation for understanding their own health and achieving positive behavior change. The multiple dimensions of health are introduced in Chapter 1 and revisited in each part opener, where they are discussed in the context of the chapters that follow. The developmental tasks are also introduced in Chapter 1, where they are applied to young, middle, and older adulthood.

Flexible Organization

The eleventh edition of *Understanding Your Health* has 21 chapters. The first stands alone as an introductory chapter that explains the focus of the book. The arrangement of the remaining chapters follows the recommendations of both the users of previous editions of the book and reviewers for this edition. Of course, professors can choose to cover the chapters in any sequence that suits the needs of their courses.

Wellness and Disease Prevention

Throughout this new edition, students are continually urged to be proactive in shaping their future health. Even the chapter titles invite students to take control of their health behavior.

Integrated Presentation of Aging

Topics of interest to midlife and older adults are integrated into appropriate chapters according to subject. This organization allows both traditional-age and nontraditional-age students to learn about the physical and emotional changes that take place as we age.

Separate Coverage of Cancer and Chronic Conditions

Rapid developments in cancer prevention, diagnosis, and treatment warrant a single comprehensive chapter on cancer, in which we present the latest research and information. In addition, *Understanding Your Health* features a separate chapter in which more than 20 of the most common chronic conditions are discussed.

Technology: The Key to Teaching and Learning

Just a quick glance through the pages of *Understanding Your Health* shows that technology is woven throughout every chapter, both in the content and in the chapter pedagogy. Similarly, the package of supplements that accompanies the text emphasizes technology. Together, the text and its supplements offer the ideal approach to teaching and learning—one that integrates the best tools that technology has to offer, challenging both instructors and students to reach higher.

Updated Coverage: New and Expanded Topics

As experienced health educators and authors, we know how important it is to provide students with the most current information available. The eleventh edition of *Understanding Your Health* has been thoroughly updated with the latest information, statistics, and findings. A summary of notable changes for each chapter follows.

Chapter 1

- New section on life roles (child, employee, parent, etc.) and their reciprocal relationships with developmental tasks and a refined definition of health
- New Star box, "Factors That Influence Health and Well-Being"
- New Figure 1-2, illustrating the role and composition of health
- New discussions that address the limitations of our current medical care system

Chapter 2

- Updated statistics and data throughout
- Former Figures 2-2 and 2-3 are now combined into one figure
- New Considering Complementary Care box on using brain waves and electrical activity to diagnose and treat mental illness

Chapter 3

- New Figure 3-4 showing what percentages of students work 20 hours or more a week, provide child-care for 11 hours or more a week, and commute more than 6 hours a week
- Revised Figures 3-5 and 3-6
- New Building Media Literacy Skills box, "Advertisers May Be Selling You Stress"

Chapter 4

- New coverage of the U.S. Department of Health and Human Services' 2008 policy recommendations on physical activity
- Updated American College of Sports Medicine (ACSM) guidelines for recommended exercise intensity levels, target heart rate levels, resistance training, and flexibility

Chapter 5

- Revised and updated Figure 5-1, Composition of Dietary Fats
- Streamlined Table 5.3, USDA Food Guide at Six Different Calorie Levels, for better readability
- Table 5.6, Nutritional Facts for Popular Fast-Food Menu Items, fully updated
- New Considering Complementary Care box, "Is Juice the Next Miracle Drink?"
- Revised Mediterranean diet pyramid in the box "Diverse Food Pyramids"
- Updated information throughout, including the latest research findings on the DASH diet, vegetarianism, and food poisoning, and discussion of recent salmonella outbreaks, artificial sweeteners, and the latest FDA regulations

Chapter 6

- Figure 6-1, Rates of Overweight and Obesity among Americans, revised to include most current statistics
- Former Table 6.2 revised and expanded to become Figure 6-2 to include the most current obesity statistics and states with the lowest obesity rates
- Coverage of recent developments related to weight-management strategies, including gastric sleeve resection and lipodissolve
- Figure 6-3 revised to include an illustration of gastric sleeve resection, which is also now discussed in the text

Chapter 7

- Updated statistics throughout, including for Figures 7-2 and 7-3.
- New discussion of process addictions
- Revised Building Media Literacy Skills box, "Do Public Service Announcements Make a Difference?"
- New Considering Complementary Care box on rapid detoxification
- Learning from Our Diversity box includes an expanded discussion of how marijuana use can affect relationships

Chapter 8

- New Table 8.1, Blood Alcohol Concentration Effects for Men and Women (replaces former Table 8.1, which showed only the effects for a 160-pound man)
- Fully updated to include the latest statistics on alcohol use and alcohol-related problems, including updated data for Figure 8-2
- Information on alcohol-related legal problems has been converted from boxed information to a section in the chapter and includes updated information on the costs associated with DUIs
- Rewritten section on responsible drinking

Chapter 9

- Updated statistics throughout, including Table 9.2
- New table on the top 10 states with the highest and lowest smoking rates
- Updated information in the section on new product development and a new photo
- Rewritten Discovering Your Spirituality and Considering Complementary Care boxes
- New section and table on medically managed smoking cessation
- New end-of-chapter Personal Assessment featuring a revised version of the Fagerström test for nicotine dependence

Chapter 10

- Updated statistics throughout, including for Figure 10-1 and Table 10.1
- New photo of an automated external defibrillator

Chapter 11

- Updated statistics throughout, including for Figure 11-2 and Table 11.1
- Updated information on breast, colorectal, and prostate screening recommendations
- New Star box on prophylactic mastectomies
- Revised and updated section on treatment for breast cancer
- Revised final section in chapter, "Cancer and a Sense of Well-Being"

Chapter 12

- New Star box, "Delivering the Very Best Medicine—No Prescription Required"
- New Considering Complementary Care box, "Busy Brains Don't Need Special Exercise"
- Revised final section in chapter, "Chronic Conditions and a Sense of Well-Being"

Chapter 13

- Coverage of the lifting of stem cell research restrictions
- Discussion of the unsubstantiated contention that the MMRP vaccine causes autism
- Updated Immunization Schedule for Adults (Figure 13-4)
- Updated information on flu medications and coverage of the swine flu epidemic of 2009
- Updated statistics on HIV/AIDS incidence, including for Table 13.3
- Discussion of syphilis moved from Star box into the chapter text
- New section on "Sexually Transmitted Diseases, Health, Role Fulfillment, and a Sense of Well-Being"

Chapter 14

- New information on low-estrogen birth control pills that have also been approved to treat PMDD symptoms

- Updated information on androgen replacement therapy

Chapter 15

- Revised section on "Same-Sex Marriage"
- Updated statistics throughout

Chapter 16

- New Star Box, "New President, New Policy"
- Updated information on the effectiveness of abstinence-only programs
- Revised section on partial-birth abortion

Chapter 17

- New discussions of the ethical questions surrounding IVF and changes to government policy regarding the use of embryonic stem cells
- Former Star box on home pregnancy tests now moved into the "Signs of Pregnancy" section

Chapter 18

- Updated information on the types and coverage of health insurance options, the pharmaceutical industry, and the current health (medical) care debate

Chapter 19

- Updated statistics throughout, including for Figure 19-1
- New Figure 19-2
- Changing for the Better box "Don't Be a Victim of Violent Crime" now includes a section for staying safe when among strangers

Chapter 20

- New Table (20.2) that consolidates information about how to minimize exposure to pollutants in the home, neighborhood, and workplace
- Expanded and updated discussions of phthalates and bisphenol A
- Revised and updated Star box, "The High-Tech Revolution and E-Waste"

Chapter 21

- New information on how to become an organ donor and how patients are linked with matching donors
- Updated discussions on near-death experiences, interacting with dying people, and funeral costs

Student-Friendly Chapter Pedagogy

Each chapter of *Understanding Your Health* is rich with pedagogical features that offer a variety of ways to address new and emerging health issues and to pique student interest in particular topics.

"What Do You Know?" Quizzes

Each chapter opens with a brief quiz to challenge students and help spark their interest in key topics. Quiz answers are found at the end of the chapter.

Building Media Literacy Skills

Face it—a student's world revolves around media of all types, especially the Web. Students get most of their health information not from instructors and textbooks but from television, self-help books, popular news magazines, the Web, and the radio. To meet students on this familiar ground, we've included Building Media Literacy Skills boxes, which take a critical look at these media sources of health information. Topics include evaluating websites and health news stories, media messages about body image, smoking in movies, anti-drug public service announcements, alcohol ads directed at young people, and interpersonal relationships as portrayed in popular TV dramas.

Discovering Your Spirituality

Spirituality has become an important focus in health courses. Discovering Your Spirituality boxes highlight the spiritual dimension of health and its effect on overall wellness. The boxes cover topics such as mindfulness, yoga, living well with cancer or a chronic infectious disease, making decisions about sex, and having an enjoyable social life without abusing alcohol or other drugs.

Considering Complementary Care

This feature highlights nontraditional approaches to health care. Topics include the use of herbal supplements, acupuncture, hypnotism, Ayurveda, and dietary aids. Students are encouraged to critique these approaches, weighing their possible advantages and disadvantages. Although methods that are known to be dangerous are clearly identified as such, students are invited to consider new approaches that are becoming more accepted because they show promising results. An underlying theme is patient responsibility coupled with a physician's advice.

Changing for the Better

These unique question-and-answer boxes show students how to put health concepts into practice. Each box begins with a real-life question, followed by helpful tips and practical advice for initiating behavior change and staying motivated to follow a healthy lifestyle. Topics include fighting depression, eating well on the go, improving one's marriage, helping the bereaved, and performing self-exams for cancer.

Learning from Our Diversity

These boxes expose students to alternative viewpoints and highlight what we can learn from the differences that make us unique. Topics include women and alcohol, diverse food pyramids, gender and body image, violence against people with disabilities, smoking patterns around the world, and relationships among race, economic status, and exposure to pollution.

Star Boxes

In each chapter, special material in Star boxes encourages students to delve into a particular topic or closely examine an important health issue. Topics covered in Star boxes include Internet addiction, suicide intervention, energy drinks, and cell phone safety.

Talking Points

Interspersed throughout each chapter, Talking Points offer students opportunities to explore how they might start a dialogue about specific health-related issues and situations.

Personal Assessments

Each chapter ends with at least one Personal Assessment inventory. These self-assessment exercises serve three important functions: to capture students' attention, to serve as a basis for introspection and behavior change, and to provide suggestions for carrying the applications further.

Taking Charge of Your Health

Located at the end of each chapter, these bulleted lists invite students to put the knowledge and information they've gleaned from the chapter to work in their everyday lives. Cross-referencing the text with Internet links and real-world situations allows students to see how what they've learned can be applied in their own lives.

Definition Boxes

Key terms are set in boldface type and defined in corresponding boxes. Pronunciation guides are provided where appropriate. Other important terms in the text are set in italics for emphasis. Both approaches facilitate student vocabulary comprehension.

Chapter Summaries

Each chapter concludes with a bulleted summary of key concepts and their significance or application. The student can then return to any topic in the chapter for clarification or study.

Review Questions

A set of questions appears at the end of each chapter to aid the student in review and analysis of chapter content.

Illustrations and Photos

The inviting look and bold colors of the eleventh edition draw the reader into the book. Appealing photographs, attractive illustrations, and informative tables help support and clarify the chapter material.

Comprehensive Health Assessment

The Comprehensive Health Assessment at the end of Chapter 1 allows students to take a close look at their current state of health, typical health behavior, and risk factors. Using this assessment, students can pinpoint trouble spots in their own health behavior and find out what they can do to reduce their risk of disease or other health conditions. At the end of the semester, they can take a look at their previous answers to see how their behavior changed as they learned more about health and wellness issues.

Comprehensive Glossary

At the end of the text, all terms defined in boxes are merged into a comprehensive glossary.

First-Aid Appendix

This updated appendix outlines important general first-aid measures, such as what to do when someone is choking, bleeding, or in shock. It includes a special section on recognition and first-aid treatment of epileptic seizures.

Supplements

An extensive supplements package is available to adopters to enhance the teaching-learning process. We have made a concerted effort to produce supplements of extraordinary utility and quality. This package has been carefully planned and developed to help instructors derive the greatest benefit from the text. We encourage instructors to examine them carefully. Many of the products can be packaged with the text at a discounted price. Beyond the following brief descriptions, additional information about these supplements is available from your McGraw-Hill sales representative.

Online Learning Center

www.mhhe.com/payne11e

The Online Learning Center (OLC) to accompany this text offers many additional resources for both students and instructors. Visit this website to find useful materials such as the following:

For the instructor

- Course Integrator Guide: This guide includes all the useful features of an instructor's manual, such as learning objectives, suggested lecture outlines, suggested activities, media resources, and Web links. It also integrates the text with all the related resources McGraw-Hill offers, such as the Online Learning Center and the HealthQuest CD-ROM. The guide also includes references to relevant print and broadcast media.
- Test Bank: This file includes more than 1,000 questions, including multiple-choice, true/false, and short essay.
- Computerized Test Bank: The test bank is available with EZ Test computerized testing software. EZ Test provides a powerful, easy-to-use test maker to create printed quizzes and exams. For secure online testing, exams created in EZ Test can be exported to WebCT, Blackboard, PageOut, and EZ Test online. EZ Test comes with a Quick Start Guide, and once the program is installed, users have access to a User's Manual and Flash tutorials. Additional help is available online at www.mhhe.com/eztest.
- PowerPoint Slides: You can modify the presentations as much as you like to meet the needs of your course.
- Image Bank: This collection of illustrations from *Understanding Your Health* can be used to highlight lecture points or be incorporated into PowerPoint slides.
- High-Definition Videos: This collection of short video clips correlates with chapter topics and is designed to engage students in class discussions and promote critical thinking. The videos feature student interviews and historical health videos on body image, depression, alcohol and drug use, stress, intimate relationships, and many other topics. Videos can be downloaded to a computer or viewed directly from the OLC. Selected video clips include Instructor Video Guides with objectives and critical thinking and discussion questions. (Longer videos, including those from Films for the Humanities, are also available; check with your sales representative for more information.)

- Classroom Performance System (CPS) questions: These questions work with the CPS wireless classroom response system, which gives instructors and students immediate feedback from the entire class.
- Links to professional resources.

For the student

- Self-scoring chapter quizzes
- Flash cards for learning key terms and their definitions
- Audio chapter summaries
- Learning objectives
- Interactive activities
- Web links for study and exploration of topics in the text
- Online self-assessments
- Articles on additional topics

HealthQuest CD-ROM, by Bob Gold and Nancy Atkinson

The HealthQuest CD-ROM (ISBN 0-07-295117-6) helps students explore their wellness behavior using state-of-the-art interactive technology. Students can assess their current health status, determine their risks, and explore options for positive lifestyle change. Tailored feedback gives students a meaningful and individualized learning experience without using valuable classroom time. Modules include the Wellboard (a health self-assessment); Stress Management and Mental Health; Fitness; Nutrition and Weight Control; Communicable Diseases; Cardiovascular Health; Cancer; Tobacco, Alcohol, and Other Drugs.

Fitness and Nutrition Log

This logbook (ISBN 0-07-734970-9) helps students track their diet and exercise programs. It serves as a diary to help students monitor their behaviors. It can be packaged with any McGraw-Hill textbook for a small additional fee.

NutritionCalc Plus

http://nutritioncalc.mhhe.com

NutritionCalc Plus is a dietary analysis program with an easy-to-use interface that allows users to track their nutrient and food group intakes, energy expenditures, and weight control goals. It generates a variety of reports and graphs for analysis, including comparisons with My-Pyramid and the latest Dietary Reference Intakes (DRIs). The database includes thousands of ethnic foods, supplements, fast foods, and convenience foods, and users can add their own foods to the food list. NutritionCalc Plus is available on CD-ROM or in an online version.

PageOut: The Course Website Development Center

www.pageout.net

PageOut, free to instructors who use a McGraw-Hill textbook, is an online program you can use to create your own course website. PageOut offers the following features:

- A course home page
- An instructor home page
- A syllabus (interactive and customizable, including quizzing, instructor notes, and links to the text's Online Learning Center)
- Web links
- Discussions (multiple discussion areas per class)
- An online gradebook
- Links to student Web pages

Contact your McGraw-Hill sales representative to obtain a password.

Course Management Systems

Instructors can combine their McGraw-Hill Online Learning Center with today's most popular course management systems. Consult your McGraw-Hill sales representative to learn what other course management systems are easily used with McGraw-Hill online materials.

CourseSmart eTextbook

This text is available as an eTextbook at www.CourseSmart.com. At CourseSmart, your students can take advantage of significant savings off the cost of a print textbook, reduce their impact on the environment, and gain access to powerful web tools for learning. CourseSmart eTextbooks can be viewed online or downloaded to a computer. The eTextbooks allow students to do full text searches, add highlighting and notes, and share notes with classmates. CourseSmart has the largest selection of eTextbooks available anywhere. Visit www.CourseSmart.com to learn more and to try a sample chapter.

Primis Online

www.primisonline.com

Primis Online is a database-driven publishing system that allows instructors to create content-rich textbooks, lab manuals, or readers for their courses directly from the Primis website. The customized text can be delivered in print or electronic (eBook) form. A Primis eBook is a digital version of the customized text (sold directly to students as a file downloadable to their computer or accessed online by a password). *Understanding Your Health*, eleventh edition, is included in the database.

Acknowledgments

The publisher's reviewers made excellent comments and suggestions that were very useful to us in writing and revising the eleventh edition of this book. Their contributions are present in every chapter. We would like to express our sincere appreciation for both their critical and comparative readings.

Christine Bouffard, *Waubonsee Community College*
Dawn Brammer, *Chadron State College*
Sandy Frazier, *Ohio Dominican University*
Monair Hamilton, *Coastal Carolina University*
Dennis Johnson, *Wingate University*
Rich Morris, *Rollins College*
Dave Oster, *Jefferson College*
Kay Perrin, *University of South Florida College of Public Health*
Janne Postma, *Wayne State University*
Tabatha Tovar, *Southwestern College*
Ashley Walker, *University of North Texas*

Special Acknowledgments

In our early years of writing, we quickly realized that we were not working alone. To publish successful textbooks, an entire team of professionals must work together for a significant amount of time. During the past three decades, we have worked with many talented people to publish nearly 25 editions of three college textbooks.

For this eleventh edition of *Understanding Your Health,* we used the professional expertise and writing talents of a team of three contributing authors, all professors at Ball State University. Lenny Kaminsky, Ph.D., Professor of Exercise Science and Coordinator, Clinical Exercise Physiology and Adult Physical Fitness Programs, took on the task of revising and updating Chapter 4 (Becoming Physically Fit) and Chapter 10 (Enhancing Your Cardiovascular Health). Robert Pinger, Ph.D., Professor in the Department of Physiology and Health Science, revised Chapter 19 (Protecting Your Safety). David LeBlanc, Ph.D., Professor of Biology, revised Chapter 20 (The Environment and Your Health). We thank these experienced contributors for their professional dedication to this book and their personal commitment to the health of college students with whom they work on a daily basis.

The sponsoring editor for this edition of *Understanding Your Health* is Chris Johnson. Chris is also the executive editor for Health and Human Performance at McGraw-Hill Higher Education. Interestingly, Chris proved his dedication to our textbooks by moving from San Francisco to the Indianapolis area just to be closer to his handful of Ball State University authors! Although we say this "tongue in cheek," it is abundantly clear to us that Chris has watched over the development of this edition with a careful eye. Chris exhibits a positive vision for the future of our personal health textbooks. With his good sense of humor and level-headed thinking, Chris is a person we hope to work with on many future editions.

New to the eleventh edition of *Understanding Your Health* is our developmental editor, Sarah Hill. We have known Sarah for a few years but, until now, we had not worked with her on a full project. Simply stated, it has been a real treat to work with Sarah. She is a great communicator with a knack for identifying knotty editorial problems and finding the best solutions for those problems. She is gentle, but persistent. Sarah tactfully seeks consensus among the authors and deals directly with issues as they come up. She refuses to let our wheels spin with indecision. For all of these traits, we are very thankful to have Sarah as the McGraw-Hill person most closely attached to this revision.

On the production end of this textbook, we interacted with many people for the first time. Two people particularly stand out. Rachel Castillo was our production editor. Rachel's duties were to oversee the entire production end of this project. Although we did not have day-to-day contact with Rachel, it was comforting knowing that our revised manuscript was being carefully watched over by Rachel's experienced eyes. Thank you for coordinating this massive effort, Rachel.

Robin Gold worked with us for the first time as our manuscript editor. We have worked with many editors in this capacity, but few were as dedicated to the manuscript as Robin. Affable and easy to work with, Robin calmly turned into a "hawk" when it came to finding better ways to get our points across in the manuscript. Much of the clarity in the writing is due to Robin's fine work. Thanks, Robin.

We were quite fortunate to have Melanie Field serve as our production manager. Melanie worked with us on our last revisions, so we had a good feel for her experience and her vision for our books. (Plus, we all have enjoyed the clever, evocative name of her company, Strawberry Field Publishing.) Melanie again did a wonderful job of juggling this book and its shorter version simultaneously. She did this with her own quiet enthusiasm, grace, and humor. Certainly, it was a challenge for her to work on two books with three authors and three contributors. Thank you for agreeing to work with us on these editions, Melanie.

Finally, we would like to thank our families for their continued support and love. More than anyone else, they know the energy and dedication it takes to write and revise textbooks. To them we continue to offer our sincere admiration and loving appreciation.

Wayne A. Payne
Dale B. Hahn
Ellen B. Lucas

Shaping Your Health

What Do You Know About Health and Wellness?

1. The label *millennial generation* encompasses all of today's traditional-age college students. True or False?

2. Society holds developmentally oriented expectations for young adults, but not for middle-aged and older adults. True or False?

3. Definitions of health derived from episodic and preventive medicine are strongly influenced by concerns related to morbidity and mortality. True or False?

4. Persons with diagnosed disabilities, both visible and hidden, compose less than 5 percent of the current college student population. True or False?

5. The loss of functionality is a reality for many older adults. True or False?

6. Males' shorter life expectancy, compared with that of females, results almost completely from males' greater genetic weakness. True or False?

7. A holistic perception of health is a perception totally focused on the structure and function of the body. True or False?

Check your answers at the end of the chapter.

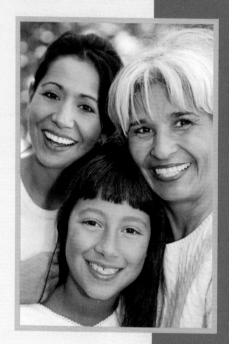

"Take care of your health, because you'll miss it when it's gone," younger people hear often from their elders. This simple and heartfelt advice is given in the belief that young people take their health for granted and assume that they will always maintain the state of health and wellness they now enjoy. Observation and experience should, however, remind all of us that youth is relatively brief, and health is always changing.

How do you imagine your life in the future? Do you ever think about how your health allows you to participate in meaningful life activities—and what might happen if your health is compromised? Consider, for example, how your health affects the following activities:

- Your ability to pursue an education or a career
- Your opportunities to socialize with friends and family
- The chance to travel—for business, relaxation, or adventure
- The opportunity to meet and connect with new people
- The ability to conceive or the opportunity to parent children
- Your participation in hobbies and recreational activities

- Your enjoyment of a wide range of foods
- The opportunity to live independently

As you will learn in this chapter, quality of life is intertwined with activities such as these—indeed, your authors will present a new definition of health specifically related to accomplishing these and the important life roles that you will assume. But first, let's review the millennial generation of which traditional-age students are a part of, the traditional developmental tasks of adulthood, and a few familiar perceptions about health. This chapter will provide you with a foundation for understanding your own health, as well as strategies for changing problematic health behaviors.

The Millennial Generation

The general period of young adulthood (ages 18–39) is often divided into subperiods: early young adulthood (ages 18–24), middle young adulthood (25–33), and later young adulthood (34–39). Traditional-age college students are what we will call "early young adults" (ages 18–24). Nontraditional-age college students are students of all other age groups—middle young adults, later young adults, as well as older individuals in middle or older adulthood and the occasional teenager and even preteenager!

"Millennial generation" is the name given to today's early young adults, 18 to 24 years old.[1] If you are a nontraditional-age student reading this textbook, you will have your own generational "name." But if you are of traditional age (18–24), you are being placed in a larger group of persons, born between 1982 and 2000 and referred to collectively by sociologists as "millennials." The majority of today's young adults (18–39 years) are all millenials; thus early young adults (18–24 years) are millenials too.

There have been some initial studies of the millennial generation's progress in mastering the developmental expectations for the transition from adolescence to early adulthood. (These expectations are discussed later in this chapter.) These studies have found that, compared to earlier generations, the millennials are[2, 3, 4]

- More inclined to drop out of college for a period of time, and take longer to finish college even if they have not dropped out
- More likely to change colleges, and to change residence while at the same college
- More likely to return home to live after completing college—the "boomerang" phenomenon
- More likely to share a residence with friends from college than to live alone or to return home
- More likely to take less-substantive jobs, often in food services and retail sales, that pay relatively low wages

- Likely to leave a job rather than deal with job-related conflict, thus not experiencing advancement within the workplace, while protecting their self-concept
- More inclined to fill leisure time with technology-based media
- Less likely to have refined communications skills, due in large part to technology-based communication
- More likely to volunteer—not to pad their résumés, but for the well-being of others
- More likely to have a more diverse group of friends, in terms of both gender and race
- Less likely to marry, less likely to marry at an younger age, and more likely to delay parenting until older

In spite of the bulleted findings regarding characteristics of millennials, some of which might seem somewhat regressive to members of the predecessor generation, the boomers, a recent report finds that a high level of self-esteem is carried into this period of life by recently arriving high school graduates.[5] In terms of their own future, will this initial high level of self-worth diminish over time or will they, as they age, be able to retain the positive perspectives on life that they are initially carrying into early young adulthood?

If you are a nontraditional-age student (particularly if you were born before 1982), take an opportunity to look back to your early young adult years and assess, from the perspective of your current age, how you handled your younger adult years. Also, speculate on how your soon-to-be-completed college education might have altered your initial progress through early young adulthood, if you had completed college at that younger age.

Developmental Tasks of Early Adulthood

Let's look next at some predictable areas of growth and development (defined as developmental expectations or tasks) that society has traditionally believed should characterize the lives of young adults. Of course, society's expectations for the next generation of early young adults are always stated in the context of permissible "uniqueness," thus allowing you a fair measure of latitude so that you can do things "your way." Your textbook will provide a brief and general view of each early young adult developmental task—note that five of these tasks are more immediate in their completion, while two are traditionally brought to fruition a bit later. Making progress in these areas contributes to a sense of well-being and life satisfaction.

Forming an Initial Adult Identity

As emerging adults, most young people want to present a personally satisfying initial adult identity as they transition from adolescence into early young adulthood. Internally they are constructing perceptions of themselves as the adults they wish to be; externally they are formulating the behavioral patterns that will project this identity to others. Completion of this first developmental task is necessary for early young adults to establish a foundation on which to nurture their identity during the later stages of adulthood.

Establishing Independence

Society anticipates that, by the time their college education is completed, younger adults should be moving away from their earlier socialization and dependent relationships, particularly with their family and adolescent peer group. Travel, new relationships, military service, marriage, and, of course, college studies have been the traditional avenues for disengagement from the family.

Assuming Responsibility

Our society's third developmental expectation for traditional-age college students is that these early young adults will assume increasing levels of responsibility. Traditional-age students have a variety of opportunities, both on and off the college campus, to begin the process of becoming responsible for themselves and for other individuals, programs, and institutions. Central at this time is the need to assume increasing levels of responsibility in one's movement through the academic curriculum and for one's own and others' health (see the box "The Internet—Your Health Superstore").

 TALKING POINTS What does being an adult mean to you at this point? How would you explain this to your best friend?

Broadening Social Skills

The fourth developmental task for early young adults is to broaden their range of appropriate and dependable social skills. Adulthood ordinarily involves "membership" in a variety of groups that range in size from a marital pair to a multiple-member community group or a multinational corporation. These memberships require the ability to function in many different social settings, with an array of people, and in many roles. Accomplishing this task particularly requires that early young adults refine their skills in communication, listening, and conflict management.

Nurturing Intimacy

The task of nurturing intimacy usually begins in early young adulthood and continues, in various forms, through much of the remainder of life. Persons of traditional college age can experience intimacy in a more mature sense, centered on deep and caring relationships, than was true

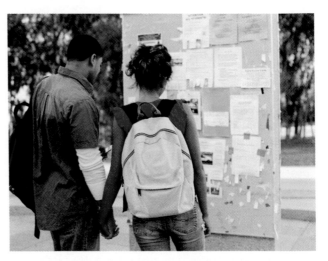

Developmental tasks for young adults include establishing independence from their families, assuming more responsibility for themselves and others, and nurturing intimate relationships, while playing the roles of student and friend.

during adolescence. Dating relationships, close and trusting friendships, and mentoring relationships are the arenas in which mature intimacy will take root. From a developmental perspective, what matters is that we have quality relationships involving persons with whom we share our most deeply held thoughts, feelings, and aspirations as we attempt to validate our own unique approach to life. Young adults who are unwilling or unable to create intimacy can develop a sense of emotional isolation.

Obtaining Entry-Level Employment and Developing Parenting Skills

In addition to the five developmental tasks just addressed, two other areas of growth and development seem applicable to early young adults, but may come into "focus" more gradually. They include obtaining entry-level employment within the field of one's academic preparation and the development of parenting skills.

For nearly three-quarters of a century (thanks in part to the GI Bill after World War II), the majority of students have pursued a college education in anticipation that its completion would open doors (entry-level opportunities) in particular professions or fields of employment. In many respects these forms of employment meet needs beyond those associated purely with money. Employment of this nature provides opportunities to build new skills that expand upon those learned in academic majors, to undertake new forms of responsibility beyond those available on campus, and to play a more diverse set of roles, including colleague, supervisor, mentor, mentee, or partner. And today, more so than in the past, intimate relationships often have their origin in the workplace.

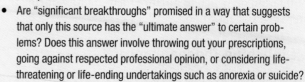
Although Americans today are having fewer children than in past generations, the fact remains that parenting-related decisions and skills are important components of the young adulthood years. Decisions regarding parenting (both biological and adoptive) involve important questions regarding age for the onset of parenting, number of children, and interval between subsequent children, as well as the manner in which parenting will be undertaken and the role it will play relative to the overall aspirations of the adults involved. In today's complex society, young adults need to more clearly than ever understand the significant differences between reproduction and parenting; thus we assign the development of parenting skills as a socially anticipated developmental task.

Developmental Tasks of Middle and Older Adulthood

For students of traditional college age, help in more fully understanding the developmental tasks of middle and older adulthood can be supplied by the nontraditional-age students with whom you are in class with, as well as by your parents, family friends, older coworkers, and grandparents.

Midlife Developmental Tasks

If you are a traditional-age student, have you wondered what it would be like to be 20 or 30 years older than you are now? What would you be doing, feeling, and thinking if you were the age of your parents? What are your parents thinking about and trying to accomplish as they move through their midlife years?

One thought that probably recurs all too often is the reality of their eventual death (see the box "Why Men Die Young"). Their awareness that they will not live forever is a subtle but profoundly influential force that can cause them to be restless, to renew attention to their spirituality, and to be more highly motivated to master the developmental tasks of middle adulthood. This motivation and the awareness of the reality of death combine to produce the dynamic concept of being at "the prime of life"—a time when there seems to be a great deal to accomplish and a diminishing amount of time in which to accomplish it.

Achieving Generativity   In a very real sense, people in middle adulthood are asked to do something they have not been expected to do previously. As a part of their development as unique people, they are expected to "pay back" society for the support it has given them. Most people in middle adulthood begin to realize that the collective society, through its institutions (families, schools, churches), has been generous in its support of their growth and development and that it is time to replenish these resources.[6, 7] Younger and older people may have needs that middle-aged people can best meet. By meeting the needs of others, people in middle adulthood can fulfill their own needs to grow and develop. *Generativity,*

Why Men Die Young

The extra longevity of women in our society is well established. In fact, the difference in life expectancy for infants born today is projected to be 80 years for females and only 75 for males. This 5-year difference has commonly been attributed to genetic factors. However, new evidence demonstrates that this discrepancy may be affected more by male behavior than by genetic traits.

Men outrank women in all of the top 15 causes of death except for Alzheimer's disease. Men's death rates are twice as high for suicide, homicide, and cirrhosis of the liver. In every age group, American males have poorer health and higher risk of mortality than do females. Common increased risks include the following:

- More men than women smoke.
- Men are twice as likely to be heavy drinkers and to engage in other risky behaviors such as abusing drugs and driving without a seat belt.
- More men work in dangerous settings than women do, and men account for 90 percent of on-the-job fatalities.
- More men drive SUVs that are rollover prone and suffer fatalities in motorcycle accidents.

Perhaps some of these increased risks are associated with deep-seated cultural beliefs, which reward men for taking risks and facing danger head-on. This "macho" attitude seems to extend to the care that men take of their own physical and mental health. Women are twice as likely as men to visit their doctor on an annual basis and explore preventive medical treatments. Men are more likely to ignore symptoms and less likely to schedule checkups or seek follow-up treatment. Psychologically, men tend to internalize their feelings or stressors, or even self-medicate to deal with stress, while women tend to seek psychological help. Almost all stress-related diseases are more common in men.

In the final analysis, men and women alike must be responsible for their own health and well-being. By making sound choices regarding diet, exercise, medical care, and high-risk behaviors, both genders can attempt to maximize the full potential of their life expectancy.

---

a term introduced into the field of adult emotional development by Erik Erikson,[8] reflects a process in which the emotional maturation needs of middle-aged people interact with society's need to support its most vulnerable members—its children and older adults, particularly the infirm and the frail.

The process of repaying society for its support is structured around familiar types of activities. Developmentally speaking, people in middle adulthood are able to select the activities that best use their abilities to contribute to the good of society.

The most traditional way in which people in middle adulthood repay society is through parenting. Children, with their potential for becoming valuable members of the next generation, need the support of people who recognize the contribution they can make. By supporting children, either directly through quality parenting or through institutions that function on behalf of children, middle-aged people repay society for the support they have themselves received. As they extend themselves outward on behalf of the next generation, they ensure their own growth and development. In a similar fashion, their support of aging parents and institutions that serve older adults provides another means to express generativity.

For people who possess artistic talent, generativity may be accomplished through the pleasure brought to others. Artists, craftspeople, and musicians have unique opportunities to speak directly to others through their talents. Volunteer work serves as another avenue for generativity. Most people in middle adulthood also express generativity through their jobs by providing quality products or services and thus contribute to the well-being of those who desire or need these goods and services.

Reassessing the Plans of Young Adulthood People in middle adulthood must also begin coming to terms with the finality of their death. In conjunction with doing this, they often feel compelled to take time to think about their goals for adulthood they formulated 25 or more years previously. Their dreams are thus revisited. This reassessment constitutes a second developmental task of people in middle adulthood.

By carefully reviewing the aspirations they had as young adults, middle-aged people can more clearly study their short- and long-term goals. Specifically, strengths and limitations that were unrecognizable when they were young adults are now more clearly seen. The inexperience of youth is replaced by the insights gained through experience. A commitment to quality often replaces the desire for quantity during the second half of the life cycle. Time is valued more highly because it is now seen in a more realistic perspective. The dream for the future is more sharply focused, and the successes and failures of the past are more fully understood as this developmental task of reassessing earlier plans of young adulthood is accomplished.

Developmental Tasks of Older Adulthood

In this section, we focus on the developmental tasks confronted by older adults. Accepting the physical changes of aging, maintaining physical functionality, and reassessing one's sense of integrity are tasks of the older adulthood period.

Accepting the Changes of Aging The general decline associated with the latter part of the life cycle is particularly serious between the seventh and ninth decades.

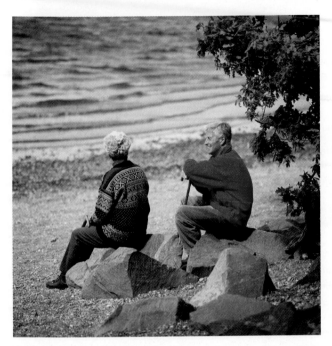

Accepting the physical changes of aging while maintaining a high level of functionality is a key developmental task for older adults.

Physically, emotionally, socially, intellectually, and occupationally, older adults must accept at least some decline. For example, a person may no longer be able to drive a car, which could in turn limit participation in social activities. Even a spiritual loss may be encountered at those times when life seems less humane. A developmental task to be accomplished by the older adult is to accept the nature and extent of these changes.

Maintaining Functionality Because each segment of the life cycle should be approached with the fullest level of involvement possible, the second developmental task of the older adult is to maintain as much functionality as possible, particularly those aspects of physical functioning that support independence.

For areas of decline in which some measure of reversal is possible, older adults are afforded an opportunity to seek *rehabilitation*. Whether through a self-designed and individually implemented program or with the aid of a skilled professional, older adults can bring back some function to a previously higher level.

The second approach, often used in combination with rehabilitation, is *remediation*, whereby an alternative to the area of loss is introduced. Examples of remediation include the use of hearing aids, audiocassettes, and caregivers or home health aids. By using alternative resources, an adequate level of functionality can be sustained.

For a growing number of older adults, rehabilitation and remediation are rarely necessary because of the high level of health that they enjoy. For most, only minor modifications are necessary to enjoy full independence.

Establishing a Sense of Integrity The third major developmental task that awaits older adults is to establish their sense of integrity, or sense of wholeness, concerning the journey that may be nearly complete.[8] The elderly must look back over their lives to see the value in what they were able to accomplish. They must address the simple but critical questions: Would I do it over again? Am I satisfied with what I managed to accomplish? Can I accept the fact that others will have experiences to which I can never return?

If older adults can answer these questions positively, then they will feel a sense of wholeness, personal value, and worth. Having established this sense of integrity, they will believe that their lives have had meaning and that they have helped society.

Because they have already experienced so much, many older adults have no fear of death, even though they may fear the process of dying. Their ability to come to terms with death thus reinforces their sense of integrity.

Like all the other developmental tasks, this critical area of growth and development is a personal and, thus, a unique experience. Older adults must assume this last developmental task with the same sense of purpose they used for earlier tasks. When older adults can feel this sense of integrity, their reasons for having lived will be more fully understood.

Roles and Their Reciprocal Relationship to Developmental Tasks

Throughout life individuals are assigned or selected to assume a variety of roles and, in doing so, to willingly assume the behavioral patterns that accompany (and define) these roles. Depending on the life cycle stage, we experience the majority of the following roles: a child, a sibling, a grandchild, a student, a peer group member, a team member, an employee, a significant other, a parent, an employer, a mentee or mentor, a neighbor, a community member, a grandparent, and so on. These roles are played out both privately and publicly, while depicting a reciprocal relationship with the major developmental tasks of each life cycle stage. For example, the development of an initial adult identity may influence and be influenced by the occupational role you are able to assume. Or, as a second example, a midlife adult's growth in generativity will have been influenced by her role as a parent and her pending role of being a grandparent. For those in older adulthood, the successful interplay of earlier developmental expectations and requirements associated with roles once (or still) played may be the basis of a salient question of this final life cycle stage: *Have I played my roles well? Was my life well lived?* Am I entitled to feel a sense of life satisfaction and the feeling of well-being that accompanies it?

Today's College Students

In the minds of most people the length of a generation has traditionally been described as 20 years. Today, however, with postponements in both the age of first marriage and the age of initial reproduction, this time frame may be too short. When discussing a "generation" of undergraduate students, however, a very different perception is required because this unique generation lasts only for approximately 5 years. This rapid turnover in students certainly keeps the college environment vibrant; it does, however, make it somewhat difficult to paint a continuously accurate picture of how the student population is composed. Some demographic trends continue rather predictably, such as female undergraduate students outnumbering male undergraduates. In other cases, a recession, such as that first officially announced in late 2008, can quickly alter the profile of the college population because loss of employment often stimulates college enrollment, particularly among the newly unemployed. You will find tables[9,10] that depict undergraduate enrollment categories based on the best evidence available at the time and based on longer range projections available on the book's Online Learning Center (www.mhhe.com/payne11e; see Tables 1 and 2). As a point of reference, **nontraditional-age students** are often defined as students who fall outside of the age range of 18 to 24 years that is typically used for **traditional-age students.**

 TALKING POINTS You are in charge of a campus event for students of various ages from several cultural groups. How would you go about finding out what would make the event attractive to students with backgrounds different from your own?

Perhaps one of the largest groups on campus, if we include those with non-obvious impairments, is disabled students. With enactment of the Americans with Disabilities Act in 1990, the opportunity for postsecondary education significantly increased. Today's students having one or more of a wide variety of disabilities, once identified, are able to enroll in virtually all of the institutions for postsecondary education to which the nondisabled have long enjoyed access and to have appropriate services available. Visit the book's Online Learning Center for a table listing the major classifications of disabilities encountered within the population,[11] some of which are clearly identifiable to the observer, while others are less obvious, as if to be "hidden" (www.mhhe.com/payne11e; see Table 3). Access to services is based on the substantiation of disability, a request for services, and the establishment of an interactive relationship with the institution's appropriate service coordination center. Faculty members are made aware of adjustments in the teaching-learning environment that are appropriate to the needs of students with particular disabilities.

As noted earlier, painting an accurate picture of the American undergraduate student population is less than a perfectly accurate process. This includes all student segments, including disabled students. The size of the disabled student portion of the student population ranges from a low of 6 percent, through 11 percent, to a percentage in the upper teens. Private colleges and universities usually have a smaller percentage of disabled students than do publicly supported schools.[12] The most prevalent disabilities are collectively encompassed by the term *specific learning disabilities.* Multiple disabilities can coexist in one particular student.

Sources of Our Traditional Definitions of Health

By the time they reach college age, most Americans are familiar with the many ways in which health care is provided. Following are some easily recognizable examples, all of which reinforce our traditional definitions of health. Note that these examples involve the cure or management of illness and the extension of life, indicated by concerns about **morbidity** and **mortality.**

Episodic Health Care

The vast majority of Americans use the services of professional health care providers during periods (*episodes*) of illness and injury, that is, when we are "unhealthy." We consult providers, seeking a diagnosis that will explain why we are not feeling well. Once a problem is identified, we expect to receive effective treatment from the practitioners that will lead to our recovery (the absence of illness) and thus a return to health. If we are willing to comply with the care strategies prescribed by our practitioners, we should soon be able to define ourselves as "healthy" once again.

The familiarity of episodic health care is evident in the 22 million times that Americans 18 or older visited

---

Key Terms
nontraditional-age students An administrative term used by colleges and universities for students who, for whatever reason, are pursuing undergraduate work at an age other than that associated with the traditional college years (18–24).
traditional-age students College students between the ages of 18 and 24.
morbidity Pertaining to illness and disease.
mortality Pertaining to death.

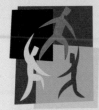
physicians during 2006.[13] Although some of these visits were for preventive health care (see the discussion in the next section), the vast majority were in conjunction with illness. When viewed according to racial group, approximately 80 percent of Whites, 79 percent of Blacks, 75 percent of Asians, 84 percent of Native Americans, 68 percent of Hispanic Americans, and 63 percent of Mexican Americans made one or more physician office visits in 2006. When viewed collectively, 13.5 percent of all Americans over the age of 18 made 10 or more visits.

Differences in the number of office visits by race are most likely related to a combination of factors, including differences in the types and extent of illnesses within specific racial groups, health insurance or ability to pay for health care services, proximity to services, availability of dependable transportation, and personal and cultural practices related to illness.

Of the 22 million office visits in 2006, women were more likely to visit physicians than were men, and infants and persons over 65 were twice as likely to visit physicians than were older children, adolescents, and adults under age 65. People living in metropolitan areas were one-third more likely to make physician visits than were people from nonmetropolitan areas. Again, no single factor accounts for these observed differences.

When office visits are viewed in terms of the types of physicians visited, primary care physicians accounted for the majority of visits while surgeons and other specialists accounted for the remainder. Usually surgeons and specialists become involved in a patient's care only after a referral from a primary care physician.

Preventive or Prospective Medicine

Simple logic would seem to suggest that it makes more sense to prevent illness than to deal with it through episodic health (medical) care. This philosophy characterizes **preventive or prospective medicine.** Unfortunately, however, many physicians say they have little time to practice preventive medicine because of the large number of episodically sick people who fill their offices every day.

When physicians do practice preventive or prospective medicine, they first attempt to determine their patient's level of risk for developing particular conditions. They make this assessment by identifying **risk factors** (and **high-risk health behaviors**) with a variety of observational techniques and screening tests, some of which may be invasive (taking tissues from the body such as a biopsy or blood draw). Additionally, an important tool in assessing risk is an accurate family health history, something that over one-third of all adults cannot adequately provide to their health care providers.[14] So important is a health history that the federal government has established a website to assist us in becoming familiar with our family's health history (www.hhs.gov/familyhistory).[15] Certainly, if you identify any of the leading causes of death, they should be shared with your primary care physician.[16]

It is disconcerting to report that important medical information, including laboratory reports, comprehensive drug inventories, and family health histories, are often missing from medical files. A 2003 study involving primary care physician medical records suggests that perhaps one out of every seven patient files is missing

What Is Complementary Medicine?

In addition to the episodic and preventive forms of medical care described earlier, a variety of other forms of health care, both curative and preventive, are moving more progressively into the medical care mainstream. Among these are chiropractic, reflexology, homeopathy, naturopathy, and herbalism (see Chapter 18), to mention but a few. Although the established medical community has long scoffed at these practices as being unscientific and ineffective, they are increasingly attractive to a growing segment of the population. Initially referred to collectively as *alternative* forms of health care, and more recently as *complementary* forms of care, today they are increasingly referred to as *integrative* forms of health care. This last term suggests a fusion (or integration) of various forms of care into traditional treatment/prevention approaches.

The increasing acceptance of integrative forms of health care is also seen in two relatively recent developments. The first is the formation in the mid-1990s of an Office of Complementary and Alternative Medicine within the National Institutes of Health. This office has been charged with the objective and systematic study of selected forms of nontraditional care. Clinical trials of various types are ongoing; they include *treatment trials, supportive care trials, prevention trials, screening trials* (early detection trials), and *diagnostic trials,* all

employing forms of alternative or complementary treatments. Subsequent assessments will be released as they are completed.

A second expression of the growing popularity of integrative forms of health care is the increasing tendency of health insurance companies and HMOs (health maintenance organizations; see Chapter 18) to provide reimbursement of services from providers of nontraditional care. Today approximately 65 percent of all HMOs and several major insurance companies provide coverage for selective forms of integrative care.

As impressive as the "rush to coverage" described previously might appear, consumers of medical care services should remember that at this time relatively little carefully controlled research is available on the *efficacy* (effectiveness) of most forms of integrative care.

In spite of cautionary notes such as this, the *popularity* of alternative medical services for improving, maintaining, or restoring health is beyond dispute. Today supplement use, relaxation breathing techniques, meditation, chiropractic, yoga, acupuncture, hypnosis, healing touch, and massage are all employed. Prayer, in various settings, was by far the most widely employed.

---

information important to providing comprehensive health care.[17]

Once they have identified levels of risk in patients, health practitioners try to lower those risk levels through patient education, lifestyle modification, and, when necessary, medical intervention. Continued compliance on the part of the patients should result in a lower level of risk that will continue over the years. Note that preventive medicine is guided by practitioners, and patients are expected to be compliant with the directions they are given.

Although preventive medical care appears to be a much more sensible approach than episodic care in reducing morbidity and mortality, third-party payers (insurance plans) traditionally have not provided adequate coverage for preventive services.

In recent years the belief that preventive or prospective medical care can reduce the incidence of chronic illnesses, and thus reduce the likelihood of premature death, has been clouded by conflicting results from studies involving prevention-oriented changes in lifestyle, including, among others, dietary practices, exercise protocols, smoking cessation, weight management strategies, the use of hormone supplementation, and the inclusion of spiritual practices in daily routines. This inconsistency in effectiveness is seen by many experts as being largely a methodological problem in research study design. However, when viewed from a cost-benefit perspective, there is now increasing concern that preventive (prospective) medicine may be less cost effective than treating some chronic conditions in a more

episodic manner.[18, 19] This concern encompasses some of the multifaceted problems mentioned earlier, in addition to the high cost of using expensive monitoring procedures over an extended number of years, as is often the case with preventive approaches to health care. Regardless, when successful, this form of health care provides some people with a personal sense of **empowerment**[20] that is always a useful resource for leading a healthy, productive, and satisfying life.

See the box "Considering Complementary Care" for more on broadening perspectives on health care.

Key Terms

preventive or prospective medicine Physician-centered medical care in which areas of risk for chronic illnesses are identified so that they might be lowered.

risk factor A biomedical index such as serum cholesterol level or a behavioral pattern such as smoking associated with a chronic illness.

high-risk health behavior A behavioral pattern, such as smoking, associated with a high risk of developing a chronic illness.

empowerment The nurturing of an individual's or group's ability to be responsible for their own health and well-being.

Health Promotion—Personal and Collective Empowerment

High-level health is more likely to be obtained by people who have been exposed to the knowledge, behavioral patterns, and attitudinal stances required in adopting a health-enhancing approach to living. Whether these "tools" for better health are sought out by an individual person or developed by a group of people working as a "learning community," they become the resources reflected in the term *empowerment*. Empowered persons, individually or collectively, are now active participants in their own health enhancement quest. Health promotion specialists have played an active role in leading people in this process.

Individually Oriented Health Promotion Throughout the United States, YMCA/YWCA-sponsored wellness programs, commercial fitness clubs, and corporate fitness centers offer risk-reduction programs under the direction of qualified instructors, many of whom are university graduates in disciplines such as exercise science, wellness management, and **health promotion.** Using approaches similar to those employed in preventive medicine, these nonphysician health professionals attempt to guide their clients toward activities and behaviors that will lower their risk of chronic illness. Unlike preventive medicine, with its sometimes invasive assessment procedures and medication-based therapies, health promotion programs are not legally defined as medical practices and thus do not require the involvement of physicians. In addition, the fitness focus, social interaction, and healthy lifestyle orientation these programs provide tend to mask the emphasis on preventing chronic illness that would be the selling point of such efforts if they were undertaken as preventive medicine. In fact, it is likely that people receiving health promotion in these settings do not recognize it as such. Rather, they are very often submitting to assessments and listening to health-related information only as incidental parts of personal goals, such as losing weight, preparing for their first marathon, or simply meeting friends for lunch-hour basketball.

Group-Oriented Health Promotion In addition to the practices just described, a group-oriented form of health promotion is offered in many communities. This approach to improving health through risk reduction is directed at empowering community groups, such as church congregations or neighborhood associations, so that they can develop, operate, and financially sustain their own programs with little direct involvement of health promotion specialists. Most often these community-based programs are initially funded by small governmental grants and, upon becoming self-funded, may have very small costs per person served. For example, one particular program, "Shape Up Somerville,"

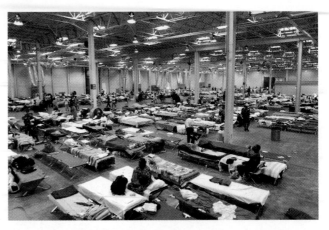

As survivors flocked to New Orleans' Superdome in the days following Hurricane Katrina, both health- and comfort-related needs of thousands were met in large part by community organizations using volunteers in a wide variety of roles.

estimates its cost of service at no more than 3 to 4 dollars per child served.[21]

Empowerment programs have produced positive health consequences for groups that traditionally have been underserved by the health care system, such as minority populations. Once such people are given needed information, inroads into the political process, and skills for accessing funding sources, they become better able to plan, implement, and operate programs tailored to their unique health needs.[22]

In virtually all areas of the country, small groups are engaged in the process of empowering people to eventually manage their own health and safety programs. These groups include neighborhood associations organizing Crime Watch programs and identifying "safe houses" for children to go to when they encounter situations they recognize as unsafe, churches sponsoring smoking abatement programs for members of their congregations, and locally organized groups of parents that petition the local school board to improve the healthfulness of the school lunch program.

Wellness

With the conclusion of an introduction to the traditionally morbidity- and mortality-based conceptions of health, your text can now introduce the most recent entry into the health care system, **wellness.** Recall that episodic health care, preventive medicine, and group-oriented health promotion are directly aligned with concerns about morbidity and mortality, whereas health promotion at the individual level is focused on aspects of appearance, weight management, body composition, and physical performance capabilities. Wellness differs from these kinds of health care concerns because it has virtually no interest in morbidity and mortality.

Factors That Influence Health and Well-Being

The schematic shown in Figure 1-1 is adapted from works undertaken by Canadian Ronald Labonte in various locations within Canada and presented in a meeting held at the University of Edinburgh, Edinburgh, Scotland. The research protocol identified four arenas from which conditions beneficial to higher-level health and a sense of well-being arose. The conclusion was that when these conditions were experienced simultaneously, they led to an enhanced quality of life, higher levels of functionality, and a sense of well-being. Although not conducted in this country, these findings would most likely mirror the same factors influencing health and wellness in the United States.

Protective Factors

Healthy conditions and environments	Psychosocial factors	Effective health services	Healthy lifestyles
Safe physical environments	Participation in civic activities and social engagement	Provision of preventative services	Decreased use of tobacco and drugs
Supportive economic and social conditions	Strong social networks	Access to culturally appropriate health services	Regular physical activity
Regular supply of nutritious food and water	Feeling of trust	Community participation in the planning and delivery of health services	Balanced nutritional intake
Restricted access to tobacco and drugs	Feeling of power and control over life decisions		Positive mental health
Healthy public policy and organizational practice	Supportive family structure		Safe sexual activity
Provision for meaningful, paid employment	Positive self-esteem		
Provision of affordable housing			

Quality of life, functional independence, well-being

Figure 1-1 The Factors Affecting Health and Well-Being

Source: Labonte, R. *A Community Development Approach to Health Promotion: A Background Paper on Practice Tensions, Strategic Models, and Accountability Requirements for Health Authority Work on the Broad Determinants of Health,* Health Education Board of Scotland, Research Unit on Health and Behaviour Change, University of Edinburgh, Edinburgh, 1998. © NHS Health Scotland, 1998.

Practitioners describe wellness as a process of extending information, counseling, assessment, and lifestyle-modification strategies leading to a desirable change in the recipients' overall lifestyle, or the adoption of a wellness lifestyle. Once adopted, the wellness lifestyle produces a sense of well-being that in turn enables recipients to unlock their full potential (see the box "Factors That Influence Health and Well-Being").

This explanation of how wellness differs from episodic health care, preventive medicine, and health promotion does, on first hearing, seem progressive and clearly devoid of interest in morbidity and mortality concerns. But in practice, wellness programs are not all that different from other kinds of health care. We have consistently noted that wellness programs, as carried out on college campuses, in local hospital well centers, and in corporate settings, routinely transmit familiar health-related information and engage in the same risk-reduction activities that characterize preventive medicine and health promotion. Given that the wellness movement indicates that its absence of programmatic concern over issues of morbidity and mortality makes it substantially different from health promotion, their observable activities seem very similar to health promotion. This similarity raises a salient question regarding the nature of a "sense of well-being" that replaces the health care system's more familiar concerns over illness and desire to live longer rather than not as long: How does the adoption of a wellness lifestyle, resulting from exposure to wellness, lead to the

Key Terms

health promotion A movement in which knowledge, practices, and values are transmitted to people for use in lengthening their lives, reducing the incidence of illness, and feeling better.

wellness A process intended to aid individuals in unlocking their full potential through the development of an overall wellness lifestyle.

eventual development of a sense of well-being? In the opinion of your textbook, until the wellness movement can more clearly identify the basis of its uniqueness, then it appears we are seeing health promotion being carried out under a different label.

Having learned about the sources of our familiar and traditional definitions of health, recall that a new and unique definition of health is presented later in the chapter.

A Health Care System or a Medical Care System?

Having now examined the origins of our traditional definitions of health (and wellness) and noted that to varying degrees they all focus on concerns over morbidity and premature mortality, the use of the term *health care system* is more, in fact, a *medical care system*. Your text will establish, by the end of the chapter, a proposition that if a true health care system did exist, it would need to be much more broadly based, and less medically oriented, than the system the American public now discusses with such fervor.

Federal Programs to Improve the Health of People in the United States

In 1991 the U.S. Department of Health and Human Services document titled *Healthy People 2000: National Health Promotion and Disease Prevention Objectives*[23] outlined a strategic plan for promoting the health of the American public. The plan included 300 health objectives in 22 priority areas. Forty-seven of the 300 objectives were defined as "sentinel" ones, that is, particularly significant goals that could be used to measure the progress of the 1990s health promotion objectives.

Progress toward achieving the objectives was assessed near the middle of the decade and reported in a document titled *Healthy People 2000: Midcourse Review and 1995 Revisions.*[24] Although progress was reported in some areas, little or no progress was reported in many. Subsequently, a new plan, called *Healthy People 2010: Understanding and Improving Health,* Volume 1,[25] was formulated, refined, and is now being implemented.

Healthy People 2010: Understanding and Improving Health, Volume 2 is a health promotion program intended to be implemented at all levels,[26] ranging from individual involvement through multinational cooperative efforts, including *Health for All in the 21st Century,* a World Health Organization health promotion initiative. Although the goals of *Healthy People 2000: National Health Promotion and Disease Prevention Objectives* and *Healthy People 2010: Understanding and Improving Health* are similar, the latter focuses on the projected needs of the United States during the first decade of the new century.

Central to the design of *Healthy People 2010: Understanding and Improving Health* are two paramount goals: (1) increasing quality and years of life and (2) eliminating health disparities in areas such as gender, race, and ethnicity, as well as income and education level. These goals in turn provide 28 more focused areas. These 28 focused goals are, in turn, broken down into 467 specific objects.

As was true with the parent program, *Healthy People 2000, Healthy People 2010* underwent a mid-course assessment in 2005. The resulting document, *Healthy People 2010—Midcourse Review,* reported that seven levels of accomplishment (exceeding target, movement toward target, no change, mixed progress, movement away from target, not assessed, and deleted at midcourse) were identified. It was concluded that 356 objectives met (70 percent), exceeded, or moved toward their target, 70 objectives (14 percent) met their target, 286 (56 percent) moved toward their target, 38 (8 percent) showed no change, and 113 (22 percent) moved away from their target. Sixty-seven objectives were dropped, generally due to a lack of baseline standards against which progress could be assessed.[27]

The success of *Healthy People 2010: Understanding and Improving Health* will not be known for a few years. However, if its goals are ultimately reached, Americans can anticipate improved quantity and quality of life.

Improving Health Through Planned Behavior Change

Although some health concerns can be successfully addressed through local, state, national, or international efforts, such as those just outlined, most are ultimately based on the willingness and ability of persons to change aspects of their own behavior. However, for many people health-related behavior change proves difficult or even impossible to make.

Why Behavior Change Is Often Difficult

Several factors can strongly influence a person's desire to change high-risk health behaviors, including these:

1. A person must know that a particular behavioral pattern is clearly associated with (or even causes) a particular health problem. For example: cigarette smoking is the primary cause of lung cancer.
2. A person must believe (accept) that a behavioral pattern will make (or has made) him susceptible to this particular health problem. For example: my cigarette smoking will significantly increase my risk of developing lung cancer.
3. A person must recognize that risk-reduction intervention strategies exist and that should she adopt

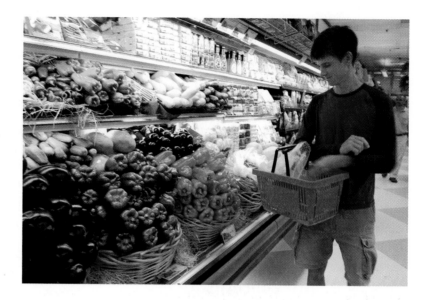

People can improve their health through planned behavior change. As part of a plan to improve his eating habits, this man shops for healthy food choices.

these in a compliant manner she too will reduce her risk for a particular health condition. For example: smoking-cessation programs exist, and following such a program could help me quit smoking.

4. A person must believe that benefits of newly adopted health-enhancing behaviors will be more reinforcing than the behaviors being given up. For example: the improved health, lowered risk, and freedom from dependence resulting from no longer smoking are better than the temporary pleasures provided by smoking.

5. A person must feel that significant others in his life truly want him to alter his high-risk health behaviors and will support his efforts. For example: my friends who are cigarette smokers will make a concerted effort to not smoke in my presence and will help me avoid being around people who smoke.

When one or more of these conditions is not in place, the likelihood that persons will be successful in reducing health-risk behaviors is greatly diminished.

Transtheoretical Model of Health Behavior Change

The process of behavioral change unfolds over time and progresses through defined stages. James Prochaska, John Norcross, and Carol DiClemente outlined six predictable stages of change. They studied thousands of individuals who were changing long-standing problems such as alcohol abuse, smoking, and gambling. While these people used different strategies to change their behavior, they all proceeded through six consistent stages of change in the process referred to as **Prochaska's Transtheoretical Model of Health Behavior Change.** [28]

Precontemplation Stage The first stage of change is called *precontemplation,* during which persons might think about making a change but ultimately find it too difficult and avoid making it. For example, during this phase a smoker might tell friends, "Eventually I will quit" but have no real intention of stopping within the next six months.

Contemplation Stage For many, however, progress toward change begins as they move into a *contemplation* stage, during which they might develop the desire to change but have little understanding of how to go about it. Typically, they see themselves taking action within the next six months. For example: when the semester is finished and my stress level is lower, I'll start the stop smoking program that I have material about.

Preparation Stage Following the contemplation stage, a *preparation* stage begins, during which change begins to appear to be not only desirable but possible as well. A smoker might begin making plans to quit during this stage, setting a quit date for the very near future (a few days to a month) and perhaps enrolling in a smoking-cessation program. For example: this is the last weekend of my "smoking career"—on Monday I plan to quit.

> ### Key Terms
>
> **Prochaska's Transtheoretical Model of Health Behavior Change** Six predictable stages—precontemplation, contemplation, preparation, action, maintenance, and termination—people go through in establishing new habits and patterns of behavior.

Action Stage Plans for change are implemented during the *action* stage, during which changes are made and sustained for a period of about six months.

Maintenance Stage The fifth stage is the *maintenance* stage, during which new habits are consolidated and practiced for an additional six months. For example: I think that I'm almost home, but I better continue paying attention to my maintenance plan for a bit longer—returning to the bar scene too soon could be my downfall.

Termination Stage The sixth and final stage is called *termination,* which refers to the point at which new habits are well established, and so efforts to change are complete.

Today's Health Concerns

Earlier in the chapter we looked at those illnesses that are the major causes of death that afflict adults in the United States (see Table 4 on the book's Online Learning Center at www.mhhe.com/payne11e). However, in spite of astonishing progress on many fronts, we continue to face a number of serious health challenges from those and other illnesses. Heart disease, cancer, accidents, drug use, and mental illness all are important concerns for each of us, even if we are not directly affected by them. Also becoming increasingly troublesome are the complex problems of environmental pollution, violence, health care costs, an Avian flu pandemic, and the international scope of HIV/AIDS and H1N1, as well as other sexually transmitted diseases. World hunger, overpopulation, and the threat of domestic and international terrorism are other health-related issues that will affect us as well as the generations that follow.

The health concerns just mentioned are by no means unmanageable. Fortunately, we as individuals can reduce the likelihood of encountering many of these conditions by making choices in the way we live our lives. On a personal level, we can decide to pursue a plan of healthful living to minimize the incidence of illness and disease and to extend life.

Health: More Than the Absence of Illness

What exactly is health? Is it simply the absence of disease and illness, as Western medicine has held for centuries—

Key Terms

holistic health A view of health in terms of its physical, emotional, social, intellectual, spiritual, and occupational makeup.

---

or does health embrace other elements we ought to consider now that the twenty-first century has begun?

Rather routinely, national news magazines (and other media) feature articles describing advances in modern medicine. These articles describe vividly in words and images the impressive progress being made in fields such as drug research, gene manipulation, robotics-aided surgery, and the role of diet in health. Because of articles like this that relate health to medical care, most of us continue to hold to our traditional perception of health as (1) the virtual absence of disease and illness (low levels of morbidity) and (2) the ability to live a long life (reduced risk of mortality). However, in striving to be fully "health educated" in the new century, perhaps we need to consider a broader definition that more accurately reflects the demands associated with becoming functional and satisfied persons as we transition through each adult stage of life—*early adulthood, middle adulthood,* and, finally, *older adulthood.* With this in mind, look forward to another definition of health—one that recognizes the importance of the more familiar definitions of health but is focused on the demands of our own growth and development.

The Multiple Dimensions of Health

In an earlier section of the chapter we promised to give you a new definition of health that would be less focused on morbidity (illness) and mortality (death) than most others are. However, before we present that new definition, we introduce here a *multidimensional concept of health* (**holistic health**)—a requirement for any definition of health that moves beyond the cure/prevention of illness and the postponement of death.

Although our modern health care community too frequently acts as if the structure and the function of the physical body are the sole basis of health, common experience supports the validity of a holistic nature to health. In this section we examine six components, or dimensions, of health, all interacting in a synergistic manner allowing us to engage in the wide array of daily role-related activities (see Figure 1-2).

Physical Dimension

Most of us have a number of physiological and structural characteristics we can call on to aid us in accomplishing the wide array of activities that characterize a typical day and, on occasion, a not-so-typical day. Among these physical characteristics are our body weight, visual ability, strength, coordination, level of endurance, level of susceptibility to disease, and powers of recuperation. In certain situations the physical dimension of health may be the most important. This importance almost certainly

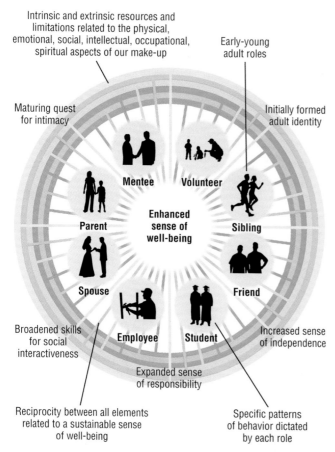

Intrinsic and extrinsic resources and limitations related to the physical, emotional, social, intellectual, occupational, spiritual aspects of our make-up

Early-young adult roles

Maturing quest for intimacy

Initially formed adult identity

Mentee
Volunteer
Parent
Enhanced sense of well-being
Sibling
Spouse
Friend
Employee
Student

Broadened skills for social interactiveness

Increased sense of independence

Expanded sense of responsibility

Reciprocity between all elements related to a sustainable sense of well-being

Specific patterns of behavior dictated by each role

Figure 1-2 Young Adult Roles, Health, and an Enhanced Sense of Well-Being Societal expectation for maturation during young adulthood requires daily role-based involvement, the acceptable completion of which serves as the basis for self-assessment, and, one hopes, results in an expanded sense of well-being. Resources needed for this process to unfold are drawn from the multiple dimensions of health. Reciprocity exists between all elements, at all levels as depicted. Source: illustration by Shaw Design, Muncie, IN. © Wayne Payne.

is why traditional medicine for centuries has equated health with the design and operation of the body.

Emotional Dimension

We also possess certain emotional characteristics that can help us through the demands of daily living. The emotional dimension of health encompasses our ability to see the world in a realistic manner, cope with stress, remain flexible, and compromise to resolve conflict.

For young adults, growth and development often give rise to emotional vulnerability, which may lead to feelings of rejection and failure that can reduce productivity and satisfaction. To some extent we are all affected by feeling states, such as anger, happiness, fear, empathy, guilt, love, and hate. People who consistently try to improve their emotional health appear to enjoy

life to a much greater extent than do those who let feelings of vulnerability overwhelm them or block their creativity.

Social Dimension

A third dimension of health encompasses social skills and cultural sensitivity. Initially, family interactions, school experiences, and peer group interactions foster development in these areas, but future social interactions will demand additional skill development and refinement of already existing skills and insights. In adulthood, including young adulthood, the composition of the social world changes, principally because of our exposure to a wider array of people and the expanded roles associated with employment, parenting, and community involvement.

The importance of the social dimension of health, in terms of a sense of well-being, cannot be understated. Most succinct is the declining number of confidants that the typical American possesses. Whether called "friends," "best friends," or "trusted friends," these may be the most important persons in one's social environment. Today one out of every four American adults has no one to play this important role.[29] In the absence of someone to confide in, both on a regular basis and during times of conflict, stress is often more frequent, of greater intensity, longer in duration, and eventually damaging to all of the dimensions of health.

Although far from being answerable, increasingly questions are being raised regarding the ramification of social networking. As today's early young adults (and some older adults) respond positively to adding yet another person to their list of "cyber friends," information once reserved for trusted friends is potentially placed in the hands of hundreds of other people. Knowing the work required in sustaining true friendships, this level of openness seems fraught with potential for misuse. Academics question whether social networking, capable of reaching so many, will prove powerfully healthful, or perhaps, will serve as a detriment to sustaining eventual traditional relationships, thus increasing the stress of living in the twenty-first century.

Intellectual Dimension

The abilities to process and act on information, clarify values and beliefs, and exercise decision-making capacity rank among the most important aspects of total health. For many college-educated persons, the intellectual dimension of health may prove to be the most important and satisfying of the six. In fact, for all of us, at least on certain occasions, this holds true. Our ability to analyze, synthesize, hypothesize, and then act on new information enhances the quality of our lives in multiple ways.

How Does Spirituality Affect Your Life?

Spirituality or faith can include religious practice, but it can also be quite distinct from it. Spirituality is the most fundamental stage in the human quest for the meaning of life. It's a developing focus of the total person that gives purpose and meaning to life.

By the time people reach college age, their spirituality or faith may have already placed them in uncomfortable situations. Taking seriously their responsibility for their own commitments, lifestyles, beliefs, and attitudes, they've had to make some difficult personal decisions. This demands objectivity and a certain amount of independence. It requires finding a balance between personal aspirations and a developing sense of service to others. Finally, actual behavioral choices can be conflicted by religiously related issues. The following examples depict such situations:

- A newly developing dating relationship that triggers religiously based intolerance on the part of one partner's parents

- The momentary uncertainty of wishing your professors either Merry Christmas or, rather, the more secular Happy Holidays, or saying nothing at all

- A decision to fast for Ramadan, or setting it aside, in fear that midday lethargy could negatively affect your energy level during the days on which you have your fullest schedule of classes

- Being the only Jewish student attending a small, church-affiliated college

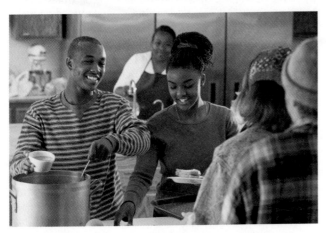

Community service—such as volunteering at a homeless shelter—can be a way to express personal values and nurture the spiritual dimension of health.

Spiritual Dimension

The fifth dimension of health is the spiritual dimension. Although certainly it includes religious beliefs and practices, many young adults would expand it to encompass more diverse belief systems, including relationships with other living things, the nature of human behavior, and the need and willingness to serve others (see the box "How Does Spirituality Affect Your Life?"). All are important components of spiritual health.

The extent to which the American public professes a personal relationship with God or some form of supernatural power source is frequently assessed by the academic community. In a recent study by sociologists at Baylor University, which utilized data supplied by the Pew Research Center, interesting findings emerged. Analysis of these data indicated that approximately 93 percent of the adults sampled attended services or participated in activities focusing on religion or the enhancement of spiritual understanding. Further, among those who reported believing in God, four prevailing perceptions of God's nature emerge—an authoritarian God, a benevolent God, a critical God, or a distant God.[30] These perceptions to a large extent influence the nature of the believers' relationship with God—and perhaps their daily relationships with others within the home, school, and community. Further, believers' views of God's personality would also affect their views on important questions regarding issues such as gay marriage, the role of faith-based programs in the delivery of government-financed services, abortion, and stem cell research—and even the question of whose side is God on during times of war.

For those persons for whom a theist-based perception of life's meaning is repugnant, lacking in validity, or just not of importance, other paths, if explored, could be capable of providing a sense of meaning of and direction for living. Typically college and university campuses are excellent arenas for finding programs, sources of information, and kindred spirits devoted to spiritual growth in the absence of religion per se.

Occupational Dimension

A significant contribution made by the currently popular wellness movement is that it defines for many people the importance of the workplace to their sense of well-being. In today's world, employment and productive efforts play an increasingly important role in how we perceive ourselves and how we see the "goodness" of the world in which we live. In addition, the workplace serves as both a testing ground for and a source of life-enhancing skills. In our place of employment we gain not only the financial resources to meet our demands for both necessities and luxuries but also an array of

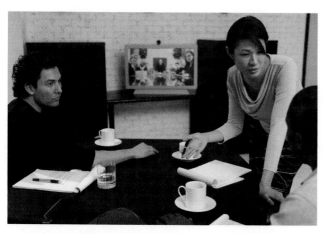

The workplace provides a setting to develop such skills as cooperation and conflict resolution. Our workplace experiences strongly affect our perceptions of ourselves and others as well as our overall sense of well-being.

useful skills such as conflict resolution, experiences in shared responsibility, and intellectual growth that can be used to facilitate a wide range of non-employment-related interactions. In turn, the workplace is enhanced by the healthfulness of the individuals who contribute to its endeavors.

Environmental Dimension

Some academics would add to the dimensions just discussed an *environmental dimension*. If this dimension is defined on the basis of land, air, and water, then it might be an additional dimension to consider. However, should the environmental dimension be extended to include all that is material and metaphysical surrounding each individual, such a concept seems beyond the scope of this chapter. Thus, we have elected not to expand the number of holistic dimensions of health beyond those traditionally discussed.

A New Definition of Health

Now we are ready to define for you a new way to view health. This new view is far less centered in morbidity and mortality concerns than are the traditional concepts of health drawn from episodic and preventive medicine, health promotion, and even wellness. The definition that we propose takes into account the differences between *what health is for* (its role) and *what health is* (its composition).

The Role of Health

The role of health in our lives is similar to the role of a car. Much as a car (or other vehicle) takes us to the

place we need or want to be at, good health enables us to accomplish the activities that transition us into and through developmental tasks associated with each stage of adulthood (pages 2–6). Recall that the process of moving through each stage of adulthood does not occur simply because of the passage of time but rather because we understand the functional intent of the roles that we assume, and we have entered into them with a commitment that they are carried out to the best of our ability.

The Composition of Health

Now that you know what the role of health is, its composition can be seen as being more than simply having a body free of illness and apparently destined for a long life. Rather, the composition of health is that of a collection of resources, from each dimension of health (pages 14–17), determined to be necessary for the successful accomplishment of activities that you need or want to do. Some of these needed resources are already within you (intrinsic), whereas others need to come from outside (extrinsic). Regardless of their origin, however, these resources must be directed toward the behavioral patterns that lead to the fulfillment of role-required behavioral patterns. To recognize what resources are needed, you must be a student of society's expectations for persons of your age, in terms of task mastery, such as those first identified on pages 14–17, and the role-related behavioral patterns that ensure both role functionality and, eventually, your honestly earned claim to task mastery. Successful completion of a decades-long trip through life requires that the predictable expectations of society have been called to your attention, so that your own unique approach to meeting these expectations is both personally satisfying and deemed adequately functional by society.

Our Definition of Health

By combining the role of health with the composition of health, we offer a new definition of **health:** Health consists of ability to use the *intrinsic* and *extrinsic* resources related to each dimension of our holistic makeup to participate fully in the role-related activities that contribute to growth and development, with the goal of feeling a

> ### Key Terms
>
> **health** A reflection of ability to use the *intrinsic* and *extrinsic* resources related to each dimension of our holistic makeup to participate fully in the role-related activities that contribute to growth and development, with the goal of feeling a sense of well-being as we evaluate our progress through life.

sense of well-being as we evaluate our progress through life. For those wondering about the "evaluation process" just alluded to, standards for you to measure your own progress against often include your own predetermined aspirations, performance demonstrated by comparable others (often peers or older siblings), the expectations of significant others (parents, employers, spouses), standards held by institutions of higher education, available demographic standards (starting salary, size and cost of first home), or even, for some, God's expectations.

Regardless, this comparative process often forms the nature of our "sense of well-being" and, later in life, a final self-assessment, "a sense of life satisfaction based on a life well-lived."

In light of this definition, do not be surprised when we ask whether you are resourceful (healthy) enough to attain the goals you wish to reach, whether you are healthy enough to sustain a particular role-based behavioral pattern that you have adopted, or whether you are experiencing the sense of well-being to which you aspire.

Taking Charge of Your Health

- Complete the Comprehensive Health Assessment on pages 21–30. Develop a plan to modify your behavior in the areas in which you need improvement.
- Take part in a new spiritual activity, such as meditating, creating art or music, or attending a religious service.

- To promote the social dimension of your health, try to meet one new person each week during the semester.
- Choose one developmental task you would like to focus on, such as assuming responsibility, and plan the steps you can follow to progress in this area.

- Volunteer to be an assistant in a community service program, such as a literacy project or a preschool program.

SUMMARY

- The millennial generation encompasses persons born between 1982 and 2000.
- Each phase of the life cycle involves a set of personal developmental tasks that are common to all people yet may be undertaken differently by each individual. Young adulthood is characterized by five key developmental tasks: forming an initial adult identity, establishing independence, assuming responsibility, broadening social skills, and nurturing intimacy.
- Generativity and integrity are developmental tasks of midlife and older adulthood, respectively.
- Today's college campus is a dynamic blend of students of both traditional and nontraditional ages and of diverse backgrounds, cultures, and attributes.
- When we seek the services of health care practitioners because of symptoms of illness or disease, we are said to be seeking episodic health care.
- Preventive medical care attempts to minimize the incidence of illness and disease by identifying early indicators of risk to bring them under control.
- Individual-centered health promotion involves risk-reduction activities similar to those used in preventive medical care, except that the techniques cannot be invasive and are directed by professionals who are not physicians. Its most visible emphasis tends to be on fitness and body composition.
- Group-centered health promotion involves the empowerment of individuals so that they can organize collectively and participate in their own health promotion activities.

- Wellness contends a disinterest in morbidity and mortality, rather emphasizing living a wellness lifestyle that leads to a sense of well-being.
- A decision to change a health behavior is often difficult to make because of the multiplicity of factors underlying the maintenace of the high-risk behavior.
- Health behavior change requires movement through a multistaged process, including precontemplation, contemplation, preparation, action, maintenance, and termination.
- A wide array of health problems (for example, cancer, cardiovascular disease, HIV/AIDS) persist despite today's highly sophisticated health care technology.
- Complementary and integrative medicine involves the integration of alternative forms of care, such as acupuncture and therapeutic massage, into traditional medical practices.
- Current multidimensional definitions of health may include many or all of the following dimensions: physical, emotional, social, intellectual, spiritual, and occupational.
- Our new definition of health includes the role of health and the composition of health. The role of health is to enable individuals to participate in the activities that collectively fulfill role requirements and, in doing so, establish reciprocity between day-to-day living and life stage developmental task mastery. The composition of health is the intrinsic and extrinsic resources on which individuals can draw to participate fully in their own growth and development.

REVIEW QUESTIONS

1. What birth years are encompassed within the label *millennial generation*?
2. What are the five developmental tasks of young adulthood, and how can the accomplishing of one influence the accomplishing of any of the remaining four?
3. What is implied by the statement "growth and development are predictable yet unique"?
4. What is the most likely route that midlife adults will take in their quest for a sense of generativity?
5. In what ways is the current U.S. college student population more diverse than any that came before?
6. What are morbidity and mortality, and how are they involved in the more traditional definitions of health?
7. In preventive medical care, who determines a person's level of risk and decides what risk-reduction techniques should be implemented?
8. What does the term *empowerment* mean, and how would it appear as a component of a community-based health promotion program?
9. What is the main reason that proponents of wellness give for being uninterested in morbidity and mortality?
10. What factors could underlie the inability or unwillingness of persons to change their health behavior?
11. What are the six stages that persons pass through as they consider and then attempt to change their health behavior?
12. What are the most frequently included dimensions of a holistically centered definition of health?
13. How does your textbook define the role of health? Composition of health?
14. How does our definition of health differ from traditional definitions?
15. Why is it necessary to understand developmental expectations before we can answer the question "Are you healthy enough to . . . ?"

ANSWERS TO THE "WHAT DO YOU KNOW?" QUIZ

1. True   2. False   3. True   4. False   5. True   6. False   7. False

Visit the Online Learning Center (**www.mhhe.com/payne11e**), where you will find tools to help you improve your grade, including practice quizzes, key terms flashcards, audio chapter summaries for your MP3 player, and many other study aids.

SOURCE NOTES

1. Strauss W, Howe N. *Generations: The History of America's Future: 1584–2069.* New York: William Morrow, 1992.
2. Furstenberg FF, Kennedy S, McLoyd VC, et al. Growing Up Is Harder to Do. *Context,* 3(3), Summer 2004.
3. Diversity in Word and Deed: Most Teens Claim Multicultural Friends. *The TRU Study.* Teen Research Unlimited (TRU), November 2004.
4. Putman RD. *Bowling Alone: The Collapse and Revival of American Community.* New York: Simon & Schuster, 2000.
5. Twenge JM, Campbell WK. Increases in Positive Self-Views Among High School Students: Birth-Cohort Changes in Anticipated Performance, Self-Satisfaction, Self-Liking, and Self-Competence. *Psychological Science,* 19(11), 1082–1086, 2008.
6. St. Aubin ED, McAdams DP, Tee-Chang K (Eds.). *The Generative Society: Caring for future generations.* Washington, DC: American Psychological Association, 2003.
7. McAdams DP. Generativity in Midlife. In Lachman M (Ed.). *Handbook of Midlife Development.* Hoboken, NJ: Wiley, 2001.
8. Erikson EH. *The Life Cycle Completed* (Extended ed.). New York: W.W. Norton, 1998.
9. Total Fall Enrollment in Degree-Granting Institutions, by Level, Age, and Attendance Status of Students: 2005. (Table 182) (2007). *Digest of Education Statistics.* National Center for Education Statistics. www.nces.ed.gov/programs/digest/d07/tables/dt07_182.asp
10. Number and Percentage of Students Enrolled in Postsecondary Institutions, by Level, Disability, and Selected Student Characteristics: 2003–2004. (Table 221) (2007) *Digest of Education Statistics.* National Center for Education Statistics. www.nces.ed.gov/programs/digest/dto7/tables/dt07_221asp.
11. Types of Disabilities. *Digest of Education Statistics: 2005.* (2006). www.nces.ed.gov/fastfacts/display.asp?id=64
12. Postsecondary Students with Disabilities: Enrollment, Services, and Persistence. Stats in Brief. (2000). *National Postsecondary Student Aid Study.* National Center for Education Statistics. www.eric.ed.gov/ERICWebPortal/custom/portlets/recordsDetails/detailmini.jsp-nf...
13. Summary Health Statistics for U.S. Adults. *National Health Interview Survey, 2006.* Vital and Health Statistics. Series 10, Number 235. December 2007.
14. Roper Center for Public Opinion Research (for Pfizer Women's Health), University of Connecticut. Adults Know Their Family History. *USA Today,* May 30, 2000. p. 5D.
15. *U.S. Surgeon General's Family History Initiative.* Washington, DC: U.S. Department of Health and Human Services, 2004, www.hss.gov/familyhistory/download.html.
16. Deaths: Final Data for 2005. *National Vital Statistics Reports,* 56(10), April 2008. Centers for Disease Control and Prevention. U.S. Department of Health and Human Services.
17. Smith PC, et al. Missing Information During Primary Care Visits. *Journal of the American Medical Association,* 293(5), 567–571, February 2, 2005.
18. Cohen T, Neumann P, Weinstein M. Does Preventive Care Save Money? Health Economics and the Presidential Candidates. *New England Journal of Medicine,* 358(7), 661–663, 2008.

19. Fielding J, Husten C, Richland J. Does Preventive Care Save Money? *New England Journal of Medicine*, 368(26), 2847, 2008.
20. Cottrell RR, Girvan JT, McKenzie JF. *Principles and Foundations of Health Promotion and Education* (3rd ed.). San Francisco: Benjamin Cummings, 2005.
21. *Shape Up Somerville: Eat Smart Play Hard*. Clinical Trials.gov. U.S. National Institutes of Health. (2005) September 7. www .clinicaltrials.gov/ct2/show/record/NCT00153322
22. McKenzie JF, Neiger BL, Smeltzer JL. *Planning, Implementing and Evaluating Health Promotion Programs* (4th ed.). San Francisco: Benjamin Cummings, 2005.
23. *Healthy People 2000: National Health Promotion and Disease Prevention Objectives* (full report with commentary). Washington, DC: U.S. Department of Health and Human Services. Public Health Services, 1991.
24. *Healthy People 2000: Midcourse Review and 1995 Revisions.* Washington, DC: U.S. Department of Health and Human Services. Public Health Services, 1995.
25. *Healthy People 2010: Understanding and Improving Health*. Volume 1. Washington, DC: U.S. Department of Health and Human Services, 2000.
26. *Healthy People 2010: Understanding and Improving Health*. Volume 2. Washington, DC: U.S. Department of Health and Human Services, 2000.
27. *Healthy People 2010—Midcourse Review. Executive Summary.* 2005. www.healthypeople.gov/Data/midcourse/execsummary/progress .htm
28. Prochaska JO, Norcross JC, Clemente CC. *Changing for Good.* New York: William Morrow, 1994.
29. Smith-Lovin L, McPherson M, Brashears M. Social Isolation in America: Changes in Core Discussion Networks over Two Decades. *American Sociologica*, 353–375, June 2006.
30. *American Piety in the 21st Century: New Insights to the Depths and Complexity of Religion in the U.S.* Baylor Institute for Studies of Religion. Baylor University, September 2006. www.baylor .edu/isreligionj/index.[ip?id=40634.

Comprehensive Health Assessment

Now that you have read the first chapter, complete the following Comprehensive Health Assessment. We strongly suggest that you retake this assessment after you have completed your health course. Then compare your responses in each section of the assessment. Have your scores improved?

Social and Occupational Health

	Not true/ rarely	Somewhat true/ sometimes	Mostly true/ usually	Very true/ always
1. I feel loved and supported by my family.	1	2	3	4
2. I establish friendships with ease and enjoyment.	1	2	3	4
3. I establish friendships with people of both genders and all ages.	1	2	3	4
4. I sustain relationships by communicating with and caring about my family and friends.	1	2	3	4
5. I feel comfortable and confident when meeting people for the first time.	1	2	3	4
6. I practice social skills to facilitate the process of forming new relationships.	1	2	3	4
7. I seek opportunities to meet and interact with new people.	1	2	3	4
8. I talk with, rather than at, people.	1	2	3	4
9. I am open to developing or sustaining intimate relationships.	1	2	3	4
10. I appreciate the importance of parenting the next generation and am committed to supporting it in ways that reflect my own resources.	1	2	3	4
11. I recognize the strengths and weaknesses of my parents' childrearing skills and feel comfortable modifying them if I choose to become a parent.	1	2	3	4
12. I attempt to be tolerant of others whether or not I approve of their behavior or beliefs.	1	2	3	4
13. I understand and appreciate the contribution that cultural diversity makes to the quality of living.	1	2	3	4
14. I understand and appreciate the difference between being educated and being trained.	1	2	3	4
15. My work gives me a sense of self-sufficiency and an opportunity to contribute.	1	2	3	4
16. I have equal respect for the roles of leader and subordinate within the workplace.	1	2	3	4
17. I have chosen an occupation that suits my interests and temperament.	1	2	3	4
18. I have chosen an occupation that does not compromise my physical or psychological health.	1	2	3	4
19. I get along well with my coworkers most of the time.	1	2	3	4
20. When I have a disagreement with a coworker, I try to resolve it directly and constructively.	1	2	3	4

POINTS _____

Spiritual and Psychological Health

	Not true/ rarely	Somewhat true/ sometimes	Mostly true/ usually	Very true/ always
1. I have a deeply held belief system or personal theology.	1	2	3	4
2. I recognize the contribution that membership in a community of faith or spirituality can make to a person's overall quality of life.	1	2	3	4

3. I seek experiences with nature and reflect on nature's contribution to my quality of life.   1   2   3   4

4. My spirituality is a resource that helps me remain calm and strong during times of stress.   1   2   3   4

5. I have found appropriate ways to express my spirituality.   1   2   3   4

6. I respect the diversity of spiritual expression and am tolerant of those whose beliefs differ from my own.   1   2   3   4

7. I take adequate time to reflect on my own life and my relationships with others and the institutions of society.   1   2   3   4

8. I routinely undertake new experiences.   1   2   3   4

9. I receive adequate support from others.   1   2   3   4

10. I look for opportunities to support others, even occasionally at the expense of my own goals and aspirations.   1   2   3   4

11. I recognize that emotional and psychological health are as important as physical health.   1   2   3   4

12. I express my feelings and opinions comfortably, yet am capable of keeping them to myself when appropriate.   1   2   3   4

13. I see myself as a person of worth and feel comfortable with my own strengths and limitations.   1   2   3   4

14. I establish realistic goals and work to achieve them.   1   2   3   4

15. I understand the differences between the normal range of emotions and the signs of clinical depression.   1   2   3   4

16. I know how to recognize signs of suicidal thoughts and am willing to intervene.   1   2   3   4

17. I regularly assess my own behavior patterns and beliefs and would seek professional assistance for any emotional dysfunction.   1   2   3   4

18. I accept the reality of aging and view it as an opportunity for positive change.   1   2   3   4

19. I accept the reality of death and view it as a normal and inevitable part of life.   1   2   3   4

20. I have made decisions about my own death to ensure that I die with dignity when the time comes.   1   2   3   4

POINTS _____

Stress Management	Not true/ rarely	Somewhat true/ sometimes	Mostly true/ usually	Very true/ always
1. I accept the reality of change while maintaining the necessary stability in my daily activities.	1	2	3	4
2. I seek change when it is necessary or desirable to do so.	1	2	3	4
3. I know what stress-management services are offered on campus, through my employer, or in my community.	1	2	3	4
4. When necessary, I use the stress-management services to which I have access.	1	2	3	4
5. I employ stress-reduction practices in anticipation of stressful events, such as job interviews and final examinations.	1	2	3	4
6. I reevaluate the ways in which I handled stressful events so that I can better cope with similar events in the future.	1	2	3	4
7. I turn to relatives and friends during periods of disruption in my life.	1	2	3	4
8. I avoid using alcohol or other drugs during periods of stress.	1	2	3	4
9. I refrain from behaving aggressively or abusively during periods of stress.	1	2	3	4

Comprehensive Health Assessment—*continued*

	Not true/ rarely	Somewhat true/ sometimes	Mostly true/ usually	Very true/ always
10. I sleep enough to maintain a high level of health and cope successfully with daily challenges.	1	2	3	4
11. I avoid sleeping excessively as a response to stressful change.	1	2	3	4
12. My diet is conducive to good health and stress management.	1	2	3	4
13. I participate in physical activity to relieve stress.	1	2	3	4
14. I practice stress-management skills, such as diaphragmatic breathing and yoga.	1	2	3	4
15. I manage my time effectively.	1	2	3	4

POINTS _____

Fitness

	Not true/ rarely	Somewhat true/ sometimes	Mostly true/ usually	Very true/ always
1. I participate in recreational and fitness activities both to minimize stress and to improve or maintain my level of physical fitness.	1	2	3	4
2. I select some recreational activities that are strenuous rather than sedentary in nature.	1	2	3	4
3. I include various types of aerobic conditioning activities among the wider array of recreational and fitness activities in which I engage.	1	2	3	4
4. I engage in aerobic activities with appropriate frequency, intensity, and duration to provide a training effect for my heart and lungs.	1	2	3	4
5. I routinely include strength-training activities among the wider array of fitness activities in which I engage.	1	2	3	4
6. I routinely vary the types of strength-training activities in which I participate in order to minimize injury and strengthen all of the important muscle groups.	1	2	3	4
7. I do exercises specifically designed to maintain joint range of motion.	1	2	3	4
8. I believe that recreational and fitness activities can help me improve my physical health and my emotional and social well-being.	1	2	3	4
9. I include a variety of fitness activities in my overall plan for physical fitness.	1	2	3	4
10. I take appropriate steps to avoid injuries when participating in recreational and fitness activities.	1	2	3	4
11. I seek appropriate treatment for all injuries that result from fitness activities.	1	2	3	4
12. I believe that older adults should undertake appropriately chosen fitness activities.	1	2	3	4
13. My body composition is consistent with a high level of health.	1	2	3	4
14. I warm up before beginning vigorous activity, and I cool down afterward.	1	2	3	4
15. I select properly designed and well-maintained equipment and clothing for each activity.	1	2	3	4
16. I avoid using performance-enhancing substances that are known to be dangerous and those whose influence on the body is not fully understood.	1	2	3	4
17. I sleep seven to eight hours daily.	1	2	3	4
18. I refrain from using over-the-counter sleep-inducing aids.	1	2	3	4

	Not true/ rarely	Somewhat true/ sometimes	Mostly true/ usually	Very true/ always
19. I follow sound dietary practices as an important adjunct to a health-enhancing physical activity program.	1	2	3	4
20. My current level of fitness allows me to participate fully and with reasonable comfort in my daily activities.	1	2	3	4

POINTS _____

Nutrition and Weight Management

	Not true/ rarely	Somewhat true/ sometimes	Mostly true/ usually	Very true/ always
1. I balance my caloric intake with my calorie expenditure.	1	2	3	4
2. I obtain the recommended number of servings from each of the food groups.	1	2	3	4
3. I select a wide variety of foods chosen from each of the food groups.	1	2	3	4
4. I understand the amount of a particular food that constitutes a single serving.	1	2	3	4
5. I often try new foods, particularly when I know them to be healthful.	1	2	3	4
6. I select breads, cereals, fresh fruits, and vegetables in preference to pastries, candies, sodas, and fruits canned in heavy syrup.	1	2	3	4
7. I limit the amount of sugar that I add to foods during preparation and at the table.	1	2	3	4
8. I examine food labels to determine the presence of trans-fats (trans-fatty acids) and select foods free of these fats.	1	2	3	4
9. I select primarily nonmeat sources of protein, such as peas, beans, and peanut butter, while limiting my consumption of red meat and high-fat dairy products.	1	2	3	4
10. I consume an appropriate percentage of my total daily calories from protein.	1	2	3	4
11. I select foods prepared with unsaturated vegetable oils while reducing consumption of red meat, high-fat dairy products, and foods prepared with lard (animal fat) or butter.	1	2	3	4
12. I carefully limit the amount of fast food that I consume during a typical week.	1	2	3	4
13. I consume an appropriate percentage of my total daily calories from fat.	1	2	3	4
14. I select nutritious foods when I snack.	1	2	3	4
15. I limit my use of salt during food preparation and at the table.	1	2	3	4
16. I consume adequate amounts of fiber.	1	2	3	4
17. I routinely consider the nutrient density of individual food items when choosing foods.	1	2	3	4
18. I maintain my weight without reliance on over-the-counter or prescription diet pills.	1	2	3	4
19. I maintain my weight without reliance on fad diets or liquid weight loss beverages.	1	2	3	4
20. I exercise regularly to help maintain my weight.	1	2	3	4

POINTS _____

Alcohol, Tobacco, and Other Drug Use

	Not true/ rarely	Somewhat true/ sometimes	Mostly true/ usually	Very true/ always
1. I abstain or drink in moderation when offered alcoholic beverages.	1	2	3	4
2. I abstain from using illegal psychoactive (mind-altering) drugs.	1	2	3	4
3. I do not consume alcoholic beverages or psychoactive drugs rapidly or in large quantities.	1	2	3	4
4. I do not use alcohol or psychoactive drugs in a way that causes me to behave inappropriately.	1	2	3	4
5. My use of alcohol or other drugs does not compromise my academic performance.	1	2	3	4
6. I refrain from drinking alcoholic beverages or using psychoactive drugs when engaging in recreational activities that require strength, speed, or coordination.	1	2	3	4
7. I refrain from drinking alcoholic beverages while participating in occupational activities, regardless of the nature of those activities.	1	2	3	4
8. My use of alcohol or other drugs does not generate financial concerns for myself or for others.	1	2	3	4
9. I refrain from drinking alcohol or using psychoactive drugs when driving a motor vehicle or operating heavy equipment.	1	2	3	4
10. I do not drink alcohol or use psychoactive drugs when I am alone.	1	2	3	4
11. I avoid riding with people who have been drinking alcohol or using psychoactive drugs.	1	2	3	4
12. My use of alcohol or other drugs does not cause family dysfunction.	1	2	3	4
13. I do not use marijuana.	1	2	3	4
14. I do not use hallucinogens.	1	2	3	4
15. I do not use heroin or other illegal intravenous drugs.	1	2	3	4
16. I do not experience blackouts when I drink alcohol.	1	2	3	4
17. I do not become abusive or violent when I drink alcohol or use psychoactive drugs.	1	2	3	4
18. I use potentially addictive prescription medication in complete compliance with my physician's directions.	1	2	3	4
19. I do not smoke cigarettes.	1	2	3	4
20. I do not use tobacco products in any other form.	1	2	3	4
21. I minimize my exposure to secondhand smoke.	1	2	3	4
22. I am concerned about the effect that alcohol, tobacco, and other drug use is known to have on developing fetuses.	1	2	3	4
23. I am concerned about the effect that alcohol, tobacco, and other drug use is known to have on the health of other people.	1	2	3	4
24. I seek natural, health-enhancing highs rather than relying on alcohol, tobacco, and illegal drugs.	1	2	3	4
25. I take prescription medication only as instructed, and I use over-the-counter medication in accordance with directions.	1	2	3	4

POINTS _____

Disease Prevention

	Not true/ rarely	Somewhat true/ sometimes	Mostly true/ usually	Very true/ always
1. My diet includes foods rich in phytochemicals.	1	2	3	4
2. My diet includes foods rich in folic acid.	1	2	3	4
3. My diet includes foods that are good sources of dietary fiber.	1	2	3	4
4. My diet is low in dietary cholesterol.	1	2	3	4
5. I follow food preparation practices that minimize the risk of foodborne illness.	1	2	3	4
6. I engage in regular physical activity and am able to control my weight effectively.	1	2	3	4
7. I do not use tobacco products.	1	2	3	4
8. I abstain from alcohol or drink only in moderation.	1	2	3	4
9. I do not use intravenously administered illegal drugs.	1	2	3	4
10. I use safer sex practices intended to minimize my risk of exposure to sexually transmitted diseases or infections, including HIV and HPV.	1	2	3	4
11. I take steps to limit my risk of exposure to the bacterium that causes Lyme disease and to the virus that causes hantavirus pulmonary syndrome.	1	2	3	4
12. I control my blood pressure with weight management and physical fitness activities.	1	2	3	4
13. I minimize my exposure to allergens, including those that trigger asthma attacks.	1	2	3	4
14. I wash my hands frequently and thoroughly.	1	2	3	4
15. I use preventive medical care services appropriately.	1	2	3	4
16. I use appropriate cancer self-screening practices, such as breast self-examination and testicular self-examination.	1	2	3	4
17. I know which chronic illnesses and diseases are part of my family history.	1	2	3	4
18. I know which inherited conditions are part of my family history and will seek preconceptional counseling regarding these conditions.	1	2	3	4
19. I am fully immunized against infectious diseases.	1	2	3	4
20. I take prescribed medications, particularly antibiotics, exactly as instructed by my physician.	1	2	3	4

POINTS _____

Sexual Health

	Not true/ rarely	Somewhat true/ sometimes	Mostly true/ usually	Very true/ always
1. I know how sexually transmitted diseases are spread.	1	2	3	4
2. I can recognize the symptoms of sexually transmitted diseases.	1	2	3	4
3. I know how sexually transmitted disease transmission can be prevented.	1	2	3	4
4. I know how safer sex practices reduce the risk of contracting sexually transmitted diseases.	1	2	3	4
5. I follow safer sex practices.	1	2	3	4
6. I recognize the symptoms of premenstrual syndrome and understand how it is prevented and treated.	1	2	3	4
7. I recognize the symptoms of endometriosis and understand the relationship of its symptoms to hormonal cycles.	1	2	3	4

	Not true/ rarely	Somewhat true/ sometimes	Mostly true/ usually	Very true/ always
8. I understand the physiological basis of menopause and recognize that it is a normal part of the aging process in women.	1	2	3	4
9. I understand and accept the range of human sexual orientations.	1	2	3	4
10. I encourage the development of flexible sex roles (androgyny) in children.	1	2	3	4
11. I take a mature approach to dating and mate selection.	1	2	3	4
12. I recognize that marriage and other types of long-term relationships can be satisfying.	1	2	3	4
13. I recognize that a celibate lifestyle is appropriate and satisfying for some people.	1	2	3	4
14. I affirm the sexuality of older adults and am comfortable with its expression.	1	2	3	4
15. I am familiar with the advantages and disadvantages of a wide range of birth control methods.	1	2	3	4
16. I understand how each birth control method works and how effective it is.	1	2	3	4
17. I use my birth control method consistently and appropriately.	1	2	3	4
18. I am familiar with the wide range of procedures now available to treat infertility.	1	2	3	4
19. I accept that others may disagree with my feelings about pregnancy termination.	1	2	3	4
20. I am familiar with alternatives available to infertile couples, including adoption.	1	2	3	4

POINTS _____

Safety Practices and Violence Prevention

	Not true/ rarely	Somewhat true/ sometimes	Mostly true/ usually	Very true/ always
1. I attempt to identify sources of risk or danger in each new setting or activity.	1	2	3	4
2. I learn proper procedures and precautions before undertaking new recreational or occupational activities.	1	2	3	4
3. I select appropriate clothing and equipment for all activities and maintain equipment in good working order.	1	2	3	4
4. I curtail my participation in activities when I am not feeling well or am distracted by other demands.	1	2	3	4
5. I repair dangerous conditions or report them to those responsible for maintenance.	1	2	3	4
6. I use common sense and observe the laws governing nonmotorized vehicles when I ride a bicycle.	1	2	3	4
7. I operate all motor vehicles as safely as possible, including using seat belts and other safety equipment.	1	2	3	4
8. I refrain from driving an automobile or boat when I have been drinking alcohol or taking drugs or medications.	1	2	3	4
9. I try to anticipate the risk of falling and maintain my environment to minimize this risk.	1	2	3	4
10. I maintain my environment to minimize the risk of fire, and I have a well-rehearsed plan to exit my residence in case of fire.	1	2	3	4
11. I am a competent swimmer and could save myself or rescue someone who was drowning.	1	2	3	4

	Not true/ rarely	Somewhat true/ sometimes	Mostly true/ usually	Very true/ always
12. I refrain from sexually aggressive behavior toward my partner or others.	1	2	3	4
13. I would report an incident of sexual harassment or date rape whether or not I was the victim.	1	2	3	4
14. I would seek help from others if I were the victim or perpetrator of domestic violence.	1	2	3	4
15. I practice gun safety and encourage other gun owners to do so.	1	2	3	4
16. I drive at all times in a way that will minimize my risk of being carjacked.	1	2	3	4
17. I have taken steps to protect my home from intruders.	1	2	3	4
18. I use campus security services as much as possible when they are available.	1	2	3	4
19. I know what to do if I am being stalked.	1	2	3	4
20. I have a well-rehearsed plan to protect myself from the aggressive behavior of other people in my place of residence.	1	2	3	4

POINTS _____

Health Care Consumerism

	Not true/ rarely	Somewhat true/ sometimes	Mostly true/ usually	Very true/ always
1. I know how to obtain valid health information.	1	2	3	4
2. I accept health information that has been deemed valid by the established scientific community.	1	2	3	4
3. I am skeptical of claims that guarantee the effectiveness of a particular health care service or product.	1	2	3	4
4. I am skeptical of practitioners or clinics who advertise or offer services at rates substantially lower than those charged by reputable providers.	1	2	3	4
5. I am not swayed by advertisements that present unhealthy behavior in an attractive manner.	1	2	3	4
6. I can afford proper medical care, including hospitalization.	1	2	3	4
7. I can afford adequate health insurance.	1	2	3	4
8. I understand the role of government health care plans in providing health care to people who qualify for coverage.	1	2	3	4
9. I know how to select health care providers who are highly qualified and appropriate for my current health care needs.	1	2	3	4
10. I seek a second or third opinion when surgery or other costly therapies are recommended.	1	2	3	4
11. I have told my physician which hospital I would prefer to use should the need arise.	1	2	3	4
12. I understand my rights and responsibilities as a patient when admitted to a hospital.	1	2	3	4
13. I practice adequate self-care to reduce my health care expenditures and my reliance on health care providers.	1	2	3	4
14. I am open-minded about alternative health care practices and support current efforts to determine their appropriate role in effective health care.	1	2	3	4
15. I have a well-established relationship with a pharmacist and have transmitted all necessary information regarding medication use.	1	2	3	4

Comprehensive Health Assessment—*continued*

16. I carefully follow labels and directions when using health care products, such as over-the-counter medications.

1	2	3	4

17. I finish all prescription medications as directed, rather than stopping use when symptoms subside.

1	2	3	4

18. I report to the appropriate agencies any providers of health care services, information, or products that use deceptive advertising or fraudulent methods of operation.

1	2	3	4

19. I pursue my rights as fully as possible in matters of misrepresentation or consumer dissatisfaction.

1	2	3	4

20. I follow current health care issues in the news and voice my opinion to my elected representatives.

1	2	3	4

POINTS _____

Environmental Health

	Not true/ rarely	Somewhat true/ sometimes	Mostly true/ usually	Very true/ always
1. I avoid use of and exposure to pesticides as much as possible.	1	2	3	4
2. I avoid use of and exposure to herbicides as much as possible.	1	2	3	4
3. I am willing to spend the extra money and time required to obtain organically grown produce.	1	2	3	4
4. I reduce environmental pollutants by minimizing my use of the automobile.	1	2	3	4
5. I avoid the use of products that contribute to indoor air pollution.	1	2	3	4
6. I limit my exposure to ultraviolet radiation by avoiding excessive sun exposure.	1	2	3	4
7. I limit my exposure to radon gas by using a radon gas detector.	1	2	3	4
8. I limit my exposure to radiation by promptly eliminating radon gas within my home.	1	2	3	4
9. I limit my exposure to radiation by agreeing to undergo medical radiation procedures only when absolutely necessary for the diagnosis and treatment of an illness or disease.	1	2	3	4
10. I avoid the use of potentially unsafe water, particularly when traveling in a foreign country or when a municipal water supply or bottled water is unavailable.	1	2	3	4
11. I avoid noise pollution by limiting my exposure to loud noise or by using ear protection.	1	2	3	4
12. I avoid air pollution by carefully selecting the environments in which I live, work, and recreate.	1	2	3	4
13. I do not knowingly use or improperly dispose of personal care products that can harm the environment.	1	2	3	4
14. I reuse as many products as possible so that they can avoid the recycling bins for as long as possible.	1	2	3	4
15. I participate fully in my community's recycling efforts.	1	2	3	4
16. I encourage the increased use of recycled materials in the design and manufacturing of new products.	1	2	3	4
17. I dispose of residential toxic substances safely and properly.	1	2	3	4
18. I follow environmental issues in the news and voice my opinion to my elected representatives.	1	2	3	4

19. I am aware of and involved in environmental issues in my local area.

| | 1 | 2 | 3 | 4 |

20. I perceive myself as a steward of the environment for the generations to come, rather than as a person with a right to use (and misuse) the environment to meet my immediate needs.

| | 1 | 2 | 3 | 4 |

POINTS _____

YOUR TOTAL POINTS _____

Interpretation

770 to 880 points—Congratulations! Your health behavior is very supportive of high-level health. Continue to practice your positive health habits, and look for areas in which you can become even stronger. Encourage others to follow your example, and support their efforts in any way you can.

550 to 769 points—Good job! Your health behavior is relatively supportive of high-level health. You scored well in several areas; however, you can improve in some ways. Identify your weak areas and chart a plan for behavior change, as explained at the end of Chapter 1. Then pay close attention as you learn more about health in the weeks ahead.

330 to 549 points—Caution! Your relatively low score indicates that your behavior may be compromising your health. Review your responses to this assessment carefully, noting the areas in which you scored poorly. Then chart a detailed plan for behavior change, as outlined at the end of Chapter 1. Be sure to set realistic goals that you can work toward steadily as you complete this course.

Below 330 points—Red flag! Your low score suggests that your health behavior is destructive. Immediate changes in your behavior are needed to put you back on track. Review your responses to this assessment carefully. Then begin to make changes in the most critical areas, such as harmful alcohol or other drug use patterns. Seek help promptly for any difficulties that you are not prepared to deal with alone, such as domestic violence or suicidal thoughts. The information you read in this textbook and learn in this course could have a significant effect on your future health. Remember, it's not too late to improve your health!

TO CARRY THIS FURTHER . . .

Most of us can improve our health behavior in a number of ways. We hope this assessment will help you identify areas in which you can make positive changes and serve as a motivator as you implement your plan for behavior change. If you scored well, give yourself a pat on the back. If your score was not as high as you would have liked, take heart. This textbook and your instructor can help you get started on the road to wellness. Good luck!

The Mind

Part One covers two topics that are closely linked to how we handle change in our lives. Chapter 2 discusses psychological health, and Chapter 3 deals with stress management. As explained below, your personal growth closely relates to each of the six health dimensions discussed in Chapter 1.

1. Physical Dimension

The physical dimension of health concerns the structure and the function of all body systems. Many of the experiences that shape your feelings about yourself are made possible by good physical health. In addition, effective coping skills often require us to draw on the physical dimension of health.

2. Psychological Dimension

Our responses to stress are primarily emotional. Feelings of uneasiness arising from the demands of college, relationships, parenting, or work are the hallmarks of stress. Fortunately, you can cope with change by using the resources of your psychological dimension of health. Your sense of humor, capacity for empathy, and attitude toward adversity will help you cope with demanding changes in your life.

3. Social Dimension

Growth and development are influenced by the people with whom you interact. When things go well with roommates, coworkers, or your spouse or children, you begin to feel capable as a social person. Occasional failures in social relationships can produce stress but can also remind you that emotional growth and coping skills take time to develop.

4. Intellectual Dimension

As you grow older, you will call on your intellectual resources with increasing frequency. These resources will help you enjoy life more fully and understand your emotional and spiritual growth. During difficult times, your mind may be your most dependable coping source. A book, a concert, or an art exhibit may be a refuge from the stress of the classroom, family, or office.

5. Spiritual Dimension

Many of today's students are searching for a deeper understanding of the meaning of life. Some students feel pressured to accept the spiritual beliefs of the majority. The uncertainties of exploring what to believe and how to express those beliefs can create stress. Your spirituality can be a valuable resource during periods of stress. Meditation, introspection, and prayer can free people from some of the stress of living in a fast-paced, sometimes uncaring world. To believe deeply in something and to act on that belief by serving others leads to personal growth.

6. Occupational Dimension

The vocation you choose will have a lasting effect on shaping the person you will become. Many people choose an occupation that allows them to serve others. However, work can be a primary source of life stress. Some of this stress is unwelcome and can be harmful. But occupational stress can also challenge you to perform at your peak, generating a sense of pride and accomplishment.

Achieving Psychological Health

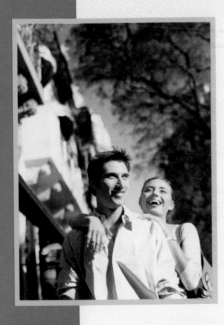

What Do You Know About Psychological Health?

1. Psychological health has been associated with having a good sense of humor. True or False?

2. Self-esteem is the highest level of psychological health on Maslow's hierarchy of needs. True or False?

3. Pessimists tend to live longer than optimists do. True or False?

4. It has been proven that personality is influenced more by heredity than by environment. True or False?

5. Mental disorders are the leading cause of disability in the United States. True or False?

6. Psychologists cannot prescribe medication such as antidepressants. True or False?

7. Schizophrenia is a mental disorder that involves having dissociative identity disorder. True or False?

Check your answers at the end of the chapter.

Defining Psychological Health

How many feelings are people capable of expressing? Happy, sad, fearful, and angry are the four primary emotions that humans universally feel. These emotions are considered to be hardwired into human neuroanatomy for survival. Permutations of these four primary emotions result in our capacity to express about 100 different emotions, such as feeling frustrated, although cultural differences do exist[1] (see the box "Cultural Differences in Emotional Expression" for more information). These feelings are all part of the psychological dimension of health. The terms *emotional wellness* and **psychological health** have been used interchangeably to describe how people function in the emotional and cognitive realms of their lives. Such functioning includes how people express their emotions; cope with stress, adversity, and success; and adapt to changes in themselves and their environment. Psychological health also addresses cognitive functioning—the ways people think and behave in conjunction with their emotions. There is some debate about whether thoughts influence feelings or feelings cause us to think and behave a certain way. However, the most accepted view is that the way we think can directly change how we feel about an event or a situation. Thus, you can change your feelings about something by changing your attitude and perspective about a situation. This ability has implications for how we can increase our self-esteem and confidence

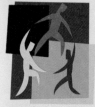

Learning from Our Diversity

Cultural Differences in Emotional Expression

Although humans share four primary emotions—happiness, fear, anger, and sadness—we do not all express them in the same way. For example, to express fear, Oriya women of Bhubaneshwar, India, extend their tongues out and downward, raise their eyebrows, and widen and cross their eyes, whereas Europeans and Americans tend to open their eyes wide, raise their eyebrows, and open their mouths wide. There are also significant cultural differences in how acceptable it is to express feelings. Some cultures (such as Asian cultures) are more emotionally restrictive, while others (such as Italians) are more emotionally intense.

Expressing anger is rare for Tahitians and Utku Eskimos; in contrast, Americans and Western Europeans tend to frequently express this emotion.

Even though cultures share the same emotions, not all situations evoke the same emotional response in all cultures. For example, people from Bali laugh in response to grief and fall asleep in reaction to unfamiliar or frightening situations. Americans tend to interpret smiling as expressing the emotion of happiness; however, in Asian cultures, smiling may be perceived as masking an unacceptable emotion such as anger or sadness.

Emotions communicate meaning and provide an interpretation of events through both nonverbal and verbal cues. Emotions are key in social interactions, as they influence behavior and elicit reactions from others. In addition, feelings convey social statements about you, others, and the situation. Therefore, to avoid miscommunication, it is important to take into consideration the cultural context of emotional expression, as this can greatly change the meaning or interpretation of an event or an emotional expression.

Sources: LeBaron M, Bridging cultural conflicts: *A New Approach for a Changing World.* San Franciso: Jossey Bass, 2003; Davidson R, Scherer K, Goldsmith H. *Handbook of Affective Sciences.* New York: Oxford University Press, 2003.

---

level, and enhance our interactions with others. You will learn more about psychological health in this chapter.

When you apply resources from the multiple dimensions of health (Chapter 1) in ways that allow you to direct your growth, assess deeply held values, deal effectively with change, and have satisfying relationships with others, you are psychologically healthy.

Research in the area of health psychology has shown that there is a mind-body connection in which biological, psychological, and social factors interact to influence health or illness. This is referred to as the **biopsychological model.**[2] We know that one's psychological state has a significant effect on physical health; stress, depression, and anxiety have been associated with how the immune system responds and can impair physical health. For example, studies have shown that terminally ill cancer patients who had good psychological health lived longer and reported having a higher quality of life than did other cancer patients.[3]

Psychological health has also been associated with developing and maintaining a positive **self-concept,** positive **self-esteem,** and a higher level of **emotional intelligence.** However, as you will see, psychological health is much more than just the absence of mental illness.

Characteristics of Psychologically Healthy People

Your self-concept is the internal picture you have of yourself and is a reflection of your psychological health. Psychologically healthy people are not perfect. They have their share of stress, problems, and flaws, and they make their share of mistakes. However, it is how they perceive themselves and how they cope with their stress and problems that separate them from unhealthy individuals. Psychologically healthy people

- Accept themselves and others
- Like themselves

Key Terms

psychological health A broadly based concept pertaining to cognitive functioning in conjunction with the way people express their emotions; cope with stress, adversity, and success; and adapt to changes in themselves and their environment.

biopsychological model A model that addresses how biological, psychological, and social factors interact and affect psychological health.

self-concept An individual's internal picture of himself or herself; the way one sees oneself.

self-esteem An individual's sense of pride, self-respect, value, and worth.

emotional intelligence The ability to understand others and act wisely in human relations and measure how well one knows one's emotions, manages one's emotions, motivates oneself, recognizes emotions in others, and handles relationships.

- Appropriately express the full range of human emotions, both positive and negative
- Give and receive care, love, and support
- Accept life's disappointments
- Accept their mistakes
- Express empathy and concern for others
- Take care of themselves
- Trust others as well as themselves
- Establish goals, both short and long term
- Can function both independently and interdependently
- Lead a health-enhancing lifestyle that includes regular exercise, good nutrition, and adequate sleep

Self-Esteem

What is self-esteem? How do you know when someone is lacking in self-esteem? Most people answer this question by saying that they define positive self-esteem as

- Having pride in yourself
- Treating yourself with respect
- Considering yourself valuable, important, worthy
- Feeling good about yourself
- Having self-confidence, being self-assured
- Accepting yourself

People with low levels of self-esteem tend to allow others to mistreat them, don't take care of themselves, have difficulty being by themselves, and have little self-confidence. In addition, people with low self-esteem tend to take things personally and are sometimes seen as overly sensitive; they tend to be perfectionists who are highly critical of themselves and others. These individuals often have a pessimistic outlook on life and see themselves as undeserving of good fortune. We explore the concepts of optimism and pessimism as they relate to psychological health in a later section of this chapter.

Where do we get our self-esteem? Most people would say from their parents, teachers, peers, siblings, religious institutions, and the media. While these factors certainly can positively or negatively affect our self-concept and self-esteem, they are all *external* factors. Self-concept refers to our *internal* self-perception. People with low self-esteem tend to have a poor self-concept, meaning that their internal picture of themselves is very negative. Because of this poor self-concept, people with low self-esteem tend to allow others to mistreat or abuse them and fail to be assertive. Many psychological problems have their underpinnings in low self-esteem, including eating disorders, substance abuse, and depression.

People who suffer from low self-esteem tend to focus on outside factors. If our self-esteem and self-concept

were based solely on external factors, then we would need to change only our environment and the people around us to raise our self-esteem. Thus, many people believe that if they had more money, a nicer car, a better relationship, and so on, they would feel better about themselves. This can become a vicious cycle, leaving these people always seeking more and being perpetually dissatisfied with themselves. This can also lead to perfectionism and not accepting yourself.

Although we don't have much control over other people, we do have control over what we internalize or accept as true and valid about ourselves. Self-esteem is not an all-or-none commodity. Most people have varying degrees of self-esteem, depending on their stage of development, events in their lives, and their environment.[4] Compared with how their parents perceived themselves 30 years ago, today's college students are more likely to have higher levels of self-esteem, perceiving themselves as better partners, parents, and workers.

Emotional Intelligence

A third aspect of psychological health is the degree of emotional intelligence you possess. Emotional intelligence refers to "the ability to understand others and act wisely in human relations."[5] Furthermore, emotional intelligence can be broken down into five primary domains:

- *Knowing your emotions.* This is considered to be the cornerstone of emotional intelligence and relates to how much self-awareness and insight you have. How quickly you are able to recognize and label your feelings as you feel them determines the level of your emotional intelligence.
- *Managing your emotions.* How well can you express your feelings appropriately and cope with your emotions? People who have trouble coping with anxiety, distress, and failures tend to have lower levels of emotional intelligence.
- *Motivating yourself.* People who can motivate themselves tend to be more highly productive and independent than are those who rely on external sources for motivation. The more you can self-motivate and engage in goal-directed activities, the higher your emotional intelligence.
- *Recognizing emotions in others.* Another aspect of emotional intelligence is the degree of empathy you have, or how sensitive you are to the feelings of others and how you relate to other people.
- *Handling relationships.* This refers to your level of social skills. The more interpersonally effective you are and the more you are able to negotiate conflict and build a social support network, the more emotional intelligence you possess.

Of course people have differing levels of emotional intelligence and may have higher levels in one domain than in another. People with overall high levels of emotional intelligence tend to take on leadership roles, are confident, are assertive, express their feelings directly and appropriately, feel good about themselves, are outgoing, and adapt well to stress.[5]

Personality

What is meant when someone says, "She has a good personality"? Is it possible to have no personality? **Personality** is generally defined as a specific set of consistent patterns of behaviors and traits that help to identify and characterize an individual. Personality includes thoughts, feelings, behaviors, motivation, instinct, and temperament.[6] Isn't it likely that you associate a "good" personality with the existence of psychological health?

There is some debate about how personality is formed and where we acquire our personality traits. A general consensus is that two factors, **nature** and **nurture,** influence the shaping of personality. *Nature* refers to the innate factors we are born with that genetically determine our personality traits. *Nurture* is the effect that the environment, people, and external factors have on our personality.[7] While it is agreed that both nature and nurture influence personality development, there is some debate about how much of a role each one plays in its formation. We all know people who are introverted or quiet or shy "by nature" or "naturally outgoing." We seem to be born with a predisposition toward certain personality traits that often resemble our parents'. "She is serious like her father" or "He is funny like his mother" are remarks people may make alluding to this genetic link. Environmental factors, such as social relationships, family harmony, financial resources, job and academic concerns, and living situations, can influence your personality.

Often assumptions are made about an individual's personality based largely on his or her appearance. Studies have shown that physically attractive people are seen as warm, friendly, and intelligent, and unattractive people are viewed as cold, humorless, and not as bright.[8] First impressions also play a major role in how we perceive other people's personalities. Research shows that we tend to make a decision about someone's personality within four minutes of meeting them. Once an impression is formed, it is difficult to change, regardless of how the person behaves or new information that you receive that might contradict what you initially perceived.[7] Thus, people can make errors in judgment because they have not taken the context into consideration or taken enough time to get to know someone over the course of several months and in a variety of settings.

The Normal Range of Emotions

You probably know people who seem happy all the time. Although some people like this may exist, they are truly the exceptions. Most people feel happy, confident, and positive at times, while at other times, they feel sad, insecure, and negative. Once you know them better, these same people may show that they feel happy, sad, pleased, uncertain, confident, excited, and afraid all in the same day or week. To outsiders, they might even appear to be moody. To the mental health professional, however, these same people would probably seem to be normal, since the feeling states that they are demonstrating all fall within a normal range of emotions.

Experiencing a range of emotions is normal and healthy. You should not expect to remain calm and rational every minute of the day. You also should not expect to adjust effectively to every situation with which you are confronted. Life has its ups and downs, and the concept of the *normal range of emotions* reflects this. It is when emotions fluctuate to an extreme level (both up and down), aren't expressed appropriately, or are out of control and overwhelming that people can become psychologically unhealthy.

Maslow's Hierarchy of Needs

Abraham Maslow has been one of the most significant contributors to the understanding of personality and emotional growth. Central to Maslow's contribution to twentieth-century American psychological thought is his view of psychological health in terms of the individual's attempt to meet inner needs, what he called *the hierarchy of needs*[9] (see Figure 2-1).

Maslow's theory is a positive, optimistic theory of human behavior. He believed that people are motivated to grow and fulfill their potential, referring to this phenomenon as **self-actualization.** He described

---

Key Terms

personality A specific set of consistent patterns of behavior and traits that helps to identify and characterize an individual; personality comprises thoughts, feelings, behaviors, motivation, instinct, and temperament.

nature The innate factors that genetically determine personality traits.

nurture The effect that the environment, people, and external factors have on personality.

self-actualization The highest level of psychological health, at which one reaches his or her highest potential and values truth, beauty, goodness, faith, love, humor, and ingenuity.

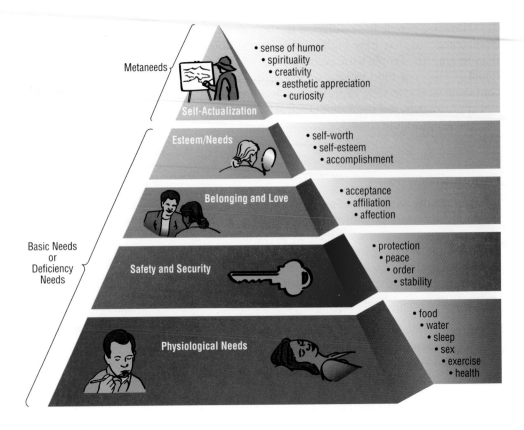

Figure 2-1 Maslow's Hierarchy of Needs Once basic needs are met, metaneeds such as creativity, spirituality, and justice come into play.

Source: Maslow, A. H., Frager, R. D. (Ed.), Fadiman, J. (Ed.). *Motivation and Personality*, 3rd ed. © 1987. By permission of Pearson Education, Inc., Upper Saddle, River, NJ.

self-actualization as "the need to become more and more what one is, to become everything that one is capable of becoming."[10] Maslow differentiated between two different categories of needs: **basic needs** and **metaneeds**. Basic needs—physiological needs, safety and security, belonging and love, and esteem needs—are the deficiency needs and are essential and urgent. Metaneeds come into play once the basic needs are met and include spirituality, creativity, curiosity, beauty, philosophy, and justice. Maslow's hierarchy of needs is arranged with the basic needs on the bottom, as they are the most fundamental and powerful needs. Lower-level needs must be met before the next level of needs can be satisfied. Maslow believed that people must fulfill their metaneeds in order to become completely developed human beings. Left unfulfilled, people can become cynical, apathetic, and lonely.[11]

Maslow arrived at this model by examining people whom he considered to be exceptionally healthy,

people he defined as having developed to their fullest potentials. People whom Maslow identified as self-actualized included Albert Einstein, Albert Schweitzer, Eleanor Roosevelt, and Abraham Lincoln. He perceived these people to share similar personality characteristics, such as being self-assured, principled, innovative, compassionate, altruistic, goal-oriented, and internally motivated.[11]

Creative Expression

Another characteristic of people who have developed their psychological health is creativity. Allowing yourself to express your thoughts, feelings, and individuality in a creative manner entails having self-confidence, self-esteem, and flexibility. Confidence and self-esteem are essential so that you feel free to share your creative side with others and don't feel embarrassed by your creativity. Children can easily do this when they draw a picture or make up a dance and say, "Look at me; look at what I made." However, as we age, some of us become inhibited and don't allow ourselves to be creative or to share this part of ourselves. If you don't exercise your creative side, it can atrophy, just as unexercised muscles do.

What are some resources that you might need to develop and foster your creativity?

- *Nonconformity.* Creative individuals aren't terribly concerned about what other people think of them. They are willing to risk looking foolish or proposing

---

Key Terms

basic needs Deficiency needs that are viewed as essential and fundamental, including physiological, safety and security, belonging and love, and esteem needs.

metaneeds Secondary concerns, such as spirituality, creativity, curiosity, beauty, philosophy, and justice, that can be addressed only after the basic needs are met.

Mindfulness: Time to Pay Attention

Have you taken a moment today to be quiet and just be with your-self? Time alone can help you step away from a busy, fragmented world and draw inward for renewal. Having strengthened awareness of yourself in both mind and body allows you to experience the full-ness of the moment, even to feel in sync with the universe. This is referred to as "mindfulness"—focusing on the present without judg-ing, just accepting.

Any time you take for this meditation will be restorative. You may start with just five minutes every morning. You will need a place where you feel comfortable to be alone with your own thoughts. For example, mindfulness could be sitting in class waiting to take a test

and observing that your heart is beating faster than usual. You perceive that you feel both ner-vous and excited to take the test, but you don't pass judgment on your emotions, you simply acknowledge them. When you are faced with a difficult project, a per-sonal crisis, or something more serious, such as sickness or death, these reflective moments will give you mental and spiritual renewal.

It's not selfish to carve out whatever time you need alone to refresh yourself. By paying attention to your thoughts and feelings, you're reconnecting to your inner self. This nourished spirit is some-thing you can share with others.

---

ideas that are divergent from others' ideas or tradi-tional ways of thinking.

- *Independence.* Highly creative people tend to work well alone and sometimes prefer this to working in a group. As children, they often were encouraged to solve problems on their own rather than having someone else do so for them.

- *Motivation.* Creative people are motivated by intrin-sic rather than external rewards, meaning they like to be creative for their own pleasure, not to please others or because it is expected of them. They enjoy creativity for creativity's sake alone, not to reap rewards or praise from others.

- *Curiosity.* Creative people have a wide range of inter-ests and a broad base of knowledge. They are open to new experiences and question things that other people ignore or take for granted.

- *Persistence.* This is seen as one of the most important traits of a creative person. As Thomas Edison said, "Genius is one-tenth inspiration and nine-tenths perspiration." Persistence requires not giving up when your first efforts are not successful and think-ing of new ways of doing something, problem solv-ing, or thinking "outside the box."[12]

Some people reviewing the preceding list may rec-ognize many of these characteristics as being already well developed in their own personalities. Others may not have demonstrated some of the traits listed, and the traits may appear far beyond their reach. Neverthe-less, most people can increase their creativity by giving themselves permission to be creative. Some people state, "I'm not a creative person," and yet they haven't explored that part of their personality, perhaps since childhood. There are many avenues of creativity, and the first step is to experiment, to be open and spontaneous. In this way, you can gain greater psychological health from accessing your inner strengths and resources.

Spiritual Health

Having a sense of purpose, direction, and awareness is a dimension of spiritual health. This aspect of psychologi-cal health also refers to how well we integrate our beliefs and values with our behavior. People with spiritual health seek meaning and purpose in their lives and have a deep appreciation for a sense of unity and community (see the box "Mindfulness"). Spiritual health also includes one's morals, ethics, intrinsic values, and beliefs. It also refers to an awareness and appreciation of the vastness of the universe, and recognition of a dimension beyond the natural and rational, involving, perhaps, a belief in a force greater than oneself.[13] Spirituality has been found to increase psychological health; people who incorporate it into their lives reported better psychological coping, increased well-being, increased satisfaction with life, lower anxiety and fewer depressive symptoms, less hos-tility and anger, and greater happiness in general.[14] Simi-larly, spirituality has also been related to better physical health. Studies have shown that no matter how *spiritual-ity* was defined or measured, it has a positive effect on reducing coronary heart disease, high blood pressure, stroke, and cancer and increasing life expectancy.[15]

As a resource in the spiritual dimension of health, the existence of spirituality provides a basis on which your belief system can mature and your expanding awareness of life's meaning can be fostered. In addition, the exis-tence of spirituality lends meaning to your career and assists you in better understanding the consequences of your vocational efforts. Further, spirituality can influence many of the experiences that you will seek throughout life and can temper the emotional relationships that you have with these experiences. In virtually all cultures, spiritual-ity provides individuals and groups with rituals and prac-tices that foster the development of a sense of community. In turn, the community provides the structure and guid-ance that nurtures the emotional stability, confidence, and sense of competence needed for living life fully.[16]

Keys to Psychological Health

Cultivating a Sense of Humor

Perhaps the most prized emotion to be experienced is a feeling of happiness about life—a feeling that is more likely to occur when day-to-day events are entered into with an underlying sense of humor. Maintaining a sense of humor is now known to be a critically important component of the psychological dimension of health.[17] People who possess this ability understand that life is not meant to be taken too seriously.

Recognizing the humor in daily situations and occasionally being able to laugh at yourself will make you feel better not only about others but also, more importantly, about yourself. Others will enjoy being associated with you, and your ability to perform physically and to recover from injuries and illnesses will also be enhanced.[18] In addition, laughter reduces stress,[19] boosts the immune system,[20] alleviates pain,[21] stabilizes mood,[22] decreases anxiety,[23] enhances communication,[24] and inspires creativity.[25] The research suggests that we need to laugh 30 minutes total in a 24-hour period in order to attain these benefits. This is an easy task for children, who on average laugh 250 times a day, but more challenging for adults, who tend to laugh only 15 times a day.[26] Employers have been putting the benefits of laughter to good use to increase productivity in factories. Factories in India have created "laughing clubs" in which people laugh together for 20 minutes a day, resulting in less absenteeism and better performance among the workers.[27]

Developing Communication Skills

When people find it difficult to initiate or even participate in conversations with others, it is likely, in part, that they have not developed some of the communication skills with which others feel comfortable. In this section we investigate how speaking and listening can foster improved social relationships. We also look at the use of unspoken communication as an aid to social interaction.

Verbal Communication   Communication between people can be viewed in terms of a particular person's role as sender or receiver. You can enhance your effectiveness as a sender of verbal information by implementing several important steps:[4]

- *Take the time to think before speaking.* Effective communication requires that you know what you want to say.
- *Focus your words on your most important thoughts and ideas.* Your main message may get lost in too many details or too long a story.

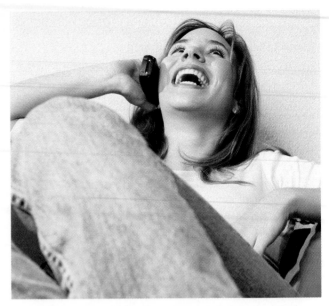

Laughing increases endorphin levels to help ease pain, decrease stress, and release tension from your body.

- *Speak clearly and concisely.* This will aid the listener, particularly when ideas are complex or new.
- *Talk with, rather than at, the listener.* Speaking with other people encourages listeners to share freely and comfortably with those speaking.
- *Start on a positive note.* Even when the message is negative, a more positive atmosphere is established when a conversation begins in this manner.
- *Seek feedback from listeners.* Provide frequent intervals between ideas to allow listeners to respond.
- *Use other forms of communication to transmit important ideas* when face-to-face conversation is not effective. Written communication or the use of a carefully selected third person is often highly effective.

Verbal communication requires that you function as skillfully as a listener, or receiver, as you do as a sender of spoken ideas. Certainly, there are skills for structuring the exchange of information. The following are a variety of listening approaches:

- *Focus on what is being said,* not on what you want to say next.
- *Ask for clarification* and summarize what you think you heard the speaker saying to ensure you have received the message accurately.
- On some occasions, *it may be necessary to guide the speaker* to ensure that excessive or confusing information is not being transmitted. This is accomplished by asking carefully worded questions intended to stay on the topic and not get off on a tangent.

Nonverbal Communication Nonverbal communication is what is communicated by your facial expressions, body posture, tone of voice, movements, and even the way you breathe, such as when you sigh or yawn. Nonverbal communication is a very powerful and sometimes more important aspect of the message than what is verbally communicated. Facial cues, particularly from the eyes, are attended to more than any other type of nonverbal communication, even when information from other sources, such as hand and body movements, may provide a more accurate picture of what the person is feeling. The following suggestions can enhance your nonverbal communication skills:

- *Facial expressions.* Facial expressions have been cited as one of the most important sources of nonverbal communication in terms of a person's emotional state.[28] When people speak with their eyebrows raised, they tend to be seen as more animated, excited, and happy. Flushing of one's face can indicate embarrassment, and crinkling one's nose can mean that you don't like something. Every part of your face can communicate some type of emotional reaction.

- *Eye contact.* Maintaining eye contact is an important component of positive nonverbal communication, while looking away or shifting your eyes can be read as seeming dishonest. But don't stare—five to seven seconds seems to be the maximum amount of time to look at someone's eyes before the person begins to feel scrutinized.

- *Personal space.* There are cultural differences in how much personal space or distance is comfortable and accepted when sitting or standing next to another person. For example, Americans' personal space—about 3 to 4 feet for a casual conversation—tends to be much greater than that of Arabs or Italians but less than for Japanese or Britons. Gender and age and degree of familiarity are other factors that can determine the amount of personal space you are comfortable having between you and another person.

- *Body posture.* Assertiveness is equated with people who carry themselves with their head up and shoulders back and maintain eye contact. Folding your arms, crossing your legs, and looking away from the speaker can indicate defensiveness and rejection.

As with verbal communication, when nonverbal components are recognized and well directed, communication is more effective.

Managing Conflict

Communication can be especially challenging when there is a conflict or disagreement. Emotions such as anger, hurt, and fear might alter your ability to communicate as effectively as you would like.

Some techniques for managing angry or upset people or conflictual situations are these:

- *Listen to and acknowledge the other person's point of view, even if it differs from your own.* To ensure that you have heard the person accurately and to let that person know you are listening, repeat back or summarize what you heard and ask if you misunderstood something that was said.

- *Use assertive communication.* Using "I" statements rather than "You" statements helps to avoid putting people on the defensive and is especially helpful when negotiating conflict or disagreements. Rather than saying "You are inconsiderate," you can say "I feel upset when you're late and don't call to let me know."

- *Focus not just on what you say but how you say it.* Pay attention to your tone of voice and speak in a conversational tone. People tend to talk louder because they think they will be better heard that way. This can result in a shouting match in which neither person hears the other.

- *Acknowledge the other person's feelings.* Use statements like "I can understand why this is so frustrating for you."

- *Watch your body posture.* Don't fold your arms in a closed, defensive posture, maintain eye contact, and be aware of your facial expression so that you are not conveying hostility nonverbally. Make sure your nonverbal communication matches your verbal communication.

- *Accept valid criticism.* If you made a mistake, admit to it and apologize for whatever you think you did to contribute to the misunderstanding or conflict. This will open the door for the other person to take responsibility for his or her part in the conflict as well.

- *Focus on the problem at hand.* If you try to resolve every disagreement you have ever had with this person, you will become overwhelmed and won't accomplish much. Stay on track by talking about the present situation.

- *Take a team approach by engaging in mutual problem solving.* Avoid the winner-versus-loser paradigm, and look for areas of compromise. Find a middle ground you can both live with.

- *Agree to disagree.* There is probably more than one right answer, and you can agree that you will not persuade the other person to change his or her point of view.

- *Agree to discuss this at a later time.* If the conversation becomes too volatile and heated, take some time to calm down and think about the situation. Some time and distance from the problem can be beneficial. Also ask yourself if this is really important enough to you to continue arguing about the situation.

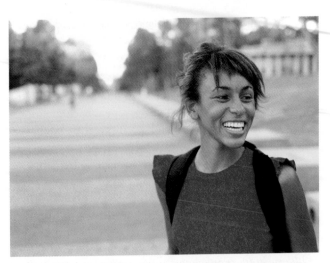

Optimists—those who see the glass as half full—interpret life's events positively and are better able to cope with setbacks and adversity.

Taking an Optimistic Approach to Life

Is your happiness within your control? Are people born naturally happy or sad? One important key to psychological health is the way you think about and interpret events in your life. For example, if you say "hello" to someone and don't get a response, do you begin to wonder if that person is angry with you? Or do you surmise that he or she didn't hear you or perhaps was distracted? Research shows that having a positive interpretation of life's events, particularly how you cope with adversity, can make a significant difference in terms of your health, academic and work performance, and how long you will live.[29] Do you see the glass half empty, as pessimists do, or half full, as optimists do? Does it matter? Again studies overwhelmingly contend that your perspective makes a tremendous difference in your psychological health. Compared with pessimists, optimists tend to

- Contract fewer infectious diseases
- Have better health habits
- Possess stronger immune systems
- Be more successful in their careers
- Perform better in sports, music, and academics

We do know that people can learn to be helpless and ultimately become depressed and even suicidal. Ivan Pavlov demonstrated the concept of **learned helplessness** in his classic study in which he administered an electric shock to dogs that were harnessed and couldn't escape the shock. When he moved the dogs to another room and delivered the shocks, the dogs lay down and whimpered and didn't try to avoid the shocks. This time the dogs were not harnessed and could have easily escaped the shocks by moving to another side of the room. This reaction has been referred to as learned helplessness. The dogs learned that there was nothing they could do to affect their situation, and they lost hope and felt trapped and powerless.[30] We have seen this same phenomenon with humans. College students volunteered for an experiment in which they were subjected to an earsplitting noise and their efforts to stop the noise were unsuccessful. Later, when they were placed in another situation in which they could have easily pulled a control lever to turn off the noise, they made no effort to do so and just suffered with the noise until the experimenter stopped it.[31] Battered women have demonstrated this same sense of powerlessness and helplessness in their inability to escape the abuse they are subjected to by their partners.

So, if people can learn to be helpless and pessimistic, can they also learn to feel more optimistic, powerful, and in control? Martin Seligman, a prominent psychologist, conducted studies to prove that this is possible, and he called this concept **learned optimism.** Learned optimism refers to your explanatory style—in other words, if you describe the glass as being half full or half empty. Seligman identified three key factors that contribute to having an optimistic or pessimistic perspective: **permanence, pervasiveness,** and **personalization.**[3]

Permanence   The first dimension is *permanence.* When something bad happens, pessimists tend to give up easily because they believe the causes of bad events are *permanent.* They say things like "Nothing ever works out for me," "That won't ever work," or "He's always in a bad mood." They use permanence language—words like *never, always,* and *forever*—which implies that this negative situation is not temporary but will continue indefinitely. Optimists tend to use language of temporariness—such words as *sometimes, frequently,* and *often*—and they blame bad events on transient conditions. Examples of optimistic language are "It didn't work out this time," "Doing it that way didn't work," and "He's in a bad mood today." Optimists see failure as a small, transitory setback and are able to pick themselves up, brush themselves off, and persevere toward their goals.

Pervasiveness   The second factor that affects our outlook is *pervasiveness.* It refers to whether you perceive negative events as universal and generalize them to everything in your life, or if you can compartmentalize and keep them defined to the specific situation. Pessimists tend to make universal explanations for their problems, and when something goes wrong in one part of their lives, they give up on everything. While pessimists would say that they are not good at math, optimists would say that they didn't perform well in that particular class with that type of math: "I'm good at algebra but not as good with geometry." The last aspect of an optimistic or pessimistic explanatory style is determined by whether you blame bad things on yourself or on other people or circumstances.

Personalization   Pessimism and low self-esteem tend to come from personalizing events—blaming oneself and having an internal explanatory style for negative events. An optimist might say, "The professor wrote a very poor exam and that is the reason I received a lower score," whereas the pessimist would say, "I am stupid" or "I didn't study enough." This is different from not taking responsibility for one's actions and blaming other people for your problems or mistakes: the idea is to have a balanced perspective and outlook on life. Pessimists tend to give credit to other people or circumstances when good things happen and blame themselves when bad events occur. For example, a pessimist would say, "That was just dumb luck" rather than taking credit for a success. However, if pessimists fail, they readily blame themselves, saying, "I messed up." In contrast, optimists tend to give themselves credit for their accomplishments, saying "I worked hard and did a good job," and they don't belittle themselves when things go wrong.

Seligman conducted many studies to test how an optimistic explanatory style might be useful in daily living. For example, he worked with a swimming team from the University of California, Berkeley, to see how optimism or pessimism might affect their performance. He had the coaches tell the athletes that their times were slower than they actually were. The swimmers were then asked to swim the event again as fast as they could. The performance of the pessimists deteriorated in their 100-yard event by two seconds, the difference between winning the event and finishing dead last. The optimists got faster by two to five seconds, again enough to be the difference between losing and winning the race.[3] So how you interpret events, your attribution style, can make a tremendous difference in the eventual success or failure in your endeavors.

Building Optimism   How can you learn to be more optimistic? Albert Ellis developed a cognitive framework for positive thinking called the ABC method. When you encounter an event, the "A" part of the formula, you try to make sense out of it and explain what has happened. For example, if you receive a notice from the bank that you have overdrawn your checking account, you start to think, "How did this happen?" These thoughts are associated with your beliefs, the "B" in ABC. Your beliefs affect your feelings, and so you can control your emotions by changing your beliefs and thoughts.[32] So, if you think, "I'm irresponsible for letting this happen. I can't manage my money," then you will feel bad about your-self. But if you said, "The bank probably made a mistake" or "I might have added something incorrectly," you will most likely feel much better about yourself and the situation.

The "C" aspect is the consequence of the event, how you end up feeling about the situation. When someone feels depressed, he or she feels hopeless, trapped, and powerless. By adopting a more positive way of reframing or thinking about events, you create options, hope, and a strategy for solving problems rather than remaining stuck, like the whimpering dogs laying down and putting up with being shocked. In the previously described scenario with the overdraft, you can generate ideas such as "I need to check with the bank, go over my bank statement, be more careful in recording and calculating my balances, and request overdraft protection to prevent this from becoming a problem again."

Everyone encounters adversity sometime in his or her life. You can become discouraged by these events, blame yourself for these problems, and feel hopeless, worthless, and cynical about the world. Or you can be persistent and become stronger by overcoming these obstacles, by having positive beliefs, and by seeing these problems as short-lived, specific, and not a flaw in your character. When you embrace an optimistic perspective, you will feel more hopeful, stronger, and confident. You will be able to accept new challenges and take risks in your life. Take the Personal Assessment at the end of this chapter to find your level of optimism and pessimism.

> **Key Terms**
>
> **learned helplessness** A theory of motivation explaining how individuals can learn to feel powerless, trapped, and defeated.
>
> **learned optimism** An attribution style regarding permanence, pervasiveness, and personalization; how people explain both positive and negative events in their lives, accounting for success and failure.
>
> **permanence** The first dimension of an individual's attribution style, related to whether certain events are perceived as temporary or long lasting.
>
> **pervasiveness** The second dimension of an individual's attribution style, related to whether events are perceived as specific or general.
>
> **personalization** The final dimension of attribution style, related to whether an individual takes things personally or is more balanced in accepting responsibility for positive and negative events.

Taking a Proactive Approach to Life

In addition to the approaches already discussed, the plan that follows is intended to give you other strategies for enhancing your psychological health. The following is a four-step process that continues throughout life: constructing perceptions of yourself, accepting these perceptions, undertaking new experiences, and reframing your perceptions based on new information.

Constructing Mental Pictures Actively taking charge of your psychological health begins with constructing a mental picture of what you're like. Use the most recent and accurate information you have about yourself—what is important to you, your values, and your abilities. You may want to ask trusted friends and family members for their input.

To construct this mental picture, set aside a period of uninterrupted quiet time for reflection. Before proceeding to the second step, you also need to construct mental pictures about yourself in relation to *other people and material objects,* including your residence and college or work environment, to clarify these relationships.

Accepting Mental Pictures The second step of the plan involves an *acceptance* of these perceptions. This implies a willingness to honor the truthfulness of the perceptions you have formed about yourself and other people.

Psychological development is an active process. You must be willing to be *introspective* (inwardly reflective) about yourself and the world around you and to apply these new perceptions.

Undertaking New Experiences The next step of the plan is to test your newly formed perceptions. This *testing* is accomplished by *undertaking* a *new experience* or by reexperiencing something in a different way.

New experiences do not necessarily require high levels of risk, foreign travel, or money. They may be no more "new" than deciding to move from the dorm into an apartment, to change from one shift at work to another, or to pursue new friendships. The experience itself is not the goal; rather, it's a means of collecting information about yourself, others, and the objects that form your material world. The goal is to "try on" or test your perceptions to see what fits you.

Reframing Mental Pictures When you have completed the first three steps in the plan, the new information about yourself, others, and objects becomes the most current source of information. Regardless of the type of new experience you have undertaken and its outcome, you are now in a position to modify the initial perceptions constructed during the first step. Then you will have new insights, knowledge, and perspectives. This is a continual process. As you grow and change, so will your perceptions.

Psychological Disorders

In the course of one year, an estimated 26 percent of Americans, about one in four, suffer from a diagnosable mental disorder. This translates to 57.7 million people being diagnosed with a mental disorder each year, with many people suffering from more than one mental disorder at a given time.[33] In addition, mental disorders are the leading cause of disability in the United States for Americans ages 15 to 44.[34] However, two-thirds of these people do not receive treatment owing to the stigma and cost associated with mental health treatment.[35] Overall, minorities and Caucasians share the same prevalence rate of mental disorders; however, there are great disparities in the rate of mental health care for minorities as compared to the nonminority population.

How common are these disorders? Quite common, as the figures just mentioned suggest. In addition, the lives of millions of other people who work, live, and have relationships with people with mental illness also suffer the effect of these disorders. While there are over 300 different types of mental illness that can be diagnosed, we will cover three major categories of mental disorder: mood disorders, including depression and bipolar disorder; anxiety disorders, including panic disorder, obsessive-compulsive disorder, and posttraumatic stress disorder; and schizophrenia.[36] (See the Considering Complementary Care box, "Can Brain Activity Diagnose and Treat Mental Illness?") We will also briefly discuss attention deficit hyperactivity disorder. Over 450 million people worldwide are affected by mental disorders at any given time, and these numbers are expected to increase in the future.[37]

In the sections that follow, we will investigate selected disorders, identify professionals who are trained to treat these conditions, and take a look at the techniques they employ to help those who are afflicted.

Mood Disorders

Mood disorders, such as depression, seasonal affective disorder, and bipolar disorder, refer to psychological problems in which the primary symptom is a disturbance in mood.[36] You might perceive someone as moody and be unable to predict if the person will be in a good or bad mood from one day to the next.

Depression   According to the World Health Organization (WHO), more than 154 million people worldwide, including 18 million of the U.S. adult population, are estimated to suffer from **clinical depression.**[37] WHO further contends that this will only worsen in the future, predicting that depression will become the second leading cause of disability worldwide by the year 2020, after heart disease, unless strides are made in prevention and treatment. We have already begun to see this trend, as the number of college students with depression has doubled over recent years.[38] About one in ten Americans suffers some form of depression, with women experiencing depression twice as often as men.[39] While depression can develop at any age, the average age of onset is the mid-20s. Figure 2-2 depicts the percentage of adult Americans who reported experiencing major depression in the past year, with the 35 to 49 age group and the 18 to 25 age group reporting the most, and the 65 and older group the least. It also shows that those who were 50 to 64 years old were the most likely to receive treatment for depression, and those who were 18 to 25 years old were the least likely. A survey of 71,860 college students nationwide revealed that 38 percent of students reported feeling so depressed they had difficulty functioning. Another study

found that working can mitigate depression because full-time workers tended to be less depressed than the unemployed did. With the economic downturn that began in mid-2007, we can anticipate an increase in the incidence of depression.

Symptoms of Depression   How can you tell the difference between having the blues and being clinically depressed? The symptoms of depression are as follows:

- Depressed mood most of the day, nearly every day
- Frequent crying
- Withdrawing, isolating yourself from others
- Lack of interest in activities that are typically enjoyable
- Increase or decrease in appetite resulting in significant weight loss or weight gain

Key Terms

clinical depression A psychological disorder in which individuals experience a lack of motivation, decreased energy level, fatigue, social withdrawal, sleep disturbance, disturbance in appetite, diminished sex drive, feelings of worthlessness, and despair.

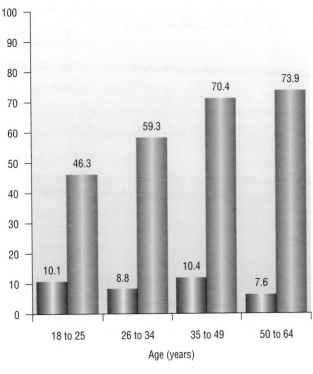

Figure 2-2 Rates of Major Depression and Treatment by Age
Percentage of American adults reporting a major depressive disorder episode and, of this group, the percentage that sought treatment in the year 2006, by age group.

Source: NSDUH Report, Depression Among Adults. Office of Applied Studies, Substance Abuse and Mental Health Services Administration (SAMHSA), July 27, 2006.

- Insomnia, disturbed or restless sleep, or sleeping more than usual
- Feeling tired most of the time, regardless of how much sleep you have had
- Low self-esteem, feelings of hopelessness and worthlessness
- Difficulty concentrating, remembering things, and focusing on a task, and indecisiveness
- Frequent thoughts of suicide

Key Terms

neurotransmitters Chemical messengers that transfer electrical impulses across the synapses between nerve cells.

Most people have experienced some of these symptoms at one point or another in their lives; however, clinically depressed individuals experience most of these symptoms every day and have felt this way for at least two weeks. Most people can find ways of pulling themselves out of feeling down, but for those suffering from clinical depression, the normal methods used to cope with the blues don't work. Clinical depression can range from mild to severe depression and can result in significant impairment in functioning, such as not being able to get out of bed to attend classes or go to work, or lacking the energy or motivation to take care of basic needs for food, hygiene, and rest. Some people tend to become irritable, negative, and uncommunicative, which can cause greater stress and conflict in their relationships. Depression has been described as constantly having a black cloud over your head, not being able to get out from underneath it no matter what you do. You might want to take the online self-assessment screening at www.depression-screening .org to assess your risk for clinical depression and to access more information on depression.

Causes of Depression There are several causes of or triggers for depression. Research suggests that if you have a family history of depression or any type of mood disorder, you are more prone to developing a depressive disorder. In fact, rates of depression for a child with a depressed parent are two to four times greater than for children without depressed parents.[40] While there is no single gene that causes depression, your genetic makeup can make you more vulnerable to depression. **Neurotransmitters** and hormone levels play a major role in the way your brain regulates your mood and emotions. Two neurotransmitters, serotonin and norepinephrine, are often found to be deficient in people with depression. (Chapter 7 includes a detailed discussion of neurotransmitters.)

However, biological processes are not the only explanation for depression. You may have a family history of depression and never develop depressive symptoms. Conversely, you may have no genetic predisposition and still become clinically depressed. Depression can be caused by many psychological factors, such as these:

- Loss of a significant relationship
- Death of a family member or friend
- Physical or sexual abuse or assault
- Response to a serious illness or health problems
- Experiencing numerous setbacks and problems simultaneously

Having a support system, effective coping strategies, and a positive attributional style can make the difference between succumbing to depression or being protected during stressful and adverse times in our lives. Some people turn to the Internet to find increased social involvement and as a way to cope with depression. While it might seem that this would be a helpful way to build your support system and cope with depression, research shows that greater use of the Internet is associated with increasing depression, social isolation, and withdrawal. (See the box "A New Problem . . . Internet Addiction.")

Treatments for Depression There are many ways to treat depression, but the most effective treatment approach is a combination of counseling and medication (see the box "Taking the First Step in Fighting Depression"). Counseling can help people develop healthy coping skills, learn stress-management strategies, focus on developing an optimistic explanatory style, and improve relationships and social skills. Medication, such as antidepressants, can be helpful in the treatment of depression because they act to increase the serotonin or norepinephrine levels to a normal and functional range. Antidepressants include fluoxetine (Prozac), paroxetine (Paxil), sertraline (Zoloft), mirtazapine (Remeron), venlafaxine (Effexor), escitalopram (Lexapro), citalopram (Celexa), and duloxetine (Cymbalta). It takes 4 to 6 weeks for an antidepressant to be fully effective, and there may be side effects such as dry mouth, decreased sexual drive, drowsiness, constipation, or diarrhea. Most of these side effects will disappear after 2 weeks of taking the medication. Most people take an antidepressant for 6 months

to a year and then are able to taper off the medication without a recurrence of symptoms. If you have had three separate episodes of depression, recovering from each episode and then relapsing, this can be a sign that your depression has a biological basis and an indication that you may need to continue taking an antidepressant medication long term. Ten percent of all Americans take an antidepressant. Interestingly, while the percentage of adults with depression taking antidepressants has almost doubled, those receiving psychotherapy has declined.[41] Until 2003, the number of children and adolescents taking antidepressants had been skyrocketing. However, after the FDA issued warnings in 2004 about the increased risk of suicide associated with this age group taking antidepressants, the trend reversed, decreasing by 20 percent.[42] In 2006, the FDA recommended extending this warning of increased suicidal risk to people taking an antidepressant who are 25 years of age and under.

Herbal supplements, such as St. John's Wort, have also been touted as a treatment for depression, although there is some debate as to how effective they truly are. Most clinicians agree that St. John's Wort can be somewhat effective in alleviating mild depression but not moderate or severe types of depression. As is the case with all herbal supplements, St. John's Wort is not subject to FDA approval, and it has not been put through the clinical trials that prescription medications have undergone to establish therapeutic dose and efficacy. A major four-year study by the National Institute of Mental Health, the National Center for Complementary and Alternative Medicine, and the Office of Dietary Supplements found that St. John's Wort was not effective in treating major depression.

Exercise and activity level also play a significant role in alleviating and insulating people from depression. Again it seems that the endorphin levels and effects on brain chemistry and hormonal levels are part of the explanation for why this is a powerful antidote for depression.[43]

Electroconvulsive therapy (ECT) is another form of treatment for depression, with 100,000 Americans receiving this treatment each year. While ECT has fallen out of favor in recent years (owing in part to depictions of it in films such as *One Flew over the Cuckoo's Nest*), it has recently enjoyed a resurgence in popularity. This is due to improved technology. The procedure involves delivering a 90-volt burst of electricity, equal to the electricity in a 40-watt light bulb, for about a minute to the brain, causing a grand mal seizure. The patient is under anesthesia and receives muscle relaxants before receiving the shock, and heart rate and oxygen level are constantly monitored during the treatment. Most patients receive 3 ECT treatments each week, for a total of 6 to 12 sessions. Proponents of ECT claim that it is an effective treatment for depression when no other antidepressant or treatment regime has worked. Critics of ECT say that it causes brain damage and memory loss and that the decrease

A New Problem . . . Internet Addiction

The Internet has certainly changed the way we work, socialize, and educate ourselves. With a few key strokes, MySpace, Facebook, and blogging have opened up a new way of meeting and interacting with people. While the Internet has provided connections that otherwise could not be made very easily with people all around the world, it has also created unique psychological problems for some individuals. There is some question about the psychological implications the Internet may be having on our society as we are moving from a world in which we used to know our neighbors and interact with people face to face to developing serious and deep relationships with people from a distance. Not all of these interactions have positive results. Marriages have broken up, and teenagers have been kidnapped by people they met over the Internet. In fact, one teenager was encouraged to overdose on drugs by his Internet friends and died while communicating over the Net to this group. Tragically, in 2006, 13-year-old Megan Meier committed suicide after receiving cruel messages on MySpace. The now defunct website JuicyCampus.com allowed students to post anonymous comments about their classmates and was used to spread malicious gossip, rumors, and information shared in confidence. Some victims of this gossip site left their campuses, became depressed, anxious, paranoid, and suicidal.

There is a feeling of anonymity that is created by talking on the Web. You can be who you want to be, reveal as much or as little as you want, and not be judged by your appearance. Of course, this also means people can be deceitful and dishonest about who they are and what they want from you. In addition, there is a blending of home and work and increased solitude. While some argue that the Internet brings people together more

now than in the past with the ease of texting and e-mailing one another throughout the day, others are concerned that Internet use decreases communication and interaction between family members and friends. For example, 25 percent of teenagers admitted to being addicted to gaming to the detriment of their school work and time with family and friends. How much time is too much online time? One study showed that using the Internet more than five hours a week resulted in less face-to-face time with friends, family, and social activities.*

In fact, there is such concern about the potential adverse effects of spending too much time on the Internet that some mental health professionals propose adding "Internet addiction" as a diagnosable mental disorder. How can you tell if you are addicted? Here are some warning signs:

1. Preoccupation with the Internet— planning and thinking about the next time you can get online.
2. Increased use of the Internet over time.
3. Repeatedly making unsuccessful attempts to curtail your use of the Internet.
4. Feeling irritable, restless, and moody when you attempt to cut down your use of the Internet or are prevented from getting online when you would like.
5. Unaware of how much time you are spending on the Internet, staying online longer than you originally intended.
6. Lying to family members and friends about your use of the Internet.
7. Jeopardizing your job or risking losing a relationship because of the time you are spending on the Web.
8. Using the Internet as a way of escaping from problems and coping with depression.

9. Declining invitations to spend time with family and friends because you would rather be online.

Of course, answering "yes" to one of these statements does not indicate a concern. However, if you can answer "yes" to more than half of them, then you may want to examine your use of the Internet. Here are some ways you can avoid being an Internet addict:

- *Decide how much time you want to spend on the Internet before you get online* and set an alarm for that time. Stick to that time allotment.

- *Take frequent breaks.* Spend at least 5 minutes out of every hour or 15 to 20 minutes of every 3 hours on unwired activity. Take a walk, get up and eat a snack, or listen to music.

- *Visit the Net with a purpose and a strategy.* Surfing the Web aimlessly can lead to being online for longer than you anticipated.

- *Interact with people in a nonwired world.* Make a commitment to socially interact at least once a day with someone who is not online.

- *Don't let the Internet be the center of your existence* or the most important, enjoyable part of your day. Remind yourself of your life goals, values, and interests. What are other ways to achieve these goals besides via the Web?

Sources: When Play Turns to Trouble, *U.S. News & World Report*, May 19, 2008; Text Messaging Taps Out A Family-Friendly Result, *USA Today*, October 20, 2008; Internet Tragedy, *People Magazine*, December 24, 2007.
*Streitfeld D, Study Finds Heavy Internet Users Are Isolated, *Washington Post*, February 16, 2000.

in depressive symptoms is only temporary.[44] Although ECT has been used for more than 60 years, no one knows exactly how it works or why it alleviates depression.

TALKING POINTS Have you ever felt depressed? If so, what did you do to cope with these feelings? What did you do that worked and/or didn't help you to feel better?

Seasonal Affective Disorder In addition to the types of depression just described, some people may be especially vulnerable to depression on a seasonal basis. **Seasonal affective disorder (SAD)** is a form of depression that develops in relation to the changes in the seasons. While most people with SAD begin to feel increasingly depressed in October and report their depression lifts in March or April, about one in six SAD sufferers experiences

The Dos and Don'ts of Suicide Intervention

Do . . .

1. If possible, stay with the person until you can get further assistance.
2. Offer support and assistance. Tell them they are not alone.
3. Remain calm and talk about the person's feelings of sadness and helplessness.
4. Encourage problem solving and taking positive steps.
5. Emphasize the temporary nature of the problem. Suicide is a permanent solution to a temporary problem.
6. Seek help and don't try to handle this problem on your own. This might involve the person's family, religious advisor, friends, and teachers, or calling a mental health agency for consultation.

7. Ask the person to promise not to hurt or kill him- or herself.

Don't . . .

1. Avoid talking about suicide or dancing around the topic. Talking about suicide doesn't upset people more. In fact, often people who are thinking about killing themselves say it is a relief to talk about it, and it helps them to let go of this idea and not pursue it further.
2. Be judgmental or argumentative. Now is not the time to debate the morality of suicide—you will lose the debate and possibly the person.
3. Assume that the person is not serious. Saying "You're not serious" or "You

don't mean that" may inadvertently encourage the person to show you how serious she or he truly is.

4. Argue that things aren't that bad or that other people have it worse and the person should be happy about his or her life. This approach can make people feel worse about themselves and guilty about their feelings of unhappiness.
5. Don't promise not to tell anyone. If you keep this promise and something happens to this person, how will you feel?

Summer SAD, beginning in May or June and ending in the fall months. Twice as many women as men are affected with SAD.[45]

SAD seems to be related to environmental factors such as amount of light, temperature, and situational stressors. Weight gain, fatigue, increased sleep, diminished sex drive, and mood swings are some of the symptoms of Winter SAD; agitation, loss of appetite, insomnia, and increased suicidal thoughts are characteristic of Summer SAD. Seasonal depression in the winter seems linked to increases in the production of melatonin, a chemical that helps set the brain's daily rhythm, set off by the decrease in light. Antidepressants, counseling, and light therapy have been used to treat SAD. Light therapy for Winter SAD involves sitting in front of a light box with about a 10,000-lux intensity bulb, housed in a plastic diffusing screen, for 20 to 90 minutes each day so that the light is falling on the eyes.[45] For Summer SAD, which tends to occur in hotter locales, individuals are instructed to travel to cooler climates, to swim in cool water, and to stay in darkened, air-conditioned rooms.

Postpartum Depression Another unique form of depression is **postpartum depression,** a more severe kind of depression than is the commonly experienced "baby blues" that many women feel following childbirth. Postpartum depression occurs in one out of eight mothers who give birth and can last from a few days to over a year, but most commonly lasts for two weeks. Postpartum depression is characterized by fatigue, frequent crying, emotional withdrawal, anxiety, and other symptoms associated with depression. This should be differentiated from postpartum psychosis, which is marked by hallucinations and delusions. Sometimes people with postpartum depression have been associated with psychotic behavior, as was the situation with the much publicized case of Andrea Yates who in 2002 drowned her five children, ages 6 months to 7 years. Reportedly, Yates suffered from postpartum depression after the birth of her fourth child, and with the birth of her fifth child along with the death of her own father, became increasingly depressed and psychotic.

Suicide Suicide is the third leading cause of death for young adults 15 to 24 years old. It is the 11th leading cause of all deaths in the United States, but the second leading cause of death for college students. More than half of college students surveyed in 2006 reported contemplating suicide at some point in their lives, with 18 percent seriously considering it. Men commit suicide four times more often than women do, and 72 percent of all suicides are committed by white men. Suicide occurs most often among middle-aged Americans.[46] However, women are three times more likely than men to attempt suicide, and middle-aged women have seen a significant increase in their rate of suicide over the past decade with an increase of hanging and suffocation as methods. The suicide rate

> **Key Terms**
>
> **seasonal affective disorder (SAD)** A type of depression that develops in relation to the changes in the seasons.
>
> **postpartum depression** A form of depression that affects women in the weeks and months following childbirth.

for women 10 to 24 years of age increased an alarming 76 percent, the biggest increase in 15 years. Hanging and suffocation were the most common suicide methods for this group. A record number of soldiers committed suicide in 2008. Men tend to employ more violent methods such as firearms, hanging, or jumping from high places, whereas women tend to use methods such as overdosing with pills or cutting their wrists, which are slower methods and allow more time for medical intervention. While using a firearm is still the most common method of committing suicide, it has decreased as a method over the years, and hanging and suffocation have increased. Most people assume suicides increase in the winter months, but actually more suicides occur in spring than during any other season. Suicide rates for African Americans have significantly decreased. Asian Americans are one of the lowest-risk groups in terms of ethnicity. The suicide rate for the Hispanic American population is higher than for Caucasians and African Americans, a reverse trend from past years.

Why do people attempt or commit suicide? The majority of suicidal people have depressive disorders and feel helpless and powerless over their lives. They say things like "I just want the pain to stop" and don't see any other options available to them. There are some risk factors associated with suicidal behavior, such as these:

- Little to no support system
- Previous suicide attempts
- Family history of mental illness, including substance abuse
- Family history of suicide
- Problems with drugs or alcohol
- Possession of a firearm
- Exposure to the suicidal behavior of others, including through the media

After the economic crisis began in 2007, there was a dramatic increase in calls to suicide hotlines and mental health centers as a result of people losing their jobs, houses, and health care and feeling hopeless because of the poor economy. It is estimated that over 300,000 suicide attempts occur each year in the United States, or one every 2 minutes. Eleven hundred of these suicides occur on college campuses. Some people say that suicidal gestures or threats are a "cry for attention" or a "cry for help" and think it is better to ignore the person. But left ignored, the person may go ahead and take the next step because no one seems to care. It is always best to take any threats or talk about suicide seriously and act accordingly. What should you do if a friend or family member talks to you about thoughts of suicide? See the box "The Dos and Don'ts of Suicide Intervention" for suggestions.

Bipolar Disorder Another important mood disorder is **bipolar disorder,** a condition that was previously known as manic depression. The term *bipolar* refers to the extreme mood swings individuals with this disorder experience, from feeling euphoric, energetic, and reckless to feeling depressed, powerless, and listless. Nearly 6 million American adults, or 3 percent, suffer from bipolar disorder, with men and women equally likely to develop this condition.[36] It is the least common of the mood disorders. The average age of onset for the first manic episode typically occurs in the early to mid-20s. This change in mood or "mood swing" can last for hours, days, weeks, or months. Bipolar disorder is found across all ages, races, ethnic groups, and social classes. When one parent has bipolar disorder, the risk to each child is estimated to be 15 to 30 percent; when both parents have bipolar disorder, the risk increases to 50 to 75 percent.[47] A recent study contended that a flawed gene appears to promote bipolar disorder. Further research is needed to examine this particular variant of the gene to better identify people at risk and develop more effective medications to treat this disorder.

We have already described depression in the previous section. Bipolar disorder involves having both depressive periods and manic episodes. **Mania** is characterized by the following:

- Excessive energy, needing little sleep, being highly excitable
- Racing thoughts, feeling as though your mind is going 50 mph
- Rapid speech, changing from topic to topic quickly in conversation
- Easily irritated and distracted
- Impulsive and reckless in behavior: for example, spending sprees, increased involvement in sexual activity, and drug and alcohol use
- Trying to do too much, feeling as though you can accomplish a great deal

Many people with bipolar disorder will tell you that they enjoy the "highs" but dread the lows. However, manic behavior can become very destructive because when

---

Key Terms

bipolar disorder A mood disorder characterized by alternating episodes of depression and mania.

mania An extremely excitable state characterized by excessive energy, racing thoughts, impulsive and/or reckless behavior, irritability, and being prone to distraction.

generalized anxiety disorder (GAD) An anxiety disorder that involves experiencing intense and nonspecific anxiety for at least six months, in which the intensity and frequency of worry is excessive and out of proportion to the situation.

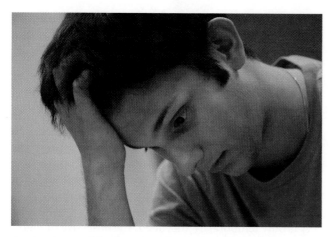

Anxiety is one of the three most frequent problems students report experiencing during college.

people are in a manic phase, they can create enormous credit card debt, abuse drugs and alcohol, drive recklessly, and often feel invincible. They stay up all night and feel very little need for rest or food, and eventually their bodies can't function and they collapse. Mood stabilizers such as lithium carbonate (Lithobid), anticonvulsant medications such as valproic acid (Depakene), gabapentin (Neurontin), topiramate (Topamax), and lamotrigine (Lamictal), and antipsychotic medications such as Abilify (aripiprazole), along with psychotherapy, have been used to treat bipolar disorder.

Anxiety Disorders

Bill, a very talented and bright 26-year-old, has a promising career as an executive in a large accounting firm. However, he is in jeopardy of losing his job because of his absenteeism and tardiness. It can take him hours to get to work even though he lives 15 minutes away, and sometimes he doesn't go to work even though he is in the car and ready to go. Bill has a routine in the morning that involves checking the windows, doors, iron, stove, and garage door five times to ensure that things are secure and safe. Sometimes he drives away and then returns to the house to check again. He feels a need to turn the handles on doors five times, and if he loses track, he starts all over again.

Susan has been having such severe panic attacks in the car while driving to work that she has needed to pull over. Her heart races, her breathing is labored, and she sometimes feels as though she is having a heart attack and might die. She is frightened of being in the car alone and having an attack and not being able to get help or having a car accident. She is beginning to be afraid to leave her house and feels safer at home. She has declined invitations to go out with her friends and on vacations and goes out only when absolutely necessary. She feels as though she is losing control of her life.

John worries constantly about what other people think of him. When he passes a group of people who are laughing, he assumes that they are laughing at him. He has trouble having conversations with people because he believes whatever he says will sound "stupid" and people will not like him. He also plays conversations over and over in his head when he is trying to go to sleep, thinking about what he should have said and worrying about how people are judging him.

Bill, Susan, and John are all suffering from *anxiety disorders*. While everyone tends to feel nervous or worry about something at some point in their lives, people with anxiety disorders feel anxious most, if not all, of the time. They also feel powerless to alleviate their anxiety, and tend to worry about becoming anxious, so their anxiety causes them even greater anxiety. Anxiety is related to fear and is part of daily life. Some anxiety can even be helpful and motivating at times. Anxiety is a physiological, adaptive response to danger or potential threat and can enhance performance and keep us out of harm's way. In Chapter 3 we discuss the fight or flight response and how the stress response is related to anxiety. Anxiety disorders are differentiated from daily stress as being

1. Intense, often debilitating, experiences during which people sometimes think they are going to die
2. Long lasting, persisting after the danger or stressful event has passed
3. Dysfunctional, causing significant interference in daily functioning

Anxiety disorders include generalized anxiety disorder, obsessive-compulsive disorder (such as Bill's problem), posttraumatic stress disorder, panic disorder (which describes Susan's symptoms), and phobias such as the social phobia John suffers from in his incessant worrying about what other people think about him. Approximately 40 million Americans, or 18 percent, have an anxiety disorder, and women are twice as likely as men to suffer from panic disorder, posttraumatic stress disorder, generalized anxiety disorder, agoraphobia, and specific phobias.[36] There are no gender differences with obsessive-compulsive disorder or social phobia.[36]

Generalized Anxiety Disorder (GAD) **Generalized anxiety disorder (GAD)** involves experiencing anxiety for at least six months in which the intensity and frequency of the worry is excessive and out of proportion to the situation. GAD can be distinguished from specific phobias in which people feel worried about a particular situation or stimulus. An individual with GAD appears to worry all the time about everything, thinks the worst, and overreacts to situations. Restlessness, fatigue, irritability, difficulty concentrating, muscle tension, and trouble sleeping are some of the symptoms associated with GAD. Physical symptoms include excessive sweating, nausea, diarrhea, being easily startled, shortness of breath, racing heart, and feeling shaky.[36] Because people with GAD are tense and anxious much of the time, they experience impairment in their relationships, work performance, and general functioning. Most people with GAD say that they are afraid of losing control, of failing, of rejection or abandonment, and of death or disease. In addition, they feel unable to cope with their fears and thus out of control in managing their anxiety.

Panic Disorder   Shortness of breath, pounding heart, dizziness, trembling, sweating, nausea, tingling in hands and feet, hot and cold flashes, chest pain, and a feeling of choking are the symptoms of **panic disorder,** exemplified by Susan's situation. Many panic disorder sufferers feel as though they are going to die, are losing control, or are going crazy, which of course makes them feel more anxious and panicked. Frequently, these individuals go to the emergency room thinking they are having a heart attack. This can seemingly occur out of the blue or because of some trigger and can last for a few minutes or for hours. Because people become fearful of having a panic attack and don't know when the next attack might occur, they may develop **agoraphobia.** Agoraphobia is a fear of being in embarrassing situations or places in which you can't escape or get help if you need it.[47]

Panic disorder can be treated with antidepressant medications such as imipramine (Tofranil) and tranquilizers such as alprazolam (Xanax). Counseling can help individuals learn to recognize when a panic attack may be starting and to minimize and ward it off before it becomes a full-blown attack, using relaxation and stress-management exercises, as well as positive self statements such as "I'm not going to die. I can get through this."

Obsessive-Compulsive Disorder (OCD)   **Obsessive-compulsive disorder,** or OCD, affects 3 million Americans and symptoms often begin during childhood or adolescence.[36] OCD involves more than just being neat and orderly: symptoms include having recurring thoughts and behaviors that seem irrational and out of control, and that can be extremely time consuming. Obsessions are intrusive thoughts, images, or impulses causing a great deal of distress. Most people recognize that their obsessions are ungrounded and senseless but can't seem to push them out of their minds. Twenty-five percent of people with OCD have only obsessive thoughts without exhibiting any compulsive behavior.[47] Compulsions are repetitive behaviors aimed at reducing the anxiety and stress that are associated with the obsessive thoughts, such as checking that the iron is off or washing your hands a certain number of times. Some compulsions seem relevant to a particular fear (such as handwashing out of a fear of germs), but others might

seem unrelated—for example, having to do something an odd number of times so that your parents will not come to any harm. The most common compulsions are washing, checking, and counting.[36]

Even though the goal of compulsive behavior is to alleviate distress brought about by obsessions, it is in itself a source of shame and anxiety. Individuals with OCD, like Bill in the earlier example, realize that their behavior is excessive and unreasonable but are unable to resist engaging in this behavior. This can cause great distress in their relationships, problems completing their work, and getting to places on time. In addition, once they have performed the compulsive behavior, their anxiety is only temporarily alleviated; the obsessive thoughts return and the cycle continues.

Treatment for OCD can include antidepressant medication such as fluoxetine (Prozac) and also counseling. Counseling might involve response prevention strategies such as exposing the individual to the situations that trigger the obsessive thoughts and then preventing the person from engaging in the compulsive behaviors to break this vicious cycle. For example, the individual might be exposed to a dirty environment and then allowed to wash his or her hands only once.

Phobias   John is suffering from one of the most common anxiety disorders, **social phobia,** previously called social anxiety disorder. Social phobia involves feelings of extreme dread and embarrassment in situations in which public speaking or social interaction is involved, because the person worries she or he will be seen as stupid, clumsy, or lacking in some way. Social phobia is the third most common mental health problem in the United States, affecting 5.3 million each year. Twice as many women as men are afflicted, and the disorder typically begins in childhood or early adolescence and rarely develops after age 25. It is sometimes confused with shyness and is misdiagnosed much of the time. The most common social phobia is fear of public speaking. Commonly called stage fright, it is the most common of all phobias; many successful actors and performers suffer from this disorder, including actor Donny Osmond, gold medalist swimmer Susie O'Neill, and actresses Kim Basinger and Barbra Streisand.

Social phobia differs from another disorder called **specific phobia** in which the person has a strong fear of and avoids one particular situation or object such as snakes, high places, or airplanes. Specific phobias affect 10 percent of the population and often begin as childhood fears that were never outgrown.[47] They are twice as common in women as in men. Sometimes a phobic reaction develops as a result of a traumatic event such as an accident or a particularly difficult visit to the doctor or dentist, or from an illness. Specific phobias tend to be easily treated with counseling in which the individual learns relaxation techniques and then is gradually exposed, first in imagery, then in real-life situations, to the feared situation.

Posttraumatic Stress Disorder (PTSD)   The essential feature of **posttraumatic stress disorder** is the development of symptoms following exposure to an extreme stressor involving threat of death or serious injury. This threat may be directly experienced or be the result of witnessing an event that is life threatening and dangerous.[36] This disorder was first identified during World War I when soldiers were observed to be suffering from anxiety, flashbacks, and nightmares. Posttraumatic stress can be the result of not only combat but any trauma that produces intense fear, horror, and feelings of helplessness, such as sexual assault, natural disasters like earthquakes or tornados, a car accident, a life-threatening illness, or a mugging. The symptoms associated with PTSD are the following:

- Recurrent and distressing thoughts about the event
- Nightmares about the event
- Flashbacks—feeling as though one is reliving the event
- Emotional numbness, feeling detached from oneself and one's feelings
- Avoidance of anything that reminds one of the event
- Detachment from others
- Difficulty expressing one's feelings
- Sleep disturbance
- Irritability, angry outbursts
- Being easily startled
- Difficulty concentrating
- Hypervigilance—extreme awareness of one's environment

People with PTSD tend to be highly anxious and depressed, to have problems with their relationships, and to have difficulty trusting people, and they may restrict their activities because of their fearfulness. It is also not uncommon to experience panic attacks when exposed to something that triggers a memory of the trauma. Again, counseling to express and resolve the feelings, losses, and negative thoughts associated with the trauma, as well as antidepressant medications or tranquilizers, may be beneficial in treating PTSD.

Attention Deficit Hyperactivity Disorder (ADHD)

Once thought to be only a childhood disorder, **attention deficit hyperactivity disorder** (ADHD) is now being diagnosed in record numbers in adults. This increase might be the result of overlooking or misdiagnosing problems in childhood that later are accurately diagnosed in adults (see the box "Television Advertisements for Psychological Medications"). With symptoms that include being fidgety, disorganized, overactive, and easily distracted, a child may be seen as simply misbehaving rather than having a diagnosable disorder. It is often the child with ADHD who is seen as "disruptive" in the classroom and "lazy, stupid, a daydreamer" by friends and family. Actually, the truth about these individuals is often the opposite: they tend to be highly intelligent, motivated, creative, and energetic individuals.

It is currently estimated that over 15 million Americans suffer from this disorder, affecting males more than females, 3:1. There is strong evidence to support a genetic cause for ADHD, although environmental factors can certainly help or hinder the problem. One of the landmark studies in ADHD was conducted on adults

---

Key Terms

panic disorder   An anxiety disorder characterized by panic attacks, in which individuals experience severe physical symptoms. These episodes can seemingly occur "out of the blue" or because of some trigger and can last for a few minutes or for hours.

agoraphobia   A fear of being in embarrassing situations from which there is no escape or in which help would be unavailable should an emergency arise; often associated with panic disorder.

obsessive-compulsive disorder   An anxiety disorder characterized by obsessions (intrusive thoughts, images, or impulses causing a great deal of distress) and compulsions (repetitive behaviors aimed at reducing anxiety or stress that is associated with the obsessive thoughts).

social phobia   A phobia characterized by feelings of extreme dread and embarrassment in situations in which public speaking or social interaction is involved.

specific phobia   An excessive and unreasonable fear about a particular situation or object that causes anxiety and distress and interferes with a person's functioning.

posttraumatic stress disorder   An anxiety disorder that sometimes develops following exposure to an extreme stressor involving threat of death or serious injury. Symptoms include recurrent and distressing thoughts or nightmares about the event, emotional numbness, feelings of detachment, sleep disturbance, hypervigilance, and irritability.

attention deficit hyperactivity disorder (ADHD)   An above-normal rate of physical movement; often accompanied by an inability to concentrate on a specified task.

and showed that there is a difference at the cellular level in energy consumption, between the parts of the brain that regulate attention, emotion, and impulse control in people with ADHD compared with those without.[48]

Following are the symptoms often seen in adult ADHD:

- A sense of underachievement, not meeting one's goals
- Difficulty getting organized
- Chronic procrastination or trouble getting started
- Trouble with follow-through and completing tasks
- Having many tasks going on simultaneously, switching from one to another
- Easily bored and frequently searching for high stimulation
- Easily distracted, trouble focusing and sustaining attention
- Creative, intuitive, highly intelligent
- Impulsive, doesn't stop to think things through
- Impatient, low tolerance for frustration
- Tendency to worry needlessly and endlessly
- Insecure
- Moody
- Restless
- Tendency toward addictive behavior
- Low self-esteem
- Inaccurate self-concept, unaware of effect on others
- Childhood history of ADHD or presence of symptoms since childhood

Psychological tests such as the Test of Variability of Attention (TOVA) and an IQ test can help substantiate a diagnosis of ADHD. The TOVA tests the subject by flashing different shapes on a screen quantifying attention, distractibility, and impulsivity based on the subject's responses. The most effective treatment for ADHD involves a multimodal approach: counseling and coaching the individual to provide strategies, techniques, and structure for daily life; education; tools such as daily planners and organizers; goal setting and time management; and medication such as methylphenidate

(Concerta, Ritalin), amphetamine-dextroamphetamine (Adderall), and atomoxetine (Strattera). (These medications are discussed in more detail in Chapter 7.)

Schizophrenia

Schizophrenia is one of the most severe mental disorders; it is characterized by profound distortions in one's thought processes, emotions, perceptions, and behavior. People with schizophrenia experience hallucinations (seeing things that are not there, hearing voices), delusions (believing that they are Jesus, the CIA is after them, or radio waves are controlling their mind), and disorganized thinking (wearing multiple coats, scarves, and gloves on a warm day, shouting and swearing at passersby, maintaining a rigid posture and not moving for hours). The movie *A Beautiful Mind* gives a glimpse into the life of one schizophrenic, John Nash, and how he managed his symptoms.

There are several types of schizophrenia: paranoid, disorganized, catatonic, and undifferentiated. This disabling illness affects 1 percent of the U.S. population, and symptoms typically surface in people in their late teens and early 20s. Men and women are equally likely to develop schizophrenia, and it seems to run in families. Schizophrenia is often confused with dissociative identity disorder (formerly called "multiple personality disorder"), which is an entirely separate and distinct mental illness. People with dissociative identity disorder display two or more distinct identities or personalities that take control of the person's life; people with schizophrenia do not have multiple, separate, enduring personalities.

There are many theories to explain what causes schizophrenia. Some research suggests that heredity accounts for about 80 percent of the cause of schizophrenia and the other 20 percent is due to environmental stressors or situations. Researchers have also identified a number of abnormalities in the brains of diagnosed schizophrenics, including smaller temporal lobes, enlargement of the ventricles, and cerebral atrophy in the frontal lobes. Research is also being done on how the variations in chromosome-22 genes may be linked to schizophrenia. Individuals with schizophrenia also seem to have nearly double the number of dopamine receptors in their brains, leading to the theory that too much dopamine is being released into the brain pathways and causing schizophrenia symptoms. The antipsychotic medications act to block the receptors and prevent the transmission of dopamine, reducing the amount of dopamine in the system that is creating this chemical imbalance.[2]

Although there is no cure for schizophrenia, certain antipsychotic medications, such as quetiapine (Seroquel), risperidone (Risperdal), olanzapine (Zyprexa),

---

Key Terms

schizophrenia One of the most severe mental disorders, characterized by profound distortions in one's thought processes, emotions, perceptions, and behavior. Symptoms may include hallucinations, delusions, disorganized thinking, and maintaining a rigid posture or not moving for hours.

aripiprazole (Abilify), and ziprasidone (Geodon), can effectively treat this illness and enable people to live functional, satisfying lives. Psychotherapy can be helpful in developing problem-solving approaches, in addition to identifying stressors and triggers, and early detection of a psychotic episode. Unfortunately, some people with schizophrenia are unable to recognize that they are delusional or irrational, and so do not get treatment or take their medications on a regular basis.

Health Providers Involved in the Treatment of Psychological Disorders

As in other areas of health care, a variety of practitioners, each of whom has unique training and uses specific therapies, treat and manage the mental health conditions just described.

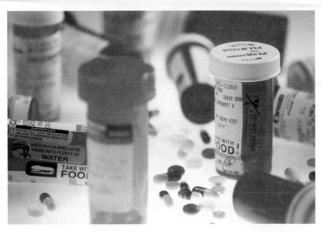

Prescription medications are a common form of treatment for psychological disorders and may be used in combination with other therapies.

Psychiatrists

A **psychiatrist** is a health care provider with a medical degree who has specialized in the field of psychiatry. Because psychiatrists are medical doctors, they may prescribe drugs and perform medical procedures such as electroshock therapy. Psychiatrists tend to treat psychological disorders through medical management and take a biological approach to addressing psychological disorders. They tend to give less focus to talking about one's problems and treat more severely and chronically ill patients.

Psychologists

A **psychologist** is a mental health care provider whose educational background includes a doctoral-level degree in the field of counseling or clinical psychology. Psychologists practice general psychology, and their clients range from those with severe pathology to those with more temporary problems of living. There is a variety of subspecialties such as children and adolescents, neurological disorders and assessments, psychological evaluations and assessments, forensic psychology, industrial psychology, health psychology, career counseling, and marriage counseling. Until recently, one difference between psychiatrists and psychologists was that psychologists did

Key Terms

psychiatrist A medical doctor with specialized training in the diagnosis and treatment of psychological disorders through the use of biological and medical interventions.

psychologist A doctoral-level practitioner with specialized training in the diagnosis and treatment of psychological disorders through the use of psychotherapy.

not have prescription privileges and so couldn't use drug therapies in their treatment interventions. However, the lines are beginning to blur, as there has been a push in many states for legislation that would allow psychologists to prescribe psychiatric medicines; such legislation exists in New Mexico and Louisiana already. In general, psychologists treat psychological disorders using behavior therapy, problem-solving approaches, and talk therapy that focuses on changing the client's attitudes, behavior, affect, and cognitions. A psychologist must be licensed in the state in which he or she practices, and this typically requires passing a national certification examination and having a specific number of hours practicing psychology under the supervision of a licensed psychologist.

Counselors

Counselors typically have a master's degree in counseling or clinical psychology. Individuals with master's degrees usually work in group counseling practices, clinics, and schools and may specialize in areas such as substance abuse, divorce recovery, vocational rehabilitation, school counseling, marriage and family therapy, sexual assault, domestic violence, and employee assistance programs. Master's-level counselors can be licensed as professional mental health counselors in all U.S. states except Nevada.

Social Workers

Social workers have a master's degree in social work and must be licensed to use the title *social worker*. Whereas psychologists, mental health counselors, and psychiatrists tend to focus on the individual's problems, social workers look at the bigger picture and take into consideration the environment, community, and system the individual is living in. Social workers provide both mental health and social services to the community and are the largest group of professionals to provide psychological services.

Social workers typically consult and counsel clients and arrange for services that can help them. Often, they refer clients to specialists in services such as debt counseling, childcare or eldercare, public assistance, or alcohol or drug rehabilitation. Social workers then follow through with the client to ensure that services are helpful and that clients make proper use of the services offered. Social workers may review eligibility requirements, visit clients on a regular basis, and provide support during crises.[49]

Approaches in Treating Psychological Disorders

There are over 200 approaches to treating psychological disorders, and new variations and models are continuing to develop. Most approaches have their foundations based on a few basic therapeutic models, which we will look at in the section that follows. These therapies can be utilized with individuals, families, or couples.

Dynamic Therapy

Dynamic therapy is based on the belief that effective treatment must focus on the psychological forces underlying the individual's problems. These forces begin in early childhood and have great significance on later behavior and personality development. Because this type of therapy focuses on the person's childhood years to uncover the source of the current problem, it usually is a long-term, intensive, and expensive form of therapy that many insurance companies refuse to cover.

Humanistic Therapy

Humanistic treatment approaches are based on the belief that people, left to their own devices, will naturally grow in positive and constructive ways. The job of the therapist is to help clients unearth their natural potential and gain greater self-awareness and self-acceptance. **Humanistic therapy** has its roots in Carl Rogers's "client-centered therapy" and in Abraham Maslow's hierarchy of needs. In client-centered therapy, the client, not the therapist, is responsible for behavior change. The task of the therapist is to facilitate in a nondirective manner the process of helping individuals resolve their problems.[7] Rogers further believed that when people accept themselves, they will also accept other people.

Behavior Therapy

Behavior therapy focuses not on one's thoughts or feelings but on behavior modification. Thus the goal of treatment is not to uncover the reasons underlying the problems an individual is having but to eliminate the symptoms and change behavior. Insight, awareness, and past history are unimportant in behavior therapy. The idea is that behavior has been learned and so can be unlearned, and different, more adaptive behavior can be taught. This can be especially effective for the treatment of phobias, panic disorder, and anxiety.

Cognitive-Behavioral Therapy

Cognitive-behavioral therapy focuses on changing an individual's thoughts or cognitive patterns in order to change his or her behavior and emotional state. Pioneered by psychologists Aaron Beck and Albert Ellis in the 1960s, cognitive therapy assumes that maladaptive behaviors and disturbed mood or emotions are the result of inappropriate or irrational thinking patterns. As with behavior therapy, cognitive-behavioral therapy does not explore why someone is thinking or behaving in a particular way, nor does it look at the client's past history. Instead, cognitive therapists attempt to make the client aware of distorted thought patterns and change them through strategies such as cognitive restructuring, cognitive reframing, challenging irrational beliefs, and thought stopping. This type of treatment has been especially effective in treating obsessive-compulsive disorder, eating disorders, anxiety disorders, and mood disorders. The learned optimism paradigm discussed earlier in this chapter was also based on cognitive-behavioral concepts.

Solution-Focused Therapy

Solution-focused therapy is a goal-oriented therapeutic approach that helps clients change by looking for solutions rather than dwelling on problems. Similar to cognitive-behavioral therapy, attention is directed to the present and the future, rather than to the past. Solution-focused therapists focus on the strength and resources within the individual. Clients are encouraged to envision a future in which their problems are no longer a dominant force in their lives, and in partnership with the therapist, treatment interventions are formulated in an effort to reach that goal.

Key Terms

social worker A professional with a master's degree in social work. Social workers provide both mental health and social services to the community and are the largest group of professionals to provide psychological services.

dynamic therapy An intensive therapy based on the belief that effective treatment must focus on the psychological forces underlying the individual's problems.

humanistic therapy A treatment approach based on the belief that people, left to their own devices, will naturally grow in positive and constructive ways.

behavior therapy A behavior modification therapy based on the learning principles of reinforcement therapy, stimulus-response, and conditioning responses to change behavior.

cognitive-behavioral therapy An action-oriented form of therapy that assumes that maladaptive, or faulty, thinking patterns cause maladaptive behavior and negative emotions; treatment focuses on changing an individual's thoughts or cognitive patterns in order to change his or her behavior and emotional state.

solution-focused therapy A goal-oriented approach that helps clients change by looking for solutions rather than dwelling on problems.

Couples and Family Therapy

Couples counseling and family therapy includes premarital counseling, marital therapy, conflict mediation, and divorce counseling. Communication skills, assertiveness skills, sexual disorders, intimacy and commitment, anger management, stepparenting, and blended families are some of the psychological issues that are typically addressed by these therapies.

Group Therapy

Group therapy usually comprises five to eight people who meet regularly with a therapist to focus on the psychological problems with which they are struggling. Often the group members share common problems such as eating disorders, childhood sexual abuse, substance abuse, or divorce recovery, and so they can support one another and understand one another's experiences. The group members can help and learn from one another and don't feel so alone in their problems. Group therapy is very beneficial in breaking your sense of isolation and challenging the belief that you are the only one having this type of problem. The idea behind group therapy is that you can learn new ways of behaving and practice these skills and behaviors in a safe, supportive atmosphere. In fact, the research strongly suggests that group therapy can be superior to individual therapy or at least a necessary next step for particular psychological problems, such as sexual abuse, eating disorders, substance abuse, and interpersonal relationship problems.

Psychological Health: A Final Thought

As you can see, psychological health involves how your emotions, thoughts, and behavior interplay with one another and with the world around you. There is an important mind-body connection in terms of your psychological health having a significant effect on your physical health and vice versa. Psychological health is not just the absence of mental illness, and there is a range or continuum of psychological health. Possessing a positive self-concept, developing high self-esteem, and cultivating an optimistic attitude toward life can promote psychological health and enhance relationships with others. While heredity plays a role in the development of personality and psychological health, environmental factors and stressors seem to have an equally important role. As people age and encounter developmental milestones, they also encounter new challenges, obstacles, and resources in continuing to maintain their psychological health.

Taking Charge of Your Health

- Take the Personal Assessment at the end of this chapter to assess your explanatory style.
- Apply the steps of a proactive approach to life to a situation in your life.
- Take the online screening assessment for depression, bipolar disorder, anxiety, or posttraumatic stress disorder at www.dbsalliance.org (look under signs and symptoms and then screenings).
- Keep a journal, and each day write down things you like about yourself or feel good about.
- Take a risk and do something you have been wanting to do, such as joining a club, trying a sport, or meeting new people.

SUMMARY

- Psychological health has also been associated with developing and maintaining a positive self-concept, positive self-esteem, and emotional intelligence.
- Personality is generally defined as a specific set of consistent patterns of behavior and traits that helps to identify and characterize an individual. Personality comprises thoughts, feelings, behaviors, motivation, instincts, and temperament.
- Two factors, nature and nurture, influence the shaping of personality. *Nature* refers to the innate factors we are born with that genetically determine our personality traits. *Nurture* is the effect that the environment, people, and external factors have on our personality.
- Nonverbal communication is what is communicated by your facial expression, body posture, tone of voice, and movements.
- Maslow's theory is a positive, optimistic theory of human behavior. He believed that people are motivated to grow and fulfill their potential, referring to this phenomenon as self-actualization.

- Having a positive interpretation of life's events, particularly how you cope with adversity, can make a significant difference in terms of your health and academic and work performance, as well as how long you will live.
- Anxiety disorders include generalized anxiety disorder, obsessive-compulsive disorder, posttraumatic stress disorder, panic disorder, and phobias.
- Schizophrenia is one of the most severe mental disorders, characterized by profound distortions in one's thought processes, emotions, perceptions, and behavior.

- A number of different health care professionals are trained to treat mental disorders, including psychiatrists, psychologists, social workers, and counselors.
- Treatments for psychological illnesses include dynamic, humanistic, behavioral, cognitive-behavioral, and solution-focused therapies, as well as drug therapies.

REVIEW QUESTIONS

1. What are three factors that have been associated with psychological health?
2. What are the characteristics commonly demonstrated by psychologically healthy people?
3. What is nonverbal communication?
4. Describe Maslow's theory of the hierarchy of needs.
5. How can having a positive interpretation of life's events make a significant difference in people's health?
6. How is clinical depression different from having the "blues"?
7. How should you respond to someone threatening or talking about committing suicide?
8. List five different types of anxiety disorders.
9. How does a psychiatrist differ from a psychologist?
10. What are five different types of therapy approaches to treat psychological disorders?

ANSWERS TO THE "WHAT DO YOU KNOW?" QUIZ

1. True   2. False   3. False   4. False   5. True   6. True   7. False

Visit the Online Learning Center (**www.mhhe.com/payne11e**), where you will find tools to help you improve your grade including practice quizzes, key terms flashcards, audio chapter summaries for your MP3 player, and many other study aids.

SOURCE NOTES

1. Turner J, Stels J. *The Sociology of Emotions.* New York: Cambridge University Press, 2005.
2. Papalia D, Olds S. *Psychology* (2nd ed.). New York: McGraw-Hill, 1988.
3. Seligman M. *Learned Optimism.* New York: Simon & Schuster, 1990.
4. McKay M, Fanning P. *Self-Esteem* (3rd ed.). Oakland, CA: New Harbinger, 1992.
5. Goleman D. *Emotional Intelligence.* New York: Bantam Books, 1997.
6. Wade C, Tavris C. *Psychology.* New York: Harper & Row, 1987.
7. Spear P, Penrod S, Baker T. *Psychology: Perspectives on Behavior.* New York: Wiley, 1988.
8. Kagan J, Segal J. *Psychology: An Introduction* (6th ed.). Orlando, FL: Harcourt Brace Jovanovich, 1988.
9. Maslow AH. *Motivation and Personality* (2nd ed.). New York: Van Nostrand, 1970.
10. Maslow AH. *The Farthest Reaches of Human Nature.* Magnolia, MA: Peter Smith, 1983.
11. Lindzey G, Thompson R, Spring B. *Psychology* (3rd ed.). New York: Worth, 1988.
12. Wade C, Tavris C. *Psychology.* New York: Harper & Row, 1987.
13. May R. Values, myths, and symbols. *American Journal of Psychiatry,* 132, 703–706, 1975.
14. Hemenway JE, et al. *Assessing Spiritual Needs: A Guide for Caregivers.* Minneapolis: Augsburg Press, 1993.
15. Ayele H, Mulligan T, Gheorghiu S, Reyes-Ortiz C. Religious activity improves life satisfaction for some physicians and older patients. *Journal of the American Geriatrics Society,* 43, 453–455, 1999.
16. Levin JS. Religion and health: Is there an association, is it valid and is it causal? *Social Science Medicine,* 38(11), 1475–1482, 1994.
17. Thorson JA, et al. Psychological health and sense of humor. *Journal of Clinical Psychology,* 53(6), 605–619, 1997.
18. Yoshino S, Fujimori J, Kohda M. Effects of mirthful laughter on neuroendocrine and immune systems in patients with rheumatoid arthritis. *Journal of Rheumatology,* 23(4), 793–794, 1996.
19. Castro B, Eshleman J, Shearer R. Using humor to reduce stress and improve relationships. *Seminar Nurse Management,* 7(2), 90–92, 1999.
20. Berk LS, et al. Immune system changes during humor-associated laughter. *Clinical Research,* 39, 124a, 1991.
21. Cogan R, et al. Effects of laughter and relaxation on discomfort thresholds. *Journal of Behavioral Medicine,* 139–144, 1987.
22. Martin RA, Lefcourt HM. Sense of humor as a moderator between stressors and moods. *Journal of Personality and Social Psychology,* 45, 1313–1324, 1983.
23. Nezu A, Nezu C, Blissett S. Sense of humor as a moderator of the relationship between stressful events and psychological distress. *Journal of Personality and Social Psychology,* 54, 520–525, 1988.

24. Miller J. Jokes and joking: A serious laughing matter. In Durant J and Miller J (Eds.), *Laughing Matters: A Serious Look at Humor.* Essex, England: Longman Scientific and Technical, 1988.
25. Lefcourt HM, Martin RA. *Humor and Life Stress: Antidote to Adversity.* New York: Springer, 1986.
26. Kuhn C. *Humor Techniques for Health Care Professionals,* Presentation at Ball Memorial Hospital, April 22, 1998.
27. Nair M. A Documentary, *The Laughing Clubs of India,* 2001.
28. Collier G. *Emotional Expression.* Hillsdale, NJ: Erlbaum, 1985.
29. Peterson C, Seligman M, Vaillant G. Pessimistic explanatory style as a risk factor for physical illness: A thirty-five-year longitudinal study. *Journal of Personality and Social Psychology,* 55, 23–27, 1988.
30. Pavlov IP. *Conditioned Reflexes.* New York: Oxford University Press, 1927.
31. Hiroto D. Locus of control and learned helplessness. *Journal of Experiential Psychology,* 102, 187–193, 1974.
32. Ellis A. *Reason and Emotion in Psychotherapy.* New York: Lyle Stuart, 1962.
33. Kessler RC, Chiu WT, Demler O, Walters EE. Prevalence, severity, and comorbidity of twelve-month DSM-IV disorders in the National Comorbidity Survey Replication (NCS-R). *Archives of General Psychiatry,* 62(6), 617–627, 2005.
34. U.S. Census Bureau population estimates by demographic characteristics. Table 2: Annual estimates of the population by selected age groups and sex for the United States: April 1, 2000 to July 1, 2004 (NC-EST2004–02). www.census.gov/popest/national/asrh/, Population Division, U.S. Census Bureau Release Data: June 9, 2005.
35. World Health Organization. *The World Health Report 2004: Changing History,* Annex table 3: Burden of disease in DALYs by cause, sex, and mortality stratum in WHO regions, estimates for 2002. Geneva: WHO, 2004.
36. American Psychiatric Association. *Diagnostic and Statistical Manual of Mental Disorders* (4th ed.) *(DSM-IV-TR).* Washington, DC: American Psychiatric Press, 2000.
37. World Health Organization. *Mental Health,* 2003.
38. Dramatic increases seen in college students' mental health problems over last 13 years. *Journal of Professional Psychology: Research and Practice,* February 2003.
39. National Institute of Mental Health, 2003.
40. Peterson K. Resilience, talking can help kids beat depression, *USA Today,* June 4, 2002.
41. Barber C. The medicated Americans: Antidepressant medications on the rise. *Scientific America,* February 2008.
42. Fewer kids taking antidepressants. *WebMD Medical News,* September 22, 2004.
43. Exercise better than drugs for depression. *British Journal of Sports Medicine,* 35, 114–117, April 2001.
44. Study puts spotlight on electroshock therapy, *USA Today,* March 13, 2001.
45. Rosenthal NE. *Winter Blues.* New York: Guilford Press, 1998.
46. U.S. Suicide Rate Increases. Johns Hopkins Bloomberg School of Public Health, October 21, 2008.
47. Bourne E. *The Anxiety and Phobia Workbook.* Oakland, CA: New Harbinger, 1995.
48. Hallowell E, Ratey J. *Driven to Distraction.* New York: Simon & Schuster, 1995.
49. *Occupational Outlook Handout,* U.S. Department of Labor Bureau of Labor Statistics, 2002–2003.

Personal Assessment

What is your explanatory style?

Instructions: For each statement, circle the response that best fits you.

1. The project you are in charge of is a great success.
   A. I kept a close watch over everyone's work. 1
   B. Everyone devoted a lot of time and energy to it. 0
2. You and your partner make up after a fight.
   A. I forgave my partner. 0
   B. I'm usually forgiving. 1
3. You get lost driving to a friend's house.
   A. I missed a turn. 1
   B. My friend gave me bad directions. 0
4. You were extremely healthy all year.
   A. Few people around me were sick, so I wasn't exposed. 0
   B. I made sure I ate well and got enough rest. 1
5. You forgot your friend's birthday.
   A. I'm not good at remembering birthdays. 1
   B. I was preoccupied with other things. 0
6. Your boss gives you too little time to finish a project, but you get it done anyway.
   A. I am good at my job. 0
   B. I am an efficient person. 1
7. They won't honor your credit card at a store.
   A. I sometimes overestimate how much money I have. 1
   B. I sometimes forget to pay my credit card bill. 0
8. Your car runs out of gas on a dark street late at night.
   A. I didn't check to see how much gas was in the tank. 1
   B. The gas gauge was broken. 0
9. You fail an important examination.
   A. I wasn't as smart as the other people taking the test. 1
   B. I didn't prepare for it well enough. 0
10. You lose your temper with a friend.
    A. My friend is always nagging me. 1
    B. My friend was in a hostile mood. 0
11. You win an athletic contest.
    A. I was feeling unbeatable. 0
    B. I trained hard. 1
12. A friend thanks you for helping her get through a bad time.
    A. I enjoy helping her through tough times. 0
    B. I am good at giving useful advice. 1

Scoring Key

Add together items 3, 5, 7, 8, 9, and 10 to get your B (bad event) score = _____

If you scored:

5 to 6—You tend to be very pessimistic and explain bad things as resulting from something you did or a personal characteristic that is lasting and extends to many areas in your life.
2 to 4—You have an average level of pessimism about negative events.
0 to 1—You tend to be very optimistic and explain bad things as resulting from something someone else did or a circumstance that is temporary and specific to only that situation.

Add together items 1, 2, 4, 6, 11, and 12 to get your G (good event) score = _____

If you scored:

5 to 6—You tend to be very optimistic and explain good things as resulting from something you did or a personal characteristic that is lasting and extends to many areas in your life.
2 to 4—You have an average level of optimism about positive events.
0 to 1—You tend to be very pessimistic and explain good things as resulting from something someone else did or a circumstance that is temporary and specific to only that situation.

TO CARRY THIS FURTHER . . .

How did you score? If your explanatory style tends to be pessimistic, try some of the strategies suggested in Chapter 2 for building optimism. When you encounter adversity, pay attention to your thinking patterns and consciously reframe them to be more positive and more focused on problem solving. Building a more optimistic approach to life can improve many dimensions of your health.

Source: Adapted from M. Seligman. *Learned Optimism*. New York: Pocket Books, 1990.

Managing Stress

3 chapter

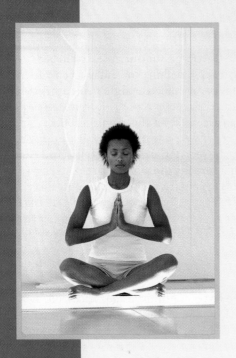

What Do You Know About Managing Stress?

1. Having stress in your life is negative. True or False?

2. Time management is the reason most college students cite for their academic success or failure. True or False?

3. Laughing is important to managing stress. True or False?

4. Different colors, sounds, and smells can affect your stress level. True or False?

5. Breathing is the key to stress management. True or False?

6. You can make up for not sleeping enough during the week by sleeping more on the weekends. True or False?

7. Exposing yourself to stressful situations can sometimes help you reduce your stress. True or False?

Check your answers at the end of the chapter.

What Is Stress?

How do you know when you are stressed? You might experience headaches, stomachaches, or back and neck aches, or you might feel irritable, tired, anxious, and depressed. Some people eat more, while others find eating difficult when they are stressed. **Stress** refers to physiological and psychological responses to a significant or unexpected change or disruption in one's life. It can be brought on by real or imagined factors or events.

Stress was first described in the 1930s by Hans Selye. During his second year of medical school, Selye observed that, although his patients suffered from a variety of illnesses, they all showed common symptoms, such as fatigue, appetite disturbance, sleep problems, mood swings, gastrointestinal problems, and diminished concentration and recall. He began developing his now-famous theory of the influence of stress on people's ability to cope with and adapt to the pressures of injury and disease. He discovered that patients with a variety of ailments manifested many similar symptoms, which he ultimately attributed to their bodies' efforts to respond to the stresses of being ill. He called this collection of symptoms—this stress disease—stress syndrome, or the **general adaptation syndrome (GAS).** He also described this as "the syndrome of being ill."[1] We will discuss Selye's discovery further later in the chapter.

Selye defines stress as "the nonspecific response of the body to any demand whether it is caused by or results in pleasant or unpleasant conditions." Stress can be positive or negative. It is our response to stress—how we manage stress—that makes a difference in terms of how it affects us. Stress resulting from unpleasant events or conditions is called **distress** (from the Greek *dys,* meaning bad, as in displeasure). Stress resulting from pleasant events or conditions is called **eustress** (from the Greek *eu,* meaning good, as in euphoria). Both distress and eustress elicit the same physiological responses in the body, as noted in Selye's GAS model.

While stress may not always be negative, our responses to it can be problematic or unhealthy. Both positive and negative stressful situations place extra demands on the body—your body reacts to an unexpected change or a highly emotional experience, regardless of whether this change is good or bad. If the duration of stress is relatively short, the overall effect is minimal and your body will rest, renew itself, and return to normal. But, as you will learn in this chapter, long-lasting stress, experiencing multiple stressors simultaneously, and not managing your stress effectively can take a toll on your body.

Stress is actually normal and healthy at a certain level. With functional, healthy levels of stress, overall physiological equilibrium is maintained at a balanced level. However, you really don't want to eliminate all stress because stress is adaptive, is functional, and can be beneficial. You need to understand how you uniquely deal with stress and what works and doesn't work well for you in coping with day-to-day pressures and problems (see the box "Different Cultures, Different Ways of Coping").

How We Respond to Stress

When we are stressed, we react in specific ways. The **stress response** is the result of learned and conditioned habits adopted early in life as a way of coping with problems, conflict, and disruptive events. But many of our responses to stress are innate, basic human survival mechanisms left over from our primordial roots. In prehistoric times, the best response to perceived danger, such as seeing a saber-toothed tiger about to attack, might be either to fight the animal or to run away. Stress in modern times remains the same except that we are responding to twenty-first-century threats and dangers rather than to saber-toothed tigers. Again, it is not the events that determine how stressed we feel but our response to these stressors. We next discuss the way that this innate stress response affects our modern lives.

Fight or Flight Response

Our response to stress involves many physiological changes that are collectively called the **fight or flight response.** In situations in which you must react immediately to danger, it is advisable to either fight off the danger or flee. For example, you are walking back from class at

night, thinking about all the studying you need to do, and you begin to cross the street. Suddenly, out of nowhere, a car's headlights are coming right at you. Since your best response is probably not to fight the car, you run as fast as you can to the other side of the road. In that split second when you see the car careening quickly toward you, your muscles tense, your heart beats faster, your adrenaline pumps faster and is released at increased levels into your bloodstream, your breathing becomes more shallow and rapid, and your pupils dilate to see the car better.

This is the fight or flight response. Receiving alert signals from the brain, the sympathetic nerves signal most of the organs of the body, and the adrenal glands are activated. Within the brain itself, neural pathways, involved in increased attention and focus, are activated. In this way, performance and learning can be heightened. Again, all these changes are adaptive and helpful to your survival in getting out of harm's way. In the preceding example, when you get to the other side of the road and realize that you are okay, your body begins to relax and return to its normal state. You take a large, deep breath, expressing a big sigh of relief. Your muscles may feel even weaker than usual, your breathing may become deeper and heavier than is typical, and you may feel shaky as your body goes from extreme arousal to relaxing very quickly. Figure 3-1a on page 63 depicts the changes from the normal state to an arousal state to a very relaxed state then back to normal.

Accompanying this fight or flight reaction is a slower response. During stressful events, the pituitary gland secretes a peptide called adrenocorticotrophin, or ACTH, into the blood. ACTH travels through the

---

Key Terms

stress The physiological and psychological state of disruption caused by the presence of an unanticipated, disruptive, or stimulating event.

general adaptation syndrome (GAS) Sequenced physiological responses to the presence of a stressor, involving the alarm, resistance, and exhaustion stages of the stress response.

distress Stress that diminishes the quality of life; commonly associated with disease, illness, and maladaptation.

eustress Stress that enhances the quality of life.

stress response The physiological and psychological responses to positive or negative events that are disruptive, unexpected, or stimulating.

fight or flight response The physiological response to a stressor that prepares the body for confrontation or avoidance.

Chapter Three Managing Stress

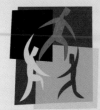

Learning from Our Diversity

Different Cultures, Different Ways of Coping

While stressful situations can affect people differently, and we all have our unique ways of coping with stress, some important cultural differences exist in the types of stress. For example, Native Americans incorporate storytelling, spirituality, dreams, and visions into their stress-management strategies. A "talking circle" may be employed to help alleviate stress. This involves sitting in a circle, connecting with others by shaking hands around the circle, sharing one's innermost feelings without interruption or response from others, burning incense and passing it around the circle, and passing a sacred object such as an eagle feather to the person who is speaking.

There are significant differences between the ways Asian and European cultures cope with stress. European cultures use social support in coping with stress; Asians tend to avoid drawing on social support for fear that they will disrupt group harmony, receive criticism about the problem, or feel ashamed. In Asian cultures people are taught to take responsibility for solving their own problems, and if they do go to others for support, they typically go to their own family. Yoga, meditation, and acupuncture are common methods for coping with stress in Asian cultures. Asian Americans focus more on logical, rational, and structured approaches, such as time management, relaxation techniques, and cognitive behavioral strategies.

African Americans tend to prefer to manage stress and problems using direct, active problem solving. In contrast to Asian cultures, African Americans tend to value social support—they tend to share their problems with others in times of stress and are more comfortable expressing feelings associated with the stress.

Hispanics tend to seek support from religion, family, and community in managing daily stressors. This culture values the present and emphasizes being rather than doing. Hispanic culture encourages accepting and enduring stress and problems rather than being assertive and provoking conflict.

Each of us needs to understand how we respond to stress and find strategies that work best to control stress levels. We should also consider issues of diversity in order to identify the unique stressors and stress-management techniques that might best fit us.

Sources: Hatfield DL, The Stereotyping of Native Americans, *Humanist*, September 2000; Native Americans of North America, Microsoft® Encarta® *Online Encyclopedia, 2005,* http://encarta.msn.com © 1997–2005 Microsoft Corporation; Sue D, Sue D, *Counseling the Culturally Different* (New York: Wiley, 1999).

---

blood to the adrenal gland, where it signals the production of a hormone called cortisol.[2] Cortisol aids the body in recovering from stressful experiences by freeing up energy stores. The logic behind the slower stress response is that the quick fight or flight response uses up a lot of the body's available energy. The slower response helps to replenish that energy. The body usually has some small amount of cortisol circulating in the blood at all times. When the stress response lasts too long or is initiated too frequently, the cortisol level is increased. After enough of these small increases, the body soon resets its control mechanism to maintain a higher constant amount of cortisol in the body.

Chronic Stress

Now let's consider a different situation. You have a test in a week that you are very concerned about. It seems to be preoccupying your every waking thought, and you have trouble sleeping as well. You are worried that you won't perform well on the test, and you really need to do better than you did on your last test. Your parents have been putting a great deal of pressure on you to do better in school in general. Because our bodies respond similarly to perceived or anticipated threat, you can have the same response to things that have and have not yet occurred. In other words, your heart races, breathing becomes labored, muscles are tense, the body sweats, and blood flow is constricted to the extremities and digestive

organs and increases to the major muscles and brain. Your body is becoming ready to fight or flee the danger. However, you cannot take any action and make a fight or flight response, because nothing has happened yet. You haven't taken the test yet, and even once you have done so, you won't know your grade. So your body remains at this high level of arousal, as depicted in Figure 3-1b.

Remaining in a continued state of physiological arousal for an extended period of time is called **chronic stress.** This high level of arousal is similar to putting your foot on the accelerator of your car while it is in park and not letting up on the gas pedal. Since the fight or flight response is meant to be a very quick, short-acting response, your body begins to wear down if kept at this physiological state of arousal for too long; eventually, you will begin to feel exhausted. This is also the reason that people cope better with anxiety by taking some action, doing something about whatever they are worried about, rather than stewing about their problems. Thus the fight or flight response can be triggered inappropriately in response to phobias, irrational beliefs, an overactive imagination, or hallucinations or delusions.

The Three Stages of Stress

Once under the influence of a stressor, people's bodies respond in remarkably similar, predictable ways. For example, when asked to give a speech for a class, your

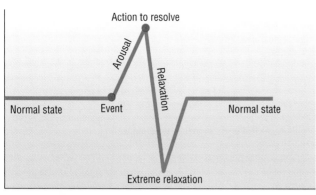

(A) Adaptive Stress Response

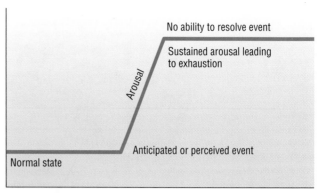

(B) Chronic Stress Response

Figure 3-1 Resolving Stress   How quickly and effectively you act to resolve stress has a significant effect on how long your body remains at a high level of physiological arousal.

Source: Selye, H. *The Stress of Life,* New York: McGraw-Hill, 1984.

heart rate may increase, your throat may become dry, your palms may sweat, and you may feel lightheaded, dizzy, and nauseous. If an individual lost her or his job or discovered that her or his partner wanted to terminate their relationship, the person might experience similar sensations. It is clear that different stressors are able to evoke common physical reactions.

Selye described the typical physical response to a stressor in his general adaptation syndrome model discussed earlier in the chapter.[3] Selye stated that the human body moves through three stages when confronted by stressors, as follows.

Alarm Stage

Once exposed to any event that is perceived as threatening or dangerous, the body immediately prepares for difficulty, entering what Selye called the **alarm stage.** These involuntary changes, shown in Figure 3-2, are controlled by the hormonal and the nervous systems, and they trigger the fight or flight response. For example, you realize that the final exam you thought was today was actually scheduled for yesterday. You may begin to experience fear, panic, anxiety, anger, depression, and restlessness.[4]

Resistance Stage

The second stage of a response to a stressor is the **resistance stage,** during which the body attempts to reestablish its equilibrium or internal balance. The body is geared for survival, and because staying in the alarm stage for a prolonged amount of time is not conducive for the body's optimal functioning, it will resist the threat or attempt to resolve the problem and reduce the intensity of the response to a more manageable level. Specific organ systems, such as the cardiovascular and digestive systems, become the focus of the body's response.[5]

During this phase, you might take steps to calm yourself down and relieve the stress on your body: You might deny the situation, withdraw and isolate yourself from others, and shut down your emotions. Thus, in the previous example, you may not tell anyone about missing the exam, may tell yourself that you don't care about that class anyway, and go back to bed.

Exhaustion Stage

Your ability to move from the alarm stage to a less damaging resistance stage determines the effect that the stressor has on your physical and psychological health. As you gain more control and balance is reestablished, you can begin to recover from the stress.

The length of time, the energy, and the effort required to accomplish recovery determines how exhausted your body becomes as a result of the stressor. Of course, the longer the body is under stress and out of balance, the more negative the effect will be on your body. Long-term exposure to a stressor or coping with

> **Key Terms**
>
> **chronic stress** Remaining at a high level of physiological arousal for an extended period of time; it can also occur when an individual is not able to immediately react to a real or a perceived threat.
>
> **alarm stage** The first stage of the stress response, involving physiological, involuntary changes that are controlled by the hormonal and the nervous systems; the fight or flight response is activated in this stage.
>
> **resistance stage** The second stage of a response to a stressor, during which the body attempts to reestablish its equilibrium or internal balance.

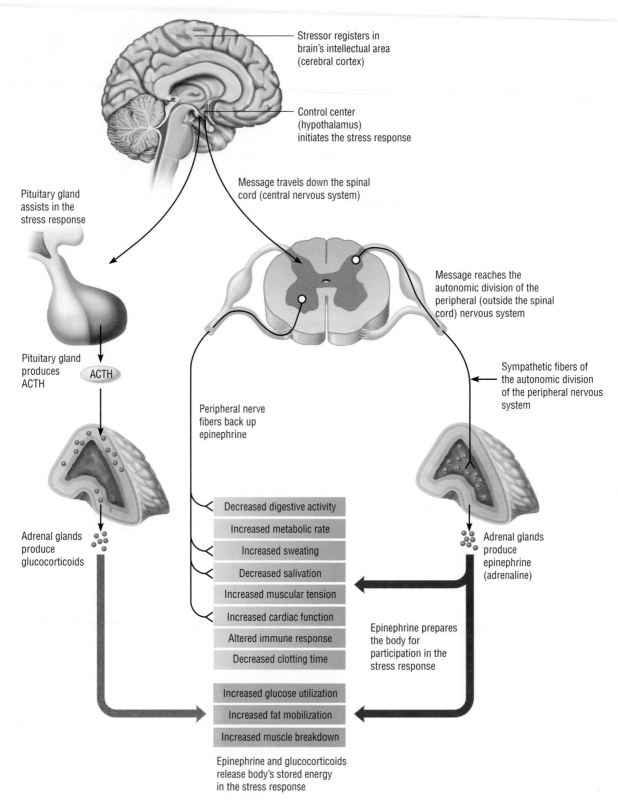

Stressor registers in brain's intellectual area (cerebral cortex)

Control center (hypothalamus) initiates the stress response

Message travels down the spinal cord (central nervous system)

Pituitary gland assists in the stress response

Message reaches the autonomic division of the peripheral (outside the spinal cord) nervous system

Pituitary gland produces ACTH

ACTH

Sympathetic fibers of the autonomic division of the peripheral nervous system

Peripheral nerve fibers back up epinephrine

Adrenal glands produce glucocorticoids

Adrenal glands produce epinephrine (adrenaline)

Decreased digestive activity

Increased metabolic rate

Increased sweating

Decreased salivation

Increased muscular tension

Increased cardiac function

Altered immune response

Decreased clotting time

Epinephrine prepares the body for participation in the stress response

Increased glucose utilization

Increased fat mobilization

Increased muscle breakdown

Epinephrine and glucocorticoids release body's stored energy in the stress response

Figure 3-2 The Stress Response   Physiological reactions to a stressor are controlled by the hormonal and nervous systems.

multiple stressors at the same time often results in overloading your system. Specific organs and body systems that were called on during the resistance stage may not be able to resist a stressor indefinitely. When all the psychological and physical resources we rely on to deal with stress are used up, an **exhaustion stage** results, and the stress-producing hormones such as adrenaline increase again.[3] This is when chronic and serious illnesses can begin to develop, and the individual may even develop clinical depression.

The Effects of Stress

If not managed well, stress can affect us in a variety of negative ways. For instance, stress can give us medical problems, interpersonal and relationship conflicts, and academic and work difficulties. However, a moderate level of stress can be beneficial.

The Physical Toll of Stress

Constant arousal and increased levels of adrenaline in your system will eventually wear down your body's immunological system. As this occurs, you will be less able to cope with stress, and so it takes less and less to cause a stress reaction. When you are chronically stressed, it takes very little to frustrate you, and you can feel easily irritated and stressed at the littlest thing. Your body is both psychologically and physically less able to cope with stress. This can compromise your immune system, and you may become ill more easily. It may also take longer for you to recover from illness.

The following medical problems have been associated with stress[6] (to examine stress indicators for your personal stress, complete the rating scale at the end of this chapter):

- Cardiovascular problems (heart attacks, strokes, hypertension)
- Gastrointestinal problems (ulcers, irritable bowel syndrome, diarrhea, constipation, diverticulitis)
- Rheumatoid arthritis
- Lupus
- Headaches and migraines
- Muscle spasms and cramps
- Sleep disorders
- Anxiety
- Jaw problems (temporomandibular joint [TMJ] syndrome)
- Allergies
- Cancer
- Back pain
- Asthma

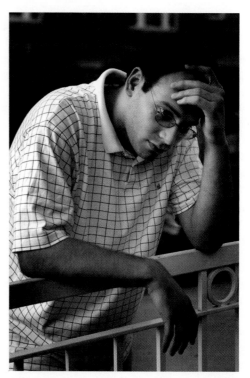

Chronic stress can contribute to headaches, anxiety, insomnia, and many other health problems.

- Kidney disease
- Sexual dysfunction
- Infertility
- Alcoholism and drug abuse

The Immune System and Stress

Corticosteroids are produced in the adrenal cortex as part of the stress response. Cortisol increases the body's fuel supply of carbohydrates, glucose, and fat, which are needed to respond to stress. It is important not to keep these levels elevated for very long, though, as too much cortisol in the system can also act to suppress the immune system. Remember that the stress response is meant to be a rapid, temporary response. Individuals who are chronically stressed are constantly pumping out a high level of corticosteroids. Over time, this can result in a breakdown of muscle, a decreased number of immune cells, and a

> **Key Terms**
>
> **exhaustion stage** The point at which the physical and the psychological resources used to deal with stress have been depleted.

Psychoneuroimmunology: Can Stress Affect Our Immune System?

The newly emerging field of psychoneuroimmunology addresses the apparent interplay of the mind, the nervous system (the hypothalamus and the autonomic nervous system), and the immune system (see Chapter 13).

On the basis of clinical observation and laboratory studies, it is recognized that feelings associated with stress (depression and anxiety) and the disruption of social support systems relate to the weakening of the immune response and the development of some illnesses. For example, a study showed that happy, relaxed people are more resistant to illness than are those who tend to be unhappy and tense. In addition, work-related or personal stress experienced for at least one month increases a person's chances of catching a cold. In other words, the longer you live in a stressful state, the more likely you are to catch a cold. People in unhappy marriages, particularly wives, also have

higher incidences of colds. Extroverts are less likely to catch a cold, as are those with diverse social roles such as spouse, parent, worker, friend, community member, student. This situation makes sense, since we know that incorporating positive social interactions into our lives helps to alleviate stress, which in turn minimizes the risk of catching a cold. In another study, immunizations were less effective in producing an immune response in students stressed by upcoming examinations than in those not scheduled to take exams.

Stress triggers the release of inflammatory particles, cytokines and histamines, that fight off infection but can also cause cold symptoms. Researchers suspect that a sense of well-being decreases the release of cytokines and eases symptoms. This phenomenon may also explain why people can get through a state of acute stress and then become ill after the crisis is over, since

stress produces adrenaline, which stimulates the immune system, releasing cortisol. This is the hormone that battles inflammation but weakens immunity.

Our growing understanding of the relationship between our thoughts, the nervous system, and the functional status of the immune system enhances our insight into illnesses and their relationship to stress. As this understanding continues to mature, we will develop more effective coping strategies that enhance the connection between our feelings and their effect on nervous system and endocrine system function and the maintenance of immune system capabilities.

Sources: Masek K, et al., Past, Present and Future of Psychoneuroimmunology, *Toxicology*, 142(3), 179–188, 2000; Elias M, In the War on Colds Personality Counts, *USA Today*, December 1, 2003; Cohen S, et al., Types of Stressors That Increase Susceptibility to the Common Cold in Healthy Adults, *Health Psychology*, 17(3), 214–223, 1998.

---

decreased inflammatory response. This can render the body less able to defend against bacteria and viruses—a stressed person is more likely to become ill. Hypertension and fluid retention are also associated with constant high levels of corticosteroids. On the other hand, if the level of corticosteroids in your system is too low, you can have an overactive immune system—this can harm healthy cells, resulting in autoimmune diseases such as lupus and rheumatoid arthritis. Therefore it is important to maintain a healthy level of corticosteroids (in other words, a moderate level of stress) to keep the body in balance. See the box "Psychoneuroimmunology" for more on the links between stress and health.

Cardiovascular Disease and Stress

Your level of stress also contributes to your risk for developing cardiovascular disease. Chronic stress exposes your body to unhealthy, persistently elevated levels of stress hormones like adrenaline and cortisol. Studies also link stress to changes in the way blood clots, which increases the risk of heart attack. Job stress, personality factors, and social isolation have all been suggested as factors contributing to cardiovascular disease. For example, one study found that people who worked more than 60 hours a week were twice as likely to have a heart attack as those working 40 hours a week.[7] High levels of stress can make other risk factors (such as high cholesterol or

high blood pressure) worse, which in turn increases the chances of developing cardiovascular disease.

Type A and Type B Personalities   Cardiologists Meyer Friedman and Roy Rosenman identified two basic types of personalities when they interviewed individuals in order to identify people who may be susceptible to stress-related heart disease.[8] In the interview, they asked individuals the following questions:

1. Does your job carry heavy responsibility?
2. Is there any time when you feel particularly rushed or under pressure?
3. When you are under pressure, does it bother you?
4. Would you describe yourself as a hard-driving ambitious type of person in accomplishing the things you want, or would you describe yourself as a relatively relaxed and easygoing person?

From the responses to these questions, Friedman and Rosenman were able to distinguish two types of personalities with respect to stress: type A and type B personalities. **Type A** individuals often feel pressured, are ambitious, impatient, competitive, walk and talk rapidly, and can be easily annoyed by delays. **Type B** individuals tend to be calm, relaxed, easygoing, and patient. Friedman and Rosenman also found that many cases of heart disease couldn't be attributed to other cardiac risk factors such as smoking or dietary habits but could be linked to stress. Type A personalities tend to share qualities of workaholism and perfectionism, such as having high expectations and feeling out of control, irritable and overwhelmed, stressed and pressured most of the time. There is a constant sense of needing to go faster and hurry through activities to get on to the next task. Thus type A people tend not to enjoy what they are doing because they are thinking about the next activity rather than enjoying the present.[9] This can cause tension in their relationships as well. Type A people tend to drive themselves to exhaustion and stop only when they collapse or become ill.

While Friedman and Rosenman didn't describe type A personalities as an illness but more as a personality type, they did find correlations with stress. Type A people sometimes need to slow down, lower their expectations of themselves, delegate responsibilities to others, and prioritize their tasks. Type A individuals often complain that they have trouble relaxing and don't know how to relax. They also don't allow themselves to have fun until all of the work is done, which rarely occurs. Scheduling social activities and time to relax is one important component in alleviating the stress that accompanies type A personalities. Exercising, meditation, massage, spiritual activities, and yoga are other ways to relax.

The Stress-Hardy Individual While some people are chronically stressed, which leads to exhaustion, other people seem to have a high stress tolerance. These "stress-hardy" individuals have a lower frequency of illness and absenteeism.[8] They view stressors as challenges and chances for new opportunities and seem to thrive with increased stress. They feel more in control of their lives and perceive themselves as having options and the power to make choices and influence situations. So it is not just the level of stress that an individual experiences that determines how he or she will respond but also the individual's ability to manage varying degrees of stress. Stress-hardy individuals who have a good social support system, exercise regularly, and maintain a healthy diet have fewer stress-related illnesses than do those who have less healthy lifestyles.

Benefits of Stress

As we have said, while too much stress can have a negative effect and cause some serious health problems, a moderate level of stress is positive and beneficial. Stress can be motivating and energizing. Without some stress, many of us may not get much accomplished in our day or even get out of bed! Look at the diagram in Figure 3-3. What do you notice? Too little and too much stress are not helpful. When you are not stressed at all, you can be apathetic and lethargic. When you are too stressed, you are paralyzed with fear, like deer in the headlights. This is referred to as the **Yerkes-Dodson Law,** which uses a

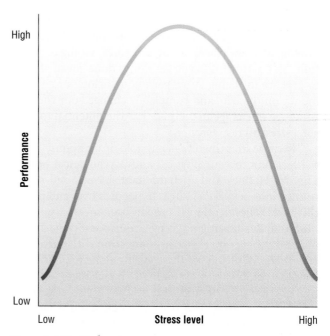

Figure 3-3 The Yerkes-Dodson Law   Too little or too much stress is not helpful, but a moderate level of stress encourages peak performance.

Source: Hebb DO. Drive and the CNS (conceptual nervous system). *Psychological Review*, 62(4), 243–254, 1955.

bell-shaped curve to demonstrate that there is an optimal level of stress for peak performance. This fact holds true for any type of performance, from academic or work activities to music or athletics.[9] Recognizing the appropriate level of stress for your ideal performance level is important in reaching your potential.

The Sources of Stress

There are other causes of stress besides experiencing positive or negative events in life.[10] What events or situations trigger stress for you? For some it is financial worries, for others it might be relationship conflict, and for still others it is work-related stress. Even positive events, such as getting married, starting a new job, or moving to a new place, can be **stressors.** Going on vacation can be stressful as you get things done ahead of time to prepare for being away, pack your belongings, spend money on the trip, and completely change your routine. Any type of change in your life has the potential to trigger a stressful response.

Because stress involves a physiological response, it has a direct link to your physical and psychological health. Thomas Holmes and Richard Rahe have found direct connections between changes in people's lives and physical illness. They developed a widely used inventory, called the Social Readjustment Rating Scale, to assess the degree of stress people experience in connection with particular life events. While one of these events alone might be tolerable, a combination of too many life changes within a short period of time may lead to illness.[10] To effectively manage your stress, you need to understand what specific sources trigger stress for you. Students experience some specific types of stress that other people do not necessarily encounter. In this next section, we will discuss stressors unique to students and how to manage them.

To assess your level of stress and potential vulnerability to illness, complete the Personal Assessment inventory at the end of this chapter.

Student Stressors

Going to college has been likened to "crossing into a new culture" where students face unique challenges and stressors.[11] Similar to going to live in another country, students must learn new customs and traditions, new ways of doing things, and a new language, and must leave comfortable and familiar surroundings. This can cause a high level of stress for students, many of whom have left their support system behind to live in a place where they know few people. In the sections that follow, we cover some of the specific stressors college students face and offer ways to manage these situations.

Interpersonal Stressors

Homesickness   Homesickness is one of the most common problems facing college students—which is understandable given that they are separated from friends and family and learning to live in an entirely new environment.[11]When you are undergoing a great deal of

change in your life, it is helpful to have the comfort and security of knowing that your home base remains stable and consistent. Moving from home to college can disrupt this sense of safety. While the college years can be an exciting and challenging time in your life, you may be missing your friends and family at home with whom you normally share these events. You may have also lost your sense of belonging while you struggle with finding a way to fit in with and navigate your new surroundings.

Often homesickness doesn't hit until a few weeks or maybe a month after you have moved, since the first few weeks are filled with meeting new people, social activities, and unpacking. After the dust settles, some people begin to feel lonely and alone. See the box "Overcoming Homesickness" for advice on how to deal with homesickness.

Relationship Problems   Along with homesickness, another very common stressor for students is relationship problems. Often students are separated by long distances from their best friends and romantic partners. While it can be difficult to maintain long-distance relationships, it is not impossible. Studies show that the key to effective long-distance relationships is communication. The quality of a long-distance relationship is improved if you both are committed to each other, you can talk openly about your concerns, feelings, and fears, and you can agree on the rules of the relationship, such as dating other people. In addition, there needs to be a strong level of trust between the partners, since trust is often tested in long-distance relationships. Both of you will change, and you must share these changes so that you can grow together, not apart. Agree on how often you will see each other, and focus on spending high-quality time together.

It can be beneficial to have your friends visit you at college (rather than you going home) so that they can interact with you in your new environment and meet your new friends. Often students feel as though they live in two worlds, home and school, and it can be stressful to negotiate going from one to the other. The more you can connect these two worlds, the less stress you will experience. So it can be helpful to share what you are doing in your day—activities around campus, details of your classes—with your friends and family back home, and ask them what they have been doing.

Balancing Work, Home, and School   It is estimated that about two-thirds of students work while going to college, and many students are working full-time to pay for the costs of tuition. In addition, it is estimated that between 5 and 10 percent of college students also have children. This, of course, adds stress to a student's life in balancing time for school, children, work, and household responsibilities (see Figure 3-4). The increase in the

---

Key Terms

stressors Factors or events, real or imagined, that elicit a state of stress.

Overcoming Homesickness

I just started college, and my family and friends are five hours away from me. I tend to be on the shy side and don't know anyone at my college. I miss my friends and family and don't feel like I belong here. I am thinking about withdrawing from school and going home. What should I do?

The following are some strategies to combat these feelings:

- *Get involved!* Become active in extracurricular social activities such as special interest clubs, student government, religious clubs, fraternities, and sororities. Clubs associated with your major are a great way to meet people, further your academic and career interests, and keep you from feeling homesick.
- *Call, e-mail, or text message* your family and friends regularly and let them know you would like to hear from them.
- *Be open to meeting new people.* Introduce yourself to people in your classes, and exchange e-mail addresses and phone numbers. This is also an excellent way to get a study partner or study group together. Keep your door open when you are in your room, and spend time in public, common areas—not just hiding away in your room when you have spare time. Strike up a conversation while doing your laundry in the common laundry room area.
- *Don't eat alone.* Ask someone to join you to eat, or ask people at a table if you can eat with them.
- *Don't go home on the weekends.* Even though it may be tempting to visit your family and friends, the weekends are the best time to meet people and participate in the activities going on around campus.
- *Be patient with yourself.* Accept that loneliness and longing for home are normal, and it will take some time for you to adjust to all the changes you are experiencing. Don't decide to throw in the towel after the first few days! It may take a month or more before you begin to feel more comfortable in your new home. Give yourself some time to face this new challenge.

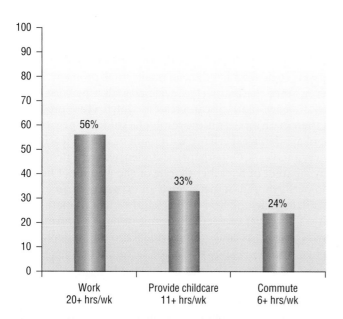

Figure 3-4 Balancing Work, School, and Home

Source: Community College Survey of Student Engagement (CCSSE). (2008). High Expectations and High Support. Austin, Texas: The University of Texas at Austin, Community College Leadership Program.

number of students who have children is partly a result of a nationwide trend of more women in their mid-20s or older starting or returning to college. In fact, a national study by the University of Michigan showed that the number of full-time female students over 25 years old grew by 500 percent over recent years.[12]

While some campuses offer child care, many do not, which leaves students having to coordinate schedules and juggle responsibilities, causing even more stress. Also, the cost of child care can be exorbitant for some and can certainly add to financial worries. Managing time well and having a strong support system are essential for students with children, particularly single parents. Often there is little to no time available for relaxation, socializing, or exercising, and so employing stress relief strategies can be challenging.

Academic Stressors

How does stress affect learning? Research suggests that people who are highly anxious tend to perform better than others do at simple learning tasks but less well than others do at difficult tasks, particularly those involving reasoning activities and time-limited tests.[14] When you are more stressed or anxious, you have a diminished ability to concentrate, to recall information, and to master problem-solving activities. You may find yourself reading the same page in your textbook over and over again, not knowing what you read.[13]

You have studied for the test you are about to take and are well prepared. You look at the first test question and suddenly your mind goes blank. The harder you try to think, the more nervous and distressed you feel. You just can't think clearly and feel as though you have some type of mental block—what is happening?

One-fifth of students experience these feelings, referred to as **test anxiety.** Exams are one of the greatest sources of stress for college students. The physical sensations associated with test anxiety are similar to those of general anxiety. People suffering from test anxiety make more mistakes on their tests, don't read the test accurately, and tend to make simple mistakes, such as spelling errors or adding something incorrectly. Many don't pace themselves well and have a hard time finishing exams. Test anxiety is a form of performance anxiety—people anticipate that they will perform poorly on the test.[13]

 TALKING POINTS What are some problems with stress described in this chapter that you have experienced?

As we have mentioned, speech anxiety, or fear of public speaking, is one of the most common anxiety disorders. Since students are frequently required to give oral presentations, expected to engage in class discussion, and graded on class-participation points, this can present a problem for some.

In addition to the basic stress-management techniques outlined in this chapter, the following strategies can be used to cope with speech anxiety:

- *Volunteer to go first.* Anxiety is dealt with best by taking action. Pressure and expectations tend to mount with each person who takes a turn so you can lessen your stress level by being the first to present. Another advantage is that your performance is judged on its own merit without being compared to anyone else's.

- *Practice in front of a mirror and for your friends.* Solicit feedback: Do you need to slow down or speak louder? Practice will also help you to remember your talk so that you don't read it word for word, which can seem less interesting to your audience.

- *Engage in positive visualization.* Take deep, comfortable breaths and imagine yourself giving your speech with confidence and receiving positive feedback and compliments about your performance.

- *Vary your presentation style and format.* Use visuals such as slides, and engage your audience in discussion so that they are an active not a passive part of your presentation. This takes some of the focus and pressure away from you.

Another common stressor for college students is math anxiety. People who suffer from math anxiety feel

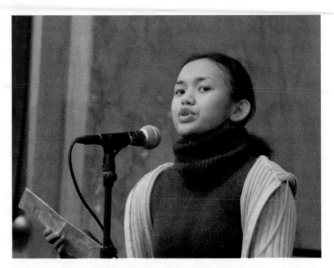

Effective behavioral and psychological interventions exist to treat speech anxiety.

that they are incapable of performing well in activities and classes that involve math. The incidence of math anxiety among college students has risen significantly over the last decade. Many students have even chosen their college major on the basis of how little math is required for the degree.

Typically, people with math anxiety have the potential to perform well in math; the anxiety is more of a psychological, rather than an intellectual, problem. However, since math anxiety interferes with a person's ability to learn math, it can create an intellectual problem. Often math anxiety is the result of a student's negative or embarrassing experience with math or a math teacher in previous years. Or perhaps the student was repeatedly told by a parent or a teacher that he or she would not be able to perform well in math. Such an experience can leave a student believing him- or herself deficient in math ability. This belief can actually result in poor performance, which serves as confirming evidence to the student. This phenomenon is known as a self-fulfilling prophecy; it is described more fully later in this chapter.[14]

Students who fear math often avoid asking questions to save embarrassment, sit in the back of the classroom, fail to seek help from the instructor, and usually put off studying math until the last moment. All these negative behaviors are intended to reduce the student's anxiety but actually result in more intense anxiety. However, there are a number of strategies to overcome math anxiety:

1. *Take an easier, slower math course* as opposed to a faster-paced, more challenging one. It is better to stack the odds in your favor than to risk reinforcing your negative experiences with math.
2. *Be aware of thoughts, feelings, and actions* as they are related to math. Develop a positive perspective toward math.

Key Terms

test anxiety A form of performance anxiety that generates extreme feelings of distress in exam situations.

3. *There is safety in numbers!* You can reduce your anxiety with the help of a tutor, studying with a friend, and talking with your instructor.

4. *Sit near the front of the class* where you will experience fewer distractions and feel more a part of what is being discussed.

5. If you have questions or can't keep up with the instructor, *ask for clarification and repetition* of whatever you missed.[15]

6. *Review the material.* Research shows that you will remember 50 percent of what you heard in class if you review it immediately after class, but only 20 percent is retained 24 hours later if you didn't review the material right away.[16]

Internal Stressors

We can also generate stress within ourselves by putting too much pressure on ourselves, procrastinating, expecting too much of ourselves, and being self-critical. These intrapsychic stressors refer to our internal worries, criticisms, and negative self-talk, which were discussed in Chapter 2. Students say that procrastination, perfectionism, and poor goal setting are common sources of stress in their lives.

Procrastination Procrastination means postponing something that is necessary to do to reach a goal.[17] Putting things off is a common problem that plagues students and can cause stress. A survey of college students found that approximately 23 percent of students said they procrastinated about half the time, and 27 percent of students said they procrastinated most of the time.[17] Procrastination has been viewed as a time-management problem, but it is really more than that, and so time-management strategies tend to be ineffective in resolving this problem. Procrastination is also different from indecision, because people can make a decision but still have trouble implementing it.

Typically there is a psychological aspect to procrastination because we tend to delay doing those things that we don't want to do. Emotions such as anxiety, guilt, and dread often accompany thinking about the task. By putting the dreaded activity off, you can temporarily alleviate your anxiety and discomfort, which is a reinforcing aspect of procrastination. In the short term, procrastination seems to be a good solution and helps you to feel better. However, in the long run, procrastination usually leads to bigger problems and more work. For example, putting off paying your bills may feel good at the moment, but when your electricity is turned off and you have to pay late fees, and your roommates are upset with you because they thought you had paid the bill, your pleasurable feelings soon turn sour.

Men and women procrastinate equally often, but people in their mid- to late-20s and 60-year-olds procrastinate more than people in any other age group do.[18] Individuals who procrastinate are frequently referred to as "lazy" or "stupid," but actually there are no differences in levels of intelligence between procrastinators and nonprocrastinators. However, students who procrastinate tend to perform less well and retain less than students who do not. You might want to take the survey at the end of this chapter to assess your risk for procrastination.

Many people who procrastinate report feeling overwhelmed and highly anxious. They have difficulty tuning out external stimulation and concentrating on the task at hand. They also worry about how their performance will be judged by others and have perfectionistic standards for themselves. We discuss perfectionism and setting unrealistic goals in the next section.

Perfectionism Perfectionism leads to undue stress because perfection is an unattainable goal. By setting the standard at perfect, you will set yourself up to fail. Perfectionists tend to be their own worst critic; they are harder on themselves than anyone else is on them, and they are also critical of others. These individuals are described as neat and organized, seeming to "have it all together" and to be able to do more than most people and do it exceptionally well. Often people envy perfectionistic people because they seem very confident and competent; however, individuals who are perfectionistic never feel good enough and often feel out of control in their lives.[19] People who are perfectionists focus on what they haven't accomplished or haven't done right rather than on what they have completed or have done well. Making mistakes feels especially humiliating to persons who are perfectionistic, and they tend to feel a strong sense of shame and low self-esteem when someone catches them in error. They have difficulty with criticism or any negative feedback because much of their self-esteem is based on being accurate, competent, and the best. While striving to do your best is an admirable quality, expecting to be perfect in everything you do and never making a mistake places a great deal of stress and pressure on you.

People with perfectionistic behavior tend to be rigid in their thinking, saying "I must be perfect or else I am a failure" and tend to put 100 percent of their effort into

---

Key Terms

intrapsychic stressors Our internal worries, self-criticisms, and negative self-talk.

procrastination A tendency to put off completing tasks until some later time, sometimes resulting in increased stress.

perfectionism A tendency to expect perfection in everything one does, with little tolerance for mistakes.

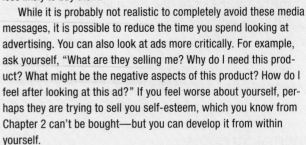

Building Media Literacy Skills

Advertisers May Be Selling You Stress

By age 18, the average American has watched television for 15,000 hours, viewed over 200,000 violent acts, and seen 350,000 commercials. As a result, media messages play a large role in our lives. Critics of the media contend that advertisers try to make us feel more anxious through media messages—in other words, they "sell anxiety" so that we feel pressured to buy their products to feel better, more confident, successful, popular, and happier. If we just were to try this diet, have this car, or meet the right person with this online service, we would feel less stressed and happier. In this way, watching television ads, and seeing ads on billboards, in magazines, and online, can create more stress in our lives. One study showed that when women looked at a women's magazine for 10 minutes, the majority of them felt more stressed, anxious, and depressed afterward than they did before looking at the magazine.

Advertisers are going to tell you the positive things about their products and not the negatives. For example, they portray cigarettes as helping to relieve stress, to manage your weight, and to feel more relaxed in social situations, but they neglect to tell you about the risk of cancer associated with smoking. Research shows that when people are exposed to the negative aspects of these products, they are less likely to buy them.

While it is probably not realistic to completely avoid these media messages, it is possible to reduce the time you spend looking at advertising. You can also look at ads more critically. For example, ask yourself, "What are they selling me? Why do I need this product? What might be the negative aspects of this product? How do I feel after looking at this ad?" If you feel worse about yourself, perhaps they are trying to sell you self-esteem, which you know from Chapter 2 can't be bought—but you can develop it from within yourself.

Sources: Maine M. *Body Wars.* Carlsbad, CA: Gurze Books, 2000; *Frontline.* Merchants of cool. November, 2005; Hersey J, Niederdeppe J, Evans W, Nonnemaker J, Holden D, Messeri P, Haviland M. The theory of "truth": How counterindustry media campaigns affect smoking behavior among teens. *Health Psychology,* 24(1), 22–31, 2005.

something or don't want to attempt it at all, which can lead to procrastination. In expecting perfection, there seems, to these individuals, to be a right and wrong way to do things. Thus, perfectionism can create a great deal of anxiety and distress.

Problems with Goal Setting and Time Management

With the rising cost of education, many students feel pressured to earn their degrees as quickly as possible, and this adds another layer of stress for them. Learning for the sake of learning can sometimes seem like a luxury because earning top grades to get into graduate programs and land well-paying jobs tends to take priority. Research shows that many students drop out of college because they don't know why they are in school, haven't found a direction or major, and feel pressured to either declare a major or quit. In addition, an overwhelming number of students identify time management as the reason for their academic success or failure. Setting priorities and goals, balancing academic life with your social life, and finding time for sleeping, eating, exercising, and working along with studying are essential aspects of managing your stress effectively; strategies will be discussed later in this chapter.

Job Stressors

Americans are spending more time at work than ever. In fact, the United States has overtaken Japan as the industrialized country with the longest working hours. Americans work 350 more hours per year than European workers.[7] What is the cost of these increased work hours? Less leisure time; less time for family, exercise, and sleep; less time for anything else but work! Seventy-five percent of workers stated that they experience job stress or burnout at work. Conflict with coworkers was the number-one source of job stress, followed by unrealistic work loads, tight deadlines, last-minute projects, and difficult bosses.

Many students are stressed about their future and possibility of finding a job once they graduate. Economic stress has recently become the most commonly experienced source of stress, and many students find that it is taking them an average of 18 months to find a job once they graduate from college. Money and the economy were at the top of the list of stressors for most Americans in a recent survey and have also been linked to an increase in irritability, anger, fatigue, insomnia, and unhealthy eating.[20] Students can also share their parents' stress as they face the possibility of losing their family home and not being able to afford to pay for college; this can place more financial burden on students to cover the cost of their college expenses.[21] Financial constraints may force people to find new ways to manage stress because they can't afford to take vacations, go out to eat, shop, go to the movies, or buy a new CD, book, or DVD as they did in the past.[22] One particular job, as a soldier in the military, has reported a tremendous increase in the number of people experiencing stress and stress-related illnesses.[23]

Environmental Stressors

Light, sounds, smells, air quality, and temperature can all affect your stress level. Some people feel more stressed if their environment is disorganized or messy and feel a

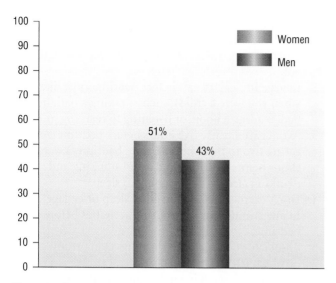

Figure 3-5 Stress and Gender 43 percent of men and 51 percent of women feel concerned about their level of stress.

Source: Only Half of Worried Americans Try to Manage Their Stress, *USA Today*, February 23, 2006.

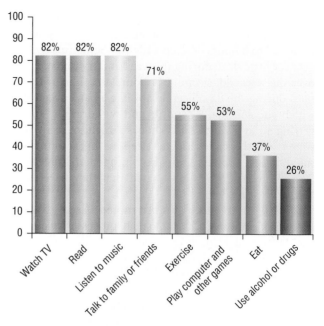

Figure 3-6 How Americans Cope with Stress People have different ways of coping with stress, such as watching TV, reading, listening to music, or playing video games. How do you cope with stress?

Source: Research Reveals Casual Games Provide Mental Balance, Stress Relief and Relaxation, www.realnetworks.com, August 14, 2006; Americans Reveal Top Stressors, How They Cope, Mental Health America, www.nmha.org, November 16, 2006.

need to clean it up before they can concentrate or relax. As you read in Chapter 2, the amount of light and type of lighting you are exposed to can affect your levels of stress and depression. Artificial light, as well as certain colors, can increase one's stress level. People tend to associate the color red with anger and hostility and blue with depression.[24] Stress has also been linked to being exposed to prolonged, daily noise such as in a factory, at a construction site, or in a crowded room.[25] Air that is too cold or too warm, or that contains mold or pollutants, can be a source of stress. Higher temperatures have been associated with an increase in violence and aggression and decreased concentration and productivity. Situations in which one does not have control over one's environment—such as being stuck in a traffic jam, in line, or in an elevator—can also be stressful. Your stress level might also increase if you don't have control over the noise, temperature level, or appearance of your environment.

Approaches to Stress Management

The research on how people cope with crisis and stress in their lives has shown that people tend to resolve problems within two weeks of experiencing a crisis. Because stress involves a disruption in equilibrium, and the body does not function well in a chronic state of unbalance, it is human nature to seek a way to alleviate the stress the body is experiencing and return to a steady state. As we discussed previously, our bodies cannot function for very long in a sustained fight or flight response without serious damage, and so a person will naturally strive to make changes to resolve the stress for survival (Figure 3-5).

However, the way that people resolve their problems and alleviate stress may be positive or negative.

A number of negative ways of dealing with stress are quite common and often quite harmful. As indicated in Figure 3-6, some people turn to alcohol and drugs to avoid their problems and numb their feelings, and cigarettes are also cited as a way of relieving stress. Many people use food to comfort themselves. Putting off distasteful tasks and avoiding stressful situations is another negative way of coping with stress. Some people use sleep as a way of escaping their problems, and certainly depression has been associated with not having the ability to effectively manage stress. In the next section, we discuss ways of effectively managing stress.

What are some positive, effective methods to cope with stress? Different strategies and methods for stress management involve the physical, social, environmental, and psychological aspects of stress. We will review techniques and strategies within each of these dimensions, and you will need to practice and experiment to find the stress-management techniques that are right for you.

Physical Aspects of Stress Management

The physical aspects of stress management involve meeting your basic needs of sleep, exercise, and nutrition as was discussed in Chapter 2 under Maslow's hierarchy of needs.[26]

Sleep As with eating, too much sleep or too little is also an ineffective way of managing stress. Most adults require 7 to 8 hours of sleep a night.[27] Sometimes people get very little sleep during the week and try to "catch up" over the weekend, sleeping 14 hours at a time or taking naps during the day. Sleep is not like a bank account in which you can make deposits and withdrawals, and so getting an average of 7 to 8 hours a night over a week's time is not the same thing as sleeping this amount each night. Sleep problems are becoming more prevalent; 70 million Americans also stated that they have problems with sleep.[28]

People also need uninterrupted sleep. Normal **circadian rhythms,** the biological processes related to the 24-hour light/dark cycle, are necessary for normal sleep and optimal daytime functioning. Our sleep patterns relate to these biological cycles, which also affect our patterns of hunger and eating, body temperature, and hormone release. These cycles must be in harmony for us to have a sense of well-being during our waking hours.[29] Sleep deprivation has been found to cause losses in higher cognitive processing tasks, decline in the performance of simple tasks, memory loss, and, with prolonged sleep deprivation, temporary psychosis, such as hallucinations and delirium.[8] Research also shows that sleeping too much can result in increased depression and decreased energy levels.

Not getting enough sleep has been related to increases in weight, depression, anxiety, cardiovascular disorders, and accidents. Problems with mood, memory, and concentration have also been linked to lack of sleep.

So how do you cope with sleep problems? Americans are turning to prescription medications in alarming numbers. The use of sleeping pills has doubled among 20- to 40-year-olds since 2000.[28] People are using more caffeine and energy drinks to wake up in the morning to compensate for morning grogginess due to hangover effects from sleep aids. Memory lapses, sleepwalking, and dependency have been associated with taking sleep medications. Sleeping pills can interfere with normal brain-wave activity during sleep and cause a rebound effect of increased insomnia when you discontinue taking them.

It is recommended that you develop healthy sleep habits so that you can get enough rest without sedatives and stimulants. Here are some tips for good sleep hygiene:

1. Establish a sleep routine. Go to bed every night at the same time and wake up at the same time every morning, regardless of how much sleep you actually got.
2. Engage in sleep rituals before bedtime (just like when you were a child), such as taking a bath before bed, reading a book, or listening to relaxing music.
3. Avoid caffeine use five hours before bedtime. Avoid eating two to three hours before bedtime. Decrease fluids before bedtime, and avoid smoking and drinking alcohol before going to sleep.
4. Don't exercise before you go to sleep or engage in any stimulating or arousing activities before bedtime.
5. Associate your bed with sleeping. Don't study, eat, or watch television in bed.
6. If you have been lying in bed for 20 minutes and haven't gone to sleep, get up and do something relaxing for 30 to 60 minutes and then try again. Keep getting out of bed after 20 minutes of no sleep and don't return to bed after your scheduled wake-up time.
7. Don't take naps during the day—this will interfere with your sleep schedule.
8. If you worry while in bed, keep a worry journal and write in it a few hours before bedtime to get these things out of your head and alleviate stress.

See the box "Alternatives for Stress Management" for more information on herbal and alternative therapies for insomnia.

Exercise Exercise is another physical aspect of stress management. Exercising aerobically at least three times a week for 20 to 30 minutes has been found to manage stress effectively for several reasons. First, exercising requires you to focus on your breathing and to breathe deeply, the key to stress management. By tensing and releasing the muscles through exercise, you are allowing your body to relax and unwind. Secondly, exercise can alleviate stress through the release of endorphins, naturally occurring chemicals in the brain. Endorphins help to counter stress, subdue pain, and increase pleasure, which is the reason people talk about the runner's high. Hitting a racquetball against the wall or playing basketball can be a great way to release the frustrations of the day and let go of tension and stress. Aerobic exercise includes walking briskly, running, bicycling, skating, and dancing. The benefits of exercise are further discussed in Chapter 4.

Nutrition In Chapter 5 you will learn about the nutrients that provide the necessary fuel the body needs to function. When people are stressed, they often skip meals or eat on the run. Since the fight or flight response requires more energy during stressful times than is normally

---

Key Terms

circadian rhythms The internal, biological clock that helps coordinate physiological processes with the 24-hour light/dark cycle.

needed, you must eat a balanced, nutritious diet. Without proper nutrition, the body will begin to break down its own tissues in an effort to obtain the energy required to survive. The immune system can then become compromised, making the body more susceptible to disease. It is not a coincidence that many people who are under a great deal of stress for prolonged periods of time become ill and that regaining their health takes longer than it does for those who are managing their stress well.

As we previously mentioned, people often use food to cope with stress and can overeat, typically eating high-sugar and high-fat foods such as chips, candy, and cookies. One study showed that women who were exposed to a high level of noise, similar to that made by a jackhammer, ate 65 to 70 grams of fat when offered snacks compared with women who were in a less stressful, quieter environment, who chose snacks with half as much fat. Eating too much or too little is not an effective way to manage stress and can eventually lead to serious health problems, such as obesity, eating disorders, diabetes, and hypertension.

Social Aspects of Stress Management

To manage stress effectively, you must also make time for fun and play. Like exercise, laughter increases the release of endorphins and requires you to breathe deeply, and so having humor in your life is an essential part of stress management.[30] Research has shown that stress can be related to having inadequate social interactions.[31] Hugging and human contact have also been demonstrated as having a significant effect in reducing the harmful physical effects of stress.[32] Participating in social activities such as social organizations, sports, or just talking with friends can give you the break you need to rest your

mind and focus on something other than work (see the box "The Fast-Growing Slow Movement").

Actually, you don't even have to have human contact to reduce stress—just owning a pet can make a difference. Studies have shown that just petting an animal produces calming effects such as lowered blood pressure and decreased heart rate. Cardiac patients who own pets tend to live much longer than do those who have no pets.[33]

Environmental Aspects of Stress Management

To effectively manage your stress, you need to take into consideration environmental stressors such as noise level, amount of light, and aesthetic quality of the space you inhabit. Natural light tends to elevate your mood.[24] Having plants or photos of friends and family around your living and work space can also alleviate stress.

Smell can also play a significant role in managing stress. As the saying goes, "Stop and smell the roses." Studies have shown that aromatherapy, using different aromas or odors therapeutically, can lower stress levels. When you breathe in the oils, they send a direct message to your brain via your olfactory nerves, where they can then affect the endocrine and the hormonal systems via the hypothalamus. Odors have an amazing effect on our emotional states because they hook into the emotional or primitive parts of our brains. Aromatherapy has been used to relieve pain, enhance relaxation and stress relief, loosen tense muscles, soften dry skin, and enhance immunity. So it is wise to pay attention to your aromatic surroundings because they may affect you much more than you realize.

While social interaction has been shown to have positive results on lessening the effects of stress, this beneficial effect depends on the type of friends with whom you

The Fast-Growing Slow Movement

Our culture has developed an increasing need for speed. We are a fast-paced society, encouraged to eat, work, play, and move faster and faster. Our addiction to speed makes us a slave to time. What is the first thing you look at in the morning when you wake up? The clock, of course. Time tells us what to do when, and how long we have to engage in that activity.

This pressure to do more in less time also causes stress in our lives. We can never be fast enough; there is never enough time. As Carrie Fisher once said, "Instant gratification takes too long." In order to beat the clock, we are consuming more caffeine and amphetamines and sleeping less. We are eating more fast food and gaining weight. We are working longer hours and taking less time to exercise, socialize, and enjoy leisure activities. The increase of road rage, relationship conflicts, and general lack of civility in our society has also been linked to our obsession with saving time. Time management and finding ways to do things more efficiently were originally intended to give us more leisure time and reduce the level of stress in our lives, but the opposite has occurred and we now pay a high price for speed.

There is a new, growing trend in the media called the "Slow movement." Books such as *In Praise of Slowness* discuss the merits of finding a balance in our lives and becoming more calm, careful, patient, and reflective

and developing real, meaningful connections with people. In fact, the author contends that slower can be better, as we can develop healthier relationships, work, and family life. We can have higher quality in our food, exercise, and other aspects of our lives if we take the time to do things well. Sometimes doing something more slowly can yield faster results, because doing things quickly can result in making mistakes and having to redo things.

We are beginning to see this trend in many facets of life. Yoga and meditation have become increasingly popular, as has the Slow Food movement. In the United States and around the world, some cities are becoming "slow cities"—which means these communities have made a commitment to create an environment that helps people slow down. The slow philosophy translates into city ordinances such as banning motorized vehicles from some streets, banning fast-food chains and neon signs, and lowering speed limits. These communities have speed bumps that read "Ready, Set, Relax," and they set aside days for "family focus night" with no school practices, no homework, and no meetings. October 24 has been designated "Take Back Your Time Day" in the United States, because by October 24 each year, Americans have worked as much as Europeans do all year.

How can you begin to break away from the cult of speediness? Here are some tips:

1. Don't overschedule yourself.
2. Don't multitask. Focus on one thing only.
3. Take time to play.
4. Do nothing. Just sit there.
5. Meditate or do yoga.
6. Make a meal from scratch.
7. Eat without watching television, reading, or doing anything else.
8. Walk and talk slower than you normally do.
9. Don't wear a watch.
10. Let someone else go before you in line.
11. Don't drink caffeinated beverages.
12. Sleep eight hours a night.

Test yourself to see how difficult it is for you to do these things. Do you have trouble relaxing and doing nothing? Are you suffering from time sickness? It is important to note that the Slow movement doesn't necessarily mean that we do everything at a snail's pace. Instead, it means finding a balance in our lives. There may be times when it is appropriate to act quickly, to be time oriented, or to multitask. The Slow movement suggests only that we take back control of our time and go at our own pace, instead of rushing around because that is what we are supposed to do.

Sources: Honore C, *In Praise of Slowness* (New York: HarperCollins, 2004); Worldwide, We Seem to Have Lost the Art of Doing Nothing, *USA Today*, May 16, 2006.

surround yourself. Spending time with negative, pessimistic people can increase your stress level rather than decrease it. It is more advantageous to surround yourself with positive, optimistic friends.[34] Feeling crowded in a room and not having enough personal space can also lead to an increase in stress.[35] Interestingly, it is not being in crowds itself but how familiar you are with the people, the activity that is taking place, and how much control you feel over your personal space that make the difference. In other words, being in a crowded room filled with your friends during a party feels subjectively different than feeling trapped in a crowded restaurant filled with strangers.

Other important aspects of managing stress in your environment include having meaningful work and challenging and interesting classes. Having work that is stimulating but not beyond your abilities helps to keep

your stress response at a moderate, optimal level for performance.

Psychological Aspects of Stress Management

Last, you can effectively cope with stress by using a variety of cognitive and psychological strategies. There are several different techniques, but as you will see, many are focused on deep breathing, which is the key to managing stress.

Relaxation and Deep Breathing The relaxation response, developed by Herbert Benson, M.D., is an effective way to ensure that you do not remain in the stress response too long. It is effective because it entails the opposite of the stress response. Rather than taking shallow breaths, you are required to breathe deeply, inhaling to a count of four and exhaling to a count of four while sitting in a comfortable position. As you breathe deeply, your muscles unwind and relax, again the opposite of the stress response. It is generally advised not to cross your legs or arms so that your muscles can relax easily. Blood flows to the extremities, and your heart rate slows. In fact, experienced users of this technique can temporarily lower their breathing rate from a typical rate of 14 to 18 breaths per minute to as few as 4 breaths per minute. Body temperature decreases, and blood pressure is lowered as well. The entire nervous system is slowed, in direct opposition to its role in the stress response. You are instructed to focus on your breathing and inner experience and become less aware of your external environment. To help tune out the outside world, you are instructed to close your eyes and let go of the worries and concerns of the day.[36]

To test this technique, take a moment to focus on your breathing and breathe in for a count of four and out for four. After doing so a few times, tighten your body, clench your hands, teeth, and jaw, close your eyes tightly, and pull your shoulders up while you are still breathing deeply. Are you able to do so? It is virtually impossible to tense your body and breathe deeply because they are mutually exclusive activities. Thus, the relaxation response is the foundation of most of the stress-management techniques described in this chapter. Deep breathing is the fundamental aspect of stress management.

Progressive Muscle Relaxation (PMR) In 1929 Edmund Jacobson, M.D., published a book describing a simple procedure of deliberately tensing and releasing major muscle groups in sequence from head to toe to achieve total relaxation of the body. His technique, called progressive muscle relaxation, still enjoys popularity.[37] By learning to recognize the difference between contracted and relaxed muscles, Jacobson believed that people would be able to have more of a sense of control over their bodies and the stress response. Progressive muscle relaxation enables you to intentionally put certain muscles into a controlled state of relaxation and reduce your overall stress level.

PMR is based on the use of positioning your body in a comfortable position, sitting or lying down, and concentrating on certain muscle groups. As you inhale, breathing in for a count of four, you contract your muscles starting with your forehead and count to four as you exhale and relax your muscles. Continue to clench and relax the muscles, using your breathing to help you to tighten and release, working your way down your body all the way to your feet and toes. Concentrate on the sensations of relaxation and how different they are from the feelings of tension and stress. Fifteen minutes, twice a day, is the recommended schedule. In one to two weeks,

you will have mastered the basics and will be aware of which muscles need more attention in order to relax. You will also be more sensitive to the buildup of tension in your body so that you will be able to decrease your stress level before it becomes overwhelming.[38]

Guided Imagery and Visualization In the early 1900s, Emil Coué, a French pharmacist, first suggested using human suggestibility to overcome the stress syndrome, to enhance recovery from illness, and to facilitate the accomplishment of positive goals.[39] By forming an image of a peaceful, serene place or seeing yourself being successful in accomplishing a task, you can use guided imagery or visualization to manage your stress. Guided imagery involves having someone describe a beautiful, relaxing scene while you focus on taking deep, comfortable breaths. While in a comfortable position, in an environment free from interruptions and distractions, you breathe deeply, relax your muscles, and imagine a pleasant scene. The imagery includes all the senses, not just what you see but pleasant smells, sounds, touch, and even taste. Guided imagery can be self-taught, or you can listen to recordings of narrated scripts.

Visualization is similar to guided imagery with the scene being more specifically focused on something you are about to do or want to accomplish, or on some performance or activity that may be causing you distress. Guided imagery and visualization techniques help you to change through positive mental images. For example, you might imagine yourself auditioning for a part in a play, seeing yourself go through your lines effortlessly and flawlessly, and feeling confident and proud of yourself. You are probably already skilled at visualization; unfortunately, we frequently engage in negative visualization and are unaware of doing so. For example, we imagine ourselves making fools of ourselves or making mistakes.

Athletes are trained in using positive visualization to improve their performance and visualize their goals.[38] Positive visualization has also been used in managing pain, especially in chronic pain management. This technique has also been effective in weight management, smoking cessation, insomnia, and for almost any type of behavior change. Some images commonly used to decrease stress are to visualize tightly twisted rope as uncoiling; hard, cold wax melting and softening; creaky hinges being oiled and becoming silent and gliding smoothly; or the feeling of sandpaper turning into silk. Again, guided imagery and visualization exercises have optimal benefit when practiced at least once a day, every day for 15 to 20 minutes.

Meditation Meditation allows the mind to transcend thought effortlessly when the person concentrates on a focal point. In transcendental meditation, a widely recognized approach to meditation, people repeat a mantra,

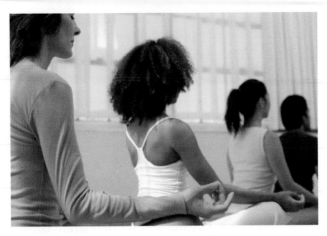
Meditation can reduce blood pressure and lower stress level.

or a personal word, while using deep-breathing and relaxation techniques. In other meditation approaches, alternative focal points are used to establish the depth of concentration needed to free the mind from conscious thought. Physical objects, music, and relaxing environmental sounds or breathing can be used as focal points. Meditation is also used in yoga. Students who meditated twice a day for 15 minutes reported lowered blood pressure and better class attendance rates, and felt less stressed during their classes.

Hypnosis Hypnosis is an artificially induced state, resembling, but physiologically distinct from, sleep. It involves a heightened state of suggestibility that creates flexible and intensified attention and receptiveness, and an increased responsiveness to an idea or to a set of ideas. The focus is on the unconscious rather than on the conscious state of mind, using deep-breathing and relaxation techniques. Hypnosis is perhaps the oldest and most misunderstood type of relaxation technique. It has been given a bad reputation by stage entertainers who use hypnosis to have unsuspecting audience members engage in embarrassing behavior.

Hypnosis is a natural state of mind that occurs spontaneously in nearly every person. It is a trancelike state, similar to those that you experience upon awakening, before falling asleep, or when you are engrossed in thought while performing other tasks—such as driving down a highway—on autopilot. It is possible to learn self-hypnosis from a trained professional or participate in hypnosis sessions with a qualified hypnotherapist.

Biofeedback The word *biofeedback* was coined in 1969 to describe procedures to teach people to alter brain activity, blood pressure, muscle tension, heart rate, and other bodily functions that are not normally controlled voluntarily. Biofeedback is a training technique in which people are taught to improve their health and performance by using signals from their own bodies. It operates on the premise that individuals can alter their involuntary responses by being "fed back" information either visually or audibly about what was occurring in their bodies. In addition, studies have shown that we have more control over so-called involuntary bodily functions than we once thought possible.

One commonly used device, for example, picks up electrical signals from the muscles and translates the signals into a form that people can detect. This device triggers a flashing light or activates a beeper every time muscles become more tense. To slow down the flashing or beeping, you need to relax tense muscles by breathing more slowly and deeply. People learn to associate sensations from the muscle with actual levels of tension and develop a new, healthy habit of keeping muscles only as tense as is necessary for as long as necessary. After treatment, individuals are then able to repeat this response at will without being attached to the sensors. Other biological functions that are commonly measured and used in a similar way to help people gain control are skin temperature, heart rate, sweat gland activity, and brain-wave activity. People can manage stress by decreasing the physiological components of the stress response.

Cognitive Aspects of Stress Management

Time Management Managing your time effectively can help you cope with your stress by feeling more in control, having a sense of accomplishment, and having a sense of purpose in your life. Establishing good time-management habits can take two to three weeks. By using specific systems, even the most disorganized persons can make their lives less chaotic and stressful.

Assess Your Habits The first step is to analyze how you are spending your time. What are your most productive and least productive times of day and night? Do you tend to underestimate how long something will take you to complete? Do you waste time or allow interruptions to take you off task? Carrying a notebook with you for a week and writing down how you spend your time might provide you with some insight into the answers to these questions and how you spend your time. You might find that you've been devoting most of your time to less important tasks. Perhaps it is tempting to do your laundry rather than to start writing that term paper, but this is probably not the best use of your time.

Use a Planner Keeping a daily planner to schedule your time is the next step in managing your time more effectively. First block off all of the activities that are consistent, regular, weekly activities, such as attending classes, eating meals, sleeping, going to meetings, exercising, and working. Then look at the open, available

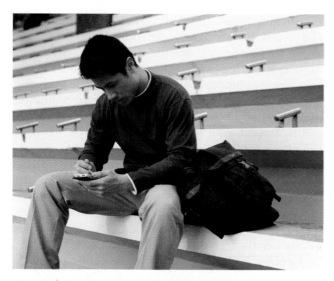

Use of a daily planner is a strategy that can help you manage your time more effectively as well as reduce your stress level.

time remaining. Schedule regular study time, relaxation time, and free time. Remember to schedule your study time during the more productive part of your waking hours. When you have a one-hour block of time, what can you realistically get done in that time? This could be a good time to review your notes from class, pay bills, or get some reading done.

Set Goals and Prioritize Set goals for the week as well as for each day. If something unexpected interferes with your time schedule, modify your plans but don't throw out the entire schedule.

Making a to-do list can be helpful, but it is only the first step. Breaking the large tasks into smaller, more manageable pieces and then prioritizing them is the key to effective time management. When you prioritize your tasks, try the ABC method of task management. The A tasks are those items that are most urgent and must be done today. Then the B tasks are those things that are important but, if need be, could wait 24 hours. The C tasks are activities that can easily wait a few days to a week. Don't fall into the C trap, which is when you do the less important tasks because they are quick and can be checked off your list with ease. This can lead to putting off the more important A activities, leaving them until you feel stressed and overwhelmed.

Stress Inoculation Working in a manner similar to a flu shot, stress inoculation involves exposing an individual to specific stressful situations, a little at a time, under controlled, safe conditions. Stress inoculation teaches individuals to relax using deep breathing and progressive muscle relaxation while they are being exposed to stressful situations.

The first step is to construct your personal list of stressful situations and arrange the list from the least to the most stressful items, and learn how to evoke each of these situations in your mind while at the same time focusing on your breathing and relaxing your muscles. The second step is to create an arsenal of stress-coping thoughts, such as "I'm going to be all right," "I've succeeded with this before," and "Getting started is the hardest part, then it will get easier for me." The third step is to practice this *in vivo*, meaning in real-life situations, while using the relaxation and cognitive techniques to minimize the stress response.[39] In addition to stress management, stress inoculation has also been helpful in anger management.

Cognitive Self-Talk What we tell ourselves, our self-talk, has a tremendous effect on how well we manage our stress. Stress can be generated from faulty conclusions, misinterpretations, and expecting the worst. Some people claim that if they expect the worst, they won't feel disappointed or hurt, but in reality, they still feel the pain from their disappointment. We need to be careful about what we expect because we may inadvertently make it happen, a phenomenon referred to as a **self-fulfilling prophecy.**[40]

Self-fulfilling prophecies can work for you or against you. If you expect that work will be boring and uninteresting, you will tend to portray a negative, unmotivated attitude and will probably have a miserable time. However, if you expect to enjoy yourself at work, you are more likely to go looking for challenge and to have fun.

If we look more closely at how we make faulty conclusions and misinterpretations, we recognize a number of cognitive distortions that lead to a more stress-filled life, such as:

1. *Filtering.* Selectively paying attention to the negative and disregarding the positive.
2. *Polarized thinking.* Putting things into absolute, all-or-nothing categories with no middle ground. For example, you have to be right or else you are wrong.
3. *Overgeneralization.* From one isolated event, you make a general, universal rule. For example, if you have failed once, you will always fail.
4. *Mind reading.* Without people saying so, you believe you know what people are feeling and the reasons

> **Key Terms**
>
> **self-fulfilling prophecy** The tendency to inadvertently make something more likely to happen as a result of one's own expectations and attitudes.

they behave the way they do. For example, if your friend seems tired, you think she doesn't really want to go out to the movies tonight as you had planned and so you cancel the plans thinking that is what she really wants.

5. *Catastrophizing.* Expecting disaster or the worst-case scenario.
6. *Personalization.* Thinking that things people do or say is in reaction to you and comparing yourself with others. For example, you walk past a group of people laughing and assume that they are laughing at you.
7. *Fallacy of fairness.* Feeling resentful when situations don't seem fair or just. Believing that good things happen to good people and bad things happen to bad people.
8. *Shoulds.* Telling yourself what you are supposed to do, what is expected of you, or what you feel obligated to do rather than what you want to do. This is often something we don't want to do but think we should do and feel somewhat pressured or forced to do.

To change these cognitive distortions, you need to generate some rebuttals to your negative self-statements. This entails finding middle ground between all-or-nothing thinking by asking yourself what evidence proves that a statement is true and identifying some exceptions to this statement. Look for balance by asking yourself what is the opposite of this negative self-statement. Rather than telling yourself what you "should" do, ask yourself what you "want" to do. Be specific instead of overgeneralizing, and avoid labeling yourself and others. Instead of telling yourself "I'm lazy," you might say, "I wish I would have studied a few more hours for that test." Stick to the facts without blaming yourself or others. Question yourself as to how you know something is true and if you might be making an assumption or "mind reading." Be mindful of your self-fulfilling prophecies. It may be wiser to acknowledge that you don't know or consider many different possible outcomes rather than to expect the worst.

Changing negative self-talk requires time, practice, and patience. We develop these patterns of thinking over years, and they become almost automatic. It takes concentrated effort to be aware of and change negative thinking. Remember that your rebuttals need to be strong, nonjudgmental, and specific. Practice developing more flexible and balanced thinking about people, behavior, and situations.

Conquering Procrastination   Some techniques for combating procrastination involve time management, stress management, assertiveness training, and increasing self-esteem and self-acceptance. Specifically with regard to time management, procrastinators tend to both over- and underestimate how much time a task will take. When they underestimate the time, they feel justified in procrastinating because they erroneously believe they have plenty of time to complete the task. When they overestimate the time needed, they feel intimidated by the magnitude of the job, feel anxious, and so have trouble getting started. So it is important to give yourself more time than you think you might need for a project and start earlier than needed in case of unforeseen delays. Breaking the task down into manageable pieces can also help it seem less daunting.

People also report procrastinating when they feel forced or pressured to do something they don't want to do. Rather than communicating assertively, they rebel by agreeing to do something but constantly put it off, which can be a passive-aggressive way of behaving. They fear the consequences of saying no or not fulfilling their obligations but are also angry about what they perceive as unfair expectations and demands on them. This is when some assertiveness training may be helpful. Finally, increasing self-esteem can solve problems with procrastination because feeling better about yourself relieves you of worrying about what others think of you and having constantly to prove yourself to them. Some people procrastinate because they think they need to do everything perfectly or not at all. With increased self-esteem, you are more accepting of mistakes and don't expect yourself to perform perfectly.

Combating Perfectionism   Perfectionism is the standard of holding yourself and others to do something 100 percent correct, with no errors or flaws. In the eyes of the perfectionist, there are also usually only two categories: perfect or flawed, success or failure, good or bad. This is an unrealistic perception because nothing is perfect. Having perfectionistic tendencies can create stress and conflict in relationships because people who interact with perfectionists feel as though nothing they do is good enough or will please that person.

To help alleviate the stress of perfectionism, base your self-esteem on who you are rather than on what you do. This involves accepting yourself and others unconditionally, including imperfections. Lowering your expectations of yourself and others and aiming for 80 percent rather than 100 percent is another strategy in battling perfectionism. Note what you are doing well and have accomplished rather than what is still left to do. Push yourself to take risks and allow yourself to make mistakes. It can be useful to make mistakes on purpose in order to get accustomed to this experience and realize that people still like and accept you and nothing bad will happen. Relaxation and stress-management techniques such as the ones described at the end of this chapter can also help alleviate the stress that comes with perfectionism. You might want to take the survey at the end of this chapter to assess your level of perfectionism.

As you can see, there are many different aspects to consider in managing stress, as well as its physical, social, environmental, and psychological components. As you think about how you can more effectively manage your stress level, you will need to practice and experiment to find the stress-management techniques most beneficial for you.

 TALKING POINTS Think back to stressful times in your life. What were some positive ways you coped, and what were some negative things you did to cope?

A Realistic Perspective on Stress and Life

The development of a realistic approach to today's fast-paced demanding lifestyle may best be achieved by fostering many of the following perspectives:[41]

Anticipate problems and see yourself as a problem solver. Although each specific problem is unique, it is most likely similar *to* past ones. Use these past experiences to quickly recognize ways of resolving new problems.

Search for solutions. Act on a partial solution, even when a complete solution seems distant. By resolving some aspects of a problem, you can gain time for more focused consideration of the remaining difficulties. In addition, some progress is a confidence builder that can help you remain committed to finding a complete solution.

Take control of your own future. Set out to accomplish your goals. Do not view yourself as a victim. Also, recall from Chapter 2 that being proactive and optimistic is an excellent way to take charge of your life and recognize capabilities that you were previously unaware of.

Be aware of self-fulfilling prophecies. Do not extend or generalize difficulties from one area into another. Further, negativity about yourself, in the form of self-doubt and self-blame, is certain to erode your feelings of success.

Visualize success. Focus on those things that are necessary and possible to ensure success. The very act

of "imaging," seeing oneself performing skillfully, has proven beneficial in a variety of performance-oriented activities.

Accept the unchangeable. Focus on taking control of what you can and letting go of the rest. The direction your life takes is only in part the result of your own doing. Cope as effectively as possible with those events over which you have no direct control; beyond a certain point, however, you must let go of those things over which you have little control.

Live each day well. Combine activity, contemplation, and a positive attitude approaching the many things that must be done each day. Celebrate special occasions. Undertake new experiences. Learn from your mistakes. Recognize your accomplishments. Most importantly, however, remember that the fabric of our lives is far more heavily influenced by day-to-day events than it is by the occasional milestones of life.

Act on your capacity for growth. Undertake new experiences and then extract from them new information about your own interests and capacities. The multiple dimensions of health identified in Chapter 1 will, over the course of your lifetime, provide a wide array of resources that will allow growth to occur throughout your entire life.

Allow for renewal. Make time for yourself, and take advantage of opportunities to pursue new and fulfilling relationships. Foster growth in each of the multiple dimensions of health—physical, psychological, social, intellectual, spiritual, and occupational. Initial renewal in one dimension may serve as a springboard for renewal in others.

Accept mistakes. Both you and others will make mistakes. Recognize that these can cause anger, and learn to avoid feelings of hostility. Mistakes, carefully evaluated, can serve as the basis for even greater knowledge and more likely success in those activities not yet undertaken.

Keep life simple. Keep the demands of life as orderly and manageable as you can. Just as adding too many appliances to an electrical circuit will quickly overload it and cause a power outage, excess demands and commitments added to our daily schedule can quickly burn out our psyches. Learning to prioritize and postpone activities is key to building a productive and enjoyable life.

Taking Charge of Your Health

- Complete the Student Stress Checklist at the end of this chapter.

- Determine if you suffer from perfectionism by completing the Perfectionism assessment at the end of this chapter.

- Join a yoga, meditation, or exercise class on campus or in the community.

- Assess your sleep hygiene and incorporate into your sleep habits some of the tips recommended in this chapter.

- Prioritize your daily goals in a list that you can accomplish, allowing time for recreational activities.

- Counteract a tendency to procrastinate by setting up imaginary (early) deadlines for assignments and rewarding yourself when you meet those dates.

- Replace a negative coping technique that you currently use, such as smoking, with an effective alternative, such as deep breathing, relaxation exercises, yoga, or exercise.

- List the positive aspects of your life, and make them the focus of your everyday thoughts.

SUMMARY

- Stress refers to physiological changes and responses your body makes in response to a situation, a real or a perceived threat.
- The fight or flight response is a physiological response to perceived, anticipated, or real threat; it causes the heart to race, breathing becomes labored, muscles are tense, the body sweats, and blood flow is decreased to the extremities and digestive organs and increased to the major muscles and brain.
- Chronic stress refers to remaining at a high level of physiological arousal too long and not being able to take immediate, effective action to alleviate the perceived or real threat.
- While too much stress can have a negative effect and cause some serious health problems, a moderate level of stress is positive and beneficial.
- Constant arousal and increased levels of adrenaline in your system will eventually wear down your body's immunological system. You will be less able to cope with stress, and so it takes less and less stress to cause a stress reaction.
- General Adaptation Syndrome is a sequenced physiological response to the presence of a stressor, involving the alarm, resistance, and exhaustion stages of the stress response.
- An overwhelming number of students identify time management as the reason for their academic success or failure. Setting priorities and goals and balancing academic life are essential aspects of managing your stress effectively.
- To effectively manage your stress, you need to take into consideration environmental stressors such as the noise level, amount of light, and aesthetic quality of the space you inhabit. It is also important to get adequate amounts of sleep, exercise, and nutrition.
- The relaxation response is effective because it entails the opposite of the stress response. Rather than taking shallow breaths, breathe deeply, inhaling to a count of four and exhaling to a count of four while sitting in a comfortable position.
- Effective psychological tools for stress management include progressive muscle relaxation, visualization, guided imagery, meditation, hypnosis, biofeedback, stress inoculation, cognitive self-talk, conquering procrastination, combating perfectionism, and setting realistic goals.

REVIEW QUESTIONS

1. What is stress?
2. How does stress relate to your physical and psychological health?
3. What is the fight or flight response?
4. What are some long-term physiological effects of chronic stress?
5. Describe the Yerkes-Dodson Law.
6. Explain the three stages of the General Adaptation Syndrome.
7. List at least five types of stressors students can experience.
8. List some environmental stressors, and explain how high levels of stress have been linked to environmental factors.
9. Describe the relaxation response and how it is effective for stress management.
10. Name seven cognitive and psychological stress-management techniques, and explain how they work.

ANSWERS TO THE "WHAT DO YOU KNOW?" QUIZ

1. False   2. True   3. True   4. True   5. True   6 False   7. True

Visit the Online Learning Center (**www.mhhe.com/payne11e**), where you will find tools to help you improve your grade including practice quizzes, key terms flashcards, audio chapter summaries for your MP3 player, and many other study aids.

SOURCE NOTES

1. Selye H. Stress *Without Distress*. New York: New American Library, 1975.
2. Scott LV, Dinan T. Vasopressin and the regulation of hypothalamic-pituitary-adrenal functions: Implications for the pathophysiology of depression. *Life Science*, 62(22), 1985–1998, 1998.
3. Selye H. *The Stress of Life*. New York: McGraw-Hill, 1984.
4. Girdano DA, Everly GS, Dusek DE. *Controlling Stress and Tension*. Boston: Allyn & Bacon, 1996.
5. Raber M, Dyck G. *Managing Stress for Mental Fitness*. Menlo Park, CA: Crisp, 1993.
6. Baucum D, Smith C, Kagan J. *Psychology: An Introduction* (9th ed.). Orlando, FL: Harcourt Brace Jovanovich, 2003.
7. Honore C. *In Praise of Slowness*. New York: HarperCollins, 2004.
8. Davis M, Eshelmar E, McKay M. *The Relaxation and Stress Reduction Workbook*. Oakland, CA: New Harbinger, 2000.
9. Robinson B. *Overdoing It. How to Slow Down and Take Care of Yourself*. Deerfield Beach, FL: Health Communications, 1992.
10. Holmes T, Rahe R. Social Readjustment Rating Scale. *Journal of Psychosomatic Research*, 11, 1967.
11. Rowh M. *Coping with Stress in College*. New York: College Board Publications, 1989.
12. Affordable Care for Kids Squeezes College Students. *Detroit News*, November 23, 2001.
13. Newman E. *No More Test Anxiety*. Los Angeles, CA: Learning Skills, 1996.
14. Lindzey G, Thompson R, Spring B. *Psychology* (3rd ed.). New York: Worth, 1988.
15. Arem C. *Conquering Math Anxiety: A Self-Help Workbook*. Pacific Grove, CA: Brooks/Cole, 1993.
16. Kahn N. *More Learning in Less Time*. Berkeley, CA: Ten Speed Press, 1992.
17. Roberts M. *Living Without Procrastination*. Oakland, CA: New Harbinger, 1995.
18. Ferrari J, Johnson J, McGown W. *Procrastination and Task Avoidance: Theory, Research and Treatment*. New York: Plenum, 1995.
19. Basco M. *Never Good Enough*. New York: Simon & Schuster, 1999.
20. Health Takes a Hit as Economy Creates More Stress. *USA Today*, October 7, 2008.
21. Financial Worries, Other Stresses Are Manifested Physically. *USA Today*, September 17, 2008.
22. Economic Pain Is a Nail Biter. *USA Today*, October 7, 2008.
23. Iraq Vets May Suffer Depression, Stress. *USA Today*, November 13, 2007.
24. Rosenthal NE. *Winter Blues*. New York: Guilford Press, 1998.
25. Goliszek AG. *Breaking the Stress Habit*. Winston-Salem, NC: Carolina Press, 1987.
26. Maslow AH. *Motivation and Personality* (2nd ed.). New York: Van Nostrand, 1970.
27. Ferber R. *Solve Your Child's Sleep Problems*. New York: Simon & Schuster, 1985.
28. Lack of Sleep Catches Up With Today's Workforce. *USA Today*, March 3, 2008.
29. Saladin KS. *Anatomy & Physiology: The Unity of Form and Function*. New York: McGraw-Hill, 2001.
30. Lefcourt HM, Martin RA. *Humor and Life Stress: Antidote to Adversity*. New York: Springer, 1986.
31. Asterita MF. *The Physiology of Stress*. 4–5. New York: Human Sciences Press, 1985.
32. Human Touch May Have Some Healing Properties. *USA Today*, September 29, 2008.
33. Allen K, Shykoff BE, Izzo JL Jr. Pet ownership but not ACE inhibitor therapy blunts home blood pressure responses to mental stress. *Hypertension*, October, 38(4), 815–820, 2001.
34. Seligman M. *Learned Optimism*. New York: Simon & Schuster, 1990.
35. Wade C, Tavris C. *Psychology*. New York: Harper & Row, 1987.
36. Benson H. *The Relaxation Response*. New York: Avon, 1976.
37. Jacobson E. *Progressive Relaxation*. Chicago: University of Chicago Press, 1942.
38. Fanning P. *Visualization for Change*. Oakland, CA: New Harbinger, 1988.
39. McKay M, Davis M, and Fanning P. *Thoughts and Feelings: The Art of Cognitive Stress Intervention*. Oakland, CA: New Harbinger, 1981.
40. Jones RA. *Self-Fulfilling Prophecies*. Hillsdale, NJ: Wiley, 1977.
41. McGinnis L. *The Power of Optimism*. New York: Harper & Row, 1990.

Personal Assessment

Student Stress Checklist

Put a check next to those stressors that apply to you.

Academic

_____ Difficulty managing time

_____ Deadlines

_____ Poor grades

_____ Competition

_____ Exams

_____ Pressure to do well (parents', own, and/or others' expectations)

_____ Study skills deficit

_____ Earned academic awards

_____ Completion of a big project

_____ Keeping scholarships

_____ Other

Interpersonal Relationships

_____ Too much or too little social activity

_____ Dating

_____ Conflict with others

_____ Few or no supportive relationships

_____ Long-distance relationship issues

_____ Sexual difficulties

_____ Beginning a new romantic relationship

_____ Negotiating relationships with professors

_____ Joining an organization

_____ Other

Personal

_____ Poor physical or psychological health

_____ Family difficulties

_____ Lack of social support

_____ Death of a loved one

_____ Financial problems

_____ Having a gay/lesbian/bisexual/transgendered identity

_____ Homesickness

_____ Change in eating or sleeping pattern

_____ Conflict in values

_____ Recent life changes (moved to a new location, new job, marriage, etc.)

_____ Becoming more independent

_____ Not belonging/fitting in

_____ Having a pet

_____ Holiday/semester breaks

_____ Dissatisfaction with appearance

_____ Peer pressure

_____ Difficulty controlling alcohol and/or drug use

_____ Other

Career

_____ Lack of career direction

_____ Unhappy with major

_____ Declaring a major

_____ Internship placement (e.g., student teaching)

_____ Graduation

_____ Other

Employment

_____ Difficulty with boss

_____ Unstable work hours

_____ Change in working conditions

_____ Job offer

_____ Promotion (more responsibility)

_____ Possible military deployment of self/friends/family

_____ Other

Environment

_____ Discrimination

_____ Unsatisfactory living environment

_____ Transportation difficulties

_____ Commuting

_____ Parking

_____ Other

_____ **Total Stressors Checked**

TO CARRY THIS FURTHER . . .

How well do you think you are managing your stress? (Make a mark on the continuum where you think you fit.)

0............. 1............. 2............. 3............ 4............. 5........... 6

Not at   Very
all   well

Keep in mind that two people with the same number of stressors may experience their stress differently. A person with a small number of stressors may feel overwhelmed by them, while a person with many stressors may feel they are manageable. As you consider the number of stressors in your life, it is important to recognize how well you manage them. Regardless of the number of stressors, if you are not managing your stress well, we encourage you to seek help in developing positive coping skills.

Personal Assessment

Am I a perfectionist?

Below are some ideas that are held by perfectionists. Which of these do you see in yourself? To help you decide, rate how strongly you agree with each of the statements below on a scale from 0 to 4.

0	1	2	3	4
I do not agree		I agree somewhat		I agree completely

_____ 1. I have an eye for details that others can miss.

_____ 2. I can get lost in details and forget the real purpose of the task.

_____ 3. I can get overwhelmed by too many details.

_____ 4. It stresses me when people do not want to do things the right way.

_____ 5. There is a right way and a wrong way to do most things.

_____ 6. I do not like my routine to be interrupted.

_____ 7. I expect a great deal from myself.

_____ 8. I expect no less of others than I expect of myself.

_____ 9. People should always do their best.

_____ 10. I am neat in my appearance.

_____ 11. Good grooming is important to me.

_____ 12. I do not like being seen before I have showered and dressed.

_____ 13. I do not like making mistakes.

_____ 14. Receiving criticism is horrible.

_____ 15. It is embarrassing to make mistakes in front of others.

_____ 16. Sharing my new ideas with others makes me anxious.

_____ 17. I worry that my ideas are not good enough.

_____ 18. I do not have a great deal of confidence in myself.

_____ 19. I'm uncomfortable when my environment is untidy or disorganized.

_____ 20. When things are disorganized, it is hard for me to concentrate.

_____ 21. What others think about my home is important to me.

_____ 22. I have trouble making difficult decisions.

_____ 23. I worry that I may make the wrong decision.

_____ 24. Making a bad decision can be disastrous.

_____ 25. I often do not trust others to do the job right.

_____ 26. I check the work of others to make certain it was done correctly.

_____ 27. If I can control the process, it will turn out fine.

_____ 28. I am a perfectionist.

_____ 29. I care more about doing a quality job than others do.

_____ 30. It's important to make a good impression.

_____ **TOTAL SCORE**

Scoring

Add all 30 items together to get your total score. If your score was less than 30, then you are probably not a perfectionist, although you may have a few of the traits. Scores from 31 to 60 suggest mild perfectionism. When you are stressed, your score may be higher. Scores of 61 to 90 suggest moderate perfectionism. This is probably means that perfectionism is causing you trouble in some specific areas, but is not out of control. Scores higher than 91 suggest a level of perfectionism that could cause you serious problems.

TO CARRY THIS FURTHER . . .

If you or a friend or family member scored in the moderate to high range for perfectionism, consider taking some of the steps described in this chapter for combating perfectionism. Allow yourself to take risks and make mistakes. General relaxation strategies can also be helpful in overcoming an unhealthy degree of perfectionism.

Source: Adapted with the permission of The Free Press, a Division of Simon & Schuster Adult Publishing Group, from *Never Good Enough: Freeing Yourself from the Chains of Perfection* by Monica Ramirez Basco, Ph.D. Copyright © 1999 by Monica Ramirez Basco. All rights reserved.

The Body

Part Two contains three chapters whose content is especially relevant to college students: fitness, nutrition, and weight management. This part will help you learn how to improve your health in these areas.

1. **Physical Dimension**
   Health experts believe that fitness, nutrition, and weight management are interrelated. How well our bodies work depends on what we eat and how we exercise. Healthy bodies allow us to participate in daily activities and recover more quickly from illness and injury.

2. **Psychological Dimension**
   When you start a fitness program or begin to pay attention to your diet, you learn about your level of motivation and commitment. You will be challenged, but the psychological rewards for your efforts, such as an improved self-concept and greater confidence, can be substantial.

3. **Social Dimension**
   The social dimension of health is closely related to fitness, nutrition, and weight management. Exercising with friends offers an opportunity for social interaction. Participation in most group fitness activities involves listening, sharing, and counseling. Food, like alcohol, can function as a "social lubricant" by bringing and holding people together. However, excessive food intake and lack of exercise can hinder social relationships when a person is significantly above his or her desirable weight.

4. **Intellectual Dimension**
   Some evidence suggests that people feel mentally sharper after they exercise. Many students report that they can study more efficiently after a workout. People deprived of adequate exercise and proper nutrition may suffer intellectual impairment. Regular physical activity, a sound diet, and effective weight management will allow you to enjoy a wide range of new experiences that can lead to improved intellectual functioning.

5. **Spiritual Dimension**
   Throughout this text we emphasize that an important part of your spiritual growth is serving others. Staying physically fit, following a healthful diet, and managing your weight can enhance your ability to serve others. You can express your own spirituality and help others find meaning in their lives when you take proper care of your health.

6. **Occupational Dimension**
   Just as you can better serve others when you feel your best, you can also pursue a career and carry out daily occupational tasks when you take care of your body. Some job functions, such as traveling and heavy lifting, require that you be in good physical condition. In addition, being fit can help you deal more effectively with the stress that inevitably accompanies employment. Taking care of your body can increase your self-esteem and improve your confidence—a definite plus when you are trying to land a job or earn a promotion.

Becoming Physically Fit

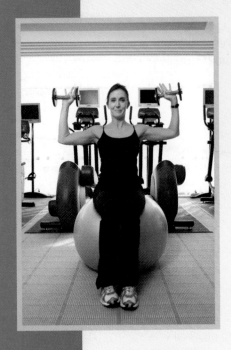

What Do You Know About Exercise and Physical Activity?

1. One of the benefits of endurance (aerobic) exercise training is that it improves both your good (HDL) and bad (LDL) cholesterol. True or False?

2. The old saying "Use It or Lose It" is correct when applied to exercise training. True or False?

3. You can estimate your maximal heart rate by subtracting your age from 200. True or False?

4. You will burn more calories in a typical aerobic exercise training session than you will in a typical resistance training session. True or False?

5. Exercise is a subcategory (that is, a specific type) of physical activity. True or False?

6. A person will obtain a greater improvement in aerobic fitness by exercising at higher intensity for a shorter duration compared with a more moderate intensity performed for a longer duration. True or False?

7. Muscle mass declines with age, beginning about age 50. True or False?

Check your answers at the end of the chapter.

For many people, the day begins early in the morning; continues with classes, assignments, study, a job, and/or recreational activities; and does not end until after midnight. This kind of pace demands that one be physically fit. Even a highly motivated college student must have a reasonably well conditioned body to maintain such a schedule.

Of course, many college students do not look at **physical fitness** as a means to a more satisfying, exciting life. Instead, many students look for the cosmetic benefits of fitness. They want to look in the mirror and see the kind of body they see in the media: one with well-toned muscles, a trim waistline, and an absence of flabby tissue, especially on the arms, legs, abdomen, and hips. Thus, many students become motivated to start exercise programs because they hope that they can build a better body. Through their efforts to do so, students usually start to feel better, physically and mentally. They realize that physical fitness can improve every aspect of their lives because they see it happening with each passing week.

Have you received mixed messages about how much exercise is necessary? Some reports tout that all you need to do is more general types of activities (raking leaves, walking the dog.) Others suggest that you can get benefits with multiple short walks throughout the day. And of course, you can go to the gym and hear that you have to feel the burn to make it worthwhile. So which message is correct? Surprisingly, all of them! It just depends on what your goal is.

Prior to the 1990s, fitness professionals recommended that you needed to exercise above certain minimal (of time, intensity, and frequency) levels to obtain fitness benefits. Their message was correct; however, many people believed that if they could not meet the minimums, they were obtaining no benefits. Thus, it was viewed as an all-or-none proposition.

In 1995 the American College of Sports Medicine (ACSM) and the Centers for Disease Control and Prevention (CDC) issued a public health statement on Physical Activity and Health. This report documented that there are clear benefits to 30 minutes a day of moderate-intensity physical activity and suggested that activities such as gardening and housework could be beneficial to health. Another important aspect of this report was

that the health benefits could be obtained by accumulating activity throughout the day (for example, three 10-minute bouts of activity: one in the morning, one in the afternoon, and one in the evening). Unfortunately, many individuals misunderstood this message and started suggesting that more vigorous forms of activity (exercise) were not really necessary and the term *exercise lite* was born.

What got confused was the difference between health benefits and fitness benefits. The Surgeon General's Report on Physical Activity and Health was issued in 1996 and helped clarify the message from the ACSM/CDC report. There are numerous health benefits to regular physical activity. Among these benefits are control of body weight, blood pressure, blood sugar, and cholesterol. The Surgeon General also operationalized the amount of activity required to obtain health benefits as 150 kilocalories per day. The report suggested that this could be achieved in a variety of ways (15 minutes of jogging, 30 minutes of walking, or 45 minutes of playing volleyball). Additionally, the report clarified that doing more than this amount would result in additional benefits. In other words, the more activity (dose), the greater the benefits (response).

In 2008, the U.S. Department of Health and Human Services released the first ever

federal policy on physical activity titled Physical Activity Guidelines for Americans. These guidelines provide the most up-to-date, research-supported recommendations about physical activity and health. The major summary points are that substantial health benefits can be derived by performing (1) at least 150 minutes per week of moderate-intensity physical activity, or (2) 75 minutes per week of vigorous-intensity physical activity, and (3) that additional and extensive health benefits can be derived by increasing to either 300 minutes per week of moderate-intensity activity or 150 minutes per week of vigorous-intensity physical activity. The guidelines also mention that an equivalent combination of moderate and vigorous physical activity can be used. More information about these guidelines can be found at the U.S. Department of Health and Human Services website: http://www.health.gov/PAguidelines/.

Because exercise is a form of physical activity, when one exercises regularly, one gets the same (or greater) health benefits as those who choose to just maintain a regularly active lifestyle. The bonus for those who exercise is that they will also derive physical fitness benefits from their program.

Fortunately, you need not become a full-time athlete to enjoy the health benefits of fitness (see the box "What Is Your Goal: Health or Fitness?"). Indeed, the Surgeon General has reported that significant health benefits can be achieved if you accumulate a moderate amount of **physical activity** on most, preferably all, days of each week.[1]

In the following sections, we discuss cardiorespiratory endurance, muscular strength, muscular endurance, flexibility, and body composition. These characteristics of physical fitness can be categorized as health-related physical fitness. Other characteristics, such as speed,

Five Components of Physical Fitness

People who engage in regular **exercise** often choose physical activities that fit their lifestyles and individual preferences. These activities have the potential for helping them achieve a state of physical fitness. Physical fitness is characterized by the ability to perform occupational and recreational activities without becoming unduly fatigued and to have the capacity to handle unforeseen emergencies.

Key Terms

physical fitness A set of attributes that people have or achieve that relates to the ability to perform physical activity.[2]

physical activity Any bodily movement produced by skeletal muscles that results in energy expenditure.[2]

exercise A subcategory of physical activity; it is planned, structured, repetitive, and purposive in the sense that an improvement or maintenance of physical fitness is an objective.[2]

---

power, agility, balance, and reaction time, are associated with what would be called performance-related physical fitness. Although the latter type is most important for competitive athletes, it is the former type that has the most relevance to the general population. Thus, this chapter focuses on health-related physical fitness.

Cardiorespiratory Endurance

If you were limited to improving only one area of your physical fitness, which would you choose—muscular strength, muscular endurance, or flexibility? Which would a dancer choose? Which would a marathon runner select? Which would an expert recommend?

The experts, exercise physiologists, would probably say that one other dimension is important for overall health. These research scientists regard improvement of heart, lung, and blood vessel function as the key focal point of a physical fitness program. **Cardiorespiratory endurance** forms the foundation for whole-body fitness. Cardiorespiratory endurance increases your capacity to sustain a given level of energy production for a prolonged period. Development of cardiorespiratory endurance helps your body to work longer and at greater levels of intensity.

Aerobic vs. Anaerobic Exercise Occasionally your body cannot continually produce the energy it needs for short-term activity. Certain activities require performance at a level of intensity that outstrips your cardiorespiratory system's ability to transport oxygen efficiently to contracting muscle fibers.

This oxygen-deprived form of energy production is called **anaerobic** (without oxygen) **energy production,** the type that fuels many intense, short-duration activities. For example, rope climbing, weight lifting for strength, and sprinting are short-duration activities that quickly cause muscle fatigue; they are generally considered anaerobic activities. The key factor is if the energy demand of the activity exceeds the aerobic energy production capability. Thus, even activities that typically are considered to be aerobic (walking or cycling) can require anaerobic energy if the intensity is high.

If you usually work or play at low intensity but for a long duration, you have developed an ability to maintain **aerobic** (with oxygen) **energy production.** As long as your body can meet its energy demands in this oxygen-rich mode, it will not convert to anaerobic energy production. Thus fatigue will not be an important factor in determining whether you can continue to participate. Marathon runners, serious joggers, distance swimmers, bicyclists, and aerobic dancers can perform because of their highly developed aerobic fitness. The cardiorespiratory systems of these aerobically fit people have developed a large capacity to take in, transport, and use oxygen.

Benefits of Cardiorespiratory Endurance Following a program of regular aerobic exercise improves the capacity of your cardiovascular and muscular systems. More specifically, regular aerobic exercise strengthens the muscles of your heart, enabling your heart to pump more blood with fewer strokes to meet the demands you place on it. As a result, your resting heart rate may become slower than in the past, indicating that you have become more physically fit. At the same time, your skeletal muscles develop improved metabolic machinery to allow them to use more oxygen and thus produce more energy. This cardiorespiratory endurance (also called cardiorespiratory fitness or aerobic fitness) enables you to deal more easily with the routine and extraordinary demands of your daily life.

In addition, improving your cardiorespiratory (aerobic) fitness has a variety of benefits that can improve nearly all parts of your life.[3] Aerobic fitness can help you gain the following physical benefits:

- Control of your weight
- Greater ability to perform a wide variety of activities throughout your life
- Ability to ward off infections
- Increased efficiency of your other body systems
- Reduced concentration of triglycerides and increased concentration of high-density lipoproteins ("good cholesterol") in your blood
- Reduced risk of heart disease and certain types of cancer (breast and colon)
- Increased capillary network
- Prevention of hypertension, type 2 diabetes, and osteoporosis
- Increased longevity
- Improved psychological health
- For women, reduced number and severity of symptoms associated with premenstrual syndrome (PMS); see Chapter 14 for more information.

Aerobic fitness also offers a variety of other benefits that, although not immediately obvious, are no less important. For example, the increased stamina that comes with cardiorespiratory fitness enables you to complete and better enjoy your daily activities. In addition, your improved fitness level may reduce the severity and shorten the duration of common illnesses. Likewise, you will find your ability to cope with stressors to be increased with your fitness level. As a result, you may find your sense of well-being and confidence to be improved (see the box "Harnessing the Spirit").

Older adults will find that improving their cardiorespiratory fitness enables them to enjoy their later years to a greater extent, giving them the energy and ability to participate in activities that they might have delayed

Harnessing the Spirit: The Saga of Lance Armstrong

In the summer of 1999, American cyclist Lance Armstrong made one of the most amazing sports comebacks in history. Armstrong won the Tour de France, the most grueling cycling event in the world. In October 1996, Armstrong had been diagnosed with advanced testicular cancer and was given less than a 50 percent chance of survival. At the time of the diagnosis, the cancer had already spread to Armstrong's abdomen, lungs, and brain.

After being diagnosed with cancer, but before starting aggressive therapy, Armstrong declared himself "a cancer survivor, not a cancer victim." He convinced himself, his family, and his medical support team that he could beat the long odds facing him. He even established the Lance Armstrong Foundation (www.laf.org) before he had surgery and chemotherapy. He battled through his therapy without giving up the hope that the cancer would be defeated.

Miraculously, Armstrong's cancer disappeared. He then stunned the cycling world by returning to active training and planning a comeback that included competing for the 1999 Tour de France title. As Armstrong's physical condition improved and his training regimen

became more demanding, cycling enthusiasts believed that Armstrong might be able to compete in—but certainly not win—the world's most famous bike race.

Armstrong proved his doubters wrong by winning the 1999 Tour de France. Perhaps even more amazingly, he has won the Tour de France *again* in the years 2000, 2001, 2002, 2003, 2004, and 2005, and he participated on the U.S. Olympic Cycling Team at the Sydney Olympics in 2000, winning a bronze medal in the Men's Individual Time Trial event. Armstrong chronicled his battle with testicular cancer in his best-selling book *It's Not About the Bike* (Putnam) and followed this with a cycling training book called *The Lance Armstrong Performance Program* (Rodale Press). His powers of the mind and spirit worked to help him overcome his physical barriers. His success story has undoubtedly inspired others to take charge of their lives by doing their best to rise above mental and physical barriers to pursue the dreams that sometimes seem impossible.

for many years, such as traveling, or even activities they might never have considered, such as joining a square dance club or learning how to line dance.

When you become aerobically fit, you may be able to achieve a long-held goal, such as hiking part of the Appalachian Trail, climbing Mt. Rainier, or bicycling through Europe. Others might find that becoming physically fit reduces their dependence on substances such as alcohol, cigarettes, or other drugs and that they sleep more soundly.

Finally, while you are pursuing your physical fitness activities, you probably will meet other healthy, active people and find that you are expanding your circle of friends. The box "A Different Kind of Fitness" takes a look at the physical and social benefits for persons with disabilities who participate in the Special Olympics.

Muscular Strength and Muscular Endurance

Muscular fitness is the term used to represent the capabilities of the skeletal muscles to perform contractions. The capacity of the muscles has two distinct yet integrated characteristics: **muscular strength** and **muscular endurance.** The strength of the muscle is related to its ability to perform at or near its maximum for a short period of time. The endurance of the muscle is related to its ability to perform at submaximal levels for a long period of time.

Both muscular strength and muscular endurance are essential for your body to accomplish work. Your ability

Key Terms

cardiorespiratory endurance The ability of the heart, lungs, and blood vessels to process and transport oxygen required by muscle cells so that they can contract over a period of time; cardiorespiratory endurance is produced by exercise that requires continuous, repetitive movements.

anaerobic energy production The body's alternative means of energy production, used when the available oxygen is insufficient for aerobic energy production; anaerobic energy production is a much less efficient use of stored energy.

aerobic energy production The body's primary means of energy production, used when the respiratory and the circulatory systems can process and transport sufficient oxygen to muscle cells to convert fuel to energy.

muscular fitness The ability of skeletal muscles to perform contractions; includes muscular strength and muscular endurance.

muscular strength The component of physical fitness that deals with the ability to contract skeletal muscles to a maximal level; the maximal force that a muscle can exert.

muscular endurance The aspect of muscular fitness that deals with the ability of a muscle or muscle group to repeatedly contract over a long period of time.

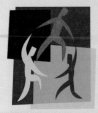

Learning from Our Diversity

A Different Kind of Fitness: Developmentally Disabled Athletes Are Always Winners in the Special Olympics

In America, as in many other countries around the world, physical fitness and athletic prowess carry a high degree of prestige, whereas lack of conditioning and poor sports performance often draw scorn and rejection. As anyone knows who's ever been picked last when sides were being chosen for a schoolyard game, few things are more damaging to youthful self-esteem than being the player nobody wants.

Some of these children blossom into accomplished athletes as they gain coordination or are inspired and guided by caring coaches. Others, lacking strong interest in sports, turn to less physical arenas in which they can excel—drama, debating, music, computers, science.

But what about people who want to be athletes at almost any cost but who have no realistic hope of attaining the standards of athletic accomplishment set for those in top physical condition? The Joseph P. Kennedy Foundation created an arena in which these athletes could compete when it established the Special Olympics in 1968. Joseph Kennedy was the father of President John F. Kennedy, whose older sister Rosemary was virtually shut away from the world when her family discovered she was mentally retarded. Many people at that time shared the Kennedys' view that the kindest way to treat family members who were developmentally disabled was to "protect" them from stares and whispers by keeping them at home or placing them in institutions or residential facilities. Spearheaded by President Kennedy's sister Eunice Kennedy Shriver, the Special Olympics was intended to change the old attitudes toward developmentally disabled people by giving them an opportunity to compete at their own level and to celebrate their victories publicly.

Now, over 40 years later, the Special Olympics holds both winter and summer games and boasts participation of more than 1 million developmentally disabled athletes in 140 countries around the world. The 2007 Special Olympics World Summer Games will be held in Shanghai, China.

The contests are open to athletes between the ages of 8 and 63, some of whom have proved wrong the specialists who claimed they would never walk, let alone compete internationally. "Mainstream" Olympic champions such as figure-skating silver medalist Brian Orser and a host of well-known entertainers have attended opening-day ceremonies to cheer and inspire the special athletes.

But medals aren't what the Special Olympics is all about. No matter where a Special Olympian finishes in a contest, he or she is applauded and celebrated for the accomplishment of playing the game and seeing it through. The oath taken by each participant in the Special Olympics aptly states the credo of this remarkable group of athletes: "Let me win. But if I cannot win, let me be brave in the attempt."

In what ways other than physical conditioning do you think a developmentally disabled person might benefit from participating in the Special Olympics? What can the rest of us learn from these athletes' courage and perseverance?

---

to maintain good posture, walk, lift, push, and pull are familiar examples of the constant demands you make on your muscles to maintain or increase their level of contraction. The stronger you are, the greater your ability to contract muscles and maintain a level of contraction sufficient to complete tasks.

Benefits of Muscular Fitness Training People who regularly perform muscular fitness exercises obtain a variety of benefits. Strength training will improve body composition, both by maintaining or increasing muscle mass and possibly by lowering body fat. Muscular fitness exercises reduce body fat largely by raising the person's resting metabolic rate, which is directly related to the amount of muscle mass a person has. Such exercises also promote improved clearance of glucose from the blood. Impaired glucose clearance can lead to diabetes.

Key Terms

flexibility The ability of joints to function through an intended range of motion.

It is also well known that people with good levels of muscular fitness can perform a variety of activities of daily living (ADLs), such as carrying a bag of groceries with more ease. These functional benefits of muscular fitness become even more important as people age. Regular resistance training can help improve balance and may increase bone mass. Thus, it may help prevent falls in the elderly, which often result in bone fractures leading to disability.

Flexibility

The ability of your joints to move through their natural range of motion is a measure of your **flexibility.** This fitness trait, like so many other aspects of structure and function, differs from joint to joint within your body and among different people. Not every joint in your body is equally flexible (by design), and, over the course of time, use or disuse will alter the flexibility of a given joint. Certainly gender, age, genetically determined body build, and current level of physical fitness affect your flexibility.

One's inability to move easily during physical activity can be a constant reminder that aging and inactivity

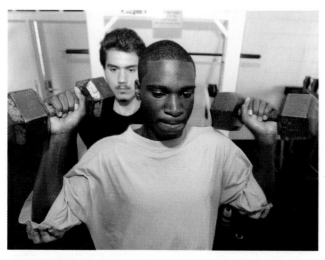

Muscular fitness training has both functional and health benefits. People with good muscular fitness can perform daily tasks more easily and enjoy more recreational activities. Muscular fitness training can also improve body composition.

are the foes of flexibility. Failure to use joints regularly will result in a loss of elasticity in the connective tissue and shortening of muscles associated with the joints. Benefits of flexibility include improved balance, posture, and athletic performance and reduced risk of low-back pain and injury.

Body Composition

Body composition refers to the different components the body is made up of (muscle, bone, fat, water, minerals).[4] Of particular interest to fitness experts are percentages of body fat and fat-free weight. Health experts are especially concerned about the large number of people in American society who are obese and with the loss of muscle as one ages. Cardiorespiratory fitness trainers increasingly are recognizing the importance of body composition and are including strength-training exercises. (See Chapter 6 for further information about body composition, health effects of obesity, and weight management.)

 TALKING POINTS Which benefits of exercise are most important to you? What would motivate you to become and stay active?

Developing a Personalized Fitness Program

Principles of Training

A personalized exercise program should meet both the needs and the preferences of the individual. The best exercise program is the one that the person will perform

regularly. However, there are a number of principles of training that need to be followed for the program to be successful.

The most basic of all the principles of exercise training is *overload*. The objective of exercise is to improve something in the body (such as heart function). To obtain this improvement, the body must be placed under a stress to make it work harder than it is usually accustomed to. When a body part or system is overloaded in an appropriate manner, that body part undergoes adaptation, increasing the capability of that body part.

A second important principle of training is *specificity*. To produce an adaptation, the exercise must be specific to the outcome that is targeted for improvement. A good example of this can be seen by considering two different types of strength training, isometric and isotonic. Over time, persons who regularly perform isometric exercises will increase their capacity to perform an isometric contraction (they will be able to generate more muscular force without lengthening their muscle); however, their ability to perform muscular contractions throughout the full range of motion will not be improved significantly. In contrast, people who prefer isotonic exercises will increase their ability to perform the muscular contraction throughout the full range of motion.

A third important principle of training is *reversibility* (sometimes referred to as regression). This is basically what is meant by the old saying "Use It or Lose It." In order for people to maintain the benefits of exercise, they must perform the exercise on a regular basis. Specific details of how to train will be discussed in the following sections.

Cardiorespiratory Endurance

For people of all ages, cardiorespiratory conditioning can be achieved through many activities. As long as the activity you choose places sufficient demand on the heart and lungs, improved fitness is possible. In addition to engaging in the familiar activities of swimming, running, cycling, and aerobic dance, many people today participate in brisk walking, rollerblading, cross-country skiing, swimnastics, skating, rowing, and even weight training (often combined with some form of aerobic activity). Regardless of age or physical limitations, you can select from a variety of enjoyable activities that will condition the cardiorespiratory system. (Complete the Personal Assessment at the end of this chapter to determine your level of fitness.)

Many people think that any kind of physical activity will produce cardiorespiratory fitness. Often people consider golf, bowling, hunting, fishing, and archery to be forms of exercise. If performed regularly and for sufficient periods of time, they may enhance your health. However, they do not meet the requirements to be called exercise and would not necessarily improve physical fitness.

The American College of Sports Medicine (ACSM), the nation's premier professional organization of exercise physiologists and sport physicians,[5] has well-accepted guidelines for exercise training.

The ACSM's most recent recommendations for cardiorespiratory conditioning were published in 2009.[6] The four major factors that are important for cardiorespiratory training are (1) mode of activity, (2) frequency, (3) intensity, and (4) duration. The ACSM has also made recommendations for muscular fitness and flexibility training. We summarize these recommendations. You may wish to compare your existing fitness program with these standards. Some have used the acronym FITT to help them remember the four factors. F represents frequency, I represents intensity, T represents time (duration), and T represents type (mode).

Mode of Activity   The ACSM recommends that the mode of activity be any continuous physical activity that uses large muscle groups and can be rhythmic and aerobic in nature. Among the activities that generally meet this requirement are continuous swimming, cycling, aerobics, basketball, cross-country skiing, rollerblading, step training (bench aerobics), hiking, walking, rowing, stair climbing, dancing, and running. Water exercise (water or aqua aerobics) has become a popular fitness mode because it is especially effective for pregnant women and older, injured, or disabled people.[7]

Endurance games and activities, such as tennis, basketball, racquetball, and handball, are fine as long as you and your partner are skilled enough to keep the ball in play; walking after the ball will do very little for you. Softball and football are generally less than sufficient continuous activities—especially the way they are played by weekend athletes. An old coaching adage applies here: You get in shape to play the game, you do not play the game to get in shape. In other words, using recreational sports is not an effective method to develop physical fitness; however, it may be a useful (and enjoyable) way to maintain fitness.

Regardless of which continuous activity you select, it should also be enjoyable. Running, for example, is not for everyone—despite what some accomplished runners say! Find an activity you enjoy. If you need others around you to have a good time, corral a group of friends to join you.

Cross-training is the use of more than one aerobic activity to achieve cardiorespiratory fitness. For example, runners may use swimming, cycling, or rowing periodically to replace running in their training routines. Cross-training allows certain muscle groups to rest and injuries to heal. In addition, cross-training provides a refreshing change of pace for the participant.

Vary your activities to keep from becoming bored. You might cycle in the summer, run in the fall, swim in the winter, and play racquetball in the spring.

Frequency of Training   **Frequency** of training refers to the number of times per week a person should exercise. The ACSM recommends three (at vigorous intensity) to five (at moderate intensity) times per week. For most people, participation in fitness activities more than five times each week does not significantly further improve their level of conditioning. Likewise, an average of only two workouts each week does not seem to produce a measurable improvement in cardiorespiratory conditioning. Thus, although you may have a lot of fun cycling twice each week, do not expect to see a significant improvement in your cardiorespiratory fitness level.

Intensity of Training   How much effort should you put into an activity? Should you run quickly, jog slowly, or swim at a comfortable pace? Must a person sweat profusely to become fit? These questions all refer to **intensity** of effort.

The ACSM recommends that healthy adults exercise at an intensity level of between 64 percent and 91 percent of their maximum heart rate, which is estimated by subtracting one's age from 220. However, be aware that there could be a considerable difference between estimated maximal heart rate and actual maximal heart rate (measured during a maximal exercise test). Or, one should exercise at an intensity level between 40 percent and 85 percent of one's heart rate range. This level of intensity is called the **target heart rate (THR)** (see the box "How to Calculate Your Target Heart Rate"). This rate refers to the minimum number of times your heart needs to contract (beat) each minute to have a positive effect on your heart, muscles, and blood vessels. This intensity produces a *training effect*. Activity at an intensity below the THR will be insufficient to make a significant improvement in your fitness level. Although intensity below the THR will still help you expend calories and thus lose weight, it will probably do little to make you more aerobically fit. However, intensity that is significantly above your THR will probably cause you to become so fatigued that you will be forced to stop the activity before the training effect can be achieved.

Choosing a particular THR depends on your initial level of cardiorespiratory fitness. If you are already in relatively good physical shape, you might feel comfortable starting exercise at 70 percent of your heart rate range. A well-conditioned person needs to select a higher THR for his or her intensity level, whereas a person with a low cardiorespiratory fitness level will still be able to achieve a training effect at a lower THR of 40 percent of heart rate range.

In the example in the box, the younger person would need to participate in a continuous activity for an extended period while working at a THR of 158 beats per minute. The older person would need to function at a THR of 150 beats per minute to achieve a positive training effect.

Determining your heart rate is not a complicated procedure. Find a location on your body where an artery passes near the surface of the skin. Pulse rates are difficult to determine by touching veins; the blood pressure is lower in veins than in arteries, making it more difficult to feel a pulse. Two easily accessible sites for determining heart rate are the carotid artery (one on each side of the windpipe at the front of your neck) and the radial artery (on the inside of your wrist, just above the base of the thumb).

Practice placing the front surface of your index and middle fingertips at one of these locations and feeling for a pulse. Once you have found a regular pulse, look at the second hand of a watch. Count the number of beats you feel in a 15-second period. Multiply this number by 4. This number is your heart rate. With a little practice, you can become proficient at determining heart rate.

Duration of Training   The ACSM recommends that the **duration** of training be between 20 and 90 minutes of continuous aerobic activity. Generally speaking, the duration can be on the shorter end of this range for people whose activities use a high intensity of training (75 percent to 85 percent of heart rate range). Those who choose activities with a low range of intensity (50 percent to 60 percent of heart rate range) should maintain that activity for a longer time. Thus a fast jog and a moderate

walk require different amounts of time to accomplish the training effect. The fast jog might be maintained for 25 minutes, whereas the brisk walk should be kept up longer—perhaps for 50 minutes. The bottom line is to achieve what the ACSM calls an adequate volume (total amount) of exercise. The ACSM recommends that individuals should expend between 1,000 and 2,000 kilocalories per week in aerobic exercises to obtain a cardiorespiratory training effect. This total volume can be achieved in a variety of ways. For example, some people may choose to exercise at a moderate intensity (50 percent to 60 percent of heart rate range) for a longer duration (40 minutes per session) and higher frequency (5 days per week), whereas others can get similar benefits by choosing higher intensity (75 percent to 80 percent of heart rate range) with a shorter duration (30 minutes per session) and lower frequency (4 days per week). Volumes of 2,000 to 3,500 kilocalories per week will result in greater health and fitness benefits.

Muscular Fitness

Recognizing that overall body fitness includes muscular fitness, the ACSM now recommends resistance training in its current standards. Some individuals are hesitant to perform resistance training because of a belief that muscle cells will turn into fat cells if they stop training. However, muscle cells are physiologically incapable of turning into fat cells. The ACSM suggests participation in resistance training two or three times a week. This training should help develop and maintain a healthy body composition—one with an emphasis on lean body mass. The goal of resistance training is not to improve cardiorespiratory endurance but to improve overall muscle strength and muscular endurance. For some people (individuals with hypertension or type 2 diabetes), resistance training with heavy weights is not recommended because it can induce a sudden and dangerous increase in blood pressure.

Key Terms

frequency   The number of exercise sessions per week; for aerobic fitness, three to five days are recommended.

intensity   The level of effort put into an activity; for aerobic fitness, 40 to 85 percent of heart rate range is recommended.

target heart rate (THR)   The number of times per minute the heart must contract to produce a cardiorespiratory training effect.

duration   The length of exercise time of each training session; for aerobic fitness, 20 to 60 minutes per session is recommended.

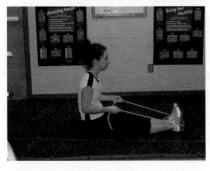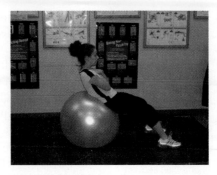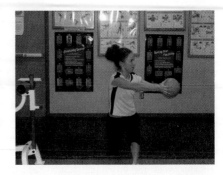

Many types of inexpensive accessory equipment are available for muscular fitness training, including resistance bands (left), stability balls (center), and weighted "medicine" balls (right).

Muscular strength can best be improved by training activities that use the **overload principle.** By overloading, or gradually increasing the resistance (load, object, or weight) your muscles must move, you can increase your muscular strength. The following three types of training exercises are based on the overload principle.

Types of Muscular Fitness Exercises   Muscular endurance can be improved by performing repeated contractions of a less than maximal level. This aspect of muscular fitness is most related to common physical activities (leaf raking, pushing a lawn mower). Although it is not as glamorous as muscular strength, muscular endurance is an important part of muscular fitness.

Key Terms

overload principle   The principle whereby a person increases the resistance load to levels above which he or she is normally accustomed to; this principle also applies to other types of fitness training.

isometric exercises   (**eye** so **met** rick) Muscular strength training exercises in which the resistance is so great that the object cannot be moved.

isotonic resistance exercises   Muscular strength training exercises in which traditional barbells and dumbbells with fixed resistances are used.

isokinetic exercises   (**eye** so kin **e** tick) Muscular strength training exercises in which machines are used to provide variable resistances throughout the full range of motion at a fixed speed.

static stretching   The slow lengthening of a muscle group to an extended stretch, followed by a holding of the extended position for 15 to 60 seconds.

ballistic stretching   A "bouncing" form of stretching in which a muscle group is lengthened repetitively to produce multiple quick, forceful stretches.

In **isometric** (meaning "same length") **exercises,** the resistance is so great that the contracting muscles cannot move the resistant object at all. For example, you could contract your muscles against an immovable object such as a wall. Because of the difficulty of precisely evaluating the training effects, isometric exercises are not usually used as a primary means of developing muscular strength and can be dangerous for people with hypertension.

Isotonic resistance exercises, also called *same-tension exercises,* are currently the most popular type of strength-building exercises and include the use of traditional free weights (dumbbells and barbells), as well as many resistance exercise machines. People who perform progressive resistance exercises use various muscle groups to move (or lift) specific fixed resistances or weights. Although during a given repetitive exercise the weight remains the same, the muscular contraction effort required varies according to the joint angles in the range of motion.[4] The greatest effort is required at one angle (sticking point) in the range of motion of the movement.

Isokinetic (meaning "same speed") **exercises** use mechanical devices that provide resistances that consistently overload muscles throughout the entire range of motion. The resistance moves only at a preset speed regardless of the force applied to it. For the exercise to be effective, a user must apply maximal force. Isokinetic training requires elaborate, expensive equipment. Thus the use of isokinetic equipment may be limited to certain athletic teams, diagnostic centers, or rehabilitation clinics. The most common isokinetic machines are Cybex, Mini-Gym, ExerGenie, KinCom, and Biodex.

Free Weights or Machines?   Which type of strength-building exercise (machines or free weights) is most effective? Take your choice, since all will help develop muscular strength. Some people prefer machines because they are simple to use, do not require stacking the weights, and are already balanced and less likely to drop and cause injury. Other people prefer free weights because they encourage the user to work harder to maintain balance during the lift. In addition, free weights can be used in a greater variety of exercises than can weight machines.

Accessory Equipment   What about other types of equipment? There are many types of equipment that can be used for strength training. Some types may focus on one part of the body (such as the abdominal muscles), while others also train additional skills, such as balance. Here are just a few of the many available types of accessory equipment:

- *Resistance tubes and bands* come in different levels of resistance and are useful for training a variety of muscle groups in movement patterns that mimic everyday activities. They are small and lightweight, making them easy to store and ideal for taking along on a trip.
- *Stability balls* come in different sizes and are useful for training the core muscle groups (principally the abdominal and back muscles).
- *Inflatable exercise discs* can be used to train both strength and balance.
- *Weighted exercise ("medicine") balls* come in different weights and are useful both for training the upper body muscles and as an added source of resistance when doing abdominal exercises. Throwing and catching the balls can also assist in balance training.
- *Abdominal isolation devices* come in a variety of different styles and are useful for training the abdominal muscles.
- *Hard foam rollers* come in different sizes and are useful for training the core muscle groups, for balance, and for therapeutic relief for some forms of muscular tension.

Talk with an exercise professional to learn what pieces of equipment might work best for you and how to properly use the equipment. The good news is that many of these exercise accessories are inexpensive enough to purchase for use at home.

Frequency, Intensity, and Duration   The resistance training recommended by the ACSM includes two to four sets of 8 to 12 repetitions (10 to 15 repetitions for individuals over age 50) of 8 to 10 different exercises performed two or three times per week. Although any weight that produces an overload will result in improvement, the greatest muscular fitness gains will be achieved if the weight lifting results in fatigue of the muscle (that is, more than 12 repetitions cannot be performed). These exercises should be geared to the body's major muscle groups (for example, legs, arms, shoulders, trunk, and back) and should not focus on just one or two body areas (Figure 4-1). Isotonic (progressive resistance) or isokinetic exercises are recommended. For the average person, resistance training activities should be done at a moderate-to-slow speed, use the full range of motion, and not impair normal breathing. With just two sets recommended for each exercise, resistance training is not very time consuming.

Flexibility Training

To develop and maintain a healthy range of motion for the body's joints, the ACSM suggests that flexibility exercises be included in one's overall fitness program. Stretching can be done in conjunction with other (cardiorespiratory or muscular fitness) training or can be performed separately. Note that if flexibility training is done separately, a general warm-up should be performed before stretching so that the muscles are warm before they are stretched.

Types of Stretching Exercises   Flexibility can be developed through static stretching, which involves the slow lengthening of a muscle group, or through ballistic stretching, which involves repetitive and forceful bouncing movements. Athletic trainers generally prefer static stretching for people who wish to improve their range of motion, because ballistic stretching carries a higher risk of soft-tissue tears and injury (however, conclusive research evidence for this is lacking). For most people, static stretching is the best type.

Frequency, Intensity, and Duration   The ACSM recommends that a flexibility program include stretches for all the major muscle and/or tendon groups. Stretching exercises should be performed at least three days per week, but stretching is an activity that can be safely performed daily. Each stretch should extend to a position where you feel mild discomfort in the muscle. Slowly extend each stretch and then hold the extended position for 15 to 60 seconds. Repeat each stretch at least three to four times per training session.

Take the following precautions to reduce the possibility of injury during stretching:

- Warm up using a slow jog or fast walk before stretching.
- Stretch only to the point at which you feel tightness or resistance to your stretching. Stretching should not be painful.
- Be sure to continue normal breathing during a stretch. Do not hold your breath.
- Use caution when stretching muscles that surround painful joints. Pain is an indication that something is wrong—it should not be ignored.

Training Considerations for Body Composition

When training to improve body composition, the goal is to increase muscle (and possibly bone) mass, decrease body fat, or a combination of both. Training to maintain

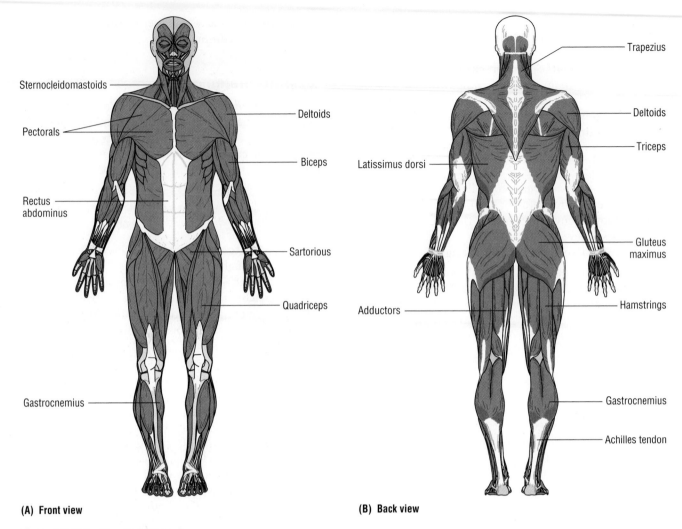

(A) Front view

Sternocleidomastoids

Pectorals

Rectus abdominus

Gastrocnemius

Deltoids

Biceps

Sartorious

Quadriceps

(B) Back view

Trapezius

Deltoids

Triceps

Latissimus dorsi

Gluteus maximus

Adductors

Hamstrings

Gastrocnemius

Achilles tendon

Figure 4-1 Major Muscle Groups

or increase muscle mass was covered earlier in this chapter in the discussion of muscular fitness. It is important to recognize that muscle mass declines with age, beginning sometime after age 35. This loss of muscle mass is called **sarcopenia.** Thus, strength training to maintain the amount and the quality of muscle is a recommended component of adult exercise programs.

The most common exercise goal related to body composition is to lose body fat. To achieve this, the exercise program should seek to maximize the caloric expenditure. Aerobic exercise activities are the best to produce relatively high rates of energy expenditure for a prolonged

period of time. The ACSM recommends that an exercise session should produce an energy expenditure of 300 to 400 kilocalories. Any combination of duration and intensity is suitable, as long as the total caloric expenditure target is achieved. Frequency should be most, if not all, days of the week.

Overtraining

The human body is an amazing piece of equipment. It functions well regardless of whether you are conscious of its processes. It also delivers clear signals when something goes wrong. You should monitor any sign that seems abnormal during or after your exercise. "Listen to your body" is a good rule for self-awareness.

However, danger signs are extremely unusual. Fear of developing these difficulties should not deter you from starting a fitness program. These risks are minimal—and the benefits far outweigh the risks. Sports injuries are discussed later in this chapter.

> **Key Terms**
>
> **sarcopenia** A reduction in the size of the muscle fibers, related to the aging process.

The Workout Routine

A training session consists of three basic parts: the warm-up, the conditioning phase, and the cooldown.[6]

Warm-Up The warm-up should last 5 to 10 minutes. During this period, you should begin slow, gradual, comfortable movements related to the upcoming activity, such as walking or slow jogging. If the upcoming activity requires specific types of movement, some range of motion exercises mimicking those movements are beneficial. All body segments and muscle groups should be exercised as you gradually increase your heart rate. Near the end of the warm-up period, the major muscle groups should be stretched. This preparation helps protect you from muscle strains and joint sprains.

The warm-up is a fine time to socialize. Furthermore, you can mentally prepare yourself for your activity or think about the beauty of the morning sky, the changing colors of the leaves, or the friends you will meet later in the day. Mental warm-ups can be as beneficial for you psychologically as physical warm-ups are physiologically.

Conditioning The second part of the training session is the conditioning phase, the part of the session that involves improving muscular fitness, cardiorespiratory endurance, and flexibility. Workouts can be tailor-made, but they should follow the ACSM guidelines discussed previously in this chapter (Table 4.1).

Cooldown The third important part of each fitness session is the cooldown. Ideally, one should not abruptly stop exercise as this could cause circulatory problems (insufficient blood returning to the heart). The cooldown consists of a 5- to 10-minute session of relaxing exercises, such as slow jogging, walking, and stretching. Note, this is the ideal time for flexibility training, since the muscles and joints are warmed from the conditioning phase. This activity allows your body to cool and return to a resting state. A cooldown period helps reduce muscle soreness.

Exercise over the Life Span

Regardless of age, exercise provides health and fitness benefits. However, there are modifications to the exercise recommendations that are age-specific.

Children's Physical Activity

Major research studies published during the last 10 years have indicated that U.S. children and teenagers lead very sedentary lives. Children ages 6 to 17 score extremely poorly in the areas of strength, flexibility, and cardiorespiratory endurance. In many cases, parents are in better shape than their children are. A major consequence of these sedentary habits in children is obesity. The 2006 health report from the Centers for Disease Control and the National Center for Health Statistics indicates that 17 percent of children and adolescents ages 6 to 19 years are overweight. Indeed, from National Health and Nutrition Examination Survey (NHANES) NHANES II (1976–80) to NHANES III (1988–1994), the prevalence of overweight nearly doubled among children and adolescents and has continued to rise. The seriousness of these data is revealed by the fact that most obese children become obese adults.

Table 4.1 Summary of Exercise Training Recommendations for Each Component of Physical Fitness

	Cardiorespiratory Endurance	Muscular Strength	Muscular Endurance	Flexibility	Body Composition
Mode	Any using large muscle groups in a rhythmic pattern	Free weights, machines, resistive devices	Free weights, machines, resistive devices	Static is recommended	Aerobic for fat loss and strength for muscle mass gains
Intensity	64–91% HR_{max} or 40–85% HRR	Amount of weight that can be moved only 12–15 times without rest	Less than maximal	To point of mild to moderate discomfort	Specific to mode of training
Duration	150 minutes per week (moderate intensity); 75 minutes per week (vigorous intensity)	2–4 sets of 8–10 using major muscle groups	2–4 sets of 10–15 using major muscle groups	≥ 4 repetitions of 15–60 seconds each, for all major joints	300–450 minutes per week
Frequency	3–5 days per week	2–3 days per week	3–5 days per week	2–3 days per week	5–7 days per week

Note: HR_{max} = maximum heart rate; HRR = heart rate range.
Source: Adapted from American College of Sports Medicine.

This situation presents a challenge to educators and parents to emphasize the need for strenuous play activity. Television watching and parental inactivity were implicated as major factors in these studies. The National Center for Chronic Disease Prevention and Health Promotion recommends that children and teenagers get at least 60 minutes per day of moderate-intensity physical activity.[8] Furthermore, they advise that part of this should be of moderate-to-vigorous intensity, 20 or more minutes per session, on 3 or more days per week.

Exercise and Aging

With aging, physical decline occurs and the components of physical fitness become more difficult to maintain. From the fourth decade onward, a gradual decline in vigor and resistance eventually gives way to various types of illnesses. In the opinion of many authorities, people do not die of old age. Rather, old age worsens specific conditions responsible for death. However, physical decline can be slowed, and the onset of illness delayed, by staying physically active. The process of aging can be described on the basis of predictable occurrences,[9] as follows:

- *Change is gradual.* In aging, gradual changes occur in body structure or function before specific health problems are identified.
- *Individual differences occur.* When two people of the same age are compared for the type and the extent of change that has occurred with age, important differences can be noted. Even within the same person, different systems decline at differing rates and to varying extents.
- *Greatest change is noted in areas of complex function.* In physiological processes involving two or more major body systems, the most profound effects of physiological aging can be noted.
- *Homeostatic decline occurs with age.* Becoming older is associated with a growing difficulty in maintaining homeostasis (the dynamic balance among body systems). In the face of stressors, the older adult's system takes longer to respond, does not respond with the same magnitude, and may take longer to return to baseline.

Like growth and development, aging is predictable yet unique for each person.

Exercise for "30-Somethings"

People who are in their 30s need to make few, if any, significant adjustments in their fitness programs. Men and women can continue physical activities they have used since their 20s—the key word being *continue*. Unfortunately, many "30-somethings" have developed sedentary habits and have suffered the consequences of gaining excess body fat and acquiring cardiac risk factors (such as high blood pressure). It is important for these individuals either to increase their activity gradually, say by walking more each day, or to seek the assistance of an exercise professional to guide them through the first one to three months of a new exercise program. See the box "Overcoming Barriers to Being Regularly Active" for ideas on how to get started on an exercise program.

Those 30-somethings who feel mired in activities that now seem boring might try a new activity. However, any new activity (or increase in the intensity of a current activity) should be undertaken gradually.

Exercise for Older Adults

Health Concerns The body experiences a number of changes as a person ages. Some of these changes are accelerated or magnified for those whose lifestyle does not include regular physical activity.

Changes in Midlife Adults The period between 45 and 64 years of age brings with it a variety of subtle changes in the body's structure and function. When life is busy and the mind is active, these changes are generally not evident. Even when they become evident, they are not usually the source of profound concern. Nevertheless, older students in your class and people with whom you work could be experiencing these changes:[9]

- Decrease in bone mass and density
- Increase in vertebral compression
- Degenerative changes in joint cartilage
- Increase in adipose tissue; loss of lean body mass

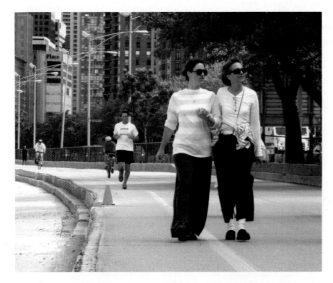

Choosing activities that are safe, convenient, and enjoyable can help people maintain an exercise program throughout the life span.

- Decrease in capacity to engage in physical work
- Decrease in visual acuity
- Decrease in resting energy requirements
- Decrease in fertility
- Decrease in sexual function

For some midlife adults these health concerns can be quite threatening, especially for those who view aging with apprehension and fear. Some middle-aged people reject these physical changes and convince themselves they are sick. Indeed, hypochondriasis is much more common among midlife people than among young people.

Changes in Older Adults In older people, it is frequently difficult to distinguish between changes caused by aging and those caused by disease. For virtually every body system, biomedical indexes for the old and young can overlap. In the respiratory system, for example, the cardiorespiratory endurance of a man of 70 may be no different from that of a man of 55 who has a history of heavy cigarette smoking. Is the level in the older man to be considered an indicator of a disease, or should it be considered a reflection of normal old age? In dealing with older adults, physicians frequently must make this kind of distinction.

In older people, as in midlife people, structural and physiological changes are routinely seen. In some cases, these are closely related to disease processes, but in most

cases they reflect the gradual decline that is thought to be a result of the normal aging process. The most frequently seen changes include the following:

- Further decrease in bone mass, resulting in changes in the structure of bone
- Decrease in muscle bulk and strength
- Decrease in cardiorespiratory endurance
- Loss of nonreproducing cells in the nervous system
- Decrease in hearing and vision abilities
- Decrease in all other sensory modalities, including the sense of body positioning
- Slower reaction time
- Gait and posture changes resulting from a weakening of the muscles of the trunk and legs

In addition to these changes, the most likely change seen in older adults is the increased sensitivity of the body's homeostatic mechanism. Because of this sensitivity, a minor infection or superficial injury can be traumatic enough to decrease the body's ability to maintain its internal balance. An illness that would be easily controlled in a young person could even prove fatal to a seemingly healthy 75-year-old person.

Continuing to follow a physical fitness plan throughout midlife and older adulthood is essential to minimizing age-related health problems. The plan should be modified as necessary to accommodate changes in physical functioning.

Safe Exercise Programs   An exercise program designed for younger adults may be inappropriate for older people, particularly those over age 50. Special attention must be paid to matching the program to the interests and abilities of the participants. Often, this is best achieved by having older individuals begin their exercise program under the supervision of a certified exercise professional. The goals of the program should include both social interaction and physical conditioning.

Older adults, especially those with a personal or family history of heart problems, should have a physical examination before starting a fitness program. This examination should include an evaluation of all the physiological systems of the body, especially the cardiovascular, respiratory, and musculoskeletal. Ideally, the evaluation should also include a maximal exercise test (a "stress" test). Participants should learn how to monitor their own cardiorespiratory status during exercise.

Well-designed fitness programs for older adults will include activities that begin slowly, are monitored frequently, and are geared to the enjoyment of the participants.[10] The professional staff coordinating the program should be familiar with the signs of distress (excessively elevated heart rate, nausea, breathing difficulty, pallor, and pain) and must be able to perform CPR and use an automated external defibrillator (AED). Warm-up and cooldown periods should be included. Activities to increase flexibility are beneficial in the beginning and ending segments of the program. Participants should wear comfortable clothing and appropriate shoes, and they should be mentally prepared to enjoy the activities.

A program designed for older adults will largely conform to the ACSM criteria specified previously in this chapter, including both cardiorespiratory and muscular fitness training. Certainly, specific modifications or restrictions to the exercise program may be required due to health concerns of the individual. For example, because of possible joint, muscular, or skeletal problems, certain activities may have to be done in a sitting position. Pain or discomfort should be reported immediately to the fitness instructor.

Fortunately, properly screened older adults will rarely have health emergencies during a well-monitored fitness program. Many fit older adults can also safely exercise alone.

Special Health Concerns

Low-Back Pain

A common occurrence among adults is the sudden onset of low-back pain. Four out of five adults develop this condition at least once in their lifetime, which can be so uncomfortable that they miss work, lose sleep, and generally feel incapable of engaging in daily activities. Many of the adults who have this condition will experience these effects two to three times per year.

Although low-back pain can reflect serious health problems, most low-back pain is caused by mechanical (postural) problems. As unpleasant as low-back pain is, the symptoms and functional limitations usually subside within a week or two. The services of a physician, physical therapist, or chiropractor are generally not required.

By engaging in regular exercise, such as swimming, walking, and bicycling, and by paying attention to your back during bending, lifting, and sitting, you can minimize the occurrence of this uncomfortable and incapacitating condition. Many commercial fitness centers and campus recreational programs are starting to offer specific exercises geared to muscular improvement in the lower back and abdominal areas.

Female Athlete Triad

In the early 1990s, the ACSM identified a three-part syndrome of disordered eating, **amenorrhea** (lack of menstruation), and osteoporosis as the female athlete triad.[11] The conditions of this syndrome appear independently in many women, but among female athletes they appear together. The female athlete triad is most likely to be found in athletes whose sport activities emphasize appearance (for example, diving, ice skating, or gymnastics) and can also be observed in women who become compulsive exercisers.

Parents, coaches, athletic trainers, teammates, and friends should be watchful for signs of the female athlete triad. This syndrome has associated medical risks, including inadequate fuel supply for activities, inadequate iron intake, reduced cognitive function, altered hormone levels, reduced mental health, early onset of menopause, increased likelihood of skeletal trauma, altered blood fat profiles, and increased vulnerability to heart disease.[11] Vitally important is an early referral to a physician who is knowledgeable about the female athlete triad. The physician will likely coordinate efforts with a psychologist, a nutritionist, and an athletic trainer to improve the health of the athlete and prevent recurrences.

Pregnancy

Pregnant women should continue to exercise.[12] During pregnancy a woman's entire body undergoes many physical changes. Muscles are stretched, joints are loosened, and tissues are subjected to stress. If a woman is in good physiological condition, she is more likely to handle these changes with few complications. The baby may also benefit. Studies have shown that women who exercise moderately during pregnancy tend to give birth to healthier babies.[13]

Some reports suggest that exercise during pregnancy can make delivery of the baby easier and faster. Exercise can also help control the woman's weight gain and improve her balance during pregnancy, and make it easier to get back to normal weight after delivery.

The types of exercises a woman should perform during pregnancy depend on the individual and the stage of pregnancy.[6] Most pregnant women should perform general exercises that increase overall fitness and stamina, as well as exercises that strengthen specific muscle groups. Muscles of the pelvic floor, for example, should be exercised regularly because these muscles will be supporting most of the extra weight of the baby.

A variety of exercises are appropriate, including walking, swimming, stretching, and strengthening exercises. Yoga and tai chi are also good forms of exercise for pregnant women. The muscles of the pelvic floor, abdomen, and back are especially subject to stress and strain during pregnancy and delivery, so certain exercises can also be performed to strengthen these muscles. Exercises can also be performed to speed up recovery after delivery. Such postpartum exercises can be started in some cases within 24 hours after delivery. Exercises can even be started before conception if a pregnancy is anticipated.

Some types of exercise can put the fetus at risk. A pregnant woman should avoid any activity in which she becomes overheated, because her elevated body temperature will warm up the fetal environment. Thus pregnant women should not use saunas or hot tubs, nor should they exercise in a hot, humid environment. During the last trimester of pregnancy, women should also avoid any strenuous or high-impact exercise that involves bouncing, jumping, or jarring motions. Pregnant women should first consult with their obstetricians to develop a safe, productive exercise routine.

Osteoporosis

Osteoporosis is a condition frequently seen in older middle-aged women. However, it is not fully understood why menopausal women are so susceptible to the increase in calcium loss that leads to fractures of the hip, wrist, and vertebral column. Approximately 80 percent of the 10 million people with osteoporosis are women. An additional 34 million people have low bone mass. Estimates from the National Osteoporosis Foundation are that half of women and one in four men over age 50 will have an osteoporosis-related fracture in their lifetime.[14]

The endocrine system plays a large role in the development of osteoporosis. At the time of menopause, a woman's ovaries begin a rapid decrease in the production of estrogen, one of two main hormones associated with the menstrual cycle. This lower level of estrogen may decrease the conversion of the precursors of vitamin D into the active

form of vitamin D, the form necessary for absorbing calcium from the digestive tract. As a result, calcium may be drawn from the bones for use elsewhere in the body.

Additional explanations of osteoporosis focus on two other possibilities—hyperparathyroidism (another endocrine dysfunction) and the below-average degree of muscle development seen in osteoporotic women. In the latter case the reduced muscle mass is associated with decreased activity, which in turn deprives the body of the mechanical stimulation needed to facilitate bone growth.

An important fact to know is that 85 to 90 percent of one's peak bone mass is obtained by age 20. Thus, it is essential to encourage lifestyle habits that promote bone building in youth. Premenopausal women have the opportunity to build and maintain a healthy skeleton through an appropriate intake of calcium. Depending on age, current recommendations are for an intake of 1,000 to 1,300 mg of calcium per day. Three to four daily servings of low-fat dairy products should provide sufficient calcium. The diet also must contain adequate vitamin D because it aids in the absorption of calcium.

Many women do not consume an adequate amount of calcium. Calcium supplements, again in combination with vitamin D, can be used to achieve recommended calcium levels. It is now known that calcium carbonate, a much-advertised form of calcium, is no more easily absorbed by the body than are other forms of calcium salts. Consumers of calcium supplements should compare brands to determine which, if any, they should buy.

In premenopausal women, calcium deposition in bone is facilitated by exercise, particularly exercise that involves movement of the extremities. Today, women are encouraged to consume at least the recommended servings from the milk group and engage in regular physical activity that involves the weight-bearing muscles of the legs, such as aerobics, jogging, and walking.

Postmenopausal women who are not elderly can markedly slow the resorption of calcium from their bones through the use of estrogen-replacement therapy. When combined with a daily intake of 1,500 mg of calcium, vitamin D, and regular exercise, estrogen therapy almost eliminates calcium loss. Of course, women need to work closely with their physicians to monitor the use of estrogen because of continuing concern over the role of estrogen-replacement therapy in the development of breast cancer and the increased risk of coronary heart disease events and stroke.

Key Terms

amenorrhea The absence of menstruation.

osteoporosis Decrease in bone mass that leads to increased incidence of fractures, primarily in postmenopausal women.

Osteoarthritis

Arthritis is an umbrella term for more than 100 forms of joint inflammation. The most common form is osteoarthritis. It is likely that as we age, all of us will develop **osteoarthritis** to some degree. Often called "wear and tear" arthritis, osteoarthritis occurs primarily in the weight-bearing joints of the knee, hip, and spine. In this form of arthritis, joint damage can occur to bone ends, cartilaginous cushions, and related structures as the years of constant friction and stress accumulate.

The object of current management of osteoarthritis (and other forms) is not to cure the disease but rather to reduce discomfort, slow the progression of the disease, and maintain or improve function in daily activities.[15] Analgesics and nonsteroidal anti-inflammatory agents are the medications most frequently used to treat osteoarthritis.

It is now believed that osteoarthritis develops most commonly in people with a genetic predisposition for excessive damage to the weight-bearing joints. Thus the condition seems to run in families. Further, studies comparing the occurrence of osteoarthritis in those who exercise and those who do not demonstrate that regular movement may decrease the likelihood of developing this form of arthritis.

Fitness Questions and Answers

Along with the major components of your fitness program, you should think about many additional issues when you start a fitness program.

Should I See My Doctor Before I Get Started?

First it is highly desirable to have regular checkups as part of your overall health plan. However, the Surgeon General has suggested that most adults can safely increase their activity level to a moderate amount without the need for a comprehensive medical evaluation.[1] Individuals with chronic diseases should consult with their physician before increasing their activity level.

If vigorous forms of exercise are desired, then a medical exam is recommended for men over 44 and women over 54. It is also recommended for individuals with more than one risk factor for coronary artery disease or with any other notable health problems. The American College of Sports Medicine also recommends an exercise ("stress") test for these individuals.[6]

> **Key Terms**
>
> **osteoarthritis** Arthritis that develops with age; largely caused by weight bearing and deterioration of the joints.

What Causes a "Runner's High"?

During or after exercise, a person occasionally experiences feelings of euphoria. Runners and joggers call these feelings the "runner's high." However, these positive feelings of relaxation, high self-esteem, and reduced stress are not limited to runners. Almost any fitness activity can leave participants with these intense positive feelings. Swimmers, aerobic exercisers, hikers, and cyclists all have reported exercise-induced highs.

Although these pleasurable feelings can be attributed in part to psychological causes, there is plenty of scientific evidence to suggest a physiological cause. During physical activity, the brain releases its own morphinelike (opiate-like) substances called *endorphins*. These chemicals are released by brain neurons and produce sensations that are pleasurable, and sometimes even numbing. Exercisers report that these episodes of euphoria are unpredictable. Sometimes they experience highs and sometimes they do not. However, endorphin highs are more likely to occur during or after a strenuous, challenging workout.

What Are Low-Impact Aerobic Activities?

Because long-term participation in some aerobic activities (for example, jogging, running, aerobic dancing, and rope skipping) may lead to injury of the hip, knee, and ankle joints, many fitness experts promote low-impact aerobic activities. Low-impact aerobic dancing, water aerobics, bench aerobics, and brisk walking are examples

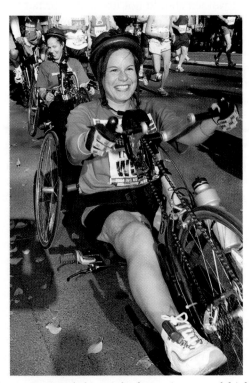

Wearing appropriate clothing and safety equipment and drinking adequate amounts of fluid are good strategies for any type of exercise.

of this kind of fitness activity. Participants still conform to the principal components of a cardiorespiratory fitness program. THR levels are the same as in high-impact aerobic activities.

The main difference between low-impact and high-impact aerobic activities is the use of the legs. Low-impact aerobics require having one foot on the ground at all times. Thus, weight transfer does not occur with the forcefulness seen in traditional, high-impact aerobic activities. In addition, low-impact activities may include exaggerated arm movements and the use of hand or wrist weights. All these variations are designed to increase the heart rate to the THR without undue strain on the joints of the lower extremities. Low-impact aerobics are excellent for people of all ages, and they may be especially beneficial to older adults.

In-line skating (rollerblading) is one of the fastest-growing fitness activities. This low-impact activity has cardiorespiratory and muscular benefits similar to those of running without the pounding effect that running can produce. However, it should be recognized that it requires both skill and balance. Rollerblading requires important safety equipment: sturdy skates, knee and elbow pads, wrist supports, and a helmet. The potential for falling makes this a higher-risk activity.

What Is the Most Effective Way to Replace Fluids During Exercise?

Despite all the advertising hype associated with commercial fluid-replacement products, for an average person involved in typical fitness activities, water is still the best fluid replacement. The availability and cost are unbeatable. However, when activity is prolonged and intense, commercial sports drinks may be preferred over water because they contain electrolytes (which replace lost sodium and potassium) and carbohydrates (which replace depleted energy stores). However, the carbohydrates in sports drinks are actually simple forms of sugar. Thus, sports drinks tend to be high in calories just like regular soft drinks. Regardless of the drink you choose, exercise physiologists recommend that you drink fluids before and at frequent intervals throughout the activity, particularly in warm, humid environments.

What Clothing Should I Wear for Exercise?

The two points of emphasis for exercise clothing are to wear clothing that is comfortable, more than stylish, and that promotes temperature regulation. Generally, loose-fitting attire that does not restrict movement is desirable. However, new materials have been developed that are more form-fitting, yet are comfortable, do not restrict movement, and do not impede temperature regulation.

In warmer temperatures the goal is to prevent the body from overheating. Generally, in a warm or hot environment, less clothing should be worn and the materials should allow for the transfer of moisture from the skin so that it can evaporate. Evaporation is what results in heat loss. Sweat that drips off or is wiped off the body does not produce any cooling. Also, for outdoor exercising, light-colored clothing should be worn to diminish radiant heat transfer to the body.

In cooler temperatures the goal is to prevent losing too much heat, which can result in hypothermia. In cold environments, a layered approach to dressing is recommended. When you exercise, even in the cold, you will produce body heat. Layering enables you to remove the outermost layer of clothing during exercise. (Note: You might need to put this layer back on if you perform your cooldown routine outdoors.) The innermost layer should be made of a material that will transfer moisture away from your skin. Cotton is not recommended because it tends to absorb and retain moisture from sweat, which can increase the amount of heat loss in cold temperatures. The outermost layer should be of a material that will shield the body from the wind but allow for moisture to be transferred away from the body. Material such as Gore-Tex is ideal for this. Additionally, you should protect your extremities by wearing a hat that covers your ears and using gloves or mittens as dictated by the outdoor temperature.

Where Can I Find Out About Proper Equipment?

College students are generally in an excellent setting to locate people who have the resources to provide helpful information about sports equipment. Contacting physical education, exercise science, or health education faculty members who have an interest in your chosen activity might be a good start. Most colleges also have a number of clubs that specialize in fitness interests—cycling, hiking, and jogging clubs, for example. Attend one of their upcoming meetings. For many activities, the only equipment you'll need is a good pair of athletic shoes.

Many types of cardiorespiratory fitness equipment are now available for home use. Home fitness equipment can be especially helpful for those who do not have access to a health or fitness club, who prefer to exercise alone and at home, or who must exercise at irregular hours. Some of the most popular devices are described following.

Stationary bicycles come in models ranging in price from about $150 to $3,500. Some upright bikes can also be used for an upper body workout because the user can pump the handlebars. Recumbent bikes, so named because the user sits back while pedaling, take the pressure off the lower back and permit the rider to exercise the hamstring muscles to a greater degree than on an upright bike. Also available are stands that allow the user to convert a regular bicycle into a stationary bike.

Treadmills consist of a moving belt stretched over rollers. Less expensive varieties, starting at a few hundred dollars, are driven manually by the walking or running action of the user. More expensive treadmills are driven by an electric motor and typically allow the user to change speeds and the incline angle of the platform to increase the intensity of the workout; top-of-the-line models can cost thousands of dollars. If you are a first-time user of a motorized treadmill, start slowly so you can become familiar with the motion. Also take special care getting on and off the moving belt.

Stair climbers simulate climbing up a series of stair steps while saving the knees from much of the pressure normally associated with stair climbing. Prices vary from about $200 for a simple level model to $5,000 for a programmable model that varies the speed and amount of resistance. Some models come with an upper-body component that allows the user to pump the arms while climbing.

Rowing machines have a sliding seat and movable handles that are similar to oars and allow the user to simulate the movements of rowing a racing scull. Users push their feet against footplates while pulling back on the handles and sliding the seat. Rowing machines can range in cost from about $300 to more than $3,000.

Elliptical trainers provide a low-impact simulation of the action of walking or running. The feet describe an ellipse, which is roughly the same pattern that we move in when we walk or run. These trainers can require more involvement of the gluteal and thigh muscles than do treadmills or stationary cycles. Prices range from several hundred to several thousand dollars.

Most forms of equipment can provide a good cardiorespiratory workout, but you may have to add strength training to your fitness program in order to obtain a complete workout. In terms of effectiveness, a *Journal of the American Medical Association* study found that treadmill users walking or running "somewhat hard" burned more calories per hour than users of five other common home exercise machines; in this study, people using regular and dual-action stationary cycles burned the fewest calories per hour.[16]

The machine that is best for you is the one that you enjoy using and that lasts. Unfortunately, many people purchase a machine and seldom use it. Using just one piece of equipment can become monotonous, and you may find yourself avoiding exercise due to boredom. It is advisable to thoroughly test out equipment before purchase. Check the quality of the equipment and its appropriateness for you. See the box "Infomercials and Advertisements for Fitness Equipment" for consumer guidelines.

How Worthwhile Are Commercial Health and Fitness Clubs?

The health and fitness club business is booming. Fitness clubs offer activities ranging from free weights to weight machines to step walking to general aerobics. Some clubs have saunas and whirlpools and lots of frills. Others have course offerings that include wellness, smoking cessation, stress management, time management, dance, and yoga. The atmosphere at most clubs is friendly, and people are encouraged to have a good time while working out.

If your purpose in joining a fitness club is to improve your cardiorespiratory fitness, measure the program offered by the club against the ACSM standards.[17] If your primary purpose in joining is to meet people and have fun, request a trial membership for a month or so to see whether you like the environment.

Before signing a contract at a health club or spa, do some careful questioning. Find out when the business was established, ask about the qualifications of the employees, contact some members for their observations, and request a thorough tour of the facilities. You might even consult your local Better Business Bureau for additional information. Finally, make certain that you read and understand every word of the contract.

What Are Steroids, and Why Do Some Athletes Use Them?

Steroids are drugs that physicians can legally prescribe for a variety of health conditions, including certain forms of anemia, inadequate growth patterns, and chronic debilitating diseases. Steroids can also be prescribed to aid recovery from surgery or burns. **Anabolic steroids** are drugs that function like the male sex hormone testosterone. They can be taken orally or by injection.

 TALKING POINTS If you suspected a young person you know was using steroids, what strategies would you use to encourage the person to change his or her behavior?

Anabolic steroids are used by athletes who hope to gain weight, muscular size and strength, power, endurance, and aggressiveness. Over the last few decades, many bodybuilders, weightlifters, track athletes, and football players have chosen to ignore the serious health risks posed by illegal steroid use. More recently, steroid use among high school and college campuses has reached epidemic levels. The mass media has begun to focus attention on the dangers of steroid use, but many young athletes choose to ignore these warnings.

The use of steroids is highly dangerous because of serious, life-threatening side effects and adverse reactions. These effects include heart problems, certain forms of cancer, liver complications, and even psychological disturbances. The side effects on female steroid users are as dangerous as those on men. Figure 4-2 shows the adverse effects of steroid use.

Steroid users have developed a terminology of their own. Anabolic steroids are called "roids" or "juice." "Roid rage" is an aggressive, psychotic response to chronic steroid use. "Stacking" means using multiple steroids at the same time.

Many organizations that control athletic competition (such as the National Collegiate Athletic Association or the NCAA, The Athletics Congress, the National Football League, and the International Olympic Committee) have banned steroids and are testing athletes for illegal use. Fortunately, some athletes finally seem to be getting the message and are steering clear of steroids. For more information on the potential health hazards of using anabolic steroids, see the National Institute on Drug Abuse's Info Facts, found on the Web (www.nida.nih .gov/infofacts/steroids.htm). For more on other supplements taken by athletes, see the box "Evaluating Nutritional Supplements Promoted to Enhance Exercise."

Exercise Injuries

At any time during your participation in fitness or sport activities, it is possible that you will become injured, even if you carefully warm up before your exercise and cool down after your exercise. If you are lucky, the injury will be only a minor one and after a short period of rest you will be able to resume your fitness interests. Sometimes, however, an injury can be significant and require you to seek medical care and undergo extensive rehabilitation.

It is beyond the scope of this textbook to provide a comprehensive discussion of the prevention, care, and treatment of sports injuries. (You can find this information in an athletic training textbook, a fitness textbook, or a sports medicine book.) However, here we provide you with some general principles related to the prevention and care of sports injuries and a table that lists many common fitness injuries.[18] (See Table 4.2 on page 110.)

Key Terms

anabolic steroids (ann uh **bol** ick) Drugs that function like testosterone to produce increases in muscle mass, strength, endurance, and aggressiveness.

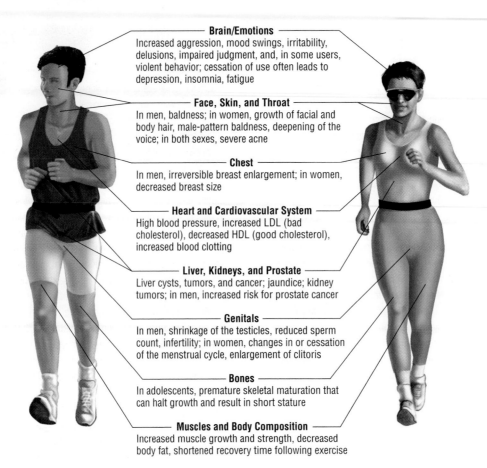

Brain/Emotions
Increased aggression, mood swings, irritability, delusions, impaired judgment, and, in some users, violent behavior; cessation of use often leads to depression, insomnia, fatigue

Face, Skin, and Throat
In men, baldness; in women, growth of facial and body hair, male-pattern baldness, deepening of the voice; in both sexes, severe acne

Chest
In men, irreversible breast enlargement; in women, decreased breast size

Heart and Cardiovascular System
High blood pressure, increased LDL (bad cholesterol), decreased HDL (good cholesterol), increased blood clotting

Liver, Kidneys, and Prostate
Liver cysts, tumors, and cancer; jaundice; kidney tumors; in men, increased risk for prostate cancer

Genitals
In men, shrinkage of the testicles, reduced sperm count, infertility; in women, changes in or cessation of the menstrual cycle, enlargement of clitoris

Bones
In adolescents, premature skeletal maturation that can halt growth and result in short stature

Muscles and Body Composition
Increased muscle growth and strength, decreased body fat, shortened recovery time following exercise

Figure 4-2 Effects of Steroids In addition to the effects listed above, people who inject steroids run the added risk of contracting or transmitting HIV infection or hepatitis.

Sources: Steroids (Anabolic-Androgenic), *NIDA InfoFacts*, National Institute on Drug Abuse, March 2007; Anabolic Steroids, *NIDA Community Drug Alert Bulletin*, National Institute on Drug Abuse, April 2000.

1. *A well-planned fitness program starts at a low level and progresses gradually and consistently.* This principle supports the concept of starting at a level of activity that can be handled comfortably. If the activity is a walking program, an unfit person should not begin with walks of five or six miles a day but should start with a shorter distance and gradually add additional distance in a consistent manner to avoid muscle, skeletal, or joint injuries.

2. *If you stop exercising for an extended time, do not restart the activity at the level at which you stopped.* Do not plan on returning to a high level of activity if you have been inactive for an extended time. Rather, reduce your activity significantly and gradually return to your earlier levels of activity.

3. *"Listen to your body."* Always be aware of the nature of your body as you are exercising. If you sense that something is wrong, stop the activity and assess the situation. For example, if you think you might be hurting your back or that a joint or muscle is being strained, stop and evaluate the situation. If you think something is wrong, by all means don't test your body by returning to the activity. (Have you ever seen a person with a suspected ankle injury "test" the ankle by hopping up and down on the injured leg? This makes no sense at all.) Pain indicates that something is wrong. If this is the case, seek a professional evaluation, perhaps from an athletic trainer or a physical therapist. A physician, especially one trained in sports medicine, can make an accurate diagnosis of the injury.

4. *Follow rehabilitation instructions carefully.* Athletic trainers and physical therapists are trained to design effective rehabilitation programs. If you are injured, it is very important that you follow the advice of these professionals. This is especially true in cases where you start to feel better before the rehabilitation program is finished. Even though you feel better, your body may not be fully recovered. A return to activity too quickly may result in an even more serious injury than your original one. (This is especially true for adults over the age of 40.) The best advice is to resist the urge to return to your activity until you are given full clearance from your trainer or therapist.

Evaluating Nutritional Supplements Promoted to Enhance Exercise

Two of the primary reasons people exercise are to lose weight (fat) and to gain muscle mass. Often people seek ways to accomplish these goals faster. Although nutritional supplements have been available for many years, common use of supplements is a relatively recent phenomenon. The reason for the popularity of supplements is not breakthrough scientific studies that have proven that they work, but instead their increased promotion by athletes and celebrities who provide testimonials about their benefits.

The most commonly used supplements fall into three categories:

1. Products that promote increased rates of energy expenditure to enhance weight loss
2. Products that promote protein synthesis to increase the growth of muscle tissue
3. Products that provide a boost of energy to allow exercise workouts to be more intense or to allow the exercise session to last longer (without fatigue)

The most burning questions that people have are, Will a supplement work for me? and Is the supplement safe to use?

Generally, most products go through extensive testing before they reach the marketplace. For supplements this testing can be done by the manufacturers or by independent laboratories. It is important to understand that, unlike for medications, there are no federal regulations that require testing on supplements to ensure that the product is effective and safe. Testing performed by manufacturers can be biased and therefore is of limited value. Consumers should be wary of claims that "research has shown . . ." unless the research has been published in a peer-reviewed scientific journal.

A second factor to consider is the value of a testimonial. Certainly it is tempting to believe that the product works when one sees convincing before-and-after pictures and hears the endorsement of a popular athlete or entertainer. However, remember that the person who is endorsing the product is being paid by the manufacturer. Furthermore, what the endorser often does not tell you in detail is the type of exercise training program that was followed and other changes that were made to the diet. It is possible that much, and possibly all, of the beneficial changes (shown in the before-and-after pictures) were the result of the exercise and dietary changes. In other words, there is little, if any, proof that the supplement used had any effect at all.

The last factor to consider is the cost and safety of the supplements. Generally speaking, these products are relatively expensive because there are few manufacturers of the products and advertising campaigns (including paying celebrities) are expensive. Safety is largely unknown because nutritional supplements are not federally regulated. Additionally, consumers often seek products at reduced cost from suppliers that sell only their own products through advertisements in the print media or over the Internet. Certainly, consumers need to be wary of these types of faceless companies that offer little in the way of assurance of the quality and purity of the products they sell.

5. *Develop a prevention approach.* After you recover from an injury, try to discover ways to prevent that injury from happening again. Learn about proper stretching exercises, effective strength-training activities, appropriate equipment, and the proper mechanics for your selected sports/fitness activities. Use this collective knowledge to prevent the injury from recurring.

For example, if you have injured your hamstring muscles while running, you will need to learn how to effectively stretch these muscles in the future. You will also need to learn how to strengthen these muscles through resistance training. If your running shoes are old and worn, they may have to be replaced. Finally, don't run too fast before warming up; start slowly and gradually increase your speed after the muscles are fully warmed up. Preventive actions such as these will allow you to have a fitness program that is not regularly interrupted by a nagging injury.

Taking Charge of Your Health

- Assess your level of fitness by completing the National Fitness Test on pages 112–113.
- Implement or maintain a cardiorespiratory fitness program that uses the most recent American College of Sports Medicine recommendations.

- Start a daily stretching program based on the guidelines in this chapter.
- Recognize that a comprehensive physical fitness program includes performing muscular fitness exercises at least twice a week.

- Monitor your physical activities for potential danger signs indicating that you should consult an athletic trainer, physical therapist, or physician.
- Make sure that you always include a warm-up and a cooldown with each exercise session.

Table 4.2 Common Injuries Associated with Physical Activity

Injury	Condition
Achilles tendinitis	A chronic tendinitis of the "heel cord" or muscle tendon, located on the back of the lower leg just above the heel. It may result from any activity that involves forcefully pushing off with the foot and ankle, such as in running and jumping. This inflammation involves swelling, warmth, tenderness to touch, and pain during walking and especially running.
Ankle sprains	Stretching or tearing of one or several ligaments that provide stability to the ankle joint. Ligaments on the outside or lateral side of the ankle are more commonly injured by rolling the sole of the foot downward and toward the inside. Pain is intense immediately after injury, followed by considerable swelling, tenderness, loss of joint motion, and some discoloration over a 24- to 48-hour period.
Groin pull	A muscle strain that occurs in the muscles located on the inside of the upper thigh just below the pubic area and that results either from an overstretch of the muscle or from a contraction of the muscle that meets excessive resistance. Pain will be produced by flexing the hip and leg across the body or by stretching the muscles in a groin-stretch position.
Hamstring pull	A strain of the muscles on the back of the upper thigh that most often occurs while sprinting. In most cases, severe pain is caused simply by walking or in any movement that involves knee flexion or stretch of the hamstring muscle. Some swelling, tenderness to touch, and possibly some discoloration extending down the back of the leg may occur in severe strains.
Patellofemoral knee pain	Nonspecific pain occurring around the knee, particularly the front part of the knee, or in the kneecap (patella). Pain can result from many causes, including improper movement of the kneecap in knee flexion and extension; tendinitis of the tendon just below the kneecap, which is caused by repetitive jumping; bursitis (swelling) either above or below the kneecap; and osteoarthritis (joint surface degeneration) between the kneecap and thigh bone. It may involve inflammation with swelling, tenderness, warmth, and pain associated with movement.
Quadriceps contusion "charley horse"	A deep bruise of the muscles in the front part of the thigh caused by a forceful impact or by some object that results in severe pain, swelling, discoloration, and difficulty flexing the knee or extending the hip. Without adequate rest and protection from additional trauma, small calcium deposits may develop in the muscle.
Shin splints	A catch-all term used to refer to any pain that occurs in the front part of the lower leg or shin, most often caused by excessive running on hard surfaces. Pain is usually caused by strain of the muscles that move the ankle and foot at their attachment points in the shin. It is usually worse during activity. In more severe cases it may be caused by stress fractures of the long bones in the lower leg, with the pain being worse after activity is stopped.
Shoulder impingement	Chronic irritation and inflammation of muscle tendons and a bursa underneath the tip of the shoulder, which results from repeated forceful overhead motions of the shoulder, such as in swimming, throwing, spiking a volleyball, or serving a tennis ball. Pain is felt when the arm is extended across the body above shoulder level.
Tennis elbow	Chronic irritation and inflammation of the lateral or outside surface of the arm just above the elbow at the attachment of the muscles that extend the wrist and fingers. It results from any activity that requires forceful extension of the wrist. Typically occurs in tennis players who are using faulty techniques hitting backhand ground strokes. Pain is felt above the elbow after forcefully extending the wrist against resistance or applying pressure over the muscle attachment above the elbow.

Source: Prentice WE, *Get Fit, Stay Fit*, 5th ed., McGraw-Hill, 2009. Reproduced with permission of The McGraw-Hill Companies.

SUMMARY

- Physical fitness allows one to avoid illness, perform routine activities, and respond to emergencies.
- The health benefits of exercise can be achieved through regular, moderate exercise.
- Fitness comprises five components: cardiorespiratory endurance, muscular strength muscular endurance, flexibility, and body composition.
- The American College of Sports Medicine's program for cardiorespiratory fitness has four components: (1) mode of activity, (2) frequency of training, (3) intensity of training, and (4) duration of training.
- Additionally, ACSM now recommends that everyone also include resistance training and flexibility training.

- The target heart rate (THR) refers to the number of times per minute the heart must contract to produce a cardiorespiratory training effect.
- Training sessions should take place in three phases: warm-up, conditioning, and cooldown.
- Static stretching is usually recommended for stretching.
- Fitness experts are concerned about the lack of fitness in today's youth.
- Street dancing, swing dancing, step aerobics, and rollerblading are currently popular aerobic activities.
- Low-impact aerobic activities have a lower risk of muscle and joint injuries than do high-impact activities.

- College students who are interested in fitness should be as knowledgeable as possible about the important topics of supplement use, cross-training, fluid replacement, and bodybuilding.

- Following a few simple principles can help prevent many common sports injuries.

REVIEW QUESTIONS

1. Identify the five components of fitness described in this chapter. How does each component relate to health?
2. What is the difference between anaerobic and aerobic energy production? What types of activities are associated with anaerobic energy production? With aerobic energy production?
3. List some of the benefits of fitness.
4. Describe the various methods used to promote muscular fitness.
5. What does the principle of overload mean in regard to fitness training programs?
6. Identify the ACSM's components of an effective cardio-respiratory conditioning program. Explain the important aspects of each component.
7. Under what circumstances should you see a physician before starting a physical fitness program?
8. Identify and describe the three parts of a training session.
9. Describe some of the negative consequences of anabolic steroid use.
10. Name three common types of nutritional supplements used that are related to exercise programs.
11. Describe the three-part female athlete triad.
12. Discuss the five basic principles important in avoiding sports injuries.

ANSWERS TO THE "WHAT DO YOU KNOW?" QUIZ

1. False   2. True   3. False   4. True   5. True   6. False   7. False

Visit the Online Learning Center (**www.mhhe.com/payne11e**), where you will find tools to help you improve your grade including practice quizzes, key terms flashcards, audio chapter summaries for your MP3 player, and many other study aids.

SOURCE NOTES

1. U.S. Department of Health and Human Services. *Physical Activity and Health: A Report of the Surgeon General.* Atlanta: U.S. Department of Health and Human Services, Centers for Disease Control and Prevention, National Center for Chronic Disease Prevention and Health Promotion, 1996.
2. Casperson C, et al. *Public Health Reports,* 100, 126, 1985.
3. American Heart Association, Councils on Clinical Cardiology and Nutrition, Physical Activity and Metabolism. Exercise and physical activity in the prevention and treatment of atherosclerotic cardiovascular disease. *Circulation,* 107, 3109, 2003.
4. Brubaker PH, Kaminsky LA, Whaley MH. *Coronary Artery Disease.* Champaign, IL: Human Kinetics, 2002.
5. American College of Sports Medicine. Position on the recommended quantity and quality of exercise for developing and maintaining cardiorespiratory and muscular fitness and flexibility in healthy adults. *Medicine and Science in Sports and Exercise,* 30(6), 975–991, 1998.
6. American College of Sports Medicine. *Guidelines for Exercise Testing and Prescription* (8th ed.). Philadelphia: Wolters Kluwer, 2009.
7. Sanders ME (Ed.). *YMCA Water Fitness for Health.* Champaign, IL: Human Kinetics, 2000.
8. National Center for Chronic Disease Prevention and Health Promotion. 2000. Healthy Youth: Promoting Better Health for Young People through Physical Activity and Sports. A Report to the President. www.cdc.gov/healthyyouth/physicalactivity/promoting_health.
9. Ferrini AF, Ferrini RL. *Health in Later Years* (2nd ed.). Guilford, CT: Brown & Benchmark, 1992.
10. American College of Sports Medicine and American Heart Association. Physical activity and public health in older adults. *Circulation,* 116, 1094–1105, 2007.
11. American College of Sports Medicine. The female athlete triad. *Medicine and Science in Sports and Exercise,* 39, 1867–1882, 2007.
12. American College of Obstetricians and Gynecologists. *Exercise During Pregnancy.* Pamphlet AP119, 2003.
13. Williams RD. Healthy pregnancy, healthy baby. *FDA Consumer,* 33(2), 18–23.
14. National Osteoporosis Foundation. Fast Facts. www.nof.org/osteoporosis/diseasefacts.htm.
15. Arthritis Foundation. Osteoarthritis treatment. www.arthritis.org/conditions/diseasecenter/OA/oa_treatment1.asp
16. Zeni AL, et al. Energy expenditure with indoor exercise machines. *Journal of the American Medical Association,* 275(18), May 8, 1996.
17. American College of Sports Medicine. *ACSM's Health/Fitness Facility Standards and Guidelines* (3rd ed). Champaign, IL: Human Kinetics, 2006.
18. Prentice WE. *Fitness for Wellness and Life* (6th ed.). New York: McGraw-Hill College Division, 1998.

Personal Assessment

What is your level of fitness?

You can determine your level of fitness in 30 minutes or less by completing this short group of tests based on the National Fitness Test developed by the President's Council on Physical Fitness and Sports. If you are over 40 years old or have chronic medical disorders such as diabetes or obesity, check with your physician before taking this or any other fitness test. You will need another person to monitor your test and keep time.

3-Minute Step Test

Aerobic capacity. Equipment: 12-inch bench, crate, block, or step ladder; stopwatch. Procedure: face bench. Complete 24 full steps (both feet on the bench, both feet on the ground) per minute for 3 minutes. After finishing, sit down, have your partner find your pulse within 5 seconds, and take your pulse for 1 minute. Your score is your pulse rate for 1 full minute.

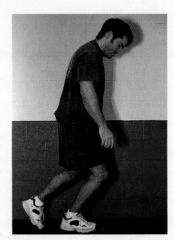

	Scoring standards (heart rate for 1 minute)									
Age	18–29		30–39		40–49		50–59		60+	
Gender	F	M	F	M	F	M	F	M	F	M
Excellent	<80	<75	<84	<78	<88	<80	<92	<85	<95	<90
Good	80–110	75–100	84–115	78–109	88–118	80–112	92–123	85–115	95–127	90–118
Average	>110	>100	>115	>109	>118	>112	>123	>115	>127	>118

Sit and Reach

Hamstring flexibility. Equipment: yardstick; tape. Positioned parallel to your legs and between them, tape a yardstick to the floor. Sit with legs straight and heels about 5 inches apart, heels even with the 15-inch mark on the yardstick. While in a sitting position, slowly stretch forward as far as possible. Your score is the number of inches reached.

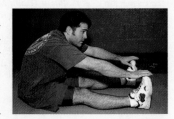

	Scoring standards (inches)									
Age	18–29		30–39		40–49		50–59		60+	
Gender	F	M	F	M	F	M	F	M	F	M
Excellent	>22	>21	>22	>21	>21	>20	>20	>19	>20	>19
Good	17–22	13–21	17–22	13–21	15–21	13–20	14–20	12–19	14–20	12–19
Average	<17	<13	<17	<13	<15	<13	<14	<12	<14	<12

Arm Hang

Upper body strength. Equipment: horizontal bar (high enough to prevent your feet from touching the floor); stopwatch. Procedure: hang with straight arms, palms facing forward. Start watch when subject is in position. Stop when subject lets go. Your score is the number of minutes and seconds spent hanging.

Scoring standards (hanging time)

Age	18–29		30–39		40–49		50–59		60+	
Gender	F	M	F	M	F	M	F	M	F	M
Excellent	>1:30	>2:00	>1:20	>1:50	>1:10	>1:35	>1:00	>1:20	>:50	>1:10
Good	:46–1:30	1:00–2:00	:40–1:20	:50–1:50	:30–1:10	:45–1:35	:30–1:00	:35–1:20	:21–:50	:30–1:10
Average	<:46	<1:00	<:40	<:50	<:30	<:45	<:30	<:35	<:21	<:30

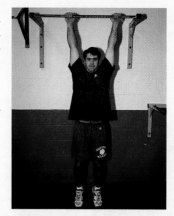

Curl-Ups

Abdominal and low back strength. Equipment: stopwatch. Procedure: Lie flat on upper back, knees bent, shoulders touching the floor, arms extended above your thighs or by your sides, palms down. Bend knees so that feet are flat and 12 inches from the buttocks. Curl up by lifting head and shoulders off the floor, sliding hands forward above your thighs or the floor. Curl down and repeat. Your score is the number of curl-ups in 1 minute.

Scoring standards (number in 1 minute)

Age	18–29		30–39		40–49		50–59		60+	
Gender	F	M	F	M	F	M	F	M	F	M
Excellent	>45	>50	>40	>45	>35	>40	>30	>35	>25	>30
Good	25–45	30–50	20–40	22–45	16–35	21–40	12–30	18–35	11–25	15–30
Average	<25	<30	<20	<22	<16	<21	<12	<18	<11	<15

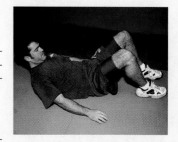

Push-Ups (Men)

Upper body strength. Equipment: stopwatch. Assume a front-leaning position. Lower your body until chest touches the floor. Raise and repeat for 1 minute. Your score is the number of push-ups completed in 1 minute.

Scoring standards (number in 1 minute)

Age	18–29	30–39	40–49	50–59	60+
Excellent	>50	>45	>40	>35	>30
Good	25–50	22–45	19–40	15–35	10–30
Average	<25	<22	<19	<15	<10

Modified Push-Ups (Women)

Upper body strength. Equipment: stopwatch. Assume a front-leaning position with knees bent up, hands under shoulders. Lower your chest to the floor, raise, and repeat. Your score is the number of push-ups completed in 1 minute.

Scoring standards (number in 1 minute)

Age	18–29	30–39	40–49	50–59	60+
Excellent	>45	>40	>35	>30	>25
Good	17–45	12–40	8–35	6–30	5–25
Average	<17	<12	<8	<6	<5

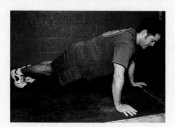

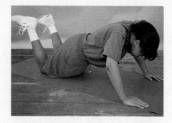

TO CARRY THIS FURTHER . . .

Note your areas of strengths and weaknesses. To improve your fitness, become involved in a fitness program that reflects the concepts discussed in this chapter. Talking with fitness experts on your campus might be a good first step.

Source: Data from the National Fitness Foundation.

Understanding nutrition and Your Diet

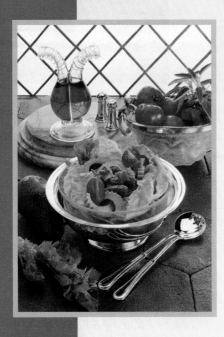

What Do You Know About Nutrition?

1. Coffee is Americans' number one source of antioxidants. True or False?

2. Whole-grain bread does not have the same nutritional benefits as wheat bread. True or False?

3. Most people get enough vitamin D from exposure to the sun. True or False?

4. Saturated fats are the same thing as trans fats. True or False?

5. The current dietary guidelines do not make recommendations for how much water you should drink each day. True or False?

6. Foods with phytochemicals are bad for you and should be avoided. True or False?

7. Fruit juice is a good way to meet the dietary recommendations for the fruit group. True or False?

Check your answers at the end of the chapter.

Healthy eating is important from the prenatal period throughout life, in order to prevent malnourishment and minimize the development of illnesses. Food supports growth and development by providing the body with the nutrients needed for energy, repair of damaged tissue, growth of new tissue, and regulation of physiological processes. Our food selections also reflect personal, familial, and cultural traditions. The preparation and serving of food at regular mealtimes and during holiday gatherings and other special occasions enhance all of the dimensions of health (see the box "Mealtime—A Chance to Share and Bond"). For example, sharing a meal with fellow parishioners after a religious service supports the spiritual dimension of health, sharing popcorn at the movies with your friends can enhance the social dimension of health, and learning about the cuisine of another culture develops the cultural dimension of health. As you read this chapter, keep in mind this balanced view of food as sustenance and food as a resource for the dimensions of health.

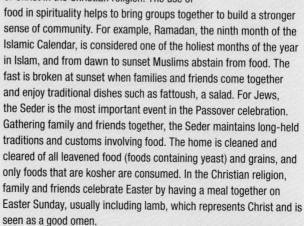
Types and Sources of Nutrients

Your body relies on seven **nutrients** to carry out its physiological functions: carbohydrates, fats, protein, vitamins, minerals, dietary fiber, and water.* The first three—carbohydrates, fats, and protein—will be discussed together because they provide **calories.** These calories are either used quickly by our bodies in energy metabolism or stored in the form of glycogen or fat for delayed use as energy sources. The other nutrients—vitamins, minerals, dietary fiber, and water—are not sources of calories for the body. However, regardless of their relationship to calories, all nutrients are essential to human health. The function of each is discussed later in the chapter.

Carbohydrates

Carbohydrates are various combinations of sugar units, or saccharides, and are the major energy source for the body.[1]

Types and Sources of Carbohydrates   Carbohydrates occur in three forms, depending on the number of saccharide (sugar) units that make up the molecule.

Carbohydrates are divided into two categories: simple (monosaccharides and disaccharides) and complex carbohydrates (polysaccharides).

- *Monosaccharides—carbohydrates with one saccharide unit.* These are the primary source of the body's energy. Examples include glucose, found in vegetables, honey, fruits, and syrup; and fructose, found in fruits and berries.

- *Disaccharides—carbohydrates with two saccharide units, one of which is always a glucose unit.* Examples include sucrose, or table sugar; maltose, which is

> ### Key Terms
>
> **nutrients** Elements in foods that are required for the growth, repair, and regulation of body processes.
>
> **calories** Units of heat (energy); specifically, 1 calorie is the amount of energy needed to raise the temperature of 1 gram of water by 1 degree C. In common usage, on food labels, and in this chapter, the term *calorie* is used to refer to a larger energy unit, *kilocalorie* (1,000 calories).
>
> **carbohydrates** The body's primary source of energy for all body functioning; chemical compounds including sugar, starches, and dietary fibers.

*Since most of our water intake comes from beverages rather than from food, some nutritionists do not consider water a nutrient, even though it is essential for life.

derived from germinating cereals; and lactose, found in human and animal milk.

- *Polysaccharides—carbohydrates with more than two saccharide units.* Polysaccharides include starches and dietary fiber. Examples are vegetables, breads, cereals, legumes, and pasta.

Both simple and complex carbohydrates contain 4 calories per gram, and both are digested into glucose. Simple carbohydrates are digested more quickly because they are composed of fewer saccharide units than complex carbohydrates. Complex carbohydrates also take longer to digest because they have more fiber, vitamins, and minerals.

How Much Carbohydrate Is Recommended? Each gram of carbohydrate contains 4 calories. Since the average person requires approximately 2,000 calories per day and about 45 to 65 percent of our calories come from carbohydrates, it is recommended that approximately 1,200 of our daily calories come from carbohydrates.[1] However, age, gender, and activity level affect the number of calories an individual requires each day; individual energy needs are discussed later in this chapter.

Simple Sugars: The American Sweet Tooth According to the USDA, the average adult American consumes approximately 156 pounds of sweeteners (sugar, corn sweetener, syrup, and honey) each year,[2] an increase of 30 percent in the past 30 years. These sugars are usually found in sodas, candy, and bakery items, which have little nutritional value. Corn sweetener consumption increased to 79 pounds in 2003, up 400 percent from 1970, largely due to the high-fructose corn syrup found in many beverages. This increase in sugar consumption is a major contributor to the more than 500-calorie-per-day increase in overall consumption since 1970.

Much of the sugar we consume is hidden; that is, sugar is a principal product we may overlook in a large number of food items. Foods such as ketchup, salad dressings, cured meat products, and canned vegetables and fruits can contain much hidden sugar. Corn syrup, frequently found in these items, is a highly concentrated sucrose solution. Whether the sugar is overt or hidden, the USDA has suggested a limit of 8 teaspoons of sugar per day for a 2,000-calorie diet, which would be equivalent to six ounces of yogurt and one cup of cereal.

Sugar Substitutes For a number of years, sugar substitutes have been used in a wide array of beverages, candy, baked goods, chewing gum, frozen desserts, gelatins and puddings, jams, toppings, and syrups. Among the most familiar of these are saccharin and aspartame (Nutrasweet), both of which are several hundred times sweeter than sucrose. Since 1977, saccharin has been linked to cancer, particularly bladder cancer, and warnings were given about its use until 2000, when Congress removed this requirement.[3] Some of the newer artificial sweeteners are sorbitol, found in ice cream; acesulfame potassium (ace K), used in Pepsi ONE; xylitol, found in some brands of chewing gum; neotame, found in candy and soft drinks; sucralose (Splenda); and tagatose, found in Slurpees. These sweeteners can be more than 600 times sweeter than sugar; neotame is 7,000 to 13,000 times sweeter than sugar. Stevia is an herbal sweetener made from the leaves of the South American shrub by this name. It is 200 to 300 times sweeter than table sugar and is sold as a dietary supplement in the United States. There has been concern that consumption of stevia could cause infertility and cancer. Stevia can be found in soft drinks under the name Truvia (in Coca-Cola) and Purevia (in Pepsi-Cola). There have been concerns about other artificial sweeteners such as aspartame and acesulfame-potassium being associated with cancer, but the USDA has deemed them safe at this point. While many people use artificial sweeteners as a way to decrease caloric intake and for weight management, studies have shown that people consuming food and beverages with artificial sweeteners actually consumed more calories than those who did not. So sugar substitutes may actually contribute to weight gain rather than weight loss.[4]

Fats

Fats (lipids, fatty acids) have been given a bad name but are an important nutrient in our diets. Fats provide a concentrated form of energy (over double that of carbohydrates—there are 9 calories per gram consumed versus 4 for carbohydrates and protein). Fats provide a sense of satiety and keep us from feeling hungry. Because fats take longer to leave the stomach than either carbohydrates or proteins do, our stomachs feel full for a longer period of time, decreasing our appetite. Fats also help to give our food its pleasing taste, and they serve as carriers of fat-soluble vitamins A, D, E, and K. Without fat, these vitamins would quickly pass through the body. Fat insulates the body and helps it retain heat.

Sources of Fat Dietary sources of fat are often difficult to identify. The visible fats in our diet, such as butter, salad oils, and the layer of fat on some cuts of meat, represent only about 40 percent of the fat we consume. Most of the fat we eat is "hidden" in food because it is incorporated into the food during preparation or used to fry the food or as a sauce.

Types of Fat Every type of dietary fat is made up of a combination of three forms of fat (saturated, mono-unsaturated, and polyunsaturated), based on its chemical composition (Figure 5-1). In each of the three forms of fat, the absence of double bonds (saturated fats) or the

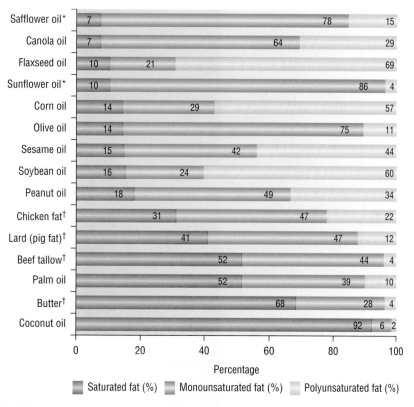

	Saturated fat (%)	Monounsaturated fat (%)	Polyunsaturated fat (%)
Safflower oil*	7	78	15
Canola oil	7	64	29
Flaxseed oil	10	21	69
Sunflower oil*	10	86	4
Corn oil	14	29	57
Olive oil	14	75	11
Sesame oil	15	42	44
Soybean oil	16	24	60
Peanut oil	18	49	34
Chicken fat†	31	47	22
Lard (pig fat)†	41	47	12
Beef tallow†	52	44	4
Palm oil	52	39	10
Butter†	68	28	4
Coconut oil	92	6	2

*Safflower and sunflower oil come in several forms; those given here are high oleic (monounsaturated) forms.
†Only animal fats contain cholesterol; per tablespoon, chicken fat has 11 mg; lard, 12 mg; beef tallow, 14 mg; and butter, 31 mg.

Figure 5-1 Composition of Dietary Fats

Note: Some fats total over 100 percent due to rounding.
Source: Data from USDA Nutrient Database for Standard Reference (Release 21), September 2008.

presence of double bonds (monounsaturated and polyunsaturated fats) and the location of the double bonds within the molecule determine the nature and degree of restructuring that the body can do in changing dietary fat into physiology-friendly forms. Today, consumers need to pay attention to the amount of each type of fat in dietary fat because of the role that each form plays in heart disease (see Chapter 10).

Saturated and Trans Fats   Not all fats are created equal. **Saturated fats,** including those found in animal sources and in vegetable oils to which hydrogen has been added (hydrogenated), becoming **trans-fatty acids,** need to be carefully limited in a modern healthy diet. The presence of trans-fatty acids (an altered form of normal vegetable oil molecule or from meat and dairy products, having formed naturally by fermentation in the intestinal tract of animals)[5] is associated with changes in the cell membrane, including those cells lining the artery wall. This possibly prevents these vessel wall cells from freeing cholesterol from their surfaces.[6] Processing can change the structure of fat, making it more saturated. As a result, the oils become semisolid and more stable at room temperature. The term *trans* describes the chemical makeup of a fatty acid. Most trans-fatty acids come from hydrogenated oil, which is found in foods such

as stick margarine, peanut butter, and crackers. They are popular in food manufacturing because they can extend the shelf life of the food: The oil stays mixed in the food and doesn't rise to the top, and the food doesn't become too soft at room temperature. The fast-food industry uses these fats to fry many foods.[7] Additionally, trans-fatty acids are associated with increases in low-density lipoprotein (LDL), the "bad" cholesterol, without corresponding increases in high-density lipoprotein (HDL), the "good" cholesterol[8] (see Chapter 10). The amount of trans-fatty acids in the diet should be limited to 2 grams or less daily.

Trans fats can act like saturated fat, potentially raising LDL blood cholesterol levels and decreasing HDL

Key Terms

satiety (suh **tie** uh tee) The feeling of no longer being hungry; a diminished desire to eat.

saturated fats Fats that promote cholesterol formation; they are in solid form at room temperature; primarily animal fats.

trans-fatty acid An altered form of an unsaturated fat molecule in which the hydrogen atoms on each side of the double bond(s) are on opposite sides; also called *trans fats.*

cholesterol. This is the reason nutritionists encourage us to use butter rather than stick margarine. To reduce your intake of trans fat, make sure you check the labels on foods to see if they list "partially hydrogenated vegetable oil" as one of the ingredients. Foods such as cakes, cookies, crackers, snack foods, stick margarine, vegetable shortening, and fried foods are most likely to contain hydrogenated vegetable oil.

Trans fat is seen as being so unhealthy it has been called a "dangerous and unnecessary ingredient" and has been banned for use in restaurants in New York City. The Cheescake Factory chain, McDonalds, Taco Bell, Kentucky Fried Chicken, and Wendy's have pledged not to use trans fat in their cooking oil. The FDA now requires food manufacturers to list trans fat on any product that contains more than 0.5 gram of trans fat per serving. However, that means products that boast they contain "no trans fat" can have less than half a gram of trans fat per serving, and if you eat multiple servings you can easily consume more than the 2 grams of trans fat a day that is the USDA's suggested daily limit. Many food producers are jumping on the no-trans-fat bandwagon, and you will see more cereals, chips, crackers, and other foods labeled "No trans fat."

Monounsaturated Fats Fortunately, the replacement of saturated fats with monounsaturated and polyunsaturated fats and oils appears to lower blood cholesterol levels and reduce the risk of heart disease. Vegetable oils tend to be low in saturated fats, with the exception of the tropical oils (coconut, palm, and palm kernel oils). Monounsaturated fats are found in high quantities in olive oil, peanut oil, and sesame oil.

Polyunsaturated Fats Polyunsaturated fats are especially prevalent in soybean oil and corn oil. Monounsaturated fats can reduce the harmful low-density lipoproteins (LDLs). Polyunsaturated fats reduce both LDLs and total cholesterol. However, polyunsaturated fats also *lower* the healthful high-density lipoproteins (HDLs), which is not a desirable outcome. Omega-3 fatty acids, found in most varieties of fish, are a type of polyunsaturated fat and have been associated with decreased risk of heart disease. Our bodies require omega-3 fatty acids, but we can't produce them on our own, and therefore we must get them from the foods we eat. Flax seed, walnuts, and olive oil are good sources for omega-3 fatty acids. You can also consume omega-3 fish oil as a dietary supplement.

Tropical Oils Although all cooking oils (and fats such as butter, lard, margarine, and shortening) have the same number of calories by weight (9 calories per gram), some oils contain high percentages of saturated fats. All oils and fats contain varying percentages of saturated,

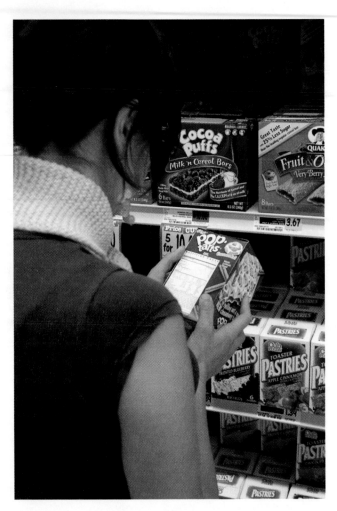

Food labels are an important source of information about the type and amount of fats, carbohydrates, and other nutrients contained in a food.

monounsaturated, and polyunsaturated fats. The tropical oils—coconut, palm, and palm kernel—contain much higher percentages of saturated fats than do other cooking oils. Coconut oil is 92 percent saturated fat. Tropical oils can still be found in some brands of snack foods, crackers, cookies, nondairy creamers, and breakfast cereals, although they have been removed from most national brands. Do you check for tropical oils on the ingredients labels of the food you select?

How Much Fat, and What Type, Is Recommended? The new dietary guidelines recommend that no more than 20 to 35 percent of our calories come from fat. In addition it is suggested that people

- Consume less than 10 percent of calories from saturated fatty acids and less than 300 mg/day of cholesterol, and keep trans-fatty acid consumption as low as possible, no more than 2 grams per day

- Get most fats from sources of polyunsaturated and monounsaturated fatty acids, such as fish, nuts, and vegetable oils.
- Make choices that are lean, low-fat, or fat-free when selecting and preparing meat, poultry, dry beans, and milk or milk products.

Cholesterol   **Cholesterol** is a white, fatlike substance found in cells of animal origin. It is not found in any vegetable product, so products such as peanut butter and margarine that claim they are cholesterol-free never had it in the first place. Cholesterol is used to synthesize cell membranes and also serves as the starting material for the synthesis of bile acids and sex hormones. Although we consume cholesterol in our diet, in such foods as shrimp and other shellfish, animal fat, and milk, we don't need to obtain cholesterol from external sources—the human liver can synthesize enough of the substance to meet the body's needs.

Cholesterol is essential for many of the body's functions. However, if you have too much cholesterol, it builds up in your bloodstream and clogs arteries, putting you at risk for heart disease, heart attack, and stroke. There are different kinds of cholesterol. LDL, often referred to as "bad" cholesterol, builds up on the walls of arteries to form artery-clogging "plaques" that contribute to the development of heart disease and stroke. HDL, or good cholesterol, helps remove excess LDL cholesterol from the blood and transports it back to the liver, where it can be eliminated from the body. You want to have lower LDL (under 130) and higher HDL (higher than 40), with total cholesterol under 200 (see Chapter 10). Almonds, oatmeal, fish, soy, and red wine (a limit of one glass daily) help lower overall cholesterol levels. Whole milk, processed meats, and foods with trans fats and tropical oils, such as fast foods and baked goods, can increase overall cholesterol levels and should be avoided.

A number of medical conditions can give rise to high blood cholesterol, such as liver disease, kidney failure, hypothyroidism, and diabetes. Certain medications, (some diuretics, for example) can also raise blood cholesterol, irrespective of diet.

Nutritionists recommend that people restrict their dietary intake of cholesterol to 300 mg or less per day. In addition, no more than 20 to 35 percent of your total caloric intake should come from fat, with most fats being monounsaturated and polyunsaturated.

Low-Fat Foods   *Low-fat* and *low-calorie* do not mean the same thing, but often people confuse the two. Fat-free, low-fat, and reduced-fat foods have been popular for many years, with people thinking they can eat as much as they want of these foods. This is far from true; a fat-free or reduced-fat product may have as many if not more calories per serving than regular products do. For example, 2 tablespoons of fat-free caramel topping have 103 calories, the same amount as homemade-with-butter caramel topping; 2 tablespoons of Skippy peanut butter have the same number of calories as 2 tablespoons of Skippy reduced-fat peanut butter, 190 calories; and 2 tablespoons of Cool Whip are equal to lite Cool Whip, 25 calories.[9]

Fatty foods make people feel fuller longer than do fat-free foods; thus people tend to eat more of the fat-free foods and so consume more calories. In general, the lower the fat, the higher the price tag because the food industry recognizes that Americans are willing to pay more for products labeled *reduced-fat* and *fat-free*. However, foods such as low-fat sour cream, yogurt, or salad dressings are healthier choices because they have less saturated fat.

Fat-Free Substitutes   Fat-free substitutes such as Z-Trim, Simplesse, Simple Pleasures, Olestra, and Trailblazer contain no cholesterol and have 80 percent fewer calories than do similar products made with fat. Although fat-free substitutes first appeared only in snack foods, today they are found in ice cream, salad dressing, cheese spreads, yogurt, cakes, pies, and French fries.

The development of Olestra (marketed as Olean), as an example, required more than 25 years and $200 million on the part of Procter & Gamble, as an array of new technologies were required. In general, fat-free substitutes are made through processes called *microparticulation*, in which several fatty acids are bonded to a sugar molecule to create a triglyceride-like molecule that imparts all the characteristics of fats but is incapable of being enzymatically broken down by the body as are the triglycerides.

In spite of the apparent desirability of the fat-free technology, concerns have been voiced regarding the inability of these "nouveau fats" to carry fat-soluble vitamins (vitamins A, D, E, and K) and their interference with nutrient absorption. Additional concern was raised over side effects in some people, such as abdominal cramping, loose stools, anal leakage, and an unpleasant aftertaste.[10]

Proteins

The word *protein* derives from the ancient Greek word *proteios,* meaning "first importance." Protein serves primarily to promote growth and maintenance of body

---

Key Terms

cholesterol A primary form of fat found in the blood; lipid material manufactured within the body, as well as derived from dietary sources.

tissue. However, when calorie intake falls, protein is broken down for glucose. This loss of protein can impede growth and repair of tissue. From this, it can be seen that adequate carbohydrate intake prevents protein from serving as an energy source.[11] Protein also is a primary component of enzyme and hormone structure; it helps maintain the *acid-base balance* of our bodies and serves as a source of energy (4 calories per gram consumed).

Sources and Types of Proteins

Proteins are manufactured in every living cell; they are composed of chains of amino acids. **Amino acids** are the "bricks" from which the body constructs its own protein. Twenty amino acids are used in various combinations to build the protein required for physiological processes to continue in a healthy manner.

The human body obtains amino acids from two sources—by breaking down protein from food (as if to take a brick wall apart for its bricks) or by manufacturing its own bricks (amino acids) within its cells. The latter process is less than fully successful because only 11 of the necessary 20 amino acids can be built by the body. The 9 amino acids that *cannot* be built by the body are called *essential amino acids* (indispensable amino acids), because they must be obtained from outside the body through the protein in food. The 11 amino acids that the body itself can make are called *nonessential amino acids* (dispensable amino acids) because the body does not have to rely solely on food protein to obtain these bricks.[11]

In terms of food sources of amino acids, foods can be classified into one of two types, depending on whether they can supply the body with the essential amino acids or not. Complete protein foods contain all nine essential amino acids and are of animal origin (milk, meat, cheese, and eggs). The incomplete protein foods do not contain all the essential amino acids and are of plant origin (vegetables, grains, and legumes [peas or beans, including chickpeas and butter beans]). Vegan vegetarians (see page 136), people with limited access to animal-based food sources, and those who have significantly limited their meat, egg, and dairy product consumption, need to understand how essential amino acids can be obtained from incomplete protein sources. When even one essential amino acid is missing from the diet, deficiency can develop.

Soybeans are a good source of protein for vegetarians. Soybeans provide the same high-quality protein as animal protein.[12] Furthermore, soybeans contain no cholesterol or saturated fat. In 1999 the FDA stated that diets low in saturated fat and cholesterol that include 25 grams of soy protein a day may reduce the risk of heart disease. The sale of soy foods doubled since that proclamation. However, the research on which that claim was based has not been replicated, and in February 2006 the American Heart Association concluded that soy doesn't lower cholesterol as much as was originally suggested. Three long-term government-funded studies currently are investigating the effects of soy on cholesterol levels and its role, if any, in the prevention of cancer and heart disease.[12]

How Much Protein Is Recommended?

The latest recommendations for protein intake are part of a set of standards known as the **Dietary Reference Intakes,** or DRIs. Protein intake recommendations are based on body weight and activity level. The current DRI for protein is 0.36 gram per pound of body weight per day, based upon a sedentary lifestyle, and is higher for athletes and those who are more active. In terms of overall energy intake, nutritionists recommend that 10 to 35 percent of our total caloric intake come from protein.[13]

Vitamins

Vitamins are organic compounds that are required in small amounts for normal growth, reproduction, and maintenance of health. Vitamins differ from carbohydrates, fats, and proteins because they do not provide calories or serve as structural elements for our bodies. Vitamins serve as *coenzymes*. By facilitating the action of **enzymes,** vitamins help initiate a wide variety of body responses, including energy production, use of minerals, and growth of healthy tissue.

Types and Sources of Vitamins

Discovered just after the beginning of the twentieth century, the 13 essential vitamins can be classified as *water-soluble* (capable of

---

Key Terms

proteins Compounds composed of chains of amino acids; primary components of muscle and connective tissue.

amino acids The building blocks of protein; can be manufactured by the body or obtained from dietary sources.

Dietary Reference Intakes (DRIs) Measures that refer to three types of reference values: Estimated Average Requirement, Recommended Dietary Allowance, and Tolerable Upper Intake Level.

vitamins Organic compounds that facilitate the action of enzymes.

enzymes Organic substances that control the rate of physiological reactions but are not altered in the process.

hypervitaminosis Excessive accumulation of vitamins within the body; associated with the fat-soluble vitamins.

---

being dissolved in water) or *fat-soluble* (capable of being dissolved in fat or lipid tissue). Water-soluble vitamins include the B-complex vitamins and vitamin C. Most of the excess of these water-soluble vitamins is eliminated from the body during urination. The fat-soluble vitamins are A, D, E, and K. These vitamins are stored in the body in the adipose tissue or fat with excessive intake.

Dietary Reference Intakes for Vitamins It is possible to consume and retain too many fat-soluble vitamins, particularly A and D. All the fat-soluble vitamins, however, hold the potential for toxicity if taken in amounts that far exceed Dietary Reference Intakes (see Table 5.1). Most toxicity results from the use of supplements by adults or through excessive food intake of particular sources in very small children. When toxicity develops, the condition is referred to as **hypervitaminosis.**

People often think taking megadoses of vitamins such as vitamin C can be health-enhancing, but the reverse is true. Taking large doses of vitamin C from a dietary supplement can put a strain on your kidneys, causing kidney stones and diarrhea. Too much niacin, vitamin B$_6$, and folate can also be harmful.[7]

Because water-soluble vitamins dissolve rather quickly in water, you should be cautious in the preparation of fresh fruits and vegetables. One precaution is to avoid overcooking fresh vegetables. The longer fresh vegetables are steamed or boiled, the more water-soluble vitamins will be lost. More vitamins are retained with microwave cooking and steaming than with boiling vegetables. Even soaking sliced fresh fruit or vegetables can result in the loss of vitamin C and B-complex vitamins.

To ensure an adequate vitamin intake, do not rely on bottled vitamins sold in grocery stores or health food stores. The best way is really the simplest and least expensive way: eat a variety of foods. Unless there are special circumstances, such as pregnancy, infancy, or an existing health problem, virtually everyone in our society who eats a reasonably well-rounded diet consumes appropriate levels of all vitamins. The validity of this was recently substantiated by a study of 42,000 women in which it was demonstrated that those women with a sustained history of eating a balanced diet were significantly less likely to die prematurely from a variety of chronic conditions than were those women who ate less balanced diets.[14]

Should I Take a Supplement? While conducting research to formulate the new dietary guidelines, the USDA found that most Americans are consuming too many calories but are not meeting their nutritional needs. How can this be? We eat too many nutrient-deficient foods such as junk food and not enough nutrient-dense foods (which will be discussed later in this chapter).

The USDA and the American Dietician Association recommend following the food pyramid guidelines, particularly eating 4½ cups of fruits and vegetables a day, rather than taking supplements to rectify this problem. Most Americans do not consume this amount of fruit and vegetables on a daily basis and don't meet their DRIs. We discuss the food pyramid guidelines in a later section.

Some believe that additional vitamin intake will prevent or delay the onset of chronic health conditions such as cancer and cardiovascular disease. To date there seems to be no absolute consensus regarding the effectiveness of most supplements in chronic disease prevention. This said, there is at least one well-established success story regarding vitamin supplementation. That success story is the effectiveness of folic acid supplementation in ensuring the appropriate closure of the neural tube during embryonic development, thus preventing the development of spina bifida.[15] In spite of widespread awareness of the necessity for folic acid, however, nearly one-third of women of childbearing age do not take this B vitamin on a daily basis.

The DRI for folic acid for adults is 300 to 400 μg daily; however, for pregnant women it is 600 μg a day and for lactating women it is 500 μg daily. There has been some debate about whether folic acid can prevent cardiovascular disease, cancer, and Alzheimer's disease. There still isn't enough evidence to make these claims. Some research suggests that folic acid can accelerate the spread of cancer in people with pre-cancerous or cancer cells. Vitamin B$_{12}$ deficiency is a concern for vegetarians because this vitamin is primarily obtained from liver, fish, cheese, and eggs. Anemia, disturbances in walking and balance, a loss of vibration sensation, confusion, and dementia can be caused by vitamin B$_{12}$ deficiencies. The body requires B$_{12}$ to make the protective coating surrounding the nerves, and inadequate B$_{12}$ can expose nerves to damage. B$_{12}$ can sometimes be difficult for the body to absorb. The DRI for vitamin B$_{12}$ is 2.4 μg daily and for B$_6$ is 1.3 to 1.7 mg per day. Vitamin B$_6$ deficiency can lead to anemia, fatigue, poor appetite, and diarrhea. Good sources of B$_6$ are meat, liver, cereal, grains, bananas, and nuts.

Who else might benefit from vitamin supplementation? In the opinion of nutritionists, this group might include vegans, people with limited milk intake and limited exposure to sunlight, people with lactose intolerance, and people on a severely restricted weight loss diet. Children and adolescents are another group that may benefit from vitamin D supplements. Physicians have been increasingly concerned about vitamin D deficiency owing to reduced outdoor activity and decreased milk consumption among children and adolescents. Stress, as well as soft drinks, fiber, and iron in foods, can decrease calcium absorption, and calcium is best absorbed when taken in frequent, small amounts

Table 5.1 Facts about Vitamins and Minerals

	Functions in the Body	Selected Food Sources	Adult Daily DRI*
Water-Soluble Vitamins			
Biotin	Supports the nervous system, helps form red blood cells, aids digestion and energy production	Liver, eggs, peas, beans, nuts, tomatoes; smaller amounts in fruits and meats	Men: 30 μg Women: 30 μg
Folate	Helps produce and maintain new cells, prevents a form of anemia and neural tube birth defects	Dark green leafy vegetables; legumes; oranges; bananas; enriched, fortified, and whole-grain products	Men: 400 μg Women: 400 μg UL: 1,000 μg from supplements
Niacin	Helps maintain the skin and the nervous and digestive systems, helps the body process protein and fats	Meat, fish, poultry; peanuts; beans; enriched, fortified, and whole-grain products	Men: 16 mg Women: 14 mg UL: 35 mg
Pantothenic acid	Helps form new red blood cells, helps the body process nutrients	Chicken, beef, potatoes, oats, tomato products, peas, beans, eggs, broccoli, whole grains	Men: 5 mg Women: 5 mg
Riboflavin	Helps maintain skin and create energy	Organ meats, milk, bread products, fortified cereals	Men: 1.3 mg Women: 1.1 mg
Thiamine	Supports the nervous system, aids in production of energy from carbohydrates	Enriched, fortified, and whole-grain cereals and other grain products	Men: 1.2 mg Women: 1.1 mg
Vitamin B_6	Helps form enzymes and maintain normal blood sugar levels, supports the nervous and immune systems, prevents a type of anemia	Fortified cereals, soybeans, meat, poultry, fish, bananas, carrots, potatoes, nuts	Men: 1.3 mg Women: 1.3 mg UL: 100 mg
Vitamin B_{12}	Maintains healthy nerve and red blood cells, prevents one type of anemia	Fortified cereals, meat, fish, poultry, eggs, milk	Men: 2.4 μg Women: 2.4 μg
Vitamin C	Helps form connective tissue, acts as an antioxidant, promotes wound healing and iron absorption	Citrus fruits, tomatoes, potatoes, cruciferous vegetables, green leafy vegetables, strawberries, bell peppers, tomato juice	Men: 90 mg Women: 75 mg UL: 2,000 mg
Fat-Soluble Vitamins			
Vitamin A	Aids in vision, bone growth, immunity, reproduction, and tissue repair; maintains healthy skin and mucous membranes; acts as an antioxidant	Liver, dairy products, tomatoes, fish, eggs, deep yellow and orange fruits and vegetables, dark green vegetables	Men: 900 μg Women: 700 μg UL: 3,000 μg
Vitamin D	Helps the body absorb calcium and phosphorous and build bone; supports immune function; regulates cell growth	Fatty fish, eggs, fortified milk products and cereals	Men: 5 μg Women: 5 μg UL: 50 μg 200 IU

(Continued)

and with meals. Vitamin C improves the absorption of calcium, as does the presence of estrogen (so women after menopause are at increased risk of calcium deficiency).

If you take a vitamin D supplement, look for vitamin D_3 (also called cholecalciferol) instead of vitamin D_2, which is 25 percent less potent. The DRI for vitamin D is 5 μg or 200 international units (IU) (higher for individuals over 50 years of age), with 50 μg or 2,000 IU as the Tolerable Upper Intake Level (UL). Too much calcium may cause kidney stones and may block absorption of other substances such as antibiotics.

Physicians also recommend supplementation to individual patients because of pregnancy, lactation, smoking, malnutrition, or recovery from specific conditions. Some recommend that supplements be taken with food, since they're really components of food and help the body metabolize other food components. The fat-soluble nutrients should be taken with a little oil or fat to enhance absorption. The water-soluble nutrients are easily absorbed without food but may work better when taken with meals. In addition, some people complain of stomach upset when they take vitamins on an empty stomach.

Phytochemicals

Certain physiologically active components are believed to deactivate carcinogens or function as **antioxidants.** Antioxidants are substances that may protect cells from the damage caused by unstable molecules known as

Table 5.1   Facts about Vitamins and Minerals (Continued)

	Functions in the Body	Selected Food Sources	Adult Daily DRI*
Vitamin E	Helps repair body tissues, supports immunity, acts as an antioxidant	Vegetable oils, fortified grains, seeds, nuts, tomato products, green leafy vegetables, avocados	Men: 15 mg Women: 15 mg UL: 1,000 mg
Vitamin K	Promotes normal blood clotting and bone health	Dark green leafy vegetables, cruciferous vegetables, vegetable oils, cheese	Men: 120 μg Women: 90 μg
Minerals (Selected)			
Calcium	Forms bone, aids in blood clotting and muscle and nerve function	Dairy products, calcium-set tofu, canned fish, dark green vegetables, fortified products	Men: 1,000 mg Women: 1,000 mg UL: 2,500 mg
Iron	Helps form red blood cells, enzymes, and proteins; supports energy production and the immune system; prevents a form of anemia	Meat, shellfish, poultry, legumes, fortified grain products, deep green leafy vegetables, pumpkin seeds	Men: 8 mg Women: 18 mg UL: 45 mg
Magnesium	Maintains normal muscle, nerve, and heart functions; supports immunity; helps the body produce energy; aids in bone health	Green leafy vegetables, whole grains, seeds, nuts, legumes, fish, soybeans, artichokes	Men: 420 mg Women: 320 mg UL: 350 mg from supplements
Potassium	Aids in nerve transmission and muscle function, helps regulate blood pressure	White and sweet potatoes, green leafy vegetables, winter squash, bananas, oranges, dried fruit, legumes, tomatoes	Men: 4,700 mg Women: 4,700 mg
Sodium	Maintains body fluid balance and blood pressure, aids in nerve transmission and muscle function	Processed foods, table salt, soy sauce, and other condiments; small amounts occur naturally in foods	Men: 1,500 mg Women: 1,500 mg UL: 2,300 mg
Zinc	Supports immunity; aids in tissue repair; maintains the senses of taste and smell; aids in reproduction, growth, development	Fortified cereals, red meat, poultry, certain seafood, milk, eggs, whole grains, legumes, seeds, nuts	Men: 11 mg Women: 8 mg UL: 40 mg

*For a complete listing of the Dietary Reference Intakes for all age groups and life stages, as well as information on the adverse effects of excessive consumption, visit the website for the Food and Nutrition Board, Institute of Medicine, National Academies (www.iom.edu/CMS/3788.aspx).

Sources: Food and Nutrition Board, Institute of Medicine of the National Academies. Dietary Reference Intakes (www.iom.edu/CMS/3788.aspx); U.S. Department of Health and Human Services and U.S. Department of Agriculture. Dietary Guidelines for Americans, 2005 (www.healthierus.gov/dietaryguidelines); NIH Office of Dietary Supplements, Vitamin and Mineral Supplement Fact Sheets (http://ods.od.nih.gov/Health_Information/Vitamin_and_Mineral_Supplement_Fact_Sheets.aspx).

free radicals, which can lead to cancer. Antioxidants may prevent cancer by interacting with and stabilizing free radicals. A few examples of antioxidants are beta carotene, lycopene, and vitamins C, E, and A. However, Americans' number one source of antioxidants is coffee. Chocolate, green tea, and nuts are other popular sources of antioxidants for Americans.[16] The different types of **phytochemicals** include the carotenoids (from green vegetables), polyphenols (from onions and garlic), indoles (from cruciferous vegetables), and the allyl sulfides (from garlic, chives, and onions). These phytochemicals may play an important role in sparking the body to fight and slow the development of some diseases, such as cancer. At this time, however, the exact mechanisms through which the various phytochemicals reduce the formation of cancer cells is not understood. Although it is generally agreed that these foods are important in planning food selections, no precise recommendations regarding the amounts of various phytochemical-rich plants have been made.

Key Terms

antioxidants Substances that may prevent cancer by interacting with and stabilizing unstable molecules known as free radicals.

phytochemicals Physiologically active components of foods that are believed to deactivate carcinogens and to function as antioxidants.

Minerals

Nearly 5 percent of the body is composed of inorganic materials, the *minerals*. Minerals function primarily as structural elements (in teeth, muscles, hemoglobin, and thyroid hormones). They are also critical in the regulation of a number of body processes, including fluid balance, nerve impulses, muscle contraction, heart function, blood clotting, protein synthesis, and red blood cell synthesis. Approximately 21 minerals have been recognized as being essential for human health.[1] Unlike vitamins, minerals are inorganic and can't be destroyed by heat or food processing.

Macronutrients (major minerals) are those minerals that are seen in relatively high amounts in our body tissues. Examples of macronutrients are calcium, phosphorus, sodium, potassium, and magnesium. Examples of *micronutrients*, minerals seen in relatively small amounts in body tissues, include zinc, iron, copper, selenium, and iodine. Although micronutrients **(trace elements)** are required only in small quantities, fewer than 20 mg daily of each, they are still essential. Active, menstruating women need at least 18 mg of iron daily; however, a well-balanced diet supplies around 12 mg of iron for 2,000 calories. Eating a food rich in vitamin C along with iron-rich foods will help your body efficiently utilize iron. Examples of this might be eating spaghetti with meat and tomato sauce, meat and potatoes, hamburger and coleslaw, fruit and iron-fortified cereal, or fruit with raisins.

Water and Fluids

Water may well be our most essential nutrient, since without water most people would die from **dehydration** effects in less than a week. People could survive for weeks and even years without some of the essential minerals and vitamins. More than half the body's weight comes from water. Water provides the medium for nutrient and waste transport and temperature control and plays a key role in nearly all of the body's biochemical reactions. A common indication of inadequate fluid intake is strained, uncomfortable bowel movements.

Key Terms

trace elements Minerals whose presence in the body occurs in very small amounts; micronutrient elements.

dehydration Abnormal depletion of fluids from the body; severe dehydration can be fatal.

fiber Cellulose-based plant material that cannot be digested; found in cereal, fruits, and vegetables.

Most people seldom think about the importance of an adequate intake of water and fluids. The average adult loses about 10 cups of water daily through perspiration, urination, bowel movements, and breathing. Physical activity and heat exposure contribute to water loss and an increased need for fluids. The Institute of Medicine's general recommendation for the average woman is approximately 2.7 liters (91 ounces) of total water (from all food and beverages) each day, and for the average man approximately 3.7 liters (125 ounces) daily. Recommendations for fluid intake vary with age, gender, metabolism, weight, and diet.

There are several ways to calculate how much water intake an individual requires. One simple rule is that for every pound of body weight, you need about half an ounce of fluid intake per day. Another method is to base your fluid need on your caloric intake, using the following formula: 0.034 ounce $\times$ Daily Caloric Intake = Daily Fluid Requirement in ounces.

About 80 percent of people's total water intake comes from drinking water and beverages, including caffeinated beverages, while the other 20 percent is derived from food. It is recommended to avoid beverages that are high in sugar, such as fruit juice, regular sodas, and flavored coffee drinks (see the box "Is Juice the Next Miracle Drink?"). For example, a Starbucks caramel frappuccino has 550 calories and a strawberries and crème frappuccino contains 750 calories.[17]

To see if you're drinking enough fluid, check your urine. A small amount of dark-colored urine can be an indication that you are not consuming enough fluid and need to drink more. Urine that is pale or almost colorless means you are most likely taking in enough fluids. Of course, people also obtain needed fluids from fruits, vegetables, fruit and vegetable juices, milk, and noncaffeinated soft drinks, although these can be high in sugar and calories. However, excessive water consumption by persons of any age, including forced consumption by infants, can lead to fatal brain edema (swelling) and aspiration pneumonia.[18, 19]

Fiber

Although not considered a nutrient by definition, **fiber** is an important component of sound nutrition. Fiber consists of plant material that is not digested but rather moves through the digestive tract and out of the body. Cereal, fruits, and vegetables all provide us with dietary fiber.

Fiber can be classified into two large groups on the basis of water solubility. *Insoluble* fibers are those that can absorb water from the intestinal tract. By absorbing water, the insoluble fibers give the stool bulk and decrease the time it takes the stool to move through the digestive tract. In contrast, *soluble* fiber turns to a "gel" within the intestinal tract and in so doing binds to liver bile, which has cholesterol attached. Thus, soluble fiber is valuable in removing (or lowering) blood cholesterol levels. Also, because foods high in soluble fiber are generally low in sugar and saturated fats, fiber may indirectly contribute to keeping blood sugar low[20] and reduce the risk of colon cancer associated with diets high in saturated fats, although today this latter contention is being seriously challenged.[21]

How much fiber do you need? Adults should eat between 21 and 38 g of fiber each day; however, most American adults eat only 11 g per day. Fiber has many benefits, including helping to curb your appetite and prevent overeating because it is filling, requires more chewing, stays in the stomach longer, and absorbs water, adding to the feeling of fullness. Fiber also helps to slow the absorption of sugar from the intestines, thus steadying the blood sugar and slowing down the absorption of fat from the foods you eat. Consuming adequate amounts of fiber has an important effect on reducing serious medical problems because soluble fiber lowers LDL cholesterol and protects against cardiovascular disease, whereas insoluble fiber protects against developing colon cancer.[22]

In recent years attention has been directed toward three forms of soluble fiber—oat bran, psyllium (from the weed plantain), and rice bran—for their ability to lower blood cholesterol levels and prevent heart disease.[23] To lower your total cholesterol by 5 or 6 points, daily consumption of oat bran equaling a large bowl of oat bran cold cereal or three or more packs of instant oatmeal would be necessary. One serving of bran plus one serving of beans each day will also give you more than half your total daily fiber needs. It is recommended to eat fiber from a variety of sources to obtain a good balance of soluble and insoluble fibers.

The Absorption of Nutrients

When we eat, the food is digested and then absorbed into and through the walls of the gastrointestinal (GI) tract, into the bloodstream, and is distributed to the cell sites at which it will be used for energy, growth, repair, and regulation. Figure 5-2 shows the GI tract and other organs of the digestive system. In terms of the absorption of nutrients, the first 18 inches of the small intestine make up the most active site for absorption, surpassing the level of activity in the remainder of the small intestine, the large intestine, and the stomach. Some portion of the alcohol contained in alcoholic drinks enters the body through the stomach wall (more in women than in men), although most is absorbed in the small intestine. Water and salts are principally regulated by the walls of the large intestine.

In light of the importance of the small intestine, any injury or disease in this location could seriously harm nutritional status by impairing the body's ability to obtain nutrients. Gastric bypass surgery involves cutting away a portion of small intestine to restrict the movement of nutrients into the body. Many nutrients needed for overall health must then be supplemented, often for the rest of the person's life (see Chapter 6).

Planning a Healthy Diet

Several tools, including USDA's MyPyramid and the Dietary Guidelines for Americans, are available to help you plan a diet that will provide adequate nutrients as

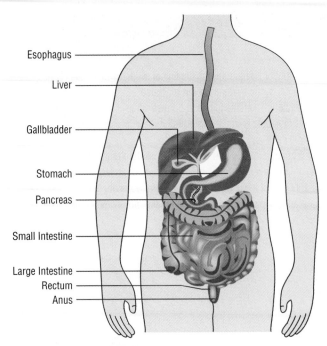

Esophagus

Liver

Gallbladder

Stomach

Pancreas

Small Intestine

Large Intestine

Rectum

Anus

Figure 5-2 The Digestive System   Food moves through the digestive tract (mouth, esophagus, stomach, large and small intestines, rectum, anus) as it is changed into substances that can be absorbed into the bloodstream for distribution to the body. The liver, pancreas, and gallbladder produce enzymes and other compounds that help digest food.

Table 5.2   Find Your Calorie Count

Gender	Age	Sedentary	Moderately active	Active
Child	2–3	1,000	1,000–1,400	1,000–1,400
Female	4–8	1,200	1,400–1,600	1,400–1,800
	9–13	1,600	1,600–2,000	1,800–2,200
	14–18	1,800	2,000	2,400
	19–30	2,000	2,000–2,200	2,400
	31–50	1,800	2,000	2,200
	51+	1,600	1,800	2,000–2,200
Male	4–8	1,400	1,400–1,600	1,600–2,000
	9–13	1,800	1,800–2,200	2,000–2,600
	14–18	2,200	2,400–2,800	2,800–3,200
	19–30	2,400	2,600–2,800	3,000
	31–50	2,200	2,400–2,600	2,800–3,000
	51+	2,000	2,200–2,400	2,400–2,800

(Activity Level spans Sedentary, Moderately active, and Active columns.)

Sedentary means a lifestyle that includes only the light physical activity associated with typical day-to-day life.
Moderately active means a lifestyle that includes physical activity equivalent to walking about 1.5 to 3 miles per day at 3 to 4 miles per hour, in addition to the light physical activity associated with typical day-to-day life.
Active means a lifestyle that includes physical activity equivalent to walking more than 3 miles per day at 3 to 4 miles per hour, in addition to the light physical activity associated with typical day-to-day life.

Source: U.S. Department of Health and Human Services and U.S. Department of Agriculture. Dietary Guidelines for Americans, 2005 (www.healthierus .gov/dietaryguidelines).

well as reduce your risk of developing heart disease, cancer, and other chronic diseases.[24]

The USDA Food Guide: MyPyramid

The most effective way to take in adequate amounts of nutrients is to eat a balanced diet as outlined by the USDA's most current guidelines.[25] The latest version of the USDA food group plan is called MyPyramid (Figure 5-3). The colors and sizes of the bands in the pyramid reflect the proportion of each food group that people generally need to consume each day. The steps signify the importance of daily exercise.

MyPyramid takes a personalized approach by acknowledging that people have different energy and nutrient needs based on their age, gender, and physical activities. Table 5.2 can help you identify a daily calorie level that is appropriate for you. Based on your calorie needs, you can apply one of MyPyramid's 12 sets of food intake recommendations (Table 5.3, page 128). For additional help in finding the MyPyramid plan that's right for you, and for online evaluation and tracking of your food intake and physical activity, visit the MyPyramid website (MyPyramid.gov). The "Rate Your Plate" Personal Assessment at the end of this chapter will also help you evaluate your current eating habits.

Each food group in MyPyramid is briefly described following, with advice on identifying portion sizes and making good choices within the group.

Fruits   The new guidelines suggest eating 2 cups of fruits per day for a 2,000 calorie/day adult diet. One medium-sized fruit, ½ cup dried fruit, or 1 cup of fresh, frozen, or canned fruit is equivalent to 1 cup. Orange fruits such as mango, cantaloupe, apricots, and red or pink grapefruit provide sources of vitamin A. Kiwi, strawberries, guava, papaya, cantaloupe, and citrus fruits are good sources of vitamin C. Oranges and orange juice also provide folate. Some good sources for potassium are bananas, plantains, dried fruits, oranges and orange juice, cantaloupe and honeydew melons, and tomato products. For the majority of your fruit intake, it is generally recommended to consume whole fruits and avoid fruit juices to ensure adequate fiber and to avoid the high sugar content associated with fruit juices. The American Cancer Society indicates that this food group may play an important role in the prevention of certain forms of cancer.[26]

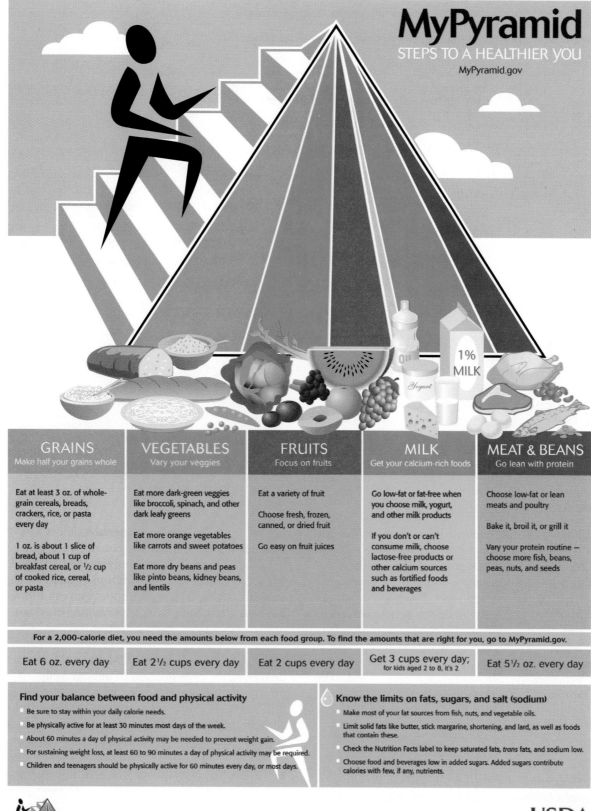

GRAINS
Make half your grains whole

VEGETABLES
Vary your veggies

FRUITS
Focus on fruits

MILK
Get your calcium-rich foods

MEAT & BEANS
Go lean with protein

Eat at least 3 oz. of whole-grain cereals, breads, crackers, rice, or pasta every day

1 oz. is about 1 slice of bread, about 1 cup of breakfast cereal, or ½ cup of cooked rice, cereal, or pasta

Eat more dark-green veggies like broccoli, spinach, and other dark leafy greens

Eat more orange vegetables like carrots and sweet potatoes

Eat more dry beans and peas like pinto beans, kidney beans, and lentils

Eat a variety of fruit

Choose fresh, frozen, canned, or dried fruit

Go easy on fruit juices

Go low-fat or fat-free when you choose milk, yogurt, and other milk products

If you don't or can't consume milk, choose lactose-free products or other calcium sources such as fortified foods and beverages

Choose low-fat or lean meats and poultry

Bake it, broil it, or grill it

Vary your protein routine — choose more fish, beans, peas, nuts, and seeds

For a 2,000-calorie diet, you need the amounts below from each food group. To find the amounts that are right for you, go to MyPyramid.gov.

| Eat 6 oz. every day | Eat 2½ cups every day | Eat 2 cups every day | Get 3 cups every day; for kids aged 2 to 8, it's 2 | Eat 5½ oz. every day |

Find your balance between food and physical activity
- Be sure to stay within your daily calorie needs.
- Be physically active for at least 30 minutes most days of the week.
- About 60 minutes a day of physical activity may be needed to prevent weight gain.
- For sustaining weight loss, at least 60 to 90 minutes a day of physical activity may be required.
- Children and teenagers should be physically active for 60 minutes every day, or most days.

Know the limits on fats, sugars, and salt (sodium)
- Make most of your fat sources from fish, nuts, and vegetable oils.
- Limit solid fats like butter, stick margarine, shortening, and lard, as well as foods that contain these.
- Check the Nutrition Facts label to keep saturated fats, *trans* fats, and sodium low.
- Choose food and beverages low in added sugars. Added sugars contribute calories with few, if any, nutrients.

U.S. Department of Agriculture
Center for Nutrition Policy and Promotion
April 2005
CNPP-15

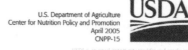

USDA is an equal opportunity provider and employer.

Figure 5-3 MyPyramid   The USDA food guide emphasizes a personal approach to healthy eating; specific pyramids at 12 different calorie levels are available at MyPyramid.gov.

Table 5.3 USDA Food Guide at Six Different Calorie Levels

Daily Amount of Food from Each Group (vegetable subgroup amounts are per week)

Calorie Level	1,200	1,600	2,000	2,400	2,800	3,200
Food Group	Food group amounts shown in cup (c) or ounce-equivalents (oz-eq), with number of servings (srv) in parentheses when it differs from the other units. Oils are shown in grams (g).					
Fruits	1 c (2 srv)	1.5 c (3 srv)	2 c (4 srv)	2 c (4 srv)	2.5 c (5 srv)	2.5 c (5 srv)
Vegetables	1.5 c (3 srv)	2 c (4 srv)	2.5 c (5 srv)	3 c (6 srv)	3.5 c (7 srv)	4 c (8 srv)
Dark green veg.	1.5 c/wk	2 c/wk	3 c/wk	3 c/wk	3 c/wk	3 c/wk
Orange veg.	1 c/wk	1.5 c/wk	2 c/wk	2 c/wk	2.5 c/wk	2.5 c/wk
Legumes	1 c/wk	2.5 c/wk	3 c/wk	3 c/wk	3.5 c/wk	3.5 c/wk
Starchy veg.	2.5 c/wk	2.5 c/wk	3 c/wk	6 c/wk	7 c/wk	9 c/wk
Other veg.	4.5 c/wk	5.5 c/wk	6.5 c/wk	7 c/wk	8.5 c/wk	10 c/wk
Grains	4 oz-eq	5 oz-eq	6 oz-eq	8 oz-eq	10 oz-eq	10 oz-eq
Whole grains	2	3	3	4	5	5
Other grains	2	2.5	3	4	5	5
Lean meat and beans	3 oz-eq	5 oz-eq	5.5 oz-eq	6.5 oz-eq	7 oz-eq	7 oz-eq
Milk	2 c	3 c	3 c	3 c	3 c	3 c
Oils	17 g	22 g	27 g	31 g	36 g	51 g
Discretionary calorie allowance	171	182	267	362	426	648

Source: U.S. Department of Health and Human Services and U.S. Department of Agriculture. Dietary Guidelines for Americans, 2005 (www.healthierus.gov/dietaryguidelines).

Vegetables Two and one-half cups of vegetables per day is the recommendation for adults following a 2,000-calorie diet. As with the fruit group, the important function of this group is to provide vitamin A, vitamin C, complex carbohydrates, and fiber. Because Americans tend to eat only a few vegetables, such as potatoes, corn, and carrots, the new guidelines give specific recommendations about the types of vegetable. One general rule is to "eat your colors," meaning you should consume a variety of vegetables over the course of a week. The USDA recommends the following:

- Dark green vegetables (such as broccoli, spinach)— 3 cups/week
- Orange vegetables (such as carrots, sweet potatoes)—2 cups/week
- Legumes (such as soy, kidney, lentil, pinto beans)— 3 cups/week
- Starchy vegetables (such as corn, potatoes, green peas)—3 cups/week
- Other vegetables (such as cauliflower, asparagus, celery)—6½ cups/week

Again, avoid drinking vegetable juices as a way of meeting these requirements because they can be high in salt and sugar and don't provide the fiber intake that whole vegetables do. **Cruciferous vegetables,** such as broccoli, cabbage, brussels sprouts, and cauliflower, may be particularly helpful in the prevention of certain forms of cancer.[26]

Milk and Milk Products MyPyramid recommends increasing the consumption of milk to 3 cups of fat-free or low-fat milk each day, or its equivalent in another milk product. Milk consumption has been associated with higher bone density and can help fight osteoporosis.[27] Calcium and high-quality protein, required for bone and tooth development, are two primary nutritional benefits provided by this food group. The guidelines further suggest that children 2 to 8 years old should consume 2 cups per day of fat-free or low-fat milk, or equivalent milk products, whereas children 9 years of age and older should consume 3 cups per day of fat-free or low-fat milk, or equivalent milk products. Milk, cheese, yogurt, and ice cream are included in this food group. For individuals who are lactose-intolerant (lactose upsets

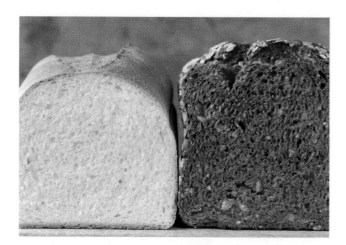

MyPyramid recommends that half of all grain servings come from whole grains. Because whole grains can't always be identified by color, it is important to check food labels for whole-grain content.

their intestines) or are vegan (vegetarians who don't consume any animal products, including dairy products), soybeans, tofu, spinach, kale, okra, beet greens, and oatmeal are good alternative sources of calcium.

Meat, Poultry, Fish, Eggs, Dry Beans, and Nuts   Our need for selections from this protein-rich group is based on our daily need for protein, iron, and the B vitamins. Meats include all red meat (beef, pork, and game), fish, and poultry. It is strongly recommended that we choose lean meats and low-fat or fat-free foods in this group. Meat substitutes include dry beans, eggs, tofu, peanut butter, nuts, and seeds. For a 2,000-calorie diet, MyPyramid recommends that adults eat 5½ ounces of meat or protein foods each day. One ounce is equivalent to the following:

- 1 ounce cooked lean meat, poultry, or fish
- 1 egg
- ¼ cup cooked dry beans
- ¼ cup tofu
- 1 tablespoon peanut butter
- ½ ounce nuts or seeds

The fat content of meat varies considerably. Some forms of meat yield only 1 percent fat, whereas others may be as high as 40 percent fat. Poultry and fish are generally significantly lower in overall fat than are red meats. Interestingly, the higher the grade of red meat, the more fat is marbled throughout the muscle fiber. People may find that higher-grade steak usually tastes better, but that is because of its higher fat content.

Meats are generally excellent sources of iron. Iron is present in much greater amounts in red meats and organ meats (liver, kidney, and heart) than in poultry and fish. Iron plays a critically important role in hemoglobin

synthesis on red blood cells and thus is an important contributor to physical fitness (see Chapter 4) and overall cardiovascular health (see Chapter 10). However, meat and fish should be fresh, stored appropriately, and cooked adequately to reduce the likelihood of serious foodborne illnesses. This will be discussed later in this chapter.

Breads, Cereals, Rice, and Pasta   The nutritional benefit from the breads, cereals, rice, and pasta group lies in its contribution of B-complex vitamins and energy from complex carbohydrates. Some nutritionists believe that foods from this group promote protein intake, since many of them are prepared as complete-protein foods—for example, macaroni and cheese, cereal and milk, and bread and meat sandwiches.

This group is referred to as the "grain group" by the USDA, and there is a particular emphasis on consuming at least 3 of the 6 ounces of this group from whole grains. Whole grains can reduce the risk of chronic disease and help with weight maintenance.

Whole grains consist of the entire grain seed, or the kernel, and can't be identified by the color of the food. The FDA requires that food contain 51 percent or more whole-grain ingredients by weight and be low-fat in order to be called "whole grain." On food labels, "whole grain" should be the first ingredient listed. Avoid refined grains because the grain-refining process typically removes most of the bran and some of the germ, resulting in the loss of dietary fiber, minerals, vitamins, and other important nutrients. Wheat flour, enriched flour, and degerminated cornmeal are not whole grains.

Reading and understanding what labels mean is important when you are trying to meet your whole-grain requirements. Optimally you would want the label to say "100% whole grain," meaning there is no refined flour in the food. If it says "Made with whole grain," then it has some whole grain but you don't know how much. "A good source of whole grain" indicates the food may have as little as 8 grams of whole grain per serving, and "An excellent source of whole grain" means as little as 16 grams per serving. "Multigrain" is a mixture of grains that is mostly refined grain with some whole grains sprinkled in. Some products are labeled **enriched,** meaning that

> **Key Terms**
>
> **cruciferous vegetables**   Vegetables, such as broccoli, whose plants have flowers with four leaves in the pattern of a cross.
>
> **enriched**   Foods that have been resupplied with some of the nutritional elements (B vitamins and iron) removed during processing.

some of the nutritional elements that were removed during processing are returned to the food; however, only three B vitamins (thiamine, niacin, riboflavin) and iron are replaced.

For a 2,000-calorie diet, MyPyramid recommends 6 ounces of grains daily, with at least 3 ounces coming from whole grains. One ounce is equivalent to

- 1 slice bread
- 1 cup dry cereal
- ½ cup cooked rice, pasta, cereal

The food industry has risen to the challenge of providing nutritious whole-grain foods with improved taste and texture. For example, ConAgra has spent millions of dollars to develop "white wheat" made from a naturally occurring albino variety of flour. It has 3½ times more dietary fiber, 11 times more vitamin E, 5 times more magnesium, and 4 times more niacin than does refined, unenriched wheat flour. It also tastes milder and sweeter than most whole grains do. It combines the best of both worlds—the nutrition of whole wheat with the taste of white flour.[28]

Oils The USDA defines oils as fats that are liquid at room temperature, such as vegetable oils used in cooking. Oils come from many different plants and from fish. Some common oils are canola oil, corn oil, cottonseed oil, olive oil, safflower oil, soybean oil, and sunflower oil. Canola and olive oil are preferred over other types of oils. Some foods, such as nuts, olives, fish, and avocados, are naturally high in oils. Foods that are mainly oil include mayonnaise, salad dressings, and soft margarine with no trans fats. A limit of 24 grams, or 6 teaspoons, of oils is the daily recommendation. One teaspoon is equal to

- 1 teaspoon margarine
- 1 tablespoon low-fat mayonnaise
- 2 tablespoons light salad dressing
- 1 teaspoon vegetable oil

Discretionary Calories Where do such items as beer, butter, candy, sodas, cookies, corn chips, and pastries fit into your diet? Most of these items contribute relatively little to healthful nutrition; they provide additional calories, generally from sucrose and significant amounts of salt and fat. Fats, salt, sugar, and alcohol are referred to as "discretionary calories" and are limited to 100 to 300 calories a day by the MyPyramid food guide. As described earlier in this chapter, the recommended total daily fat intake should be 20 to 35 percent of total calories, with most fats coming from sources of polyunsaturated and monounsaturated fatty acids. Less than 10 percent of total calories should be from saturated fats, and less than 300 mg/day should come from cholesterol. Trans-fatty acid consumption is to be kept to 2 grams or less daily.

Table 5.4 Sample Menu for a 2,000-Calorie Food Plan
Breakfast
1 cup cold cereal topped with 1 cup fat-free milk and 1 small banana
1 slice whole-wheat toast with 1 teaspoon soft margarine
1 cup orange juice
Lunch
Tuna sandwich (2 slices rye bread, 3 ounces water-packed tuna, 2 teaspoons mayonnaise, 1 tablespoon diced celery, ¼ cup romaine lettuce, and 2 tomato slices)
1 medium pear
1 cup fat-free milk
Dinner
3-ounce boneless, skinless chicken breast
1 baked sweet potato
½ cup peas with onions with 1 teaspoon soft margarine
1 whole-wheat dinner roll (1 ounce) with 1 teaspoon soft margarine
1 cup leafy greens salad with 1 tablespoon sunflower oil and vinegar dressing
Snacks
1 cup low-fat fruited yogurt
¼ cup dried apricots
Source: MyPyramid.gov.

The USDA also suggests that we choose and prepare foods and beverages with little added sugars or caloric sweeteners. The new food guide recommends no more than 8 teaspoons of added sugars per day, which is equivalent to ½ ounce of jelly beans or an 8-ounce glass of lemonade. Eating too much sugar has been thought to be a major contributor to the increase in obesity in Americans.

Table 5.4 provides a sample 2,000-calorie menu based on the MyPyramid food guide.

Dietary Guidelines for Americans 2005

The Dietary Guidelines for Americans are science-based and summarize the analysis of the most current information regarding nutrition, health, physical activity, and food safety. The goal of these guidelines is to lower the risk of chronic disease and promote health through diet and physical activity. Taken together, these guidelines encourage Americans to eat fewer calories, make wiser food choices, and be more physically active.

Focus on Nutrient Density Many Americans consume too many calories and too much saturated and trans fat, cholesterol, added sugar, and sodium. At the same time, many people do not meet the recommended intakes for

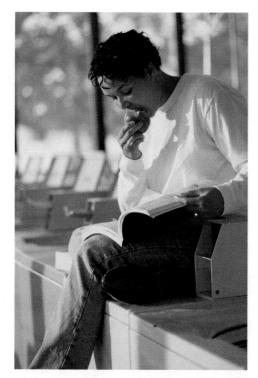

The Dietary Guidelines for Americans recommend that we increase our intake of fruits, vegetables, whole grains, and fat-free or low-fat dairy products. Fruit can be easily incorporated into the daily diet as part of a meal or as a snack.

fiber and a number of vitamins and minerals. Therefore, people should choose mostly **nutrient-dense foods,** which provide substantial amounts of vitamins and minerals and comparatively few calories. Junk foods typically are not nutrient-dense because they are high in sugar and saturated and trans fat, high in calories, and low in vitamins and minerals. Choosing nutrient-dense foods can be especially challenging when eating out.

Following the recommendations in the MyPyramid plan can help you choose nutrient-dense foods. In general, Americans are advised to consume more dark green and orange vegetables, legumes, fruits, whole grains, and low-fat milk and milk products. These choices can be substituted for refined grains and foods high in fat (especially saturated and trans fats), added sugars, and calories. Meet your dietary needs by consuming healthy food choices, not dietary supplements.

Physical Activity Of course, part of managing your weight in a healthy manner includes physical activity. The Dietary Guidelines have emphasized the important role that physical activity plays in our lives by including it in the food pyramid. It is proposed that Americans engage in at least 30 minutes of moderate-intensity physical activity, in addition to the usual activities of daily life, at work or home on most days of the week to reduce the risk of chronic disease. However, to prevent gradual, unhealthy weight gain in adulthood, we are advised to engage in approximately 60 minutes of moderate- to vigorous-intensity activity on most days of the week while not exceeding caloric intake requirements. To lose weight, you need to spend 60 to 90 minutes each day in physical fitness activities, which include cardiovascular conditioning, stretching exercises for flexibility, and resistance exercises or calisthenics for muscle strength and endurance (see Chapter 4).

Weight Management The Dietary Guidelines for Americans define weight management as meaning "to maintain body weight in a healthy range, balance calories from foods and beverages with calories expended, and to prevent gradual weight gain over time, make small decreases in food and beverage calories and increase physical activity." The dietary guidelines were designed with the goal of weight management in mind, and the recommendations for the different food groups were developed to reach this goal. Chapter 6 will go into further detail on how to identify a healthy weight and manage your weight effectively.

Food Groups to Encourage: Fruits, Vegetables, and Milk Americans are advised to consume more fiber-rich whole grains, fruits and vegetables, and milk products. Specifically, it is suggested that we consume 3 to 6 ounce-equivalents of whole-grain products per day, with the rest of the recommended grains coming from enriched or whole-grain products. In general, at least half the grains should come from whole grains. Americans are also encouraged to choose a variety of fruits and vegetables, selecting from all four vegetable subgroups: dark green, orange, legumes, and starchy vegetables. Drinking three cups of fat-free or low-fat milk or the equivalent is also encouraged, especially because milk consumption has been decreasing over the past 30 years.

Foods to Limit: Fats, Sugars, Sodium, and Alcohol

Choose Your Fats Wisely According to the USDA, we should limit our total fat intake to 20 to 35 percent of calories, with most fat calories coming from polyunsaturated and monounsaturated fatty acids. Less than 10 percent of our calories should come from saturated fatty acids, keeping our consumption of trans-fatty acids to 2 grams or less daily. Also, we need to limit our cholesterol intake to less than 300 mg/day, getting our protein from low-fat, fat-free, or lean meat, poultry, milk, and bean products.

> **Key Terms**
>
> **nutrient-dense foods** Foods that provide substantial amounts of vitamins and minerals and comparatively few calories.

Sugar Consumption   The Dietary Guidelines for Americans suggest that we choose and prepare foods and beverages with little added sugar or noncaloric sweeteners. Shopping for foods that limit sugar (and fat) can be a challenge, however; see the box "If You See It, You Will Buy It."

Sodium Intake   Something new to the USDA guidelines is the limitation on salt intake. They advise consuming less than 2,300 mg, or 1 teaspoon, of sodium each day and to choose and prepare foods with little salt. Most of our salt intake comes from processed or prepared foods. Many people are unaware of the high sodium content in prepared foods, sauces, soups, and canned foods, and so reading the labels for ingredients is extremely important. You might be surprised by some of the foods that contain salt—cookies, minute rice, canned green beans, soft drinks, and cereal. It is also difficult to know how to make healthy choices when eating out if you don't know the sodium content in the menu items. Too much sodium is linked to hypertension, and about 30 percent of Americans have sodium-sensitive high blood pressure, which can lead to heart attack or stroke. A study showed that a low-sodium diet reduced the risk of cardiovascular disease by 25 to 30 percent.[29] It is estimated that about 150,000 deaths each year are caused by consumption of too much salt.

Alcohol Consumption   Another difference in the current dietary guidelines is the recommendation concerning alcohol consumption. The USDA states that "those who choose to drink alcoholic beverages should do so sensibly and in moderation." *Moderation* is defined as the consumption of up to one drink per day for women and up to two drinks per day for men. One drink is defined

Table 5.5 DASH Eating Plan

Food Groups	Servings/day		
	1,600 calories/day	2,600 calories/day	3,100 calories/day
Grains*	6	10–11	12–13
Vegetables	3–4	5–6	6
Fruits	4	5–6	6
Fat-free or low-fat milk and milk products	2–3	3	3–4
Lean meats, poultry, and fish	3–6	6	6–9
Nuts, seeds, and legumes	3/week	1	1
Fats and oils	2	3	4
Sweets and added sugars	0	Less than 2	Less than 2

*Whole grains are recommended for most grain servings as a good source of fiber and nutrients.

Source: National Heart, Lung, and Blood Institute. Your Guide to Lowering Your Blood Pressure with DASH, 2006 (www.nhlbi.nih.gov/health/public/heart/hbp/dash/how-make-dash.html).

as either 12 fluid ounces of regular beer, 5 fluid ounces of wine, or 1½ fluid ounces of 80-proof distilled spirits. Because alcoholic beverages tend to contribute calories but little nutrition, they are counterproductive to taking in sufficient nutrients while not going over the daily caloric allotment. However, there are some indications that moderate alcohol consumption, such as having a glass of red wine each day, decreases the risk of coronary heart disease.

Food Safety   Food safety has become a more prominent issue with the recent *E. coli* outbreaks, mad cow disease, and concerns about bird flu in poultry. The dietary guidelines suggest commonsense safety measures, such as making sure your hands and work surfaces are clean before you prepare food. Food should be cooked or chilled at appropriate temperatures (see the section on food safety on page 143). It is further suggested that we *not* wash meat or poultry prior to preparing them, which is the opposite of what has been advised in the past. Avoid unpasteurized juices, milk, and milk products; raw or partially cooked eggs, or foods containing raw eggs; undercooked meat and poultry; and raw sprouts. This will be discussed in more detail in the food safety section later in this chapter.

Recommendations for Special Populations   There are also some special recommendations for specific population groups. For people over 50, consuming vitamin B_{12} in its crystalline form (such as fortified foods or supplements) is recommended. Women of childbearing age need to eat iron-rich plant food or iron-fortified food with an enhancer for iron absorption, such as vitamin-C-rich foods. Taking in adequate amounts of folic acid daily from fortified foods or supplements is important

for pregnant women and women who may become pregnant. Older adults, people with dark skin, and those not exposed to enough sunlight need to consume extra vitamin D from vitamin-D-fortified foods or supplements.

Dietary modifications may also be recommended for athletes and other active individuals.

Additional Eating Plans and Recommendations

Other eating plans are consistent with the Dietary Guidelines for Americans and appropriate for different groups. This section describes the DASH diet, introduces different types of vegetarian diets, and provides nutritional guidelines for older adults. The box "Diverse Food Pyramids" describes food group plans based on different ethnic dietary patterns.

Dietary Approaches to Stop Hypertension (DASH)
The DASH diet is not a weight loss program but an example of how to eat in accordance with the Dietary Guidelines for Americans. The DASH diet is constructed across a range of calorie levels to meet the needs of various age and gender groups. Originally developed to study the effects of an eating pattern on the prevention and treatment of hypertension, DASH is a balanced eating plan consistent with the USDA's dietary guidelines. You can view examples of the DASH program on the National Institutes of Health website at www.nhlbi.nih.gov/health/public/heart/hbp/dash. Table 5.5 also shows how the DASH diet varies by caloric intake requirements. A 25-year study of 88,000 women showed that those who followed the DASH diet were 24 percent less likely to have a stroke than were those women who didn't follow it.

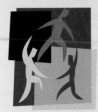

Learning from Our Diversity

Diverse Food Pyramids

Besides MyPyramid discussed earlier in this chapter, other food pyramids exist. The Mediterranean food pyramid emphasizes fruits, beans, legumes, nuts, vegetables, whole grains, and breads. In fact, the latest version of the USDA pyramid and dietary guidelines are in keeping with what had already been suggested by the Mediterranean food pyramid—for example, using more olive oil, limiting consumption of alcohol, eating more whole grains, fruits, and vegetables, choosing lean meat, eating fish and shellfish, and exercising daily.

The Asian food pyramid limits meat consumption even more by recommending consumption of meat on a monthly basis and daily consumption of fish, shellfish, and dairy products. The Asian diet,

like the Mediterranean diet, encourages daily intake of fruit, legumes, vegetables, and whole grains. In addition, the Asian diet includes rice and noodles and suggests eating poultry, eggs, and sweets only once a week.

The Latin American food pyramid also advises consumption of meat, sweets, and eggs only once a week. Like the Asian diet, it encourages eating fish and shellfish on a daily basis, and, unlike the Mediterranean and Asian diets, it advises consumption of poultry on a daily basis. As in the other food pyramids, fruit, vegetables, beans, and whole grains are to be consumed every day, and physical exercise is emphasized by all three food pyramids.

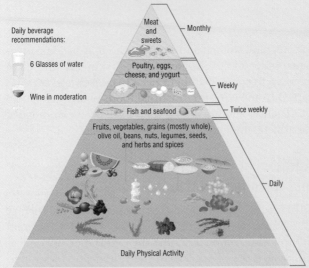

Source: © 2000 Oldways Preservation & Exchange Trust. www.oldwayspt.org

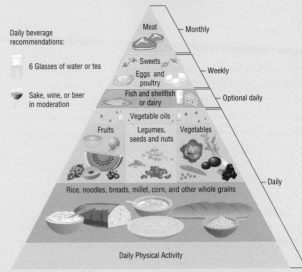

Source: © 2000 Oldways Preservation & Exchange Trust. www.oldwayspt.org

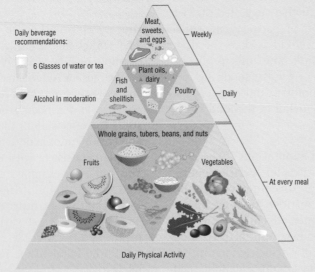

Source: © 2000 Oldways Preservation & Exchange Trust. www.oldwayspt.org

Vegetarian Diets

For some, vegetarianism is a way of eating, and for others, it is a way of life. In the sections that follow, various forms of vegetarianism will be addressed. The MyPyramid food guide described earlier in this chapter can be used as a guide for all types of vegetarian diets.

A *vegetarian diet* relies on plant sources for most of the nutrients the body needs. Studies show that vegetarians who eat a balanced diet don't seem to have any more iron-deficiency problems than do meat eaters. Although the iron in plant food is not as well absorbed as the iron in animal food is, vegetarians tend to eat more iron-containing foods and more vitamin C foods, which help with the absorption of the iron.[22] In addition, vegetarians tend to get enough calcium from dairy foods, tofu, beans, soybeans, calcium-fortified cereals, and vegetables such as broccoli. There has been some concern about a vitamin B_{12} deficiency because animal foods are the best source for B_{12} and plant foods don't naturally contain this vitamin. However, soy foods may contain vitamin B_{12}, although it is not as biologically active as the source in animal foods. Many soy products are fortified with vitamin B_{12} as well. Note also that the liver stores so much B_{12} that it would take years to become deficient in this vitamin.[22] Vegetarians tend to eat healthier diets, have lower rates of cardiovascular disease, lower blood pressure, lower levels of LDL cholesterol, less incidence of diabetes, and weigh 15 percent less than do those who eat meat. Vegetarian diets encompass a continuum from diets that allow some animal sources of nutrients to those that exclude all animal sources. We briefly describe three vegetarian diets, beginning with the least restrictive in terms of food sources.

Ovolactovegetarian Diet Depending on the particular pattern of consuming eggs (*ovo*) and milk (*lacto*) or using one but not the other, ovolactovegetarianism can be an extremely sound approach to healthful eating during the entire course of the adult years. An **ovolactovegetarian diet** provides the body with the essential amino acids while limiting the high intake of fats seen in more conventional diets. The exclusion of meat as a protein source lowers the total fat intake, while the consumption of milk or eggs allows for an adequate amount of saturated fat to remain in the diet. The consistent use of vegetable products as the primary source of nutrients supports the current dietary recommendations for an increase in overall carbohydrates, an increase in complex carbohydrates, and an increase in fiber. Most vegetarians in the United States fit into this category.

Meatlike products composed of textured vegetable protein are available in supermarkets. Nonmeat bacon strips, hamburger and chicken patties, and link sausage can be used by people who want to restrict their meat intake but still want a meatlike product. Soybeans are a primary source of this textured vegetable protein.

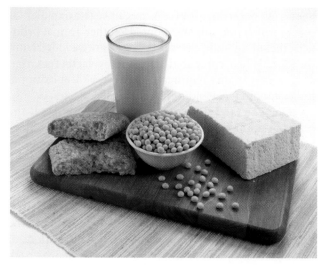

Soy foods are an important source of protein and other nutrients for vegetarians.

Vegetarians who do consume dairy products face challenges when making food choices if they wish to avoid other animal products in their food. Because most cheese is made with rennet, a coagulating agent that usually comes from stomachs of slaughtered newly born calves, many vegetarians eliminate cheese from their diet or opt for rennetless cheese. Vegetarian cheeses are manufactured using rennet from either fungal or bacterial sources. Similarly, yogurt is often made with gelatin derived from animal ligaments, skins, tendon, and bones (gelatin is also found in marshmallows, candy such as jelly beans, and candy corn, poptarts, and a variety of other foods).

It has become easier to follow a vegetarian diet since stores have begun offering organic vegetarian items that do not contain these animal products. However, it can be difficult to avoid all animal products without being an avid and knowledgeable label reader.

Lactovegetarian and Ovovegetarian Diets People who include dairy products in their diet but no other animal products, such as eggs and meat, are *lactovegetarians*. In contrast, people who exclude dairy products such as milk and cheese, yet consume eggs, are *ovovegetarians*. Both diets carry the advantages of ovolactovegetarianism.

> ### Key Terms
>
> **ovolactovegetarian diet** (**oh** voe **lack** toe veg a **ter** ee in)
> A diet that excludes all meat but does allow the consumption of eggs and dairy products.

Vegan Vegetarian Diet A **vegan vegetarian diet** is one in which not only meat but also other animal products, including milk, cheese, and eggs, are excluded from the diet. When compared with the ovolactovegetarian diet, the vegan diet requires a higher level of nutritional understanding to avoid nutritional inadequacies.

One potential difficulty is that of obtaining all the essential amino acids. Since a single plant source does not contain all the essential amino acids, the vegan must learn to consistently employ a complementary diet. By carefully combining various grains, seeds, and legumes, amino acid deficiency can be prevented.

In addition to the potential amino acid deficiency, the vegan could have some difficulty in maintaining the necessary intake of vitamin B_{12}. Possible ramifications of inadequate B_{12} intake include depression, anemia, back pain, and menstrual irregularity. Vegans often have difficulty maintaining adequate intakes of iron, zinc, and calcium.[1] Calcium intake must be monitored closely by the vegan. In addition, vitamin D deficiencies can occur. Supplements and daily exposure to sunshine will aid in maintaining adequate levels of this vitamin.

A final area of potential difficulty for the vegan is that of an insufficient caloric intake because of the satiation resulting from the nature of the diet. Early satiation caused by a large amount of fiber may lower carbohydrate intake to the point that protein stores (muscle mass) are used for energy.

When practiced knowledgeably, vegan vegetarianism is sound for virtually all people, including pregnant and breast-feeding women, infants and children, older adults, and athletes.

Semivegetarian Diets People become vegetarians for many reasons. Some avoid meat and animal products for ethical or spiritual reasons. Others choose vegetarianism for health or environmental reasons. In recent years, however, some people have found a middle ground between the two eating styles. These so-called **semivegetarians,** also referred to as "flexitarians," are increasing their intake of vegetables and cutting back greatly on meat consumption but not necessarily eliminating meat entirely. Semivegetarians add occasional servings of fish and poultry to the ovolactovegetarian diet, and some even eat red meat on occasion. **Pesco-vegetarians** eat fish, dairy products, and eggs along with plant foods.

A semivegetarian diet is much healthier than the typical meat-laden Western diet. The American Cancer Society, the American Heart Association, and the National Academy of Science all recommend dietary changes that are closely related to the typical semivegetarian diet. The health benefits of such a diet are well documented.

The semivegetarian diet may be desirable to some people because the limited consumption of meat products may help ward off some nutrient deficiencies, and such a diet can be healthier than that of the typical American.

Nutrition and the Older Adult

Nutritional needs change as adults age. Age-related alterations to the structure and function of the body are primarily responsible for this. Included among the changes that alter nutritional requirements and practices are changes in the teeth, salivary glands, taste buds, oral muscles, gastric acid production, and peristaltic action (movement of food through the gastrointestinal tract). Older adults can find food less tasteful and harder to chew. Chronic constipation resulting from changes in gastrointestinal tract function can also decrease interest in eating.[30]

The progressive lowering of the body's basal metabolism is another factor that eventually influences dietary patterns of older adults. As energy requirements fall, the body gradually senses the need for less food. This gradual recognition of lower energy needs results in a lessened food intake and loss of appetite in many older adults. Because of this decreased need for calories, nutrient density—the nutritional value of a food relative to the number of calories supplied—is an important factor for older adults. The USDA dietary guidelines make some specific suggestions for people over 50. They include consuming more vitamin B_{12}, because older people tend to have difficulty absorbing this vitamin. Older adults are also encouraged to consume extra vitamin D–fortified foods, since this vitamin may be lacking in this group.

Besides the physiological factors that influence dietary patterns among the elderly, several psychosocial factors alter the role of food in the lives of many older adults. Social isolation, depression, chronic alcohol consumption, loss of income, transportation limitations, and housing restrictions are factors in lifestyle patterns that can alter the ease and enjoyment associated with the preparation and consumption of food.

Special Nutrition Concerns: Challenges and Tools for Consumers

Food Labels

Since 1973, food manufacturers have been required by the FDA to provide nutritional information (labels) on products to which one or more nutrients have been added or for which some nutritional claim has been made. Despite the presence of these labels, there was concern about whether the public could understand the labels as they appeared and whether additional information was required. Accordingly, the FDA, in consultation with individual states and public interest groups, developed new labeling regulations. Revised labels began appearing on food packages in 1993. The currently used label is shown in Figure 5-4. Specific types of information contained on the new label are highlighted. Additionally, newly developed definitions for nutrition-related terms are shown in the box "Speaking Label-ese" on page 140.

Proposals for the labeling of raw foods, including fresh produce, meat, and seafood, are now being studied. Concern for consumer protection stems from recent disclosures regarding inadequate meat inspection, undercooking of hamburgers, and the risk of contaminated seafood. Processed meat, fish, and poultry products, such as hot dogs, fish sticks, and chicken patties, must be labeled. Produce, such as vegetables and fruit, is not required to be labeled. Currently, single-ingredient meat, fish, and poultry products are not required to have a label. In 2008 the "Country of Origin" legislation took effect requiring all fresh or frozen meats, fish, fruits, and vegetables to be identified by their country of origin. This identification may be made by using a sticker, sign, placard, or label to indicate the country of the product's origin. However, cooked and processed foods, such as frozen or cooked shrimp and smoked ham or fish, are exempt. Also exempt are foods packaged together such as frozen peas and carrots.

As of January 1, 2006, foodmakers are required by the FDA to put the amount of trans fat on food labels, sparking some companies such as Frito-Lay and Kraft to start reducing and even eliminating trans fat from their products. The FDA has further recommended that food labels list calories in larger print, list the percentage of the consumer's daily allotment of calories, and list the total amount of calories in the container, not just the calories per serving. For example, pretzels might be listed as having 100 calories per serving and approximately 15 servings per bag, leaving it up to you to compute how many servings and calories you have consumed. The FDA prohibits any nutrient claim that it has not defined. For example, the FDA redefines *low-fat* as containing 3 grams or less of fat per serving. The FDA has not yet defined what can be considered to be low-carb even though many foodmakers and restaurants use this term in their advertising. Consumers need to know what is meant by claims such as *low-calorie, low-fat,* and *low-carb;* having a standard definition makes it much easier to make healthy and informed nutritional choices.

The FDA is considering whether to add symbols to food labels to indicate whether the product is a healthy choice. PepsiCo already uses its "Smart Choice" symbol on Diet Pepsi and baked Lays' potato chips. The FDA is also urging restaurants to list calories on their menus. California and New York have passed legislation that requires restaurant chains with at least 15 stores to prominently display calorie information on their menus. Ten other states including Indiana, Maine, and Hawaii have legislation pending to follow suit. Wendy's, Taco Bell, KFC, and Pizza Hut announced they plan to post product calorie information on indoor menu boards in all of their stores by January 1, 2011, and some stores have already done so.

On January 1, 2006, the FDA began requiring food labels to clearly state if food products contain any proteins derived from any of the eight major food allergens. In addition, the Food Allergen Labeling and Consumer Protection Act of 2004 (FALCPA) requires manufacturers to clearly identify the presence of ingredients that contain protein derived from milk, eggs, fish, crustacean shellfish, tree nuts, peanuts, wheat, or soybeans in the list of ingredients or to say "contains" followed by name of the food allergen after or adjacent to the list of ingredients. This is very important for those who suffer from food allergies, and there is a discussion of this topic later in this chapter.

Fast Foods

Fast foods are convenience foods usually prepared in walk-in or drive-through restaurants. The nutritional values of fast foods can vary considerably (see Table 5.6 on page 139), and **fat density** remains a serious limitation of fast foods. In comparison to the recommended standard (20–35 percent of total calories from fat), 40 to 70 percent of the calories in fast foods are obtained from fats. The restaurant and fast-food industry has received strong criticism lately for its contribution to creating overweight Americans. In response, Wendy's, Olive Garden, Applebee's, Chili's, and some other national restaurant chains are going trans-fat-free. Table 5.6 shows how many fast foods are high in sodium and saturated and trans fat.

> ### Key Terms
>
> **vegan vegetarian diet (vee** gun *or* **vay** gun) A vegetarian diet that excludes the consumption of all animal products, including eggs and dairy products.
>
> **semivegetarian diet** Also called "flexitarian," a diet that significantly reduces but does not eliminate meat consumption and allows consumption of dairy products and eggs.
>
> **pesco-vegetarian diet** A vegetarian diet that includes fish, dairy products, and eggs along with plant foods.
>
> **fat density** The percentage of a food's total calories that are derived from fat; above 30 percent reflects high fat density.

Nutrition Facts

Serving Size 1 cup (228g)
Servings Per Container 2

Amount Per Serving

Calories 250	Calories from Fat 110

	% Daily Value*
Total Fat 12g	18%
Saturated Fat 3g	15%
Trans Fat 3g	
Cholesterol 30mg	10%
Sodium 470mg	20%
Potassium 700mg	20%
Total Carbohydrate 31g	10%
Dietary Fiber 0g	0%
Sugars 5g	
Protein 5g	
Vitamin A	4%
Vitamin C	2%
Calcium	20%
Iron	4%

* Percent Daily Values are based on a 2,000 calorie diet. Your Daily Values may be higher or lower depending on your calorie needs.

	Calories:	2,000	2,500
Total Fat	Less than	65g	80g
Sat Fat	Less than	20g	25g
Cholesterol	Less than	300mg	300mg
Sodium	Less than	2,400mg	2,400mg
Total Carbohydrate		300g	375g
Dietary Fiber		25g	30g

Check the serving size and number of servings.

• The Nutrition Facts Label information is based on ONE serving, but many packages contain more. Look at the serving size and how many servings you are actually consuming. If you double the servings you eat, you double the calories and nutrients, including the % DVs.

• When you compare calories and nutrients between brands, check to see if the serving size is the same.

Calories count, so pay attention to the amount.

• Fat-free doesn't mean calorie-free. Lower-fat items may have as many calories as full-fat versions.

• If the label lists that 1 serving equals 3 cookies and 100 calories, and you eat 6 cookies, you've eaten 2 servings, or twice the number of calories and fat.

Know your fats and reduce sodium for your health.

• The % DV for total fat includes all different kinds of fats.

• Trans fat doesn't have a % DV, but consume as little as possible because it increases your risk of heart disease.

• To help lower blood cholesterol, replace saturated and trans fats with monoun-saturated and polyunsaturated fats found in fish, nuts, and liquid vegetable oils.

• Limit sodium to help reduce your risk of high blood pressure.

Reach for healthy, wholesome carbohydrates.

• Whole grain foods can't always be identified by color or name, such as multi-grain or wheat. Look for the "whole" grain listed first in the ingredient list, such as whole wheat, brown rice, or whole oats.

• There isn't a % DV for sugar, but you can compare the sugar content in grams among products.

• Limit foods with added sugars, which add calories but not other nutrients. Make sure that added sugars are not one of the first few items in the ingredients list.

For protein, choose foods that are lower in fat.

• When choosing a food for its protein content, such as meat, poultry, dry beans, milk and milk products, make choices that are lean, low-fat, or fat-free.

Look for foods that are rich in these nutrients.

• Some Americans don't get enough vitamins A and C, potassium, calcium, and iron, so choose the brand with the higher % DV for these nutrients.

• Get the most nutrition for your calories—compare the calories to the nutrients you would be getting to make a healthier food choice.

The % Daily Value is a key to a balanced diet.

The % DV is a general guide to help you link nutrients in a serving of food to their contribution to your total daily diet. It can help you determine if a food is high or low in a nutrient—5% or less is low, 20% or more is high. You can use the % DV to make dietary trade-offs with other foods throughout the day. The * is a reminder that the % DV is based on a 2,000-calorie diet. You may need more or less, but the % DV is still a helpful gauge.

Figure 5-4 Nutrition Facts Label
Source: U.S. Department of Agriculture, Nutrition Facts Label, August 2006.

Although many fast-food restaurants have broadened their menus to include whole-wheat breads and rolls, salad bars, fruit, and low-fat milk, a recent study showed that those who said they ate out at fast-food restaurants at least twice a week gained 10 pounds more than those who did not. Another study showed that most people underestimate how many calories they have eaten when they eat fast food, often by as much as 681 calories. Also, sit-down chain restaurants such as Applebee's, Outback Steakhouse, Chili's, Cracker Barrel, Denny's, Olive Garden, and Red Lobster offer children's meals that are adult-sized in calories and fat content. For example, Ruby Tuesday's Colossal burger has 1,940 calories and 141 grams of fat. Applebee's Southwest Philly roll-up with fries contains 2,231 calories with 160 grams of fat.

Table 5.6 Nutritional Facts for Popular Fast-Food Menu Items

	Calories	Total Fat (g)	Saturated Fat (g)	Trans Fat (g)	Sodium (mg)
Burgers					
McDonald's Hamburger	250	9	3.5	0.5	520
McDonald's Cheeseburger	300	12	6	0.5	750
McDonald's Quarter Pounder	410	19	7	1	730
McDonald's Quarter Pounder with Cheese	510	26	12	1.5	1,190
McDonald's Double Quarter Pounder with Cheese	740	42	19	2.5	1,380
McDonald's Big Mac	540	29	10	1.5	1,040
Burger King Hamburger	290	12	4.5	0.5	550
Burger King Cheeseburger	340	16	7	0.5	770
Burger King Whopper with Cheese	770	48	16	1.5	1,450
Burger King Veggie Burger	420	16	2.5	0	1,090
Burger King Double Stacker	920	58	19	2.5	1,090
Burger King Triple Stacker	1,160	76	27	3	1,170
Burger King Quad Stacker	1,010	70	30	3	1,800
Wendy's Single with Everything	430	20	7	1	870
Wendy's Double with Everything	700	40	16	2	1,440
Wendy's Triple with Everything	960	60	27	3.5	2,010
Chicken					
McDonald's McChicken	360	16	3	0	830
McDonald's Premium Grilled Chicken Classic Sandwich	420	10	2	0	1,190
McDonald's Premium Crispy Chicken Club Sandwich	530	17	6	0	1,470
Burger King TenderGrill Chicken Sandwich	490	21	4	0	1,220
Burger King TenderCrisp Chicken Sandwich	800	46	8	0.5	1,640
Burger King Chicken Tenders (8 piece)	370	21	4.5	0	980
Wendy's Ultimate Chicken Grill Sandwich	320	7	1.5	0	950
Wendy's Crispy Chicken Sandwich	330	14	2.5	0	680
Wendy's Chicken Nuggets (10 piece)	460	30	6	0	1,040
Fish					
McDonald's Filet-O-Fish	380	18	3.5	0	640
Burger King BIG FISH Sandwich	640	32	5	0.5	1,540
Long John Silver's Fish Sandwich	470	23	5	4.5	1,210
Long John Silver's Ultimate Fish Sandwich	530	28	8	5	1,400
Salads (without dressing)					
McDonald's Southwest Salad with Grilled Chicken	320	9	3	0	960
McDonald's Southwest Salad with Crispy Chicken	430	20	4	0	920
McDonald's Caesar Salad with Chicken	220	6	3	0	890
Burger King TenderGrill Chicken Garden Salad	220	7	3.5	0	790
Burger King TenderCrisp Chicken Garden Salad	420	23	6	0	1,080
Wendy's Mandarin Chicken Salad	550	25.5	3	0	890
Wendy's Chicken Caesar Salad	370	19.5	4	0	1,735
Wendy's Southwest Taco Salad	645	38.5	16.5	1	1,565
French Fries					
McDonald's Medium French Fries	380	19	2.5	0	270
Burger King Medium French Fries	480	23	5	0	820
Wendy's Medium French Fries	430	20	3	0	370
Desserts and Shakes					
McDonald's Chocolate Triple Thick Shake (16 ounces)	580	14	8	1	250
Burger King Chocolate Milk Shake (Medium)	670	21	13	0.5	510
Wendy's Chocolate Frosty (large)	540	13	8	0.5	370
McDonald's Fruit'n Yogurt Parfait	160	2	1	0	85
McDonald's McFlurry with M & M's Candies	620	20	12	1	190
McDonald's McFlurry with OREO Cookies	550	17	9	1	250

Visit the company websites for the most current menu items and nutritional information.

Sources: McDonald's USA Nutritional Facts for Popular Menu Items, www.mcdonalds.com, April 20, 2007; Burger King Nutritional Information, www.burgerking.com, 2009; Long John Silver's Nutritional Analysis, www.ljsilvers.com, January 2009; Wendy's U.S. Nutrition Information, www.wendys.com, February 2009.

Speaking Label-ese

Food labels constitute a language all their own, defined by government regulation. You need to learn this language and understand its terms. Here are some translations of what is meant by the labels you read:

- Calorie-free = contains less than 5 calories per serving
- Low-calorie = contains 40 calories or less per serving
- Reduced-calorie = contains at least 25 percent fewer calories than regular versions of the food do
- Lite or light = contains one-third fewer calories than do regular versions of the product or no more than half the fat of the regular version of the product
- Fat-free = contains less than 0.5 g of fat per serving
- Free = contains none or trivial amounts of a substance such as sodium, fat, cholesterol, calories, or sugars

- Low-fat = contains 3 g or less per serving
- Reduced-fat = at least 25 percent or less fat than regular versions of the food
- Cholesterol-free = contains no more than 2 mg of cholesterol and 2 g or less of saturated fat per serving
- Low saturated fat = contains 1 g or less of saturated fat per serving
- Lean = contains fewer than 10 g of fat, 4 g of saturated fat, and 95 mg of cholesterol per serving or per 100 g of food
- Fresh = unprocessed, uncooked, unfrozen
- Healthy = contains no more than 3 g of fat, including 1 g of saturated fat and 60 mg of cholesterol per serving and must also contain at least 10 percent of RDA of one of these: vitamin A, vitamin C, calcium, iron, protein, fiber. Must

contain no more than 300 mg of sodium, but there is no limit on sugar content

- Good source = serving must contain 10 to 19 percent of RDA of a particular nutrient
- High = serving contains 20 percent or more of the RDA of a particular nutrient
- More = serving contains 10 percent or more of the RDA of a particular nutrient than does the regular food to which it is being compared
- Less = contains at least 25 percent less of the nutrient to which it is being compared
- Energy = refers to any product that contains calories; so any drink, except water, can meet this definition

---

Some fast-food restaurants seem to be turning away from their healthy food offerings and reinstating high-fat and high-calorie meals. For example, Burger King has a Double Whopper with cheese containing 960 calories and 60 grams of fat, 22 of these being from trans fat. Add King Fries and a Coke for a "Meal Deal," and this totals 1,271 calories and 82 grams of fat, 68 grams from trans fat.

Hardee's has a Country Breakfast Burrito with 1,020 calories and 66 grams of fat and a Monster Thickburger with 1,400 calories and 107 grams of fat. Even Hardee's chicken salad has 1,100 calories and 83 grams of fat. Many of the "meal deals" offered by restaurants, such as Burger King's King Value Meal and Wendy's Triple with Everything and Cheese plus Great Biggie Fries and a Biggie Cola, supply more than a day's worth of calories and sodium and two days of saturated and trans fats.

Who are these restaurants appealing to with these menu items? Research shows that men ages 18 to 24 make fast-food choices based on getting the most for the least amount of money, not on nutritional value. And don't be fooled by thinking that if it's salad, it's healthy; that can be far from the truth. Wendy's Southwest Taco Salad and Chicken BLT Salad, for example, have half the daily fat allowance and one-half of the day's sodium. McDonald's Southwest Salad with Crispy Chicken has 430 calories and 20 grams of fat.

On the other side of the coin, some healthy fast-food choices are Burger King's Chicken Bites with 252 calories, Wendy's Grilled Chicken Go Wrap with 260 calories, and McDonald's Hamburger with 250 calories, and McDonald's Fruit and Yogurt Parfait (160 calories).

See the box "Eating on the Run" on page 142 for more suggestions on healthier fast-food choices.

 TALKING POINTS What fast-food restaurants are your favorites? Are you surprised at any of the information in this chapter regarding your favorite meals? Will you change your order next time you visit a fast-food restaurant?

Functional Foods

At the forefront of healthful nutrition is the identification and development of foods intended to affect a particular health problem or to improve the functional capability of the body. **Functional foods** contain not only recognized nutrients but also new or enhanced elements that impart medicinelike properties to the food. Alternative labels also exist for various subclasses of functional foods, such as *nutraceutics,* or food elements that may be packaged in forms appearing more like medications (for example, pills or capsules), and *probiotics.*[31] **Probiotics,** "for life," are living bacteria (good bugs) that are thought to help prevent disease and boost the immune system. Probiotic bacteria have been associated with the alleviation of allergies, irritable bowel, respiratory infections, and urinary infections, and with cancer prevention. They make the environment in the digestive system inhospitable for harmful bacteria (the bad bugs). More than 400 types of bacteria reside in and on our bodies and outnumber human cells 10 to 1. Yogurt is one example of a food that gives you a dose of these good bugs—*Lactobacillus bulgaricus.*

Examples of functional foods include garlic (believed to lower cholesterol), olive oil (thought to prevent heart disease), foods high in fiber (which prevent constipation and lower cholesterol), and foods rich in calcium (which help prevent osteoporosis). In addition, foods that contain high levels of vitamins A, C, and E—primarily fruits and vegetables—and provide the body with natural sources of antioxidants are functional foods.

Other functional foods are those that contain or are enriched with folic acid. These vitamin B–family foods aid in the prevention of spina bifida and other neural tube defects (see Chapter 12) and the prevention of heart disease. Foods that are rich in selenium are sometimes categorized as functional foods because of selenium's potential as an agent in cancer prevention. The FDA approved a "heart healthy" label for foods that are rich in soy protein,[32] although there is some debate about the impact soy protein has in the prevention of cardiovascular disease. All the functional foods discussed here are approved to carry **health claims** on the basis of current FDA criteria.[33] Phytosterols are another example of a functional food. Phytosterols are found in plants and help lower cholesterol levels. In the past they had been found only in margarine spreads such as Benecol and Take Control, but now they are found in Yoplait Heart Healthy Yogurt, Rice Dream Heartwise Rice Drink, and Lifetime Low-Fat Cheese.[33]

One category of functional foods being researched is vegetables that are genetically engineered to produce a specific biological element that is important to human health. An example is tomatoes that are high in lycopene. Food technologists are interested in expanding the functional food family to include a greater array of health-enhancing food items.

Dietary Supplements

Americans spend $22 billion annually on a wide array of over-the-counter (OTC) products known collectively as *dietary supplements.* These unregulated, nonprescription products are legally described as

- Products (other than tobacco) that are intended to supplement the diet, including vitamins, amino acids, minerals, glandular extracts, herbs, and other plant products such as fungi.

- Products that are intended for use by people to supplement the total daily intake of nutrients in the diet.

- Products that are intended to be ingested in tablet, capsule, soft gel, gelcap, and liquid form.

- Products that are not in themselves to be used as conventional foods or as the only items of a meal or diet.

Unlike prescription medications, dietary supplements have been available in the marketplace for years almost without restriction. However, dietary supplements now must be deemed safe for human use on the basis of information supplied to the FDA by the manufacturers. In addition, the labels on these products cannot make a direct claim, with the exception of calcium and folic acid supplements, that they can cure or prevent illnesses. However, other materials with such claims may be displayed close to the dietary supplements themselves. Further, the labels on dietary supplements must remind consumers that the FDA has not required these products to undergo the rigorous research required of prescription medications, and so the FDA cannot attest to their effectiveness. Beyond this, consumers are left to themselves to decide whether to purchase and use dietary supplements.

As we mentioned, probiotic products, dietary supplements with live bacteria, are gaining in popularity, with total sales of $937 million to date. Actimel is one of the biggest sellers, claiming to "help to strengthen your body's natural defenses" and enhance your immune system.[34]

Easily accessible to anyone, over 15,000 different dietary supplements can be purchased in grocery stores, drugstores, and discount stores, through mail-order catalogs, and over the Internet. Because of the great demand for these products, major pharmaceutical companies are now entering the dietary supplement field. Whether this trend leads to the development of more effective products, or to a greater effort on the part of the FDA to demand proof of effectiveness, remains to be seen. By definition,

---

> **Key Terms**
>
> **functional foods** Foods capable of contributing to the improvement/prevention of specific health problems.
>
> **probiotics** Living bacteria ("good bugs") that help prevent disease and strengthen the immune system.
>
> **health claims** Statements authorized by the FDA as having scientific proof of claims that a food, nutrient, or dietary supplement has an effect on a health-related condition.

Eating on the Run

I am always in a hurry and don't have time to cook, and so a lot of my meals end up being fast food. Are there better choices I can make when eating on the run?

The typical American eats about three hamburgers and four orders of French fries each week so you aren't alone. With over 300,000 fast-food restaurants in the United States, fast food is definitely part of the American lifestyle. Here are some things to consider when eating at fast-food restaurants:

- Don't supersize! Go for the "small" or "regular" size.
- Don't wait until you are starving because that leads to overeating and supersizing!
- Decide what you want to order ahead of time, and don't be swayed by "value meal" or what "looks good."
- Ask for a nutritional guide for the menu. Look at the calories, fat grams, and sodium when making your selection.
- Order grilled instead of fried chicken or fish.

- Look for the "light" choices.
- Limit your condiments. Mustard, ketchup, salsa, or low-fat or fat-free condiments and dressing are preferable to regular mayonnaise or high-fat dressings.
- For breakfast, choose cereal and milk or pancakes rather than a breakfast sandwich (which can have about 475 calories, 30 grams of fat, and 1,260 mg of sodium).
- Bring fast food from home! Buy portable foods at the grocery store to take with you that can be eaten quickly and easily such as portable yogurt, banana, apple, low-fat granola bar, or breakfast bar.
- Order low-fat or skim milk or water instead of soda.
- Go to a variety of different kinds of fast-food restaurants so you aren't eating hamburgers every day, and set a limit on how many meals you are going to eat out each week.

---

supplements are not foods but simply "supplements." Therefore, they remain free from requirements to substantiate their claims of effectiveness (as is now required for functional foods).

 TALKING POINTS A friend asks you about the advantages and disadvantages of taking a dietary supplement. What would you point out to your friend?

Food Allergies

Foods enjoyed by the vast majority of people may be harmful and even deadly to others because of their unique food allergies. For some people, peanuts, the familiar snacks once served on many plane flights, are such a food. Today, U.S. airlines are replacing peanuts with pretzels in order to provide "peanut-free" flights and to protect people known to be allergic to peanuts and peanut-based products. Many schools have already established peanut-free tables in their lunchrooms for the same purpose.

Being intolerant to certain foods is not the same as being allergic to particular foods. **Food intolerance** means that a food upsets your intestines, usually because of an enzyme deficiency. A lactase deficiency, for example, causes lactose intolerance. Lactose intolerance affects 20 percent of Caucasian Americans, 75 percent of Native Americans and African Americans, 90 percent of Asian Americans, and 50 percent of Hispanic Americans. Intolerance of gluten (found in wheat, rye, barley, and

perhaps oats) affects 1 of every 150 Americans and can cause malnutrition, premature osteoporosis, colon cancer, thyroid disease, diabetes, arthritis, miscarriage, and birth defects.

A **food allergy** mistakenly calls the body's disease-fighting immune system into action, creating unpleasant and sometimes life-threatening symptoms. Peanuts, milk, eggs, shellfish, tree nuts, fish, soy, and wheat account for 90 percent of food allergies. Food allergies in American children have increased 18 percent in the past few years, with African American and Caucasian children having more food allergies than Hispanic children have. Eight percent of children and 2 percent of adults have food allergies. For some members of this group, food-based allergies may be serious or even life threatening.

Because food allergies generally develop slowly, initial symptoms may not be fully recognized or even associated with the food. It takes three exposures to the allergic food to obtain a significant food allergy reaction. The first time a person eats a food she is allergic to, she may have little or no reaction. The second time she eats this food, she will most likely have a more observable reaction, such as breaking out in hives, itching, runny nose, burning in the mouth, and wheezing. The third exposure can bring on a full-blown reaction, which, for peanut allergies among others, can result in death within minutes. There is no cure for food allergies, and the treatment is for the food-allergic person to avoid these foods and carry an EpiPen (epinephrine) at all times.

For the first time, an experimental drug has proven highly effective against potentially deadly peanut allergies. The once-a-month shots don't cure peanut allergy, which affects about 1.5 million Americans and kills 50 to 100 people each year. Xolair, a drug currently patented for patients with asthma, may hold promise in preventing or reducing the severity of reactions for people who suffer from peanut allergy. Xolair, an anti-IgE therapy, blocks a protein called *immunoglobulin E* from causing an asthmatic reaction. Genentech and Novartis Pharmaceuticals are currently conducting clinical trials for use with people who suffer from peanut allergy in hope that anti-IgE therapy can be used to diminish or eliminate the reaction caused by peanut allergy in the same way it treats asthma. However, Xolair is not a cure or a vaccine. It just adds protection against a fatal reaction in case of accidental ingestion of peanut-containing food. Scientists also are working on treatments that could suppress peanut allergy permanently, but those developments are probably 5 to 10 years in the future.

Food Safety

Technological advances in food manufacturing and processing have done much to ensure that the food we eat is fresh and safe. Yet concern is growing that certain recent developments may also produce harmful effects on humans. For example, the preparation, handling, and storage of food; irradiation of foods; and genetic engineering of foods all contribute to the safety of our food.

Preventing Foodborne Illness

Foodborne illness or food poisoning is the result of eating contaminated food. The symptoms of food poisoning can be easily mistaken for the flu—fatigue, chills, mild fever, dizziness, headaches, upset stomach, diarrhea, and severe cramps. Illness develops within one to six hours following ingestion of the contaminated food, and recovery is fairly rapid.[35] However, new research suggests that 10 percent of people who contract food poisoning from ingesting food with *Escherichia coli* develop a life-threatening illness, hemolytic uremic syndrome, which can cause kidneys and other major organs to eventually fail. Bacteria are the culprits in most cases of food poisoning, which can be the result of food not being cooked thoroughly to destroy bacteria or not keeping food cool enough to slow their growth. In addition, nearly half of all cases of food poisoning can be prevented with proper hand washing so as to not contaminate food by viruses, parasites, or toxic chemicals. Food safety is such an important issue that the USDA incorporated it into the new dietary guidelines. Food should be refrigerated below 40°F or kept warm above 140°F. Between 40°F and 140°F, bacteria can double in number in as little as 20 minutes, so it is important to keep food at safe temperatures. (See Figure 5-5 on temperature rules for safe cooking and handling of foods.)

It is estimated that 1 of every 4 Americans is the victim of food poisoning each year, and about 5,000 of these people die. Salmonella bacteria are the most common cause of foodborne illness and are found mostly in raw or undercooked poultry, meat, eggs, fish, peanut butter, fruit, vegetables, unpasteurized milk, and even pet food. *Clostridium perfringens*, also called the "buffet germ," grows where there is little to no oxygen and grows fastest in large portions held at low or room temperatures. For this reason, buffet table servings should be replaced often and leftovers should be refrigerated quickly. Refrigerated leftovers may become harmful to eat after 3 days (Table 5.7). The old adage "If in doubt, throw it out" applies to any questionable leftovers. A third type of food poisoning is botulism, which is rare but often fatal. It is caused by home-canned or commercially canned food that hasn't been processed or stored properly. Some warning signs are swollen or dented cans or lids, cracked jars, loose lids, and clear liquids turned milky. Can you tell if meat is spoiled by looking at it? Not necessarily. Some supermarkets package their meat with carbon monoxide, which reacts with the pigment in the meat to make it redder.

The Center for Science in the Public Interest found that fruits and vegetables account for the majority of foodborne illnesses. Salads are by far the biggest culprit. The reason for this seems to be because some of the water used to irrigate and wash produce is contaminated with human and animal feces. *Escherichia coli* has historically been a harmless bacterium that resides in the guts of animals, including humans. A new and pathogenic strain called *E. coli* O157:H7 was identified in 1982 and now causes an estimated 73,000 cases of infection and 60 deaths in the United States each year. *E. coli* can be found in uncooked produce, raw milk, unpasteurized juice, contaminated water, and meat. Dozens of people contracted food poisoning from the green onions in food served at some Taco Bell restaurants in 2006. This same strain of *E. coli* was linked to the spinach that sickened 200 people in 2006. In 2009, over 600 people in 43 states were sickened by tainted peanut butter produced by the Peanut Corp of America (PCA). Twenty-three percent of these people were hospitalized and at least nine died as a result of salmonella poisoning. In its report on the PCA, the FDA found poor sanitation such as bird feces, tainted

> ### Key Terms
>
> **food intolerance** An adverse reaction to a specific food that does not involve the immune system; usually caused by an enzyme deficiency.
>
> **food allergy** A reaction in which the immune system attacks an otherwise harmless food or ingredient; allergic reactions can range from mildly unpleasant to life threatening.

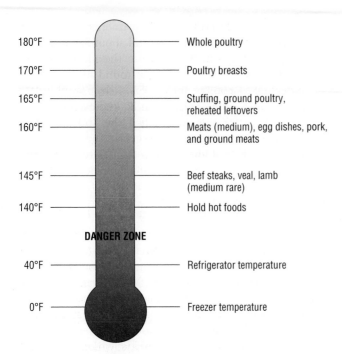

180°F	—	Whole poultry
170°F	—	Poultry breasts
165°F	—	Stuffing, ground poultry, reheated leftovers
160°F	—	Meats (medium), egg dishes, pork, and ground meats
145°F	—	Beef steaks, veal, lamb (medium rare)
140°F	—	Hold hot foods
DANGER ZONE		
40°F	—	Refrigerator temperature
0°F	—	Freezer temperature

Figure 5-5 Temperature Rules for Cooking and Safe Handling of Food Keep food out of the danger zone between 40 degrees F and 140 degrees F, in which bacteria can multiply rapidly.

Source: U.S. Department of Health and Human Services and U.S. Department of Agriculture. Dietary Guidelines for Americans, 2005 (www.healthierus. gov/dietaryguidelines).

Table 5.7 Cold Storage Limits

Apples	3 weeks
Apricots, peaches, nectarines, pears	3–4 days
Bacon	1 week
Beans, green	3–4 days
Berries, cherries	1–2 days
Butter	1–3 months
Carrots	2 weeks
Cheese, hard	3–4 weeks
Cheese, soft	1 week
Chicken or turkey (fresh)	1–2 days
Chicken or turkey (cooked)	3–4 days
Citrus fruit	1–2 weeks
Deli and vacuum-packed products	3–5 days
Eggs (fresh, in shell)	3–5 weeks
Eggs (hard cooked)	1 week
Fish or seafood (fresh)	1–2 days
Fish (cooked)	3–4 days
Fish (canned, after opening)	3–4 days
Gravy and meat broth	1–2 days
Hot dogs (after opening)	1 week
Lettuce, leaf	3–7 days
Luncheon meat (after opening)	3–5 days
Margarine	4–5 months
Mayonnaise (after opening)	2 months
Milk (after opening)	5 days
Meat (fresh, ground)	1–2 days
Meat (fresh; steak, chops, roasts)	3–5 days
Meat (cooked)	3–4 days
Pizza (cooked)	3–4 days
Soups and stews	3–4 days
Spinach	1–2 days
Yogurt	7–14 days

Sources: Food Safety and Inspection Service, U.S. Department of Agriculture. Basics for Handling Food Safely, September 2006; Food Marketing Institute. A Consumer Guide to Food Quality and Safe Handling.

water, and cockroaches accounted for the salmonella. In addition, the FDA contended that there were substandard food inspections so that the problem was not discovered and corrected quickly. In fact, the FDA issued a recall of the company's production of peanut butter from the previous two years, involving over 432 different products such as crackers, cookies, and ice cream.

This problem can be difficult to regulate or correct, because produce comes from all over the world, not just from the United States, leading to the "Country of Origin" labeling on certain foods. Even the ready-to-eat bags of produce that boast they have been "thoroughly" or "triple" washed cannot be guaranteed to be bacteria-free. Washing the produce yourself may not solve the problem, either. Produce washes such as veggie wash don't claim to kill *E. coli* but only to clean off wax, pesticides, and dirt. The best way to avoid getting sick from produce is to cook it so that you kill any remaining bacteria.

What do you do if you suspect food poisoning?

1. Contact a medical professional immediately. Don't wait to see if you feel better.
2. Report the incident to your local health department as soon as possible if the suspected food came from a public place.
3. Preserve the suspected food including any packaging to give to the health department for investigation and possible prevention of further poisoning.

Handle food properly to avoid food poisoning. Frequent handwashing is at the top of the list of food safety tips (see the box "Dos and Don'ts for Food Safety"). Bacteria live and multiply on warm, moist hands, and hands can inadvertently transport germs from one surface to another. It is also important to clean work surfaces with hot, soapy water and keep nonfood items such as the mail, newspapers, and purses off the countertops. Some people advocate the use of antibacterial products, whereas others maintain that if they are overused, these products can lose their effectiveness, and bacteria then become resistant to them. Utensils, dishes, cutting boards, cookware, and towels and sponges need to be washed in hot, soapy water and rinsed well.[36]

Food Irradiation

Because of the increasing concern about contaminated meat and meat products, the first irradiated meat, ground beef, arrived in American supermarkets in early 2000. Irradiated frozen chicken was introduced more recently. Irradiation is a process that causes damage to the DNA of

Dos and Don'ts for Food Safety

1. Do wash your hands.
2. Do put groceries away as soon as you get home and don't make other stops first.
3. Do use two different plates for raw and grilled meat.
4. Do use different spoons to stir and taste the food, and use each tasting spoon only once.
5. Do refrigerate leftovers from restaurants immediately.
6. Do use different knives to cut raw meat and chop vegetables.
7. Do store food in an airtight container. Don't store food in open cans or on uncovered dishes.
8. Do wash fresh fruits and vegetables, even if you are throwing away the rind or peels, because cutting through the produce can carry bacteria from the outside surface to the inside of the produce.
9. Don't rinse poultry or meat in water, because this can cause cross-contamination.
10. Don't thaw food on the countertop—keep it in a covered container in the refrigerator.
11. Don't leave food out of the refrigerator for too long.
12. Don't use wooden cutting boards with deep grooves or knife scars.
13. Don't marinate food at room temperature.

Source: R. Duyff, *American Dietetic Association Complete Food and Nutrition Guide*, 2nd ed. © John Wiley and Sons. This material is used by permission of John Wiley and Sons, Inc.

---

disease-causing bacteria such as salmonella and *E. coli* as well as of insects, parasites, and other organisms so that they can't reproduce. While irradiated meat has much lower bacteria levels than regular meat does, irradiation doesn't destroy all bacteria in meat. In fact, irradiation actually destroys fewer bacteria than does proper cooking.[37] The FDA recently approved irradiation of spinach and lettuce to kill *E. coli* and other germs. There is also some concern that irradiation will lull consumers into a false sense of security so that they erroneously believe that they don't have to take the usual precautions in food handling and preparation. For example, undercooking, unclean work surfaces or cooking utensils, and improper storage can still contaminate meat. Some also claim that irradiated meat has a distinct off-taste and a smell like "singed hair."

Safe Farming Techniques

In recent decades, there has been an increased push toward ensuring better treatment of animals raised for slaughter and for dairy production in the United States. As a result of recent reforms, more than half of beef cattle in North America meet their end at slaughterhouses based on innovative designs that consider the fears and inclinations of herd animals. The cages of laying hens are nearly one-third larger than the old ones were, and the practice of starving hens for weeks at a time to stimulate egg production is beginning to be phased out. These reforms are important to ensure more humane treatment of these animals, but they are also proving beneficial to human health and food quality. It has been suggested that there is an increase in the quality of meat when animals are treated humanely, with less bruising, improved tenderness, lower incidence of dark-cutting beef, and lessened occurrence of pale, soft, and dry pork. Furthermore, the taste of eggs is said to be significantly better if they come from humanely treated hens.

One important component in these reforms—some of which have been government mandated and others voluntarily adopted by the agricultural industry—relates to the feed given to beef cattle. The spread of bovine spongiform encephalopathy, more commonly known as mad cow disease, has largely been attributed to the use of animal feed containing the protein-rich by-products of slaughtered cows, including nerve tissue, the tissue most likely to harbor the disease. Such feed—which is believed to be the primary, if not the only, way the disease can be transmitted—was banned in the United States and Canada in August 1997.[35] However, from August 1997 to March 2004, 52 companies recalled 410 feed products because of suspected infectious prions, the proteins thought to spread mad cow disease. While the disease had been restricted to European cows, a number of cases of mad cow detected in American cattle in late 2003 encouraged the U.S. government to impose even stricter rules to protect the nation's beef supply from the disease, including banning the butchering of sick or injured cows, banning certain animal parts from the food supply, and increased testing on suspect animals.[38] Mad cow disease is still problematic as Canada reported its 13th case in 2008.

Eliminating animal products from feed has also proven beneficial in hens. Many consumers choose to eat only poultry and eggs from free-range, vegetarian-fed chickens, for health and safety reasons. Several companies (such as Eggland's Best) claim that their vegetarian-fed hens produce eggs that have seven times more vitamin E, are lower in cholesterol, have a higher unsaturated/saturated fat ratio, and contain more omega-3 fatty acids than do factory-farmed eggs.[39]

There has also been increasing concern about giving chickens Roxarsone (3-Nitro) because it contains arsenic. It is given to chickens to fatten the birds faster and kill microbes. Human antibiotics are also fed to chickens to increase growth, but the bacteria in the chickens' intestines can develop resistance to the antibiotics. This can result in the antibiotic-resistant bacteria being passed along to people who consume this poultry, causing them to become ill and not respond to drugs typically prescribed to treat this illness.

Organic Foods

The current USDA organic food labels went into effect in October 2002 to standardize regulations for foods grown without synthetic pesticides or other chemicals. Under the current USDA rules, organic means the following:

- Meat, poultry, and eggs are from animals given no growth hormones or antibiotics. Vitamin and mineral supplements are allowed. Livestock are given organic feed and live in conditions that allow for "exercise, freedom of movement, and reduction of stress."

- Products are not genetically engineered or irradiated to kill germs.

- Crops are grown on land that has not been fertilized with sewage sludge or chemical fertilizers.

- Pests and plant diseases are treated primarily with insect predators, traps, natural repellants, and other nonchemical methods.

- Weeds are controlled by mulching, mowing, hand weeding, or mechanical cultivation, not chemical herbicides.

There are different types of organic foods: "100 percent organic," meaning the food contains all organic ingredients; "organic," which means at least 95 percent of the product is organic; and "made with organic ingredients," which means at least 70 percent of the food is organic as previously defined.[40]

In recent years, the 24-billion-dollar organic food industry has enjoyed a 20 percent annual growth rate, much higher than that of the rest of the food industry. Almost 70 percent of people said they bought organic food at least once in the past three months. While organic foods have been found to have fewer pesticides, to create less damage to the environment, and possibly to have more nutrients, they can still contain some pesticide residue and chemical contaminants from the environment and have risk of *E. coli* contamination. See Chapter 20 for more information on the benefit of organic foods for health and food safety.

Food Additives

Food additives are substances added to food to preserve and improve its taste and appearance. Some additives are thickening agents, and some add color and prevent food from spoiling. Food additives are found in all types of foods and beverages such as meat, soup, salad dressings, peanut butter, chips, cakes, cookies, and soda. Vinegar, food coloring, artificial sweeteners, white sugar, salt, monosodium glutamate (MSG), and antioxidants are some common examples of additives. For example, emulsifiers help give peanut butter a more consistent texture and prevent separation, while stabilizers and thickeners

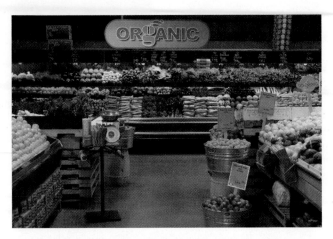

Organic products have grown in popularity in recent years and are now available in many major grocery stores.

give ice cream a smoother, more uniform texture. The three most common additives are sugar, salt, and corn syrup.[41] Food additives must undergo FDA testing and approval to ensure that the benefits outweigh any risks associated with these additives. There has been some debate about how safe some additives are despite their FDA approval. Some of the ones in question are aspartame (NutraSweet); red, blue, yellow, and green food coloring; saccharin; propyl gallate; potassium bromate; sodium nitrate; and stevia. Many of these additives have been linked with an increased risk of cancer.

Genetically Modified Foods

Biotech crops increased 20 percent in 2004, with the United States, Argentina, and Canada being the front-runners.[42] The success of American agriculture, in terms of food quality and marketability, has been based on the ability to genetically alter food sources to improve yield, reduce production costs, and introduce new food characteristics. Today, however, genetic technology is so sophisticated that changes are being introduced faster than scientists can fully evaluate their effects. For example, the genetic makeup of plant seeds and animals is being modified while scientists are still trying to determine whether human consumption of these products will be safe over extended periods. Concerned individuals and agencies in the United States and abroad are calling for more extensive long-term research into safety issues and stricter labeling requirements for genetically altered foods.[43] The label *GM* (for genetically modified) is appearing on some food items. Some food manufacturers have announced that they will discontinue the use of genetically modified ingredients in their products. The American public appears about equally divided in believing that genetically modified foods are safe (44 percent) or unsafe (20 percent) or that they are uncertain (36 percent) about the safety of such foods.[44]

In 2008 the FDA finally decided after seven years of discussion to allow the commercial use of genetically engineered animals. The FDA stated it would allow animals to be genetically altered if such animals produce drugs, serve as models for human disease, produce industrial or consumer products, or have improved food-use qualities such as being more nutritious. Animals are considered genetically altered when either their genes are changed or genes from another animal are added for a specific purpose. This regulation is consistent with legislation concerning giving drugs to animals for similar reasons.[43]

Taking Charge of Your Health

- Take the Personal Assessment "Are you feeding your feelings?" at the end of this chapter to determine if you are an emotional eater.
- Look on MyPyramid.gov to find your personal food pyramid.

- Assess your physical activity level using MyPyramid.gov.
- Keep track of your food intake for a week, using the pyramid tracker on MyPyramid.gov, and see how well your intake reflects the current dietary guidelines.

- Make one change per week in your eating patterns, such as drinking skim milk or including a new fruit or vegetable.

SUMMARY

- Carbohydrates are composed of sugar units and are the major source of energy for the body. About 45 to 65 percent of our calories should come from carbohydrates.
- Fats provide a concentrated source of energy for the body and keep us from feeling hungry. No more than 20 to 35 percent of our calories should come from fats, and most of these fats should be polyunsaturated or monounsaturated.
- Foods containing trans fats should be avoided as much as possible, and less than 10 percent of our calories should come from saturated fats, according to the current dietary guidelines.
- Protein primarily promotes growth and maintenance of body tissue, and is also a source of energy.
- Vitamins serve as catalysts for the body and are found in either water-soluble or fat-soluble forms.
- Minerals are incorporated into various tissues of the body and also participate in regulatory functions within the body.

- Adequate water and fluids are required by the body on a daily basis and are obtained from a variety of food sources, including beverages.
- Fast foods should play a limited role in daily food intake because of their high fat density, as well as their high levels of sugar and sodium.
- Preventive strategies such as hand washing and proper preparation, cooking, and storage of food can help to decrease foodborne illnesses.
- The USDA Dietary Guidelines for Americans focus on the role that trans fat, saturated fat, sugar, sodium, and alcohol play in weight management and health and disease. The current Dietary Guidelines for Americans address the importance of daily physical activity.

REVIEW QUESTIONS

1. What unique contributions do carbohydrates, fats, and protein each make to overall nutrition?
2. What role do vitamins play in the body? What is the most current perception regarding the need for vitamin supplementation?
3. What roles do minerals play in the body? What is a trace element?
4. What is the current recommendation regarding daily fluid intake? Why is water considered an essential nutrient?
5. What are the two principal forms of fiber, and how does each of them contribute to health?
6. What are functional foods, and what contribution do they make to health beyond supplying various nutrients as do all foods?

7. Identify each of the food groups in the current food pyramid. What is the additional group? Explain the nutritional benefit of each food group and the recommended daily adult allotments. What are discretionary calories?
8. What are the specific areas of nutritional concern addressed by the current Dietary Guidelines for Americans?
9. What do the current dietary guidelines suggest in terms of physical activity, and what are the benefits of such physical activity?
10. What is the principal concern regarding excessive fast-food consumption? How can food selection at a fast-food restaurant be made nutritionally healthier?

ANSWERS TO THE "WHAT DO YOU KNOW?" QUIZ

1. True   2. True   3. False   4. False   5. True   6. False   7. False

Visit the Online Learning Center (**www.mhhe.com/payne11e**), where you will find tools to help you improve your grade including practice quizzes, key terms flashcards, audio chapter summaries for your MP3 player, and many other study aids.

SOURCE NOTES

1. Wardlaw GM. *Perspectives in Nutrition* (5th ed.). New York: McGraw-Hill, 2002.
2. USDA Dietary Health. Washington DC: U.S. Department of Agriculture, August 2008.
3. *USDA Agricultural Outlook.* Washington, DC: U.S. Department of Agriculture, April 2000.
4. Can sugar substitutes make you fat? *Time Magazine,* February 2008.
5. Lichtenstein AH. Dietary trans fatty acid. *Journal of Cardiopulmonary Rehabilitation,* 20(3), 143–146, 2000.
6. Willer WC, Ascherio A. Trans Fatty Acids: Are the Effects Only Marginal? *American Journal of Public Health,* 84, 722, 1994.
7. Duyff R. *American Dietetic Association Complete Food and Nutrition Guide* (2nd ed.). Hoboken, NJ: Wiley, 2002.
8. Katan MB. Trans Fatty Acids and Plasma Lipoproteins. *Nutrition Review,* 58(6), 188–191, 2000.
9. National Institutes of Health. *Practical Guide to the Identification, Evaluation and Treatment of Overweight and Obesity in Adults.* Bethesda, MD: Author, 2001.
10. Cheskin LJ, et al. Gastrointestinal Symptoms Following Consumption of Olestra or Regular Triglyceride Potato Chips Score. *Journal of the American Medical Association,* 279(2), 150–152, 1998.
11. Wardlaw GM. *Contemporary Nutrition: Issues and Insights.* New York: McGraw-Hill, 1999.
12. Soyonara: Tough times for the miracle bean. *Nutrition Action,* October 2006.
13. National Academy of Sciences, *Dietary Reference Intakes.* Washington, DC: National Academies Press, 2004.
14. Kant AK. A Prospective Study of Diet Quality and Mortality in Women. *Journal of the American Medical Association,* 283(16), 2109–2115, 2000.
15. Czeizel AE, Dudaz I. Prevention of the First Occurrence of Neural-tube defects by Periconceptional Vitamin Supplementation. *New England Journal of Medicine,* 327(26), 1832–1835, 1992.
16. Antioxidants: Still Hazy After All These Years. *Nutrition Action,* November 2005.
17. Good Cup, Bad Cup: How to Survive in Latte Land. *Nutrition Action,* September 2006.
18. Garigan TP, Ristedt DE. Death from Hyponatremia as a Result of Acute Water Intoxication in an Army Basic Trainee. *Military Medicine,* 164(3), 234–238, 1999.
19. Arieff AI, Kronlund BA. Fatal Child Abuse by Forced Water Intoxication. *Pediatrics,* 103(6 Pt 1), 1292–1295, 1999.
20. Chandalia M, et al. Beneficial Effects of High Dietary Fiber Intake in Patients with Type 2 Diabetes Mellitus. *New England Journal of Medicine,* 342(19), 1392–1398, 2000.
21. Schatzkin A, et al. Lack of Effect of a Low-Fat, High-Fiber Diet on the Recurrence of Colorectal Adenomas. Polyp Prevention Trial Study Group. *New England Journal of Medicine,* 342(16), 1149–1215, 2000.
22. Sears W, Sears M. *The Family Nutrition Book.* New York: Little, Brown Co, 1999.
23. FDA Allows Whole Oat Foods to Make Health Claim on Reducing the Risk of Heart Disease. *FDA Talk Paper,* January 1998.
24. The Changing American Diet. *Nutrition Action,* April 2006.
25. www.health.gov/dietaryguidelines/dga, 2005.
26. American Cancer Society. *Cancer Facts and Figures—2001.* The Association, 2001.
27. Marcus E. On the Fast Track to Health. *Newsday,* p. B14, January 7, 2004.
28. Flour Power: A Slice of Multigrain Can Taste Like Bread. *USA Today,* August 9, 2004.
29. Cook N, Cutler J, Osborzanck E, Buring J, Rexrode K, Kumanyika S, et al. Long-Term Effects of Dietary Sodium Reduction on Cardiovascular Disease Outcomes: Observational Follow-Up of Trials of Hypertension Prevention (TOHP). *British Medical Journal,* 334, 385, April 2007.
30. Williams S, Schlenker E. *Essentials of Nutrients and Diet Therapy* (8th ed.). St. Louis, MO: Mosby, 2003.
31. Some Bacteria for Brunch? *U.S. News and World Report,* December 10, 2007.
32. FDA Approves New Health Claim for Soy Protein and Coronary Heart Disease [FDA talk paper]. U.S. Food and Drug Administration Center for Food Safety and Applied Nutrition. October 1999, www.fda.gov/fdac/bbs/topics/ANSWERS/ANS00980.html.
33. 10 Mega-Trends in the Supermarket. *Nutrition Action,* May 2003.
34. A Bug for What's Bugging You. *USA Today,* July 9, 2003, D-1.
35. Oppel RA, Jr. Infected Cow Old Enough to Have Eaten Now-Banned Feed. *New York Times,* December 30, 2003.
36. Rinzler C. *Nutrition for Dummics* (3rd ed.). Hoboken, NJ: Wiley, 2004.
37. The Truth About Irradiated Meat. *Consumer Reports,* 34–37, August 2003.
38. Grady D. U.S. Imposes Stricter Safety Rules for Preventing Mad Cow Disease. *New York Times,* December 31, 2003.
39. Corporate website, www.eggland.com.
40. USDA Gives Bite to Organic Label. *USA Today,* October 16, 2002.
41. Insel P, Turner E, Ross D. *Nutrition.* Sudbury, MA: Jones and Bartlett, 2002.
42. Biotech Crops Gained Ground Across Globe. *USA Today,* January 13, 2005.
43. FDA Moves on Genetically Altered Animals. *USA Today,* September 19, 2008.
44. Americans Are Iffy on Genetically Modified Foods. *USA Today,* September 18, 2003.

Personal Assessment

Rate Your Plate

Take a closer look at yourself, your current food decisions, and your lifestyle. Think about your typical eating pattern and food decisions.

Do You . . .

	Usually	Sometimes	Never
Consider nutrition when you make food choices?	❑	❑	❑
Try to eat regular meals (including breakfast), rather than skip or skimp on some?	❑	❑	❑
Choose nutritious snacks?	❑	❑	❑
Try to eat a variety of foods?	❑	❑	❑
Include new-to-you foods in meals and snacks?	❑	❑	❑
Try to balance your energy (calorie) intake with your physical activity?	❑	❑	❑

Now for the Details

Do You . . .

	Usually	Sometimes	Never
Eat at least 6 ounces of grain products daily?	❑	❑	❑
Eat at least 2½ cups of vegetables daily?	❑	❑	❑
Eat at least 2 cups of fruits daily?	❑	❑	❑
Consume at least 3 cups of milk, yogurt, or cheese daily?	❑	❑	❑
Go easy on higher fat foods?	❑	❑	❑
Go easy on sweets?	❑	❑	❑
Drink 8 or more cups of fluids daily?	❑	❑	❑
Limit alcoholic beverages (no more than 1 daily for a woman or 2 for a man)?	❑	❑	❑

Score Yourself

Usually = 2 points
Sometimes = 1 point
Never = 0 points

If you scored . . .

24 or more points—Healthful eating seems to be your fitness habit already. Still, look for ways to stick to a healthful eating plan—and to make a "good thing" even better.

16 to 23 points—You're on track. A few easy changes could help you make your overall eating plan healthier.

9 to 15 points—Sometimes you eat smart—but not often enough to be your "fitness best."

0 to 8 points—For your good health, you're wise to rethink your overall eating style. Take it gradually—step by step!

TO CARRY THIS FURTHER . . .

Whatever your score, make moves for healthful eating. Gradually turn your "nevers" into "sometimes" and your "sometimes" into "usually." Try some of the suggestions from the discussion of MyPyramid and the Dietary Guidelines for Americans.

Source: Adapted from R. Duyff, *The American Dietetic Association's Monthly Nutrition Companion: 31 Days to a Healthier Lifestyle*, Chronimed Publishing, 1997. Copyright ©1997 American Dietetic Association. Reproduced with permission of John Wiley & Sons, Inc.

Personal Assessment

Are you feeding your feelings?

Sometimes people use food as a way of coping with their emotions and problems. To identify how you might be using food as a coping strategy and what feelings you tend to associate with eating, complete the following inventory.

0 = Never
1 = Rarely
2 = Occasionally
3 = Often
4 = Always

1. ____Do you eat when you are angry?
2. ____When you feel annoyed, do you turn to food?
3. ____If someone lets you down, do you eat to comfort yourself?
4. ____When you are having a bad day, do you notice that you eat more?
5. ____Do you eat to cheer yourself up?
6. ____Do you use food as a way of avoiding tasks you don't want to do?
7. ____Do you view food as your friend when you are feeling lonely?
8. ____Is food a way for you to comfort yourself when your life seems empty?
9. ____When you are feeling upset, do you turn to food to calm yourself down?
10. ____Do you eat more when you are anxious, worried, or stressed?
11. ____Does eating help you to cope with feeling overwhelmed?
12. ____Do you eat more when you are going through big changes or transitions in your life?
13. ____Do you reward yourself with food?
14. ____When you think you have done something wrong, do you punish yourself by eating?
15. ____When you are feeling badly about yourself, do you eat more?
16. ____When you feel discouraged about your efforts to improve yourself, do you eat more, thinking "what's the use of trying"?

____TOTAL SCORE

Interpretation

If your total score is . . .

0 to 16—You don't eat to cope with your emotions. Your eating may not be related to your emotional state. However, you may avoid eating when you are upset or having trouble coping with your feelings. You may run away from food rather than running to food to cope.

17 to 47—Although you fall in the average range, you may use food to deal with specific situations or feelings such as anger, loneliness, or boredom. See the breakdown of scores below to identify how you may be using food to cope with particular feelings.

48 to 64—You run to food to cope with your emotions, and you may want to consider developing other ways of appropriately expressing your feelings.

Next, look more closely at your specific responses . . .

If you answered "3" or "4" to most of questions #1–#4, this can be indicative of eating when you are angry.

If you answered "3" or "4" to most of questions #5–#8, this can be indicative of eating when you are lonely or bored.

If you answered "3" or "4" to most of questions #9–#12, this can be an indication that you are a stress eater.

If you answered "3" or "4" to most of questions #13–#16, this can be an indication that you are using food to cope with feelings of low self-esteem and self-worth.

TO CARRY THIS FURTHER . . .

- Use the assessment scores to help you learn to recognize the triggers for your emotional eating.
- Make a list of things to do when you get the urge to eat and you're not hungry. Try going for a walk or calling a friend to distract yourself.
- Do something fun if you are tempted to eat to avoid work or a dreaded task.
- Reward yourself with things other than food.

Source: Adapted from *Nutrition for a Healthy Life*. Courtesy of March Leeds.

Maintaining a Healthy Weight

What Do You Know About Weight Management?

1. The number of Americans who are overweight or obese has been increasing over the past few years. True or False?

2. Body mass index (BMI) is a good way to assess body composition to determine if you are under- or overweight or in the normal weight range. True or False?

3. Socioeconomic status is not a contributing factor to developing obesity. True or False?

4. Most diets are effective for long-lasting weight management if you follow them correctly. True or False?

5. A goal of losing 5 pounds per week is a reasonable goal. True or False?

6. Diet pills and supplements are effective methods to manage your weight. True or False?

7. Bulimia nervosa is more common than anorexia nervosa. True or False?

Check your answers at the end of the chapter.

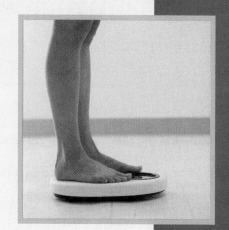

Body Weight and Wellness

Weight management has become an obsession in American culture as well as a significant health problem. In the United States, obesity has risen at an epidemic rate during the past 20 years (Figure 6-1). One of the national health objectives for the year 2010 is to reduce the prevalence of obesity among adults to less than 15 percent.[1] Research indicates that the situation is worsening rather than improving. According to the National Center for Chronic Disease Prevention and Health Promotion, an estimated 66 percent of adult Americans are either overweight or obese.[2] Currently 30 percent, or 72 million, adult Americans are obese with more women (35 percent) than men (33 percent) meeting the criteria for obesity. Obesity was highest for people 40 to 59 years of age for both men and women. Rates were higher for African American women (53 percent) than for Mexican American women (51 percent) or Caucasian women (39 percent). Up 74 percent since 1991, the number of overweight children and adolescents has tripled in the past 20 years.[3] These people face an increased risk of developing serious health problems, independent of other risk factors not directly related to weight. People who are overweight are 40 percent more likely to die prematurely than those of average weight. Obesity may account for as many as 400,000 deaths annually.[4]

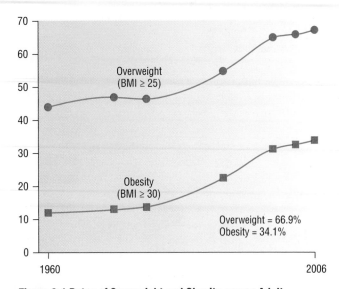

Figure 6-1 Rates of Overweight and Obesity among Adult Americans The proportion of overweight Americans has increased significantly in recent decades.

Source: National Center for Health Statistics, Centers for Disease Control and Prevention.

Defining Overweight and Obesity

How can people tell the difference between overweight and obesity? Doctors usually define **overweight** as a condition in which a person's weight is 1 to 19 percent higher than normal, as defined by a standard height/weight chart. **Obesity** is usually defined as a condition in which a person's weight is 20 percent or more above normal weight (see Figure 6-1). *Morbid obesity* refers to being 50 to 100 percent above normal weight, more than 100 pounds over normal weight, or sufficiently overweight to interfere with health or normal functioning.[5] Of course, an exception to this relationship between overweight and obesity is excessive weight caused by extreme muscularity, such as that seen in many athletes.[5]

Being most familiar with the weight guidelines used in the past, most clinicians and the general public continue to use standard height/weight tables to determine the extent to which scale weight exceeds **desirable weight** and, thus, the existence of mild, moderate, or severe obesity. However, other techniques are now available that can be used to determine body composition. The next section describes several of these techniques, including waist-to-hip ratio, body mass index, hydrostatic weighing, "Bod Pod" assessment, skinfold measurements, and electrical impedance.

Most recently the scientific community has issued guidelines for determining obesity for purposes of medical intervention. People with a **body mass index (BMI)** over 25 are considered overweight. Individuals are considered obese when BMI is 30 or above. Severe or morbid

obesity is when the BMI is greater than 40.[6] Aggressive medical intervention is necessary for people who, in addition to being obese, have a waist circumference of 40 or more inches (males) or 35 or more inches (females) and two or more of the following risk factors: diabetes, high blood pressure, high blood cholesterol, and **sleep apnea.**[7] For obese people who demonstrate fewer risk factors, less aggressive treatment may suffice.

Obesity and Disease

Among the health problems caused by or complicated by excess body fat are increased surgical risk, hypertension, various forms of heart disease, arthritis, stroke, type 2 diabetes, several forms of cancer, deterioration of joints, complications during pregnancy, gallbladder disease, and an overall increased risk of mortality.[4] So closely is obesity associated with chronic conditions that medical experts now recommend that obesity itself be defined and treated as a chronic disease.[4] In fact, the combination of type 2 diabetes, hypertension, and atherosclerosis along with obesity is so common that it is now referred to as metabolic syndrome, or *Syndrome X.*[8]

In comparison with the "spare tire" pattern of fat distribution seen in men, women more often demonstrate an excessive accumulation of fat in the hips, thighs, and buttocks. This lower body obesity is less closely associated with chronic health problems. Research shows that women who have more fat concentrated around the waist, as opposed to their hips, have a greater risk of cardiovascular disease and diabetes. This has been referred to as the "apple versus pear shape" phenomenon. Whether you're an apple or pear depends on where your body stores its excess fat. If fat tends to gather high around your abdomen, you're an apple. If it collects more around your hips and thighs, you're a pear.

Sociocultural Standards for Weight

While the definition of overweight is clearly delineated in terms of being above the norm according to the standards for height, weight, and gender, there still remains a great deal of confusion about who fits into this category. What is normal? Sociocultural ideals of body image, as discussed in the box "Mirror, Mirror on the Wall" on page 154, vary significantly from the standards set in the height/weight charts. **Body image** refers to the subjective perception of how one's body appears to oneself and others. Current Western cultural standards suggest that women should be tall and very thin and men should be tall and muscular. People often compare themselves to actors and models and look to them for the standards for beauty. However, the average actress or model is thinner than 95 percent of the female population and weighs 23 percent less than the average woman.[9]

The current cultural ideal body types for women is a tall, thin, athletic look in which the hips, waist, and shoulders line up vertically. The once-popular emphasis on an "hourglass" figure has given way to a more angular, athletic appearance, somewhat similar to the body build of many young men. The ideal body type for men is a V-shaped body with a full chest, muscular legs, well-defined abdominal muscles, and a thin waist. However, men with eating disorders strive for the lean, toned, thin shape.[10] Men, in fact, make up approximately 10 percent of those with eating disorders, for which body image concerns is an important component.[11]

Body Image and Self-Concept

In light of these standards, people may become dissatisfied and concerned about their inability to resemble ideal images. The scope of this dissatisfaction is evident in a study of more than 800 women, which revealed that nearly half were unhappy with their weight, muscle tone, hips, thighs, buttocks, and legs.[12] Not surprisingly, when this dissatisfaction exists, people can question their own attractiveness, and eventually their self-concept and self-esteem declines.

Whether the body image desired can realistically be achieved seems irrelevant to many people. Some spend hours each week in weight rooms and reduce or increase their food intake dramatically in a quest to attain the desired body image. For those who are ultimately unsuccessful, disappointment, frustration, and serious medical and psychological problems, such as eating disorders, can result.

Overall, men report feeling more comfortable with their weight and perceive less pressure to be thin than women do. A national survey showed that 41 percent of men were dissatisfied with their weight, with many of these men wanting to gain weight and increase muscle mass. While the average American woman wants to lose 11 pounds, the average American man wants to lose 1 pound or is happy with his weight.[13]

See the box "Gender, Clothing Sizes, and Body Image Around the World" on page 155 for more on issues related to weight and self-concept.

Measuring and Assessing Weight and Body Fat Composition

A wide array of techniques exist to determine weight and body fat composition. Some techniques are, of course, much more accurate and more expensive than others. The following section describes a variety of these techniques.

Body Mass Index

As we mentioned in the previous section, one means of assessing healthy body weight is the body mass index (BMI). The BMI indicates the relationship of body weight (expressed in kilograms) to height (expressed in meters) for both men and women. The BMI does not reflect body composition (fat versus lean tissue) or consider the degree of fat accumulated within the central body cavity. It is, nevertheless, widely used in determining obesity (see Table 6.1 on page 156). BMI is calculated metrically as weight divided by height squared (kg/m^2).

A BMI chart is also available for children and adolescents. The importance of having a BMI chart appropriate for age 2 years through 20 years was stimulated by the increasing percentage of children and adolescents who are now classified as being overweight (20 percent). Because of the availability of this chart, pediatricians and parents have the ability to more quickly and more accurately determine the risk of potential obesity in children and take appropriate action to minimize its occurrence. Additional information on this BMI chart can be obtained at www.cdc.gov/growthcharts.

You can also determine your healthy body weight by using the weight guidelines in the 2005 Dietary Guidelines of Americans[14] (see Chapter 5). This assessment involves two body measurements: BMI and waist circumference (see Table 6.1).

Key Terms

overweight A condition in which a person's excess fat accumulation results in a body weight that exceeds desirable weight by 1–19 percent.

obesity A condition in which a person's body weight is 20 percent or more above desirable weight as determined by standard height/weight charts.

desirable weight The weight range deemed appropriate for people, taking into consideration gender, age, and frame size.

body mass index (BMI) A mathematical calculation based on weight and height; used to determine desirable body weight.

sleep apnea A condition in which abnormalities in the structure of the airways lead to periods of greatly restricted air flow during sleep, resulting in reduced levels of blood oxygen and placing greater strain on the heart to maintain adequate tissue oxygenation.

body image One's subjective perception of how one's body appears to oneself and others.

Mirror, Mirror on the Wall

Television, magazines, billboards, movies, and a variety of other sources constantly bombard us with messages about how we should look. How realistic are these images? While the average woman's measurements are 37-29-40 (chest, waist, hips), store mannequins measure 38-18-28. The average American woman is 5 feet 4 inches tall, weighs 140 pounds, and wears a size 12–14. The average American female model is 5 feet 11 inches, weighs 117 pounds, and wears a size 2. Very early in our lives, we receive messages about how we should aspire to look, with unrealistic models such as the Barbie doll—whose measurements would be equivalent to a woman who is 5 feet 9 inches, weighs 110 pounds, and measures 39-18-33. G.I. Joe in life-size form would have a 55-inch chest and 27-inch biceps; Batman would be 7 feet tall with a 57-inch chest, a 30-inch waist, and 27-inch biceps. Fairy tales reinforce these messages as the thin, beautiful heroine becomes a princess and finds true love while the ugly, larger-bodied women are the villains, evil stepmothers, or stepsisters. Beauty is the most important quality for women, the evil queen in *Snow White* tells us as she asks her magic mirror each day, "Who is the fairest of us all?" Men are not immune to these messages—the strong, handsome men are the princes who have the wealth and the beautiful women, while men who are not as attractive are seen as weak, pitiful, or evil.

Do we really buy into these messages? Researchers found that girls in middle school who read dieting articles were two to three times more likely to develop eating-disordered behaviors than those who didn't. While 44 percent of girls reported reading diet articles, only 14 percent of boys did—and this didn't seem to translate into these boys developing eating problems later in life. Another study showed that after women looked at a fashion magazine for three minutes, 70 percent of them became significantly more depressed and felt guilty and ashamed. A recent poll of 1,000 women showed that they would take extreme measures to attain their ideal weight, as 21 percent said they would give up 10 years of their lives, 23 percent said they would spend a week in jail, 23 percent said they would shave their head, and 22 percent said they would wear a bikini on television in order to do so. Eighty-five percent said they would rather have an extra toe than weigh 50 pounds more than they currently weigh. Certainly it appears that these media messages have a strong negative influence on women's self-esteem, body image, and behavior.

Dove's campaign for "Real Beauty" broke out of this mold and took an advertising risk by featuring real women, not models, sizes 6 to 14, to advertise their beauty and soap products. Rather than advertising beauty products as substances that will morph purchasers into a smaller, thinner, unrealistic image of themselves, Dove is suggesting in their ads that people who buy their products will feel more self-accepting and confident. While Dove is moving in the right direction in portraying beauty as coming in all shapes and sizes, some wonder if Dove is also trying to sell self-esteem in a bottle.

Bath & Body Works is focusing on preteens and teens in its line of shampoos and lotions under the American Girl brand, and their advertising addresses beauty "inside and out." Nike has also employed this type of advertising campaign with its use of a mixture of real women and pro athlete models showing their "big butts" and "thunder thighs." Wal-Mart's ads use real women to show that "fashion is reachable for everybody," and Wal-Mart has been using employees and their families in their ads since 1989. There was a great furor in Spain's top fashion show in 2006 when 30 percent of the models were ejected from the show for being too thin, having a body mass index under 18 when under 18.5 is considered underweight and unhealthy. This is quite a reverse from the trend of models being anorexic-looking and being rejected if they are not underweight.

What can you do as a consumer? Support companies, such as Dove, Nike, and Wal-Mart, that are moving in the right direction in terms of allowing for a broader definition of beauty. Don't read magazines that will quickly make you feel bad about yourself. Choose not to watch television programs like *Dr. 90210, America's Next Top Model*, or *Extreme Makeover* and instead watch programs, such as *Ugly Betty*, that send the message that being smart, genuine, and passionate about life is more important than appearance. Focus on accepting your body and attaining self-esteem and self-worth from all aspects of yourself, not just appearance.

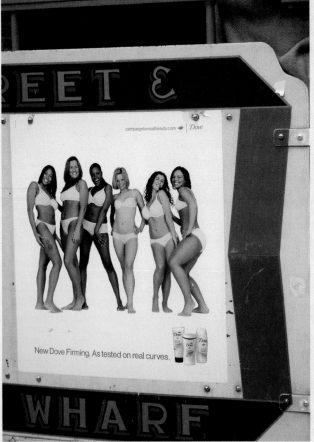

What do you think about the message in this outdoor ad from the Dove "Real Beauty" campaign?

Sources: What's a Girl to Do? Hot and Brainy Brings Mixed Emotions, *USA Today*, July 25, 2006; Ad Campaigns Tell Women to Celebrate Who They Are, *The Star Press*, July 10, 2005; Unhealthy Obsession: Girls Who Read Diet Articles Show Later Signs of Eating Disorders, *The Star Press*, January 2, 2007; Real Curvy Women Betray Media Image of Beauty, *The Star Press*, August 27, 2005; Dove Ads Enlist All Shapes, Styles and Sizes, *USA Today*, August 29, 2005; Would You Trade 10 Years of Life to Be an Ideal Weight? *USA Today*, January 7, 2008.

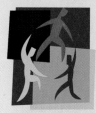

Learning from Our Diversity

Gender, Clothing Sizes, and Body Image Around the World

You are in London, England, and decide to buy some of the latest British fashions. You find a pair of pants you like and try them on. They don't fit. In fact nothing in your size fits. Why not? Because not all sizes are the same for women.

As you can see from the table below, if you wear a size 12 in American stores, you will need to find a size 14 in British stores or an 11 in Japanese stores or a 42 in Parisian boutiques.* Is this true for men's clothing? No, you will find that a waist size of 38 is the same in American, British, and Japanese clothing. Why is this? Well, it is the same reason that you will find that not all women's size-12 clothing is the same even in the same country! What you will find is that the more expensive the clothing, the smaller the size compared to its true size. In other words, you can compare a pair of jeans from a discount store to the identical pair of pants in an expensive department store and find that the expensive pants are labeled one to two sizes smaller than the pants in the discount store. You will also discover that the smaller size

pants have a much larger size price tag. Again, does this hold true for men's clothing? No, it doesn't. The reason is that women will pay more for a smaller size, a lot more, while most men will not. There is not a market for smaller size clothing for men the way there is for women. The fashion industry calls this "faith-based sizing" because consumers want to believe that they are the size the label tells them they are, even if the scale says something different. This is also referred to as "vanity sizing."[†]

Men, however, are not immune to the trend of rising obesity around the world. In Cyprus, the Czech Republic, Finland, Germany, Greece, Malta, and Slovakia, more men are overweight or obese than American men are. Although the Mediterranean diet has been touted as a healthy diet, obesity is also higher in the Mediterranean countries.[‡]

Eating disorders and distorted eating are more prevalent in cultures adopting Westernized values. One startling example of how quickly and significantly Western ideals of beauty can influence others was seen when television first came to the island of Fiji in 1995. Before the introduction of television, a common compliment given to someone was "you've gained weight," and dieting was almost nonexistent. Telling someone that he or she looked thin was a way of saying that the person didn't look well. Within three years of having television, the number of teenagers at risk for eating disorders more than doubled; 74 percent of teens said they felt too big or too fat, and 62 percent reported that they had been dieting in the past month.[§]

In the United States and other Westernized societies, the cultural ideal for beauty is becoming thinner and thinner. A generation ago, a model weighed 8 percent less than the average woman did, but she now weighs 23 percent less. With the models wearing clothing of size 00, there is a message for women to aspire to nothingness.[§] What can be done about this alarming trend? Women can refuse to buy more expensive clothes just because they are labeled with smaller sizes, as men have done for years. We can glorify all sizes and shapes of women. As Angel, a 17-year-old high school basketball player from West Los Angeles, stated, "I'm 5 feet 8 inches and 165 pounds. I'm not a size 4. I'm tall. I'm muscular. I'm a thick girl. I accept that."**

Clothing Size Comparisons

Women's Clothing

USA	4	6	8	10	12	14	16	18	20
UK	6	8	10	12	14	16	18	20	22
Russia	40	42	44	46	48	50	52	54	56
Spain/France	34	36	38	40	42	44	46	48	50
Italy	38	40	42	44	46	48	50	52	54
Germany	32	34	36	38	40	42	44	46	48
Japan	3	5	7	9	11	13	15	17	19

Men's Clothing

Suits, Sweaters, Jackets, and Pants

USA	34	36	38	40	42	44	46	48
UK	34	36	38	40	42	44	46	48
Europe	44	46	48	50	52	54	56	58
Japan	S	–	M	–	–	L	–	–

Shirt Collars

USA	14	14½	15	15½	16	16½	17	17½
UK	14	14½	15	15½	16	16½	17	17½
Europe	36	37	38	39	40	41	42	43
Japan	36	37	38	39	40	41	42	43

Source: www.hostelscentral.com/hostels-article-34.html.

*International Clothes Sizes Compared, www.hostelscentral.com.
[†]Faith Based Sizing, *Newsweek*, October 18, 2006.
[‡]Some European Countries More Obese Than in U.S., *USA Today*, March 28, 2005.
[§]Kilbourne, J. *Can't Buy My Love.* New York: Simon & Schuster, 1999.
**The New Girls, *Oprah Magazine*, May 2004.

Height/Weight Tables

Traditionally the 1983 Metropolitan Life Insurance Height and Weight Table has been the basis for determining the desirable or ideal weight for your gender, height, and frame size. However, the use of this table and others like it is no longer considered the best way to determine whether body weight is acceptable. It is now

recognized that this table excludes uninsurable people, disregards the influence of age, fails to consider other causes of mortality (such as smoking), and relies on subjective determinations of frame size to express the influence of body composition on weight. In addition, people have failed to take into consideration that the Metropolitan Life Insurance Height and Weight Table was based

Table 6.1 Body Mass Index (BMI)

BMI	Normal (18.5–24.9)						Overweight (25–29.9)					Obese (≥ 30)										Extreme Obesity
	19	20	21	22	23	24	25	26	27	28	29	30	31	32	33	34	35	36	37	38	39	40
Height (inches)	Body Weight (pounds)																					
58	91	96	100	105	110	115	119	124	129	134	138	143	148	153	158	162	167	172	177	181	186	191
59	94	99	104	109	114	119	124	128	133	138	143	148	153	158	163	168	173	178	183	188	193	198
60	97	102	107	112	118	123	128	133	138	143	148	153	158	163	168	174	179	184	189	194	199	204
61	100	106	111	116	122	127	132	137	143	148	153	158	164	169	174	180	185	190	195	201	206	211
62	104	109	115	120	126	131	136	142	147	153	158	164	169	175	180	186	191	196	202	207	213	218
63	107	113	118	124	130	135	141	146	152	158	163	169	175	180	186	191	197	203	208	214	220	225
64	110	116	122	128	134	140	145	151	157	163	169	174	180	186	192	197	204	209	215	221	227	232
65	114	120	126	132	138	144	150	156	162	168	174	180	186	192	198	204	210	216	222	228	234	240
66	118	124	130	136	142	148	155	161	167	173	179	186	192	198	204	210	216	223	229	235	241	247
67	121	127	134	140	146	153	159	166	172	178	185	191	198	204	211	217	223	230	236	242	249	255
68	125	131	138	144	151	158	164	171	177	184	190	197	203	210	216	223	230	236	243	249	256	262
69	128	135	142	149	155	162	169	176	182	189	196	203	209	216	223	230	236	243	250	257	263	270
70	132	139	146	153	160	167	174	181	188	195	202	209	216	222	229	236	243	250	257	264	271	278
71	136	143	150	157	165	172	179	186	193	200	208	215	222	229	236	243	250	257	265	272	279	286
72	140	147	154	162	169	177	184	191	199	206	213	221	228	235	242	250	258	265	272	279	287	294
73	144	151	159	166	174	182	189	197	204	212	219	227	235	242	250	257	265	272	280	288	295	302
74	148	155	163	171	179	186	194	202	210	218	225	233	241	249	256	264	272	280	287	295	303	311
75	152	160	168	176	184	192	200	208	216	224	232	240	248	256	264	272	279	287	295	303	311	319
76	156	164	172	180	189	197	205	213	221	230	238	246	254	263	271	279	287	295	304	312	320	328

Note: At any BMI, a waist circumference of more than 40 inches for men and 35 inches for women is associated with a significantly increased risk of chronic disease.

Source: Adapted from *Clinical Guidelines on the Identification, Evaluation, and Treatment of Overweight and Obesity in Adults: The Evidence Report*, National Institutes of Health.

on height that included 1-inch heel shoes and allowed 3 pounds of clothing. The tables were also designed for adults ages 25 to 59 years of age and were not intended for use with children.[13] Fortunately, the newer tables are intended for use with the guidelines describing healthy body weight and body mass index (BMI).

Waist and Hip Measurement

The size of your waist is a surprisingly accurate measure of your abdominal fat. Among people who have an acceptable waist-to-hip ratio (WHR), female "healthy weight" is near the lower end of each weight range, whereas male "healthy weight" is at the higher end of each weight range.

To use these weight ranges, the following procedure must be performed:

1. Measure around your waist near your navel while you stand relaxed, not pulling in your stomach.
2. Measure around your hips, over the buttocks where your hips are the largest.
3. Divide the waist measurement by the hip measurement.

Women with a WHR of 0.80 or less generally have a body weight that falls within the healthy range for their age and height as depicted in Table 6.1; men with a WHR of 0.90 or less will also probably fall within the range that is considered healthy for their age and height.

This assessment procedure was developed in response to the growing concern over the relationship between the amount of fat in the central abdominal cavity (upper body obesity) and the development of several serious health problems. As we mentioned earlier, the risk of health problems such as heart disease and diabetes increases at a waist measurement of 35 inches for women and 40 inches for men, regardless of height.[15]

As a point of interest, the guidelines found in the Dietary Guidelines for Americans do not use waist-to-hip ratio as a clinical marker for the treatment of obesity but rather use only waist circumference, believing it to be a better predictor of risk. Only time will tell about the continued use of healthy body weight in assessing risk for cardiovascular disease and other chronic conditions.

Appearance

While it may seem as though the simplest method of determining one's body size is to look in the mirror, for most people this is not an accurate measure. Research shows that most women are dissatisfied with their appearance or body image and perceive themselves as needing to lose an average of 10 to 15 pounds when in actuality they are in a healthy weight range. Body dissatisfaction is endemic to young women in Western culture as evidenced by the rate of dieting in the United States, starting at a young age. In fact, on any given day, 50 percent of 10-year-olds are on a diet, and two-thirds of high school women and one-third of all adult women are dieting.[16] There is also an important difference between one's internal concept of one's body and actual body perception, and this is particularly problematic for people with eating disorders.

Home Scale

Most people use scales at home or in a gym to determine their weight, but scales can be highly inaccurate, as evidenced by weighing yourself on a variety of scales and weighing different amounts. Also, you will probably weigh less in the morning when you first wake up and more in the evening, after having eaten during the day. So, if you are using a scale to monitor your weight, you need to do so on the same scale, at the same time of day, and with approximately the same weight of clothing. Also, remember that muscle weighs more than fat, which explains why some toned and muscular athletes can weigh as much as someone who is sedentary and overweight. In general, risk of disease increases with a higher percentage of body fat, not weight.

Body Fat Measurement

A number of techniques are available to measure the relative proportion of the body's weight that is fat. Young adult men normally have a body fat percentage of 10 to 15 percent. The normal range for young adult women is 22 to 25 percent. When a man's body fat percentage exceeds 25 percent and a woman's body fat percentage exceeds 30 percent, these people are classified as obese.

The relatively higher percentage of fat found in women compared to men is related to the female's capacity for pregnancy and lactation. Women require a sufficient amount of body fat in order to ovulate, menstruate, and become pregnant. In fact, some experts suggest that lack of sex drive can be related to the adverse changes in hormonal level owing to insufficient body fat. The danger zone begins when a woman's BMI is about 18 or below. Women tend to store fat in their pelvic region, around their hips and thighs ("pears"). Not only does this fat help to protect vital reproductive organs, it also acts as a source of stored energy for pregnancy and breast-feeding. As women enter menopause, they produce less estrogen. This leads to a change in body shape and fat distribution. During a woman's fertile years, the female hormones estrogen and progesterone are responsible for maintaining the female shape of a narrow waist and rounded hips. During and after menopause, the female waist thickens

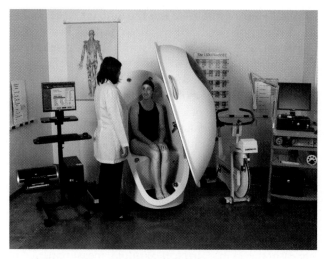

The Bod Pod measures air displacement, which can be used to calculate percentage of body fat.

and fat is deposited around the stomach area similar to the male's pattern of fat distribution ("apples"). In addition, as in men, the metabolic rate slows and fewer calories are required. So if a woman continues to eat the same amount of food as she has throughout her fertile years, without increasing her exercise, weight and fat gain are likely to occur.[17]

Electrical impedance, the Bod Pod, skinfold measurement, and hydrostatic weighing are some of the most common methods for assessing body fat composition.

Electrical Impedance **Electrical impedance** is a relatively new method to determine body composition. This assessment procedure measures the electrical impedance or resistance to a weak electrical flow directed through the body. Because adipose tissue resists the passage of the electrical current more than muscle tissue does, electrical impedance can be used to calculate the percentage of body fat. However, in addition to high cost and limited availability, psychological variables, such as fear or discomfort associated with the electrical current flow, can reduce the practicality of electrical impedance.

Bod Pod (Body Composition System) The Bod Pod is an egg-shaped chamber that uses computerized pressure sensors to determine the amount of air displaced by the person's body (larger people displace more air than smaller people). The person is allowed to breathe

> **Key Terms**
>
> **electrical impedance** A method used to measure the percentage of body fat using a harmless electrical current.

normally during the test, and the amount of air in the lungs can either be measured directly in the Bod Pod or is estimated. A complete test, with printed results, can be achieved in less than 4.5 minutes.[18] Body density can itself be used to determine the percentage of the subject's body that is composed of fat. Upon knowing the percent body fat, the percent of lean body mass can be calculated, again using a mathematical formula.[19] The Bod Pod is highly accurate and much more comfortable for subjects than is hydrostatic weighing.

Skinfold Measurements A skinfold measurement provides another way to measure body fat percentage. Skinfold measurements rely on constant-pressure calipers to measure the thickness of the layer of fat beneath the skin's surface. Skinfold measurements of subcutaneous fat are taken at several key places on the body. Measurements of skinfold thickness can then be used to calculate the percentage of body fat, and then a relatively simple conversion can be made to determine desired body weight.[18] There are some drawbacks to this type of measure: First, a second person may be required to perform the test, because it is sometimes difficult to get an accurate measurement on yourself. Second, skinfolds are notoriously hard to locate precisely, and being just a few millimeters off can make a significant difference. Research recommends that 50 to 100 tests are needed before an examiner can be classified as "competent" with body fat calipers. Body fat calipers used correctly are accurate to within 4 percent at best.[5]

Hydrostatic Weighing Hydrostatic weighing (underwater weighing) is a precise method for determining the relative amounts of fat and lean body mass that make up body weight. A person's percentage of body fat is determined by comparing the underwater body weight with the body weight out of the water and dry. The necessity for expensive equipment and trained technicians makes the use of this method impractical for the average person. Traditionally, hydrostatic weighing has been considered the most accurate or sensitive means of determining body composition, with a 97 percent accuracy rate. The Bod Pod appears to be just as accurate and certainly more comfortable to use than underwater weighing.

Additional techniques used to determine body composition include computerized axial tomography (CT) scans, magnetic resonance imaging (MRI), infrared light transmission, and neutron activation. These techniques have limited application because of cost and availability.

Causes of Obesity

Genetic, physiological, metabolic, environmental, psychological, and other factors may all play a part. In the past decade, the overall prevalence of obesity has increased so that currently one-third of all Americans are obese. Moreover, in the last 20 years, the number of overweight children in the United States has tripled to one in five children.[20] Genetics, dietary practice, and activity level seem to all play a role in this dramatic increase.

Four additional factors seem to play a significant role in the prevalence of obesity: sex, age, socioeconomic status, and race. Biology accounts for only 33 percent of the variation in body weight, so the environment can also exert an enormous influence. Among women, obesity is strongly associated with socioeconomic status, being twice as common among those with lower socioeconomic status as it is among those with higher status.[21] Although prevalence among Black and White men does not differ significantly, obesity is far more common among Black than among White women, affecting 51 percent of Black women compared with 39 percent of White women aged 40 to 59.

While the precise cause of obesity remains unclear, we do know that obesity is a complex condition caused by a variety of factors. Until we are sure what causes obesity, it will remain difficult to develop effective ways of managing weight.

Calorie Balance: Energy Intake Versus Energy Output

What accounts for the high percentage of Americans defined as overweight or obese? Experts point to two salient factors: greater daily caloric consumption and a relatively low level of consistent physical activity. Women eat 335 more calories, and men eat 168 more calories, per day than they did 30 years ago. In addition, nearly two-thirds of Americans are not physically active on a regular basis and 25 percent are completely sedentary.[22] (See Chapter 4.)

The increase in weight occurs, of course, when the body is supplied with more energy than it can use and the excess energy is stored in the form of adipose tissue, or fat. This is called a positive caloric balance. Consuming about 3,500 calories a week more than is needed results in a weight gain of 1 pound of fat per week.[23] Weight remains constant when caloric input and caloric output are equal. This is called caloric balance. To maintain a specific weight, people must balance their energy intake with the energy expenditure. To lose weight, an individual must achieve a negative caloric balance, which involves expending more calories than are taken in. A negative caloric balance can be created by reducing caloric intake, increasing physical activity, or both. The key to losing weight and keeping it off is engaging in regular aerobic exercise and eating a balanced diet that is consistent with the current dietary guidelines as described in Chapter 5. In other words, eat healthfully and exercise regularly.

What are our energy needs? How many calories should we consume (or expend) to achieve a healthy weight? There is no single answer for everyone. The USDA dietary guidelines are based on consuming 2,000 calories a day.[24] (See Chapter 5.) Age and gender both affect the amount of calories people need. In addition, people may need fewer or more calories than the USDA recommendation depending on these three factors: (1) basal metabolism, (2) activity requirements, and (3) the thermic effect of food. Of these factors, basal metabolism is the most important determinant of the total calories required by an individual.

Basal Metabolic Rate **Basal metabolic rate (BMR)** is a measure of resting energy expenditure that is taken upon awakening, 10 to 12 hours after eating, or 12 to 18 hours after significant physical activity. A closely related construct, resting metabolic rate (RMR), is often used interchangeably with BMR. In comparison with the BMR, the RMR is measured at rest, without the stringent controls on physical activity required as with measuring BMR. RMR measures the calories needed for functioning such as blood circulation, respiration, brain activity, muscle function, body temperature, and heartbeat.[25]

Basal metabolism changes as people age. For both males and females, the BMR is relatively high at birth and continues to increase until the age of 2. Except for a slight rise at puberty, the BMR gradually declines throughout the remainder of life. A variety of other variables also affect BMR, including body composition (muscular bodies are associated with higher BMRs), physical condition (fit people have higher BMRs), gender (males have 5 percent higher BMRs), hormone secretions (people with excessively active thyroid and adrenal glands have higher BMRs), sleep (BMRs are about 10 percent lower during sleep), pregnancy (a 20 percent increase in BMR is typical, especially in the last trimester), body temperature (a 1 degree rise in body temperature increases BMR about 7 percent), and environmental temperature (deviations above and below 78 degrees F result in increased BMRs).[26]

The most important variables related to BMR are age, body composition, activity level, and caloric intake. For example, if people fail to recognize that BMR declines with aging, they might fail to adjust food intake accordingly, and weight gain will occur. Also, for those who are thinner, the presence of lean tissue favors a higher basal metabolic rate with greater resistance to weight gain. Finally, an increase in physical activity fosters a faster BMR, which contributes to weight loss. In contrast, in those people with above-average levels of body fat, BMR rates are lower, thus providing the body with excess calories that will be stored as fat.

Activity Requirements Each person's caloric *activity requirements* vary directly according to the amount of daily physical work completed. When weight management experts are asked to identify the single most important reason that obesity is so high in today's society, they are most certain to point to inactivity. People of all ages tend to be less active and burn fewer calories than did their ancestors only a few generations ago (see the box "The Growing Problem of Obesity"). Both adults and children spend less time devoted to exercise as a result of longer work hours at sedentary jobs, a decline in physical education programs in school, and increased participation in sedentary recreational activities, such as browsing the Internet, playing video games, and watching television. In addition, many of the laborsaving devices and increased automation in the home and workplace have contributed to increased inactivity. Physical activity uses between 20 and 40 percent of caloric intake. According to some studies, nearly two-thirds of Americans are not physically active on a regular basis, and 25 percent are completely sedentary.[22] It is not surprising that as inactivity becomes the norm so does overweight.

Thermic Effect of Food **Thermic effect of food (TEF)** refers to the amount of energy our bodies require for the digestion, absorption, and transportation of food. This energy breaks down the bonds that hold complex food

---

Key Terms

skinfold measurement A measurement to determine the thickness of the fat layer that lies immediately beneath the skin; used to calculate body composition.

calipers A device used to measure the thickness of a skinfold from which percentage of body fat can be calculated.

hydrostatic weighing Weighing the body while it is submerged in water.

adipose tissue Tissue made up of fibrous strands around which specialized cells designed to store liquified fat are arranged.

positive caloric balance Caloric intake is greater than caloric expenditure, resulting in weight gain.

caloric balance Caloric intake and caloric expenditure are equal and body weight remains constant.

negative caloric balance Caloric intake is less than caloric expenditure, resulting in weight loss.

basal metabolic rate (BMR) The amount of energy, expressed in calories, that the body requires to maintain basic functions.

thermic effect of food (TEF) The amount of energy our bodies require for the digestion, absorption, and transportation of food.

The Growing Problem of Obesity

Children are 9 pounds heavier today, and teens are 12 to 16 pounds heavier than they were in the early 1960s. This can lead to greater chances of developing type 2 diabetes, high cholesterol, and a host of other health problems. The trend doesn't stop with the adolescent years. Obesity doubles from the teen years to the mid-20s.

One of the reasons American children and adolescents gain weight over the generations is that children expend significantly less energy on a daily basis than their parents or grandparents did at their age. Today's youth spend endless hours engaged in sedentary play—watching television and playing computer and handheld electronic games. Schools have not helped the situation by cutting back on physical education classes and recess.

In our fast-paced society, we are eating more and more fast food and vending machine food than we have in the past. Again, schools have come under attack for providing high-sugar and high-fat foods, as well as sodas, in the cafeterias and vending machines. College students frequently complain about the food at the college dining hall being loaded with fat and sugar; however, it is often the midnight delivery of pizza or study breaks to the vending machines that lead to weight gain. College students also say that they have trouble finding time to exercise regularly and rely on walking to and from classes and on physical education classes to provide their exercise. Unfortunately, this does not typically add up to at least 30 minutes of daily physical activity as suggested by the current USDA dietary guidelines.

Americans are working more hours than they have in the past, usually well beyond the 40-hour work week, leaving little to no time for daily exercise. Many adults perceive themselves as working hard at their jobs and have no energy reserves left for exercise when they come home. The majority of Americans' jobs are sedentary and don't involve manual labor or have great physical demands.

So, what can we do to curb the growing trend toward obesity? Some factors that seem important are to

1. *Get out and play!* Go for a bike ride, play golf, take a walk, shoot some baskets.
2. *Limit screen time.* Decrease television, computer, and electronic game time to one to two hours a day maximum. Don't hit the couch or the computer as soon as you get home because it is likely you will spend the evening there.
3. *Avoid vending machines and fast-food restaurants.* Pack nutritious snacks such as apples, carrots, nuts, and yogurt.
4. *Downsize your dishes.* Studies have repeatedly shown that we eat more when we are offered more food. Use narrower glasses, and smaller bowls and plates.
5. *Quit the clean plate club!* Researchers have also shown that we tend not to feel more full even if we eat more. In one study, a bowl automatically refilled itself with soup, unbeknownst to the subjects, and they ate almost double the amount as the group with normal bowls, and yet they didn't report feeling more full.
6. *Eat weighty food.* We tend to eat the same amount or weight in food each day. Eating food that is high in fiber and water, such as fruits and vegetables, helps us to consume fewer calories. Nutrient-dense food fills you up faster, so you eat fewer calories but get more nutrition compared to eating foods that are less nutrient dense.
7. *Water yourself.* Drink water instead of juice and sodas.

---

molecules together, resulting in smaller nutritional units that can be distributed throughout the body. The amount of TEF burned varies for different types of food, with some food such as fat requiring less energy to convert to energy stores and others such as protein and carbohydrates requiring more. The TEF peaks in about 1 hour after eating and accounts for approximately 10 percent of total energy expenditure.[26]

Genetic Factors

Through years of research, we do know that heredity plays a major role in the development of body size and obesity.[5] Based on studies comparing both identical and fraternal (nonidentical) twins raised together and separately, it's evident that both environment and genetics influence obesity. In fact, it is estimated that heredity accounts for 25 to 40 percent of the development of obesity.[5] Women have a higher percentage of body fat than do men, and this seems stable across cultures and dietary habits.[5] While some scientific research has explored whether the X chromosome may be linked to fat distribution, no conclusive evidence has substantiated this link.

There is also some speculation about population differences and prevalence of obesity suggesting that some groups possess a "thrifty genotype."[27] For example, the differences in diabetes and obesity rates in Native Americans compared with European Americans prompted some researchers to consider that some groups of people have survived periods of feast and famine by increased efficiency in energy storage and expenditure through a particular genotype. However, no specific thrifty gene or genotype has been identified.

A complex interplay of genetic factors very likely influence the development of obesity, since more than 250 genes may play a role in obesity. Promising research has explored how the leptin gene influences obesity. Discovered in the mid-1990s, the leptin gene, referred to as the "fat gene," was thought to influence satiety, or the feeling of fullness, in mice.[28] When the leptin gene was faulty in mice, it produced lower leptin levels, and the mice experienced excessive weight gain. However, when the leptin gene was normal, the leptin levels were higher and the mice were able to maintain normal weight. It has been theorized that leptin resistance may be involved in weight gain and the maintenance of excessive weight, but much more research needs to be conducted in this area.[29] While we know that leptin helps to regulate fat storage and energy efficiency in humans, it still remains unclear as to how this research can be utilized in the treatment of obesity.

Physiological and Hormonal Factors

Building on the new information about the genetic and neuropsychological basis of obesity, researchers have identified centers for the control of eating within the hypothalamus of the central nervous system (CNS). These centers—the feeding center for hunger and the satiety center for fullness—tell the body when it should begin consuming food and when food consumption should stop. It takes 20 minutes on average for these signals to go from the stomach to the brain to relay the message "stop eating." These centers are thought to continuously monitor a variety of factors regarding food intake.[29]

Hormonal factors also influence obesity. Obesity can be caused by a condition called **hypothyroidism,** in which the thyroid gland produces an insufficient amount of thyroxin, a hormone that regulates metabolism. Over 5 million Americans have this common medical condition, and as many as 10 percent of women may have some degree of thyroid hormone deficiency. In such individuals, the underactive thyroid makes burning up food difficult, and so weight gain is common. As we acquire greater understanding of the hormones and neurotransmitters that influence hunger and satiety, drugs designed to influence their actions will be developed. Some of these drugs already exist and will be described later in this chapter.

The effects of hormonal changes on eating can be seen each month just before a woman's menstrual cycle; many women say that they crave salty and sugary foods during this time. Pregnancy brings about another host of hormonal and metabolic changes. During a normal pregnancy, a woman requires an extra 300 calories a day to support the developing fetus and supportive tissues, and to fuel her elevated maternal metabolic rate. In addition, pregnant women will develop approximately 9 extra pounds of adipose tissue that will be used as an energy source during lactation. The average woman is expected to gain 25 to 35 pounds during pregnancy.[30] Many women express concern about their ability to lose this weight following the birth of the child, and some women do gain much more than the recommended amount of weight. However, the majority of women lose their pregnancy weight within 6 months to a year after having a baby. Nevertheless, obesity is one of the most frequent causes for complications in pregnancy. Women who are obese during pregnancy have a much higher risk of hypertension and gestational diabetes. Obesity has also been associated with infertility, poor pregnancy outcomes, and miscarriage.[31]

Typically, breast-feeding can help women to burn more calories and return to their prepregnancy weight, although extra fat may linger, since nature intended this to be a store of energy for breast-feeding. Breast-feeding requires an additional 500 calories a day.[31] Mothers who breast-feed tend to lose more weight when their babies are 3 to 6 months old than do formula-feeding mothers who consume fewer calories. Infants who are breast-fed also have a lower chance of developing obesity and asthma in childhood and adolescence.[32, 33]

Many researchers believe that the number of fat cells a person has is initially determined during the first two years of life. Babies are born with about 10 billion fat cells and if they are overfed, they will develop a greater number of fat cells than will babies who receive a balanced diet of appropriate, infant-sized portions. Overfed babies, especially those with a family history of obesity, tend to develop **hypercellular obesity.** When these children reach adulthood, they will have more fat cells. An increase in fat cells during infancy and childhood can increase the chances of developing obesity. Individuals at a healthy weight have 10 to 20 billion fat cells, while an obese person can have up to 100 billion. An overweight person doesn't have an excess number of fat cells but rather increasingly larger fat cells. Dieting reduces only the size of fat cells, not the number of fat cells. People who have hypercellular obesity have an abnormally high number of fat cells and are biologically limited in their ability to lose weight.[34]

Hypercellular obesity in adulthood can also result from excessive weight gain in late childhood and adolescence. If an individual's weight is 75 percent above the desirable weight, this can stimulate an increase in the number of fat cells, resulting in eventual obesity.

Hypertrophic obesity is the result of a pattern of overeating for a long period of time. Over a period of years, the existing fat cells increase in size to accommodate

---

Key Terms

hypothyroidism A condition in which the thyroid gland produces an insufficient amount of the hormone thyroxin.

hypercellular obesity A form of obesity that results from having an abnormally high number of fat cells.

hypertrophic obesity A form of obesity in which there is a normal number of fat cells, but the individual fat cells are enlarged.

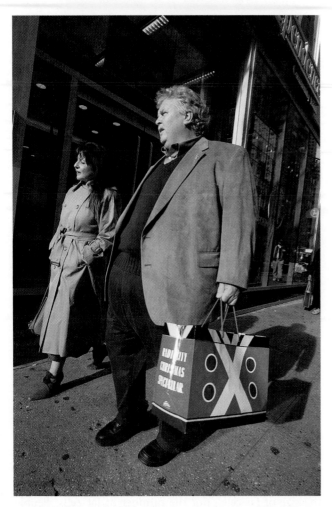

A variety of genetic, physiological, metabolic, social, environmental, and lifestyle factors contribute to the development of obesity.

excess fat intake. Note that, after puberty, as your body stores more fat, the number of fat cells remains the same but each fat cell can get bigger. Hypertrophic obesity is generally associated with excessive fat around the waist and is thought to contribute to conditions such as type 2 diabetes, high levels of fat in the blood, high blood pressure, and heart disease. Hypertrophic obesity generally appears during middle age when physical activity tends to decline, whereas caloric intake remains the same.[34]

> **Key Terms**
>
> **set point** A genetically programmed range of body weight, beyond which a person finds it difficult to gain or lose additional weight.
>
> **adaptive thermogenesis** The physiological response of the body to adjust its metabolic rate to the presence of food.

Metabolic Factors

Traditional theory has suggested that the energy expenditure and energy storage centers of the body possess a genetically programmed awareness of the body's most physiologically desirable weight, called **set point.**[35] However, the term *set point* is somewhat misleading in that it does not refer to a certain number or point but a weight range that the body is genetically programmed to maintain. When the body falls below its natural set point, one's metabolism reacts by slowing down the body's functioning in order to conserve energy. In other words, the body senses that it is not receiving enough calories to maintain healthy functioning and so it sends calories to essential areas of the body and uses the energy as efficiently as possible. Alternatively, when someone consumes more calories than are needed, the body begins to increase the rate of metabolism in an effort not to gain weight above the set point. The process of storing or burning more energy to maintain the body's "best" weight is called **adaptive thermogenesis.** This process also explains the reason that 90 percent of people who go on any diet gain all the weight back plus more within a year of going off the diet. When dieting, people reduce their caloric intake, which in turn lowers their metabolism. When they discontinue the diet, they typically eat more calories and foods with higher fat content on a lowered metabolism. This is a good formula for weight gain. In addition, dieters tend to lose muscle and regain their weight as fat.

It has also been found that weight as early as infancy is predictive of obesity in adulthood. Babies who gain weight rapidly tend to develop obesity in childhood as well. In fact, a study found that by age 2 babies who gained weight more quickly from birth than what is typical were overweight regardless of what and how much they were fed. Babies born smaller than the norm are more likely to be obese, as are children who are overweight by age 2. Some believe that there may be a metabolic switch activated in the fetus during pregnancy that causes babies to be born small and store extra calories efficiently as a way to survive.[36]

There is a great deal of debate on how an individual's set point can be altered. The number of fat cells in the body, the blood level of insulin, and regions of the brain such as the hypothalamus all seem to play a role in determining the set point. Certain drugs such as amphetamines and other diet pills and herbal supplements can act on the brain to temporarily lower the set point. However, once these drugs are discontinued, the set point returns to the previous level or perhaps an even higher level and weight increases as a result. Healthier and more permanent methods of changing one's set point are through regular exercise and healthy eating patterns. In fact, a study of 8,000 successful dieters found that the majority of them used "my own diet and exercise regimen" and did not follow any formal weight reduction program.[37]

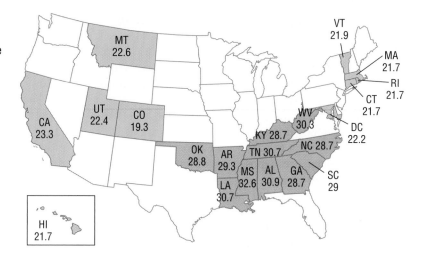

Figure 6-2 Top States with the Highest and Lowest Obesity Rates States in orange have the higest obesity rates in the country, and states in green have the lowest rates.

Source: Centers for Disease Control and Prevention (CDC). Behavioral Risk Factor Surveillance System Survey Data. Atlanta, Georgia: U.S. Department of Health and Human Services, Centers for Disease Control and Prevention, 2008.

The body's requirement for energy to maintain basic physiological processes decreases progressively with age. This change reflects the loss of muscle tissue as both men and women age. This loss of muscle mass eventually alters the ratio of lean body tissue to fat. As the proportion of fat increases, the energy needs of the body are more strongly influenced by the lower metabolic needs of the fat cells.[38] This excess energy is then stored in the fat cells of the body. A gradual decrease in caloric intake and a conscious effort to expend more calories can effectively prevent this gradual increase in weight leading to obesity.

Family, Social, and Cultural Factors

Ethnic and cultural differences also relate to the incidence of obesity and what is considered to be a healthy weight. The statistics are startling: 66 percent of African American women are overweight, and 33 percent are obese. For Mexican Americans, 75 percent of women and 76 percent of men are overweight or obese. Fifty-eight percent of Caucasian women and 70 percent of Caucasian men are overweight or obese.[39] Until recently Asian Americans had a lower rate of obesity than the general population; however, new figures now show that 8 percent of Chinese children 10 to 12 years of age are obese and 15 percent are overweight, which is closer to the overall 19 percent of 6- to 11-year-old American children who are overweight.

Obesity is second only to tobacco as the leading cause of premature deaths and disproportionately affects women of color and women of lower socioeconomic classes. On the positive side, African American women report less pressure to be thin than do their white counterparts and tend to be less self-conscious about their weight.[40] Acculturation also has a significant effect on the rates of obesity—the more an ethnic group has adapted to and absorbed Western culture, the higher the rate of obesity within that group.[41]

Socioeconomic status is also an important influence on obesity. Upper socioeconomic women tend to be thinner than lower socioeconomic women; however, among men there is not such a pattern.[42] Limited access to health care, lower education levels, lower income levels, and increased stress are some of the reasons cited for this disparity. African American and Mexican American children, as well as those living below the poverty level and in rural areas, have a higher incidence of obesity. Interestingly, higher obesity levels are also related to marriage, parenthood, and geographical location; married men, parents, and people living in rural areas tend to have a higher incidence of obesity.[43] Figure 6-2 lists the states with the highest percentages of obese Americans, citing hunger and lack of accessibility to healthy, safe food as the major reasons for this.

The information, values, traditions, and messages you receive from your family also have a significant impact on your dietary habits. If an infant's cries for food are immediately responded to, that child will likely learn what the sensation of hunger is and what the appropriate response is. If crying unrelated to hunger is responded to by the offer of a cookie or candy, the child will learn to soothe himself or herself with food. Studies show that children become confused about what hunger is and how to satisfy it if their hunger needs are neglected or overindulged in infancy.[44]

Some of the first power struggles between parents and their children revolve around issues of food. A child who has little power in her life can exert some power and control through refusing to eat certain foods and demanding other foods and determining when she wants to eat. Parents who use food as a reward for good behavior ("If you get an 'A' on your test, I will treat you to ice cream"); as punishment ("You weren't behaving so you can't have dessert"); or as a guilt trip ("Don't waste food. Clean your plate. Children are starving in the world") may inadvertently be creating negative dietary practices that will continue throughout the child's life. Interestingly, research has shown that children are extraordinarily adept at meeting their nutritional needs when left to their own devices. One study allowed children to eat whatever they wanted for a week. Did they always pick high-fat, high-sugar foods? No. Actually, when we look at each day's intake, they didn't eat a balanced diet. However, when one takes the full week into consideration, they met their nutritional needs perfectly.

What your parents say to you not only has a tremendous influence on your eating behavior; what they do, their own eating practices, can have even a greater impact. Children are exposed to different foods and model what their parents eat. If a parent makes comments such as "I shouldn't eat that because I will get fat" or doesn't eat fruits or vegetables, or sits down with a bag of chips in front of the television every night, the child will probably do the same. In the same vein, when parents exercise regularly, eat a balanced diet, and make positive comments about their weight, children tend to mimic this behavior. See the box "The Growing Problem of Obesity" on page 160.

 TALKING POINTS What were the messages you received in childhood regarding food? What positive and negative eating habits have you learned from your family?

Environmental Factors

Certainly environmental factors such as the smell or sight of freshly made cookies, or an advertisement for a candy bar, can affect your eating habits. Even the clock signaling it is "time to eat" can encourage us to eat when we aren't hungry. While this may seem adaptive and helpful in regulating our food intake, Dr. Kelly D. Brownell, a professor of psychology at Yale and an expert on eating disorders, has gone so far as to label American society a "toxic environment" when it comes to food. Researchers contend that the local environment has a powerful effect on eating. Factors such as portion size, price, advertising, the availability of food, and the number of food choices presented all can influence the amount the average person consumes. For example, moviegoers will eat 50 percent more popcorn if given an extra-large tub of popcorn instead of a container one size smaller, even if the popcorn is stale. If a tabletop in the office is stocked with cookies and candy, coworkers tend to nibble their way through the workday, even if they are not hungry. One study showed that when the candy was in plain sight on workers' desks, they ate an average of nine pieces each. Storing the candy in a desk drawer reduced consumption to six pieces, compared with putting the candy a couple of yards from the desk, which cut the number to three pieces per person.[45]

Another study found that half of children stop on their way to and from school each day to spend about $2 a day on junk food, increasing their caloric intake by 610 calories each day. Hamburgers, pizza, French fries,

cookies, candy, and pastries are the top-selling foods for school-age children. In response to these and other findings, many public schools have begun offering only healthy foods in their cafeterias, replacing soft drinks, candy, and chips with juice, milk, fruit, and granola bars.

Packaging and price can also influence the amount people consume, a concept of which advertisers, restaurants, and grocery stores are well aware. Dropping the price of the low-fat snacks by even a nickel resulted in dramatically increased sales. In contrast, stickers signaling low-fat content or cartoons promoting the low-fat alternatives had little influence over which snacks were more popular. This is true not only of food but also of beverages: people tend to drink *more* from short, wide glasses than from thin, tall ones, thinking they are drinking less.[45]

Having more choices also appears to make people eat more. In one study, people ate more when offered sandwiches with four different fillings than they did when they were given sandwiches with their single favorite filling. In another study, participants who were served a four-course meal with meat, fruit, bread, and a pudding ate 60 percent more food than did those served an equivalent meal of only their favorite course. Note that these findings apply to people of all body sizes not just people who are overweight or obese, as is often the misconception. However, one difference seems to relate to the age of the individuals studied. One study found that 3-year-olds who were served three different portion sizes of macaroni and cheese for lunch on three different days ate the same amount each time. Five-year-olds, however, ate more when more was put in front of them.[46]

This phenomenon is referred to as unit bias, or the tendency to think that a single unit of food is the right amount to eat or drink, no matter what size it is. So we often don't make a conscious decision about how much to eat, as the choice is made for us by the portion size that is offered to us. We mindlessly eat food without questioning the amount.[45] We also tend to eat or drink whatever is offered to us, one large cookie or a small one, and still think of it as the same amount of calories because it is one cookie.

Psychological Factors

Psychological factors related to overeating concern the reasons people eat other than physiological hunger. Individuals with eating disorders often report that they don't know when they are hungry and often eat when they are not hungry and don't eat when they have a biological reason for doing so. Why do people eat if not in response to hunger? Frequently people eat in response to their emotions—for example, to comfort themselves or when bored, tired, stressed, or depressed. Some people say they use food as a way of coping with hurt, sadness, and anger, "swallowing" their feelings and putting food on top of them. Others

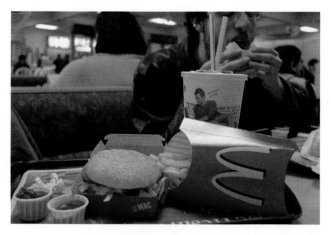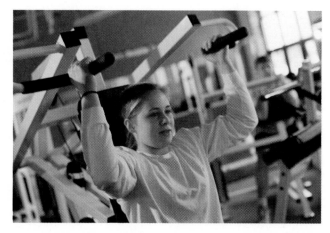

Lifestyle approaches to weight management address two key components of energy balance—energy in as food and energy out as physical activity. Strategies for creating a negative energy balance include reducing your intake of large portions of high-calorie foods (such as fast food) and increasing your level of physical activity.

eat out of habit and associate food with certain activities, such as eating popcorn at a movie, eating chips in front of the television, and having dessert after dinner. Certainly many people think of chocolate when they want to cheer themselves up. Food is also part of celebrations, holidays, and family bonding, as well as a mainstay of socialization. It is difficult to think about social activities we engage in that don't involve food in some way.

Some people develop relationships with food that substitute for real human relationships or to fill other psychological or spiritual needs. Comments such as "Food is my best friend" and "A great meal is better than sex" are indicative to the degree to which many people rely on food to fill their needs. As we'll learn in our discussion of eating disorders later in the chapter, psychological issues with food can become serious, even life-threatening problems.

Weight-Management Strategies

Weight loss occurs when the calories consumed are fewer than required by the body for physiological maintenance and activity. This may sound overly simplified, and certainly the $50 billion-a-year weight loss industry would like us to think it is much more complicated than this.

Weight loss followed by weight gain may be less healthy and certainly more frustrating than maintaining body weight, even at weight above the desirable levels. When a diet or weight loss strategy fails, the person, not the diet, is blamed. This causes people to jump to another weight loss method and then another, and a vicious cycle has begun. However, a commitment to a lifestyle change of eating in healthy ways and engaging in regular exercise seems to be the most effective strategy for weight loss and weight maintenance.

Lifestyle Approaches for Lifetime Healthy Weight Management

In order to maintain a healthy weight, you will need to eat a balanced diet supported by portion control, participate in regular physical activity, get consistent, sufficient sleep, and develop healthy ways of coping and problem solving.

Balanced Diet Supported by Portion Control A diet that reduces caloric intake is the most common approach to what seems to be a national obsession with weight loss. The choice of foods included in the diet and the amount of food that can be consumed are the two factors that distinguish the wide range of diets currently available. However, dieting alone usually does not result in long-term weight loss. Effective and long-lasting weight management requires a lifestyle change, not just going on a diet for a specific time period only to return to your old patterns of eating. This is the problem many people face when they go on strict diets and overly restrict their calories. Because the diet is so restrictive and demanding, they are unable to continue to follow it for very long and return to their previous eating patterns. In addition, people tend to overeat the foods they denied themselves while dieting because they feel deprived and the forbidden food seems even more alluring. This can also lead to binge eating. Thus diets tend not to work in the long run.

A healthy and successful approach to weight loss and subsequent management of that loss is to establish a nutritionally sound balanced diet (see Chapter 5) that controls portions. The food pyramid outlines the breakdown of daily caloric intake for each food group. You can get a personalized dietary guideline by inputting your gender, age, and activity level at MyPyramid.gov. One

Table 6.2 Calories Expended During Physical Activity

To determine the number of calories you have spent in an hour of activity, simply multiply the *calories per hour per pound* column by your weight (in pounds). For example, after an hour of archery, a 120-pound person will have expended 209 calories; a 160-pound person, 278 calories; and a 220-pound person, 383 calories.

Activity	Calories/Hour/Pound	Activity	Calories/Hour/Pound
Archery	1.74	Marching (rapid)	3.84
Baseball	1.86	Painting (outside)	2.10
Basketball	3.78	Playing music (sitting)	1.08
Boxing (sparring)	3.78	Racquetball	3.90
Canoeing (leisure)	1.20	Running (cross-country)	4.44
Cleaning	1.62	Running	
Climbing hills (no load)	3.30	11 min 30 sec per mile	3.66
Cooking	1.20	9 min per mile	5.28
Cycling		8 min per mile	5.64
5.5 mph	1.74	7 min per mile	6.24
9.4 mph	2.70	6 min per mile	6.84
Racing	4.62	5 min 30 sec per mile	7.86
Dance (modern)	2.28	Scrubbing floors	3.00
Eating (sitting)	0.60	Sailing	1.20
Field hockey	3.66	Skiing	
Fishing	1.68	Cross-country	4.43
Football	3.60	Snow, downhill	3.84
Gardening		Water	3.12
Digging	3.42	Skating (moderate)	2.28
Mowing	3.06	Soccer	3.54
Raking	1.44	Squash	5.76
Golf	2.34	Swimming	
Gymnastics	1.80	Backstroke	4.62
Handball	3.78	Breaststroke	4.44
Hiking	2.52	Free, fast	4.26
Horseback riding		Free, slow	3.48
Galloping	3.72	Butterfly	4.68
Trotting	3.00	Table tennis	1.86
Walking	1.14	Tennis	3.00
Ice hockey	5.70	Volleyball	1.32
Jogging	4.15	Walking (normal pace)	2.16
Judo	5.34	Weight training	1.90
Knitting (sewing)	0.60	Wrestling	5.10
Lacrosse	5.70	Writing (sitting)	0.78

Source: From Bannister and Brown, The Relative Energy Requirements of Physical Activity. In H. B. Falls, editor. *Exercise Physiology*, Academic Press, 1988, Table 6.5. Used with permission by Elsevier.

study showed that people cut 256 calories a day just by trimming their portion sizes by 25 percent.

Maintaining a balanced diet and watching your portion sizes is especially important on the weekends. Many people throw their good eating habits out the window on the weekends, as evidenced by a recent study that found that Americans eat an average of 115 extra calories per day from Friday to Sunday compared with the rest of the week. Most of these calories came from alcohol and increased fat consumption. These extra calories can result in a gain of 5 pounds over the course of a year.

Physical Activity Many experts now believe that the most important component of weight management is regular physical activity. Physical activity contributes to weight loss and the maintenance of weight loss because activity burns calories (Table 6.2). Remember, the need for calories decreases with age and with decreased activity.

An additional benefit derived from physical activity is that proportionately more fat is lost than is lost through dieting alone. Studies suggest that the weight loss achieved through physical activity is 95 percent fat and 5 percent lean tissue, such as muscle, in comparison with a loss of 75 percent fat and 25 percent lean tissue when dieting alone is used. Exercise also offers the benefits of increased heart and lung endurance, muscular strength, and flexibility.

How much exercise is enough? The current USDA dietary guidelines (see Chapter 5) advise American adults to engage in at least 60 minutes of moderately intense aerobic exercise almost every day for weight maintenance and 90 minutes of this type of exercise for weight loss. Weight training has become a more important factor in weight management. (See Chapter 4 for further recommendations on physical fitness.)

As with most things, too much or too little exercise is not beneficial and can be unhealthy. As will be discussed in a later section, some people with eating disorders tend to overexercise, resulting in diminishing returns.

Sleep Research has recently discovered that not getting enough sleep doesn't just make you grumpy and sluggish—it can make you gain weight as well! People who sleep 2 to 4 hours a night have been found to be 73 percent more likely to be obese than those who sleep 7 to 9 hours. Sleeping 5 hours a night results in a 50 percent chance of being obese compared to those consistently sleeping 7 to 9 hours. Twenty-three percent of people who sleep 6 hours tend to be obese. In other words, the higher the BMI, the less sleep the person got.[47]

Why does less sleep equal more weight? We used to think that sleeping too much made us gain weight and staying up meant we were more active and so burned calories, but this has been disproved. People tend to watch television, read, or be online late at night, and so they are not active. In addition, people tend to eat high-fat, high-sugar foods while they are engaging in these activities. Some people say that they eat sugary foods in order to give themselves more energy to stay up late to study or to get work done.

Two hormones, ghrelin and leptin, have been found to regulate both sleep and hunger. A sleep study at the University of Chicago found that leptin levels were 18 percent lower and ghrelin levels 28 percent higher after subjects slept 4 hours. Sleep-deprived subjects reported feeling the most hungry and craved carbohydrates, the energy food. Ghrelin has been referred to as the accelerator for eating. When ghrelin levels are up, people feel hungrier. Leptin is the brake for eating; higher levels are associated with feeling full and decreased appetite.

These sleep studies seem to indicate that a hormonal relationship exists between sleep and hunger. The ghrelin level in people who routinely slept 5 hours a night was 15 percent higher, compared to 15 percent lower leptin levels in people who slept 8 hours a night. The first group had higher BMIs than did individuals sleeping 8 hours at night. Studies have also found that children are not getting the 10 to 11 hours of sleep a night they require, which may also help explain the increase in childhood obesity.[48]

So, one way for us to manage our weight is to manage our sleep better. This means managing our time better—prioritizing our commitments and activities and not overloading our schedules, so that we can get the rest we need.

Lifestyle Support and Problem Solving Not only do you need to be committed to a lifestyle of regular physical activity and healthy food choices, but you also need to build a support group that will encourage you in these endeavors. Inform family, friends, classmates, and coworkers about your intent to rely on them for support and encouragement. Perhaps you will inspire others to make similar lifestyle changes.

Successful dieters have consistently reported that having a coach, counselor, or someone that they can meet with on a regular basis to be accountable with has made a tremendous difference in their weight loss efforts and in maintaining a healthy weight.

It may be helpful for you to reevaluate your perception of food and eating. Do you use food as a way of coping with stress, boredom, or other feelings? Consider, instead, coping with stressors with nonfood options such as talking with friends or family, exercising, or journaling. You may want to take the Personal Assessment at the end of this chapter to see if you are eating mindlessly (see also the box "Learning to Eat Mindfully"). Additionally, if you tend to use food as a way to reward yourself for hard work or completing something, you might want to choose other types of rewards, such as engaging in a hobby or another activity you enjoy. Take care that you don't adopt other unhealthy methods of coping.

The lifestyle choices suggested here will significantly help reduce your chances of developing a weight problem or a weight-related health problem in your lifetime. Again, genetics will exert its effects to some degree on weight and body composition, but you can counteract these effects by employing the methods discussed here.

Specific Dietary Approaches

There are many different strategies for losing weight, and they vary in effectiveness, harmfulness, cost, and ease of use. The next section will cover the most popular weight loss methods: temporary caloric restriction, low-calorie foods and controlled serving sizes, controlled fasting, formal or commercial weight reduction programs, weight loss drugs, herbal supplements, and surgical interventions.

Temporary Calorie Restriction   People use a variety of fad diets in an attempt to achieve rapid weight loss. Currently there are over 150 popular diets, often promoted by celebrities or people who claim to be nutrition experts. With few exceptions, these approaches are both ineffective and potentially dangerous. In addition, some require far greater expense than would be associated with weight loss or management techniques using portion control and regular physical activity. (See Table 6.3.)

The main problem with dieting is that it is a temporary, quick fix. Most diets will result in temporary weight loss if followed correctly, and they usually make the promise of losing weight rapidly. Of course, much of the weight lost initially is water weight and not fat. Research shows that 90 percent of all people who diet gain back their weight, plus more, within a year. Oprah Winfrey is a good example of what happens to most dieters. She lost 67 pounds in four months consuming only Optifast. She kept this weight off for only one day. The first day she went off her diet and went back to her old eating patterns, she began gaining weight. She weighed 211 pounds pre-diet and she weighed 226 pounds post-diet. Look at Figure 6-3 to see why people struggle with losing weight.

Table 6.3   Rating the Diets

	Overall Score	Nutritional Analysis	Short-Term Weight Loss	Long-Term Weight Loss
Volumetrics	Good	Excellent	Good	Good
Weight Watchers	Good	Excellent	Fair	Fair
Jenny Craig	Good	Excellent	Good	Good
Slim Fast	Good	Excellent	Good	Good
eDiets	Good	Excellent	Below Avg	Below Avg
Zone Diet	Good	Excellent	Fair	Below Avg
Ornish Diet	Fair	Fair	Fair	Fair
Atkins Diet	Below Avg	Poor	Good	Fair

Source: New Diet Winners, *Consumer Reports*, June 2007.

Diets don't teach us how to eat; they teach us how not to eat! The restriction of calories is the basis of all diets. Some suggest limiting the consumption of fat, others sugar, or the caloric intake is dangerously low for all food groups. Many diet plans, such as the South Beach diet and the Atkins diet, advocate the restriction of carbohydrates, which can cause ketosis. Ketosis can cause the blood to become too acidic, and dehydration can occur. The body requires a minimum of 50 to 100 grams of carbohydrate per day to avoid ketosis.[26] Low-carbohydrate diets are characterized by initial rapid weight loss, which is appealing to most people, but this is primarily due to water loss, not fat loss. Complications associated with low-carbohydrate, high-protein diets include dehydration, hypertension, heart disease, cancer, electrolyte loss, calcium depletion, weakness due to inadequate dietary carbohydrates, nausea due to ketosis, vitamin and mineral deficiencies, and possible kidney problems. Gout (painful inflammation of the joints) and kidney failure are potential side effects. The risk of coronary heart disease may be higher in those who stay on the diet a long time, owing to the increased consumption of foods high in saturated fat and cholesterol.

Most diets are temporary in nature because they are medically unhealthy and potentially harmful. They are also too restrictive, and people end up craving the very foods they are being told to avoid. Dieters begin feeling deprived and resentful, and respond by retaliating against the diet and bingeing on the "forbidden" foods.

Low-Calorie Foods and Controlled Serving Sizes   Recently, a variety of familiar foods have been developed in a reduced-calorie form. By lowering the carbohydrate content with the use of nonnutritive sweeteners, reducing the portion size, reducing the fat content of the original formulations, or removing fat entirely (see the discussion of Olestra in Chapter 5), manufacturers

Figure 6-3 Why Weight Loss Is Often Pie-in-the-Sky   *USA Today* surveyed 126 of the nation's top registered dietitians about trends in obesity and weight loss. Selected findings are shown here.

Source: From *USA Today,* December 29, 2004. Reprinted with permission.

What's the major reason people want to lose weight?

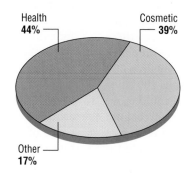

Health
44%

Cosmetic
39%

Other
17%

What's the main reason people resist changing their eating habits?

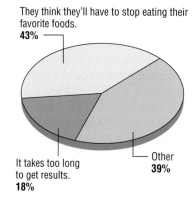

They think they'll have to stop eating their favorite foods.
43%

It takes too long to get results.
18%

Other
39%

What's the biggest mistake people make when trying to lose weight?

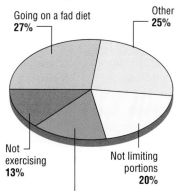

Going on a fad diet
27%

Other
25%

Not exercising
13%

Not limiting portions
20%

Setting inappropriate goals, such as wanting to lose quickly
15%

What's the main reason people don't exercise or increase physical activity to manage weight?

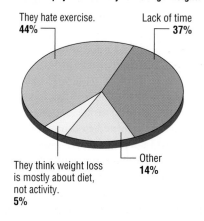

They hate exercise.
44%

Lack of time
37%

They think weight loss is mostly about diet, not activity.
5%

Other
14%

have produced "lite" versions of many food products. For example, many frozen entrees, such as Healthy Choice Five-Spice Beef and Vegetables (310 calories), Weight Watchers Lasagna Florentine (290 calories), and Healthy Choice Fettucine Alfredo (240 calories), are low in calories. Because fat helps us to feel satiated or not hungry, these low-fat, low-calorie meals tend not to satisfy our hunger for very long, and we may find ourselves wanting to snack or binge by late afternoon.

TALKING POINTS   Your best friend is trying to follow a low-fat, low-calorie diet in order to lose weight but is finding herself constantly hungry. What can you tell her about the diet plan she's chosen? What changes might she make to increase her chances of success?

Controlled Fasting   In cases of extreme obesity, some patients are placed on a complete fast in a hospital setting. The patient consumes only water, electrolytes, and vitamins. Weight loss is substantial because the body is forced to begin **catabolizing** its fat and muscle tissue.

Complete fasting is such an extreme approach to weight loss that it must be done in an institutional setting so that the patient can be closely monitored. Inadequate protein and sodium and potassium loss are particular health concerns.

Today some people regularly practice short periods of modified fasting. Solid foods are removed from the diet for a number of days. Fruit juices, water, supplements, and vitamins are used to minimize the risks associated with total fasting. However, unsupervised short-term fasting can be dangerous and is not recommended.

In addition to the controlled fasting just discussed, a somewhat different version of this practice is appearing

Key Terms

catabolizing   The metabolic process of breaking down tissue for the purpose of converting it to energy.

with the long-term use of readily available, low-calorie, nutrient-dense food supplementation products such as Ensure, Boost, SlimFast, and Sustical. Regardless of whether they are marketed as nutrient-dense supplements for older adults or as adjuncts to weight loss diets, these drinks should not be viewed, or used, as meal replacements. Because these products contain no more than 400 calories (and the lite versions contain as few as 200 calories), their routine use as meal replacements could move even a young, healthy adult dangerously close to caloric inadequacy in a short time. Perhaps if used in place of a high-calorie snack or as a very occasional substitute for breakfast, these supplements may not present the dangers that their routine use does.

Formal or Commercial Weight Reduction Programs

In virtually every area of the country, at least one version of the popular weight reduction programs, such as Take Off Pounds Sensibly (TOPS), Jenny Craig, and Nutri-System Weight Loss Centers, can be found. Pioneered by Weight Watchers, these programs generally feature a format consisting of (1) a well-balanced diet emphasizing portion control and low-fat, low-saturated fat, and high-complex carbohydrate foods, (2) specific weight loss goals to be attained over a set period of time, (3) encouragement from supportive leaders and fellow group members, (4) emphasis on regular physical activity, and (5) a maintenance program (follow-up program).

Although in theory these programs offer an opportunity to lose weight for people who cannot or will not participate in a physical activity program, their effectiveness is very limited. The minimal success of these programs and the difficulty that working adults have in attending meetings has resulted in falling enrollment and the development of home-based programs, such as those developed by hospital-based wellness programs, many YMCAs and YWCAs, and even Weight Watchers. Further, these programs can be costly when compared with self-directed approaches, especially when the program markets its own food products. The pros and cons of a variety of weight loss programs are presented in Table 6.3.

The Weight Loss Industry In response to our nation's near obsession with thinness, a thriving weight loss industry exists to assist us in our attempts to lose weight.

The weight loss industry has capitalized and profited on the meaning that thinness has in the American culture, including a bias against large people. These programs are promising not just weight loss but happiness and success in life as well. Thinness is associated not only with beauty but also with one's ability to have successful relationships, careers, and self-worth. A study was conducted asking 32,000 women what they would choose: a successful career, a satisfying romantic relationship, or a loss of 10 to 15 pounds. The majority of these women chose to lose weight, believing that they would also have a successful career and relationship if they lost 10 to 15 pounds.[9]

Another study showed children pictures of a minority child, a disabled child, and an overweight child and asked them to choose who they would like to be their friend. Overwhelmingly, the overweight child was their last choice. The American Association of University Women conducted a study to examine the changing attitudes children and adolescents have of themselves in terms of their body image. While 60 percent of elementary school girls said, "I am always happy with the way I am," only 29 percent of high school girls said the same thing. For boys, 67 percent of elementary school boys liked how they looked, and 46 percent of high school boys continued to feel this way. It is these attitudes that play into the measures to which individuals will go and the price they will pay to achieve the cultural ideal.

The financial success of the weight loss industry in this country has in part been because of its effective television advertising. Skillfully produced commercials featuring successful program members suggest likely success for the viewer willing to sign on. Before 1994, these commercials were regular fare on daytime television. Today, however, commercials for diet programs such as Jenny Craig, NutriSystem, Weight Watchers, and others are considerably more restrained in their messages about success. Under directives issued by the Federal Trade Commission (FTC), today's advertisements cannot misrepresent program performance. They must disclose that most weight loss is temporary, and they now inform the viewer that their loss will most likely not approximate that of the successful subjects featured in their commercials.

Most recently some nationally franchised weight loss programs have added a "medical" component to their format that involves prescribing medications. Consumers should find out if medical supervision will be a regular component of the program or a brief, one-time physician visit involving little more than basic screening.

Weight Loss Drugs

Another approach to weight loss involves over-the-counter weight loss drugs, herbal supplements, and prescription drugs. These are designed to either suppress hunger, increase metabolism, or block fat absorption in order to manage weight.

Over-the-Counter (OTC) Weight Loss Drugs and Herbal Supplements

Most OTC and herbal supplements are designed to suppress hunger and increase metabolism. None of them are recommended for long-term use, as they can cause serious health problems and can be addictive. It is difficult to stop taking these pills because weight loss occurs only while taking them and weight gain usually occurs once the drug or supplement is discontinued. Most of these contained ephedra or ephedrine until it was banned by the FDA in 2003.[49] Ephedra has been associated with at least 155 deaths and dozens of heart attacks and strokes, and it can cause high blood pressure, seizures, heart irregularities, insomnia, anxiety, and tremors.

Herbal weight loss supplements come as pills, bars, teas, and powders to mix in liquids. Some people see herbal supplements such as stackers, mini thins, hoodia, and fat burners as safe because they are "natural," and yet they can be more dangerous and deadly than prescription medications because they are not inspected for purity and accuracy of the contents or the potency of the ingredients. The Dietary Supplement Health and Education Act (DSHEA) of 1994 relegated herbal supplements to the category "dietary supplements," limiting the FDA's power to regulate these products to ensure that they meet certain standards or are safe and effective. In fact, it is difficult to stop the sale of dietary supplements that appear dangerous because there must be enough proof to substantiate the health risks.

However, there is some evidence linking these diet pills to heart attacks, strokes, hepatitis, headaches, tremors, anxiety, extreme irritability, and insomnia in consumers of all ages. After the FDA banned ephedra, other supplements with questionable safety took its place. For example, supplements with bitter orange contain the compound syndephrine, which is chemically similar to ephedrine and affects blood pressure and heart rate in ways similar to ephedra.[50] Aristolochia fangchi, another herb used in weight loss pills, has been associated with kidney damage, renal failure, and kidney cancer.

Some diet supplements, such as cascara and aloe, act as strong stimulant laxatives; others, often derived from caffeine, act as diuretics. Juniper seeds, dandelion, equistine, horsetail, and shave grass are examples of these and have been linked to renal damage, brain damage, and convulsions. Some diet pills sold on the Internet contain phenolphthalein, a laxative that has been associated with risk of cancer.[51] Other diet pills, such as glucomannan and guar gum, create a feeling of fullness because of their dietary fiber content and have been associated with gastrointestinal and esophageal obstructions.

There is also a danger in the potential interactions between prescription medications and herbal agents. Most people are unaware of these and physicians may overlook them because 70 percent of patients do not disclose their use of herbal supplements to their physicians. Chromium, pyruvate, 5-hydroxytryptophan (5-HTP), chitosan, and carnitine are some common herbal supplements used for weight loss; however, there are hundreds of herbal supplements, and so it is impossible to list them all. It is important to look at the labels and read the ingredients in diet pills to see what you are really ingesting and to know how these herbs may affect your body. In addition, these dietary supplements have not been shown to be effective in helping to lose weight!

One particular over-the-counter weight loss medication containing **phenylpropanolamine (PPA)** merits mentioning, as drug companies making these products were asked to stop manufacturing them in 2000 because of PPA's association with an increased risk for stroke. The FDA issued a public health advisory telling consumers not to use any products containing PPA for this reason. PPA was also found in OTC cough and cold medications.

Prescription Weight Loss Drugs Some prescription medications have also been shown to produce serious side effects. Two such medications, *phentermine* and *fenfluramine*, have been prescribed for patients who wanted to lose weight. Both drugs affect levels of serotonin, the neurotransmitter associated with satiety. This combination, referred to as *phenfen*, gradually raised concern among health experts because of the side effects it produced in people with angina, glaucoma, and high blood pressure. In addition, reports began to surface that some patients had developed a rare but lethal condition called *pulmonary hypertension.*

In September 1997, the FDA requested voluntary withdrawal of fenfluramine and dexfenfluramine from the market because of reports of heart valve damage in those using these drug combinations.[52] Manufacturers responded by ceasing all distribution of the drugs.

At the same time of the initial concern over the use of phentermine and fenfluramine, the FDA approved yet another obesity drug, *sibutramine* (brand name Meridia), even though an advisory committee within the FDA recommended against approving it. Meridia acts on serotonin in the body and has been linked to heart attacks, high blood pressure, strokes, and death; however, it remains on the market in the United States. Italy recently pulled Meridia from the market following reports of death linked to this drug.

Fat-Blocking Drugs *Orlistat* (brand name Xenical) has also been used for weight loss. Unlike phentermine and sibutramine, which influence the neurotransmitter serotonin, orlistat reduces fat absorption in the small intestine by about 30 percent. The drug is intended for use among people who are 20 percent or more over their

> **Key Terms**
>
> **phenylpropanolamine (PPA)** (**fen** ill **pro** puh **nol** uh meen) The active chemical compound found in some over-the-counter diet products and associated with increased risk of stroke.

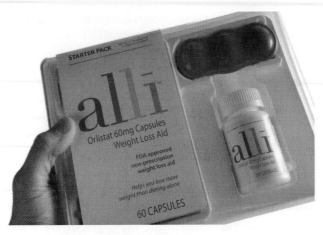

An over-the-counter version of the prescription drug orlistat (Xenical) was approved by the FDA in 2007.

ideal weight. In persons who tolerate the drug's side effects, a 10 percent reduction of weight without significant dietary restriction is possible.

For the first time, the FDA has approved a prescription diet pill, Xenical (orlistat), as an OTC medication called Alli.[53] Costing about $50 for a two-month supply, Alli contains half the dosage of Xenical. Alli is not without its risks, as it has the same problematic side effects as Xenical, including sudden diarrhea, commonly referred to as "alli-oops" because of the lack of warning and soiled pants Alli users have reported experiencing. Some have intense stomach pain when taking this pill, and it has also been linked with precancerous lesions in the colon.[53]

Some concerns related to the use of orlistat include anal leakage, severe abdominal cramping, excessive flatulence, and inhibition of the absorption of vitamins and minerals in the body. Olestra has been used in fat-free chips such as "Wow!" potato chips, and there have been complaints of stomach discomfort among people who ate them. In addition, people erroneously believe that they can eat as much as they want since it is fat-free, but it is not calorie-free and so they may end up gaining weight as a result.

Surgical Interventions

It used to be that surgical measures were undertaken only if the person's weight was severely endangering his or her health and other less invasive methods had been unsuccessful. Now surgeries such as liposuction, tummy tucks, gastric bypass surgery, and gastric band surgeries are becoming increasingly popular and commonplace, especially among teenagers. Gastric bypass surgery, vertical banded gastroplasty, and laparoscopic adjustable gastric banding all involve major surgery. They can also

be very expensive, costing upward of $25,000, and some insurance companies will not pay for this, claiming it is cosmetic surgery even though there are significant medical risks associated with obesity. Even so, the number of obesity surgeries being performed has increased 600 percent over the past five years.[54] Although obesity surgeries are not approved for patients under age 18, in 2007 there were almost 1,000 of them performed on children as test cases. With the increase in obesity among children, along with improved surgical techniques, there has been a push for the FDA to approve these surgeries for children.

All four operations limit the amount of food a person can eat at one time, because overeating results in vomiting or severe diarrhea. Because the stomach is made smaller, individuals who have undergone these procedures must limit their food intake to half a cup to a cup of food at each "meal." Individuals lose weight because this type of surgery limits the amount of food that can be digested, therefore decreasing the amount of calories that they can eat at one time. However, it is possible to regain weight by eating small portions of high-calorie foods on a consistent basis.

Gastric Bypass Surgery   Gastric bypass is the most common type of weight loss surgery, and it has gained interest since celebrities such as singer Carnie Wilson, Sharon Osbourne, author Anne Rice, *American Idol* judge Randy Jackson, and weatherman Al Roker have gone public about their experiences with this surgery. It is a major operation and involves dividing the stomach into two compartments to create a pouch, the size of a thumb, for food to enter. The small intestine is cut below the stomach and connected to a smaller portion of the stomach, bypassing the larger stomach and a section of the intestine, which are no longer used (see Figure 6-4 A–C). An average of 205,000 people each year now undergo gastric bypass surgeries (also referred to as *bariatric surgeries*), compared to just 16,800 people in 1993. The average cost per surgery is $26,000 to $35,000, and the average death rate is 1 in 200. Candidates for this surgery typically have a BMI above 40 or are 100 pounds or more (men) or at least 80 pounds (women) overweight. People with a BMI between 35 and 40 who suffer from type 2 diabetes or life-threatening cardiopulmonary problems may also be candidates for surgery.

Gastric sleeve resection is the newest option for weight loss surgery. It is typically used for individuals whose BMI is over 60 as part of a two-stage bypass surgical procedure. It involves removing two-thirds of the stomach by stapling, resulting in the stomach becoming tube shaped (see Figure 6-4D). It is not reversible.

Gastric bypass surgery tends to result in greater weight loss (93.3 pounds on average) than does gastroplasty (67 pounds on average) after one year. Over two years, gastric bypass surgery patients have been shown to

Gastric bypass surgery

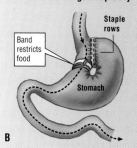

Small intestine connected to stomach compartment

Staple rows

Stomach

A

Done by an open surgery or laparoscopically. The stomach is divided into two compartments, each closed by several rows of staples, creating a thumb-size pouch at the top. A small outlet is created in the smaller portion of the stomach, and the small intestine is connected to it. Food entering the small stomach causes a sensation of fullness, then slowly empties into the intestine through the small outlet.

Vertical banded gastroplasty

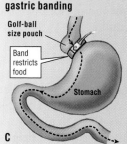

Staple rows

Band restricts food

Stomach

B

Four rows of staples are placed vertically in the upper part of the stomach. The outlet at the lower end of the pouch created by these staples is restricted by a ring that limits the passage of food into the rest of the stomach. The person feels full after a few bites of food.

Laparoscopic adjustable gastric banding

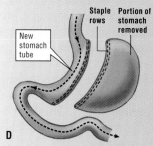

Golf-ball size pouch

Band restricts food

Stomach

C

An inflatable band is placed around the outside of the upper stomach to create a small pouch with a narrow outlet to the rest of the digestive tract.

Gastric sleeve resection

Staple rows

Portion of stomach removed

New stomach tube

D

The left side of the stomach is removed and the portion of the stomach that is left is stapled. The result is a 3–6 ounce stomach that is the size and shape of a banana. The procedure does not involve the reconnection of the intestines or the implantation of an artificial device.

Figure 6-4 Four Types of Obesity Surgery
Source: A–C from *USA Today*, May 5, 2004. Reprinted with permission.

lose two-thirds of excess weight. These surgeries are not without their risks: hernias, ulcers, liver damage, infection, internal leaks, and even death. They are not a cure-all for weight management; individuals who have these operations must continue to exercise regularly, take

nutritional supplements, eat small portions very slowly, and decrease intake of high-sugar foods in order to maintain their weight loss.

Gastric Band Surgery There are two types of gastric band surgery: vertical banded gastroplasty and laparoscopic adjustable gastric banding. Vertical banded gastroplasty uses both a band and staples to create a small stomach pouch, limiting the passage of food into the rest of the stomach. This results in a feeling of fullness after only a few mouthfuls of food. This used to be the most common weight loss surgery, but it has decreased in popularity with the rise of gastric bypass surgery. Weight loss is not as rapid as with gastric bypass surgery. However, some insurance companies will pay for gastric band surgery because it costs half as much as gastric bypass. Laparoscopic adjustable gastric banding, a less invasive procedure, involves an inflatable band being placed around the upper end of the stomach, again creating a small pouch. A narrow passage is also made into the rest of the stomach. The band is inflated with a salt solution through a tube that connects the band to an access port positioned under the skin. In this way, the band can be tightened or loosened over time to change the size of the passageway into the stomach.

This procedure is reversible. It too can involve complications following surgery, such as band slippage, erosion and deflation, obstruction of the stomach, dilation of the esophagus, infection, nausea, stomach wall deterioration, ulcers, vomiting, heartburn, and difficulty swallowing.

Cosmetic Surgeries and Procedures Cosmetic surgeries have increased 38 percent since 2000, with over 11 million Americans undergoing these surgeries. Some call it "addictive," because once they have one procedure, they notice other parts of their bodies that they want to change. In her book *Beauty Junkies: Inside Our $15 Billion Obsession With Cosmetic Surgery,* Alex Kuczynski talks about her pursuit of perfection through plastic surgery. Some believe that changing their bodies will improve their body image and their overall satisfaction with their lives. With the convenience and ease of being able to do some of the more minor procedures over the lunch hour, some people now view cosmetic surgery as being similar to getting a haircut. The most common cosmetic surgeries are liposuction, breast augmentation, eyelid surgery, abdominoplasty (tummy tuck), and breast reduction.

Liposuction and Abdominoplasty Liposuction is the most frequent cosmetic operation in the United States in which fat tissue is removed. Liposuction involves removing unwanted fat from specific areas, such as the abdomen, hips, buttocks, thighs, knees, upper arms, chin, cheeks, and neck. A small tube is inserted through the skin, and adipose tissue is vacuumed out. This is more of a sculpting or contouring operation than a weight loss surgery because little weight is lost. Potential risks and outcomes include infection; the formation of fat clots or blood clots, which may travel to the lungs and cause death; excessive fluid loss, which can lead to shock or fluid accumulation that must be drained; friction burns or other damage to the skin or nerves; numbness; skin discoloration; irregular body contours; and sagging skin. Approximately 400,000 people undergo liposuction each year. The cost of liposuction ranges from $3,000 to $8,500, depending upon the part of the body receiving the surgery and the size of the patient.

People considering these procedures should carefully investigate all aspects, including the training and experience of the surgeon, to determine whether they are appropriate for them.

There exists a growing concern regarding the safety of liposuction based on a comparison of surgery-related deaths during liposuction and the death rates for all surgery, including trauma-based cases. In the case of all types of surgery, the mortality rate is reported to be between 1 death for every 100,000 cases and 1 death for every 300,000 surgical cases, whereas for liposuction the rate may be 20 to 60 times higher.[55] In spite of these figures, the Society of Plastic and Reconstructive Surgeons believes the procedure is still acceptably safe, explaining that an office-based procedure often carries a higher mortality rate than do procedures conducted in hospitals.

Abdominoplasty, known more commonly as a tummy tuck, is a major surgical procedure to remove excess skin and fat from the middle and lower abdomen and to tighten the muscles of the abdominal wall. It leaves a permanent scar, which can extend from hip to hip. Infection and blood clots are some of the potential risks. A balanced diet and regular exercise are required to maintain the results from this surgery.

Lipodissolve   Similar to liposuction with fewer risks, lipodissolve, also referred to as mesotherapy, is a non-surgical procedure. Soy lecithin and bile salt are injected directly into problem areas such as the hips, waist, thighs, and buttocks, purportedly destroying the fat cells' walls and metabolizing and excreting the cells' contents. This process necessitates six to eight visits every two weeks and

costs approximately $2,000 for each area treated. Allergic reactions, skin ulcerations, scarring, and infections are some of the reported side effects of this procedure.

Body Wrapping   Although not a surgical procedure or weight loss technique, *body wrapping* is another form of body contouring. In this procedure, various areas of the body are tightly wrapped with 6-inch strips of material soaked in a solution of amino acids that are claimed to draw toxins out of the underlying tissue, shrink fatty deposits, diminish **cellulite,** lighten stretch marks, and eliminate inches of fat. Once the wrapping is removed, the newly contoured body area may remain this way for 4 to 10 weeks. Although the secret to the success of a particular spa's body wrapping approach is supposed to lie in its uniquely formulated soaking solution, the contouring effect probably results from dehydration of the underlying tissue and redistribution of extracellular fluids through pressure from the wrapping.

Regarding cellulite, note that no product or noninvasive procedure currently in the marketplace has been shown to be effective in removing or reducing this tissue. Thus, the dimpled appearance of the buttocks, back of the arm, and upper leg seems destined to remain, despite cosmetic companies' advertisements of lotions and creams that claim to eliminate cellulite.

Approaches for Weight Gain

For some, the lack of adequate body weight, called **underweight,** can be a serious concern. These people would likely fall into a BMI category of less than 18.5 and be 10 to 20 percent below normal on a standard height/weight table. One population that tends to struggle more with being too thin is the elderly. The CDC found that extreme thinness is associated with death in people over the age of 70. Also significant, unintentional weight loss has been associated with later development of Alzheimer's disease. A weight loss of 5 percent or more in a month is considered significant.

Nutritionists believe that the healthiest way to gain weight is to increase the intake of "calorie-dense" food (see the box "Weight Management Tips"). These foods are characterized by high fat density resulting from high levels of vegetable fats (polyunsaturated fats). Particularly good foods in this regard are dried fruits, bananas, nuts, granola, and cheeses made from low-fat milk. The current recommendation is to eat three calorie-dense meals of moderate size per day, interspersed with two or three substantial snacks. Using MyPyramid in Chapter 5, one should increase intake for each group.[56]

A second component of weight gain for those who are underweight is an exercise program that uses weight training activities intended to increase muscle mass. For all the reasons detailed in Chapter 4, the use of anabolic drugs in the absence of highly competent medical

---

Key Terms

cellulite   Tissue composed of fat cells intertwined around strands of fibrous connective tissue.

underweight   A condition in which the body is below the desirable weight.

supervision has no role in healthful weight gain. In addition, carefully monitored aerobic activity should be undertaken in sessions adequate to maintain heart-lung health, while at the same time one should restrict unnecessary activity that expends calories.

For those who cannot gain weight in spite of having tried the preceding approaches, a medical evaluation could supply an explanation for being underweight. If no medical explanation can be found, the person may be among the 5 percent of the population that are naturally underweight. However, when individuals fall below 80 percent of their desirable weight on standard height/weight tables and have BMIs below 16, it is highly probable that they are not only underweight but, more important, undernourished.[57] This condition suggests clinically significant dietary deficiencies in both the quantity and the quality of the food being consumed. Whether the undernourishment is associated with anorexia nervosa, other medical conditions characterized by weight loss (such as inflammatory bowel disease), or poverty or famine, affected people are in danger of death from starvation.

Eating Disorders

Given the pressure most people feel to maintain the cultural ideal of beauty, and being bombarded with images of very thin actresses and models, such as Portia de Rossi, Victoria Beckham, Mary-Kate Olsen, and Nicole Richie, it is no wonder that some people develop serious medical and psychological disorders associated with body image, weight, and food. It is also not surprising that many of the very models we are trying to emulate also have eating disorders, as they succumb to the pressure to be ever thinner. Anorexia nervosa, bulimia nervosa, binge eating, and disordered eating are frequently found in college populations. We have included these topics in the chapter on weight management because most eating disorders begin with dieting. However, most eating disorders also involve inappropriate food choices, as well as psychological issues. Those issues are discussed in Chapters 2 and 5.

A recent survey showed that dieting has become the norm for females starting at an early age. Fifty percent of

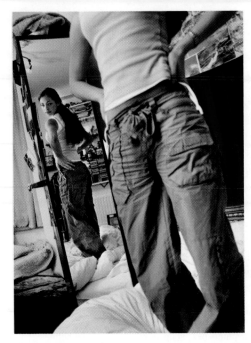

Preoccupation with weight and shape, inappropriate dieting, and perfectionism are factors associated with the development of eating disorders.

9-year-olds and 80 percent of 10-year-olds have reported dieting.[22] While eating disorders involve a preoccupation with food and weight, much deeper psychological issues underlie these conditions.

In the United States, conservative estimates indicate that after puberty 5 to 10 million females and 1 million males struggle with eating disorders such as anorexia, bulimia, or binge eating disorder. It is estimated that approximately 8 percent of college women will develop an eating disorder, and the population most at risk for developing bulimia is college freshman women. Ninety to ninety-five percent of people with eating disorders are women, although the prevalence of eating disorders in men is on the rise. Athletes such as dancers, gymnasts, swimmers, runners, and wrestlers are at risk for developing eating disorders because of the focus on weight and appearance for successful performance. In fact, any group in which success is influenced by weight or

attractiveness is at risk for the development of an eating disorder, such as those involved in the performance arts, theatre, television, and modeling.

Anorexia Nervosa

Anorexia nervosa is an eating disorder in which a person denies his or her own feelings of hunger and avoids food, with marked weight loss occurring. Anorexics tend to run from food in the relentless pursuit of thinness, although they never perceive themselves as thin enough. To meet the diagnostic criteria for anorexia nervosa, the individual has an intense fear of gaining weight, even though he or she weighs less than 85 percent of the expected weight for his or her age, gender, and height, and, in females, menstruation ceases for at least three consecutive months.[58] In addition, people with anorexia perceive themselves as overweight and much larger than they really are. Anorexics lose their ability to recognize when they are hungry and have difficulty eating even if they want to do so. Depression, irritability, withdrawal, perfectionism, and low self-esteem are some of the psychological problems associated with anorexia. In addition, anorexics tend to feel cold most of the time because they have very little body fat (2–10 percent) and also suffer from lightheadedness, dizziness, insomnia, hair loss, muscle cramps, stress fractures, fatigue, decreased memory and concentration, and gastrointestinal problems. More serious complications include heart and kidney failure, hypothermia, osteoporosis, infertility, and, in 25 percent of cases, death. See the box "Recognizing Anorexia Nervosa and Bulimia Nervosa" for more information.

As with other eating disorders, anorexia nervosa also involves a sense of feeling out of control in one's life and attempting to find control through food and weight loss. It is not a coincidence that anorexia nervosa typically begins around puberty: Most individuals with anorexia have a fear of growing up and all that goes with being an adult, such as financial responsibility, sexual relationships, leaving one's family, and becoming more autonomous and independent.

Anorexia often begins with dieting but may also begin as a result of an illness such as the stomach flu, a relationship that breaks up, or after dental surgery, when it might be expected that one would temporarily eat less. However, anorexics will tell you that the disorder begins to take on a life of its own after what started as wanting to lose a few pounds turns into losing 15 percent or more of body weight and still not feeling satisfied with one's appearance. Friends and family might initially encourage the person on his or her weight loss and say complimentary things about his or her appearance but soon become concerned when the person's weight continues to dramatically decrease.

Anorexia has become more common as changing cultural ideals for beauty have changed. Our standards

Recognizing Anorexia Nervosa and Bulimia Nervosa

The American Psychological Association uses the following diagnostic criteria to identify anorexia nervosa and bulimia nervosa.

Anorexia	Bulimia
• Body weight is 15 percent or more below desirable weight	• Binge eating two or more times a week for at least three months
• Fear of weight gain	• A lack of control over bingeing
• Distorted body image	• Engaging in inappropriate compensatory behavior, purging two or more times a week for at least three months to prevent weight gain
• In women, the absence of three or more menstrual periods (younger girls may not start menstruating at the appropriate age); in men, sex hormones decrease	• Overly concerned about body image

Characteristic symptoms include the following. Note that it is unlikely that all the symptoms will be evident in any one individual.

Anorexia	Bulimia
• Looks thin and keeps getting thinner	• Bathroom use immediately after eating
• Skips meals, cuts food into small pieces, moves food around plate to appear to have eaten	• Eating in secret
• Loss of menstrual periods and possible infertility	• Excessive time (and money) spent food shopping
• Wears baggy clothes in an attempt to disguise weight loss and to keep warm	• Shopping for food at several stores instead of one store
• Significant hair loss; lanugo (fine downy body hair)	• Menstrual irregularities and possible fertility problems
• Extreme sensitivity to cold	• Excessive constipation
• Dizziness, lightheadedness, headaches	• Swollen and/or infected salivary glands, sore throat
• Withdrawn, irritable, depressed	• Bursting blood vessels in the eyes
• Insomnia, fatigue, loss of energy	• Dental erosion in teeth and gums
• Decreased sex drive	• Dehydration and kidney dysfunction
• Dehydration, kidney dysfunction	• Significant hair loss; dry, brittle hair and nails
• Decreased concentration	• Increased acne and skin problems
• Heart irregularities, heart failure	• Heart irregularities, heart failure

have gone from Marilyn Monroe, who was a voluptuous 5 feet 4 inches and 140-pounds, to Kate Moss, who has been reported to be 5 feet 7 inches and 105 pounds.[9] Now the "lollipop look" is considered the "in look" in Hollywood, with actresses and models having stick-thin bodies, making their heads seem huge. More attention has been drawn to this disorder since Mary-Kate Olsen went public with her battle with anorexia. She is not alone; other stars have admitted to having anorexia—for example, Tracey Gold (*Growing Pains* sitcom), Spice Girl Victoria Beckham, singer Whitney Houston, and actresses Christina Ricci and Portia de Rossi. Because many of these stars are seen as the standard for the American body ideal, they may be inadvertently increasing the number of women with eating disorders.

Recently researchers have found a significant difference in the brain chemistry of anorexics, compared to those who don't have this disorder. Anorexics have a higher level of serotonin activity in their brains, which is believed to be linked to feelings of anxiety and obsessional thinking. It is further believed that starvation may act to decrease the amount of serotonin in the brain, creating a sense of calm for anorexics. Further research is being done to investigate this biochemical link to anorexia, which will have implications for treatment and recovery.

Denial of problems plays a major role in eating disorders in that the individual refuses to acknowledge that there is anything wrong, even though she is becoming thinner and wasting away, and family and friends are expressing great concern. Anorexia nervosa is considered a serious medical and psychological disorder; however, some anorexics argue, "Anorexia is a lifestyle not a disorder." Heated debates and discussions often occur on pro-anorexia websites. With names like "Thinspiration," "Stick Figures," and "Anorexic and Proud," these pro-anorexia forums have become very popular and deadly in the past few years. These websites show computer-enhanced pictures of models and actresses such as Calista Flockhart and Lara Flynn Boyle making them appear thinner and more skeletal than they really are.[59] Messages on these websites include tips on how to starve, how to purge, and ways of hiding one's disorder, as well as encouragement to lose more weight. There has been a push among health providers, educators, and health organizations to eliminate these types of websites, and they have been somewhat successful. However, these sites still do exist, although somewhat disguised and underground.[60]

Three groups that have traditionally been overlooked in the incidence of anorexia are women of color, female athletes (see "Female Athlete Triad" in Chapter 4), and men. The research shows a significant increase in the incidence of anorexia among these three groups. More focus has been given to anorexia among women of color, and it has been proposed that this group might be more vulnerable to developing eating disorders than Caucasian women are because of ethnocultural identity issues. It has been suggested that the more pressure women of color feel to fit into the dominant culture's standards of beauty and thinness, the more likely they are to develop eating disorders.

Often female athletes are not diagnosed with eating disorders because the symptoms of anorexia—absence of menses, low body fat and weight, and osteoporosis—are referred to as the female athlete triad and are not uncommon among athletes, and so they don't necessarily signify the presence of an eating disorder.

The incidence of anorexia nervosa (as well as bulimia nervosa, which we'll cover next) has traditionally been much lower in men than in women. Today, however, the incidence of both conditions is increasing in men as they begin to feel some of the same pressures that women feel to conform to the weight and body composition standards imposed by others. The "lean look" of young male models serves as a standard for more and more young men. *Mananorexic* is not a clinical term but is commonly used as a slang term for a very thin-looking man who may have struggles with anorexia nervosa. The requirement to "make weight" for various sports drives others such as runners, jockeys, swimmers, and gymnasts to lose weight quickly to meet particular standards for competition or the expectations of coaches and trainers. Researchers report that men are less inclined than women are to admit that they may have an eating disorder, thinking it is a "woman's illness." Thus they are less likely to seek treatment. In addition, physicians tend not to suspect men of having eating disorders, and so they go untreated.

Fortunately, psychological treatment in combination with medical and dietary interventions can return the person with anorexia nervosa to a more life-sustaining pattern of eating. The person with anorexia needs to receive the care of professionals experienced in the treatment of this disorder. It is not uncommon for this treatment to take three to five years. If others, including friends, coworkers, roommates, and parents, observe this condition, they should consult a health care provider for assistance.

Bulimia Nervosa

Whereas anorexics are underweight, people with **bulimia nervosa** often are of a normal weight. These individuals use food and weight as a way of coping with stress, boredom, conflict in relationships, and low self-esteem. It is not uncommon in our society to comfort ourselves with food, to have social activities based on food, and to eat as a way of procrastinating a dreaded activity. However, people with bulimia take this to the extreme, engaging in recurrent bingeing, consuming unusually large amounts of food, and feeling out of control with their eating.[58]

While anorexics run away from food, bulimics run to food to cope with their emotions, problems, and stress. Because they feel so guilty, ashamed, and anxious about the food they have consumed, people with bulimia **purge** by self-induced vomiting, taking an excessive number of laxatives and diuretics, or excessively exercising or fasting. There is a strong preoccupation with weight, calories, and food among sufferers of bulimia. Most people with bulimia constantly count calories, weigh themselves throughout the day, and frequently make negative statements concerning different parts of their bodies, primarily focusing on the thighs, stomach, and waist. As with anorexia, bulimia is associated with depression, isolation, anxiety, perfectionism, and low self-esteem. Dental erosion, hair loss, esophageal lesions, blood in the vomit and stools, loss of voluntary gag reflex, kidney damage, heart failure, gastrointestinal problems, ketosis, edema, infertility, parotid gland swelling, depression, and insomnia are just some of the medical problems associated with bulimia nervosa.

The publicity surrounding Terri Schiavo's death highlights the lethality of this disorder—she entered a persistent vegetative state following a heart attack possibly caused by bulimia. She had developed a potassium deficiency that was reportedly caused by bulimia nervosa. Many public figures have acknowledged struggling with this disorder, including singer Kelly Clarkson, Cheryl "Salt" James of the rap group Salt n' Peppa, Maureen McCormick (*The Brady Bunch*), Paula Abdul, Katharine McPhee (*American Idol*), Felicity Huffman (*Desperate Housewives*), Joan Rivers, and the late Princess Diana. All these individuals have talked about the pressures to be thin in order to be successful in their careers and how they succumbed to this pressure by developing an eating disorder.

Bulimia often begins around 17 to 18 years of age when young adults are separating from their families and are forging lives of their own; some conflict arises around issues of independence, autonomy, and relationships with family. There is a higher incidence of bulimia than anorexia, although some bulimics may have had anorexia in the past. There is also a higher rate of bulimia among female college students compared with their peers who are not attending college. Treatment for bulimia nervosa involves nutritional counseling, psychological counseling, and consultation with a physician. Often people with bulimia recover from this disorder within a year of beginning treatment.

Binge Eating Disorder

Binge eating disorder is the newest term for what was previously referred to as compulsive overeating. It is also the most common of all of the eating disorders, affecting 3.5 percent of women and 2 percent of men. It is also strongly linked to obesity. Binge eaters use food to cope in the same way that bulimics do and also feel out of control and unable to stop eating during binges. People with this disorder report eating rapidly and in secret or may snack all day. They tend to eat until they feel uncomfortably full, sometimes hoarding food and eating when they aren't physically hungry.[58] Like people with bulimia, they feel guilty and ashamed of their eating habits and have a great deal of self-loathing and body hatred. People who have binge eating disorder do not engage in purging behavior, which differentiates them from people with bulimia nervosa. Typically, binge eaters have a long history of diet failures, feel anxious, are socially withdrawn from others, and are overweight. Heart problems, high blood pressure, joint problems, abnormal blood sugar levels, fatigue, depression, and anxiety are associated with binge eating. The treatment of this eating disorder involves interventions similar to those described for treating bulimia nervosa.

Chewing and Spitting Out Food Syndrome

Chewing and spitting out food without swallowing it has also been used as a method for weight loss or weight management. This is a common eating disorder and falls within the "Eating Disorder Not Otherwise Specified" diagnosis. It differs from bulimia nervosa, and researchers contend that chewing and spitting out food without swallowing may indicate a more severe eating disorder.[61]

Night Eating Syndrome

Night eating syndrome has not yet been formally defined as an eating disorder. The signs and symptoms of this syndrome include eating more than half of one's daily food intake after dinner and before breakfast; feeling tense, anxious, and guilty while eating; difficulty falling or staying asleep at night; and having little to no appetite in the morning. Unlike binge eating, night eating involves eating throughout the evening hours rather than in short episodes. There is a strong preference for carbohydrates among night eaters. Some researchers speculate that night eating may be an unconscious attempt to self-medicate mood problems because eating carbohydrates can trigger the brain to produce so-called "feel good" neurochemicals. About 60 percent of women and 40 percent of men suffer from night eating syndrome. It is also related to obesity. Research is underway in examining the underlying causes of this syndrome and developing subsequent treatment interventions. It seems likely that a combination of biological, genetic, and psychological factors contribute to this problem.

Body Dysmorphic Disorder

Body dysmorphic disorder (BDD) is a secret preoccupation with an imagined or slight flaw in one's appearance. Sometimes, people become almost completely fixated on concerns regarding body image, leading to repeatedly weighing themselves and checking mirrors throughout the day, compulsively dieting, exercising, and undergoing cosmetic surgery.[62] Perceptions of an imperfect body may lead to psychological dysfunction, such as not wanting to leave the house because of imagined defects. People with this disorder are 45 times more likely to commit suicide than the general population, demonstrating how their self-loathing can take a devastating toll on them.

Key Terms

bulimia nervosa An eating disorder in which individuals engage in episodes of bingeing, consuming unusually large amounts of food and feeling out of control, and then engaging in some compensatory purging behavior to eliminate the food.

purging Using vomiting, laxatives, diuretics, enemas, or other medications, or means such as excessive exercise or fasting, to eliminate food.

binge eating disorder An eating disorder formerly referred to as compulsive overeating disorder; binge eaters use food to cope in the same way that bulimics do and also feel out of control, but do not engage in compensatory purging behavior.

body dysmorphic disorder (BDD) A secret preoccupation with an imagined or slight flaw in one's appearance.

Bigorexia

Bigorexia has been characterized as a "reverse anorexia nervosa" in which people want to be more muscular but see themselves as puny and scrawny.[63] Some say a better term for this would be "muscle dysmorphia" because they can never be muscular enough to satisfy their self-esteem. It has also been referred to as the "Adonis complex," but women also suffer from this disorder, though not as frequently as men. Many people take anabolic steroids (see Chapter 4) or diet supplements to get bigger and more buff. People with this preoccupation obsessively lift weights for hours each day, sometimes sacrificing important social relationships, jobs, or physical health. They can also become preoccupied with decreasing fat as they increase muscle and may develop eating disorders. Similar to people with anorexia, they tend to wear bigger clothes to hide their bodies, tend not to be seen in public, and avoid social situations because they see themselves in a distorted, negative way.

Treating Eating Disorders

The treatment for eating disorders is multimodal and multidimensional involving nutritionists, psychologists, physicians, family, and friends. There are different treatment modalities, such as individual, group, and family counseling. Sometimes treatment requires inpatient hospitalization to medically stabilize the individual. In extreme cases, a feeding tube may be inserted to treat starvation, especially if the person refuses to eat. Behavioral modification and cognitive therapy are utilized in counseling people with eating problems. Medications such as antidepressants are often used to decrease obsessive-compulsive behavior, reduce anxiety, alleviate depression, and improve mood. Some medications can stimulate or reduce appetite as well. There is some debate over the efficacy of using an addictions model, similar to the 12-step Alcoholics Anonymous philosophy, with eating disorders. Overeaters Anonymous utilizes this model in helping people with eating problems, and many hospital programs employ this model in their treatment programs. While there seems to be some overlap of eating disorders with substance abuse problems, such as denial of problems, feeling out of control of one's behavior, and using food or drugs or alcohol to cope with problems, this is where the similarities end—one needs food to live, which is not the case with drugs and alcohol.

A Final Thought About Health and Weight Management

Recognizing the attention placed on physical attractiveness and its relationship to thinness, ask yourself if you are healthy enough to accept your unique body even if it does not match the cultural ideal. As you recall from Chapter 1, it is important to develop every dimension of health, not simply the physical dimension. We hope that focusing on all dimensions of health, including the psychological aspects outlined in Chapter 2, will balance the pressure most of us feel to strive for a body image that is unrealistic and obtainable by only a few.

> **Key Terms**
>
> **bigorexia** An obsession with getting bigger and more muscular, and thinking that your body is never muscular enough.

Taking Charge of Your Health

- Investigate the resources available on your campus that you could use to determine your healthy weight and body composition profile.

- Evaluate your eating behaviors to find out if you are using food to cope with stress. If you are, develop a plan to use nonfood options, such as exercise or interaction with friends or family members, to deal with stress.

- Formulate a realistic set of goals for changing your weight and body composition in a time frame that allows you to do so in a healthful way.

- Establish a daily schedule that lets you make any necessary dietary and physical activity adjustments.

- Keep a daily journal of your weight-management efforts.

- Monitor your progress toward meeting your weight-management goals.

- Design a reward system for reaching each goal.

- Learn to accept your body including the imperfections.

- Focus on other aspects of yourself that you like that are not related to appearance.

SUMMARY

- Weight management has become an obsession in American culture as well as a significant health problem; an estimated 66 percent of U.S. adults are either overweight or obese.
- Doctors usually define "overweight" as a condition in which a person's weight is 1 to 19 percent higher than "normal," as defined by a standard height/weight chart. Obesity is usually defined as a condition in which a person's weight is 20 percent or more above normal weight. "Morbid obesity" refers to being 50 to 100 percent over normal weight, more than 100 pounds over normal weight, or sufficiently overweight to interfere with health or normal functioning.
- Some of the methods for assessing one's weight are body mass index, current height/weight tables, waist-to-hip ratios, electrical impedance, the Bod Pod, skinfold measurements, hydrostatic weighing, and home scales.
- Basal metabolic rate (BMR) is a measure of resting energy expenditure that is taken upon awakening, 10 to 12 hours after eating, or 12 to 18 hours after significant physical activity.
- Four factors seem to play a significant role in the prevalence of obesity: sex, age, socioeconomic status, and race.
- Weight loss occurs when the calories consumed are fewer than the energy the body needs for physiological maintenance and activity.
- The primary types of weight-management technique include dietary alterations, surgical interventions, medications, weight loss programs, and physical activity.
- A commitment to a lifestyle change of eating in healthy ways and engaging in regular aerobic exercise seems to be the most effective strategy for weight loss and weight maintenance.
- Anorexia nervosa is a psychological condition in which the individual weighs less than 85 percent of his or her expected weight for his or her age, gender, and height.
- People with bulimia nervosa use food and weight as a way of coping with stress, boredom, conflict in relationships, and low self-esteem. They engage in recurrent bingeing and purging to eliminate the food from their bodies.
- Binge eaters use food to cope in the same way that bulimics do and also feel out of control and unable to stop eating during binges, but they do not engage in purging behaviors.

REVIEW QUESTIONS

1. What percentage of U.S. adults are either overweight or obese?
2. How has the average caloric intake and physical activity level for Americans changed over the past two decades?
3. Define overweight, obesity, and morbid obesity.
4. List at least four of the methods used for assessing weight.
5. Define basal metabolic rate (BMR).
6. What are four factors that seem to play a significant role in the prevalence of obesity?
7. Give four examples of how environmental factors can influence the amount the average person consumes.
8. Give examples of four different types of weight-management techniques.
9. What is the most effective strategy for weight loss and weight maintenance?
10. Describe the symptoms of anorexia nervosa, bulimia nervosa, and binge eating disorder.

ANSWERS TO THE "WHAT DO YOU KNOW?" QUIZ

1. True   2. True   3. False   4. False   5. False   6. False   7. True

Visit the Online Learning Center (**www.mhhe.com/payne11e**), where you will find tools to help you improve your grade including practice quizzes, key terms flashcards, audio chapter summaries for your MP3 player, and many other study aids.

SOURCE NOTES

1. National Research Council. *Healthy People 2010.* www.healthypeople.com.
2. National Center for Chronic Disease Prevention and Health Promotion. *Defining Overweight and Obesity.* October 2006.
3. National Center for Health Statistics, Centers for Disease Control and Prevention. *Obesity Still a Major Problem, New Data Show.* October 6, 2004.
4. Field AE et al. Impact or Overweight on the risk of developing common chronic disease during a 10-year period. *Archives of Internal Medicine,* 161 (13), 1581–1586, 2001.
5. Brownell KD, Fairburn CG. *Eating Disorders and Obesity: A Comprehensive Handbook.* New York: Guilford Press, 1995.
6. Pope M, Phillips K, Olivardia T. *The Adonis Complex.* New York: Simon & Schuster, 2000.
7. National Institutes of Health. Clinical guidelines on the identification, evaluation, and treatment of overweight and obesity in adults. As reported in *First Federal Obesity Clinical Guidelines* (NIH News Advisory). June 17, 1998.
8. American Heart Association. *Heart and Stroke Facts.* 2003.
9. Poulton T. *No Fat Chicks.* Secaucus, NJ: Carol Publishing Group, 1997.

10. Anderson A. *Males with Eating Disorders.* Philadelphia: Brunner/Mazel, 1990.

11. Anderson A, Cohn L, Holbrook T. *Making Weight: Men's Conflicts with Food, Weight, Shape, and Appearance.* Carlsbad, CA: Gurze Books, 2000.

12. Cash T, Henry P. Women's Body Images: The Results of a National Survey in the U.S.A. *Sex Roles Research,* 33 (1), 19–29, 1995.

13. Gaesser G. *Big Fat Lies.* Carlsbad, CA: Gurze Books, 2002.

14. U.S. Department of Agriculture/U.S. Department of Health and Human Services. Nutrition and Your Health: Dietary Guidelines for Americans. *Home and Garden Bulletin,* 232, 2000.

15. Waist Management: Gauging Your Risks. *Consumer Reports,* p. 48. August 2003.

16. Thelen MH, Powell AL, Lawrence C, Kuhnent ME. Eating and Body Image Concerns Among Children. *Journal of Consulting and Clinical Psychology,* 21, 41, 46. 1992

17. Lindzey G, Thompson R, Spring B. *Psychology* (3rd ed.). New York: Worth, 1988.

18. International Health Racquet and Sportsclub Association. BOD POD Body Composition System to Descend on San Francisco's IHRSA Convention. As Reported in the 29th Anniversary Exhibition in San Francisco's Moscone Convention Center, March 22–24, 2001.

19. Dempster P, Aitkens S. A New Air Displacement Method for the Determination of Human Body Composition. *Medicine and Science in Sports and Exercise,* 27 (2), 1692–1697, 1995.

20. U.S. Department of Health and Human Services. *The Surgeon General's Call to Action to Prevent and Decrease Overweight and Obesity.* Rockville, MD: USDHHS, Public Health Service, Office of the Surgeon General. 2001. www.surgeongeneral.gov/topics/obesity/calltoaction/CalltoAction.pdf.

21. America the Fit. *Time Magazine,* June 23, 2008.

22. Harvard Women's Health Watch: Panel Issues New Guidelines for Healthy Eating. *Harvard Medical School,* 10 (3), November 2002.

23. Kirby J. *Dieting for Dummies* (2nd ed). New York: Wiley, 2004.

24. *Dietary Guidelines for Americans,* www.health.gov/dietaryguidelines. 2005.

25. Insel P, Turner RE, Ross D. *Nutrition* (3rd ed.). Sudbury, MA: Jones & Bartlett, 2007.

26. Wardlaw GM. *Perspectives in Nutrition* (7th ed.). New York: McGraw-Hill, 2006.

27. Halaas J et al. Weight-Reducing Effects on the Plasma Protein Encoded by the Obese Gene. *Science,* 269 (5223): 543–546, 1995.

28. Folsom AR et al. Serum Leptin and Weight Gain over Eight Years in African American and Caucasian Young Adults. *Obesity Research,* 7 (1), 1–8. 1999.

29. Sakurai T et al. Orexins and Orexin Receptors: A Family of Hypothalamic Neuropeptides and G Protein-Coupled Receptors That Regulate Feeding Behavior. *Cell,* 92 (4): 573–585, 1998.

30. La Leche League International. *The Womanly Art of Breastfeeding.* (7th ed). 2004.

31. Pettigrew R, Hamilton FD. Obesity and Female Reproductive Function. *British Medical Bulletin,* 53:2, 341–358, 1997.

32. Dell S, To T. Breastfeeding and Asthma in Young Children. *Arch Ped Adol Med* 155:1261–65, 2001.

33. Hediger ML, et al. Association Between Infant Breast-Feeding and Overweight in Young Children. *Journal of the American Medical Association,* 285 (19), 2453–60, 2001.

34. Gillman MW, et al. Risk of Overweight Among Adolescents Who Were Breastfed as Infants. *Journal of the American Medical Association,* 285 (19): 2461–67, 2001.

35. Set point: What Your Body Is Trying to Tell You. *National Eating Disorders Information Centre Bulletin,* 7 (2), June 1992.

36. Stettler N, Zemel BS, Kumaniyika S, Stallings VA. Infant Weight Gain and Childhood Overweight Status in a Multicenter, Cohort Study. *Pediatrics,* 109 (2), 194–199, February 2002.

37. The Truth About Dieting. *Consumer Reports.* June 26–31, 2002.

38. Saladin KS. *Anatomy and Physiology: The Unity of Form and Function.* Dubuque, IA: William C. Brown/McGraw-Hill, 1998.

39. Statistics Related to Overweight and Obesity. National Institutes of Health, August 2005.

40. Sorbara M, Geliebter A. Body Image Disturbance in Obese Out-patients Before and After Weight Loss in Relation to Race, Gender and Age of Onset of Diabetes. *International Journal of Eating Disorders,* 416–423, May 2002.

41. Sobal J, Stunkard AJ. Socioeconomic Status and Obesity: A Review of the Literature. *Psychological Bulletin,* 105, 260–75, 1989.

42. Stunkard AJ, Wadden TA. *Obesity: Theory and Therapy.* New York: Raven Press, 1993.

43. Sobal J, Rauschenbach B, Frongillo E. Marital Status, Fatness and Obesity. *Social Science and Medicine,* 35, 915–923, 1992.

44. Weight Watchers. *Stop Stuffing Yourself: Seven Steps to Conquering Overeating.* New York: Wiley, 1988.

45. Study: People Taking Eating Clues from Portion Size. *Star Press,* July 31, 2006.

46. Goode E, Obesity in America: The Gorge Yourself Movement. *New York Times,* August 19, 2003.

47. Sleep Loss May Equal Weight Gain. *USA Today,* December 7, 2004.

48. One More Reason to Get Enough Sleep. *Harvard Women's Health Watch,* May 2005.

49. Ephedra Ban Puts Herb Industry on Notice. *New York Times,* December 31, 2003.

50. Ephedra-Free Doesn't Mean Risk-Free. WebMD Health, September 9, 2005.

51. FDA Warns Against Some Diet Pills Sold on the Web. *USA Today,* December 22, 2008.

52. Center for Drug Evaluation and Research, FDA. FDA Announces Withdrawal of Fenfluramine and Dexfenfluramine. News Release no. 97–32. September 15, 1997.

53. Taking the Diet Pill . . . Alli. *People,* July 9, 2007.

54. Obesity Surgery Increases 600 Percent. ABC News. May 31, 2006.

55. Grazer FM, de Jong RH. Fatal Outcomes from Liposuction: Census Survey of Cosmetic Surgeons. *Plastic Reconstructive Surgery,* 105 (1), 436–446, 2000.

56. American Dietetic Association. Gaining Weight: A Healthy Plan for Adding Pounds. *Hot Topics,* www.eatright.org/nfs10html. 1998.

57. Ferro-Luzzi A, James WP. Adult Malnutrition, Simple Assessment Techniques for Use in Emergencies. *British Journal of Nutrition,* 75(1), 3–10, 1996.

58. *Diagnostic and Statistical Manual of Mental Disorders IV-TR.* Washington, DC: American Psychiatric Association. 2000.

59. Gotthelf M. The New Anorexia Outrage. *Self Magazine,* August 2001, 82–84.

60. Lilenfeld L. Academy Members Debate Over Pro-Anorexia Websites. *Academy of Eating Disorders Newsletter,* June 2001.

61. Update: Chewing and Spitting Out Food. *Eating Disorders Review,* July/August 2002.

62. A dangerous Duo: Body Dysmorphic Disorder with Anorexia Nervosa. *Eating Disorders Review,* November/December 2002, 4–5.

63. Pope H, Phillips K, Olivardia R, *The Adonic Complex.* New York: Simon & Schuster, 2000.

Personal Assessment

Do you eat mindlessly or mindfully?

Below is a collection of statements about your everyday experiences. Using the 1–6 scale, indicate how frequently or infrequently you currently have each experience. Answer according to what really reflects your experience rather than what you think your experience should be. Treat each item separately from every other item.

1	2	3	4	5	6
Almost always	Very frequently	Somewhat frequently	Somewhat infrequently	Very infrequently	Almost never

1. I could be experiencing some emotion and not be conscious of it until sometime later.   1 2 3 4 5 6
2. I break or spill things because of carelessness, not paying attention, or thinking of something else.   1 2 3 4 5 6
3. I find it difficult to stay focused on what's happening in the present.   1 2 3 4 5 6
4. I tend to walk quickly to get where I'm going without paying attention to what I experience along the way. 1 2 3 4 5 6
5. I tend not to notice feelings of physical tension or discomfort until they really grab my attention.   1 2 3 4 5 6
6. I forget a person's name almost as soon as I've been told it for the first time.   1 2 3 4 5 6
7. It seems I am "running on automatic," without much awareness of what I'm doing.   1 2 3 4 5 6
8. I rush through activities without being really attentive to them.   1 2 3 4 5 6
9. I get so focused on the goal I want to achieve that I lose touch with what I'm doing right now to get there. 1 2 3 4 5 6
10. I do jobs or tasks automatically, without being aware of what I'm doing.   1 2 3 4 5 6
11. I find myself listening to someone with one ear, doing something else at the same time.   1 2 3 4 5 6
12. I drive places on "automatic pilot" and then wonder why I went there.   1 2 3 4 5 6
13. I find myself preoccupied with the future or the past.   1 2 3 4 5 6
14. I find myself doing things without paying attention.   1 2 3 4 5 6
15. I snack without being aware that I'm eating.   1 2 3 4 5 6

Interpretation

To get your score, add up the numbers you circled for the 15 items and divide the total by 15. (This gives you the mean.) The higher your mean score, the higher your level of mindfulness.

TO CARRY THIS FURTHER . . .

If you scored low on this assessment, try some of the suggestions in the box "Learning to Eat Mindfully" to become a more mindful eater.

Source: From K. W. Brown and R. M. Ryan. The Benefits of Being Present: The Role of Mindfulness in Psychological Well-Being, *Journal of Personality and Social Psychology*, 84, 822–848. Copyright © 2003 by the American Psychological Association. Adapted with permission.

Personal Assessment

Body love or body hate?

When you catch a glimpse of yourself in a mirror, do you smile or grimace at what you see? The following quiz will help you to assess your body self-esteem associated with your appearance. Please answer using the following rating scale:

1 = Rarely or never
2 = Sometimes
3 = Almost always or always

Add up your scores to determine your total score, and look at the interpretation of your scores.

_____ 1. I worry about my weight and weighing "too much."

_____ 2. I prefer to eat by myself and not with other people.

_____ 3. My mood is determined by the scale and how I feel about my appearance.

_____ 4. I make negative comments about my appearance to myself and others.

_____ 5. I think I look less attractive on days that I haven't exercised.

_____ 6. I have a difficult time accepting compliments about my appearance from others.

_____ 7. I compare myself to other women and find myself lacking.

_____ 8. I ask other people how I look.

_____ 9. I avoid social situations, activities, and events involving food.

_____ 10. I feel more anxious about my body in the summertime because of the need to wear bathing suits and clothing suitable for warmer temperatures.

_____ **TOTAL POINTS**

Interpretation

If you scored between 10 and 15, you have positive body self-esteem and are accepting of yourself and your appearance.

If you scored between 16 and 23, you scored in the average range.

If your score was between 24 and 30, you have poor or low body self-esteem.

TO CARRY THIS FURTHER . . .

If you scored in the average range: While you are in good company, feeling about your body the way most people do, you may want to reframe your body image and develop more of an appreciation for your body and appearance.

If you have poor body self-image: Your self-esteem in general is probably driven by how you see yourself, and you may be putting too much emphasis on your appearance and are too self-critical. You may feel as though you never are thin enough or look good enough and can always find a flaw when looking in the mirror. To improve your body self-esteem, focus on other aspects of yourself, focus on the positive aspects of your body, and be more accepting of yourself and less perfectionistic.

Preventing Drug Abuse and Dependence

Health educators have no doubt that the use, misuse, and abuse of many drugs can impair health. These substances not only alter the functioning of the body and mind but also affect the other dimensions of health. In Part Three, we take a look at addictive substances and their effects on the user.

1. **Physical Dimension**
   The effects of substance use, especially the long-term use of tobacco and alcohol, are well understood. These substances cause illness and death. Alcohol abuse can destroy the structure and function of many body systems. Tobacco use damages the cardiovascular system and the tissues of the respiratory tract and can cause cancer in many sites throughout the body. Chronic abuse of psychoactive drugs impairs many central nervous system functions. Even the experimental use of these drugs carries the danger of toxic overdose.

2. **Emotional Dimension**
   Because psychoactive drugs alter nervous system functioning, many users experience depression and mood swings. Some people use drugs to avoid emotional expression or to numb their feelings. When psychological dependence combines with physical dependence, the addict may begin to lose touch with reality.

3. **Social Dimension**
   Psychoactive drug use often takes place in social settings. For some people, drinking or using other drugs is perceived as a necessary first step toward enjoying the company of others. However, most people have little tolerance for inappropriate substance use, such as use of illegal drugs, excessive alcohol intake, and smoking in public places where tobacco use is banned.

4. **Intellectual Dimension**
   Intellectual impairment is one consequence of chemical abuse. People cannot perform well intellectually when they are feeling high or low or when their senses are dulled. Some people prefer to disregard information about the dangers of substance abuse, a choice that could prove extremely harmful to their health.

5. **Spiritual Dimension**
   Although drug use has long played a role in the religious practices of people throughout the world, the nonceremonial use of drugs conflicts with the principles of service to others. Substance abuse can hinder spiritual growth by turning a person's focus inward, making it difficult to develop the other-directedness that is part of a rich spiritual life.

6. **Occupational Dimension**
   Use of both legal and illegal drugs clearly stands in the way of occupational health. Most workplaces are smoke-free, forcing smokers to stand outside or walk to the smoker's lounge to have a cigarette. These continual interruptions lower a worker's productivity. Illegal drug use can keep a job candidate from being hired and can result in being fired. And use of illegal drugs or alcohol on the job can be dangerous and will certainly lower a worker's level of performance.

7 Making Decisions About Drug Use

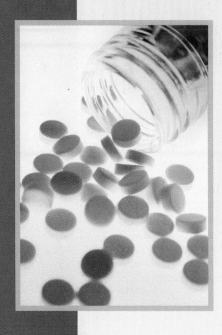

What Do You Know About Drug Use?

1. Intravenous drug injection is the most efficient and fastest way to administer a drug. True or False?

2. Socioeconomic status is not predictive of drug use. True or False?

3. Drug use is highest for 18- to 25-year-olds, compared with any other age group. True or False?

4. The use of all drugs has been increasing over the years. True or False?

5. Marijuana can be legally used for medical reasons in some states. True or False?

6. Energy drinks such as Red Bull can have dangerous effects on the heart. True or False?

7. Self-help groups are the most popular type of drug treatment. True or False?

Check your answers at the end of the chapter.

Each of us may have different ideas about what a **drug** is. Although a number of definitions are available, we consider a drug to be "any substance, natural or artificial, other than food, that by its chemical or physical nature alters structure or function in the living organism."[1] Included in this broad definition is a variety of psychoactive drugs, medicines, and substances that many people do not usually consider to be drugs.

Psychoactive drugs alter the user's feelings, behavior, perceptions, or moods when using stimulants, depressants, hallucinogens, opiates, or inhalants. Prescribed medications function to heal unhealthy tissue as well as ease pain, prevent illness, and diagnose health conditions. Although some psychoactive drugs are used for medical reasons, as in the case of tranquilizers and some narcotics, the most commonly prescribed medicines are antibiotics, hormone replacement drugs, sulfa drugs, diuretics, oral contraceptives, and cardiovascular drugs. Legal substances are also considered to be drugs (such as caffeine, tobacco, alcohol, aspirin, and other over-the-counter (OTC) drugs). These common substances are used so frequently in our society that they are rarely perceived as true drugs.

People can also be addicted to behaviors that are detrimental to their lives and relationships such as gambling, shopping, gaming, and sexual activity. These are referred to as **process addictions.** Similar to the dependency upon drugs, process addictions can cause serious financial, emotional, social, and health problems. People believe that they have control over their shopping, gambling, and gaming activities, but it becomes apparent after a while to others around them that they are out of control and their behavior is excessive and unhealthy. People with process addictions feel a compulsion to engage in this behavior and use the behavior as a stress reliever and coping strategy.

Addictions can be tremendously disruptive in many people's lives, from causing tragic deaths or the loss of employment opportunities (most Fortune 500 companies use preemployment drug testing) to causing personal relationships to deteriorate and babies to be born with profound birth defects. Perhaps realizing this, college students have generally moved away from using the most dangerous illegal drugs.

For organizational reasons, this chapter primarily focuses on psychoactive drugs. Alcohol is covered in Chapter 8. The effects of tobacco are delineated in Chapter 9. Prescription and OTC drugs and medicines are discussed at length in Chapter 18. Anabolic steroids, drugs used primarily for increasing muscle growth, are discussed in Chapter 4.

Addictive Behavior

This chapter explores the health consequences of drug use, misuse, and abuse. Before we talk about specific drugs, however, we need to put drug use in the broader context of addictive behavior. The use and abuse of drugs is just one of the many forms of addictive behavior. Addictive behavior includes addictions to shopping, gambling, sex, television, video games, Internet use, or work, as well as addictions to alcohol or other drugs.

The Process of Addiction

The process of developing an addiction has been a much-studied topic. Addictive behavior seems to have three common aspects: exposure, compulsion, and loss of control.

Exposure   An addiction can begin after a person is exposed to a drug (such as alcohol) or a behavior (such as gambling) that he or she finds pleasurable. Perhaps this drug or behavior temporarily replaces an unpleasant feeling or sensation. This initial pleasure gradually (or in some cases quickly) becomes a focal point in the person's life.

Compulsion   Increasingly more energy, time, and money are spent pursuing the drug use or behavior. At this point in the addictive process, the person can be said to have a compulsion for the drug or behavior. Frequently, repeated exposure to the drug or behavior continues despite negative consequences, such as the gradual loss of family and friends, unpleasant physical symptoms after taking the drug, and/or problems at work.

During the compulsion phase of the addictive behavior, a person's "normal" life often degenerates while she or he searches for increased pleasures from the drug or

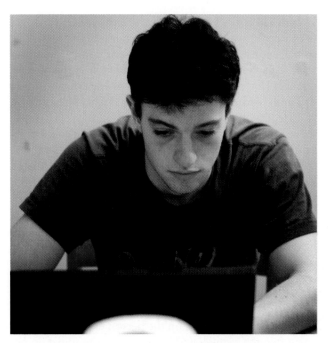

Addictive behaviors are characterized by a loss of control over one's behavior despite negative social, health, and/or financial consequences. Use of the Internet as well as online shopping or gambling can become problematic behaviors for some people.

the behavior. An addicted person's family life, circle of friends, work, or study patterns become less important than does the search for more and better "highs." The development of tolerance and withdrawal are distinct possibilities. (These terms will be discussed later in the chapter.)

Why some people develop compulsions and others do not is difficult to pinpoint, but addiction might be influenced by genetic makeup, family dynamics, physiological processes, personality type, peer groups, and available resources for help.

> ### Key Terms
>
> **drug** Any substance, natural or artificial, other than food, that by its chemical or physical nature alters structure or function in the living organism.
>
> **psychoactive drug** Any substance capable of altering feelings, moods, or perceptions.
>
> **process addictions** Addictions in which people compulsively engage in behaviors such as gambling, shopping, gaming, or sexual activity to such an extreme degree that these addictions can cause serious financial, emotional, social, and health problems similar to drug and alcohol addictions.

Loss of Control   Over time, the search for highs changes to a desire to avoid the effects of withdrawal from the drug or behavior. Addicted people lose their ability to control their behavior. Despite overwhelming negative consequences (for example, deterioration of health, alienation of family and friends, or loss of all financial resources), addicted people continue to behave in ways that make their lives worse. The person addicted to alcohol continues to drink heavily, the person addicted to shopping continues to run up large debts, and the person addicted to sex continues to have sex indiscriminately. What once may have seemed within an individual's control, or even a way someone tried to exert control over his or her life, now has control over that person. Frequently, a person has addictions to more than one drug or behavior, or may switch from one addiction to another.

Codependence

With all the focus placed on the person with a drug problem, often the families and loved ones of the addict do not receive the attention and help they need. You may already be familiar with the term *codependent,* but you might have assumed that this term applies only to those close to an alcoholic. In fact, this term can apply to anyone who is close to an individual addicted to any type of behavior, including addiction to drugs, sex, gambling, or other behaviors. Codependent behavior refers to someone who enables an addict to continue with the addiction via behaviors such as making excuses for the addict, calling in sick to work for the person, and relieving that person of any consequences that occur as a result of the addictive behavior.

Codependent people typically become unaware of their own feelings, needs, and boundaries in their preoccupation with the addicted individual. They become focused on protecting or coping with the addict and often lose their own sense of identity. This stress often results in chaotic behaviors, addictions, and physical illnesses in the codependent person.

Private and public programs are also available to help the codependent person learn new behaviors. (See Chapter 8 for more information about codependent behavior and resources.)

Basic Drug Terminology and Concepts

Before we move on to discussing specific types of drugs, it is important to review general principles of how psychoactive drugs affect the body and how different methods and patterns of use influence drug effects.

Actions of Drugs on the Central Nervous System

To better understand the disruption caused by the actions of psychoactive drugs, a general knowledge of the normal functioning of the nervous system's basic unit, the **neuron,** is required.

First, stimuli from the internal or external environment are received by the appropriate sensory receptor, perhaps an organ such as an eye or an ear. Once sensed, these stimuli are converted into electrical impulses. These impulses are then directed along the neuron's **dendrite,** through the cell body, and along the **axon,** toward the synaptic junction near an adjacent neuron.[2] On arrival at the **synapse,** the electrical impulses stimulate the production and release of chemical messengers called **neurotransmitters.** These neurotransmitters transmit the electrical impulses from one neuron to the dendrites of adjoining neurons. Thus neurons function in a coordinated fashion to send information to the brain for interpretation and to relay appropriate response commands outward to the tissues of the body.

The role of neurotransmitters is critically important to the relay of information within the system. A substance that has the ability to alter some aspect of neurotransmitter function has the potential to seriously disrupt the otherwise normally functioning system. Psychoactive drugs are capable of exerting these disruptive influences on the neurotransmitters. Drugs change the way neurotransmitters work, often by blocking the production of a neurotransmitter or forcing the continued release of a neurotransmitter (see Figure 7-1).

> **Key Terms**
>
> **neuron** A nerve cell.
>
> **dendrite** The portion of a neuron that receives electrical stimuli from adjacent neurons; neurons typically have several such branches or extensions.
>
> **axon** The portion of a neuron that conducts electrical impulses to the dendrites of adjacent neurons; neurons typically have one axon.
>
> **synapse (sinn** aps**)** The location at which an electrical impulse from one neuron is transmitted to an adjacent neuron; also referred to as a *synaptic junction.*
>
> **neurotransmitters** Chemical messengers that transfer electrical impulses across the synapses between nerve cells.
>
> **dose-response curve** The size of the effect of a drug on the body related to the amount of the drug administered.
>
> **threshold dose** The smallest amount of a drug to have an observable effect on the body.

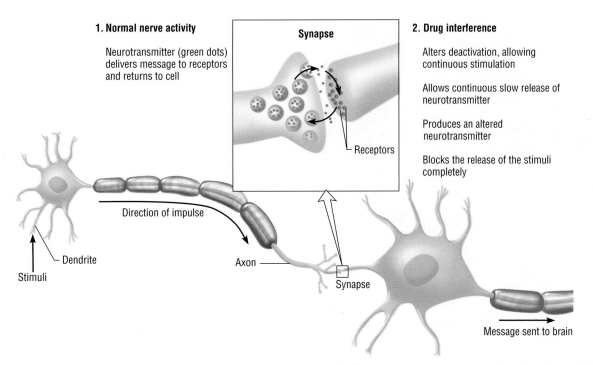

1. Normal nerve activity

Neurotransmitter (green dots) delivers message to receptors and returns to cell

Synapse

Receptors

2. Drug interference

Alters deactivation, allowing continuous stimulation

Allows continuous slow release of neurotransmitter

Produces an altered neurotransmitter

Blocks the release of the stimuli completely

Direction of impulse

Dendrite

Stimuli

Axon

Synapse

Message sent to brain

Figure 7-1 The Action of Psychoactive Drugs on the Central Nervous System   Neurotransmitters are chemical messengers that transfer electrical impulses across the synapses between nerve cells. Psychoactive drugs interrupt this process, thus disrupting the normal functioning of the nervous system.

Routes of Administration

A drug generally enters the body through one of four methods: ingestion, injection, inhalation, or absorption. Once in the body, drugs reach the brain through the bloodstream. A drug that is ingested, or administered orally, enters the body through the mouth and then is absorbed into the digestive tract. Once in the bloodstream, drugs are metabolized by the liver, some more quickly than others, as metabolic rates differ for various drugs. Injection refers to the use of a needle to insert a drug into the body. With intravenous (IV) injection, a drug can be put directly into the bloodstream, making the rate of absorption more rapid than with ingestion or even other means of injection. A very high concentration of a drug can be delivered in this way, increasing the potential for danger. Intravenous drug use also carries the risk of contracting infections and diseases, such as HIV (see Chapter 13). With inhalation, the drug enters the body through the lungs and can have the most rapid rate of absorption, even more so than with IV injections—the blood leaving the lungs moves directly to the brain in 5 to 8 seconds, compared to the 10 to 15 seconds it typically takes IV injections to reach the brain.[3] Topical application, or absorption, refers to the administration of a drug through the skin or mucous membranes. This is not a common route of administration because most drugs are not absorbed well this way, although absorption through the mucous

membranes is quicker than through the skin. Drugs that are absorbed more quickly into the brain are also more likely to lead to dependence.

With some drugs, the higher the dose, the stronger the effect on the body. For other drugs there is an all-or-none response, so when the body responds it is at the maximum level and further additions of the drug have no effect. This is called the **dose-response curve,** in which the size of the response is related to the amount of the drug administered.

The smallest amount of a drug that produces a response is referred to as the **threshold dose,** meaning any amount less than that would not have an observable effect on the body. For example, a very low dose of a sedative may have no observable effect, while a moderate dose might cause drowsiness and feelings of relaxation; a high dose of a sedative would result in loss of consciousness.

Drug Misuse and Abuse

So far in this chapter we have used the term *use* (or *user*) in association with the taking of psychoactive drugs. At this point, however, it is important to define use and to introduce the terms *misuse* and *abuse*.[1] By doing so, we can more accurately describe how drugs are used.

The term *use* is all-encompassing and describes drug-taking in the most general way. For example, Americans use drugs of many types. The term *use* can also refer

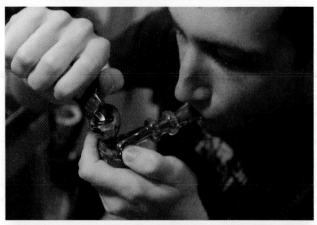

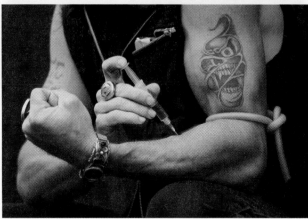

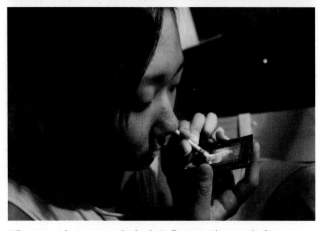

The way a drug enters the body influences the speed of its effects, and more rapid effects are associated with a higher risk of dependence. A drug reaches the brain quicker when administered by inhalation (top) than by injection (middle), because blood reaches the brain more quickly from the lungs than from a more distant injection site. Absorption through the mucous membranes (bottom) is a slower method of drug administration.

more narrowly to misuse and abuse. We often use the word in this latter regard.

The term **misuse** refers to the inappropriate use of legal drugs intended to be medications. Misuse may occur when a patient misunderstands the directions for use of a prescription or OTC drug or when a patient shares a prescription with a friend or family member for whom the drug was not prescribed. Misuse also occurs when a patient takes the prescription or OTC drug for a purpose or condition other than that for which it was intended or at a dosage other than that recommended.

The term **abuse** applies to any use of a drug when it is detrimental to health and well-being. The costs of drug abuse to the individual are extensive and include absenteeism and underachievement, loss of job, marital instability, loss of self-esteem, serious illnesses, and even death.

Dependence

Misuse and abuse of drugs over time can result in **dependence.** Psychoactive drugs have a strong potential for the development of dependence. In this chapter the term **addiction** is used interchangeably with physical dependence. When users take a psychoactive drug, the patterns of nervous system function are altered. If these altered functions provide perceived benefits for the user, drug use may continue, perhaps at increasingly larger dosages. If persistent use continues, the user can develop a dependence on the drug. Pharmacologists have identified two types of dependence—physical and psychological.

A person can be said to have developed a *physical dependence* when the body cells have become reliant on a drug. Continued use of the drug is then required because body tissues have adapted to its presence.[4] The person's body needs the drug to maintain homeostasis, or dynamic balance. If the drug is not taken or is suddenly withdrawn, the user develops a characteristic **withdrawal illness.** The symptoms of withdrawal reflect the attempt by the body's cells to regain normality without the drug. Withdrawal symptoms are always unpleasant (ranging from mild to severe irritability, depression, nervousness, digestive difficulties, and abdominal pain) and can be life threatening, as in the case of abrupt withdrawal from barbiturates or alcohol. Misuse or abuse of drugs can lead to **intoxication,** which literally means poisoning by a drug or toxic substance. Drug intoxication usually involves dysfunctional and disruptive changes in physiological and psychological functioning, mood, and cognitive processes, resulting from the consumption of a psychoactive substance.

Continued use of most drugs can lead to **tolerance.** Tolerance is an acquired reaction to a drug in which continued intake of the same dose has diminishing effects.[4] The user needs larger doses of the drug to receive previously felt sensations. The continued use of depressants, including alcohol, and opiates can cause users to quickly develop a tolerance to the drug.

Tolerance developed for one drug may carry over to another drug within the same general category. This

Table 7.1 Reported Substance Use Among Students in the Past 30 Days

Substance	Never used (%)	Have used but Not used in past month (%)	Used in past month—duration of use in days (%)					
			1–2	3–5	6–9	10–19	20–29	All 30
Alcohol	17.2	13.2	18.8	19.0	16.3	12.2	2.9	0.5
Cigarettes	64.9	17.5	5.4	2.3	1.5	2.0	2.1	4.3
Smokeless tobacco	89.6	7.1	1.2	0.5	0.4	0.4	0.3	0.5
Cigars	74.5	20.2	3.9	0.7	0.3	0.2	0.1	0.1
Marijuana	65.5	20.1	6.0	2.3	1.7	1.8	1.5	1.2
Amphetamines	92.8	4.8	0.7	0.5	0.3	0.3	0.2	0.3
Cocaine	93.9	4.5	0.9	0.3	0.2	0.1	0.0	0.1
Rohypnol, GHB,* or liquid X (intentional use)	99.0	0.9	0.1	0.0	0.0	0.0	0.0	0.0
Ecstasy (MDMA)	95.1	4.4	0.4	0.1	0.0	0.0	0.0	0.0

Based on [survey] question 9: "Within the last 30 days, on how many days did you use the following substances?"

*GHB = gamma-hydroxybutyrate acid.

Source: Used with permission by American College Health Association. American College Health Association—National College Health Assessment: Reference Group Data Report Spring 2006. Baltimore: American College Health Association, 2006.

phenomenon is known as **cross-tolerance.** The heavy abuser of alcohol, for example, might require a larger dose of a preoperative sedative to become relaxed before surgery than the average person would. The tolerance to alcohol "crosses over" to the other depressant drugs.

A person who possesses a strong desire to continue using a particular drug is said to have developed **psychological dependence.** People who are psychologically dependent on a drug believe that they need to consume the drug to maintain a sense of well-being. They crave the drug for emotional reasons despite having persistent or recurrent physical, social, psychological, or occupational problems that are caused or worsened by the drug use. Abrupt withdrawal from a drug by such a person would not trigger the fully expressed withdrawal illness, although some unpleasant symptoms of withdrawal might be felt. The term *habituation* is often used interchangeably with the term *psychological dependence*.

Drugs whose continued use can quickly lead to both physical and psychological dependence are depressants (barbiturates, tranquilizers, and alcohol), narcotics (the opiates, which are derivatives of the Oriental poppy: heroin, morphine, and codeine), and synthetic narcotics (oxycodone and methadone). Drugs whose continued use can lead to various degrees of psychological dependence and occasionally to significant (but not life-threatening) physical dependence in some users are the stimulants (amphetamines, caffeine, and cocaine), hallucinogens (LSD, peyote, and mescaline), marijuana, and inhalants (glues, gases, and petroleum products). See Table 7.1 for rates of substance abuse among college students.

Key Terms

misuse The inappropriate use of legal drugs intended to be medications.

abuse Any use of a drug in a way that is detrimental to health or well-being.

dependence A general term that refers to the need to continue using a drug for psychological or physical reasons or both.

addiction Compulsive, uncontrollable dependence on a substance, habit, or practice to such a degree that cessation causes severe emotional or physiological reactions.

withdrawal illness An uncomfortable, perhaps toxic response of the body as it attempts to maintain homeostasis in the absence of a drug; also called *abstinence syndrome*.

intoxication Dysfunctional and disruptive changes in physiological and psychological functioning, mood, and cognitive processes, resulting from the consumption of a psychoactive substance.

tolerance An acquired reaction to a drug in which the continued intake of the same dose has diminished effects.

cross-tolerance Transfer of tolerance from one drug to another within the same general category.

psychological dependence Craving a drug for emotional reasons and to maintain a sense of well-being; also referred to as *habituation*.

Dynamics of Drug Abuse

Many factors influence drug-taking behavior, including individual factors, immediate environmental factors, and societal factors. Specific aspects of each are discussed in the following sections.

Individual Factors

Genetic predisposition, personality traits, attitudes and beliefs, interpersonal skills, and unmet developmental needs can lead to drug use.

Genetic Predisposition The importance of genetic predisposition (inherited vulnerability) to drug use has not been fully determined. However, studies of alcoholics have demonstrated that genetic factors do play some role in the development of alcoholism. Research on genetic predisposition to the abuse of other drugs is much farther behind than for alcohol abuse.

Personality Traits, Attitudes, and Beliefs Although drug-taking behavior cannot be predicted strictly on the basis of personality type, correlations have been noted with certain aspects of personality (or temperament). For example, children who are easily bored and need continual activity and challenge are more likely to take drugs when they are older. A similar tendency is seen in children who are driven to avoid negative consequences for their actions and who crave immediate external reward for their efforts. Personality traits such as rebelliousness, rejection of behavioral norms, resistance to authority, and high tolerance for deviance have been reported in drug abusers.

However, a cause-and-effect relationship between personality profile and drug abuse is difficult to prove. Perhaps the abuse of drugs actually creates the personality traits, rather than the other way around.

Interpersonal Skills and Self-Esteem Drug abusers are often deficient in interpersonal skills. They are likely to score lower on tests that measure well-being, tolerance of others, and achievement. They also often have lower self-esteem than do those who do not abuse drugs. Again, the question of cause and effect is raised.

When people lack positive experiences in school, work, relationships, and varied aspects of community involvement, they may attempt to compensate through chronic heavy drug use. Of course, drug abuse creates further barriers for productive and satisfying growth and development, thus increasing the desire for the compensatory use of drugs.

Environmental Factors

Drug use can be fostered by factors within the immediate environment, which includes home and family, school, peers, and the community.

Home and Family Drug abuse that begins in childhood is often associated with the home and family.[4] Children seem to be at greater risk when parents exhibit poor management skills, antisocial behavior, and even criminality. These families are often disorganized and have poorly defined roles for parenting and being a productive member of society. In many cases, adult family members abuse drugs themselves or tolerate those who do. As with tobacco use, parents can be the best or worst models children can have.

School Children from disorganized or socially maladjusted families often have difficulty adjusting to the organized environment of the school. The following chain of events has been suggested to explain the relationship of a poor home environment and weak academic performance to drug abuse: An undesirable home environment contributes to poor school performance and poor social development; failure at school leads to loss of self-esteem, aggressive behavior, and loss of interest in school; these factors in turn may foster truancy and drug experimentation.

Peers A clear relationship exists between peer group drug abuse and drug abuse among individual members. It is unusual for a student to remain an active member of a peer group and abstain from drug use while other members abuse drugs. The pressure to "join in" can be just too powerful to resist.

Community Drug availability, drug education, and drug treatment and rehabilitation vary among communities. As a result, drug abuse rates differ from one community to another.

Societal Factors

Societal factors such as the existence of a youth subculture, modeling and advertising, and the self-medication

---

> ### Key Terms
>
> **gateway drug** An easily obtainable legal or illegal drug that represents a user's first experience with a mind-altering drug; this drug can serve as the "gateway" to the use of other drugs.
>
> **modeling** The influence others have on us by example of their own behavior.

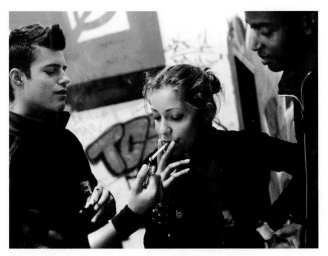

Drug use by peers, identification with youth subculture, weak academic performance, and truancy are all associated with higher rates of drug use and abuse.

movement affect drug use. Socioeconomic status is not predictive of drug use.

Youth Subculture

Many people assume that the rate of drug abuse is higher among youths 12 to 17 years old than in any other segment of American society. However, this belief is not supported by research. A recent study indicates that a higher rate of drug abuse occurs among 18- to 25-year-olds.[5] Nevertheless, the drug abuse that does occur among those in the younger age group is of concern because patterns that are established at an early age can carry over into later life. In fact, 13 percent

of those who first tried marijuana at age 14 abused or were dependent on illicit drugs after age 18, compared with 2 percent of those who first tried marijuana after age 18.[6] In fact, during this period, experimentation with a **gateway drug** (alcohol, nicotine, or marijuana) often begins, which may lead to heavier drug use later (see Table 7.1).[1]

Modeling and Advertising

Modeling of drug use within the peer group and family has already been presented. However, celebrities, musicians, and athletes also serve as models of behavior.

When models are employed by the media to sell products, advertising becomes an important factor in fostering drug use. The marketing of tobacco and alcohol products is perhaps the best example. "Beautiful people" are depicted enjoying a social drug, such as alcohol, coffee, tea, or tobacco, in opulent surroundings that most viewers can only dream of being in. Celebrities participate in events sponsored by alcohol or tobacco companies.

The Self-Medication Movement

People's ability to engage in medical self-management makes drug use easier and more socially acceptable than in the past. In a society conditioned by the effectiveness and availability of OTC and prescription medications, the use of other drugs, both legal and illegal, to make ourselves feel better seems more acceptable than ever before. This attitude can foster drug misuse and, for some, drug abuse. See the box "Improving Your Mood Without Drugs" for nondrug strategies for reducing stress and negative feelings.

Changing for the Better

Improving Your Mood Without Drugs

It's tempting to reach for a pill when I feel stressed, but I don't want to get into that habit. What can I do to improve my mood without using drugs?

Talk with a trusted friend. Confide your feelings to a close, trusted friend or family member. By opening up to another person, you'll gain insights into how you can get beyond your negative feelings without resorting to drug use.

Get moving. Go for a walk, ride your bike, or swim a few laps. Physical activity is a natural way to enhance your mood. Nearly every college provides recreation programs such as aerobics, swimming, dancing, or weight lifting.

Give yourself a break. If you're tired, take a quick power nap. If you're overworked, set aside some personal time—just for yourself. Read, watch TV, surf the Net, or call a friend. Decide what you like to do, and then do it. You'll return to your responsibilities with renewed enthusiasm.

Reexamine your spiritual health. Many people find comfort by making connections to their spiritual life. Through activities such as

meditation, spiritual reflection, and renewal of faith, people often gain reassurance and a sense of calmness.

Restructure your daily activities. If you have one hectic day after another but feel as though you're not accomplishing anything, try reorganizing your daily activities. Experiment with new patterns. Plan to get sufficient sleep, eat regular meals, and set aside specific times for work, family activities, and pleasure. Find out what works best for you.

Seek professional guidance. If you've tried these strategies but your mood still isn't improving, consider seeking professional help. This important first step is up to you. Visit your college health center or counseling center, and talk with people who are trained to help you learn how to become a happier person.

Do volunteer work. One way to feel good is to help others. Teach reading to adults, become a Big Brother or Big Sister, work in a soup kitchen, or drive a van for the elderly in your community.

Table 7.2 Psychoactive Drug Categories

Drugs and Examples of Commercial (Street) Names	Intoxication Effects	Potential Health Consequences
Stimulants		
Amphetamine Dexedrine (speed, uppers) **Cocaine** (blow, coke, crack, snow) **Methamphetamine** (crank, crystal, ice, meth) **MDMA** (Ecstasy, X, lover's speed, Adam) **Methylphenidate** Ritalin (vitamin R) **Nicotine**	Increased heart rate, blood pressure, breathing rate, metabolism; feelings of energy, exhilaration; increased mental alertness; reduced appetite *Additional specific effects:* *For cocaine*—increased temperature *For methamphetamine*—aggression, violence, psychotic behavior *For MDMA*—mild hallucinogenic effects, increased empathy and tactile sensitivity	Tolerance, dependence; rapid or irregular heart beat; weight loss; irritability, nervousness, impulsiveness, insomnia; panic, paranoia; heart failure *For cocaine*—chest pain, respiratory failure, seizures, strokes; withdrawal symptoms *For methamphetamine*—cardiac and neurological damage, impaired memory/learning, violent behavior, stroke, teeth and organ damage *For MDMA*—impaired memory and learning, hyperthermia, cardiac and liver toxicity, kidney failure *For nicotine*—see Chapter 9
Depressants		
Alcohol **Barbiturates** (downers, barbs, reds, yellow jackets) **Flunitrazepam** Rohypnol (forget-me pill, roofies, R2) **GHB** (G, Georgia home boy, liquid X, grievous bodily harm) **Methaqualone** Quaalude (ludes, quay) **Tranquilizers** Ativan, Valium, Xanax (downers, tranks)	Slowed heart rate, breathing rate, blood pressure; reduced anxiety; lowered inhibitions; impaired judgment; mood changes (feelings of well-being or euphoria or irritability and abusiveness); slurred speech; reduced concentration, reflexes, coordination; sedation, drowsiness, loss of consciousness	Tolerance, dependence; respiratory depression and arrest; injuries due to reduced coordination and judgment; coma, death; some depressants have life-threatening withdrawal symptoms *For flunitrazepam*—visual disturbances, memory loss for the time under the drug's effects *For GHB*—headache, loss of consciousness and reflexes, seizures
Hallucinogens		
LSD (acid, blotter, yellow sunshines) **Mescaline** (buttons, mesc, peyote) **Psilocybin** (shrooms, magic mushroom)	Altered states of feeling and perception; nausea; increased body temperature, heart rate, blood pressure; loss of appetite; sleeplessness; weakness, numbness; tremors; nervousness, paranoia	Persisting perception disorder (flashbacks), memory loss, depression

(continued)

Drug Classifications

Drugs can be categorized according to the nature of their physiological effects. Most psychoactive drugs fall into one of six general categories: stimulants, depressants, hallucinogens, cannabis, narcotics, and inhalants (Table 7.2). According to the 2007 National Survey on Drug Use and Health (NSDUH), American Indians had the highest rate of substance abuse and dependence (13.4 percent) while Asians had the lowest rate (4.7 percent). Eight percent of Hispanics, 9.9 percent of Pacific Islanders, and 8.5 percent of African Americans reported substance abuse or dependence in 2007; these were similar to 2006 rates. Marijuana was the most commonly used illegal drug, followed by nonmedical use of prescription drugs (Figure 7-2 on page 196).

Stimulants

In general, **stimulants** excite or increase the activity of the central nervous system (CNS). Also called "uppers," stimulants alert the CNS by increasing heart rate, blood pressure, and the rate of brain function. Users feel uplifted and less fatigued. Examples of stimulant drugs include caffeine, amphetamines, and cocaine. Most stimulants produce psychological dependence and tolerance relatively quickly, but they are unlikely to produce significant physical dependence when judged by life-threatening withdrawal symptoms. The important exception is cocaine, which seems to be capable of producing psychological dependence and withdrawal so powerful that continued use of the drug is inevitable for some users.

Table 7.2 Psychoactive Drug Categories (continued)

Drugs and Examples of Commercial (Street) Names	Intoxication Effects	Potential Health Consequences
Cannabis		
Hashish *(hash, hemp, soles)* ***Marijuana*** *(pot, dope, weed, reefer, Mary Jane, grass, ganja)*	Euphoria, slowed thinking and reaction time, confusion, impaired balance and coordination See Table 7.3.	Cough, frequent respiratory infections; impaired memory and learning; increased heart rate, anxiety; panic attacks; tolerance and dependence
Narcotics (Opiates)*		
Heroin *(dope, H, junk, smack, brown sugar)* ***Morphine*** *(M, morph, Miss Emma)* ***Opium*** *(big O, gum)* ***Oxycodone*** *(Oxy, OC, killer)*	Pain relief, euphoria, reduced pulse and blood pressure, pinpoint pupils, drowsiness, confusion, staggering gait, sedation, nausea, constipation	Tolerance, dependence; respiratory depression and arrest; unconsciousness, coma, death; unpleasant but not life-threatening withdrawal *For injection use*—risk of skin infections and transmission of HIV, hepatitis
Inhalants		
Solvents, gases, petroleum products Paint thinner, gasoline glues, propane, aerosol propellant, nitrites *(laughing gas, poppers, snappers, whippets)*	Stimulation; loss of inhibition; headache; nausea, vomiting; slurred speech; loss of motor coordination; wheezing; hallucinations, delusions; possible aggressiveness	Muscle weakness; depression, memory impairment; damage to the cardiovascular and nervous systems; unconsciousness; sudden death
Dissociative Anesthetics		
Ketamine Ketalar SV *(cat Valium, K, Special K, vitamin K)* ***PCP*** Phencyclidine *(angel dust, hog)*	Increased heart rate and blood pressure, impaired motor function, rapid and involuntary eye movements, memory loss, numbness, nausea, vomiting *For PCP*—possible acute anxiety, aggression, violence	Delirium; depression; decreased respiration, blood pressure, heart rate

*Additional narcotics with similar effects include codeine, fentanyl, meperidine (Demerol), methadone, and hydrocodone (Vicodin).

Sources: National Institute on Drug Abuse, Commonly Abused Drugs, www.drugabuse.gov/DrugPages/DrugsofAbuse.html, March 2007; U.S. Drug Enforcement Agency, Drug Briefs and Backgrounds, www.usdoj.gov/dea/concern/concern.htm, March 2007.

Caffeine The methylxanthines are a family of chemicals that includes three compounds: caffeine, theophylline, and theobromine. Of these, caffeine is the most heavily consumed.

Caffeine is a tasteless drug found in coffee, tea, chocolate, many soft drinks, energy drinks, and several groups of over-the-counter drugs (see the box "Energy Drinks"). It is a relatively harmless CNS stimulant when consumed in moderate amounts. Fifty percent of Americans drink coffee daily, drinking 330 millions cups per day, earning the United States the name "Caffeine Nation."[7]

The chronic effects of long-term caffeine use are less clear. Chronic users show evidence of tolerance and withdrawal, indicating that they are physically dependent. Researchers have attempted to link caffeine to coronary heart disease, pancreatic cancer, and fibrocystic breast disease. So far, the results have been inconclusive.

For the average healthy adult, moderate consumption of caffeine is unlikely to pose any serious health threat. However, excessive consumption, also called caffeine intoxication, can occur when consuming more than 500

mg/day of caffeine. Consuming more than this amount of caffeine can lead to anxiety, diarrhea, restlessness, delayed onset of sleep or frequent awakening, headache, and heart palpitations. Most experts agree that 400 mg/day of caffeine, which is equivalent to 4 cups of coffee, is a moderate amount of caffeine consumption. Energy drinks, an increasingly popular source of caffeine, can range in caffeine content; an 8-ounce can of Red Bull contains 80 mg of caffeine and a 16-ounce can of Monster Zero Carb contains 240 mg of caffeine (see the box "Energy Drinks"). Pregnant women are advised to avoid caffeine consumption.

> **Key Terms**
>
> **stimulants** Psychoactive drugs that stimulate the function of the central nervous system.

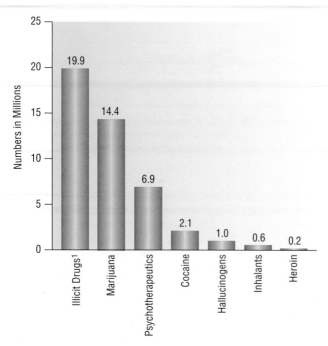

¹ Illicit Drugs include marijuana/hashish, cocaine (including crack), heroin, hallucinogens, inhalants, or prescription-type psychotherapeutics used nonmedically.

Figure 7-2 Past Month Use of Selected Illicit Drugs among Americans Ages 12 and Older, 2005 Marijuana is the most commonly used illicit drug, followed by nonmedical use of prescription drugs (psychotherapeutics).

Source: Substance Abuse and Mental Health Services Administration, Office of Applied Studies (2008). *Results from the 2007 National Survey on Drug Use and Health: National Findings* (NSDUH Series H-34, DHHS Publication No. SMA 08-4343). Rockville, MD.

Energy Drinks

Sales of energy drinks have skyrocketed in the past few years, with over 500 new energy drinks on the market in 2006 alone. It is a $3.4 billion per year industry. Thirty-one percent of American teens say that they drink them daily, more than double the percentage from 3 years ago. Energy drinks have risen in popularity owing to the increased effect in alertness they give consumers. Energy drinks contain caffeine, sugar, vitamins, amino acids, and a mixture of herbs. The energy in these drinks comes primarily from caffeine and then sugar. For example, Red Bull contains 80 mg of caffeine, Rockstar has 160 mg, No Fear has 174 mg, Monster has 160 mg, and Wired X505 has a whooping 505 mg of caffeine. Students and athletes consume energy drinks to pull all-nighters or to boost performance, while party-goers mix them with alcohol. Dizziness, light-headedness, rapid heartbeat, and numbness and tingling in the hands and feet are some of the effects these drinks can have, especially when consumed in large amounts. Health experts strongly advise consumers not to mix alcohol and energy drinks because of the dangerous effect it can have on the heart. Caffeine, like alcohol, is also a diuretic and can cause dehydration. There have been reports of caffeine overdose from drinking these beverages. Habitual users also reported problems with withdrawal, including feeling irritable, jittery, tired, and experiencing headaches.

Sources: Cohen, E. Energy Drinks Pack a Punch, but Is It Too Much? *CNN.com*, May 29, 2001; Associated Press, "Energy Drinks" Stir Health Debate, *USA Today,* December 21, 2001; CBS News, Caffeine Nation, September 7, 2003; Caffeine Labels Urged for Energy Drinks. *Indianapolis Star,* September 28, 2008.

Amphetamines Amphetamines produce increased activity and mood elevation in almost all users. The amphetamines include several closely related compounds: amphetamine, dextroamphetamine, and methamphetamine. These compounds do not have any natural sources and are completely manufactured in the laboratory. Medical use of amphetamines is limited primarily to the treatment of obesity, **narcolepsy,** and attention deficit hyperactivity disorder (ADHD).

Amphetamines can be ingested, injected, or snorted (inhaled). At low-to-moderate doses, amphetamines elevate mood and increase alertness and feelings of energy by stimulating receptor sites for two naturally occurring neurotransmitters. Amphetamines also slow the activity of the stomach and intestine and decrease hunger. In the 1960s and 1970s, amphetamines were commonly prescribed for dieters, but when it was discovered that the appetite suppression effect of amphetamines lasted only a few weeks, most physicians stopped prescribing them. At high doses, amphetamines can increase heart rate and blood pressure to dangerous levels. As amphetamines are eliminated from the body, the user becomes tired.

When chronically abused, amphetamines produce rapid tolerance and strong psychological dependence. Other effects of chronic use include impotence and episodes of psychosis. When use is discontinued, periods of depression may develop.

Methamphetamine Today the abuse of amphetamines is a more pressing concern than it has been in the recent past because of the sharp increase in the abuse of methamphetamine. Known by a variety of names and forms, including "crank," "ice," "crystal," "meth," "speed," "crystal meth," "chalk," "fire," "glass," and "zip," methamphetamine has a high potential for abuse and is produced in illegal home laboratories with over-the-counter ingredients.[8]

Methamphetamines can be smoked, ingested orally, snorted, or injected. **Crystal methamphetamine,** glass or ice, is among the most dangerous forms of methamphetamine. Ice is a very pure form of methamphetamine that looks like rock candy.[9] When ice is smoked or injected, its effects are felt in about seven seconds as a wave of intense physical and psychological exhilaration.

This effect lasts for several hours (much longer than the effects of crack), until the user becomes physically exhausted. The user experiences a rush of pleasure that is the result of the drug telling the brain to release large amounts of dopamine.[10] When ingested orally or snorted, methamphetamine induces euphoria, which may result in quick addiction for the user.

Abuse can lead to memory loss, violence, anxiety, paranoia, euphoria, hyperthermia, convulsions, increased wakefulness and physical activity, and cardiac and neurological damage. Chronic use can result in Parkinson-like symptoms, rotten teeth ("meth mouth"), stroke, anorexia, increased heart rate and blood pressure, death,[11] nutritional deficiencies, weight loss, reduced resistance to infection, and damage to the liver, lungs, and kidneys. Psychological dependence is quickly established. Withdrawal causes acute depression and fatigue but not significant physical discomfort. Tweaking refers to a dangerous stage when a methamphetamine abuser hasn't slept for 3 to 15 days, craves more of the drug, but no dosage will create the desired euphoric high. Tweakers are uncontrollable, frustrated, dangerous, unpredictable, and violent. Meth users often report experiencing hallucinations during this time, such as seeing "shadow people," which is thought to be caused by sleep deprivation.[12]

Recent data from the National Survey on Drug Use and Health (NSDUH) show that use of methamphetamine declined between 2002 and 2007 among persons 12 years old and older. Those living in the western United States were more likely to have used methamphetamine in the past year than those living in any other part of the country.

Adderall and Ritalin   There is an increasing concern about misuse and abuse of psychostimulants such as methylphenidate (Ritalin) and dextroamphetamine (Adderall), as the number of children and teens taking these medications increased 311 percent over the past 15 years. The number of girls taking these medications increased 72 percent from 2001 to 2007. Adderall, Ritalin, Strattera (atomoxetine), Concerta (methylphenidate), and Vyvanse (lisdexamfetamine) are typically prescribed to help focus attention in those who have attention deficit disorder (ADD) or ADHD. However, many people misuse these medications, using them to stay awake longer, control weight, and increase concentration (see the box "Ritalin and Adderall Abuse on College Campuses"). Strattera and Vyvanse don't have the tendency for abuse because they don't have the same stimulating effects as other medications for ADD and ADHD do.

Cocaine   Cocaine, perhaps the strongest of the stimulant drugs, has received much media attention. Cocaine is the primary psychoactive substance found in the leaves of the South American coca plant.[13] The effects of cocaine last only briefly—from 5 to 30 minutes. Regardless of the form in which it is consumed, cocaine produces an immediate, near-orgasmic "rush," or feeling of exhilaration. This euphoria is quickly followed by a period of marked depression. Used only occasionally as a topical anesthetic, cocaine is usually inhaled (snorted), injected, or smoked (typically as crack). There is overwhelming scientific evidence that users quickly develop a strong psychological dependence on cocaine. Considerable evidence suggests that physical dependence also rapidly develops. Cocaine users risk a weakened immune system making them "more susceptible to infections, including HIV."[14] However, physical dependence on cocaine does not lead to death upon withdrawal.

Crack Cocaine   Crack is made by combining cocaine hydrochloride with common baking soda. When this pastelike mixture is allowed to dry, a small rocklike crystalline material remains. This crack is heated in the bowl of a small pipe, and the vapors are inhaled into the lungs.[13] Some crack users spend hundreds of dollars a day to maintain their habit.

The effect of crack is almost instantaneous. Within 10 seconds after inhalation, cocaine reaches the CNS and influences the action of several neurotransmitters at specific sites in the brain. As with the use of other forms of cocaine, convulsions, seizures, respiratory distress, and cardiac failure have been reported with this sudden, extensive stimulation of the nervous system.

Within about 6 minutes, the stimulating effect of crack has been completely expended, and users frequently become depressed. Dependence develops within a few weeks because users consume more crack in response to the short duration of stimulation and rapid onset of depression.

Intravenous administration has been the preferred route for cocaine users who are also regular users of heroin and other injectable drugs. Intravenous injection results in an almost immediate high, which lasts about 10 minutes. A "smoother ride" is said to be obtained from a "speedball," the injectable mixture of heroin and cocaine (or methamphetamine). However, such a mixture can be volatile and even fatal.[4]

Key Terms

narcolepsy A sleep-related disorder in which a person has a recurrent, overwhelming, and uncontrollable desire to sleep, often at inappropriate times.

crystal methamphetamine A dangerous form of methamphetamine that quickly produces intense physical and psychological exhilaration when smoked.

Chapter Seven   Making Decisions about Drug Use

Ritalin and Adderall Abuse on College Campuses

Ritalin and Adderall abuse on college campuses continues to rise. Studies have shown that one in every five college students has used Ritalin illegally. Adderall is a fairly new drug similar to Ritalin, and it is being abused like Ritalin. Students who take Ritalin or Adderall without a prescription are using these drugs to help enhance concentration during late-night study sessions, to obtain a cocainelike high, or to suppress their appetites. However, students may not realize the serious side effects they can experience from misusing these drugs.

Side effects of Ritalin can include nervousness, insomnia, loss of appetite, headaches, increased heart and respiratory rates, dilated pupils, dry mouth, perspiration, and feelings of superiority. Higher doses can result in tremors, convulsions, paranoia, and/or a sensation of bugs crawling under the skin. These health risks are considerably higher if Ritalin is snorted. Death can occur from abusing Ritalin.

Side effects of Adderall are similar to those of Ritalin. These effects include loss of appetite, weight loss, insomnia, headache, and dizziness. Owing to a longer-lasting dose, Adderall has been growing in popularity. Adderall abuse can also result in death.

Sources: The Johns Hopkins News-Letter, *Ritalin Abuse Is Increasing*, www.jhunewsletter.com/vnews/display.v/ART/2002/11/22/3ddd766faebeb, February 21, 2005; The Johns Hopkins News-Letter, *Hopkins Students Turning to Drugs to Keep Grades Up*, www.jhunewsletter.com/vnews/display.v/ART/2004/04/02/406cd1793dfb2?in_archive=1, February 21, 2005; Attention Deficit Disorder Help Center, *Adderall Side Effects*, www.add-adhd-help-center.com/ adderall_side_effects.htm, February 21, 2005.

Freebasing As inhaling crack did, freebasing developed as a technique for maximizing the psychoactive effects of cocaine. Freebasing first requires that the common form of powdered cocaine (cocaine hydrochloride) be chemically altered (alkalized). This altered form is then dissolved in a solvent such as ether or benzene. This liquid solution is heated to evaporate the solvent. The heating process leaves the freebase cocaine in a powder form that can then be smoked, often through a water pipe. Because of the large surface area of the lungs, smoking cocaine facilitates fast absorption into the bloodstream.

One danger of freebasing cocaine is the risk related to the solvents used. Ether is a highly volatile solvent capable of exploding and causing serious burns. Benzene is a known carcinogen associated with the development of leukemia. Neither solvent can be used without increasing the level of risk typically associated with cocaine use.

Depressants

Depressants (or sedatives) sedate the user, slowing down CNS function. Drugs included in this category are alcohol (see Chapter 8), barbiturates, and tranquilizers. Depressants produce tolerance in abusers, as well as strong psychological and physical dependence.

Barbiturates Barbiturates are the so-called sleeping compounds that function by enhancing the effect of inhibitory neurotransmitters. They depress the CNS to the point where the user drops off to sleep or, as is the case with surgical anesthetics, the patient becomes anesthetized. Medically, barbiturates are used in widely varied dosages as anesthetics and for treatment of anxiety, insomnia, and epilepsy.[1] Regular use of a barbiturate quickly produces tolerance—eventually such a high dose is required that the user still feels the effects of the drug throughout the next morning. Some abusers then begin to alternate barbiturates with stimulants, producing a vicious circle of dependence. Other misusers combine alcohol and barbiturates or tranquilizers, inadvertently producing toxic or even lethal results. Abrupt withdrawal from barbiturate use frequently produces a withdrawal syndrome that can involve seizures, delusions, hallucinations, and even death.

Methaqualone (Quaalude, Sopor, "ludes") was developed as a sedative that would not have the dependence properties of other barbiturates.[1] Quaaludes were occasionally prescribed for anxious patients. Today, compounds resembling Quaaludes are manufactured in home laboratories and sold illegally so that they can be combined with small amounts of alcohol for an inexpensive, drunklike effect.

Tranquilizers Tranquilizers are depressants that are intended to reduce anxiety and to relax people who are having problems managing stress. Because of their sedating effects, tranquilizers have also been prescribed to treat insomnia. Lorazepam (Ativan), alprazolam (Xanax), diazepam (Valium), and chlordiazepoxide (Librium) are some of the most commonly prescribed. Unfortunately, some people become addicted to these and other prescription drugs.[15] All tranquilizers can produce physical and psychological dependence and tolerance.

"Date Rape" Drugs "Date rape" drugs or **club drugs** are commonly used on college campuses. These drugs are usually slipped into the drink of an unsuspecting person and can result in a coma or even death.

Common "date rape" drugs include GHB (gamma-hydroxybutyrate), also known as G, Liquid Esctasy, Easy Lay, Georgia Home Boy, and Rohypnol ("roofies"). When these drugs are consumed, they cause a drunklike or sleepy state that can last for hours. It is during this time when unsuspecting individuals are taken advantage of, against their will and without their knowledge. GHB acts quickly, within 10 to 20 minutes of ingestion, and lasts about 4 hours.

As a rule, it is wise not to accept drinks from people you do not know or leave your drink unattended. This recommendation extends to all parties where drinkers do not know what has been added to the punch or other drinks.[16]

Hallucinogens

As the name suggests, hallucinogenic drugs produce hallucinations—perceived distortions of reality. Also known as *psychedelic drugs* or *phantasticants,* **hallucinogens** reached their height of popularity during the 1960s. At that time, young people were encouraged to use hallucinogenic drugs to "expand the mind," "reach an altered state," or "discover reality" (see the box "Drugs and Spirituality"). Not all the reality distortions, or "trips," were pleasant. Many users reported "bad trips," or trips during which they perceived negative, frightening distortions.

Hallucinogenic drugs include laboratory-produced lysergic acid diethylamide (LSD), mescaline (from the peyote cactus plant), and psilocybin (from a particular genus of mushroom). Consumption of hallucinogens seems to produce not physical dependence but mild levels of psychological dependence. The development of tolerance is questionable. **Synesthesia,** a sensation in which users report hearing a color, smelling music, or touching a taste, is sometimes produced with hallucinogen use.

The long-term effects of hallucinogenic drug use are not fully understood. Questions about genetic abnormalities in offspring, fertility, sex drive and performance, and the development of personality disorders have not been fully answered. One phenomenon that has been identified and documented is the development of flashbacks—the unpredictable return to a psychedelic trip that occurred months or even years earlier. Flashbacks are thought to result from the accumulation of a drug within body cells.

LSD The most well-known and powerful hallucinogen is lysergic acid diethylamide (LSD). LSD was first isolated in 1938 by Albert Hoffmann, who was studying a group of chemicals that were extracted from a fungus that infects rye and other cereal grains. Five years later, he accidentally discovered its hallucinogenic effects. Dr. Timothy Leary helped to spread the popularity of LSD in the 1960s by promoting the use of LSD in mind expansion and experimentation. LSD helped define the counterculture movement of the 1960s. During the 1970s and the 1980s, this drug lost considerable popularity. LSD use peaked in 1996, with an annual prevalence of 8.8 percent.[17] There was sharp decline in the use of LSD between the years 2002 and 2003, which was attributed

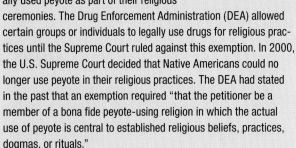

Discovering Your Spirituality

Drugs and Spirituality

Some drugs, such as mescaline from peyote, have been used in religious practices. For example, Native Americans have traditionally used peyote as part of their religious ceremonies. The Drug Enforcement Administration (DEA) allowed certain groups or individuals to legally use drugs for religious practices until the Supreme Court ruled against this exemption. In 2000, the U.S. Supreme Court decided that Native Americans could no longer use peyote in their religious practices. The DEA had stated in the past that an exemption required "that the petitioner be a member of a bona fide peyote-using religion in which the actual use of peyote is central to established religious beliefs, practices, dogmas, or rituals."

Opponents to the Supreme Court ruling claim that it violated First Amendment rights and has "far reaching implications especially for religious minorities" who have less political power. Another example occurred in 2005 when the Supreme Court was asked by the Bush administration to challenge a Christian group's ceremonial drinking of a tea called "hoasca" containing dimethyltryptamine, as this practice is in violation of the Controlled Substances Act. Both peyote and dimethyltryptamine are Schedule 1 drugs, meaning that their use is prohibited in all circumstances except for research.

What is your stance on religious freedom in terms of drug use? Would you advocate for prohibiting illicit drug use for any reason, or do you believe that certain exceptions should be made?

to the increase in Ecstasy use, and the rates have continued to decreased since that time.[18] Part of the appeal of LSD is its low cost and easy availability.

LSD is manufactured in home laboratories and frequently distributed in absorbent blotter paper or gelatin squares. It is odorless, colorless, and tasteless.[18] Users place the paper on their tongues or chew the paper to

Key Terms

depressants A category of drugs that sedate the user by slowing CNS function; they produce tolerance and strong psychological and physical addiction in users.

club drug One of a variety of psychoactive drugs typically used at raves, bars, and dance clubs.

hallucinogens Psychoactive drugs capable of producing hallucinations (distortions of reality).

synesthesia A sensation of combining of the senses, such as perceiving color by hearing it or perceiving taste by touching it.

ingest the drug. LSD is similar in structure to the neurotransmitter serotonin and produces psychedelic effects by interfering with the normal activity of this neurotransmitter. Although the typical doses ("hits") today are about half as powerful as those in the 1960s, users still tend to rapidly develop a high tolerance of LSD. The effects of LSD depend upon the dose. Physical dependence does not occur. The effects can include altered perception of shapes, images, time, sound, and body form. Synesthesia is common to LSD users. LSD is metabolized in the liver and excreted. Its effects last an average of six to nine hours.

Users may describe LSD experiences as positive and "mind-expanding," or negative and "mind-constricting," depending on the user's mood and the social setting in which the drug is taken. Positive sensations include feelings of creativity, deep understanding of oneself and the universe, and feelings of grandeur. Although LSD users report feelings of increased insight and creativity, a real increase in these skills has not been demonstrated. At the same time, some reports of bad trips on LSD are thought to have been caused by other substances, such as PCP, that were sold to the user as LSD. Deaths resulting from bizarre behavior after taking LSD have been reported. Dangerous side effects include panic attacks, flashbacks, and occasional prolonged psychosis.

Ecstasy and Designer Drugs In recent years, chemists who produce many of the illicit drugs in home laboratories have designed versions of drugs listed on **FDA Schedule 1.** Under the Controlled Substances Act, substances regulated by the Food and Drug Administration are placed in one of five schedules. Schedule 1 contains the most dangerous drugs that have no medical use.[19] Designer drugs are similar to the controlled drugs on the FDA Schedule 1 but are sufficiently different so that they escape governmental control. The designer drugs are either newly synthesized products that are similar to already outlawed drugs but against which no law yet exists, or they are reconstituted or renamed illegal substances. Designer drugs are said to produce effects similar to those of their controlled drug counterparts.

People who use designer drugs do so at great risk because the manufacturing of these drugs is unregulated. The neurophysiological effect of these homemade drugs can be quite dangerous. So far, a synthetic heroin product (MPPP) and several amphetamine derivatives with hallucinogenic properties have been designed for the unwary drug consumer.

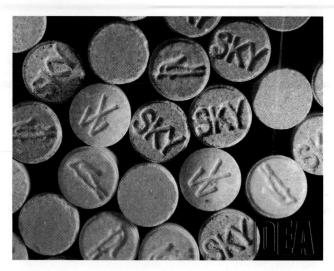

MDMA (Ecstasy) is a designer drug that has both stimulant and hallucinogenic effects. Heavy or long-term use has a number of negative effects, including memory impairment, possibly caused by depletion of the neurotransmitter serotonin.

DOM (STP), MDA (the "love drug"), and MDMA ("Ecstacy" or "XTC") are examples of amphetamine-derivative, hallucinogenic designer drugs. These drugs produce mild LSD-like hallucinogenic experiences, positive feelings, and enhanced alertness. They also have a number of potentially dangerous effects. These dangers include increased heart rate and blood pressure, muscle tension, involuntary teeth clenching, nausea, blurred vision, faintness, and chills or sweating. MDMA use can also cause hyperthermia from a sharp increase in body temperature, which can result in kidney, liver, and cardiovascular system failure.[20] Experts are particularly concerned that MDMA can produce strong psychological dependence and can deplete serotonin, an important excitatory neurotransmitter associated with a state of alertness and mood. Heavy or long-term users can experience depression, anxiety, paranoia, hallucinations, panic attacks, and hostility. Memory loss is commonly experienced in heavy MDMA users, who are therefore sometimes called "E-tards."[21] Permanent brain damage is possible.[3] As with LSD, there has been a decline in MDMA use since 2003. On average, people first tried this drug at age 20.[22]

Phencyclidine Phencyclidine (PCP, "angel dust") is a complicated drug because it not only produces hallucinogenic effects but also acts as an analgesic, a depressant, a stimulant, and an anesthetic. This makes the typical PCP experience impossible to predict or describe. The physical effects of PCP begin a few minutes after consumption and continue for four to six hours. PCP was studied for years during the 1950s and 1960s and was found to be an unsuitable animal and human anesthetic.[23]

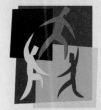
Manufactured in tablet or powder form, PCP can be injected, inhaled, taken orally, or smoked. Some users report mild euphoria, although most report bizarre perceptions, paranoid feelings, and aggressive behavior. It can increase blood pressure and body temperature and decrease coordination. People also report feeling an increased state of drowsiness, a decreased sensitivity to pain, and a sense of disconnection from reality. PCP overdose may cause convulsions, cardiovascular collapse, and damage to the brain's respiratory center.

In a number of cases, the aggressive behavior caused by PCP has led users to commit brutal crimes against both friends and innocent strangers. PCP accumulates in cells and may stimulate bizarre behavior months after initial use.

PCP is an extremely unpredictable and dangerous drug. Although PCP has been blamed in many reports of bizarre, even homicidal, behavior, it continues to be abused. Because PCP is easily and cheaply manufactured in home laboratories, authorities have difficulty limiting its availability.

Cannabis

Cannabis (marijuana) is the most widely used illicit drug among college students (see the box "Who Uses Marijuana?"). Marijuana has been labeled a mild hallucinogen for a number of years. However, most experts now consider it to be a drug category in itself. Marijuana produces mild effects like those of stimulants and depressants. Marijuana has been implicated as contributing to a large number of traffic fatalities. It has also been found that using marijuana increases the chances of developing a mental disorder by 40 percent and that users were three times more likely to have suicidal thoughts.

Products and Potency Marijuana is actually a wild plant (*Cannabis sativa*) whose fibers were once used in the manufacture of hemp rope. When the leafy material and small stems are dried and crushed, users can smoke the mixture in rolled cigarettes ("joints"), cigars ("blunts"), or pipes. The resins collected from scraping the flowering tops of the plant yield a marijuana product called hashish, or hash, commonly smoked in a pipe.[24]

The potency of marijuana's hallucinogenic effect is determined by the percentage of the active ingredient, tetrahydrocannabinol (THC), present in the product. The concentration of THC averages about 3.5 percent for regular grade marijuana, 7 to 9 percent for higher quality marijuana (sinsemilla), 8 to 14 percent for hashish, and as high as 50 percent for hash oil.[1] Today's marijuana has THC levels that are higher than in past decades.

Short-Term Effects THC is a fat-soluble substance and thus is absorbed and retained in fat tissues within the body. Before being excreted, THC can remain in the body for up to a month. With the sophistication of today's drug tests, trace metabolites of THC can be detected for up to 30 days after consumption.[3]

Once marijuana is consumed, its effects vary from person to person (see Table 7.3). Being "high" or "stoned" means different things to different people. Many people report heightened sensitivity to music, cravings for particular foods, and a relaxed mood. There is widespread consensus that marijuana's behavioral effects include four probabilities: (1) Users must learn to recognize what a marijuana high is like, (2) marijuana impairs short-term memory, (3) users overestimate the passage of time, and (4) users lose the ability to maintain attention to a task.[3]

Long-Term Effects The long-term effects of marijuana use are still being studied. Chronic abuse may lead to an amotivational syndrome in some people. Heavy marijuana users have trouble paying attention and retaining new information for at least a day after last using the drug, according to a recent study.

Table 7.3 Effects of Marijuana

Short-Term Effects	Long-Term Effects
• Increased heart rate and blood pressure • Feeling of elation • Drowsiness and sedation • Increased appetite • Red eyes • Food cravings • Slow reaction time • Feelings of depression, excitement, paranoia, panic, and euphoria • Problems with attention span, memory, learning, problem-solving, and coordination • Sleeplessness*	• Lung damage • Increased risk of bronchitis • Emphysema • Lung cancer • Heart attack[†] • Loss of motivation and short-term memory • Increased panic or anxiety • May become tolerant to marijuana • Damage to lungs, immune system, and reproductive organs • Can remain in the body for up to a month • Can cause birth defects • Five times more damaging to the lungs than tobacco products*

*National Institute on Drug Abuse. National Institutes of Health, *NIDA Research Report—Marijuana Abuse,* www.nida.nih.gov/ResearchReports/Marijuana/default.html, February 15, 2005.

[†]"Stronger Marijuana Is Major Health Risk," *The Independent,* February 1, 2001.

The irritating effects of marijuana smoke on lung tissue are more pronounced than those of cigarette smoke, and some of the more than 400 chemicals in marijuana are now linked to lung cancer development. In fact, one of the most potent carcinogens, benzopyrene, is found in higher levels in marijuana smoke than in tobacco smoke. Marijuana smokers tend to inhale deeply and hold the smoke in the lungs for long periods. It is likely that at some point the lungs of chronic marijuana smokers will be damaged.

Long-term marijuana use is also associated with damage to the immune system and to the male and female reproductive systems and with an increase in birth defects in babies born to mothers who smoke marijuana. Chronic marijuana use lowers testosterone levels in men, sometimes resulting in enlarged breast size and decreased sperm count. For women who are chronic marijuana users, their testosterone level increases, which can cause irregular menstrual cycles and infertility.

Medical Uses Marijuana has been used to relieve the nausea caused by chemotherapy, to improve appetite in AIDS patients, and to ease the pressure that builds up in the eyes of glaucoma patients. However, a variety of other drugs, many of which are nearly as effective, are also used for these purposes. The U.S. Supreme Court struck a blow to the proponents of the medical use of marijuana when, in 2005, it outlawed the use of medical marijuana. However, 13 states have state laws that allow terminally ill patients to legally use marijuana for medical purposes.

Narcotics

The **narcotics,** or opiates, are among the strongest dependence-producing drugs. Overdose can be lethal and can occur the first time taking the drug. People using narcotics experience a rush of pleasure followed by a dreamy, drowsy state in which they feel little pain. Breathing slows, sometimes to the point of respiratory failure. Users also report that their skin flushes, their pupils become pinpointed, and they feel nauseous and may vomit. Depending upon how quickly the drug is metabolized in the liver, the effects of most narcotics are experienced for 4 to 6 hours. The effects from taking methadone can last 12 to 24 hours.[21] Medically, narcotics are used to relieve pain and induce sleep. On the basis of origin, narcotics can be subgrouped into the natural, quasisynthetic, and synthetic narcotics.

Natural Narcotics Naturally occurring substances derived from the Oriental poppy plant include opium (the primary psychoactive substance extracted from the Oriental poppy), morphine (the primary active ingredient in opium), and thebaine (a compound not used as a drug). Morphine and related compounds have medical use as analgesics in the treatment of mild to severe pain.

Quasisynthetic Narcotics Quasisynthetic narcotics are compounds created by chemically altering morphine. These laboratory-produced drugs are intended to be used as analgesics, but their benefits are largely outweighed by a high dependence rate and a great risk of toxicity. The best known of the quasisynthetic narcotics is heroin. Although heroin is a fast-acting and very effective analgesic, it is extremely addictive. Heroin can be inhaled ("snorted"), smoked, injected into a vein, or "skin-popped" (injected beneath the skin surface). Heroin produces dreamlike euphoria and, like all narcotics, strong physical and psychological dependence and tolerance.

Most new heroin users are smoking or snorting heroin, rather than injecting the drug. One-quarter of the new users of heroin are under age 18, and nearly half are ages 18 to 25.[25]

Heroin users who inject the drug face an additional risk. As with the use of all other injectable illegal drugs, the practice of sharing needles increases the likelihood of transmission of various communicable diseases, including hepatitis C and HIV (see Chapter 13). Fifteen percent of users contract chronic liver disease and 17% die from heroin overdose. Abrupt withdrawal from heroin use is rarely fatal, but the discomfort during cold turkey withdrawal is reported to be excruciating.

Synthetic Narcotics Meperidine (Demerol) and propoxyphene (Darvon), common postsurgical painkillers, and methadone, the drug prescribed during the rehabilitation of heroin addicts, are synthetic narcotics. These opiatelike drugs are manufactured in medical laboratories. They are not natural narcotics or quasi-synthetic narcotics because they do not originate from the Oriental poppy plant. Like true narcotics, however, these drugs can rapidly induce physical dependence. One important criticism of methadone rehabilitation programs is that they merely shift the addiction from heroin to methadone.

Inhalants

Inhalants constitute a class of drugs that includes a variety of volatile (quickly evaporating) compounds that generally produce unpredictable, drunklike effects in users and feelings of euphoria.[26] Users of inhalants may also have some delusions and hallucinations. Some users may become quite aggressive. Drugs in this category include anesthetic gases (chloroform, nitrous oxide, and ether), vasodilators (amyl nitrite and butyl nitrite), petroleum products and commercial solvents (gasoline, kerosene, plastic cement, glue, typewriter correction fluid, paint, and paint thinner), and certain aerosols (found in some propelled spray products, fertilizers, and insecticides). Inhaling these substances has been referred to as "huffing," "sniffing," "dusting," and "chroming."

Most of the danger in using inhalants lies in the damaging, sometimes fatal effects on the respiratory and cardiovascular systems.[26] Death, or "sudden sniffing death syndrome," can occur after only 1, 20, or 100 times of inhaling a substance. Inhalants can also dissolve the myelin sheath that protects the cells in the brain, resulting in cell death and brain damage. Furthermore, users may unknowingly place themselves in dangerous situations because of the drunklike hallucinogenic effects. Aggressive behavior might also make users a threat to themselves and others.

For more information about inhalants, contact the National Inhalant Prevention Coalition at www .inhalants.org.

Combination Drug Effects

Drugs taken in various combinations and dosages can alter and perhaps intensify effects.

A synergistic effect is a dangerous consequence of taking different drugs in the same general category at the same time. The combination exaggerates each individual drug's effects. For example, the combined use of alcohol and tranquilizers produces a synergistic effect greater than the total effect of each of the two drugs taken separately. In this instance, a much-amplified, perhaps fatal sedation will occur. In a simplistic sense, "one plus one equals four or five."

When taken at or near the same time, drug combinations produce a variety of effects. Drug combinations have additive, potentiating, or antagonistic effects. When two or more drugs are taken and the result is merely a combined total effect of each drug, the result is an additive effect. The sum of the effects is not exaggerated. In a sense, "one plus one plus one equals three."

When one drug intensifies the action of a second drug, the first drug is said to have a potentiated effect on the second drug. One popular drug-taking practice during the 1970s was the consumption of Quaaludes and beer. Quaaludes potentiated the inhibition-releasing, sedative effects of alcohol. This particular drug combination produced an inexpensive but potentially fatal drunklike euphoria in the user. More recently, the combined use of various "club drugs" results in unpredictable potentiated drug effects.

An antagonistic effect, on the other hand, is a drug's action in reducing another drug's effects. Knowledge of this principle has been useful in the medical treatment of certain drug overdoses, as in the use of tranquilizers to relieve the effects of LSD or other hallucinogenic drugs.

Key Terms

narcotics Opiates; psychoactive drugs derived from the Oriental poppy plant. Narcotics relieve pain and induce sleep.

cold turkey Immediate, total discontinuation of use of a drug; associated with withdrawal discomfort.

inhalants Psychoactive drugs that enter the body through inhalation.

synergistic effect A heightened, exaggerated effect produced by the concurrent use of two or more drugs.

antagonistic effect The effect produced when one drug reduces or offsets the effects of a second drug.

additive effect The combined (but not exaggerated) effect produced by the concurrent use of two or more drugs.

potentiated effect A phenomenon whereby the use of one drug intensifies the effect of a second drug.

Because of these possible synergistic drug effects, patients should always inform their doctors and dentists of any illegal drugs they have taken.

Society's Response to Drug Use

During the last 25 years, society has responded to illegal drug use with growing concern. Most adults see drug abuse as a clear danger to society. This position has been supported by the development of community, school, state, and national organizations interested in the reduction of illegal drug use. These organizations have included such diverse groups as Parents Against Drugs, Parents for a Drug-Free Youth, Drug Abuse Resistance Education (DARE), Mothers Against Drunk Driving (MADD), Narcotics Anonymous, and the federal Drug Enforcement Administration. Certain groups have concentrated their efforts on education, others on enforcement, and still others on the development of laws and public policy.[27]

The personal and social issues related to drug abuse are very complex. Innovative solutions continue to be devised. Some believe that only through early childhood education will people learn alternatives to drug use. Starting drug education in the preschool years may have a more positive effect than waiting until the upper elementary or junior high school years. The focus on reducing young people's exposure to gateway drugs (especially tobacco, alcohol, and marijuana) may help slow down the move to other addictive drugs. Some people advocate much harsher penalties for drug use and drug trafficking.

Others support legalizing all drugs and making governmental agencies responsible for drug regulation and control, as is the case with alcohol. Advocates of this position believe that drug-related crime and violence would virtually cease once the demand for illegal products is reduced.

Unless significant changes in society's response to drug use take place soon, families and communities will continue to be plagued by drug-related tragedies. Law enforcement officials will be pressed to the limits of their resources in their attempts to reduce drug flow. Our judicial system will be heavily burdened by thousands of court cases. Health care facilities could face overwhelming numbers of patients.

Currently, approximately $19.2 billion is spent to fight the drug war in the United States—$13 billion on law enforcement (supply reduction) and $6.2 billion on education, prevention, and treatment (demand reduction).[28] In comparison with other federally funded programs, the "war on drugs" is less expensive than farm support, food stamps, Medicare, and national defense. However, it remains to be seen whether any amount of money spent on enforcement, without adequate support for education, treatment, and poverty reduction, can reduce the illegal drug demand and supply.

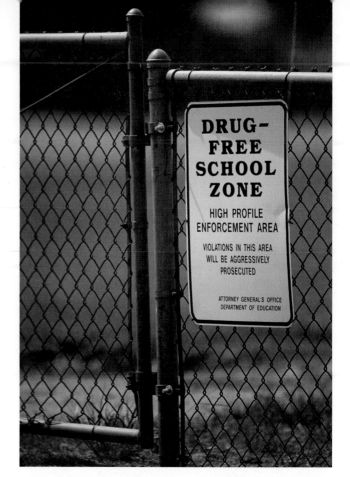

A drug-free school program is an example of a primary prevention measure designed to prevent potential drug users from ever trying drugs.

Prevention: The Best Solution

We combat the drug problem in the United States on two fronts: the demand side and the supply side. The U.S. government attempts to reduce the supply of illegal (illicit) drugs through drug interdiction efforts at our borders, through joint efforts with countries such as Mexico and Colombia, and through law-enforcement measures within our own borders.

However, the best way to avoid the immense costs of drug abuse is simply to reduce the demand. We do this by helping people develop the tools needed to avoid the use of illegal drugs. Experts are currently mounting prevention efforts on three levels: primary, secondary, and tertiary.

Primary Prevention By **primary prevention** we mean reaching people who have not yet used drugs and reducing their desire to try drugs. Primary prevention programs can target individuals, families, peer groups, neighborhoods, schools, workplaces, colleges, and the community. Examples of primary prevention include the DARE program, teaching assertiveness and refusal skills to children and teens, having drug-free schools, using student leaders from schools as role models and as presenters of peer programs, debunking the myths associated with drug use (such as that smoking is cool), and

Building Media Literacy Skills

Do Public Service Announcements Make a Difference?

The scene opens with a male teen on a basketball court shooting hoops by himself. The camera shifts and shows a black shadow behind him resembling him and mimicking his movements. He continues dribbling the ball, shoots, and scores. He then looks back and sees another teen standing at the fence of the court offering him a joint. The teen leaves the basketball court to smoke a joint with the second teen. The shadow of the basketball player is left, alone, dribbling the ball by itself on the court. The narrator asks, "If you smoke weed, how much of yourself are you leaving behind?" This television commercial is one of the "Above the Influence" public service announcements geared to decrease drug use. Some of the ads depict rats and slugs using drugs made to resemble rat and slug poison, with the question "What's the worst that could happen?" The print materials also include mock ads that "advertise" TV remote controller and couch security guard jobs with captions that read, "Hey not trying to be your mom, but there aren't many jobs out there for potheads."

Public service announcements (PSAs) have been used to prevent drug abuse since World War II. A PSA is "any announcement (including network) for which no charge is made and which promotes programs, activities, or services of federal, state, or local governments (e.g., recruiting, sale of bonds, etc.) or the programs, activities, or services of nonprofit organizations (e.g., United Way, Red Cross blood donations, etc.) and other announcements regarded as serving community interests, excluding time signals, routine weather announcements, and promotional announcements."* But how effective are they?

Research suggests that some PSAs have a positive effect, some have no effect, and some actually do the opposite of what they intend in that they result in encouraging people to use drugs. It is important to know your target audience in terms of their attitudes, beliefs about the consequences of some behavior, perceived norms, and self-efficacy.* Unfortunately this type of research is rarely done.

One study did find that viewers paid more attention to PSAs related to methamphetamine and heroin than to PSAs about marijuana or drugs in general. The PSAs that specifically pointed out negative consequences of drug use were more effective than ones with messages such as "Just Say No [because we say so]." PSAs that used humor had negative consequences (increased the likelihood of drug use). Those that were more realistic and were related to perceptions of harm, danger, or violating social norms were most effective in preventing drug use. The "Friends Don't Let Friends Drive Drunk" series of PSAs presented more realistic depictions of how allowing friends to drink and drive violates social norms and has negative consequences.

Also, the more print and air time effective PSAs receive, the more likely they are to have an impact in changing behavior. Studies have shown that when media time and space were devoted to PSAs, smoking, drinking, and drug use declined—and when less PSA advertising was donated, these rates increased.* Unfortunately, with demands for greater profit margins, less print and air time have been given to PSAs in recent years. What PSAs do you remember? Did they influence your behavior? Why or why not?

*"Avoiding the Boomerang: Testing the Relative Effectivenss of Antidrug Public Service Announcements Before a National Campaign," *American Journal of Public Health* 92(2), February 2002.

community programs for drug education. The key to primary prevention is to keep potential users from starting to use drugs. See the box "Do Public Service Announcements Make a Difference?"

Secondary Prevention   Secondary prevention targets those who are beginning to experiment with drugs and uses detection, screening, intervention, and treatment of early drug abuse to help avoid further drug use and identify people at risk for developing addictions. These programs do not prevent initial drug use but instead involve detection and early treatment of drug problems before they become severe. Popular methods include crisis telephone hotlines, peer counseling, individual and family counseling, school and worksite drug screening programs, and student and employee assistance programs.[29]

Tertiary Prevention   Tertiary prevention (third-level prevention) targets drug-dependent people, such as cocaine abusers, heroin addicts, or alcoholics. These individuals require specialized, intensive help that includes rehabilitation and maintenance. Such intensive treatments may require temporary hospitalization. Additional treatment methods include intensive outpatient care, support groups, and after-care programs. Relapse prevention is designed to help people recovering from drug abuse maintain their drug-free lifestyles.[29]

Key Terms

primary prevention Measures intended to deter first-time drug use.

secondary prevention Measures aimed at early detection, intervention, and treatment of drug abuse before severe physical, psychological, emotional, or social consequences can occur.

tertiary prevention Treatment and rehabilitation of drug-dependent people to limit physical, psychological, emotional, and social deterioration or prevent death.

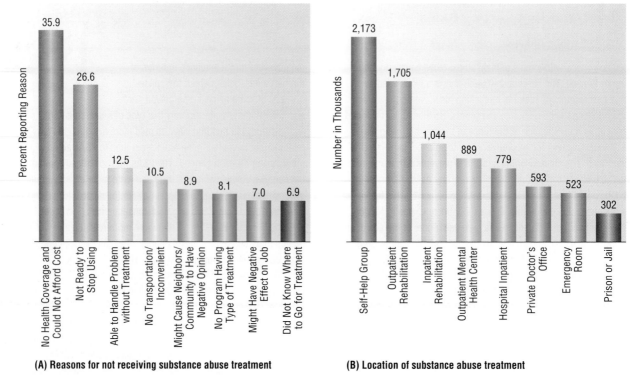

(A) Reasons for not receiving substance abuse treatment

(B) Location of substance abuse treatment

Figure 7-3 Facts about Substance Abuse Treatment (a) Among people who tried and failed to obtain drug abuse treatment, lack of insurance and cost were cited as the top barrier. (b) Among people who did obtain treatment, self-help groups and outpatient programs were the most commonly reported treatment locations.

Source: Substance Abuse and Mental Health Services Administration, Office of Applied Studies (2008). *Results from the 2007 National Survey on Drug Use and Health: National Findings* (NSDUH Series H-34, DHHS Publication No. SMA 08-4343). Rockville, MD.

Drug Testing

Drug testing is one of society's responses to drug use and is becoming an increasingly popular prevention tool. In 1986 the federal government instituted drug-testing policies for federal employees in safety-sensitive jobs. In 1988 the Drug Free Workplace Act extended the drug-free federal policy to include all federal grantees (including universities) and most federal contractors. Although this act did not mandate drug testing, it encouraged tougher approaches to prevent and deal with drug problems at the work site.

Private companies have developed drug-testing procedures similar to those used with federal agencies. Most Fortune 500 companies use drug testing to screen applicants or monitor employee drug use.

Drug tests commonly search for amphetamines, barbiturates, benzodiazepines (the chemical bases for prescription tranquilizers such as Valium and Librium), cannabinoids (THC, hashish, and marijuana), methaqualone, opiates (heroin, codeine, and morphine), and PCP. With the exception of marijuana, most traces of these drugs are eliminated by the body within a few days after use. Marijuana can remain detectable for up to 30 days after use.

How accurate are the results of drug testing? At typical cutoff standards, drug tests are likely to identify 90 percent of recent drug users. This means that about 10 percent of recent users will pass undetected. (These 10 percent are considered *false negatives.*) Nonusers whose drug tests indicate drug use (*false positives*) are quite rare. (Follow-up tests on these false positives would nearly always show negative results.) Human errors are probably more responsible than technical errors for inaccuracies in drug tests.

Recently, scientists have been refining procedures that use hair samples to detect the presence of drugs. These procedures seem to hold much promise, although certain technical obstacles remain. Watch for refinements in hair-sample drug testing in the near future.

Treatment and Intervention

The good news for people with drug addictions is that help is available through inpatient hospitalization or intensive outpatient care, self-help groups such as Narcotics Anonymous, and medical health professionals. The bad news is that treatment can be costly. Methadone treatment averages $7,400 for outpatient treatment, and alcohol treatment averages $1,500. Inpatient hospital treatment can cost thousands per day. Figure 7-3 shows the barriers people report for not getting treatment for

ANSWERS TO THE "WHAT DO YOU KNOW?" QUIZ

1. False   2. True   3. True   4. False   5. True   6. True   7. True

Visit the Online Learning Center (**www.mhhe.com/payne11e**), where you will find tools to help you improve your grade including practice quizzes, key terms flashcards, audio chapter summaries for your MP3 player, and many other study aids.

SOURCE NOTES

1. Ray O, Ksir C. *Drugs, Society, and Human Behavior* (10th ed.). New York: McGraw-Hill, 2004.
2. Shier D, Butler J, Lewis R. *Hole's Essentials of Human Anatomy and Physiology* (9th ed.). New York: McGraw-Hill, 2002.
3. Ksir C, Hart C, Oakley R. *Drugs, Society and Human Behavior* (12th ed). New York: McGraw-Hill, 2008.
4. Pinger RR, Payne WA, Hahn DB, Hahn EJ. *Drugs: Issues for Today* (3rd ed.). New York: McGraw-Hill, 1998.
5. Substance Abuse and Mental Health Services Administration (SAMHSA). *Overview of Findings from the 2005 National Survey on Drug Use and Health*, http://oas.samhsa.gov/nhsda/2k3nsduh/2k3overview.htm, February 12, 2007.
6. Results from the 2005 National Survey on Drug Use and Health, NSDUH: National Findings. SAMHSA report 2007.
7. Caffeine Nation. CBS News, September 7, 2003.
8. National Institute on Drug Abuse. National Institutes of Health. *NIDA InfoFacts—Methamphetamine*, www.nida.nih.gov/Infofax/methamphetamine.html, 2007.
9. U.S. Department of Justice. Drug Enforcement Administration. *Methamphetamine*, www.usdoj.gov/dea/concern/meth.htm, December 31, 2001.
10. Frackelmann K. Breaking Bonds of Addiction: Compulsion Traced to Part of the Brain, *USA Today*, April 18, 2002.
11. National Institute on Drug Abuse. National Institutes of Health. *NIDA Research Report—Methamphetamine Abuse and Addiction*, www.nida.nih.gov/ResearchReports/Methamph/Methamph.html .NIH Publication, No. 02-4210, January 2002.
12. National Drug Intelligence Center, U.S. Department of Justice Heavy Meth Use and Safety, www.stopdrugs.org.
13. U.S. Department of Justice. Drug Enforcement Administration. *Drugs of Abuse*, www.dea.gov/pubs/abuse/5-stim.htm, 2005 Edition.
14. Cocaine Weakens Immune System, *Boston Herald*, March 7, 2003.
15. National Institute on Drug Abuse. National Institutes of Health. *NIDA Research Report, Prescription Drugs Abuse and Addiction*, www.drugabuse.gov/ResearchReports/Prescription/Prescription.html, NIH Publication No. 01-4881, July 2001.
16. National Institute on Drug Abuse. National Institutes of Health. *NIDA InfoFacts—Rohypnol and GHB*, www.nida.nih.gov/Infofax/RohypnolGHB.html, 2007.
17. Johnston LD, O'Malley PM, Bachman JG, Schulenberg JE. *Monitoring the Future: National Survey Results on Drug Use: 1975–2003. Volume I: Secondary School Students*, www.monitoringthefuture.org/pubs/monographs/voll_2003.pdf. NIH Publication No. 04-5507. Bethesda, MD: 2004.
18. National Institute on Drug Abuse. National Institutes of Health. *NIDA InfoFacts—LSD*, www.nida.nih.gov/Infofax/lsd.html, 2007.
19. U.S. Department of Justice. Drug Enforcement Administration. Controlled Substances Act, www.usdoj.gov/dea/agency/csa.htm, 2007.
20. National Institute on Drug Abuse. National Institutes of Health. *NIDA InfoFacts—MDMA (Ecstasy)*, www.nida.nih.gov/Infofax/ecstasy.html, 2007.
21. Kuhh C, Swartzwelder S, Wilson W. *Buzzed: The Straight Facts About the Most Used and Abused Drugs from Alcohol to Ecstasy*. New York: W. W. Norton, 2003.
22. Johnston LD, O'Malley PM, Bachman JG, Schulenberg, JE. National Press Release, *Overall Teen Drug Use Continues Gradual Decline; but Use of Inhalants Rises*. Ann Arbor, MI: University of Michigan News and Information Services, December 21, 2004.
23. National Institute on Drug Abuse. National Institutes of Health. *NIDA InfoFacts—PCP (Phencyclidine)*, www.nida.nih.gov/Infofax/pcp.html, 2007.
24. National Institute on Drug Abuse. National Institutes of Health. *NIDA InfoFacts—Marijuana*, www.nida.nih.gov/Infofax/marijuana.html, 2007.
25. Leinwand D. Heroin's Resurgence Closes Drug's Traditional Gender Gap: Teenage Girls are Increasingly Falling Prey to Narcotic in Purer, "More Mainstream," Sniffable Form, *USA Today*, May 9, 2000.
26. Frackelmann K. Inhalants' Hidden Treat: Access Makes Huffing Popular But Kids Can Recover with Help, *USA Today*, June 25, 2002.
27. SADD History. Students Against Drunk Driving, www.saddonline.com, March 1, 2005, www.bacchusgamma.org/, March 1, 2005.
28. www.whitehousedrugpolicy.gov/publications/policy/04budget/exec_sum.pdf, May 21, 2003.
29. Tricker R. *Preventing Substance Use in Young Athletes*, www.tpronline.org, February 11, 2005.

Personal Assessment

Risk Assessment for Marijuana Dependence or Abuse

You may wonder if your use or a friend's use of marijuana fits the criteria for being at risk for developing marijuana dependence or abuse. The following questions may help you determine if there is cause for you to be concerned.

1. Have you tried to cut down or stop smoking marijuana and not been able to do so?
2. Do you use daily?
3. Is it hard for you to imagine life without marijuana?
4. Do you find that who your friends are is determined by your marijuana use?
5. Do you use marijuana to avoid dealing with your problems?
6. Do you use marijuana to cope with your feelings?
7. Has your marijuana use created conflict in your relationships?
8. Has your marijuana use created problems for you at work?
9. Has your marijuana use decreased your academic performance?
10. Has your use of marijuana caused problems with memory or concentration?
11. When your stash is nearly empty, do you feel anxious or worried about how to get more?
12. Do you plan your life around your marijuana use, thinking about the next time you will use?
13. Have friends or relatives ever complained that your marijuana use is damaging your relationship with them?
14. Have you or others noticed a decrease in your overall motivation level?
15. Do you find that your marijuana use has increased over time?

Interpretation

Any yes answer could indicate problematic use of marijuana.

TO CARRY THIS FURTHER . . .

If you answered yes to any of these questions, you may want to reevaluate your marijuana use and talk to a medical or mental health care provider about a further assessment for drug abuse or dependence. If you are concerned about a friend's use, you might point to these specific behavioral criteria in sharing your concerns and encourage your friend to seek professional assistance.

Source: Adapted from Ball State University Health Questionnaire, 2006.

Personal Assessment

Getting a Drug-Free High

Experts agree that drug use provides only short-term, ineffective, and often destructive solutions to problems. We hope that you have found (or will find) innovative, invigorating drug-free experiences that make your life more exciting. Circle the number for each activity that reflects your intention to try that activity. Use the following guide:

1 No intention of trying this activity
2 Intend to try this within 2 years
3 Intend to try this within 6 months
4 Already tried this activity
5 Regularly engage in this activity

1. Juggle	1	2	3	4	5
2. Go backpacking	1	2	3	4	5
3. Complete a marathon race	1	2	3	4	5
4. Start a vegetable garden	1	2	3	4	5
5. Ride in a hot air balloon	1	2	3	4	5
6. Snow ski or water ski	1	2	3	4	5
7. Donate blood	1	2	3	4	5
8. Go river rafting	1	2	3	4	5
9. Play a musical instrument	1	2	3	4	5
10. Cycle 100 miles	1	2	3	4	5
11. Go skydiving	1	2	3	4	5
12. Go rockclimbing	1	2	3	4	5
13. Play a role in a theater production	1	2	3	4	5
14. Build a piece of furniture	1	2	3	4	5
15. Solicit funds for a worthy cause	1	2	3	4	5
16. Swim	1	2	3	4	5
17. Overhaul a car engine	1	2	3	4	5
18. Compose a song	1	2	3	4	5
19. Travel to a foreign country	1	2	3	4	5
20. Write the first chapter of a book	1	2	3	4	5

TOTAL POINTS _____

Interpretation

61–100—You participate in many challenging experiences.
41–60—You are willing to try some challenging new experiences.
20–40—You take few of the challenging risks described here.

TO CARRY THIS FURTHER . . .

Looking at your point total, were you surprised at the degree to which you are aware of alternative activities? What are the top five activities, and can you understand their importance? What activities would you add to this list?

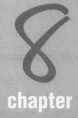
Taking Control of Alcohol Use

What Do You Know About Alcohol?

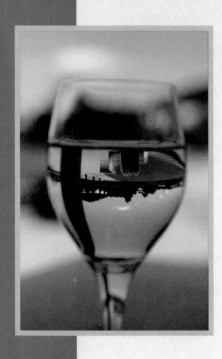

1. Women absorb alcohol into their bloodstream faster than men do. True or False?

2. Alcohol dependence is less severe than alcohol abuse. True or False?

3. The vomiting reflex can help to prevent an individual from becoming poisoned by alcohol. True or False?

4. A drink is defined as 12 ounces of beer, 5 ounces of wine, or a shot (1.5 ounces) of liquor. True or False?

5. A way to treat a hangover is by taking acetaminophen, such as Tylenol. True or False?

6. A 12-ounce bottle of beer provides about 150 calories. True or False?

7. Putting someone in a cold shower, giving him coffee, and walking him around are good ways to sober him up. True or False?

Check your answers at the end of the chapter.

The push for zero tolerance laws, the tightening of standards for determining legal intoxication, and the growing influence of national groups concerned with alcohol misuse show that our society is more sensitive than ever to the misuse of alcohol. People are concerned about the consequences of drunk driving, alcohol-related crime, and lowered job productivity. Alcohol use remains quite high among young people in the United States, and national data indicate that per-capita alcohol consumption has slowly decreased in the United States since the 1980s.[1] Alcohol use remains the preferred form of drug use for most adults (including college students), but as a society, we are increasingly uncomfortable with the ease with which alcohol can be misused.

Alcohol and Its Immediate Effects on the Body

As described in Chapter 7, alcohol is a depressant that slows the function of the central nervous system (CNS). Like for other depressants, consuming too much alcohol can lead to intoxication, sedation, and even death. Its effects on the user depend on the type of beverage, the circumstances under which it is consumed, and factors related to the individual user.[1]

The Nature of Alcoholic Beverages

Alcohol (also known as *ethyl alcohol* or *ethanol*) is the principal product of **fermentation.** In this process, yeast cells act on the sugar content of fruits and grains to produce alcohol and carbon dioxide.[2]

The alcohol concentration in beverages such as whiskey, gin, rum, and vodka is determined through a process called **distillation.** These distilled beverages are expressed by the term *proof,* a number that is twice the percentage of alcohol by volume in a beverage. Thus 70 percent of the fluid in a bottle of 140-proof gin is pure alcohol. Most proofs in distilled beverages range from 80 to 160. The pure grain alcohol that is often added to fruit punches and similar beverages has a proof of almost 200. Beer, wine, and hard liquor contain different concentrations of ethanol, which means they affect an individual in different ways. The alcohol content in beer is about 4 percent, for wine it is 10 to 14 percent, and for port and sherry it is 20 percent because they have alcohol added to them.

Lite and Ice Beers   "Lite" beer and low-calorie wines have been introduced in response to concerns about the number of calories in alcoholic beverages. These beverages are not low-alcohol beverages but merely low-calorie beverages. Only beverages marked "low alcohol" contain a lower concentration of alcohol than do the usual beverages of that type.

Ice beers actually contain a higher percentage of alcohol than do other types of beer. Most regular and light beers contain less than 5 percent alcohol, whereas ice beer generally contains 5 to 6 percent alcohol.

Nutritional Content: Empty Calories   The nutritional value of alcohol is extremely limited. Alcoholic beverages produced today through modern processing methods contain nothing but empty calories—about 100 calories per fluid ounce of 100-proof distilled spirits and about 150 calories per each 12-ounce bottle or can of beer. Therefore, alcohol consumption can significantly contribute to your weight and little else. Pure alcohol contains only simple carbohydrates; it has no vitamins and minerals, and no fats or protein.

Researchers have suggested that drinking red wine (no more than two glasses for men and one glass for women, daily) can increases levels of HDL cholesterol (the good cholesterol), reduce LDL (the bad cholesterol), and reduce blood clotting. This is because of the antioxidants in the flavonoids. Resveratrol, another antioxidant found in the skin of red grapes, is thought to help fight cancer, Alzheimer's disease, and Parkinson's disease.[3]

Physiological Effects of Alcohol Consumption

First and foremost, alcohol is classified as a drug—a very strong CNS depressant. The primary depressant effect of

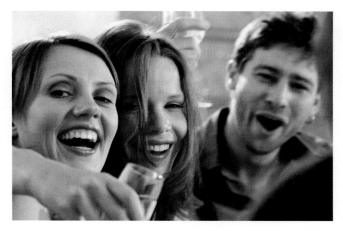

Alcohol is a strong central nervous system depressant. In social situations, it may appear to act as a stimulant because it depresses the inhibitory centers of the brain.

alcohol occurs in the brain and spinal cord. Many people think of alcohol as a stimulant because of the way most users feel after consuming a serving or two of an alcoholic beverage. Any temporary sensations of jubilation, boldness, or relief are attributable to alcohol's ability as a depressant drug to release personal inhibitions and provide temporary relief from tension.

How Is Alcohol Absorbed in the Body?   Eighty percent of alcohol is absorbed by the small intestine, and the stomach absorbs the other 20 percent. Then the alcohol enters the bloodstream, where it is carried throughout the body to all the organs. More than 90 percent of the alcohol is **metabolized** in the liver. Less than 2 percent of alcohol is excreted unchanged through the skin, breath, and urine.

Factors That Influence the Absorption of Alcohol   The rate of **absorption** of alcohol is influenced by several factors, most of which can be controlled by the individual.

Key Terms

fermentation A chemical process whereby plant products are converted into alcohol by the action of yeast cells on carbohydrate materials.

distillation The process of heating an alcohol solution and collecting its vapors into a more concentrated solution.

metabolism The chemical process by which substances are broken down or synthesized in a living organism to provide energy for life.

absorption The passage of nutrients or alcohol through the walls of the stomach or the intestinal tract into the bloodstream.

Type of Beverage and Circumstances of Consumption

- *Alcohol concentration.* The stronger the concentration of alcohol in the beverage, the more alcohol is absorbed. Also, carbonated liquids such as sodas or champagne speed up absorption, whereas water will dilute the concentration and slow the rate of absorption.[4]

- *Number of drinks consumed.* As more drinks are consumed, more alcohol is absorbed.

- *Speed of consumption.* If consumed rapidly, even relatively few drinks will result in a large concentration gradient that leads to high blood alcohol concentration.

- *Presence of food.* Food can compete with alcohol for absorption into the bloodstream, thus slowing the absorption of alcohol. When you slow your alcohol absorption, your body can remove alcohol already in the bloodstream. Your peak blood alcohol level can be three times higher when your stomach is empty than when you consume alcohol after eating something.

- *Degree of hydration.* Having more body water will help to dilute alcohol.

Individual Body Chemistry Each person has an individual pattern of physiological functioning that may affect the ability to process alcohol. For example, in some conditions, such as that marked by "dumping syndrome," the stomach empties more rapidly than is normal, and alcohol seems to be absorbed more quickly. The emptying time may be either slowed or quickened by anger, fear, stress, nausea, and the condition of the stomach tissues.

Race/Ethnicity Research suggests that alcohol tolerance levels may range from weak to strong based on an individual's race/ethnic origin. These ethnic differences may have a genetic link. Genetics may also help protect some Asians from developing alcoholism. About half of all Far East Asians produce low levels of an important enzyme that helps metabolize alcohol. These people cannot tolerate even small amounts of alcohol. In addition, genetic factors influencing the absorption rates of alcohol in the intestinal tract have been hypothesized to predispose some Native Americans to alcoholism. More research is needed about the role of genetic factors in all forms of chemical dependence.

Gender Women absorb about 30 percent more alcohol into the bloodstream than men do, despite an identical number of drinks and equal body weight. The reason for this is that women produce much less alcohol dehydrogenase than men do.[5] This enzyme is responsible for breaking down alcohol in the stomach—less alcohol dehydrogenase means more alcohol absorption.

Other reasons also help explain why women tend to absorb alcohol more quickly than do men of the same body weight: (1) Women have proportionately more body fat than men do. Since alcohol is not stored easily in fat, it enters the bloodstream relatively quickly. (2) Women's bodies have proportionately less water (52 percent) than do men's bodies of equal weight (61 percent); thus consumed alcohol does not become as diluted as it does in men. (3) Alcohol absorption is influenced by a woman's menstrual cycle. Alcohol is more quickly absorbed during the premenstrual phase of a woman's cycle. Also, there is evidence that women using birth control pills absorb alcohol more quickly than usual.[5]

With the exception of a person's body chemistry, race/ethnicity, and gender, all factors that influence absorption can be moderated by the alcohol user.

Blood Alcohol Concentration The amount of alcohol that can be metabolized is the same no matter how much alcohol is in the blood. This rate is about 0.25 to 0.30 ounce per hour. As previously mentioned, the activity of the enzyme alcohol dehydrogenase is the major factor in determining the rate of alcohol metabolism.[4] So, doing things like drinking coffee or exercising has no effect on alcohol metabolism. A person's **blood alcohol concentration (BAC)** rises when alcohol is consumed faster than it can be removed (oxidized) by the liver.[6] A fairly predictable sequence of events takes place when a person drinks alcohol at a rate faster than one drink every hour. When the BAC reaches 0.05 percent, initial measurable changes in mood and behavior take place. Inhibitions and everyday tensions appear to be released, while judgment and critical thinking are somewhat impaired. This BAC would be achieved by a 160-pound person drinking about two drinks in an hour (see Table 8.1).

At a level of 0.10 percent (one part alcohol to 1,000 parts blood), the drinker typically loses significant motor coordination. Voluntary motor function becomes quite clumsy. At this BAC, most states consider a drinker legally intoxicated and thus incapable of safely operating a vehicle. Although physiological changes associated with this BAC do occur, certain users do not feel drunk or appear impaired.

As a person continues to elevate the BAC from 0.20 to 0.50 percent, the health risk of **acute alcohol intoxication** increases rapidly. A BAC of 0.20 percent is characterized by the loud, boisterous, obnoxious drunk person who staggers. A 0.30 percent BAC produces further depression and stuporous behavior, during which time the drinker becomes so confused that he or she may not be capable of understanding anything. The 0.40 percent or 0.50 percent BAC produces unconsciousness. At this BAC, a person can die because brain centers that control body temperature, heartbeat, and respiration may virtually shut down.

Table 8.1 **Blood Alcohol Concentration Effects for Men and Women**

BAC Table for Men

Drinks	Body Weight in Pounds								Condition
	100	120	140	160	180	200	220	240	
0	.00	.00	.00	.00	.00	.00	.00	.00	Only Safe Driving Limit
1	.04	.03	.03	.02	.02	.02	.02	.02	Driving Skills Significantly Affected
2	.08	.06	.05	.05	.04	.04	.03	.03	
3	.11	.09	.08	.07	.06	.06	.05	.05	Possible Criminal Penalties
4	.15	.12	.11	.09	.08	.08	.07	.06	
5	.19	.16	.13	.12	.11	.09	.09	.08	
6	.23	.19	.16	.14	.13	.11	.10	.09	Legally Intoxicated
7	.26	.22	.19	.16	.15	.13	.12	.11	
8	.30	.25	.21	.19	.17	.15	.14	.13	Criminal Penalties
9	.34	.28	.24	.21	.19	.17	.15	.14	
10	.38	.31	.27	.23	.21	.19	.17	.16	Death Possible

Subtract .01% for each 40 minutes of drinking.
1 drink = 1.5 oz. 80 proof liquor, 12 oz. beer, or 5 oz. wine.

BAC Table for Women

Drinks	Body Weight in Pounds									Condition
	90	100	120	140	160	180	200	220	240	
0	.00	.00	.00	.00	.00	.00	.00	.00	.00	Only Safe Driving Limit
1	.05	.05	.04	.03	.03	.03	.02	.02	.02	Driving Skills Significantly Affected
2	.10	.09	.08	.07	.06	.05	.05	.04	.04	
3	.15	.14	.11	.10	.09	.08	.07	.06	.06	Possible Criminal Penalties
4	.20	.18	.15	.13	.11	.10	.09	.08	.08	
5	.25	.23	.19	.16	.14	.13	.11	.10	.09	
6	.30	.27	.23	.19	.17	.15	.14	.12	.11	Legally Intoxicated
7	.35	.32	.27	.23	.20	.18	.16	.14	.13	
8	.40	.36	.30	.26	.23	.20	.18	.17	.15	Criminal Penalties
9	.45	.41	.34	.29	.26	.23	.20	.19	.17	
10	.51	.45	.38	.32	.28	.25	.23	.21	.19	Death Possible

Subtract .01% for each 40 minutes of drinking.
1 drink = 1.5 oz. 80 proof liquor, 12 oz. beer, or 5 oz. wine.

Source: Virginia Tech Alcohol Abuse Prevention Center. © 2006

An important factor influencing the BAC is the individual's blood volume. The larger the person, the greater the amount of blood into which alcohol can be distributed. Conversely, the smaller person has less blood into which alcohol can be distributed, and as a result, a higher BAC will develop. To find out what a BAC level would be for your age and gender and the type and number of alcoholic drinks, go to this website: www.healthstatus.com/calculate/bac.

Alcohol Oxidation: Sobering Up Alcohol is removed from the bloodstream principally through the process of **oxidation.** Oxidation occurs at a constant rate (about one-fourth to one-third ounce of pure alcohol per hour) that cannot be appreciably altered. Because each typical drink of beer, wine, or distilled spirits contains about one-half ounce of pure alcohol, it takes about 2 hours for the body to fully oxidize one typical alcoholic drink.[4]

After a night of drinking alcohol, the next morning people may experience uncomfortable symptoms such as headache, nausea, fatigue, diarrhea, loss of appetite, or an overall feeling of being sick. These symptoms are commonly known as a *hangover* and are the result of the body reacting to too much alcohol in its system. These symptoms may be intensified by dehydration, poor nutrition, an empty stomach, lack of sleep, poor health, or increased physical activity while drinking.

Although people have attempted to sober up by drinking hot coffee, taking cold showers, or exercising, the oxidation rate of alcohol is unaffected. Thus far the FDA has not approved any commercial product that can help people achieve sobriety. Since alcohol causes dehydration, rehydration and the passage of time remain the only effective way to sober up.

Alcohol Poisoning

Not everyone who goes to sleep, passes out, or even becomes unconscious after drinking has a high BAC. People who are already sleepy, have not eaten well, are sick, or are bored may drink a little alcohol and quickly fall asleep. However, people who drink heavily in a short

---

Key Terms

blood alcohol concentration (BAC) The percentage of alcohol in a measured quantity of blood; BAC can be determined directly, through the analysis of a blood sample, or indirectly, through the analysis of exhaled air.

acute alcohol intoxication A potentially fatal elevation of BAC, often resulting from heavy, rapid consumption of alcohol.

oxidation The process that removes alcohol from the bloodstream.

time may be setting themselves up for an extremely unpleasant, toxic, potentially life-threatening experience because of their high BAC.

What are the danger signs of alcohol poisoning (also referred to as acute alcohol intoxication)? The first sign is **shock,** signaling that the body is not getting enough blood flow. The drinker will already have become unconscious. He or she cannot be aroused from a deep stupor. A person's BAC level can continue to rise even when she or he has stopped drinking, is sleeping, or is unconscious. The person will probably have a weak, rapid pulse (over 100 beats per minute). The skin will be cool and damp, and breathing will be increased to once every three or four seconds. These breaths may be shallow or deep but will certainly occur in an irregular pattern. The skin will be pale or bluish. (In a person with dark skin, these color changes will be more evident in the fingernail beds or in the mucous membranes inside the mouth or under the eyelids.) Whenever any of these signs are present, seek emergency medical help immediately.

Involuntary regurgitation (vomiting) can be another potentially life-threatening emergency for a person who has drunk too much alcohol. When a drinker has consumed more alcohol than the liver can oxidize, the pyloric valve at the base of the stomach tends to close. Additional alcohol remains in the stomach. This alcohol irritates the lining of the stomach so much that involuntary muscle contractions force the stomach contents to flow back through the esophagus. By removing alcohol from the stomach, vomiting may be a life-saving mechanism for conscious drinkers.

An unconscious drinker who vomits, however, may be lying in such a position that the airway becomes obstructed with the vomitus from the stomach. This person is at great risk of dying from **asphyxiation.** As a first-aid measure, unconscious drinkers should always be rolled onto their sides to minimize the chance of airway obstruction. If you are with a person who is vomiting, make certain that his or her head is positioned lower than the rest of the body. This position minimizes the chance that vomitus will obstruct the air passages. People who are unconscious from alcohol intoxication may "swallow their tongue." While it is physically impossible to swallow your tongue, when someone is unconscious the muscles relax and the tongue can fall backward into the throat, obstructing the airway. Again, rolling the person on his or her side can help prevent this from happening.

Also keep a close watch on anyone who passes out from drinking. This is the reason you don't want to let a drunk friend "sleep it off," as the BAC can rise during sleep or unconsciousness, resulting in death. Instead, you need to constantly monitor the physical condition of anyone who becomes unconscious from drinking or take the person to the emergency room if you are unable to monitor him or her or are uncertain about the physical condition of that person.

Alcohol's Interaction with Other Drugs

Consuming alcohol when you have taken other drugs can change how these drugs normally act in your system. Some of these interactions, like those that occur when sedatives are taken with alcohol, can be potentially dangerous. Because sedatives and alcohol are both depressants, taken together they can induce coma, unconsciousness, and death. Anti-anxiety medications, anti-convulsants, benzodiazepines, and antihistamines are also sedating and cause increased drowsiness. Alcohol taken with some antibiotics can cause nausea, vomiting, and seizures. Acetaminophen, such as Tylenol, can interact in a dangerous manner with alcohol, causing liver damage. Ibuprofen and aspirin can be taken with alcohol but may cause stomach upset. Antidepressants combined with alcohol can impair both mental and physical skills. The action of some antidepressants is increased with alcohol; others have decreased action when taken with alcohol. Antipsychotic medications, such as Thorazine, taken with alcohol can cause drowsiness, impaired coordination, and potentially fatal respiratory suppression. It is advisable to avoid consuming alcohol if taking any other type of drugs or medications.

Patterns of Alcohol Use

Although alcohol is a widely used drug, many people choose not to drink. Among drinkers, there is a great deal of variation in the amount and circumstances of their alcohol consumption. It is important to distinguish between light, responsible drinking and patterns of alcohol use that are potentially harmful in the short or long term.

Reasons People Choose to Drink

People drink for many different reasons. Most people drink because alcohol is an effective, affordable, and legal substance for altering the brain's chemistry. As **inhibitions** are removed by the influence of alcohol, behavior that is generally held in check is expressed (Figure 8-1). At least temporarily, drinkers become a different version of themselves—more outgoing, relaxed, and uninhibited.

How Much Do People Drink?

Before we discuss how much alcohol people drink, we first need to define some terms. What counts as a **drink?** The National Survey on Drug Use and Health (NSDUH) defines "one drink" as "a can or bottle of beer, a glass of wine or a wine cooler, a shot of liquor, or a mixed drink with liquor in it."[7] (More precisely, this means 8 ounces

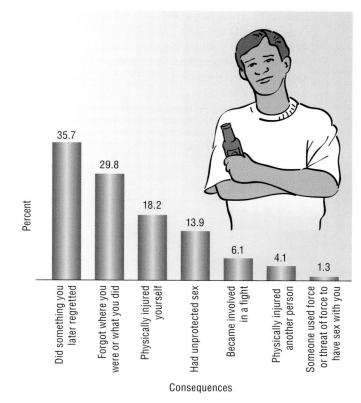

Figure 8-1 Negative Consequences of Alcohol and Drug Use
Reported consequences experienced by college students after drinking alcohol in the past school year.

Source: American College Health Association Spring 2006 Survey, *Journal of American College Health* 55 (January/February 2007).

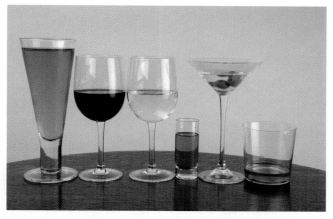

"One drink" is equivalent to 12 ounces of beer, 5 ounces of wine, or 1.5 ounces of liquor (in a mixed drink or as a shot). Moderate drinking is defined as no more than two drinks per day for men and no more than one drink per day for women.

of beer, 5 ounces of wine, 1.5 ounces of hard liquor, or a mixed drink containing 1.5 ounces of liquor.) Over half of Americans aged 12 and over (over 126 million people) reported being current drinkers in the 2007 survey. **Current use** is defined as "at least one drink in the past 30 days." This is an increase in usage since 2002. Twenty-three percent of people 12 and older (57.8 million Americans) reported having engaged in binge drinking at least once in the past month. **Binge drinking** is defined as "five or more drinks on the same occasion (at the same time or within a couple of hours of one another) on at least 1 day in the last 2-week period." These rates have not changed much since 2002. In 2005, 6.9 percent of Americans 12 and older (17 million) reported heavy drinking, again comparable to the rates since 2002. Heavy use is considered "five or more drinks on the same occasion on each of 5 or more days in the past 30 days."

Who Drinks?

As Figure 8-2 shows, current use, binge use, and heavy use were highest for the 21–25 age group and then decreased with increasing age. However, drinking can be a problem at any age (see the box "Alcohol and Older Adults"). On average, more men than women drink. However, for the 12- to 17-year-old age range, more females than males reported drinking. Caucasians had the highest drinking rate (56.1 percent) of any racial group, followed by American Indians and Alaskan Natives (44.7 percent) and 42.1 percent for Hispanics; 39.3 percent of African Americans and 35.2 percent of Asians reported alcohol use. In the United States, drinking rates are lowest in the South (46.8 percent) and highest in the Northeast (56 percent); however, this may be changing, as the South was the only U.S. region that showed a significant increase in alcohol use since 2002. Almost 55 percent (54.6) of midwesterners and

Key Terms

shock Profound collapse of many vital body functions; evident during acute alcohol intoxication and other serious health emergencies.

asphyxiation Death resulting from lack of oxygen to the brain.

inhibitions Inner controls that prevent a person from engaging in certain types of behavior.

drink 12 ounces of beer, 5 ounces of wine, or 1.5 ounces of liquor.

current use At least one drink in the past 30 days.

binge drinking Five or more drinks on the same occasion (at the same time or in the span of a couple of hours) on at least 1 day in the last 2-week period.

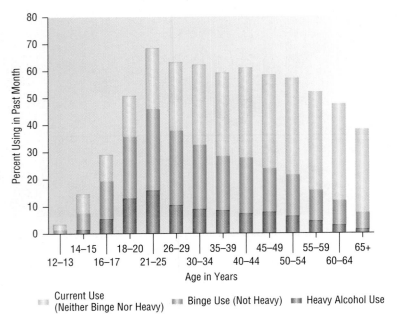

Figure 8-2 Current, Binge, and Heavy Alcohol Use among Persons Ages 12 and Older Alcohol use is highest among Americans 21–25 years old. Binge use is having five or more drinks on the same occasion in the past month. Heavy use is having five drinks on the same occasion on five or more days during the past month.

Source: Substance Abuse and Mental Health Services Administration. (2008). *Results from the 2007 National Survey on Drug Use and Health: National Findings* (Office of Applied Studies, NSDUH Series H-34, DHHS Publication No. SMA 08-4343). Rockville, MD.

50.8 percent of westerners reported drinking. Current use and heavy drinking were most frequent in large metropolitan areas, but binge drinking was more common in small metropolitan areas. Current drinkers tended to be employed; heavy drinkers tended to be unemployed. There was no difference in employment rates for binge drinkers. Heavy drinkers also reported tobacco use (58 percent).

College Drinking

The National College Health Assessment 2006 reported that 78.5 percent of college students drank at the last party they attended. However, students thought that more of their peers drank than actually did, guessing that 96 percent of students drink. The NSDUH study actually found that college students were more likely to drink than their age peers who weren't in college and that drinking increased with level of education. Rates of binge and heavy drinking were also higher among college students than among their age peers who were not in college.[9]

TALKING POINTS If alcohol did not make people more outgoing, relaxed, and adventuresome, do you think they would consume as much?

Binge Drinking Binge drinking refers to the consumption of five drinks in one sitting at least once during the previous 2-week period. One large study of more than 17,000 students on 89 campuses found that 49.7 percent of students engaged in binge drinking.[9] The strongest

predictors for bingeing were living in a fraternity or sorority, adopting a party-centered lifestyle, and engaging in other risky behavior. The study also suggested that many college students began binge drinking in high school.

By its very nature, binge drinking can be dangerous. Drunk driving, physical violence, property destruction, date rape, police arrest, and lowered academic performance are all highly associated with binge drinking. Besides the role that heavy drinking may play in the aggressor in date rape, a recent study found that more than half the victims in sexual assaults also were at least somewhat drunk.

The direct correlation between the amount of alcohol consumed and lowered academic performance results in impaired memory, verbal skill deficiencies, and altered perceptions.[10] Frequently, the social costs of binge drinking can be very high.

For large numbers of students who drink, the college years are a time when they drink more heavily than at any other period during their lifetimes (Figure 8-3). Some will suffer serious consequences as a result. For some, their college years will also mark the entry into a lifetime of problem drinking.

Drinking Games Drinking games are a form of binge drinking in which individuals consume large amounts of alcohol in a short period of time. Drinking games and pregame drinking are especially risky for inexperienced drinkers who are unfamiliar with changes associated with heavy alcohol consumption. Many college students also report engaging in "pre-gaming," or drinking, before

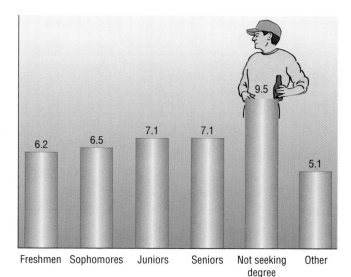

Figure 8-3 How much alcohol do college students drink?
Research shows that 20- to 24-year-olds drink more alcohol than any other age group. How many drinks per week do you have?

Source: Data from Core Institute: *2003 Statistics on Alcohol and Other Drug Use on American Campuses,* Center for Alcohol and Other Drug Studies, Student Health Programs, Southern Illinois University at Carbondale, 2003.

going out to a party or football game to save money on drinks and as a social lubricant. They place themselves at increased risk for drinking-related problems, such as alcohol poisoning, injuries, property destruction, legal problems, and sexual assaults.

Alcohol and Wellness

Alcohol use can contribute to a variety of medical, psychological, social, legal, and family problems.

Alcohol-Related Medical Problems

The relationship of chronic alcohol use to the structure and function of the body is reasonably well understood. Heavy alcohol use causes a variety of changes in the body that lead to an increase in morbidity and mortality. Figure 8-4 describes these changes.

Research shows that chronic alcohol use also damages the immune system and the nervous system. Thus chronic users are at high risk for a variety of infections and neurological complications.

Effects of Chronic Alcohol Use on the Body   Because alcohol goes to every organ in the body, with chronic use it can negatively affect every organ in your body. Chronic malnutrition can result from consuming alcohol instead of calories with nutritional value. This in turn can result in brain damage, such as **Wernicke-Korsakoff syndrome,**

> **Key Terms**
>
> **Wernicke-Korsakoff syndrome** A syndrome that results from vitamin B$_1$ deficiency, often the result of alcoholism. Symptoms include impaired short-term memory, psychosis, impaired coordination, and abnormal eye movements.

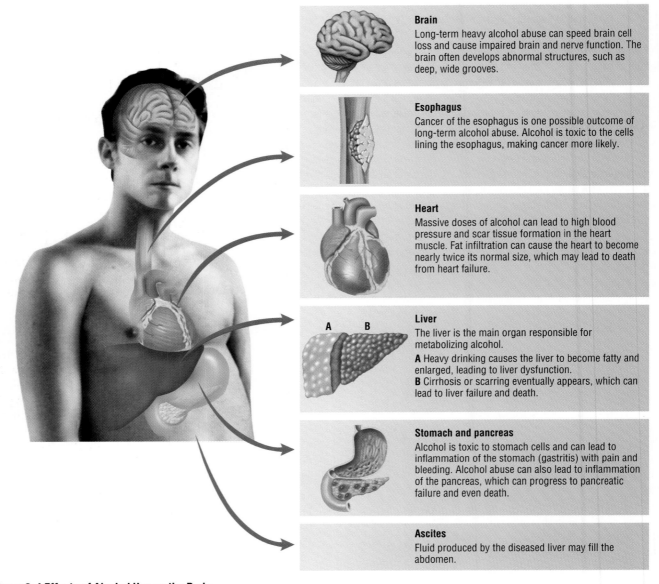

Brain
Long-term heavy alcohol abuse can speed brain cell loss and cause impaired brain and nerve function. The brain often develops abnormal structures, such as deep, wide grooves.

Esophagus
Cancer of the esophagus is one possible outcome of long-term alcohol abuse. Alcohol is toxic to the cells lining the esophagus, making cancer more likely.

Heart
Massive doses of alcohol can lead to high blood pressure and scar tissue formation in the heart muscle. Fat infiltration can cause the heart to become nearly twice its normal size, which may lead to death from heart failure.

Liver
The liver is the main organ responsible for metabolizing alcohol.
A Heavy drinking causes the liver to become fatty and enlarged, leading to liver dysfunction.
B Cirrhosis or scarring eventually appears, which can lead to liver failure and death.

Stomach and pancreas
Alcohol is toxic to stomach cells and can lead to inflammation of the stomach (gastritis) with pain and bleeding. Alcohol abuse can also lead to inflammation of the pancreas, which can progress to pancreatic failure and even death.

Ascites
Fluid produced by the diseased liver may fill the abdomen.

Figure 8-4 Effects of Alcohol Use on the Body

Source: Wardlaw G, Hampl J. *Perspectives in Nutrition,* 7th ed. Copyright © 2007 The McGraw-Hill Companies, Inc. Reproduced by permission of The McGraw-Hill Companies.

which results from vitamin B₁ deficiency. This syndrome is characterized by symptoms such as impaired short-term memory, psychosis, impaired coordination, and abnormal eye movements, and is often irreversible. Liver disorders such as cirrhosis of the liver are related to chronic drinking and are the seventh leading cause of death in the United States.[4] Heart disease, hypertension, stroke, and cancer are also commonly associated with chronic alcohol use. Infectious diseases such as tuberculosis, pneumonia, yellow fever, cholera, and hepatitis B have also been linked with chronic alcohol use.

Fetal Alcohol Syndrome and Fetal Alcohol Effects
A growing body of scientific evidence shows that alcohol use by pregnant women can cause birth defects in unborn children. When alcohol crosses the **placenta,** it enters the fetal bloodstream in a concentration equal to that in the mother's bloodstream. Because the fetal liver is underdeveloped, it oxidizes this alcohol much more slowly than the alcohol is oxidized in the mother. During this time of slow detoxification, the developing fetus is certain to be overexposed to the toxic effects of alcohol. Mental retardation frequently develops.

This exposure has additional disastrous consequences for the developing fetus. Low birth weight, mental retardation, facial abnormalities such as a small head and widely spaced eyes, and heart problems are often seen in such children (Figure 8-5). This combination of

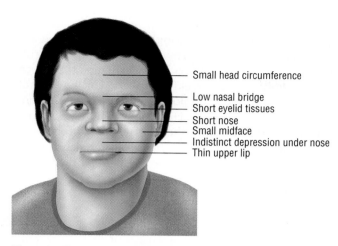

- Small head circumference
- Low nasal bridge
- Short eyelid tissues
- Short nose
- Small midface
- Indistinct depression under nose
- Thin upper lip

Figure 8-5 Fetal Alcohol Syndrome   The facial features shown are characteristic of affected children. Additional abnormalities in the brain and other internal organs accompany fetal alcohol syndrome but are not obvious in the child's appearance.

effects is called **fetal alcohol syndrome (FAS).** Recent studies estimate that the full expression of this syndrome occurs at a rate of 1 to 3 per 1,000 births. Partial expression (*fetal alcohol effects [FAE]*) can be seen in 3 to 9 per 1,000 live births. In addition, it is likely that many cases of FAE go undetected.[11]

Is there a safe limit to the number of drinks a woman can consume during pregnancy? No, because no one can accurately predict the effect of drinking even small amounts of alcohol during pregnancy. The wisest plan is to avoid alcohol altogether.

Because of the critical growth and development that occur during the first months of fetal life, women who have any reason to suspect they are pregnant should stop all alcohol consumption. Furthermore, women who are planning to become pregnant in the near future and women who are not practicing effective contraception should also keep their alcohol use to a minimum, or avoid consuming alcohol altogether.

Alcohol-Related Psychological Problems

Depending on the amount and pattern of alcohol use, inappropriate or chronic drinking may be classified as alcohol dependence (alcoholism) or problem drinking (alcohol abuse).

Alcohol Dependence (Alcoholism)   **Alcohol dependence** is a primary, chronic disease with genetic, psychosocial, and environmental factors influencing its development and manifestations. The disease is often progressive and fatal. It is characterized by impaired control over drinking, preoccupation with the drug alcohol, use of alcohol despite adverse consequences, and

distortions in thinking, most notably denial. Each of these symptoms may be continuous or periodic.[12]

This definition incorporates much of the knowledge gained from addiction research during the last two decades. It is well recognized that alcoholics drink to escape life's problems. For alcoholics, alcohol helps them cope with stress and pain.

Alcoholism involves a physical addiction to alcohol that develops over time (see the box "Progressive Stages of Alcohol Dependence"). For an alcoholic, when the body is deprived of alcohol, physical and mental withdrawal symptoms become evident. These withdrawal symptoms can be life threatening. **Delirium tremens (DTs)** can progress to nausea, vomiting, hallucinations, shock, and cardiac and pulmonary arrest. Delirium tremens are an occasional manifestation of alcohol withdrawal.[13]

The complex reasons for the physical and emotional dependence of alcoholism have not been fully explained. Why, when more than 100 million adults use alcohol without becoming dependent on it, do 10 million or more others become unable to control its use?

Could alcoholism be an inherited disease? Studies in humans and animals have provided strong evidence that genetics plays a role in some cases of alcoholism. We do know that individuals with a family history of alcoholism are five times more likely to develop alcoholism due to this predisposition. Two forms of alcoholism are thought to be inherited: type 1 and type 2. Type 1 is thought to take years to develop and may not surface until midlife. Type 2 is a more severe form and appears to be passed primarily from fathers to sons. This form of alcoholism frequently begins earlier in a person's life and may even start in adolescence.

The role of personality traits as conditioning factors in the development of alcoholism has received considerable attention. Factors ranging from unusually low

Key Terms

placenta   The structure through which nutrients, metabolic wastes, and drugs (including alcohol) pass from the bloodstream of the mother into the bloodstream of the developing fetus.

fetal alcohol syndrome (FAS)   Characteristic birth defects noted in the children of some women who consume alcohol during their pregnancies.

alcohol dependence   Tolerance, withdrawal, and a pattern of compulsive use of alcohol. A primary, chronic disease with genetic, psychosocial, and environmental factors influencing its development. Also referred to as *alcoholism.*

delirium tremens (DTs)   Uncontrollable shaking combined with irrational hallucinations, caused by abstinence from alcohol following habitual alcohol use.

Progressive Stages of Alcohol Dependence

Early
- Escape drinking
- Binge drinking
- Guilt feelings
- Sneaking drinks
- Difficulty stopping after beginning to drink
- Increased tolerance
- Preoccupation with drinking
- Occasional blackouts

Middle
- Loss of control
- Self-hate
- Impaired social relationships
- Changes in drinking patterns (more frequent binge drinking)
- Temporary sobriety
- Morning drinking
- Dietary neglect
- Increased blackouts

Late
- Prolonged binges
- Alcohol used to control withdrawal symptoms
- Alcohol psychosis
- Nutritional disease
- Frequent blackouts

self-esteem to an antisocial personality have been implicated. Additional factors making people susceptible to alcoholism may include excessive reliance on denial, hypervigilance, compulsiveness, and chronic levels of anxiety. Complicating the study of personality traits is the uncertainty of whether the personality profile is a predisposing factor (perhaps from inheritance) or is caused by alcoholism.

Alcohol Abuse (Problem Drinking) Alcohol abuse, or problem drinking, is considered less severe than alcohol dependence. School and job performance suffers, responsibilities are neglected, and interpersonal conflicts arise when individuals abuse alcohol. Individuals who abuse alcohol might drive while intoxicated, have legal problems, experience **blackouts,** and know that their drinking is causing them problems, but they persist in drinking. Instead of helping them cope with their stress, alcohol is now creating problems in their lives. One major difference between dependence and abuse is that tolerance, withdrawal, and a pattern of compulsive use are part of the definition of dependence but not of abuse. Abuse refers to experiencing harmful consequences from repeated use of alcohol.[14]

For college students, two clear indications of **problem drinking** are missing classes and lowered academic performance caused by alcohol involvement. Problem drinkers are not always heavy drinkers; they might not be daily or even weekly drinkers. Unlike alcoholics, problem drinkers do not need to drink to maintain "normal" body functions. However, when they do drink, they (and others around them) experience problems—sometimes with tragic consequences. It is not surprising that problem drinkers are more likely than other drinkers to eventually develop alcoholism.

Alcohol-Related Social Problems

Alcohol abuse is related to a variety of social problems. These problems affect the quality of interpersonal relationships, employment stability, and the financial security of both the individual and the family. Alcohol's negative social consequences lower our quality of life. In financial terms the annual cost of alcohol abuse and dependence has been estimated at more than $185 billion.[15]

Accidents The four leading causes of accidental deaths in the United States (motor vehicle collisions, falls, drownings, and fires and burns) have significant statistical connections to alcohol use.

Motor Vehicle Collisions Data from the National Highway Traffic Safety Administration (NHTSA) indicate that in 2007, approximately 13,000 alcohol-related vehicular crash deaths occurred. Thirty-five percent of car accidents with aged 21 to 24 drivers involve alcohol-impaired fatalities, higher than for any other age group. This total represented a 3.7 percent decrease over the previous year.[16]

Presently in the United States, an alcohol-related car crash fatality occurs every 31 minutes. Forty percent of all fatal car accidents are alcohol related. Every 2 minutes, an alcohol-related car crash injury happens. More than 275,000 people were injured in such crashes. The NHTSA reported that approximately 1.5 million drivers were arrested for drunk driving, reflecting an arrest rate of 1 for every 130 licensed drivers in the United States.[16]

One response to drunk driving has been for all states to raise the minimum legal drinking age to 21 years. This was accomplished in the mid-1980s. In October 2000, President Clinton signed into law a federal bill that required all states to lower the legal BAC to 0.08 percent by the year 2003 or risk losing federal highway funds. All states have lowered the driving standard to 0.08 percent BAC. You can search the Mothers Against Drunk Driving (MADD) website at www.madd.org to find out current 0.08 percent BAC law information.[17]

Other programs and policies are being implemented that are designed to prevent intoxicated people from

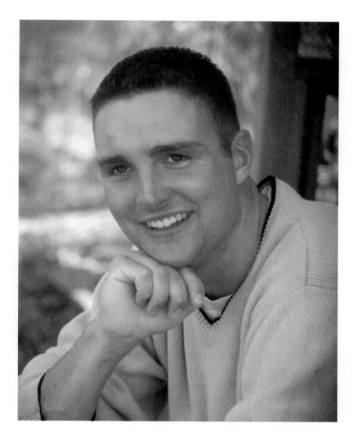

On August 4, 2000, 23-year-old Casey Ray Beaver was driving with two friends along U.S. Highway 71 near Goodman, Missouri, when an oncoming vehicle crossed the center line and collided with his car. Casey, a recent graduate of the University of Kansas, was pronounced dead at the scene, as was the driver of the other vehicle. The offender, who had seven prior convictions of driving under the influence and whose driver's license had been revoked seven years earlier, had a BAC above 0.10 percent. Casey was due to begin classes at the Illinois College of Optometry 10 days after the accident occurred.

Drownings Drownings are the third leading cause of accidental death in the United States. Studies have shown that alcohol use is implicated in 21 to 47 percent of these deaths.[18] High percentages of recreational boaters have been found to drink alcohol while boating.[18] Alcohol can impair judgment and swimming ability and reduce body temperature.[20]

Fires and Burns Fires and burns are responsible for an estimated 5,000 deaths each year in the United States, the fourth leading cause of accidental death. This cause is also connected to alcohol use: studies indicate that half of burn victims have BACs above the legal limit.[18]

Crime and Violence Have you noticed that most of the violent behavior and vandalism on your campus is related to alcohol use? The connection of alcohol to crime has a long history. Prison populations have large percentages of alcohol abusers and alcoholics: people who commit crimes are more likely to have alcohol problems than are people in the general population. This is especially true for young criminals. Furthermore, alcohol use has been reported in 53 to 66 percent of all homicides, with the victim, the perpetrator, or both found to have been drinking. In rape situations, rapists are intoxicated 50 percent of the time and victims 36 percent of the time.[20]

Because of research methodological problems, pinpointing alcohol's connection to family violence is difficult. However, it seems clear that among a large number of families, alcohol is associated with violence and other harmful behavior, including physical abuse, child abuse, psychological abuse, and abandonment.[21]

The difficult question that arises when discussing the relationship between alcohol use and violence is whether a cause-effect link can be proven. Not everyone who drinks becomes violent, but in many violent crimes, at least one person involved has been drinking. The answer perhaps is that alcohol use by itself is not enough to cause violence, but use of alcohol may be one of several factors

driving. Many states have enacted **zero-tolerance laws** to help prevent underage drinking and driving. Also included have been efforts to educate bartenders to recognize intoxicated customers, to use off-duty police officers as observers in bars, to place police roadblocks, to develop mechanical devices that prevent intoxicated drivers from starting their cars, and to encourage people to use designated drivers.

Falls Many people are surprised to learn that falls are the second leading cause of accidental death in the United States. Alcohol use increases the risk for falls. Various studies suggest that alcohol is involved in 21 to 77 percent of deadly falls and 18 to 53 percent of nonfatal falls.[18]

> **Key Terms**
>
> **blackout** An inability to remember events that occurred during a period of alcohol use, including things that a person said or did during that time.
>
> **problem drinking** An alcohol use pattern in which a drinker's behavior creates personal difficulties or difficulties for other people.
>
> **zero-tolerance laws** Laws that severely restrict the right to operate motor vehicles for underage drinkers who have been convicted of driving under the influence of alcohol or any other drug.

that act in combination to cause violent behavior in some instances.

Suicide   Alcohol use has been related to large percentages of suicides. Alcoholism plays a large role in 30 percent of completed suicides.[22] Also, alcohol use is associated with impulsive suicides rather than with premeditated ones. Drinking is also connected with more violent and lethal means of suicide, such as the use of firearms.[22]

For many of these social problems, alcohol use impairs critical judgment and allows a person's behavior to quickly become reckless, antisocial, and deadly. Because most of us wish to minimize problems associated with alcohol use, acting responsibly when we host a party is a first step in this direction.

Alcohol-Related Legal Problems

People who drink and drive often fail to consider the aftermath of their behavior before it is too late. Many college students admit to having driven a car after drinking alcohol. Some even admit that they have left a party after drinking and then driven to another location, but could not remember actually driving the car. This behavior reflects an alcoholic blackout. These dangerous activities are serious for the driver, the passengers, and anyone else on (or near) the road.

Although laws vary from state to state, here is the general sequence of events: If you are driving a car and are stopped by a police officer who suspects you may have been driving under the influence of alcohol, you will be asked to get out of your car and undergo a field test for sobriety. This test could include tests of motor coordination, such as walking in a line in a heel-to-toe fashion. You may even be given an alcohol breath test on the spot.

If you appear to fail the field test, you could be arrested and frisked, read your Miranda rights, and taken to the local jail. A more precise blood alcohol test may be given. Depending on local or state law, you will either spend some hours in jail (until your BAC is lowered) or be immediately eligible for bail (if you, a family member, or a friend can come up with the money to post bond).

You will be required to face a judge in court and answer the charges against you. By this time, you probably will have hired an attorney to help you in this process. If you are convicted or decide to plead guilty to misdemeanor charges of driving while intoxicated (DWI), you will receive a fine, be required to pay court costs, and probably be required to attend alcohol education classes and be placed on probation. You will generally be required to see your probation officer once a month, and you may be required to take random drug tests. Besides the costs for the attorney, court fees, and fines, you will be required to pay other fees, such as those for license reinstatement, probation, mandatory alcohol education and counseling, drug testing, and community

drug prevention programs. The average cost of a DWI conviction is between $5,000 and $20,000. Additionally, your automobile insurance rates will likely be raised, and a DWI will be on your driving record, which may prevent you from pursuing your chosen career in many professions, such as teaching, nursing, and aviation, for which employers will not consider applicants with this type of record.

Alcohol-Related Family and Relationship Problems

Alcohol abuse can have a tremendous impact on the abuser's friends and family. The effects of dysfunctional family life can be significant and long-lasting, and those close to an alcoholic may develop unhealthy codependent relationships. Adult children of alcoholics are at greater risk for becoming alcohol abusers and may have problems developing healthy relationships and coping skills.

Alcohol and the Family   The alcohol abuser hurts more than just himself or herself. Everyone around the addicted person suffers. Alcoholism is a family disease, and a family can be defined as a person, a family, a fraternity, a sorority, a dormitory floor, even a therapy group or a 12-step group. Sometimes people deny there is an alcohol problem in their family. They may feel embarrassed, have suffered from physical, sexual, or mental abuse, and may not want to deal with or think about their personal situation.

As a result of these constant dysfunctional behaviors, the person living with an alcoholic can become[23]

- Isolated and afraid of people and authority figures.
- An approval-seeker and lose his or her identity in the process.
- Frightened by angry people and any criticism.
- An alcoholic, marry one, or find another compulsive personality such as a workaholic.
- Attracted to people in need of assistance or rescuing.
- Extremely responsibile and focused on others to the detriment of himself or herself.
- Guilty when being assertive or saying no.
- Addicted to excitement, conflict, and chaos.
- Confused about the difference between abuse and love.
- Unable to feel or express feelings.
- Terrified of abandonment and willing to tolerate abuse to hold on to a relationship.
- Similar in behavior to an alcoholic without actually drinking.

The good news is that many resources, such as recovery and support groups, are now available for both the alcoholic and those who live with the alcoholic. Those who have lived with an alcoholic will face their own issues as they work through their own recovery. They may find that they learned compulsions from the alcoholic, or they may transfer the compulsions to other behaviors, such as excessive eating, gambling, house cleaning, or taking up lost causes or people. Those who know, or are still living with, an active alcoholic also can consider intervention to urge the alcoholic to seek help.

Enabling and Codependance For family and friends of chemically dependent people, denial is part of a process known as *enabling*. In this process, people close to the problem drinker or alcoholic inadvertently support drinking behavior by denying that a problem really exists. Enablers unconsciously make excuses for the drinker, try to keep the drinker's work and family life intact, and in effect make the continued abuse of alcohol possible. For example, college students enable problem drinkers when they clean up a drinker's messy room, lie to professors about a student's class absences, and provide class notes or other assistance to a drinker who cannot perform academically. Even the use of designated drivers has been criticized as enabling behavior.

Alcohol counselors contend that enablers can significantly delay the onset of effective therapy. Do you know of a situation in which you or others have enabled a person with alcohol problems?

A new term was coined in the 1980s to describe the relationship between drug-dependent people and those around them—*codependence*. This term implies a kind of dual addiction. The alcoholic and the person close to the alcoholic are both addicted, one to alcohol and the other to the alcoholic. People who are codependent often find themselves denying the addiction and enabling the alcohol-dependent person.

Unfortunately, this kind of behavior damages both the alcoholic and the codependent. The alcoholic's intervention and treatment may be delayed for a considerable time. Codependent people often pay a heavy price as well. They often become drug or alcohol dependent themselves, or they may suffer a variety of psychological consequences related to guilt, loss of self-esteem, depression, and anxiety. Codependents may be at increased risk for physical and sexual abuse.

Fortunately, researchers continue to explore this dimension of alcoholism. Many students have found some of the sources listed at the end of this chapter to be especially helpful. (To determine whether you could benefit from a support program such as Al-Anon or Alateen, answer the questions in the Personal Assessment "Does Someone's Drinking Trouble You?" at the end of this chapter.)

Adult Children of Alcoholic Parents In recent years a new dimension of alcoholism has been identified—the unusually high prevalence of alcoholism among adult children of alcoholics (ACOAs). It is estimated that these people are about four times more likely to develop alcoholism than are persons whose parents are not alcoholics. Even the ACOAs who do not become alcoholics may have a difficult time adjusting to everyday living.

In response to this concern, support groups have been formed to prevent the adult sons and daughters of alcoholics from developing the condition that afflicted their parents. If a stronger link for an inherited genetic predisposition to alcoholism is found, these groups may play an even greater role in the prevention of alcoholism.

Women and Alcohol For decades, women have consumed less alcohol and had fewer alcohol-related problems than men. Evidence is mounting that a greater percentage of women are choosing to drink and that some subgroups of women, especially young women, are drinking more heavily. A greater number of admissions of women to treatment centers may also reflect that alcohol consumption among women is on the rise. Special approaches for women to use for staying sober are discussed in the box "Women and Alcohol."

Studies show that there are now almost as many female as male alcoholics. However, differences appear to exist between men and women when it comes to alcohol abuse.[20] Some of the more pronounced differences are: (1) More women than men can point to a specific triggering event, such as a divorce, death of a spouse, a career change, or children leaving home, that started them drinking heavily. (2) Alcoholism among women often starts later and progresses more quickly than alcoholism among men. (3) Women tend to be prescribed more mood-altering drugs than men are; thus, women face a greater risk of drug interaction or cross-tolerance. (4) Nonalcoholic men tend to divorce their alcoholic spouses nine times more often than nonalcoholic women divorce their alcoholic spouses; thus, alcoholic women are not as likely to have a family support system to aid them in their recovery attempts. (5) Female alcoholics do not tend to receive as much social support as men in their treatment and recovery. (6) Although men outnumber women entering treatment programs by almost four to one, women alcoholics tend to come into treatment earlier than men. (7) Women alcoholics are more likely than male alcoholics to have medical complications. This may result from the differences in the metabolism of alcohol between men and women. Women are particularly susceptible to diseases of the liver. (8) Unmarried or divorced single-parent women often have economic problems that make entry into treatment programs especially difficult. In light of the generally recognized educational, occupational, and social gains made by women during the last two decades, it will be interesting to see whether these male-female differences continue.

Chapter Eight   Taking Control of Alcohol Use

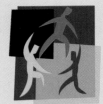

Do women drink for the same reasons men do? The research says no—there are some important differences in alcohol use for men and women. Women with low self-esteem are twice as likely to drink alcohol, whereas no such relationship exists for men. This was true for teenage girls as well as for college women. Women who were sexually or physically abused in childhood are much more likely than men to have alcohol-related problems. Peer pressure, a family history of alcohol abuse, and maternal drinking during pregnancy are more predictive of a likelihood to have alcohol problems for women than for men. Genetics plays a role to some degree in the variation between the genders; however, this does not account for all of these differences.

There are critical periods in women's lives where they are more likely to develop alcohol-related problems. For instance, more female college freshmen than female high school seniors reported binge drinking. Compared to men, women have more late-onset alcoholism (developing alcoholism after age 59). Life transitions, stressful life events, experiencing a crisis or a loss, loneliness, and boredom are triggers for women to develop problems with alcohol.

Because women have different triggers for their alcohol-related problems, they require different treatment approaches for alcohol treatment. We are now beginning to see specialized groups and treatment facilities that focus on women's issues related to alcohol abuse and dependence. One such group, Women for Sobriety (WFS), is a mutual aid organization for women with alcohol problems that was founded in 1975 by Dr. Jean Kirkpatrick. The WFS program focuses on improving self-esteem; members achieve sobriety by taking responsibility for their actions and by learning not to dwell on negative thoughts. Another alternative, Rational Recovery (RR), is open to both men and women. RR, which is based on the theories of psychologist Albert Ellis's Rational Emotive Therapy, also uses a cognitive, nonspiritual approach that fosters cohesiveness and provides the emotional support sought by people who seek to gain and maintain sobriety.

Particularly for "marginalized" alcoholic women such as lesbians, members of racial and ethnic minorities, and those of non-Christian religious backgrounds, alcoholism treatment professionals increasingly are being encouraged to present the full range of support-group options, including but not emphasizing the approach of Alcoholics Anonymous.

Sources: Galanter M, et al., Rational Recovery: Alternative to AA for Addiction? *American Journal of Drug and Alcohol Abuse,* 19, 499, 1993; Hall J, Lesbians' Participation in Alcoholics Anonymous: Experience of Social, Personal, and Political Tensions, *Contemporary Drug Problems,* 23(1), 113, Spring 1996; Kaskutas L, A Road Less Traveled: Choosing the "Women for Sobriety" Program, *Journal of Drug Issues,* 26(1), 77, Winter 1996; Women for Sobriety, Inc., www .womenforsobriety.org/, March 10, 2005; The National Center on Addiction and Substance Abuse at Columbia University, *Women Under the Influence* (Baltimore: Johns Hopkins University Press, 2006).

Responsible Use of Alcohol

The responsible use of alcohol involves keeping your own drinking safe and moderate as well as being a responsible host. On a social and community level, we all need to be concerned about the messages sent about alcohol in both advertisements and public service announcements. A number of organizations work to prevent the potentially dangerous effects of alcohol use, including some that focus specifically on drinking among college students.

Responsible Drinking

Drinking alcohol in a responsible way means reducing the potential negative consequences of drinking and increasing your safety and the safety of others around you. It involves some practical strategies such as these:

- Don't make getting drunk the goal or drinking the focus of your activity.
- Eat food before drinking.
- Set a limit on the number of drinks you will consume.
- Limit alcoholic drinks to one an hour and drink water or soda in between.

- Don't use alcohol to manage your feelings such as stress, boredom, anger, or loneliness.
- When going to a party or bar, have a designated driver.
- Don't leave your drinks unattended.

Drinking responsibly helps you to avoid the negative legal, social, and medical problems that can be associated with alcohol use.

Hosting a Party Responsibly

Fortunately, an increasing awareness of the value of responsible party hosting seems to be spreading among college communities. The impetus for this awareness has come from various sources, including respect for an individual's right to choose not to drink alcohol, the growing recognition that many automobile crashes are alcohol related, and the legal threats posed by **host negligence.** Responsibly hosting parties at which alcohol is served is becoming a trend, especially among college-educated young adults. For guidelines for hosting a social event at which alcoholic beverages are served, see the box "Partying 101."

In addition to these suggestions, the use of a **designated driver** is an important component of responsible alcohol use. By planning to abstain from alcohol or

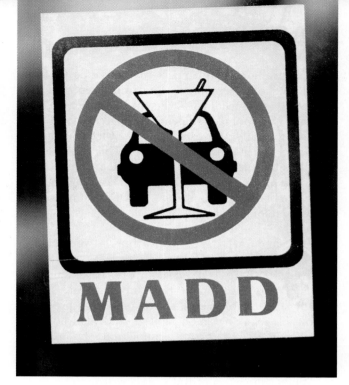

Mothers Against Drunk Driving is one of many organizations working against the irresponsible use of alcohol.

to carefully limit their own alcohol consumption, designated drivers are able to safely transport friends who have been drinking. Designated drivers have indisputably saved many lives. However, there may be a downside. Some health professionals are concerned that the use of designated drivers allows the nondrivers to drink more heavily than they might otherwise. In effect, designated drivers "enable" drinkers to be less responsible for their own behavior. This freedom from responsibility might eventually lead to further problems for the drinkers.

 TALKING POINTS Have you noticed an increased use of designated drivers in your community? Would you be willing to be a designated driver?

Organizations That Support Responsible Drinking

The serious consequences of the irresponsible use of alcohol have led to the formation of a number of concerned-citizen groups. Although each organization has a unique

approach, all attempt to deal objectively with two indisputable facts: Alcohol use is part of our society, and irresponsible alcohol use can be deadly.

Mothers Against Drunk Driving   MADD is a national network of over 600 local chapters in the United States and Canada. This organization attempts to educate people about alcohol's effects on driving and to influence legislation and enforcement of laws related to drunk drivers. For more information about MADD, visit its website at www.madd.org.[17]

Students Against Destructive Decisions   Many students have known the acronym *SADD* to stand for the youth group Students Against Driving Drunk or Students Against Destructive Decisions. Recently, the group has restructured itself to expand beyond drunk driving to include other high-risk activities that are detrimental to youth, such as underage drinking, drug use, and failure to use seat belts. Founded in 1981, this organization

Key Terms

host negligence   A legal term that reflects the failure of a host to provide reasonable care and safety for people visiting the host's residence or business.

designated driver   A person who abstains from or carefully limits alcohol consumption to be able to safely transport other people who have been drinking.

now has millions of members in thousands of chapters throughout the country. Remaining central to the drunk driving aspect of SADD is the "Contract for Life," a pact that encourages students and parents to provide safe transportation for each other if either is unable to drive safely after consuming alcohol. This contract also stipulates that no discussions about the incident are to be started until both can talk in a calm and caring manner. For more information about SADD, visit its website at www.saddonline.com.[24]

BACCHUS and GAMMA Peer Education Network Boost Alcohol Consciousness Concerning the Health of University Students (BACCHUS) began in 1975 as an alcohol-awareness organization at the University of Florida. Run by student volunteers, this organization promoted responsible drinking among college students who chose to drink. It was not an anti-alcohol group, but a "harm reduction" group. Over the years, hundreds of chapters were formed on campuses across the country.

When supporters of BACCHUS realized that many students interested in alcohol awareness were from fraternities and sororities, they developed Greeks Advocating Mature Management of Alcohol (GAMMA) to join BACCHUS to form a peer education network. Campuses are now able to choose BACCHUS, GAMMA, or any other acronym or name for their groups.

With the broadening of the original BACCHUS organization has come an expansion of the health issues this group addresses. Originally, the focus was on alcohol abuse and prevention. Now the BACCHUS and GAMMA Peer Education Network confronts a variety of student health and safety issues. For additional information about this organization, check out its website at www.bacchusgamma.org.[25]

Other Approaches Other responsible approaches to alcohol use are surfacing nearly every day. Even among college fraternity organizations, attitudes toward the indiscriminate use of alcohol are changing. Many fraternity rush functions are now conducted without the use of alcohol, and growing numbers of fraternities are alcohol-free.

Another encouraging sign on college campuses is the increasing number of alcohol-use task forces. Although each of these groups has its own focus and title, many are meeting to discuss alcohol-related concerns on their particular campus. These task forces often try to formulate detailed, comprehensive policies for alcohol use across the entire campus community.

Alcohol Advertising

Every few years, careful observers can see subtle changes in the ways the alcoholic beverage industry markets its products. Recently, the marketing push appears to be directed toward minorities (through advertisements for malt liquor and fortified wines), women (through wine and wine cooler ads), and youth (through trendy, young adult-oriented commercials). See the box "Do Alcohol Ads Target Young People—and Does It Matter?" for more on the issue of targeted marketing campaigns.

On the college campus, aggressive alcohol campaigns have used rock stars, beach party scenes, athletic event sponsorships, and colorful newspaper supplements to encourage the purchase of alcohol. Critics claim that most of the collegiate advertising is directed at minors and that the prevention messages are not strong enough to offset the potential health damage to this population. It is not just radio and television that are the culprits; Facebook and Google now permit alcohol companies to advertise on their websites and search results.

Some beer and liquor companies have begun using websites on the Internet to promote their products. Critics contend that the colorful graphics, hip language, games, chat rooms, and "virtual bars" are designed to recruit underage drinkers.

Alcohol Advertising in Ethnic Communities A literature review by the Trauma Foundation at San Francisco General Hospital reports some interesting facts concerning alcohol availability and alcohol advertising in ethnic communities.[26] In the United States, low-income Latino and African American communities have a disproportionate number of alcohol outlets compared with White communities. This concentration of alcohol outlets seems to be related to an increase in traffic injuries and assaults. Additionally, as the number of alcohol outlets increases, the likelihood of increased crime and violence rises. Crime and violence drive out existing business establishments and discourage new businesses from locating in the area. Economic development can become thwarted.

The Trauma Foundation also reports that alcohol is more heavily advertised in low-income African American and Latino communities than in other neighborhoods. The advertisements are found on billboards as well as the displays inside and around the alcohol outlets. Advertising frequently exploits important cultural symbols, and promotions are targeted toward specific ethnic groups. For example, malt liquor is marketed especially to African Americans. Thus, rap singers are frequently featured in promotions and advertisements for malt liquor.

Alcohol Prevention Messages

The first successful national campaign against drunk driving, "Designated Driver," began in 1998. Besides targeting specific audiences and using well-timed and strategically placed public service announcements, its developers convinced TV producers and writers to work references to the designated driver into the dialogue of

Do Alcohol Ads Target Young People—and Does It Matter?

Recent studies have shown that television and radio advertisements have a disproportionate amount of alcohol ads aimed at youth (defined as 12- to 20-year-olds) compared to any other age group. Youths drink alcohol more than they smoke or use other drugs, so there is a growing concern that these ads are contributing to an increase in underage drinking. Researchers at the Center on Alcohol Marketing and Youth (CAMY) evaluated the placement of radio and television advertisements for the most-advertised U.S. alcohol brands and found that alcohol advertising is common on programs that have disproportionately large youth audiences. In addition, this advertising accounts for a substantial proportion of all alcohol radio advertising heard by underage youth. This contradicts the alcohol industry's voluntary standard to not advertise alcohol on radio or television programs that have an audience that is 30 percent or more youth. This study also found that almost half of the 67,404 alcohol ads were placed in youth-oriented programming. More than 40 percent of the alcohol ads youth see are on youth-oriented television programs such as those on *VH1, Lost, Desperate Housewives, Monday Night Football,* and *CSI.* The Grammy Awards allowed alcohol ads for the first time in 2009.

Does it really make a difference if youth are exposed to ads selling alcohol? Yes. Studies show that, compared to people who started drinking later in their lives, people who start drinking before age 15 are 4 times more likely to become alcohol dependent, 7 times more likely to be involved in an alcohol-related motor vehicle crash, and at least 10 times more likely to experience alcohol-related violence at some point in their lives. Numerous studies have shown that the more alcohol advertising young people are exposed to, the more likely they are to drink or drink more.

Alcohol advertising to youth has increased 38 percent since 2001. The National Research Council and the Institute of Medicine (NRC/IOM) recommend that the alcohol industry voluntarily restrict its advertising to programs for which the audience is 25 percent or less youth, with the goal of decreasing this to programs with 15 percent or less youth instead of its current 30 percent threshold. The Federal Trade Commission (FTC) reviewed the alcohol industry's efforts at self-regulation of its marketing practices in 1999 and 2003, and will examine these efforts again in 2007. If the alcohol industry does not start complying with its own standards, the FTC may begin efforts to force them to do so.

Sources: CAMY: Alcohol Ads on the Radio Continue to Reach Youth, Georgetown University, September 2006; The Center for Alcohol Marketing for Youth, Georgetown University Executive Summary, Still Growing After All These Years: Youth Exposure to Alcohol Advertising on Television, 2001–2005, December 2006.

their shows. Gradually, the message got through to young people.

In contrast, the "Campaign for Alcohol Free Kids" relied heavily on dramatic graphics, such as grisly photos of car crash scenes on prom night.[27] Although the overall visual impact was powerful, the campaign lacked a practical element. Worse, the ads seemed to be preaching.

The Ad Council's "Friends Don't Let Friends Drive Drunk" is based on the idea that we all have responsibility for one another. If someone is your friend, you want to take care of that person, so don't let your friend do something dangerous.

The "You Drink & Drive, You Lose" campaign, a part of the National Public Education Campaign, targets two high-risk groups, 21- to 34-year-olds and repeat offenders. The message is simple: make the right choice—don't drink and drive. The "Buzzed Driving Is Drunk Driving" and "Over the Limit, Under Arrest" campaigns have similar messages that if you make the wrong choice—having a BAC over the legal limit—you risk being arrested.

What the successful campaigns have in common is a message that is simple, to the point, and believable. Rather than scolding or preaching, the ads emphasize the fact that you have a choice and ask you to make the right one. They also reinforce the consequences of using poor judgment.

Treatment for Alcohol Problems

Similar to the treatment approaches for drug use described in Chapter 7, treatments for problem drinking, alcohol abuse, and alcohol dependence can involve outpatient individual counseling, group counseling, intensive outpatient treatment, or even nontraditional approaches (see the box "Acupuncture as Treatment for Alcoholism"). Inpatient hospitalization may be required for those with alcohol dependence, particularly in addressing the physical withdrawal symptoms. Counseling focuses on understanding the triggers and high-risk situations and developing healthier ways of coping with stress and life's problems. However, alcohol recovery can often require lifestyle changes as well, including finding new friends, social activities, and habits, drinking soda or water if at a social event, playing golf or watching sports without drinking, and rewarding yourself with something other than a drink when relaxing at the end of a long week.

Often people who have been in treatment are considered in recovery rather than cured. This comes from a belief that once an alcoholic, always an alcoholic, as the individual can never drink alcohol without risking relapse. There is another philosophy about treatment, called "harm reduction," that suggests that people with alcoholism or alcohol-related problems can decrease their drinking to a moderate level and don't have to abstain from alcohol to recover. There is debate about which is more effective, whether abstinence or moderation should be the goal of alcohol treatment. However, most people don't recover the first time they go into treatment. In fact, the average number of times an alcoholic goes into treatment is five times before recovery is successful and lasting.

Helping the Alcoholic: Rehabilitation and Recovery

It is estimated that as many as two-thirds of people can recover from alcoholism. Recovery is especially improved when the addicted person has a good emotional support system, including concerned family members, friends, and employer. When this support system is not well established, the alcoholic's chances for recovery are considerably lower.

Alcoholics Anonymous (AA) is a voluntary support group of recovering alcoholics who meet regularly to help one another get and stay sober. There are over 100,000 groups in 150 countries worldwide.[28] AA encourages alcoholics to admit their lack of power over alcohol and to turn their lives over to a higher power (although the organization is nonsectarian; see the box "The Spiritual Component in Alcoholics Anonymous"). Members of AA are encouraged not to be judgmental about the behavior of other members. They support anyone with a problem caused by alcohol.

Al-Anon and Alateen are parallel organizations that give support to people who live with alcoholics. Al-Anon is geared toward spouses and other relatives, whereas Alateen focuses on children of alcoholics. Both organizations help members realize that they are not alone and that successful adjustments can be made to nearly every situation. AA, Al-Anon, and Alateen chapter organizations are usually listed in the telephone book or in the classified sections of local newspapers. You can locate Al-Anon and Alateen on the Web at www.al-anon.alateen.org.[29]

For people who feel uncomfortable with the concept that their lives are controlled by a higher power, secular recovery programs are becoming popular. These programs maintain that sobriety comes from within the alcoholic. Secular programs strongly emphasize self-reliance, self-determination, and rational thinking about one's drinking. Secular Organizations for Sobriety (SOS) and Rational Recovery are examples of secular recovery programs.

The Spiritual Component in Alcoholics Anonymous

Alcoholics Anonymous (AA) is a self-help support group for people with problems with alcohol. It was started in 1935 by Bill Wilson and Dr. Robert Smith, who were recovering alcoholics themselves. Together they also wrote the "Big Book," a 400-page book outlining the 12 steps to recovery. Fellowship and "spiritual awakening" are important components of this program.

Following are the 12 steps that AA believes an individual must go through to gain sobriety:

1. We admitted we were powerless over alcohol—that our lives had become unmanageable.
2. Came to believe that a power greater than ourselves could restore us to sanity.
3. Made a decision to turn our will and our lives over to the care of God as we understood Him.
4. Made a searching and fearless moral inventory of ourselves.
5. Admitted to God, to ourselves and to another human being the exact nature of our wrongs.
6. Were entirely ready to have God remove all these defects of character.
7. Humbly asked Him to remove our shortcomings.
8. Made a list of all persons we had harmed, and became willing to make amends to them all.
9. Made direct amends to such people wherever possible, except when to do so would injure them or others.
10. Continued to take personal inventory and when we were wrong promptly admitted it.
11. Sought through prayer and meditation to improve our conscious contact with God as we understood Him, praying only for knowledge of His will for us and the power to carry that out.
12. Having had a spiritual awakening as the result of these steps, we tried to carry this message to alcoholics, and to practice these principles in all our affairs.

As you can see, 6 of the 12 steps refer to *God,* and there are religious references and overtones throughout the steps. While AA does have roots in evangelical Christianity, the modern-day AA groups claim that it is a nonreligious organization and is not affiliated with any specific religion. AA certainly has a spiritual component, but people can choose their own definitions of their greater power, including their own personal power or the power of the AA group.

Abstaining from alcohol, finding support with a group of people who share similar struggles, taking an honest introspective look into one's flaws, and finding ways to make peace within oneself and with others are part of the AA process of spiritual awakening. Having a sense of a community and connecting to a higher power can provide alcoholics with strength and help them not to feel alone. AA has helped millions of people recover from alcoholism, and AA groups are found all over the world.

Source: The Twelve Steps are reprinted with permission of Alcoholics Anonymous World Services, Inc. Permission to reprint the Twelve Steps does not mean that A.A.W.S. has reviewed or approved the contents of this publication or that A.A.W.S. necessarily agrees with the views expressed herein. A.A. is a program of recovery from alcoholism only—use of the Twelve Steps in connection with programs and activities which are patterned after A.A., but which address other problems, or in any other non-A.A. context, does not imply otherwise.

Medical Treatment for Alcoholism

Could there be a medical cure for alcoholism? For nearly 50 years, the only prescription drug physicians could use to help drinkers stop drinking was antabuse. Consuming alcohol after taking antabuse can cause drinkers to become extremely nauseated and can even be life threatening.

In 1995 the Food and Drug Administration approved a drug called naltrexone that works by reducing the craving for alcohol and the pleasurable sensations felt when drinking. Combining naltrexone with conventional behavior modification has been shown to reduce alcohol relapse significantly. A more recent medication, Campral, helps to reduce alcohol cravings and decrease withdrawal symptoms.

Taking Charge of Your Health

- Determine whether you are affected by someone's drinking by doing the Personal Assessment "Does someone's drinking trouble you?" at the end of this chapter.
- Determine how you use alcohol by taking the first assessment at the end of the chapter.

- Assess your level of social responsibility by reviewing the box "Partying 101."
- If you think that you are a problem drinker or an alcoholic, join a support group to get help.
- Enter into a "Contract for Life" with your parents or closest friends, a pact that says that you will provide safe transportation for one another if any of you are unable to drive safely after consuming alcohol.
- Make a commitment to responsible alcohol use by joining a campus group that works toward this goal.

SUMMARY

- As BAC rises, predictable depressant effects take place, and the risk of acute alcohol intoxication increases; people with this condition are in danger and must receive first aid immediately.
- Federal legislation has pushed all states to lower the legal BAC standard to 0.08 percent.
- Alcohol is removed from the bloodstream through the process of oxidation.
- Chronic alcohol use causes a variety of serious health problems for the drinker and can cause fetal alcohol syndrome in infants when a woman drinks during pregnancy.
- Alcohol-related social problems include accidents (motor vehicle crashes, falls, drownings, and fires and burns), crime and violence, and suicide.

- Problem drinking is an alcohol use pattern in which a drinker's behavior creates personal difficulties or problems for others.
- Alcoholism, or alcohol dependence, is a primary, chronic disease characterized by addiction to alcohol; it has a variety of possible causes and manifestations.
- Enabling is a behavior pattern in which people close to the problem drinker or alcoholic make the continued use of alcohol possible by keeping the drinker's work and family life intact.
- Alcoholics Anonymous and other support groups can help an alcoholic recover from the disease.
- The drugs Antabuse, naltrexone, and Campral are sometimes prescribed to treat alcoholism.

REVIEW QUESTIONS

1. What is the definition of an alcoholic drink?
2. What is binge drinking?
3. What is meant by the term *proof*?
4. What is the nutritional value of alcohol?
5. Identify and explain the various factors that influence the absorption of alcohol. Why is it important to be aware of these factors?
6. What is BAC? Describe the general sequence of physiological events that takes place when a person drinks alcohol at a rate faster than the liver can oxidize it.
7. What are the signs and symptoms of acute alcohol intoxication? What are the first-aid steps you should take to help a person with this problem?
8. Describe the characteristics of fetal alcohol syndrome and fetal alcohol effects.
9. Explain the differences between problem drinking, alcohol abuse, and alcoholism.
10. List some ways you can drink responsibly.

ANSWERS TO THE "WHAT DO YOU KNOW?" QUIZ

1. True   2. False   3. True   4. True   5. False   6. True   7. False

Visit the Online Learning Center (**www.mhhe.com/payne11e**), where you will find tools to help you improve your grade including practice quizzes, key terms flashcards, audio chapter summaries for your MP3 player, and many other study aids.

SOURCE NOTES

1. U.S. Department of Health and Human Services. *Alcohol and Health: Tenth Special Report to the U.S. Congress*, NIH Publication No. 00-1583. Washington, DC: U.S. Government Printing Office, 2000.
2. Zest for Life. *Alcohol and Ethanol Information Page*, www.anyvitamins.com/alcohol-ethanol-info.htm, March 9, 2005.
3. Gaziano JM, et al. Light-to-Moderate Alcohol Consumption and Mortality in the Physicians' Health Study Enrollment Cohort. *Journal of the American College of Cardiology*, 35(1), 96–105, 2000.
4. Ksir C, Hart C, Oakley R. *Drugs, Society and Human Behavior* (12th ed.). New York: McGraw-Hill, 2008.
5. Be Responsible About Drinking. *Women and Alcohol*, www.brad21.org/alcohol_and_women.html, March 9, 2005.
6. Pinger RR, et al. *Drugs: Issues for Today* (3rd ed.). New York: McGraw-Hill, 1998.
7. Substance Abuse and Mental Health Services Administration. (2006). *Results from the 2005 National Survey on Drug Use and Health: National Findings* (Office of Applied Studies, NSDUH Series H-30, DHHS Publication No. SMA 06-4194). Rockville, MD.
8. Walking the Tightrope of the 20's, *USA Today*, August 15, 2007.
9. American College Health Association Spring 2006 Survey, *Journal of American College Health*, 55 (January–February 2007).
10. Brown SA, Tapert SF, Granholm E, et al. Neurocognitive Functioning of Adolescents: Effects of Protracted Alcohol Use, *Alcoholism, Clinical and Experimental Research*, 24(2), 164–171, 2000.
11. ADA: Division of Drug and Alcohol Abuse. *As a Matter of Fact . . . Fetal Alcohol Syndrome*, www.well.com/user/woa/fsfas.htm, March 9, 2005.
12. Morse RM, et al. The Definition of Alcoholism, *Journal of the American Medical Association*, 268(8), 1012–1014, 1992.
13. Burns M. *Delirium Tremens*, emedicine.com, Inc., November 8, 2004.
14. *Diagnostic and Statistical Manual of Mental Disorders* (4th ed). Washington, DC: American Psychiatric Association, 2000.
15. National Institute on Alcohol Abuse and Alcoholism. *Tenth Special Report to the U.S. Congress on Alcohol and Health*, Chapter 6. NIH Publication No. 00-1583. Rockville, MD: U.S. Department of Health and Human Services, 2000.

16. *Traffic Safety Facts 2006: Alcohol.* U.S. Department of Transportation National Highway Traffic Safety Administration.

17. Mothers Against Drunk Driving. *About Us,* www.madd.org, March 9, 2005.

18. *Alcohol and Unintentional Injury: A Brief Review of the Literature,* The Trauma Foundation. www.tf.org/tf/alcohol/ariv/reviews/injurev5.html, June 16, 2003.

19. *Training Guide for USLA Safety Tips: General Information on Drowning.* USLA Lifeguards for Life, www.usla.org/PublicInfo/Safety.asp, June 16, 2003.

20. Kinney J. *Loosening the Grip: A Handbook of Alcohol Information* (7th ed.). New York: McGraw-Hill, 2003.

21. Vaughn C. *Children of Alcoholics: At Risk for Family Violence.* U.S. Department of Health and Human Services and SAMHSA's National Clearinghouse for Alcohol and Drug Information, February 10, 2003.

22. *Facts about Suicide.* Centers for Disease Control and Prevention, National Center for Health Statistics, 1998.

23. Adult Children Educational Foundation Computer Bulletin Board. *Sick Families,* www.recovery.org/acoa/families.html, December 24, 1997.

24. SADD History. *Students Against Drunk Driving,* www.saddonline.com, March 1, 2005.

25. Organization History and Mission. The BACCHUS and GAMMA Peer Education Network, www.bacchusgamma.org/, March 1, 2005.

26. Trauma Foundation at San Francisco General Hospital. *The Effects of Alcohol on Different Ethnic Communities: Fact Sheet,* www.tf.org/tf/alcohol/ariv/facts/ethfct25.html, June 20, 2003.

27. Campaign for Alcohol Free Kids: Who We Are, www.alcoholfreekids.com Ad Council, March 8, 2005.

28. Alcoholics Anonymous. *AA At a Glance,* www.alcoholics-anonymous.org, March 1, 2005.

29. Al-Anon/Alateen Web Site Information, www.al-anon.alateen.org/, March 1, 2005.

Personal Assessment

How do you use alcoholic beverages?

Answer the following questions about your own alcohol use. Record your number of yes and no responses at the end of the questionnaire.

Do you: Yes   No

1. Drink more often than you did a year ago?
2. Drink more heavily than you did a year ago?
3. Plan to drink, sometimes days in advance?
4. Gulp or "chug" your drinks, perhaps in a contest?
5. Set personal limits on the amount you plan to drink but then consistently disregard these limits?
6. Drink at a rate greater than one drink per hour?
7. Encourage or even pressure others to drink with you?
8. Frequently want a nonalcoholic beverage but then end up drinking an alcoholic drink?
9. Drive your car while under the influence of alcohol or ride with another person who has been drinking?
10. Use alcoholic beverages while taking prescription or OTC medications?
11. Forget what happened while you were drinking?
12. Have a tendency to disregard information about the effects of drinking?
13. Feel embarrassed because of your alcohol use?

   TOTAL

Interpretation

If you answered yes to any of these questions, you may be using alcohol irresponsibly. Two or more yes responses indicate an unacceptable pattern of alcohol use and may reflect problem drinking behavior.

TO CARRY THIS FURTHER . . .

Ask your friends or roommates to take this assessment. Are they willing to take this assessment and then talk about their results with you? Be prepared to discuss any follow-up questions they might have about their (or your) alcohol consumption patterns. Your willingness to talk about drinking behavior might help someone realize that this topic can and should be discussed openly. Finally, be aware of how people in your area can get professional help with drinking or other drug concerns.

   Use the space below to write down important phone numbers where you can find alcohol-related assistance for you or your friends and relatives.

_____

_____

_____

_____

_____

_____

_____

_____

_____

Personal Assessment

Does someone's drinking trouble you?

The following questions are designed to help you decide whether you are affected by someone's drinking and could benefit from a program such as Al-Anon. Record your number of yes and no responses on the total lines at the end of the questionnaire.

	Yes	No
1. Do you worry about how much someone else drinks?	_____	_____
2. Do you have money problems because of someone else's drinking?	_____	_____
3. Do you tell lies to cover up for someone else's drinking?	_____	_____
4. Do you feel that if the drinker loved you, he or she would stop drinking to please you?	_____	_____
5. Do you blame the drinker's behavior on his or her friends?	_____	_____
6. Are plans frequently upset or meals delayed because of the drinker?	_____	_____
7. Do you make threats, such as "If you don't stop drinking, I'll leave you"?	_____	_____
8. Do you secretly try to smell the drinker's breath?	_____	_____
9. Are you afraid to upset someone for fear it will set off a drinking bout?	_____	_____
10. Have you been hurt or embarrassed by a drinker's behavior?	_____	_____
11. Are holidays and gatherings spoiled because of someone's drinking?	_____	_____
12. Have you considered calling the police for help in fear of abuse?	_____	_____
13. Do you search for hidden alcohol?	_____	_____
14. Do you often ride in a car with a driver who has been drinking?	_____	_____
15. Have you refused social invitations out of fear or anxiety that the drinker will cause a scene?	_____	_____
16. Do you sometimes feel like a failure when you think of the lengths to which you have gone to control the drinker?	_____	_____
17. Do you think that if the drinker stopped drinking, your other problems would be solved?	_____	_____
18. Do you ever threaten to hurt yourself to scare the drinker?	_____	_____
19. Do you feel angry, confused, or depressed most of the time?	_____	_____
20. Do you feel there is no one who understands your problems?	_____	_____
TOTAL	_____	_____

Interpretation

If you answered yes to three or more of these questions, Al-Anon or Alateen may be able to help. You can contact Al-Anon or Alateen by looking in your local telephone directory or by writing to Al-Anon Family Group Headquarters, Inc., 1600 Corporate Landing Parkway, Virginia Beach, VA 23454–5617, or you may call (888) 4AL-ANON.

TO CARRY THIS FURTHER . . .

Sometimes the decision to seek help from a support group is a difficult one. If you answered yes to any of the questions, spend a few moments reflecting on your responses. How long have you been experiencing problems because of someone else's drinking? How would sharing your feelings with others—people who have dealt with very similar problems—help you cope with your own situation? Knowing you're not alone can often be a great relief; it's up to you to take the first step.

Source: From *Are You Troubled by Someone's Drinking?* © 1980 by Al-Anon Family Group Headquarters, Inc. Reprinted with permission.

Rejecting Tobacco Use

9

chapter

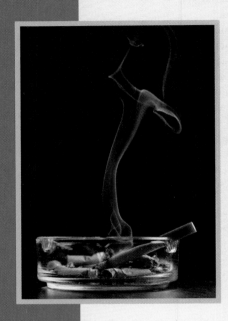

What Do You Know About Tobacco Use?

1. Until recently there was an inverse relationship between the level of education completed and the level of cigarette smoking. True or False?

2. Internal documents of the tobacco industry demonstrate that the tobacco industry neither knew of the health risks associated with its products nor intentionally marketed its products to young adolescents. True or False?

3. Nicotine dependency is easily (and quickly) established in the majority of people who begin cigarette use. True or False?

4. Carbon dioxide, produced during the combustion of tobacco, is the gaseous element in tobacco smoke that reduces the oxygen-carrying capacity of the blood. True or False?

5. When homicide and suicide are removed from death-related statistics, the life expectancy of smokers is virtually the same as that of their nonsmoking peers. True or False?

6. When assessed at the end of one year, well over half of the people who successfully completed a 10- to 12-week smoking cessation program will still be tobacco-free. True or False?

7. In public places, today's smokers are more likely to be asking, "Where can I smoke?" rather than "Where can't I smoke?" True or False?

Check your answers at the end of the chapter.

Tobacco Use in American Society

If you were to visit certain businesses, entertainment spots, or sporting events in your community, you might leave convinced that virtually every adult is a tobacco user. Certainly, for some segments of society, tobacco use is the rule rather than the exception. You may be quite surprised, however, to find out that the great majority of adults do not use tobacco products.

Table 9.1 indicates that only three states have a percentage of smokers above 25 percent, with Kentucky having the highest percentage at 28.2 percent, whereas Utah, a state in which nearly three-fourths

Table 9.1 The Top 10 States with the Highest and Lowest Smoking Rates

Highest Smoking Prevalence		Lowest Smoking Prevalence	
1. Kentucky	28.2%	1. Utah	11.7%
2. West Virginia	26.9%	2. California	14.3%
3. Oklahoma	25.8%	3. Connecticut	15.4%
4. Missouri	24.5%	4. Massachusetts	16.4%
5. Tennessee	24.3%	5. Minnesota	16.5%
6. Indiana	24.1%	6. Washington	16.8%
7. Mississippi	23.9%	7. Oregon	16.9%
8. Ohio	23.1%	8. Rhode Island	17.0%
9. North Carolina	22.9%	9. Hawaii	17.0%
10. Louisiana	22.6%	10. New Jersey	17.1%
National Average: 22.2%			

Source: Centers for Disease Control and Prevention (CDC). *Current Cigarette Smoking among Adults*—United States, 2007. *Morbidity and Mortality Weekly,* 57(45), November 14, 2008.

of the residents are Mormons and thus refrain from tobacco and alcohol use, reports the smallest percentage of tobacco use (11.7 percent).[1] How does your home state compare?

Only 8.5 percent of the population of the U.S. Virgin Islands are smokers.[2] Whether this reflects the influences of cultural practices, cigarette prices and availability, or preferences for other forms of tobacco is not known. Also, when 14 states were asked what percentage of their households were "totally smoke-free," reports ranged from 63.6 percent in Kentucky to 82.9 percent in Arizona; "totally smoke-free workplaces" ranged from a low of 54.8 percent in Kentucky to a high of 85.5 percent in West Virginia.[3]

Following the Surgeon General's 1964 report (the first official statement of concern by the federal government regarding the dangers of smoking), the prevalence of smoking began a decline that lasted until 1991, when a leveling off was noted that lasted for the next three years. Since 1994 the percentage of the population who smoke has declined slowly but progressively.

Cigarette Smoking Among College Students

Until very recently, the rate of cigarette smoking among college graduates was lower than that reported for the population as a whole, and it was significantly lower than the rate for persons with very little formal education. In fact, the prevalence of smoking among college students decreased progressively from 21 percent in 1964 to 14 percent in 1995. However, an upward trend in cigarette use by college students was noted during the later years of the 1990s into the early years of the 2000s, with 30.6 percent of full-time enrolled students reporting that

they had smoked, and 42.7 percent of part-time students had smoked within the preceding months.[4] In contrast, smoking among high school 12th graders during 2007 reached its lowest level in several years with only 6 percent smoking daily.[5] Since today's college students have matriculated to college from the high school class of 2007 and even more recent classes, a corresponding low level of daily smoking will hopefully be reflected in the collegiate population. However, factors that more likely reflect college life, in comparison to high school, may well intervene in a negative direction.

When a college community is viewed as a whole regarding which segments of the student body are most likely to smoke, there appears to be a direct relationship between the level of alcohol consumption and cigarette smoking. Additional direct relationships appear between smoking and other drug use and in housing where smoking is permitted. Similar, although perhaps less influential, relationships are seen among tobacco use and coping style, depression, and perceptions of life satisfaction.

The historically predictable relationship between higher levels of completed education and the lessened likelihood of smoking remains clearly evident even today.

Demographic Trends in Smoking

A number of different factors appear to influence smoking rates among Americans (Table 9.2). Among the most important are the following:

- *Gender.* Men have higher rates of smoking than women, a pattern that is consistent for people of different ages and ethnicities.

- *Race/ethnicity.* American Indians and Alaska Natives have the highest smoking rate, while people of Asian descent have the lowest rate.

- *Level of education.* Higher levels of education have historically been associated with lower rates of smoking, a trend that continues today. People with undergraduate or graduate degrees are far less likely to smoke than those with lower levels of education. However, today's college students may be reversing this trend.

- *Age.* The rate of smoking goes down as age goes up; among those age 65 and over, the rate drops below 10 percent. Over the course of time, it is likely that both quitting and premature death reduce the percentage of smokers in the population.

- *Geographical residence.* The Midwest has the highest percentage of smokers, while the West has the lowest percentage.

- *County population density.* People who live outside metropolitan areas are most likely to be smokers, and small metropolitan areas have a higher percentage of smokers than large metropolitan areas.

Table 9.2 Patterns of Cigarette Smoking

	Percentage of Smokers
	Total
All adults*	19.8
Race/ethnicity*	
White	21.4
Black	19.8
Hispanic	13.3
American Indian/ Alaskan Native	36.4
Asian	9.6
Education*	
9–11 years	33.3
GED diploma	44.0
High school graduate	23.7
Associate degree	19.9
Some college	20.9
Undergraduate degree	11.4
Graduate degree	6.2
Age (years)*	
18–24	22.2
25–44	22.8
45–64	21.0
65+	8.3
Geographical division†	
Midwest	27.2
South	25.5
Northeast	22.1
West	21.1
Geographical Area†‡	
Large metropolitan areas	22.7
Small metropolitan areas	24.8
Urbanized nonmetropolitan areas	28.0
Less urbanized nonmetropolitan areas	29.5
Rural counties	23.6

* Percentage of people who report smoking at least 100 cigarettes during their lifetimes and current smoking every day or some days.

† Percentage of people who report past-month smoking.

‡ A metropolitan area is defined as an area of high population density and its socially and economically related surrounding counties. Large metropolitan areas have a population of 1 million or more. Small metropolitan areas have a population of fewer than 1 million. Nonmetropolitan areas are areas outside metropolitan areas. "Urbanized" counties have a population of 20,000 or more in urbanized areas, "less urbanized" counties have at least 2,500 but fewer than 20,000 population in urbanized areas, and "completely rural" counties have fewer than 2,500 population in urbanized areas.

Sources: Centers for Disease Control and Prevention, Cigarette Smoking Among Adults—United States, 2007. 57 (42), November 14, 2008; U.S. Substance Abuse and Mental Health Services Administration, *Results from the 2007 National Survey on Drug Use and Health: National Findings* (NSDUH Series H-34, DHHS Publication No. SMA 08-4343). (Rockville, MD: U.S. Department of Health and Human Services, Office of Applied Statistics, 2008).

- *Recent homelessness or incarceration.* People who have spent more than 24 hours on the street or who have lived in a shelter or prison have a high smoking rate (56.2 percent).[6]

- *Place of birth.* In comparison to native-born Americans, people living in the United States who are foreign-born are among the least likely to be current smokers (14.1 percent).[7] For information on smoking rates outside the United States, see the box "Smoking Around the World."

Marketing of Tobacco Products

Shredded plant material, wrapped in paper or leaf, ignited with a flame, and then placed on or near the delicate tissues of the mouth . . . what other human behavior does this resemble? If you answered *None!* to this question, then you appreciate that smoking is unique and, therefore, that it must be learned. How it is learned is currently a less than fully understood process that most likely requires a variety of stimuli ranging from modeling to actual experimentation. The role of advertising as a source of models has long been suspected and intensely debated. Today, as in the past, controversy surrounds the intent of the tobacco industry's advertising. Are the familiar logos seen in a variety of media intended to challenge the brand loyalty of those who have already decided to smoke, as the industry claims? Or are the ads intended to entice new smokers, older children and young adolescents, in sufficient numbers to replace the 3,000 smokers who die each day from the consequences of tobacco use? This latter objective is now known, by admission of the tobacco industry, to have been pursued for decades.

Master Tobacco Settlement Agreement A significant roadblock to the tobacco industry's success in addicting another generation of cigarette smokers began in the early 1990s when previously secret documents of the five largest cigarette manufacturers were leaked to the public. The fortuitous availability of these documents gave rise to a massive suit by all of the attorneys general of the 50 states. Using information regarding the tobacco industry's decades-old knowledge of the health risks of their products, the states brought suit against the industry to recoup Medicaid money paid by the states in treating illness due to smoking. This huge class-action suit was promulgated in 1998, leading to a Master Tobacco Settlement Agreement in 1999.

Although the settlement is multifaceted and is far too complex to detail in this text, two significant components of the settlement are the monetary award to the states of $246 billion, to be paid to the states over 25 years, and the implementation of restrictions on the tobacco industry regarding multiple aspects of their marketing of cigarettes and other tobacco products. The following is a highly abbreviated list of restrictions placed on the tobacco industry's marketing:[8]

- Prohibits brand-name sponsorship of concerts, events with significant youth attendance, and

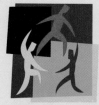

Learning from Our Diversity

Smoking Around the World

People in less-developed areas of the world are becoming increasingly exposed to the cultural influences of the postindustrial world, including behavioral patterns and access to products. Among the most insidious of these behavioral patterns is cigarette smoking, which is supported by access to imported cigarettes or the technology to manufacture indigenous brands. As the postindustrial countries of the world turn away from cigarette smoking and move toward improved health, the people in less-developed areas of the world are progressing toward levels of smoking exceeding the highest levels ever seen in the United States or Western Europe.

According to the American Cancer Society, the following levels of adult smoking for males and females were reported for 2005. In the United States the rates of cigarette smoking hover slightly above 20 percent—so we can easily imagine the level of smoking-related illnesses being experienced in and projected for the future in less-developed areas of the world.

The data indicate that heavy smoking is more common in males, although levels of smoking for women are distressingly high, particularly in the first countries listed. China has a large effect on the demand for imported and indigenous tobacco—30 percent of all of the world's cigarettes are smoked in China. Needless to say, American tobacco companies consider China one of the "bright spots" in the future economic well-being of their industry.

Countries Reporting Heavy Levels of Smoking for Males and Females

Males (%)		Females (%)	
Russian Federation	70.1	Nauru	52.4
Ukraine	63.8	Serbia & Montenegro	43.8
Belarus	63.7	Austria	40.1
Greece	63.6	Greece	39.8
Indonesia	62.1	Bosnia & Herzegovina	35.1
Tonga	61.8	Hungary	33.9
Lao People's Democratic Republic	61.1	Portugal	31.0
China	59.5	Chile	30.5
Korea, Democratic People's Republic of Korea	58.6	Nive	30.4
Georgia	57.1	Netherlands	30.3

Source: Shafey O, Eriksen M, Ross H, Mackay J, *The Tobacco Atlas* (3rd ed.), 2009, American Cancer Society

---

team sports (basketball, football, auto racing, and so on)

- Limits tobacco companies from sponsoring more than one public event per year (music, cultural, artistic events—the tobacco product's brand name cannot appear)

- Bans the use of tobacco product names for stadiums and arenas

- Bans the use of cartoon characters in tobacco advertisements and promotions

- Bans the paid placement of tobacco products in movies, videos, and theater productions; smoking can still be featured in movies (see the box "Smoking in Film")

- Prohibits the distribution and sale of nontobacco products (such as caps and T-shirts) with brand-name logos

- Bans future tobacco products from using previous product names (such as Wings and Old-Golds) or trade names of other products (such as Harley-Davidson and Nike)

- Bans outdoor billboards and transit ads and restricts other indoor advertisements to poster dimensions

- Prevents the tobacco industry from attempting to stop outdoor advertising that discourages tobacco use

After the Master Tobacco Settlement Agreement In spite of the marketing restrictions just listed, the industry continues to be active and innovative in other aspects of the media to which it has access. For example, Philip Morris contemplated the introduction of an upscale lifestyle magazine to be provided free to over 1 million smokers. Interestingly, the magazine would feature articles about healthful activities that many longtime smokers would be unable to engage in because of the effects of smoking.

In the 9 months following the 1999 settlement, the tobacco industry increased its magazine advertising budget by 30 percent over presettlement levels in magazines with 15 percent or more youth (under 18 years of age) readership. Most recently, increased tobacco advertising has been noted in magazines that appeal specifically to younger women, working women, fans of hip-hop music, and women of color.

The development of nonmarket brands of cigarettes for free distribution to patrons of bars and restaurants

Smoking in Film

It is well established that most smokers began using cigarettes during their early years of adolescence, and that adolescent smoking is influenced by an interplay of environmental factors including parental smoking and parental supervision of media exposure, as well as the adolescent's personality and group affiliations. Particularly influential is the extent to which adolescents see movies in which cigarette use is portrayed and the attractiveness of the film characters who are seen smoking.

In a series of studies in which hundreds of G-, PG-13-, and R-rated films were assessed, literally thousands of scenes depicted smoking by one or more characters. The percentage of characters who smoked closely approximated the percentage of adult smokers in the general population (approximately 23 percent), with men smoking a bit more often than women (approximately 25 percent versus 20 percent). Further, of the film characters who smoke in comparison to those who do not, White male antagonists (often favored by young adolescents) from lower socioeconomic class backgrounds and with little apparent education were the most likely to smoke. Interestingly, largely independent of the socioeconomic background of the youthful movie attendees, characters in today's films meeting the "smoker-profile" described seem to hold a near-universal attractiveness to pre- and early-adolescent viewers. Certainly, the tobacco industry might "prefer" that film scripts would use characters representing a broader demographic palette, but they also know that they are well served by having these marginalized yet strangely attractive characters introduce their products to a susceptible audience.

Adding to the tobacco-positive message portrayed by the highly attractive smokers is the cumulative power of characters' presence. Consider, for example, that in a single financially successful film, the number of scenes in which smoking occurs multiplied by the number of preteens and younger adolescents seeing the films easily equals billions of worldwide "hits" beneficial to the tobacco industry. This amazing reality fuels the tobacco industry's willingness to spend tens of thousands of dollars per film on product placement.

On a positive note, in 2007 Disney announced that it will ban depictions of tobacco use in its films. Additionally, new websites such as www.smokefreemovies.ucsf.edu and www.screenit.com allow parents to determine the suitability of films. Efforts are also underway to require films in which smoking is depicted to be rated R.

Parents and others who worry about the continued trend of early-onset smoking among today's younger adolescents would do well to pay attention to the role movies play in the lives of their children. Certainly, parents must discuss the intentions of the tobacco industry and why film production companies purposely let some of a film's characters be depicted engaging in a practice that is so dangerous to real people.

Sources: Charlesworth A, Glanz S, Smoking in the Movies Increases Adolescent Smoking: A Review, *Pediatrics*, 116, 1516–1528, December 2005; Sargent JD, Tanski SE, Gibson J, Exposure to Movie Smoking Among U.S. Adolescents Aged 10 to 14 Years: A Population Estimate, *Pediatrics*, 119(5), 31167–e1176, May 2007; Hanewinkel R, Sargent JD, Exposure to Smoking in Internationally Distributed American Movies and Youth Smoking in Germany, *Pediatrics*, 121(1), e108–117, January 2008; Davis R, *The Role of the Media in Promoting and Reducing Tobacco Use* (Bethesda, MD: U.S. Department of Health and Human Services, National Institutes of Health, National Cancer Institute).

---

who are attempting to "bum" cigarettes represents a second form of "advertising." This "premarketing" introduction of a prototype brand technically does not violate the law regarding the distribution of samples. To date, several hundred establishments in several major cities have participated.

Perhaps the most unanticipated form of "pro-smoking" advertisements that seem to be encouraging young adolescents to experiment with smoking are the public service messages being aired by the tobacco industry as a part of the 1999 settlement. In these television spots, parents are directed, "Talk with your children about the negative consequences of smoking," or children are told, "Think, don't smoke" and "Tobacco is whacko if you're a teen." However potentially "positive" these ads appear to adults, experts now suggest that they might actually be delivering the opposite message to young adolescent viewers, as if they unintentionally "highlight" the mystique of a product used by many adults but legally denied to younger people. Additionally, adolescents seem to hold the companies that "sponsor" these messages (or at least their brand-name products) in higher esteem than companies not associated with the televised message.[9]

Tobacco Use and the Development of Dependence

Although not true for every tobacco user (see the discussion of "chippers" later in this section), the vast majority of users, particularly cigarette smokers, will develop a dependency relationship with the nicotine contained in tobacco. This state of **dependence** causes users to consume greater quantities of nicotine over extended periods of time, further endangering their health.

Laboratory tests, using newer technology, have indicated that nicotine content in cigarettes has increased by approximately 11 percent from the year 2000 to the present—a finding that the tobacco industry rejects.

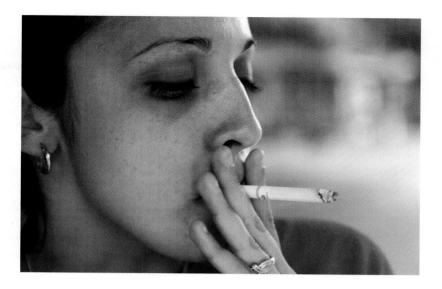

Dependence can imply both a physical and psychological relationship. Particularly with cigarettes, *physical dependence* or *addiction,* with its associated *tolerance, withdrawal,* and **titration,** is strongly developed by 40 percent of all smokers. The development of addiction reflects a strong genetic predisposition to physical dependence. Most of the remaining population of smokers will experience lesser degrees of physical dependence. Psychological *dependence* or *habituation,* with its accompanying psychological components of *compulsion* and *indulgence,* is almost universally seen.

Compulsion is a strong emotional desire to continue tobacco use despite restrictions on smoking and the awareness of health risks. Very likely, users are "compelled" to engage in continual tobacco use in fear of the unpleasant physical, emotional, and social effects that result from discontinuing use. In comparison to compulsion, indulgence is seen as "rewarding" oneself for aligning with a particular behavior pattern—in this case, smoking. Indulgence is made possible by the existence of various reward systems built around the use of tobacco, including a perceived image, group affiliation, and even appetite suppression intended to foster weight control.

Much to the benefit of the tobacco industry, dependence on tobacco is easily established. Many experts believe that physical dependence on tobacco is far more easily established than is physical dependence on alcohol, cocaine (other than crack), or heroin. Of all people who experiment with cigarettes, 85 percent develop various aspects of a dependence relationship.

A small percentage of smokers, known as "chippers," can smoke on occasion without becoming dependent. Most likely, chippers respond differently to environmental cues than do more dependent smokers, thus smoking less frequently. Chippers, once described as "social smokers," smoke in a wide variety of settings, including when alone, when socializing, during indulgent activities, and when eating and consuming alcohol, just as heavy smokers do. The primary difference is that chippers have a highly developed level of stimulus control, whereas heavy smokers lack a large measure of such control.[10] Unfortunately, many inexperienced smokers feel that they too are only social smokers; however, a few months or even a few days of this type of occasional smoking could be a transitional period into a dependence pattern of tobacco use.

Sandwiched between regular smokers and chippers is a newly emerging group of smokers—part-time smokers. Today these smokers constitute about 20 percent of all smokers. Also called nondaily smokers, these part-time smokers show many of the same types of negative health effects as those seen in daily smokers, although in part-time smokers they are not as well established or as debilitating. Thus these smokers receive less encouragement from physicians to enter smoking cessation programs.[11] Perhaps nondaily smokers exist in part because of the reality of the high cost of cigarettes and restrictions in the workplace.

> **Key Terms**
>
> **dependence** A physical or psychological need to continue the use of a drug.
>
> **titration** (tie **tray** shun) The particular level of a drug within the body; adjusting the level of nicotine by adjusting the rate of smoking.

Theories of Nicotine Addiction

The establishment and maintenance of physical dependence or addiction is less than fully understood. Most experts, however, believe that for a specific individual, addiction has a multifaceted etiology, or cause, with increasing attention being directed toward a genetic basis for addiction. Accordingly, several theories have been proposed to explain the development of dependence. We present a brief account of some of these theories. Readers are reminded that many of these theories are technically sophisticated and only a most basic description can be provided in a personal health textbook. The more emotional aspects of dependence formation are discussed later in the chapter.

Genetic Influences Although the specific genetic pathways that influence both the initiation and maintenance of smoking (or other forms of tobacco use) are less than fully understood, a role for genetic influence is evident. Applying new statistical techniques to earlier studies of smoking patterns in families and between identical twins, it is now believed that initiation and maintenance of initial smoking is 60 percent driven by genetic influences.[12]

Recent research studies have identified specific chromosomes that contribute to the genetic susceptibility of developing nicotine dependence. These include chromosomes 1, 3, 4, 7, 8, 9, 11, 16, 17, and 20,[13] with chromosomes 5 and 10 contributing to dependence in African Americans.[14, 15] Most likely, additional genetic markers will soon be included in this lengthening list.[16, 17]

Of course, the smoking of the first few cigarettes is a choice made by beginning smokers. In a yet-to-be-determined percentage of beginning smokers, the *initiation* of smoking, or the desire to continue with this new behavior, is underlined by a genetic predisposition to neurohormonally "appreciate" the stimulating effects of nicotine. Once smoking has been so easily and successfully initiated, the continuation of smoking is then *maintained* by the same, or closely related, genetic predisposition for neurohormonal excitation of the central nervous system. The "hook" for a lifetime of smoking is, thus, set in large part by a genetic susceptibility.[18] The remaining influence needed for initiation and maintenance of initial smoking is 20 percent environmental and 20 percent the unique needs of individuals.[19]

Once the relatively brief period of initial exposure (initiation) and early maintenance is passed, the role of genetic influences may be even more powerful—providing 70 percent of the maintenance stimulus required over decades of smoking. Environmental and personality factors subside accordingly.[19]

Bolus Theory In the **bolus theory** of nicotine addiction, one of the oldest and most general theories of addiction, each inhalation of smoke releases into the blood a concentrated quantity of nicotine (a ball or bolus) that reaches the brain and results in a period of neurohormonal excitement. The smoker perceives this period of stimulation as pleasurable but, unfortunately, short-lived. Accordingly, the smoker attempts to reestablish this pleasurable feeling by again inhaling and sending another bolus of nicotine on its way to the brain. The 70,000 or more inhalations during the first year of smoking serve to condition the novice smoker, resulting in a lifelong pattern of cigarette dependence. The level needed for arousal is different for each individual smoker, depending on the length of addiction, the level of tolerance, genetic predisposition, and environmental and personal stimuli.

Recognition of two types of smokers emerges from an understanding of the bolus theory of smoking. *Peak smokers* are those smokers who become dependent on the arousal of pleasure centers in the brain (see page 243) that are stimulated by the rapid increase of nicotine levels following inhalation and distribution of nicotine within the CNS. In contrast, *trough maintenance smokers* maintain an even, consistently higher level of nicotine titration in order to avoid the negative consequences of withdrawal. In other words, some smokers enjoy the consequences (arousal) caused by arrival of the bolus, whereas others so dislike the feelings caused by dissipation of the bolus that they inhale to avoid these unpleasant feelings.

Adrenocorticotropic Hormone (ACTH) Theory Yet another theory of dependence suggests that nicotine stimulates the release of adrenocorticotropic hormone (ACTH) from the anterior pituitary, or "master gland" of the endocrine system (see Chapter 3), causing the release of **beta endorphins** (naturally occurring opiate-like chemicals) that produce mild feelings of euphoria. Perhaps this stresslike response mechanism involving ACTH accounts for the increased energy expenditure seen in smokers and thus their tendency to maintain a lower body weight.

When these physiological responses are viewed collectively, nicotine may be seen as biochemically influencing brain activity by enhancing the extent and strength of various forms of "communication" between different brain areas and even glands of the endocrine system. If this is the case, it is apparent why, once addicted, the functioning of the smoker's control system is much altered in comparison with that of nonsmokers.

Self-Medication Theory Another explanation of the addiction to smoking, called *self-medication,* suggests that nicotine, through the effects of mood-enhancing dopamine, may allow smokers to "treat" feelings of tiredness, lack of motivation, or even depression. In other words, a smoke lifts the spirits, if only briefly. Eventually, however, smokers become dependent on tobacco as a "medication" to make themselves feel better. Recent research, however, challenges the role of self-medication (purposeful stimulating of dopamine release) as a causative factor in establishing and maintaining smoking behavior. Some now suggest that, instead, the removal of the depressed level of arousal (being in a period of withdrawal) is the primary player in the establishment of nicotine dependence.

Regardless of the mechanism involved, as tolerance to nicotine develops, smoking behavior is adjusted to either maintain arousal or prevent the occurrence of withdrawal symptoms. At some point, however, the desire for constant arousal is probably superseded by the smoker's desire not to experience withdrawal.

The importance of nicotine as the primary factor in establishing dependence on tobacco is supported by research that demonstrates that smokers will not select a nontobacco cigarette if a tobacco cigarette is available. Even tobacco cigarettes with a very low level of nicotine seem to be unacceptable to most smokers, as do cigarettes with very low nicotine but with high tar content. Interestingly, users of low-nicotine cigarettes tend to inhale more frequently and deeply to obtain as much nicotine as possible.

Even more impressive (and alarming) than the power of nicotine to cause dependence is the small amount of time needed for it to do so. Instruments designed to assess the time required for the onset of dependence on nicotine—such as Development and Assessment of Nicotine Dependency in Youths (DANDY)[20] and Hooked On Nicotine Checklist (HONC)[21]; see the Personal Assessment at the end of this chapter—have established that beginning smokers (recall that most smokers begin during adolescence) become dependent on cigarettes within 3 weeks to 3 months of smoking as few as two cigarettes per day. Males are more likely to be a bit more resistant to dependence, taking a month or two, whereas females can become dependent in a matter of a very few days of initial experimentation. Additionally, it is now known that for children who try smoking on a very limited basis and then stop, a "sleeper effect" may be put into place that increases their vulnerability to becoming a smoker within the next three years, in comparison with peers who did not experiment with smoking.[22]

A newly recognized variable in understanding dependence formation in young, light smokers (1 to 6 cigarettes per day) is influence by the rate of nicotine metabolism. Dependence, reflected in withdrawal symptoms, occurs much sooner in individuals whose rate of nicotine breakdown was faster than in those with slower rates.[23]

TALKING POINTS A smoker says that she does not consider smoking to be a form of drug use. She becomes angry at the suggestion that cigarettes are part of a drug-delivery system. How would you respond to her position?

Nicotine Dependence and Traumatic Brain Injury

Recent findings related to the consequence of strokes occurring in a very specific area of the brain called the insula provide an interesting aside to the discussion of the brain and nervous system's role in nicotine dependence. Located in the brain at ear level, the insula is a small area that plays a critical role in the communication of information to the prefrontal cortex, where behavioral decisions are formulated. In a smoker whose insula has been damaged by the disruption of blood flow (stroke), nicotine dependence often disappears instantly and the individual can immediately stop smoking. In other words, damage to this specific area of the brain appears to disrupt the flow of information from other nicotine-sensitive areas of the brain, disrupting the reward system that would otherwise result in the act of smoking. Perhaps in the future there will be a smoking-cessation technology centered on insula function.

Acute Effects of Nicotine on Nervous System Function

In comparison with the more chronic effects of nicotine on the central nervous system (CNS) that may eventually result in physical dependence or addiction, nicotine also produces changes of short duration. In the CNS, nicotine activates receptors within the nucleus accumbens (a reward center) and the locus caeruleus (a cortical activating center) of the brain. Through the use of electroencephalography (EEG) and magnetic resonance imaging (MRI) technology, the location and extent of brain activity can be assessed. Upon reaching the brain areas mentioned, nicotine induces increased brain activity in a consistent and predictable manner. This is part of a general arousal pattern signaled by the release of the neurotransmitter **norepinephrine,** dopamine, acetylcholine, and serotonin. Heavy use of tobacco products, resulting in high levels of nicotine in the bloodstream, eventually produces a blocking effect as more and more receptor sites for these neurotransmitters are filled. The result is a generalized depression of the CNS.

| Key Terms |

bolus theory A theory of nicotine addiction based on the body's response to the bolus (ball) of nicotine delivered to the brain with each inhalation of cigarette smoke.

beta endorphins Mood-enhancing, pain-reducing, opiatelike chemicals produced within the smoker's body in response to the presence of nicotine.

norepinephrine (nor epp in **eff** rin) An adrenaline-like neurotransmitter produced within the nervous system.

The level of plasma nicotine associated with normal levels of heavy smoking (one to two packs per day) would not likely produce the depressive effect just described. However, in chain smokers (four to eight packs per day), plasma nicotine levels would be sufficient to have a depressive influence on nervous system function. In fact, it has been suggested that chain smoking is driven by the fruitless effort to counter the depressive influence of chronically excessively high levels of nicotine. In contrast to chain smokers, inexperienced smokers, lacking tolerance, can quickly reach a blood level of nicotine sufficient to activate the brain's vomiting centers. This response is a built-in protective mechanism against nicotine poisoning.

In carefully controlled studies involving both animals and humans, nicotine increased the ability of subjects to concentrate on a task. However, the duration of this improvement was limited. Most people would agree that this brief benefit is not enough to justify the health risks associated with chronic tobacco use.

Non–Nervous-System Acute Effects of Nicotine

Outside the CNS, nicotine affects the transmission of nerve signals at the point where nerves innervate muscle tissue (called the *neuromuscular junction*) by mimicking the action of the neurotransmitter acetylcholine. Nicotine occupies receptor sites at the junction and prevents the transmission of nerve impulses from nerve cell to muscle cell.

Nicotine also causes the release of epinephrine from the adrenal medulla (see Chapter 3), which results in an increase in respiration rate, heart rate, blood pressure, and coronary blood flow. These changes are accompanied by the constriction of the blood vessels beneath the skin, a reduction in the motility in the bowel, loss of appetite, and changes in sleep patterns.

Although a lethal dose of nicotine could be obtained through the ingestion of a nicotine-containing insecticide, to "smoke oneself to death" in a single intense period of cigarette use would be highly improbable. In humans, 40 to 60 mg (0.06–0.09 mg/kg) is a lethal dose. A typical cigarette supplies 0.05 to 2.5 mg of nicotine, and that nicotine is relatively quickly broken down for removal from the body.

Psychosocial Factors Related to Dependence

Recall that a psychological aspect of dependence (habituation) exists and is important in maintaining the smoker's need for nicotine. Both research and general observation support many of the powerful influences this aspect of dependence possesses, especially for beginning smokers, before the onset of physical addiction. Consequently, in the remainder of this section, we explore nonphysiological factors that may contribute to the development of this aspect of dependence.

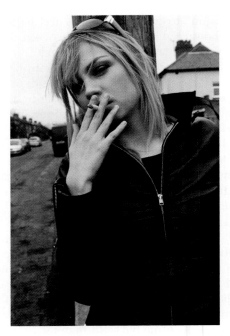

Most smokers pick up the habit as young teens, possibly influenced by older smoking peers and by widespread tobacco advertising and promotions.

Modeling Behavior   Because tobacco use is a learned behavior, it is reasonable to accept that modeling acts as a stimulus to experimental smoking. Modeling suggests that susceptible people smoke to emulate, or model their behavior after, smokers whom they admire or with whom they share other types of social or emotional bonds. Particularly for young adolescents (ages 11 to 16), smoking behavior correlates with the smoking behavior of slightly older peers and very young adults (ages 18 to 22), older siblings, and, most important, parents. Negative parental influences on cigarette smoking by their children include their own smoking status, their failure to clearly state their disapproval of smoking, and their reluctance to openly criticize the tobacco industry.[24] Further, for parents who smoke, it is important that they cease smoking before their children turn 8 years of age if they wish to maximize an anti-smoking message.

Modeling is particularly evident when smoking is a central factor in peer group formation and peer group association and can lead to a shared behavioral pattern that differentiates the group from others and from adults. Further, when risk-taking behavior and disregard for authority are common to the group, smoking becomes the behavioral pattern that most consistently identifies and bonds the group. Particularly for those young people who lack self-directedness or the ability to resist peer pressure, initial membership in a tobacco-using peer group may become inescapable. The ability to counter peer pressure is a salient component of successful anti-smoking programs for use with older children and younger adolescents.

In addition, when adolescents have lower levels of self-esteem and are searching for an avenue to improve self-image, a role model who smokes is often seen as tough, sociable, and sexually attractive. These three traits have been played up by the tobacco industry in their carefully crafted advertisements. In fact, young teens from any background may see the very young and attractive models used in tobacco (and beer) advertisements as being more peerlike in age than they really are. FCC regulations require that models for both products be 21 years of age or older, regardless of how youthful they might (and the advertisers hope they do) appear to older children and young adolescents.

Manipulation In addition to modeling as a psychosocial link with tobacco use, cigarette use may meet the beginning smoker's need to manipulate something and at the same time provide the manipulative "tool" necessary to offset boredom, feelings of depression, or social immaturity. The availability of affordable smoking paraphernalia provides smokers with ways to reward themselves. A new cigarette lighter, a status brand of tobacco, or a cap or jacket with a cigarette's logo are all reinforcements to some smokers. Fortunately, the last two items will become increasingly harder to find since logos can no longer be placed on items such as these. For others, the ability to take out a cigarette or fill a pipe adds a measure of structure and control to situations in which they might otherwise feel somewhat ill at ease. The cigarette becomes a readily available and dependable "friend" to turn to during stressful moments.

Susceptibility to Advertising The images of the smoker's world portrayed by the media can be particularly attractive. For adolescents, women, minorities, and other carefully targeted groups of adults, the tobacco industry has paired suggestions of a better life with the use of its products. To these users and potential users, the self-reward of power, liberation, affluence, sophistication, or adult status is achieved by using the products that they are told are associated with these desired states. Thus the self-rewarding use of tobacco products becomes a means of hoped-for achievement.

With this multiplicity of forces at work, we can understand why so many who experiment with tobacco use find that they quickly, in combination with genetic predisposition, become emotionally dependent on tobacco. Human needs, both physiological and psychosocial, are many and complex. Tobacco use meets the needs on a short-term basis, whereas dependence, once established, replaces these needs with a different, more immediate set of needs.

For those who question whether tobacco promotion leads to the initiation of smoking in children and young adolescents, a recent meta-analysis of current research indicates that the power of tobacco promotion is so pervasive that, when other environmental factors associated with initiation, such as smoking by parents and peer

group and the socioeconomic background of the young persons, are controlled for, exposure to tobacco promotion is the single most powerful factor underlying adolescent smoking. In fact, the association between high exposure to tobacco promotion and a high probability of smoking is so strong that causality is assigned.[25] Once smoking is initiated, dependence in some is almost a certainty and will prove difficult to overcome.

Preventing Teen Smoking

An attempt by the federal government to prevent the onset of smoking by minors has a long history that included both public service television spots during the 1970s that were intended to inform parents that their smoking habits could easily be "transferred" to their children and nearly universally ignored requirements that cigarettes could not be sold to minors.

As noted in the discussion of the Master Tobacco Settlement Agreement (see page 238), the tobacco industry agreed to a number of restrictions regarding formally used "enticement techniques" (such as logos on clothing, use of cartoon characters, and sponsorship of concerts). Today these restrictions remain in place, although the tobacco industry has made subtle adjustments in marketing to short-circuit, where possible, the requirements of the settlements. Additionally, more strenuous enforcement of restrictions on sales to minors remains in effect.

Perhaps the most innovative attempt to prevent tobacco sales to minors was inherent in requests made by the FDA to allow it to define cigarettes as a drug delivery device (nicotine being the drug). This reclassification would have led to strict requirements on the "authorization to purchase" cigarettes—requirements similar to those needed in order to obtain a prescription (Rx) for pharmaceuticals, and to a major reduction in the number and types of locations where sales could occur. This plan, widely supported by anti-smoking advocates, was routinely blocked by the pro-smoking lobby's strong association with the Republican-controlled houses of Congress during George W. Bush's presidential terms. Today, with the political tables turned in Congress, FDA control of cigarettes has been approved, and its first action was to ban flavored and mentholated cigarettes.

In a different vein, the current anti-tobacco advertisements sponsored by the several national-level tobacco-free groups that feature extremely gross depictions of smoking's harmful effects, is making a positive impact on decisions regarding smoking experimentation by pre-adolescent and young adolescents.

Early Childhood Intervention

Although significant concern centers on the onset of smoking behavior by adolescents in the 11- to 14-year-old age group and later teen years, the decision to smoke (or use other forms of tobacco) may be made at a much earlier age. Accordingly, parents (and other adults) who do not want their children to smoke or use tobacco in other forms should begin educating their children as preschoolers and certainly by school age. The following recommendations, and many additional ones as well, can be found in *A Parent's Guide to Prevention,* available from the National Clearinghouse for Alcohol and Drug Information.

When dealing with preschool children, it should be remembered that facts are unlikely to be comprehended. Accordingly, the following activities are suggested:

- Set aside regular time when you can give your child your full attention. Playing and reading together builds a strong parent-child bond.
- Point out poisonous and harmful substances that can be found in the home.
- Explain how medicines can be harmful if used incorrectly.
- Provide guidelines that teach the child what kind of behavior is expected.
- Encourage the child to follow instructions.
- Help the child learn decision-making skills; give positive feedback when appropriate decisions have been made.

For children in kindergarten through third grade, new skills and insights need to be developed to deal with drugs, including tobacco products. Adults should attempt to

- Help the child recognize and understand family rules.
- Discuss how television advertisements try to persuade people to buy their products.
- Practice ways in which the child can say no to other people.
- Develop a "helper" file made up of the names and phone numbers of people the child can turn to when confronted by others who want them to try smoking or smokeless tobacco.

As children approach the preteen years, more focused presentations can be made regarding the dangers associated with smoking and the use of other substances. Adults working with children in grades four through six should focus on the following activities:

- Create special times when an adult is available to talk with the child about whatever he or she wants to talk about.
- Encourage participation in a variety of activities that are both fun and allow the child to meet new friends.

- Teach the child how drugs, including tobacco products, are promoted and how their messages can be "defused."
- Continue to assist the child in learning how to say no.
- Become acquainted with the parents of the child's friends so that you will be able to work with them in support of a smoke-free community.
- Participate in providing support for supervised activities for children of this age.

Although nothing is certain regarding the decision that older preadolescents or teens make about beginning to smoke, the activities just listed may be effective in countering the influences of the peer group and the mass media.

Tobacco Smoke: The Source of Physiologically Active Compounds

When burned, the tobacco in cigarettes, cigars, and pipe mixtures is the source of an array of physiologically active chemicals, many of which are closely linked to significant changes in normal body structure and function. At the burning tip of the cigarette, the 900°C (1,652°F) heat oxidizes tobacco (as well as paper, wrapper, filter, and additives). With each puff of smoke, the body is exposed to approximately 4,700 chemical compounds, hundreds of which are known to be physiologically active, toxic, and carcinogenic. These chemicals have their origins in the tobacco or have been introduced as additives, pesticides, and other agricultural chemicals. An annual 70,000 puffs taken in by the one-pack-a-day cigarette smoker results in an environment that makes the most polluted urban environment seem clean by comparison.

Table 9.3 presents a partial list of toxic and carcinogenic compounds of tobacco smoking. In addition to tobacco smoke, these materials, and hundreds of others not listed, are routinely found within many materials used in industrial and residential settings.

Particulate Phase

Cigarette, cigar, and pipe smoke can be described on the basis of two phases. These phases include a particulate phase and a gaseous phase. The **particulate phase** includes **nicotine,** water, and a variety of powerful chemicals known collectively as tar. **Tar** includes phenol, cresol, pyrene, DDT, a benzene-ring group of compounds that includes benzo[a]pyrene, and hundreds of additional compounds. A person who smokes one pack of cigarettes per day collects four ounces of tar in his or her lungs in a year. Only the gases and the smallest particles reach the small sacs of the lungs, called the *alveoli,*

Table 9.3 Partial Listing of Toxic and Carcinogenic Components of Cigarette Smoke

Agent in Tobacco Smoke	Nontobacco Sources of Chemical Compounds
Carbon Monoxide	Released by internal combustion engines (cars, trucks, buses, etc.)
Nitrogen Oxides (NO_x)	Released by internal combustion engines
Hydrogen Cyanide	Burning of polyurethane foam (insulating material)
Formaldehyde	Released by internal combustion engines and the burning of many forms of building materials
Acrolein	Burning of fat (e.g., barbecuing of meats)
Acetaldehyde	Released by internal combustion engines
Ammonia	Found in fertilizers, many cleaning agents, and released during decomposition of organic material
Hydrazine	Rocket fuel exhaust
Vinyl Chloride	Released by burning plastics
Benzo[a]pyrene	Produced when grilling meats and found in wood smoke and soot
Aromatic Amines	Released during the decomposition of organic material
Aromatic Nitrohydrocarbons	Found in fumes produced by the incineration of municipal wastes
Polonium-210	Released into air during radioactive decay
Nickel	Leakage from/burning of nickel-cadmium batteries
Arsenic	Found in localized ground-water areas
Cadmium	Found in pesticides and batteries, and released by municipal waste incineration

Source: Mulcahy S. *The Toxicology of Cigarette Smoke and Environmental Tobacco Smoke,* A Review of Cigarette Smoke and Its Toxicological Effects, www.csn.ul.ie/nstephen/reports/bc4927.html. Used with permission by Stephen Mulcahy.

where oxygen exchange occurs. The carcinogen-rich particles from the particulate phase are deposited somewhere along the air passage leading to the lungs.

Gaseous Phase

The **gaseous phase** of tobacco smoke, like the particulate phase, is composed of a variety of physiologically active compounds, including carbon monoxide, carbon dioxide, ammonia, hydrogen cyanide, isopyrene, acetaldehyde, and acetone. At least 60 of these compounds in the gaseous phase have been determined to be **carcinogens,** or co-carcinogenic promoters, thus capable of stimulating the development of cancer. Carbon monoxide is, however, the most damaging compound found in this component of tobacco smoke. Its effect is discussed next.

Carbon Monoxide   Like every inefficient engine, a cigarette, cigar, or pipe burns (oxidizes) its fuel with less than complete conversion into carbon dioxide, water, and heat. As a result of this incomplete oxidation, burning tobacco forms **carbon monoxide (CO)** gas. Carbon monoxide is one of the most harmful components of tobacco smoke.

Carbon monoxide is a colorless, odorless, tasteless gas that possesses a very strong physiological attraction for hemoglobin, the oxygen-carrying pigment on each red blood cell. When CO is inhaled, it quickly bonds with hemoglobin and forms a new compound, carboxyhemoglobin. In this form, hemoglobin is unable to transport oxygen to the tissues and cells where it is needed.

Although it is true that normal body metabolism always keeps an irreducible minimum of CO in our blood (0.5–1 percent), the blood of smokers may have levels of 5 to 10 percent CO saturation.[26] We are exposed to additional CO from environmental sources such as automobiles and buses and other combustion of fossil fuels. When we consider the combination of a smoker's CO with environmental CO, we are not surprised that smokers more easily become out of breath than nonsmokers do. The half-life of CO combined with hemoglobin is approximately four to six hours. Most

---

Key Terms

particulate phase The portion of tobacco smoke composed of small suspended particles.

nicotine A physiologically active, dependence-producing drug found in tobacco.

tar A chemically rich, syrupy, blackish-brown material obtained from the particulate matter within cigarette smoke when nicotine and water are removed.

gaseous phase The portion of the tobacco smoke containing carbon monoxide and many other physiologically active gaseous compounds.

carcinogens Environmental agents, including chemical compounds within cigarette smoke, that stimulate the development of cancerous changes within cells.

carbon monoxide (CO) A chemical compound that can "inactivate" red blood cells.

smokers replenish their level of CO saturation at far shorter intervals than this.

As mentioned, the presence of excessive levels of carboxyhemoglobin in the blood of smokers leads to shortness of breath and lowered endurance. Because an adequate oxygen supply to all body tissues is critical for normal functioning, any oxygen reduction can have a serious impact on health. Brain function may be eventually reduced, reactions and judgment are dulled, and cardiovascular function is impaired. Fetuses are especially at risk for this oxygen deprivation (hypoxia) because fetal development is so critically dependent on a sufficient oxygen supply from the mother.

Illness, Premature Death, and Tobacco Use

For people who begin tobacco use as adolescents or young adults, smoke heavily, and continue to smoke, the likelihood of premature death is virtually ensured. Two-pack-a-day cigarette smokers can expect to die seven to eight years earlier than their nonsmoking counterparts will. (Only nonsmoking-related deaths that can afflict smokers and nonsmokers alike keep the difference at this level rather than much higher.) Not only will these people die sooner, but they will also probably be plagued with painful, debilitating illnesses for an extended time. Smoking is responsible for nearly 438,000 premature deaths each year.[27] Figure 9-1 presents an overview of illnesses known to be caused or worsened by tobacco use.

Cardiovascular Disease

Although cancer is now the leading cause of death for Americans under 80 years of age, cardiovascular disease is the leading cause of death among all adults, accounting for 829,072 deaths in the United States in 2006.[28] Tobacco use, and cigarette smoking in particular, is one of the major factors contributing to this cause of death.

Key Terms

myocardial infarction Heart attack; the death of heart muscle as a result of a blockage in one of the coronary arteries.

cardiac arrest Immediate death resulting from a sudden change in the rhythm of the heart causing loss of heart function.

angina pectoris (an jie nuh **peck** tor is) Chest pain that results from impaired blood supply to the heart muscle.

platelet adhesiveness The tendency of platelets to clump together, thus enhancing the speed at which the blood clots.

Although overall progress is being made in reducing the incidence of cardiovascular-related deaths, tobacco use impedes these efforts. So important is tobacco use as a contributing factor in deaths from cardiovascular disease that the cigarette smoker more than doubles the risk of experiencing a **myocardial infarction,** the leading cause of death from cardiovascular disease. Smokers also increase their risk of **cardiac arrest** by two to four times. Fully one-third of all cardiovascular disease can be traced to cigarette smoking.

The relationship between tobacco use and cardiovascular disease is centered on two major components of tobacco smoke: nicotine and carbon monoxide.

Nicotine and Cardiovascular Disease The influence of nicotine on the cardiovascular system occurs when it stimulates the nervous system to release norepinephrine. This powerful stimulant increases the heart rate. In turn, an elevated heart rate increases cardiac output, thus increasing blood pressure. The extent to which this is dangerous depends in part on the coronary circulation's ability to supply blood to the rapidly contracting heart muscle. The development of **angina pectoris** and the possibility of sudden heart attack are heightened by this sustained elevation of heart rate, particularly in those individuals with existing coronary artery disease (see Chapter 10).

Nicotine is also a powerful vasoconstrictor of the peripheral blood vessels. As these vessels are constricted by the influence of nicotine, the pressure against their walls increases. Research shows that irreversible atherosclerotic damage to major arteries also occurs with smoking.

For over a decade it has been known that nicotine also increases blood **platelet adhesiveness.** As the platelets become more and more likely to "clump," a person is more likely to develop a blood clot. In people already prone to cardiovascular disease, more rapidly clotting blood is an unwelcome liability. Heart attacks occur when clots form within the coronary arteries or are transported to the heart from other areas of the body.

In addition to other influences on the cardiovascular system, nicotine possesses the ability to decrease the proportion of high-density lipoproteins (HDLs) and to increase the proportion of low-density lipoproteins (LDLs) and very-low-density lipoproteins that constitute the body's serum cholesterol. Low-density lipoproteins appear to support the development of atherosclerosis and are clearly increased in the bloodstreams of smokers. (See Chapter 10 for further information about cholesterol's role in cardiovascular disease.)

Carbon Monoxide and Cardiovascular Disease A second substance contributed by tobacco influences the type and extent of cardiovascular disease found among tobacco users. Carbon monoxide interferes with oxygen transport within the circulatory system.

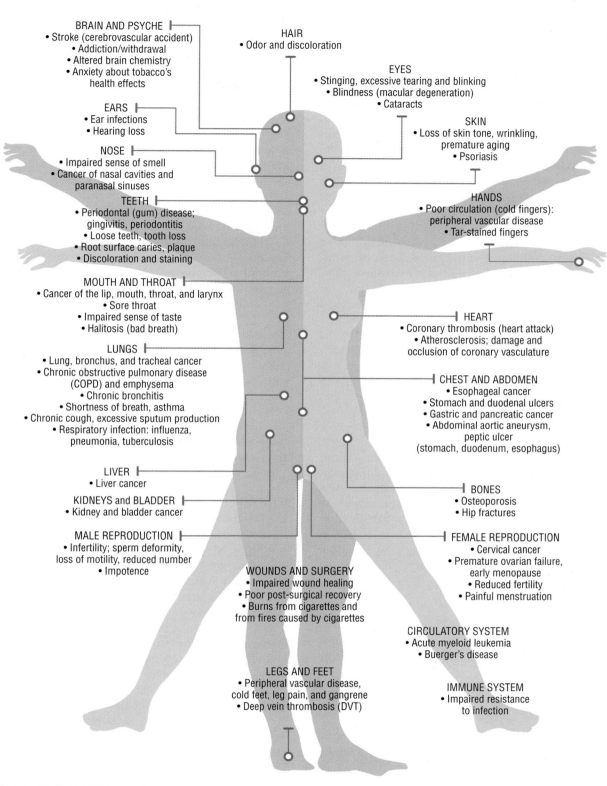

BRAIN AND PSYCHE
- Stroke (cerebrovascular accident)
- Addiction/withdrawal
- Altered brain chemistry
- Anxiety about tobacco's health effects

HAIR
- Odor and discoloration

EYES
- Stinging, excessive tearing and blinking
- Blindness (macular degeneration)
- Cataracts

EARS
- Ear infections
- Hearing loss

SKIN
- Loss of skin tone, wrinkling, premature aging
- Psoriasis

NOSE
- Impaired sense of smell
- Cancer of nasal cavities and paranasal sinuses

HANDS
- Poor circulation (cold fingers): peripheral vascular disease
- Tar-stained fingers

TEETH
- Periodontal (gum) disease; gingivitis, periodontitis
- Loose teeth, tooth loss
- Root surface caries, plaque
- Discoloration and staining

MOUTH AND THROAT
- Cancer of the lip, mouth, throat, and larynx
- Sore throat
- Impaired sense of taste
- Halitosis (bad breath)

HEART
- Coronary thrombosis (heart attack)
- Atherosclerosis; damage and occlusion of coronary vasculature

LUNGS
- Lung, bronchus, and tracheal cancer
- Chronic obstructive pulmonary disease (COPD) and emphysema
- Chronic bronchitis
- Shortness of breath, asthma
- Chronic cough, excessive sputum production
- Respiratory infection: influenza, pneumonia, tuberculosis

CHEST AND ABDOMEN
- Esophageal cancer
- Stomach and duodenal ulcers
- Gastric and pancreatic cancer
- Abdominal aortic aneurysm, peptic ulcer (stomach, duodenum, esophagus)

LIVER
- Liver cancer

BONES
- Osteoporosis
- Hip fractures

KIDNEYS and BLADDER
- Kidney and bladder cancer

MALE REPRODUCTION
- Infertility; sperm deformity, loss of motility, reduced number
- Impotence

FEMALE REPRODUCTION
- Cervical cancer
- Premature ovarian failure, early menopause
- Reduced fertility
- Painful menstruation

WOUNDS AND SURGERY
- Impaired wound healing
- Poor post-surgical recovery
- Burns from cigarettes and from fires caused by cigarettes

CIRCULATORY SYSTEM
- Acute myeloid leukemia
- Buerger's disease

LEGS AND FEET
- Peripheral vascular disease, cold feet, leg pain, and gangrene
- Deep vein thrombosis (DVT)

IMMUNE SYSTEM
- Impaired resistance to infection

Figure 9-1 Health Risks of Tobacco Use

Source: Mackay J, Eriksen M, Shafey O. *The Tobacco Atlas* (3rd ed.). 2009. American Cancer Society. Modified and reprinted by the permission of the American Cancer Society, Inc. All rights reserved.

As described earlier in the chapter, carbon monoxide is a component of the gaseous phase of tobacco smoke and readily joins with the hemoglobin of the red blood cells. Carbon monoxide has an affinity for hemoglobin 206 times that of oxygen. Once the hemoglobin of a red cell has accepted carbon monoxide molecules, the hemoglobin is transformed into carboxyhemoglobin. Thereafter, the carboxyhemoglobin permanently weakens the red blood cell's ability to transport oxygen. So long as smoking continues, these red blood cells remain relatively useless during the remainder of their 120-day lives. Levels of carboxyhemoglobin in heavy smokers are associated with significant increases in the incidence of myocardial infarction.

When a person has impaired oxygen-transporting abilities, physical exertion becomes increasingly demanding on both the heart and the lungs. The cardiovascular system will attempt to respond to the body's demand for oxygen, but these responses are themselves impaired as a result of the influence of nicotine on the cardiovascular system. If tobacco does create the good life, as advertisers claim, it also unfortunately lessens the ability to participate actively in that life.

Smoking and Oral Contraceptive Use Women who smoke and use oral contraceptives, particularly after age 35, are placing themselves at a much greater risk of experiencing a fatal cardiovascular accident (heart attack, stroke, or an **embolism**) than are oral contraceptive users who do not smoke. This risk of cardiovascular complications increases further for oral contraceptive users 40 years of age or older. Women who both smoke and use oral contraceptives are four times more likely to die from myocardial infarction (heart attack) than are women who only smoke. Because of this adverse relationship, *it is strongly recommended that women who smoke not use oral contraceptives.*

Cancer

Over the past 60 years, research from the most reputable institutions in this country and abroad has consistently concluded that tobacco use is a significant factor in the development of virtually all forms of cancer and the most significant factor in cancers involving the respiratory system.

In describing cancer development, the currently used reference is 20 pack-years, or an amount of smoking equal to smoking one pack of cigarettes a day for 20 years. Thus the two-pack-a-day smoker can anticipate cancer-related tissue changes in as few as 10 years, while the half-pack-a-day smoker may have 40 years to wait. Regardless, the opportunity is there for all smokers to confirm these data by developing cancer as predicted. It is hoped that most people will think twice before disregarding this evidence.

Data supplied by the American Cancer Society (ACS) indicate that during 2007 an estimated 1,494,920 Americans developed cancer.* These cases were nearly equally divided between the sexes and resulted in approximately 559,650 deaths. In the opinion of the ACS, 30 percent of all cancer cases are heavily influenced by tobacco use. Lung cancer alone accounted for about 213,380 of the new cancer cases and 160,390 deaths in 2007. Fully 87 percent of men with lung cancer were cigarette smokers.[27] A genetic "missing link" between smoking and lung cancer was established, when mutations to an important tumor suppressor gene were identified. If it was necessary to have a final "proof" that smoking causes lung cancer, that proof appears to be in hand.

Cancer of the entire respiratory system, including lung cancer and cancers of the mouth and larynx, accounted for about 229,400 new cases of cancer and 174,480 deaths.[27] Despite these high figures, not all smokers develop cancer.

Respiratory Tract Cancer Recall that tobacco smoke produces both a gaseous and a particulate phase. As noted, the particulate phase contains the tar fragment of tobacco smoke. This rich chemical environment contains more than 4,000 known chemical compounds, hundreds of which are known to be carcinogens.

In the normally functioning respiratory system, particulate matter suspended in the inhaled air settles on the tissues lining the airways and is trapped in **mucus** produced by specialized *goblet cells*. This mucus, with its trapped impurities, is continuously swept upward by the beating action of hairlike **cilia** of the ciliated columnar epithelial cells lining the air passages (Figure 9-2). On reaching the throat, this mucus is swallowed and eventually removed through the digestive system.

When tobacco smoke is drawn into the respiratory system, however, its rapidly dropping temperature allows the particulate matter to accumulate. This brown, sticky tar contains compounds known to harm the ciliated cells, goblet cells, and the basal cells of the respiratory lining. As the damage from smoking increases, the cilia become less effective in sweeping mucus upward to the throat. When cilia can no longer clean the airway, tar accumulates on the surfaces and brings carcinogenic compounds into direct contact with the tissues of the airway.

At the same time that the sweeping action of the lining cells is being slowed, substances in the tar are stimulating the goblet cells to increase the amount of mucus they normally produce. The "smoker's cough" is the body's attempt to remove this excess mucus.

With prolonged exposure to the carcinogenic materials in tar, predictable changes will begin to occur within the respiratory system's basal cell layer (Figure 9-2). The

*Excluding cases of nonmelanoma skin cancer.

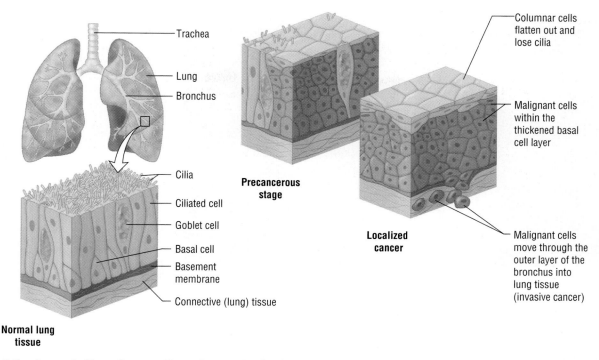

Figure 9-2 Development of Lung Cancer   Tissue changes associated with lung cancer (bronchogenic carcinoma).

basal cells begin to display changes characteristic of all cancer cells. In addition, an abnormal accumulation of cells occurs. When a person stops smoking, preinvasive lesions do not repair themselves as quickly as once thought.

By the time lung cancer is usually diagnosed, its development is so advanced that the chance for recovery is very poor. Still today, only 16 percent of all lung cancer victims survive for five years or more after diagnosis.[27] Most die in a very uncomfortable, painful way.

Two primary forms of lung cancer are seen in smokers: squamous cell carcinoma and adenocarcinoma. The former is declining in prevalence as the level of smoking in this country declines, but the latter form of lung cancer is increasing. Some experts attribute this increase, in the face of declining smoking, to a change in the chemical nature of cigarette smoke due to subtle changes in the formulation of cigarette tobacco and the ventilation of filters.

Cancerous activity in other areas of the respiratory system, including the larynx, and within the oral cavity (mouth) follows a similar course. In the case of oral cavity cancer, carcinogens found within the smoke and within the saliva are involved in the cancerous changes. Tobacco users, such as pipe smokers, cigar smokers, and users of smokeless tobacco, have a higher (4 to 10 times) rate of cancer of the mouth, tongue, and voice box.

Other Tobacco-Enhanced Cancers   In addition to drawing smoke into the lungs, tobacco users swallow saliva that contains an array of chemical compounds from tobacco. This saliva is retained in the stomach and then passes into the small intestine, where carcinogenic and toxic compounds in the saliva are absorbed into the blood. Contact between this material and the walls of the digestive organs leads to an enhanced risk of cancer in these areas of the gastrointestinal system. Additionally, the breakdown of carcinogens and toxic substances in the liver greatly increases the development of cancer in this critically important organ. Filtering of the blood by the kidneys eventually concentrates toxic materials in the urinary bladder, leading to increases in kidney and bladder cancer. Smoking may also accelerate the rate of pancreatic cancer development.

As reported earlier in the chapter, documents released in 1997 from within the tobacco industry clearly

---

Key Terms

embolism   A potentially fatal condition in which a circulating blood clot lodges in a smaller vessel.

mucus   Clear, sticky material produced by specialized cells within the mucous membranes of the body; mucus traps much of the suspended particulate matter within tobacco smoke.

cilia (sill ee uh**)**   Small, hairlike structures that extend from cells that line the air passages.

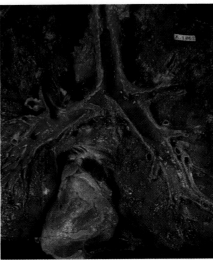

A healthy lung (right) versus the lung of a smoker (left). Smoking causes shortness of breath and "smoker's cough" and can lead to chronic obstructive lung disease.

show that the major tobacco companies were aware of tobacco's role in the development of cancer and had made a concerted effort to deprive the American public access to such knowledge.

Chronic Obstructive Lung Disease

Chronic obstructive lung disease (COLD), also known as chronic obstructive pulmonary disease (COPD), is a disorder in which the amount of air that flows in and out of the lungs becomes progressively limited. COLD is a disease state that is made up of two separate but related diseases: **chronic bronchitis** and **pulmonary emphysema.**

With chronic bronchitis, excess mucus is produced in response to the effects of smoking on airway tissue, and the walls of the bronchi become inflamed and infected. This produces a characteristic narrowing of the air passages. Breathing becomes difficult, and activity can be severely restricted. With cessation of smoking, chronic bronchitis is reversible.

Emphysema causes irreversible damage to the tiny air sacs of the lungs, the **alveoli.** Chest pressure builds when air becomes trapped by narrowed air passages (chronic bronchitis) and the thin-walled sacs rupture.

Key Terms

chronic bronchitis Persistent inflammation and infection of the smaller airways within the lungs.

pulmonary emphysema An irreversible disease process in which the alveoli are destroyed.

alveoli (al vee oh lie) Thin, saclike terminal ends of the airways; the sites at which gases are exchanged between the blood and inhaled air.

Emphysema patients lose the ability to ventilate fully. They feel as though they are suffocating. You may have seen people with this condition in malls and other locations as they walk slowly by, carrying or pulling their portable oxygen tanks.

More than 10 million Americans suffer from COLD. It is responsible for a greater limitation of physical activity than any other disease, including heart disease. COLD patients tend to die a very unpleasant, prolonged death, often from a general collapse of normal cardiorespiratory function that results in congestive heart failure (see Chapter 10).

Smoking and Body Weight

Although not perceived as a health problem by people who continue smoking in order to control weight, smoking does appear to minimize weight gain. In studies using identical twins, twins who smoked were six to eight pounds lighter than their nonsmoking siblings. Current understanding about why smoking results in lower body weight is less than complete. One factor may be an increase in basal metabolic rate (BMR) (see Chapter 6) brought about by the influence of nicotine on sympathetic nervous system function. However, in spite of the modest level of weight management provided by regular cigarette smoking, the overall increase in morbidity and premature death experienced by smokers is in no way "worth" the benefit of weighing a few pounds less.

Additional Health Concerns

In addition to the serious health problems stemming from tobacco use already described, other health-related changes are routinely seen. These include a generally poor state of nutrition, a decline in insulin sensitivity, a decline in short-term memory, the gradual loss of the sense of smell, and premature wrinkling of the skin. Tobacco users are also more likely to experience strokes (a potentially fatal condition), lose bone mass leading to osteoporosis, experience more back pain and muscle injury, and find that fractures heal more slowly. Further, smokers who have surgery spend more time in the recovery room. Additionally, smokers have a fourfold greater risk of developing serious gum (periodontal) disease, now thought to be a risk factor for cardiovascular disease. Also, smokers may need supplementation for two important water-soluble vitamins, vitamin C and vitamin B.

Combining Tobacco and Alcohol Use

Although there are exceptions to every generalization, it is very common to see tobacco and alcohol being used by the same people, often at the same time. Younger people who use both tobacco and alcohol are also more likely to use additional drugs. Accordingly, both tobacco and alcohol are considered *gateway drugs* because they are often introductory drugs that "open the door" for a more broadly based polydrug use pattern (see Chapter 7).

Beyond the potential for polydrug use initiated by the use of tobacco and alcohol is the simple reality that the use of both tobacco products and alcoholic beverages is associated with a wide array of illnesses and with premature death. As you have seen in this chapter and in Chapter 8 regarding alcohol use, the negative health impact of using both is significant. When use is combined, of course, the risks of living less healthfully and dying prematurely are accentuated.

Risks from Specific Tobacco Products

Most tobacco used today in the United States is in the form of standard machine-produced cigarettes. However, there are other forms of tobacco and variations on the standard cigarette in use by Americans. Tobacco products such as bidis, cigars, mentholated cigarettes, and smokeless tobacco have their own special health risks and regulatory challenges. New products developed by the tobacco industry have been marketed as being safer in some way than standard cigarettes, but there is no such thing as a safe cigarette.

Nonmanufactured Forms of Cigarettes

Although the vast majority of American cigarette smokers use familiar brand-name manufactured cigarettes produced in this country, segments of the smoking population use, to some degree, nonmanufactured cigarettes. Nonmanufactured cigarettes (or the supplies for

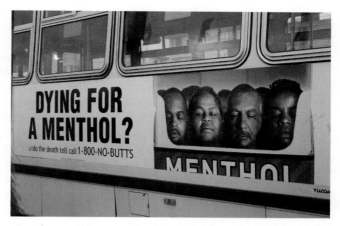

Mentholated cigarettes have been heavily marketed to African American smokers.

making them) generally are sold in places that might not enforce the legal age restrictions on purchasing manufactured cigarettes. Of course, in terms of dependence and harmfulness, these kinds of cigarettes are no better, if not worse, than manufactured cigarettes. Nonmanufactured cigarettes include roll-your-own cigarettes, bidis, and kreteks.

Bidis   Most often imported from the Indian subcontinent, bidis are small, handmade cigarettes consisting of a small amount of tobacco wrapped in a dried temburni or tendu leaf tied with a small length of colorful string. These cigarettes are particularly dangerous to health because the tobacco used is high in tar and nicotine and these cigarettes' inefficient combustion delivers a high level of carbon monoxide.

Kreteks   A popular cigarette from Indonesia, kreteks are hand-wrapped cigarettes made from clove-flavored tobacco or other highly flavored tobacco. A particular health danger of kreteks is that they contain an additive, eugenol, that produces an anesthetic effect in the throat, resulting in a tendency to inhale more deeply, thus delivering more tar and nicotine.

Mentholated Cigarettes

Of the 599 approved additives for use in the manufacturing of cigarettes, one of the most familiar, and most popular, is menthol—which imparts a unique taste and "cooling" sensation in the throat. Menthol-flavored cigarettes have been on the market for decades and have proven highly attractive to African American male smokers. Fortunately, the FDA is now preventing the sale of mentholated brands.

Health researchers have speculated that there is a relationship between the long-term smoking of mentholated cigarettes among African American males and

Water Pipes (Hookahs)

With origins in the Middle East, the hookah consists of a head into which prepackaged shredded tobacco leaves are combined with sweetened flavoring agents (collectively called shisha) and set atop lit charcoal. When one draws a breath through the end of the pipe, the shisha is ignited and smoke travels down a tube-like body of the pipe into a partially filled bowl of water where the smoke is cooled, released into the airspace above the water, and continues upward through the flexible hose's mouthpiece for movement into the airways. Multiple users may alternately use a single hose/mouthpiece or their own if the water pipe is designed accordingly.

Although the hookah has been in use for centuries, research into its unique potential for serious health-related consequences is a relatively new field of study. One of the many concerns surrounding hookah use is that single periods of use as long as 40 to 45 minutes can lead to a tobacco smoke exposure period approximating the smoke generated by nearly 100 cigarettes. This hyper-extended period of tobacco-based exposure generates nicotine levels 2.5 times higher than those associated with one episode of cigarette use. An analysis of hookah-generated smoke suggests a chemical composition very similar to that of cigarette smoke. When hookah users also smoke cigarettes, the combined use of both sources of tobacco leads to even higher levels of exposure to carcinogenic chemicals, carbon monoxide, and nicotine. The contribution of contaminants from the charcoal or woodchip-based fuel used to heat the tobacco mixture is unknown. The transmission of infectious agents through shared use of mouthpieces has also been reported.

Although hookah use may be socially integrative, it is far from being safer than cigarettes, and when combined with cigarette

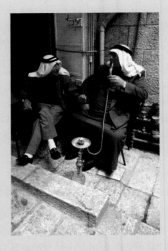

use the stage is set for potentially serious negative health consequences.

Source: American Lung Association, Tobacco Policy Trend Alert, 2007. An Emerging Deadly Trend: Waterpipe Tobacco Use. www.lungusa.org

---

the high level of lung cancer in this population. A meta-analysis of five large epidemiological studies of African American smokers concluded that the menthol in cigarette tobacco was not a factor in the higher rate of lung cancer in this population. Additionally, menthol did not increase puff number or puff volume, or result in elevated heart rates, higher levels of carbon monoxide in the blood, higher tar intake, or high levels of nicotine-breakdown by-products.

Despite the lack of association between mentholated cigarettes and lung cancer just reported, a recent study of cessation among African American light smokers indicates that it was more difficult to quit smoking mentholated brands than those without menthol. The underlying reason, however, is not fully understood.[29]

Pipe and Cigar Smoking

Many people believe that pipe or cigar smoking is a safe alternative to cigarette smoking. Unfortunately, this is not the case. All forms of tobacco present users with a series of health threats (see the box "Water Pipes [Hookahs]").

When compared with cigarette smokers, pipe and cigar smokers have cancer of the mouth, throat, larynx (voice box), and esophagus at the same frequency. Cigarette smokers are more likely than are pipe and cigar smokers to have lung cancer, cancer of the larynx, COLD, COPD, and heart disease. The cancer risk of death to pipe and cigar smokers is 4 times greater from lung cancer and 10 times greater from laryngeal cancer than it is for nonsmokers.

In comparison to cigarette smokers, pipe and cigar smokers are considerably fewer in number. Interestingly, cigar smoking enjoyed a resurgence through much of the 1990s. During 1998–1999 there was a substantial decline in sales of premium cigars, but beginning in 1999 an upward trend in cigar imports began. By 2005, 319.4 million cigars were imported into the United States. In comparison with the 2005 total, imports of cigars into the United States declined to 204.39 million in 2007.[30] Because many people smoke cigars only on occasions, it is difficult to determine the number of regular cigar smokers. That said, use is known to be highest among persons with only a high school diploma (4.4 percent) and lowest among college graduates (2.1 percent).[31]

Perhaps because of the increase in cigar smoking noted previously, the National Cancer Institute commissioned the first extensive study of regular cigar smoking. That report confirmed and expanded on the health risks identified in earlier smaller studies.

In response to the recognition of these risks, the FTC now requires that cigar manufacturers disclose the tobacco content and additives in their products. Most recently the FTC announced its intention of requiring five rotating health warnings to appear on cigars, including two that are currently agreed on by the FTC and major cigar manufacturers: *Cigars Are Not a Safe Alternative to Cigarettes* and *Cigar Smoking Can Cause Cancer of the Mouth and Throat, Even If You Don't Inhale.*

The federal government has also imposed a tax on premium cigars based on price and weight, which can be as high as $0.40.

Smokeless Tobacco Use

As the term implies, smokeless tobacco, such as Skoal and Copenhagen, is not burned; rather, it is placed into the mouth. Once in place, the physiologically active nicotine and other soluble compounds are absorbed through the mucous membranes and into the blood. Within a few minutes, chewing tobacco and snuff generate blood levels of nicotine in amounts equivalent to those seen in cigarette smokers.

Chewing tobacco is taken from its foil pouch, formed into a small ball (called a "wad," "chaw," or "chew"), and placed into the mouth. Once in place, the bolus of tobacco is sucked and occasionally chewed, but not swallowed.

Snuff, a more finely shredded smokeless tobacco product, is marketed in small round cans. Snuff is formed into a small mass (or "quid") for dipping or used in prepackaged pouches. The quid or pouch is placed between the jaw and the cheek; the user sucks the quid or pouch, then spits out the brown liquid. Snuff, as once used, was actually a powdered form of tobacco that was inhaled through the nose.

Although smokeless tobacco would seem to free the tobacco user from many of the risks associated with smoking, chewing and dipping are not without their own substantial risks. The presence of *leukoplakia* (white spots) and *erythroplakia* (red spots) on the tissues of the mouth indicate precancerous changes. In addition, an increase in **periodontal disease** (with the pulling away of the gums from the teeth, resulting in later tooth loss), the abrasive damage to the enamel of the teeth, and the high concentration of sugar in processed tobacco all contribute to dental problems among users of smokeless tobacco. In those who develop oral cancer, the risk is dramatically heightened if the cancer metastasizes from the site of origin in the mouth to the brain.

In addition to the damage done to the tissues of the mouth, the need to process the inadvertently swallowed saliva that contains dissolved carcinogens places both the digestive and urinary systems at risk of cancer.

In the opinion of health experts, the use of smokeless tobacco and its potential for life-threatening disease is very real and should not be disregarded. Consequently, television advertisements have been banned, and the following warnings have been placed in rotation on all smokeless tobacco products:

WARNING: THIS PRODUCT MAY CAUSE
MOUTH CANCER

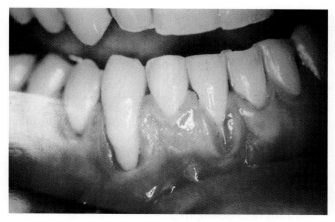

Use of smokeless tobacco leads to gum disease, tooth loss, and oral cancer.

WARNING: THIS PRODUCT MAY CAUSE GUM
DISEASE AND TOOTH LOSS

WARNING: THIS PRODUCT IS NOT A SAFE
ALTERNATIVE TO CIGARETTE
SMOKING

Smokeless tobacco is a dangerous product, and little doubt exists that continued use of tobacco in this form is a serious problem to health in all its dimensions. Fortunately, however, the percentage of adults using smokeless tobacco during the previous month is slightly less than reported for cigar use, and this figure too is inversely related to education level. Among high school graduates, 4.4 percent use smokeless tobacco, while only 2.1 percent of college graduates reported use during the previous month.

New Product Development

The old adage "When going gets tough, the tough get going" reflects the response the tobacco industry has undertaken given the restrictions placed on it through the Master Tobacco Settlement Agreement (see page 238). Additionally, the restrictions on places to smoke, smoking cessation due to health concerns, and the deaths of long-time users have added to its problems. However, in response to these hurdles, in addition to aggressive marketing and product placement, the industry has brought out countless new products in hopes of sustaining or building its nicotine-dependant customer base. The list of products that follows reflects a sample of their efforts:

> **Key Terms**
>
> **periodontal disease** Destruction of soft tissue and bone that surround the teeth.

1. Eclipse: A cigarette that uses a ceramic capsule to heat, rather than burn, tobacco. This product is advertised as being "the next best thing to quitting."
2. Accord: A "smoking system" that uses a battery-powered holder that reduces the production of sidestream smoke.
3. Omni, Quest, and Advance: Cigarettes with new or improved filtering systems that result in nearly nicotine-free or low carcinogenic smoke.
4. Reduced-ignition propensity (RIP) cigarettes: Cigarettes that are self-extinguishing if not actively smoked after a predetermined interval. Today three states require this technology for cigarettes sold within their boundaries.
5. Exotic blend cigarettes: Cigarettes flavored with "pleasing flavors" such as lime or mocha that are intended to mask the taste and smell of traditionally formulated blends of tobacco.
6. Menthol light cigarettes: Cigarettes with reduced levels of menthol developed to attract young adult smokers (YAS). Today mentholated brands, such as Marlboro Milds, account for slightly over one-fourth of all cigarette sales.
7. Superslim cigarettes: Long, very slim, cigarettes that are skillfully packaged in purse-sized packages (see photo on this page). This packaging innovation is clearly focused on the women's market segment. Similarly, Camel No 9 cigarettes feature a stylishly colored package that is, itself, a selling feature.

New FDA restrictions on the availability of exotic blends and mentholated cigarettes will likely rally the tobacco industry to heightened innovation.

Nontobacco Sources of Nicotine

Regardless of whether they are intended as aids to smoking cessation or only supplemental forms of nicotine for use when smoking is not permitted, numerous new forms of nicotine delivery systems have appeared in the marketplace in recent years. An area of growing concern is, of course, that these nontobacco delivery sources of nicotine could provide introductory exposure to nicotine, at a tragically early age, for the next generation of nicotine-dependent youth. Included among these nontobacco sources of nicotine are multiple flavors of nicotine suckers, nicotine-flavored gum, nicotine straws, nicotine-enhanced water (Nico Water), inhalers, sprays, drops, lozenges, and transdermal patches. To date, the pharmacological aspects of these products have yet to be addressed. As a result, these products currently enter the market as over-the-counter (OTC) products that are scrutinized with far less rigor than prescription medications and medical devices.

E-cigarettes are designed to look like and produce a similar experience to regular cigarettes, yet they contain

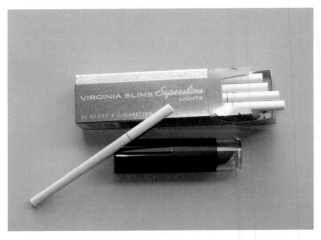

Always innovative, Virginia Slims modified its packaging to again remind women that smoking and thinness are synonymous, as well as salient components of the good life—although likely a shortened life.

no tobacco and produce no smoke. An e-cigarette comprises a battery chamber with a glowing indicator light on the end, followed by an atomizer, and an inhalation tip that contains a nicotine cartridge. When the user inhales, warmed air passes through the atomizer where liquid propylene glycol is vaporized into a fine mist that resembles tobacco smoke, then on through the inhalation tip, where synthetic nicotine is released into the "smoke." On exhalation, the purportedly nicotine-free vaporous "smoke" is released into the air. Early testing of e-cigarettes found some familiar carcinogenic agents of regular cigarettes within the vapor, in addition to a nicotine content that is higher than that of traditional tobacco cigarettes. Because these devices can be sold to anyone, including children, the product's appearance and nicotine content suggest a clear gateway device to the future use of real cigarettes, although their price is high at $50 to $200 for a starter kit. So far, the Food and Drug Administration has attempted to prevent foreign-manufactured versions of the product from entering the country, but they are still being sold domestically.

Nicotine Bridge Products In light of the rapidly expanding restrictions on smoking, how do smokers survive long hours in smoke-free environments? The answer, a nicotine bridge product: a gel, cream, or candy-like piece that contains nicotine for absorption through a body surface to maintain an adequate level of titration until cigarettes can be smoked. These OTC products, bearing names such as Ariva and Stonewall, are more convenient, affordable, tasty, or pleasant smelling than the nicotine step-down products used for smoking cessation. Of course, there is concern that these products enable smokers to continue their nicotine dependence in place of seeking cessation, and that they may be nicotine-introductory products if they become too readily available to children.

Whether defined as another form of smokeless tobacco or as a bridge product, the Swedish-developed product snus (sounds like *noose*) is being successfully marketed as Camel Snus. The use of snus closely resembles the use of other smokeless tobacco products that feature small pouches inserted between the gum line and the cheek. The attractive features of snus include a flavored taste (available in three flavors), an apparent lack of odor on the breath, and an absence of the need to spit the juicy extract that is common to other forms of spit tobacco. The tobacco used in snus is steam-pasteurized, a process that alters the nature of fluid extract in a manner allowing it to be "safely" swallowed. Although legally sold in this country, the European Union banned the sale of snus in 2004 over concerns about its potential for adverse health influences.

Yet to come to the market but reportedly under development are dissolvable nicotine-containing strips (akin to breath-freshening strips), as well as a variety of delivery devices that will, most likely, serve the tobacco industry well as it attempts to toughen its hold on the current nicotine-dependent population and build its base for the future.

Smoking and Reproduction

In all its dimensions, the reproductive process is impaired by the use of tobacco, particularly cigarette smoking and environmental tobacco smoke in close proximity to pregnant women.[32, 33] Problems can be found in association with infertility, problem pregnancy, breast-feeding, and the health of the newborn. So broadly based are reproductive problems and smoking that the term *fetal tobacco syndrome* or *fetal smoking syndrome* is regularly used in clinical medicine. Some physicians even define a fetus being carried by a smoker as a "smoker" and, upon birth, as a "former smoker."

Infertility

Recent research indicates that cigarette smoking by both men and women can reduce levels of fertility. Among men, smoking adversely affects blood flow to erectile tissue, reduces sperm motility, and alters sperm shape, and it causes an overall decrease in the number of viable sperm. Among women, the effects of smoking are seen in terms of abnormal ovum formation, including a lessened ability on the part of the egg to prevent polyspermia, or the fertilization by multiple sperm. Smoking also negatively influences estrogen levels, resulting in underdevelopment of the uterine wall and ineffective implantation of the fertilized ovum. Lower levels of estrogen may also influence the rate of transit of the fertilized egg through the fallopian tube, making it arrive in the uterus too early for successful implantation or, in some cases, restricting movement to the point that an **ectopic, or tubal, pregnancy** may develop. Also, the early onset of menopause is associated with smoking.

Although causative pathways remain somewhat unclear, the influences of smoking are noted in two aspects of male infertility, sperm degradation and erectile dysfunction. In the former case, several chemicals in tobacco smoke are able to cross the blood-testis barrier and structurally alter the DNA of the genetic material within the sperm. The presence of abnormal sperm in the male compromises the chances of fertilization. In erectile dysfunction, smoking, most likely through the effects of nicotine on blood-flow dynamics, decreases blood flow into the erectile tissues of the penile shaft, resulting in the inability to obtain or sustain an erection.[34, 35]

Problem Pregnancy

The harmful effects of tobacco smoke on the course of pregnancy are principally the result of the carbon monoxide and nicotine to which the mother and her fetus are exposed. Carbon monoxide from the incomplete oxidation of tobacco is carried in the maternal blood to the placenta, where it diffuses across the placental barrier and enters the fetal circulation. Once in the fetal blood, the carbon monoxide bonds with the fetal hemoglobin to form fetal carboxyhemoglobin. As a result of this exposure to carbon monoxide, the fetus is progressively deprived of normal oxygen transport and eventually becomes compromised by chronic **hypoxia.**

Nicotine also exerts its influence on the developing fetus. Thermographs of the placenta and fetus show signs of marked vasoconstriction within a few seconds after inhalation by the mother. This constriction further reduces the oxygen supply, resulting in hypoxia. In addition, nicotine stimulates the mother's stress response, placing the mother and fetus under the potentially harmful influence of elevated epinephrine and corticoid levels (see Chapter 3). Any fetus exposed to all of these agents is more likely to be miscarried, stillborn, or born prematurely. Even when carried to term, children born to mothers who smoked during pregnancy have lower birth weights and may show other signs of a stressful intra-uterine life.

Key Terms

ectopic (tubal) pregnancy Pregnancy resulting from the implantation of the fertilized ovum within the inner wall of the fallopian tube.

hypoxia Oxygenation deprivation at the cellular level.

Breast-Feeding

Women who breast-feed their infants and continue to smoke continue to expose their children to the harmful effects of tobacco smoke. It is well recognized that nicotine appears in breast milk and thus is capable of exerting its vasoconstricting and stress-response influences on nursing infants. Mothers who stop smoking during pregnancy should be encouraged to continue to refrain from smoking while they are breast-feeding.

Neonatal Health Problems

Babies born to women who smoked during pregnancy are, on average, shorter and have a lower birth weight than do children born to nonsmoking mothers. During the earliest months of life, babies born to mothers who smoke experience an elevated rate of death caused by sudden infant death syndrome (SIDS). Statistics also show that infants are more likely to develop chronic respiratory problems, have more frequent colic, be hospitalized, and have poorer overall health during their early years of life. Problems such as those just mentioned may also be seen in children of nonsmoking mothers, when they were exposed prenatally to environmental tobacco smoke. In addition, environmental tobacco smoke exposure extending beyond the home and into the workplace may increase the probability of problem pregnancies and neonatal health problems. Recently, the interest in the effects of tobacco smoke on pregnancy has been extended to include behavioral differences in children born to women who smoked during pregnancy.

Parenting, in the sense of assuming responsibility for the well-being of children, does not begin at birth, but during the prenatal period. In the case of smoking, this is especially true. Pregnant women who continue smoking are disregarding the well-being of the children they are carrying. Other family members, friends, and coworkers who subject pregnant women to cigarette, pipe, or cigar smoke are, in a sense, exhibiting their own disregard for the health of the next generation.

Key Terms

mainstream smoke Smoke inhaled and then exhaled by a smoker.

sidestream smoke Smoke that comes from the burning end of a cigarette, pipe, or cigar.

environmental tobacco smoke Tobacco smoke, regardless of its source, that stays within a common source of air.

Involuntary (Passive) Smoking

The smoke generated by the burning of tobacco can be classified as either **mainstream smoke** (the smoke inhaled and then exhaled by the smoker) or **sidestream smoke** (the smoke that comes from the burning end of the cigarette, pipe, or cigar that simply disperses into the air without being inhaled by the smoker). When either form of tobacco smoke is diluted and stays within a common source of air, it can eventually be referred to as **environmental tobacco smoke.** All three forms of tobacco smoke lead to involuntary or passive smoking and can present health problems for both nonsmokers and smokers.

Surprisingly, mainstream smoke makes up only 15 percent of our exposure to the harmful substances associated with involuntary smoking. Sidestream smoke is responsible for 85 percent of the harmful substances associated with secondhand smoke exposure. Because it is not filtered by the tobacco, the filter, or the smoker's body, sidestream smoke contains more free nicotine and produces higher yields of carbon dioxide and carbon monoxide. Much to the detriment of nonsmokers, sidestream smoke has a much higher quantity of highly carcinogenic compounds, called *N-nitrosamines,* than mainstream smoke has.

Current scientific opinion suggests that smokers and nonsmokers are exposed to very much the same smoke when tobacco is used within a common airspace. The important difference is the quantity of smoke inhaled by smokers and nonsmokers. It is likely that for each pack of cigarettes smoked by a smoker, nonsmokers who must share a common air supply with the smokers involuntarily smoke the equivalent of three to five cigarettes per day. Even today, because of the small size of the particles produced by burning tobacco, environmental tobacco smoke cannot be completely removed from a workplace, restaurant, or shopping mall by the most effective ventilation system.

Health Risks of Passive Smoking

Recently reported research indicates that involuntary smoke exposure may be responsible for 35,000 to 40,000 premature deaths per year from heart disease among nonsmokers in the United States.[36] Other estimates range upward to 53,000 premature deaths when lung cancer and COPD are included. In addition, large numbers of people exposed to involuntary smoke develop eye irritation, nasal symptoms, headaches, and a cough. Furthermore, most nonsmokers dislike the odor of tobacco smoke.

Involuntary smoking poses some threats to nonsmokers within residential settings. Spouses and children of smokers are at greatest risk for involuntary smoking. Scientific studies suggest that nonsmokers married to

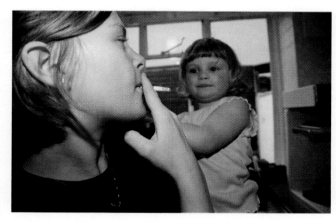

Children exposed to environmental tobacco smoke are at increased risk for wheezing, ear infections, bronchitis, and pneumonia.

smokers are more likely to experience heart attacks than nonsmoking spouses of nonsmokers. This said, a recent meta-analysis of earlier meta-analyses concludes that involuntary smoking carries an increased risk for cardiovascular disease, though the risk for a nonsmoking spouse is less than was once reported.

In spite of what may or may not be the effects of passive smoking on the nonsmoking partners of smokers, the effects of environmental tobacco smoke on the health of children seems well established. The children of parents who smoke are twice as likely as children of nonsmoking parents to experience bronchitis or pneumonia during the first year of life. In addition, throughout childhood these children will experience more wheezing, coughing, and sputum production than will children whose parents do not smoke. Otitis media (middle-ear infection), one of the most frequently seen conditions in pediatric medicine, is also significantly more common in children under age 3 who reside with one or more adults who smoke.

Regarding the relationship between exposure to environmental tobacco and SIDS, a comprehensive reassessment (meta-analysis) raised important issues about the methodology of nearly 60 earlier studies on this issue. In particular, research needs to better separate the influences of maternal smoking during pregnancy, maternal smoking after pregnancy (in the months immediately following delivery), and other sources of environmental tobacco during the prenatal and postnatal periods.[37]

The Cost of Smoking

The 20 percent of the U.S. population that smoke inflict a substantial cost on their nonsmoking neighbors in a multiplicity of ways. However, in more personal ways,

smokers also accrue costs that are less easily documented. Smokers lose some independence (nicotine-based needs will structure many aspects of day-to-day living) and may be socially rejected by the nonsmoking majority, including the significant number of young adults who do not want smokers as their life partners (see the box "The Hidden Cost of Smoking"). Smokers may experience subtle forms of discrimination when they search for employment (smokers miss more days of work, waste an hour per day on smoking breaks, and eventually raise their employer's health insurance expenditures). Smokers often receive lower trade-ins on their vehicles (double detailing is expensive to the dealer) and have a harder time selling their smoke-saturated houses (even freshly baked bread won't hide the odorous evidence that smokers have lived in the house).

Smokers' contention that "smoking only hurts smokers" is patently untrue. In fact, the economic costs alone should stimulate those smokers reading this chapter to pay close attention to the discussion of quitting at the end of this chapter.

Stopping What You Started

Experts in health behavior contend that before people will discontinue harmful health behaviors, such as tobacco use, they must appreciate fully what they are expecting of themselves. This understanding grows in relation to the following:

1. *Knowledge* about the health risks associated with tobacco use
2. *Recognition* that these health risks are applicable to all tobacco users
3. *Familiarity* with steps that can be taken to eliminate or reduce these risks
4. *Belief* that the benefits to be gained by no longer using tobacco will outweigh the pleasures gained through the use of tobacco
5. *Certainty* that one can start and maintain the behaviors required to stop or reduce the use of tobacco

These steps combine both knowledge and desire (or motivation). Being knowledgeable about risks, however, will not always stop behaviors that involve varying degrees of psychological and physical dependence. The 75 percent failure rate thought to be common among tobacco-cessation programs suggests that the motivation is not easy to achieve or maintain. In fact, on the basis of information reported by the Hazelden Foundation, for persons who are successful in quitting, approximately 18.6 years elapse between the first attempt to stop and actual quitting. The many health benefits of quitting smoking are shown in Figure 9-3.

In an introductory college course, such as your personal health course, instructors sometimes must set aside certain chapters in the interest of time, or by the time you have reached this chapter, an earlier chapter's content may be less than clearly recalled. Regardless, consideration of Figure 1-2 on page 15 will be helpful.

Note and recall that the figure focuses on the development of an *earned* sense of well-being resulting from an individual's ability to engage in activities that fulfill role obligations, while making progress in meeting the developmental expectations held by society for persons in that particular life cycle stage. It is, in fact, a central contention of your textbook that this quest for a sense of well-being (or, later in life, referred to as a *sense of life satisfaction*) results in a positive emotional state and, more succinctly, relates to an individual's search for life's meaning, or in meeting a supreme being's or supernatural personality's intentions for your life.

Assuming that the figure's contention seems plausible to you, then raise for serious consideration this question: In what ways can anyone contend that smoking makes the quest for a sense

of well-being, the fulfillment of role obligations, and meeting of society's developmental expectations more easily accomplished or less detrimental to one's self and the well-being of others? More specifically, are children well served by their parents' smoking? Are employers pleased with the increased demands that smokers will eventually make on their business costs? Are smokers more ideal life partners than similar persons who do not smoke? Is a frantic midnight search for a 24-hour convenience store at which to buy cigarettes a reflection of the independence that young adults are in search of? Is purposely shortening one's life a positive reflection of a maturing sense of self-responsibility that society expects from early young adults? Is a belief that we are created in God's image well articulated by the smoker's dependency and damaging influence on others? The list could go on and on, but common sense suggests that smokers are in a minority with whom the majority wants less and less direct or even indirect physical contact.

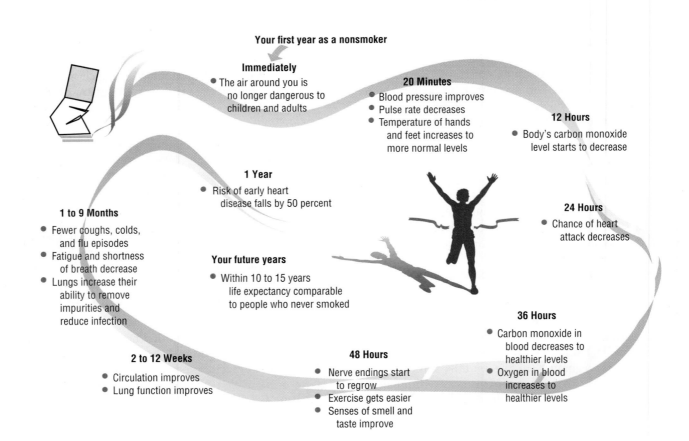

Your first year as a nonsmoker

Immediately
- The air around you is no longer dangerous to children and adults

20 Minutes
- Blood pressure improves
- Pulse rate decreases
- Temperature of hands and feet increases to more normal levels

12 Hours
- Body's carbon monoxide level starts to decrease

1 Year
- Risk of early heart disease falls by 50 percent

1 to 9 Months
- Fewer coughs, colds, and flu episodes
- Fatigue and shortness of breath decrease
- Lungs increase their ability to remove impurities and reduce infection

Your future years
- Within 10 to 15 years life expectancy comparable to people who never smoked

24 Hours
- Chance of heart attack decreases

36 Hours
- Carbon monoxide in blood decreases to healthier levels
- Oxygen in blood increases to healthier levels

2 to 12 Weeks
- Circulation improves
- Lung function improves

48 Hours
- Nerve endings start to regrow
- Exercise gets easier
- Senses of smell and taste improve

Figure 9-3 Benefits of Quitting   The health benefits of quitting smoking begin immediately and become more significant the longer you stay smoke-free.

Sources: Adapted from American Cancer Society, Guide to Quitting Smoking, http://www.cancer.org/docroot/PED/content/PED_10_13X_Guide_for_Quitting_Smoking.asp. October 2006; American Lung Association, Quit Smoking Benefits. http://www.lungusa.org/site/pp.asp?c=dvLUK900&b=33568, October 2007.

Countdown to Quit Day: A Plan for Smoking Cessation

I started smoking at parties to feel more relaxed. Now I smoke at least a pack a day, and I'm afraid I'm hooked for life. How do I get myself off tobacco?

Make a decision to quit smoking on a particular day during the next week. Then use the following steps to begin preparing yourself for that day.

Five Days Before Quit Day

- Keep a daylong record of each cigarette you smoke. List the time you smoked, whom you were with, and why you decided to light up (for example, for stimulation, tension reduction, or social pleasure, or because you had a craving or wanted something to do with your hands). Once you know why you smoke, you can plan intervention strategies for use during the two-minute periods of craving you will feel during the first weeks of your smoke-free life.
- Contact your physician to help you decide whether to use prescription or OTC nicotine-replacement therapy. Make sure you understand all directions for its safe and effective use.
- Draw up a contract in which you formally state your intention to quit smoking. Sign and date the contract and clearly display it in your home or workplace.

Four Days Before Quit Day

- Solicit support from family, friends, and coworkers by sharing your intention with them and asking for their help and encouragement.
- Organize your intervention strategies and assemble needed supplies, such as gum, bottled water, diet soda, handwork (for example, needlepoint or wood carving), and walking shoes.

Three Days Before Quit Day

- Review your quitting contract and touch bases with several people in your support group to bolster your resolve.
- Study all nicotine-replacement-therapy product information and any material supplied by your physician.
- Continue preparing your intervention supplies.

- Reschedule your personal calendar and work schedule to minimize situations that could tempt you to smoke during the first several days of your smoke-free life.

Two Days Before Quit Day

- Continue or revisit any earlier tasks that you have not yet finished.
- Practice your intervention strategies as appropriate. For example, map out a safe walking route and practice your deep-breathing exercises.
- Obtain a large glass or other container, such as an empty milk jug, that will serve as a bank into which you will deposit daily the money that you would have otherwise spent on cigarettes.
- If you feel comfortable doing so, construct a yard sign to inform outsiders that your home is a smoke-free environment and to report your daily success toward a smoke-free life.
- Smoke-proof your home and workplace by removing and destroying all materials and supplies associated with tobacco use, saving only enough tobacco products needed for today and tomorrow.

One Day Before Quit Day

- Complete all preparations described, including the almost total removal and destruction of smoking-related materials.
- As the end of the day approaches, review your contract and call a few people in your support network for last-minute words of encouragement.
- Smoke your last cigarette and flush any remaining cigarettes down the toilet.
- Begin your nicotine-replacement therapy as directed by your physician or by product insert information.
- Publicly display your yard sign, if you decided to make one.
- Retire for the night and await your rebirth in the morning as a former smoker.

InfoLinks

www.smokefree.gov

Smoking Cessation Programs

A variety of smoking cessation programs exist, including those using highly organized formats, with or without the use of prescription or OTC nicotine replacement systems. In past years, most people who managed to quit smoking each year did so by throwing away their cigarettes (going cold turkey) and paying the physical and emotional price of waiting for their bodies to adjust to life without nicotine. Today, however, the use of nicotine replacement products in combination with external smoking cessation approaches, such as those

described later in this chapter, or the use of prescription medication is more common. The box "Countdown to Quit Day" highlights strategies to help smokers prepare to quit.

Programs to help people stop their tobacco use are available in a variety of formats, including educational programs, behavior modification, aversive conditioning, hypnosis, acupuncture, and various combinations of these approaches (see the box "Hypnotism" on page 262). Programs are offered in both individual and group settings and are operated by hospitals, universities,

Hypnotism: A Solution for Smokers?

In addition to all of the other aids to smoking cessation that are discussed in this chapter, what is the role of hypnosis in helping smokers break away from their dependence on nicotine? Unfortunately, the question is not easily answered because hypnosis is a relatively minor player in smoking cessation aids, and research to date is relatively small and often conflicting. Additionally, there is uncertainty and disagreement within the hypnotic community itself, in terms of both technique and the underlying psycho-physiological dynamic that occurs, further clouding an understanding of the nature of hypnosis and the hypnotic state. This said, today, when practiced by medically trained practitioners, such as psychiatrists, hypnosis can be placed among the various other forms of psychotherapy currently practiced. In addition, self-hypnosis techniques using various approaches can move hypnosis out of the clinical realm and into the confines of the self-care movement.

Although great variability in theory and technique exists today, the basis of hypnosis can be traced back to at least the late eighteenth century and the eye-fixation method of hypnosis pioneered by James Braid. In this approach to induction, the subject is instructed to concentrate on a bright shiny object that is positioned by the hypnotist between 10 and 15 inches away, with or without a pendulum-like movement. As the subject becomes increasingly fixated on the object, the hypnotist, using eye pupil changes in the subject's eyes as a guide, slowly moves the hand, with fingers extended, closer and closer to the subject's eyes. In the hypnotically susceptible adult, the eyelids slowly close as the subject moves into hypnotic sleep. If capable of reaching this state, the subject is determined to be hypnotized and, thus, susceptible to suggestions for changes in behavior or perception, in this case the discontinued need for nicotine-containing products. If the subject is initially incapable of reaching this highly relaxed state, another attempt may be made, but multiple attempts are rarely undertaken.

As noted earlier, the efficacy of hypnosis is consistently in question. A host of potential problems exist in designing well-controlled studies, including the tendency to rely on self-reporting of continued cessation of smoking, the limited use of laboratory-based assessments such as blood serum measurements of carbon monoxide levels or other nicotine substrates, and the unreported uses of other cessation techniques in addition to having been hypnotized. In other studies, however, hypnosis has been shown to be equal to or better than other recognized approaches.

Sources: Ahijevych K, et al. Descriptive Outcomes of the American Lung Association of Ohio Hypnotherapy Smoking Cessation program. *International Journal of Clinical and Experimental Hypnosis,* 48(4), 374–387, October 2000; Elkins G, et al. Intensive Hypnotherapy for Smoking Cessation: A Prospective Study. *International Journal of Clinical and Experimental Hypnosis,* 54(3), 303–315, July 2006.

health departments, voluntary health agencies, churches, and private practitioners. The better programs will have limited success rates—20 to 50 percent as measured over one year (with self-reporting), whereas the remainder will have even poorer results. If results are monitored using the assessment of nicotine-breakdown products in the blood, the effectiveness rate of these programs falls even lower, as some "successful" self-reporters are not completely honest in their reporting of cessation. When followed beyond one year, the success of smoking cessation efforts continues to drop, particularly with self-directed efforts (without directed involvement of physicians or group-based leadership), often reaching levels as low as 5 percent.

Although lying outside of most smoking cessation programs, two additional resources found effective in aiding smokers to both attempt and succeed at cessation are increased taxes on cigarettes and the involvement of family, friends, and coworkers. In a study of attrition from ongoing cessation programs, it was noticed that when a spouse (67%), friend (36%), coworker in a small firm (34%), or sibling (25%) has quit or will join a program with a smoker, completion of the program increased.[38]

A second effective tool for moving smokers into cessation programs was clearly effective in New York state when the per pack state tax on cigarettes was increased from $1.25 per pack to $2.75, raising the price of cigarettes in some areas of the state into the $6.00 to $7.00 range and to nearly $10 per pack in New York City. Further, during the first month of President Obama's administration, a 62-cent increase in the federal tobacco tax was imposed on each pack of cigarettes. This was done to gain revenue to expand the provision of affordable health care insurance for 11 million children. We can hope this additional layer of taxation will encourage yet more potential smokers and young smokers to reconsider a trip into dependency.

In a recent meta-analysis of smoking cessation program success involving African Americans, it was found that there is no statistically significant difference between the success of this racial group and others. Of interest, however, was a finding that church-based programs might be more successful for smoking cessation than previously recognized.

Medically Managed Smoking Cessation

Having given a general overview of smoking cessation, your text will give more detailed attention to medically managed cessation programs, such as those conducted

Table 9.4 R$_x$ and OTC Medications for Smoking Cessation

	Advantages	Disadvantages	Dosing Schedule
Non-nicotine-based therapy			
Bupropion HCl Wellbutrin Zyban	Nonnicotine. May be used in combination with patch for greater efficacy. Provides therapy for comorbid depression (anti-smoking effect independent of this).	Use relatively contraindicated in smokers with a history of seizures, head trauma, heavy alcohol abuse, or anorexia. Multiple drug-drug interactions, esp. with anti-HIV meds.	300 mg/day (in 2 divided doses to minimize side effects). Start **two weeks** before anticipated quit date and continue for 7 to 12 weeks. Optimal duration of treatment not well defined.
Varenicline Chantix	Nonnicotine	Not assessed in combination with other medications. Cautionary labeling due to suicidal thoughts and vivid dreams.*	One 0.5 mg tablet daily for three days, one 0.5 mg tablet twice daily for the next four days, one 1 mg tablet twice daily starting at day seven.
Nicotine replacement			
Nicotine polacrilex (gum or lozenge)	Accessible over-the-counter. May satisfy oral behavior.	Low nicotine levels. Requires multiple dosing, thus, compliance may be affected.	Start on quit date <25 cigarettes/day use: 2 mg tab. ≥25 cigarettes/day use: 4 mg tab. 1 to 2 tab/hour for 6 weeks, taper over 6 weeks.
Nicotine patch	Easy dosing (QD) may improve compliance over-the-counter.	Local skin irritation in up to 50 percent of users. Insomnia with 24-hour dosing. Requires 30 to 60 minutes for maximum effect.	Precaution: pregnant women (Category D), smokers with recent MI (within 4 weeks), or serious arrhythmia. Nicoderm CQ: 21 mg/day for 6 weeks, then 14 mg/day for 2 weeks, then 7 mg/day for 2 weeks (may be used for either 24 or 16 hours to avoid insomnia). Nicotrol: Use single-dose patch for 16 hours/day for 6 weeks (no tapering recommended).
Nicotine nasal spray	Higher/quicker nicotine levels.	Initial adverse effects (nasal and throat irritation, sneezing, rhinorrhea, coughing, and eye irritation) may discourage users before tolerance occurs.	1 to 2 doses per hour for 3 months. Most patients require from 7 to 40 sprays over 24 hours.
Nicotine inhaler	Substitutes for behavioral aspects of smoking.	Low nicotine levels similar to those achieved with gum.	10 mg cartridges used over 20 minutes. Six to 16 cartridges per day.

* Chantix (varenicline) label update to include warning for neuropsychiatric symptoms.
Doctor's Guide (Personal Edition), January 18, 2008. Supplied news release by Pfizer, Inc.
Source: Up To Date, Inc. © 2009

by clinics, hospitals, or your university's student health center. Because they have a medical affiliation, these programs have access to prescription medication, in addition to OTC products, nutritional and exercise expertise, and affiliated behavior therapy. The prescription medications are a key component to these programs and can be found (by classification) in Table 9-4.

Nonnicotine-based medications are those medications that influence the production, diffusion, or reuptake of neurotransmitters with the central nervous system (CNS) that are associated with feelings of hunger, satiety, and the CNS's neurological reward centers. A simple description of synaptic function can be found in Chapter 7. Medication influencing neurotransmitter function includes many antidepressants, including Zyban, Wellbutrin, and Prozac, among others.

A relative newcomer to this group (brand name Chantix) is not a neurotransmitter-influencing medication, such as those just described, but rather a drug that blocks the ability of nicotine receptors in various tissues of the body to recognize the presence of nicotine, thus depriving it of exerting its dependence-producing potential. Although Chantix is effective in cessation from nicotine, potentially serious issues related to suicidal

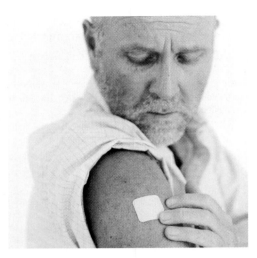

Nicotine patches are one form of nicotine replacement therapy available to help smokers quit.

thoughts and vivid dreams have resulted in Pfizer, Inc. adding cautionary information to the drug's labeling regarding the need to more fully assess its appropriateness for particular individuals.

Nicotine replacement medications, the second category in Table 9.4, comprise a variety of products, some obtainable only by prescription and others available as OTC products, intended to allow a controlled and less harmful relationship with nicotine than that associated with tobacco products. This form of nicotine replacement therapy (NRT) facilitates a gradual turning down of nicotine dependence, until the individual is virtually free of a tissue-based dependence on tobacco products. A variety of delivery systems are used in NRT, including gum, lozenge, transdermal patches, nasal sprays, and inhalers.

People who are concerned that NRT is simply a trade-off of dependences should remember that while using the therapy the former smoker is no longer being exposed to carbon monoxide and carcinogens, and the step-down feature allows for a gradual return to a totally nicotine-free lifestyle. Therefore, a short period of cross-addiction should be seen as an acceptable cost to recovery.

Prescription Medications Based on Nicotine Receptor Inhibitors

Several newer medications have been recently approved or are still in controlled trials. One such medication,

developed in Europe, is marketed in the United States as Chantix (varenicline). Chantix influences nervous system receptors for nicotine to level out the peaks and valleys normally associated with smoking. This leveling-out aids cessation by diminishing the "highly satisfying" character of the first inhalation following a low-nicotine valley, and by minimizing the discomfort experienced while in a state of nicotine depletion (a valley). Recall that earlier in the chapter the potential for suicidal thoughts and vivid dreams with the use of Chantix led the FDA to require a black box label to be added to the packaging of this smoking cessation drug.

A second medication, now on the first track for approval, is another European drug, rimonabant, that will be marketed in the United States as Acomplia. This medication initially was developed to aid in weight loss, but it has shown efficacy in aiding smoking cessation.

Anti-Smoking Vaccines

The goal of anti-smoking vaccines is to prevent nicotine from reaching nicotine receptors in the brain by conditioning the immune system to attack the nicotine molecules. Research in vaccine development has begun to bear fruit. Clinical trials are currently under way on a vaccine named NicVAX.[39] In these trials, subjects will receive four or five immunization shots over a period of many weeks. In response, the immune system should eventually begin producing antibodies (see Chapter 12) against nicotine. At the 2008 meeting of the American Heart Association, a report on the far from complete clinical trials of NicVAX indicated that the experimental groups displayed higher levels of antibodies to nicotine than did those given placebo injections, leaving the researchers cautiously optimistic about longer-term trials. Still, NicVAX and other vaccines in development need extensively more assessment. At least four other vaccines are in earlier stages of development.

Despite the satisfaction of the dependence that continued smoking brings, approximately 80 percent of adult smokers have, on at least one occasion, expressed a desire to quit, and the majority of these have actually attempted to become nonsmokers. Today, with the over-the-counter availability of transdermal nicotine patches, nicotine-containing gum, prescription medications such as antidepressants, nicotine inhalers, and nicotine receptor inhibitors, the number of smokers making concerted and repeated attempts to stop smoking is up considerably over that seen in the past. It therefore seems apparent that tobacco use is a source of **dissonance.** This dissonance stems from the need to deal emotionally with a behavior that is both highly enjoyable and highly dangerous but known to be difficult to stop. The degree to which this dissonance exists probably varies from user to user.

Tobacco Use: A Question of Rights

For those readers who have found themselves involved (or nearly so) in confrontation situations involving smokers' versus nonsmokers' rights, we hope the following section allows you to see more clearly the positions that you have taken. For those who have somehow remained removed from this discussion, consideration of these issues now may be good preparation for the future. Regardless, consider these two important questions:

1. To what extent should smokers be allowed to pollute the air and endanger the health of nonsmokers?
2. To what extent should nonsmokers be allowed to restrict the personal freedom of smokers, particularly since tobacco products are sold legally?

At this time, answers to these questions are only partially available, but one trend is developing: the tobacco user is being forced to give ground to the nonsmoker. Today, in fact, it is becoming more a matter of where the smoker will be allowed to smoke, rather than a matter of where smoking will be restricted. Smoking is currently becoming less and less tolerated. The health concerns of the majority are prevailing over the dependence needs of the minority.

 TALKING POINTS You're having a discussion with a friend about life insurance and mention that you get a 10 percent reduction in your annual premium because you're a nonsmoker. Your friend, who is a smoker, becomes annoyed and says that this is just one example of how smokers are penalized. How would you respond?

Taking Charge of Your Health

- Commit yourself to establishing a smoke-free environment in the places where you live, work, study, and recreate.

- Support friends and acquaintances who are trying to become smoke-free.

- Support legislative efforts, at all levels of government, to reduce your exposure to environmental tobacco smoke.

- Be civil toward tobacco users in public spaces, but respond assertively if they infringe on smoke-free spaces.

- Support agencies and organizations committed to reducing tobacco use among young people through education and intervention.

SUMMARY

- The percentage of American adults who smoke is continuing to decline.
- In spite of a reversal on the part of more recent college graduates, cigarette smoking has traditionally been inversely related to the level of formal education.
- A number of demographic variables influence the incidence of tobacco use.
- The tobacco industry continues to aggressively market its products to potential smokers.
- Multiple theories regarding nicotine's role in dependence have been advanced, including a better understanding of the proportional influences of genetics, environment, and personality.
- Nicotine exerts acute effects both within the central nervous system and on a variety of other tissues and organs.
- Tobacco smoke can be divided into gaseous and particulate phases. Each phase has its unique chemical composition.
- Thousands of chemical components and hundreds of carcinogenic agents are found in tobacco smoke.
- Nicotine and carbon monoxide have predictable effects on the function of the cardiovascular system.

- The development of nearly one-third of all cancers can be attributed to tobacco use, and virtually every form of cancer is found more frequently in smokers than in nonsmokers.
- Chronic obstructive lung disease (COLD), also called chronic obstructive pulmonary disease (COPD), is a likely consequence of long-term cigarette smoking, with early symptoms appearing shortly after beginning regular smoking.
- Smoking alters normal structure and function of the body, as seen in a wide variety of noncardiovascular and noncancerous conditions, such as infertility, problem pregnancy, and neonatal health concerns. Additional health concerns include the diminished ability to smell, periodontal disease, vitamin inadequacies, and bone loss leading to osteoporosis.
- The use of smokeless tobacco carries its own health risks, including oral cancer.
- The presence of secondhand smoke results in involuntary (or passive) smoking by those who must share a common air source with smokers.
- Stopping smoking can be undertaken in several ways.

REVIEW QUESTIONS

1. What percentage of the American adult population smoke? In what direction has change been occurring?
2. What is the current direction that adolescent smoking is taking?
3. What was the outcome of the class action suit brought by all states, and what was the effect of the Master Settlement Agreement (1999) on the ability of the tobacco industry to market its products?
4. What are the two principal dimensions of nicotine dependence? What are specific aspects seen within physical dependence?
5. Identify each of the theories of nicotine dependence discussed in the chapter.
6. How do modeling and manipulation explain the development of emotional dependence on tobacco?
7. In the amount consumed by the typical smoker, what is the effect of nicotine on central nervous system function? How does this differ in chain smokers?
8. What effects does nicotine have on the body outside of the central nervous system? How does the influence of nicotine resemble that associated with the stress response?
9. What is the principal effect of carbon monoxide on cardiac function?
10. What influences does passive smoking have on nonsmoking adult partners of smokers? On their children?
11. How is the federal government attempting to limit the exposure that children and adolescents currently have to tobacco products and tobacco advertisements?
12. In comparison to cigarettes, what health risks are associated with pipe and cigar smoking?
13. How might concerned parents begin to "tobacco proof" their children to keep them from becoming smokers in the future?
14. What prescription and OTC products are now available to assist smokers in quitting?
15. What percentage of smokers are able to quit, and what is the best way to confirm that quitting has occurred?

ANSWERS TO THE "WHAT DO YOU KNOW?" QUIZ

1. True   2. False   3. True   4. False   5. False   6. False   7. True

Visit the Online Learning Center (**www.mhhe.com/payne11e**), where you will find tools to help you improve your grade including practice quizzes, key terms flashcards, audio chapter summaries for your MP3 player, and many other study aids.

SOURCE NOTES

1. Centers for Disease Control and Prevention (CDC). *Behavioral Risk Factor Surveillance System Survey Data, 2007.* Atlanta: Department of Health and Human Services, 2007.
2. *Adult Smoking by Sex, 2007—Virgin Islands.* Kaiser State Health Facts. www.statehealthfacts.org/profileind.jsp?rgn=56@cat=2&ind=81
3. State-Specific Prevalence of Current Cigarette Smoking Among Adults and Second-Hand Rules and Policies in Home and Workplaces—United States, 2005. *Morbidity and Mortality Weekly,* 55(42), 1148–1151, Table 2, October 27, 2006.
4. Aldworth J, et al. 2006. *Results from the 2005 National Survey on Drug Use and Health: National Findings.* SAMHSA. Department of Health and Human Services, DHHS Publication No. SMA 06-4194.
5. Centers for Disease Control and Prevention (CDC). Your Risk Behavior Surveillance—United States, 2007. *Morbidity and Mortality Weekly,* 57 (22–4), June 6, 2008.
6. QuickStats: Cigarette Smoking Prevalence Among Adults Aged 18 Years Who Have Ever Spent 24 Hours on the Streets, in a Shelter, or in a Jail or Prison, by Sex—United States, 2004. *Morbidity and Morality Weekly,* 55(10), 287, March 17, 2006.
7. QuickStats: Percentage of U.S.-Born and Foreign-Born Adults Aged 18 Years Reporting Selected Health Risk Factors and Conditions, 1998–2003. *Morbidity and Morality Weekly,* 55(11), 313, March 24, 2006.
8. Wilson, JJ. *Summary of the Attorneys General Master Tobacco Settlement Agreement.* 1999. National Conference of State Legislators. March; pages 1–44. www.academic.idayton.edu/health/syllabi/tobacco/summary.htm.
9. Henriksen L, et al. Industry Sponsored Anti-Smoking Ads and Adolescent Reactance: Test of a Boomerang Effect. *Tobacco Control,* 15(1), 13–18, February 2006.
10. Shiffman S, Paty J. Smoking Patterns and Dependence: Contrasting Chippers and Heavy Smokers. *Journal of Abnormal Psychology,* 115(3), 509–523, August 2006.
11. Tong EK, et al. Nondaily Smokers Should Be Asked and Advised to Quit. *American Journal of Preventive Medicine,* 30(1), 23–30, January 2006.
12. Maes HH, et al. A Twin Study of Genetic and Environmental Influences on Tobacco Initiation, Regular Tobacco Use, and Nicotine Dependence. *Psychological Medicine,* 34(7), 1251–1261, October 2004.
13. Wang D, Ma JZ, Li MD. Mapping and Verification of Susceptibility Loci for Smoking Quantity Using Permutation Linkage Analysis. *Pharacogenomics,* 5(3), 166–172, 2005.
14. Li MD, et al. A Genomewide Search Finds Major Susceptibility Loci for Nicotine Dependence on Chromosome 10 in African Americans. *American Journal of Human Genetics,* 79(4), 745–751, October 2006.
15. Gelernter J, et al. Genomewide Linkage Scan for Nicotine Dependence: Identification of a Chromosome 5 Risk Loci. *Biological Psychiatry.* October 31, 2006. (e-publication ahead of print).
16. Spitz MR, et al. The CHRNA5-A3 Region on Chromosome 15q24-25.1 Is a Risk Factor Both for Nicotine Dependence and for Lung Cancer. *Journal of the National Cancer Institute,* 100(21), 1552–1556, November 5, 2008.
17. Boardman JD. State-Level Moderation of Genetic Tendencies to Smoke. *American Journal of Public Health,* January 15, 2009.
18. Sullivan PF, et al. Candidate Genes for Nicotine Dependence via Linkage, Epistasis, Bioinformatics. *American Journal of Medical Genetics. Part B, Neuropsychiatric Genetics,* 126(1), 23–36, April 1, 2004.
19. Sullivan PF, Kendler KSW. The Genetic Epidemiology of Smoking. *Nicotine & Tobacco Research,* Suppl. 2:51, 1999.

20. DiFranza JR, et al. Trait Anxiety and Nicotine Dependence in Adolescents: A Report from the DANDY Study. *Addictive Behaviors,* 29(5), 911–919, July 2004.

21. Wheeler KC, et al. Screening Adolescents for Nicotine Dependence: The Hooked On Nicotine Checklist. *Journal of Adolescent Health,* 35(3), 225–230, September 2004.

22. Fidler JA, et al. Vulnerability to Smoking After Trying a Single Cigarette Can Lie Dormant for Three Years. *Tobacco Control,* 15(3), 205–209, June 2006.

23. Rubinstein ML, et al. Rate of Nicotine Metabolism and Withdrawal Symptoms in Adolescent Light Smokers. *Pediatrics,* 122(3), e643–e647, September 2008.

24. Bernat DH, et al. Adolescent Smoking Trajectories: Results from a Population-Based Cohort Study. *Adolescent Health,* 43(4), 334–340, October 2008.

25. DiFranza JR, et al. Tobacco Consortium, Center for Child Health Research of the American Academy of Pediatrics. *Pediatrics,* 117(6), e1237–1248, June 2006.

26. Saladin KS. *Anatomy and Physiology: The Unity of Form and Function* (4th ed.). New York: McGraw-Hill, 2007.

27. American Cancer Society. *Cancer Facts and Figures—2008.* Atlanta: American Cancer Society, 2008.

28. American Heart Association/American Stroke Association. Heart Disease and Stroke Statistics—2009 Update. *Circulation,* 119(3), e21–181, January 27, 2009.

29. Okuyemi KS, et al. Relationship Between Menthol Cigarettes Cessation Among African American Light Smokers. *Addiction,* 102(12), 1979–1986, December 2007.

30. Cigar Imports Down in 2008, Although It's Too Early to Call This a "Cigar Recession." Heard In The Humidor: November 10–14, 2008. www.cigarreportdaily.com

31. U.S. Substance Abuse and Mental Health Services Administration. *Results from the 2007 National Survey on Drug Use and Health: National Findings* (Figure 4.6). Rockville, MD: U.S. Department of Health and Human Services, Office of Applied Statistics.

32. Weaver K, et al. Pregnancy Smoking in Context: The Influence of Multiple Levels of Stress. *Nicotine and Tobacco Research,* 10(6), 1065–1073, June 2008.

33. Jedrychowski W, et al. Fetal Exposure to Secondhand Tobacco Smoke Assessed by Maternal Self-Reports and Cord Blood Cotinine: Prospective Cohort Study in Krakow. *Maternal and Child Health Journal,* April 25, 2008.

34. Hassa H, et al. Effect of Smoking on Semen Parameters of Men Attending an Infertility Clinic. *Clinical and Experimental Obstetrics & Gynecology,* 33(1), 19–22, 2006.

35. Elhanbly S, et al. Erectile Dysfunction in Smokers: A Penile Dynamic and Vascular Study. *Journal of Andrology,* 25(6), 991–995, November–December 2004.

36. Centers for Disease Control and Prevention. Annual Smoking-Attributed Mortality, Years of Potential Life Lost, and Productivity Losses—United States, 1997–2001. *Morbidity and Mortality Weekly Report,* 54(25), 625–628, 2005.

37. Adgent MA. Environmental Tobacco Smoke and Sudden Infant Death Syndrome: A Review. *Birth Defects Research. Part B, Developmental and Reproductive Toxicology,* 77(1), 69–85, February 2006.

38. Christakis NA, Fowler JH. The Collective Dynamics of Smoking in a Large Smoking Network. *New England Journal of Medicine,* 358(21), 2249–2258, May 22, 2008.

39. Maurer P, Bachmann MF. Vaccination Against Nicotine: An Emerging Therapy for Tobacco Dependence. *Expert Opinion on Investigational Drugs,* 16(11), 1775–1783, November 2007.

Personal Assessment

A Simple Dependency Test: Your Relationship with Cigarettes

To nonsmokers it must seem that smokers would realize the existence of their dependency on cigarettes; however, such might not be the case. Responding to the following survey (a revised version of the Fagerström Tolerance Questionnaire) is a simple way to determine whether a cigarette-based dependence exists. If you are a smoker, answer each question in an honest manner, add up your total point value, and then give careful consideration to your findings. If you are a nonsmoker, ask a smoker to complete the survey and share responses to each item with you—a good discussion could ensue.

1. How many cigarettes a day do you smoke?
   a. Over 26 cigarettes a day (2)
   b. About 16–25 cigarettes a day (1)
   c. About 1–15 cigarettes a day (0)
   d. Less than 1 a day (0)

2. Do you inhale?
   a. Always (2)
   b. Quite often (1)
   c. Seldom (1)
   d. Never (0)

3. How soon after you wake up do you smoke your first cigarette?
   a. Within the first 30 minutes (1)
   b. More than 30 minutes after waking but before noon (0)
   c. In the afternoon (0)
   d. In the evening (0)

4. Which cigarette would you hate to give up?
   a. First cigarette in the morning (1)
   b. Any other cigarette before noon (0)
   c. Any other cigarette in the afternoon (0)
   d. Any other cigarette in the evening (0)

5. Do you find it difficult to refrain from smoking in places where it is forbidden (church, library, movies, etc.)?
   a. Yes, very difficult (1)
   b. Yes, somewhat difficult (1)
   c. No, not usually difficult (0)
   d. No, not at all difficult (0)

6. Do you smoke if you are so ill that you are in bed most of the day?
   a. Yes, always (1)
   b. Yes, quite often (1)
   c. No, not usually (0)
   d. No, never (0)

7. Do you smoke more during the first two hours than during the rest of the day?
   a. Yes (1)
   b. No (1)

TOTAL SCORE: _____

Interpretation

Scores of 0–2: No dependence
Scores of 3–5: Moderate dependence
Scores of 6–9: Substantial dependence

TO CARRY THIS FURTHER . . .

Think about it! A score of 3 or more is your own honest self-assessment that you have already lost the freedom and ability to simply and effortlessly walk away. Two-thirds of all teens whom you see smoking regularly will spend their entire life as slaves to nicotine.

Source: Prokhorov AV, Pallonen UE, Fava JL, Ding L, & Niaura R. Measuring Nicotine Dependence Among High-Risk Adolescent Smokers. *Addictive Behaviors*, 21(1), 117–127, 1996. Used with permission from Elsevier.

Preventing Diseases

Part Four consists of four chapters that focus on disease prevention. Each illness you contract or develop can harm your health in each of its dimensions; therefore, prevention should be a high priority. There are many positive personal health choices you can make to reduce your risk of developing many diseases.

1. Physical Dimension

We usually associate illness with pain, fear, discomfort, and limitations. But paradoxically, health problems can also improve the physical dimension of health. For example, exposure to certain infectious diseases may allow your body to develop immunity. Illness can also force you to rest, reduce your workload, and reconsider your health behavior. Weight loss, smoking cessation, improved dietary practices, genetic counseling, or a renewed commitment to fitness may follow your recovery from an illness.

2. Emotional Dimension

Emotionally healthy people feel good about themselves and others and are able to cope with most of life's demands. Being diagnosed with an illness or disease can jeopardize your emotional resources. You may feel anxious, isolated, and vulnerable. Fortunately, many diseases can be prevented or at least managed or treated successfully.

3. Social Dimension

People rarely face an illness or manage a chronic health condition alone. People who have heart disease, cancer, diabetes, or HIV infection often join support groups or establish friendships with others who have the same condition. In addition, you probably interact with people during activities aimed at preventing diseases. For example, you might exercise with a partner or meet people at a weight-loss group.

4. Intellectual Dimension

We can best use our intellect when we are free from health problems. In some cases, diseases or medications can impair our intellectual functioning. However, managing a condition or recovering from an illness can allow you to learn about your body, your personality, and the health care system. Learning how to reduce your risk of certain diseases will also require you to draw on your intellectual resources.

5. Spiritual Dimension

Your ability to serve others can be hindered by an illness or chronic condition. In addition, your faith can be shaken when a family member falls ill or when you are diagnosed with a serious disease. For most people, however, this initial questioning leads to an even stronger faith or spirituality than they had before the experience.

6. Occupational Dimension

Diseases and your efforts to prevent them can have a significant effect on your job performance. If you have an acute illness, you probably will not be able to work temporarily. If you have a chronic condition or disease, you must try to manage it well enough that you are still able to work. Some conditions are so severe that employment becomes impossible. However, your efforts to prevent illness, such as fitness activities, will enhance your job performance.

Enhancing Your Cardiovascular Health

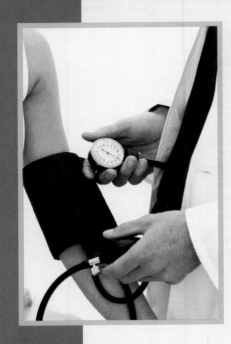

What Do You Know About Keeping Your Heart Healthy?

1. About one in every three American adults has some form of cardiovascular disease. True or False?

2. There are more cardiovascular disease risk factors that you can change (such as your cholesterol levels) than those you cannot change (such as your age). True or False?

3. The risk for a heart attack is the same for a person who smoked a pack a day of cigarettes for 20 years and quit more than a year ago as for the person who has smoked for 20 years and is continuing to smoke a pack a day. True or False?

4. You do not need to have your cholesterol checked until you are 30 years old. True or False?

5. Only health care professionals should use an automated external defibrillator (AED) to assist a person experiencing a cardiac arrest. True or False?

6. African Americans have a greater risk of stroke than Caucasians do. True or False?

7. Individuals with diabetes have a greater risk of developing cardiovascular disease than do people of the same age without diabetes. True or False?

Check your answers at the end of the chapter.

Great progress has been made with respect to **cardiovascular** disease (CVD), the focus of this chapter. Although heart disease continues to be the top killer overall and the number-two killer of Americans under the age of 85 (behind cancer), between 1995 and 2005 the death rates from CVD declined 26.4 percent.[1] Still, CVD claimed about 864,480 lives in 2005.[1] (By comparison, cancer caused 559,312 deaths, accidents caused 117,809, Alzheimer's disease caused 65,829, and HIV/AIDS caused 12,995.) CVD directly caused 34.2 percent of all deaths, or 1 out of every 2.9 deaths in 2005; it contributed to another 22 percent of deaths. The prevalence of CVD—the number of Americans currently living with one or more forms of CVD—is even higher, with about 1 in 3 adults affected (Table 10.1).

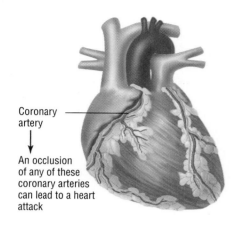

Coronary artery

An occlusion of any of these coronary arteries can lead to a heart attack

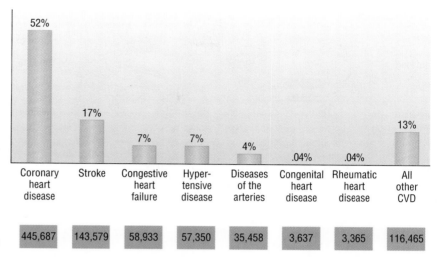

	Coronary heart disease	Stroke	Congestive heart failure	Hypertensive disease	Diseases of the arteries	Congenital heart disease	Rheumatic heart disease	All other CVD
Percent	52%	17%	7%	7%	4%	.04%	.04%	13%
Number of deaths	445,687	143,579	58,933	57,350	35,458	3,637	3,365	116,465

Figure 10-1 Deaths from Cardiovascular Disease Of the 864,480 deaths in the United States in 2005* resulting from cardiovascular diseases, nearly half were attributable to heart disease.

*The most recent year for which statistics are available.

Source: National Center for Health Statistics, reproduced in American Heart Association. Heart Disease and Stroke Statistics—2009 Update, *Circulation*, 119(3e), e21–e181.

Table 10.1 Estimated Prevalence of Major Cardiovascular Diseases

Hypertension	73,600,000
Coronary heart disease	16,800,000
Stroke	6,500,000
Congestive heart failure	5,700,000
Congenital heart disease*	1,300,000
TOTAL (people)	80,000,000

Note: The sum of the individual estimates exceeds 80,000,000 because so many people have more than one cardiovascular disorder.

*The prevalence of congenital cardiovascular defects is estimated to range from 650,000 to 1.3 million.

Source: National Heart, Lung, & Blood Institute, reproduced in American Heart Association, Heart Disease and Stroke Statistics—2009 Update, *Circulation* 119(3e), e21–e181.

Today, nearly 2,400 Americans die each day of CVD, an average of 1 death every 37 seconds. Cardiovascular diseases claim more lives each year than the next four leading causes of death combined. If all major forms of CVD were eliminated, life expectancy in the United States would increase by almost seven years. Figure 10-1 shows the number of deaths from major forms of CVD each year; more information on these specific diseases is presented later in this chapter.

Fortunately, there are many concrete steps you can take to reduce your personal risk for cardiovascular disease. In this chapter, we explain how the heart works and help you identify your CVD risk factors. Prevention efforts are most effective when started in childhood, but it is never too late to adopt a wellness lifestyle.

Quitting smoking, becoming physically active, following a nutritious diet, and controlling your blood pressure are important ways of reducing your risk of heart disease and improving your overall health.

Normal Cardiovascular Function

The cardiovascular system, also called the *circulatory system,* uses a muscular pump to send a complex fluid on a continuous trip through a closed system of tubes. The pump is the heart, the fluid is blood, and the closed system of tubes is the network of blood vessels.

The Vascular System

The term *vascular system* refers to the body's blood vessels. Although we might be familiar with the arteries (vessels that carry blood away from the heart) and the veins (vessels that carry blood to the heart), arterioles, capillaries, and venules are also part of the vascular system. Arterioles are the smaller-diameter extensions of arteries. These arterioles lead eventually to capillaries, the smallest extensions of the vascular system. At the

Key Terms

cardiovascular Pertaining to the heart (*cardio*) and blood vessels (*vasculara*).

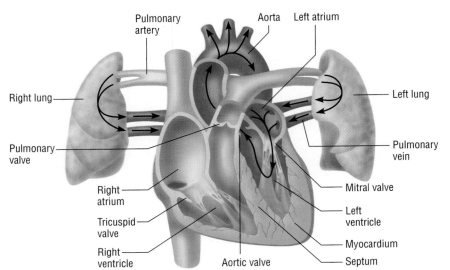

Pulmonary artery · Aorta · Left atrium · Right lung · Left lung · Pulmonary valve · Pulmonary vein · Right atrium · Mitral valve · Tricuspid valve · Left ventricle · Right ventricle · Myocardium · Aortic valve · Septum

Figure 10-2 Circulation Through the Heart
The heart functions like a complex double pump. The right side of the heart pumps deoxygenated blood to the lungs. The left side of the heart pumps oxygenated blood through the aorta to all parts of the body. Note the thickness of the walls of the ventricles. These are the primary pumping chambers.

capillary level, oxygen, food, and waste are exchanged between cells and the blood.

After the blood leaves the capillaries and begins its return to the heart, it drains into small veins, or venules. The blood in the venules flows into increasingly larger vessels called *veins.* Blood pressure is highest in arteries and lowest in veins, especially the largest veins, which empty into the right atrium of the heart.

The Heart

The heart is a four-chambered pump designed to create the pressure required to circulate blood throughout the body. Usually considered to be about the size of a clenched fist, this organ lies slightly tilted between the lungs in the central portion of the **thorax.** The heart does not lie completely in the center of the chest. Rather, approximately two-thirds of the heart is to the left of the body midline and one-third is to the right.

Two upper chambers, called *atria,* and two lower chambers, called *ventricles,* form the heart.[2] The thin-walled atrial chambers are considered collecting chambers, whereas the thick-walled muscular ventricles are considered the pumping chambers. The right and left sides of the heart are divided by a partition called the

septum. Study Figure 10-2 and follow the flow of blood through the heart's four chambers.

To function well, the heart muscle must receive adequate amounts of oxygen. The two main **coronary arteries** (and their many branches) accomplish this. These arteries are located outside of the heart. If the coronary arteries are diseased, a heart attack (myocardial infarction) is possible.

Heart Stimulation The heart contracts and relaxes through the delicate interplay of **cardiac muscle** tissue and cardiac electrical centers, called *nodes.* Nodal tissue generates the electrical impulses necessary to contract heart muscle.[3] The heart's electrical activity is measured by an instrument called an *electrocardiograph* (*ECG* or *EKG*), which provides a printout called an *electrocardiogram* that can be evaluated to determine cardiac electrical functioning.

Blood

The average-size adult has approximately 5 quarts of blood in his or her circulatory system. Blood's functions, which are performed continuously, are quite similar to the overall functions of the circulatory system and include the following:

- Transportation of nutrients, oxygen, wastes, hormones, and enzymes.
- Regulation of water content of body cells and fluids.
- Buffering to help maintain appropriate pH balance of body fluids.
- Regulation of body temperature; the water component in the blood absorbs heat and transfers it.
- Prevention of blood loss; by coagulating or clotting, the blood can alter its form to prevent blood loss through injured vessels.

Key Terms

thorax The chest; portion of the torso above the diaphragm and within the rib cage.

coronary arteries Vessels that supply oxygenated blood to heart muscle tissues.

cardiac muscle Specialized muscle tissue that forms the middle (muscular) layer of the heart wall.

- Protection against toxins and microorganisms, accomplished by chemical substances called *antibodies* and specialized cellular elements circulating in the bloodstream.

Cardiovascular Disease Risk Factors

As you have just read, the heart and blood vessels are among the most important structures in the human body. By protecting your cardiovascular system, you lay the groundwork for a more exciting, productive, and energetic life. The best time to start protecting and improving your cardiovascular system is early in life, when lifestyle patterns are developed and reinforced. Of course, it is difficult to move backward through time, so the second-best time to start protecting your heart is today. Improvements in certain lifestyle activities can pay significant dividends as your life unfolds. (Complete the Personal Assessment at the end of this chapter to estimate your risk for heart disease.)

The American Heart Association encourages people to protect and enhance their heart health by examining the 10 cardiovascular risk factors that are related to various forms of heart disease (Table 10.2). A *cardiovascular risk factor* is an attribute that a person has or is exposed to that increases the likelihood that he or she will develop some form of heart disease. Three risk factors are non-modifiable (you will be unable to change). An additional six risk factors are those you can clearly change. One final risk factor is thought to be a contributing factor to heart disease. Let's look at these three groups of risk factors separately.

Risk Factors That Cannot Be Changed

The risk factors that you cannot change are increasing age, male gender, heredity, and race. Despite the fact that these risk factors cannot be changed, your knowledge that they might be an influence in your life should encourage you to make a more serious commitment to the risk factors you *can* change.

Increasing Age   Heart disease tends to develop gradually over the course of one's life. Although we may know of a few people who experienced a heart attack in their 20s or 30s, most of the serious consequences of heart disease become evident as we age. For example, nearly 84 percent of people who die from heart disease are age 65 and older.

Male Gender   Before age 55, men have a greater risk of heart disease than women do. Yet when women move through menopause (typically in their 50s), their rates of heart disease become similar to men's rates (see the box "Women and Heart Disease"). It is thought that women have a degree of protection from heart disease because of

Table 10.2   Risk Factors for Cardiovascular Disease
Factors You Cannot Change
• Increasing age
• Male gender
• Heredity (including race)
Factors You Can Change ("Big Six" Risk Factors)
• Cigarette smoking and secondhand smoke
• Physical inactivity
• Abnormal blood cholesterol levels
• High blood pressure
• Diabetes mellitus
• Abdominal obesity
Contributing Factor
• Individual response to stress

their natural production of the hormone estrogen during their fertile years.

Heredity   You have no input in determining who your biological parents are. Like increasing age and male gender, this risk factor cannot be changed. By the luck of the draw, some people are born into families where heart disease has never been a serious problem, whereas others are born into families where heart disease is quite prevalent. In this latter case, children are said to have a genetic predisposition (tendency) to develop heart disease as they grow and develop throughout their lives. These people have every reason to be highly motivated to reduce the risk factors they can control.

Race is also a consideration related to heart disease. The prevalence of hypertension among African Americans is among the highest in the United States.[1] More than 40 percent of African Americans have hypertension (two out of every three over age 65).[4] Hypertension significantly increases the risk of heart disease, stroke, and kidney disease. Fortunately, as you will soon read, hypertension can be controlled through a variety of methods. It is especially important for African Americans to take advantage of every opportunity to have their blood pressure measured so that preventive actions can be started immediately if necessary. See the box "Cardiovascular Disease Is Not Necessarily an Equal Opportunity Disease" on page 275 for more on CVD risk among different population groups.

Risk Factors That Can Be Changed

Six cardiovascular risk factors are influenced, in large part, by our lifestyle choices. These risk factors are tobacco smoke, physical inactivity, high blood cholesterol level, high blood pressure, diabetes mellitus, and obesity and overweight.[3] Healthful behavior changes you

Women and Heart Disease

Is heart disease mainly a problem for men? According to the American Heart Association, the answer is no. In fact, data indicate that 53 percent of all cardiovascular disease deaths occur in women.* Sixty-four percent of women who died suddenly of coronary heart disease had no previous symptoms. On average, one woman dies every minute from heart disease in the United States. More women die from heart disease each year than from the next five leading causes of death (cancer, diabetes, lung disease, Alzheimer's disease, and accidents) combined.

For many years, it was thought that men were at much greater risk than women were for the development of cardiovascular problems. Today it is known that young men are more prone to heart disease than young women are, but once women reach menopause (usually in their early to middle 50s), their rates of heart-related problems quickly equal those of men. See the box "Heart Attack Warning Signs" on page 282 for heart attack symptoms that are unique to women.

The protective mechanism for young women seems to be the female hormone estrogen. Estrogen appears to help women maintain a beneficial profile of blood fats. When the production of estrogen is severely reduced at menopause, this protective factor no longer exists. Prescribing postmenopausal hormone replacement therapy (HRT) was a common practice by many physicians in treating a number of factors in postmenopausal women. One of the benefits of HRT was considered to be prevention of cardiovascular diseases. However, in 2002 a major clinical research trial was stopped owing to the finding that more women on HRT were experiencing heart attacks and strokes. Thus, the American Heart Association now recommends that HRT should not be used for the purpose of preventing cardiovascular diseases. Certainly, HRT may still be utilized for other purposes (i.e., relief of menopausal symptoms or osteoporosis prevention). Women prescribed HRT need to be aware of the increased risk for cardiovascular disease in evaluating its value. Certainly, much more research is under way that may influence the use of HRT in the future.†

Young women should not rely solely on naturally produced estrogen to prevent heart disease. The general recommendations for maintaining heart health—good diet, adequate physical activity, monitoring blood pressure and cholesterol levels, controlling weight, avoiding smoking, and managing stress—will benefit women at every stage of life. The American Heart Association has a "Go Red for Women" campaign to promote increased awareness of the seriousness of this disease for women's health.†

*American Heart Association. Heart Disease and Stroke: Statistics—2007 Update.
†American Heart Association: www.americanheart.org/presenter.jhtml?identifier=1928.

---

make concerning these "big six" risk factors can help you protect and strengthen your cardiovascular system.

Tobacco Smoke   Approximately, 48.5 million adults (21 percent) in the United States smoke cigarettes and 20 percent of high school students are smokers.[5] Smokers have a heart attack risk that is more than twice that of nonsmokers. Smoking cigarettes is the major risk factor associated with sudden cardiac death. In fact, smokers have two to four times the risk of dying from sudden cardiac arrest than do nonsmokers. Smokers who experience a heart attack are more likely to die suddenly (within an hour) than are those who don't smoke.

Smoking also adversely affects nonsmokers who are exposed to environmental tobacco smoke. Studies suggest that the risk of death caused by heart disease is increased about 30 percent in people exposed to secondhand smoke in the home. The risk of death caused by heart disease may even be higher in people exposed to environmental tobacco smoke in work settings (for example, bars, casinos, enclosed offices, some bowling alleys and restaurants), since higher levels of smoke may be present at work than at home. Because of the health threat to nonsmokers, restrictions on indoor smoking in public areas and business settings are increasing in every part of the country.

For years it was commonly believed that if you had smoked for many years, it was pointless to try to quit; the damage to one's health could never be reversed. However, the American Heart Association now indicates that by quitting smoking, regardless of how long or how much you have smoked, your risk of heart disease declines rapidly.

This news is exciting and should encourage people to quit smoking, regardless of how long they have smoked. Of course, if you have started to smoke, the healthy approach would be to quit now . . . before the nicotine controls your life and leads to heart disease or damages your lungs or leads to lung cancer. (For additional information about the health effects of tobacco, see Chapter 9.)

Physical Inactivity   Lack of regular physical activity is a significant risk factor for heart disease. Regular aerobic exercise (discussed in Chapter 4) helps strengthen the heart muscle, maintain healthy blood vessels, and improve the ability of the vascular system to transfer blood and oxygen to all parts of the body. In addition, physical activity helps lower overall blood cholesterol levels for most people, encourages weight loss and retention of lean muscle mass, and allows people to moderate the stress in their lives.

With all the benefits that come with physical activity, it amazes health professionals that so many Americans refuse to become regularly active. In 2008, the National Health Interview Survey reported that only 31.7 percent

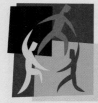

Learning from Our Diversity

Cardiovascular Disease Is Not Necessarily an Equal Opportunity Disease

Although cardiovascular disease is a significant problem for people of all races and ethnic backgrounds in the United States, there are distinct differences between some segments of our population. For example, did you know that African Americans have the highest rate of hypertension of any group of people throughout the world? Compared to white Americans, African Americans develop hypertension at an earlier age and have higher average blood pressure values. This is partly responsible for African Americans' higher death rates from stroke and heart disease and their higher rates of end-stage renal (kidney) disease.

Other racial and ethnic groups also have some notable differences in factors related to cardiovascular disease. American Indians and Alaskan Natives develop diabetes at a rate that is more than double that of the rest of the U.S. population. Mexican Americans have the highest rates of metabolic syndrome, and the rate is 57 percent higher in women than in men in this population group. Similarly, African American women have a 26 percent higher rate of metabolic syndrome compared to African American men. Asians are far less likely to have two or more risk factors for coronary heart disease compared to other population groups.

What are the factors that contribute to these differences between different groups of people? The answers are not entirely clear, but it is likely that the differences result from a combination of factors. Certainly genetics could play a role. For example, it has been theorized that African Americans may have some nervous system differences that would cause their blood pressure to be higher. However, as with the population at large, cultural, environmental, and socioeconomic factors probably contribute to the increased rates of cadiovascular complications in some racial and ethnic groups.

The good news is that preventive approaches and treatment programs can work equally well for all people. So, regardless of what racial or ethnic group you belong to, learn the lifestyle factors that contribute to good heart health and lead that type of lifestyle. Also, tune in to risk factors that are more prevalent for your specific racial group, and make sure you monitor them for yourself. For example, if you are an African American, make sure you have your blood pressure checked regularly.

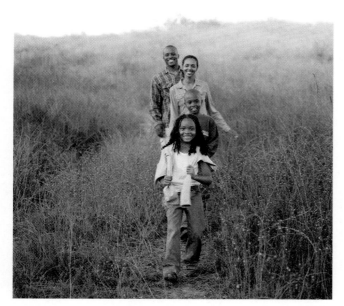

Regular physical activity throughout life helps prevent heart disease and has many other health and functional benefits.

of American adults achieve the recommended amount of physical activity each week.[6] In terms of relative risk for developing CVD, physical inactivity is comparable to high blood pressure, high blood cholesterol, and cigarette smoking.

Critical findings reported in the year 2000 from the highly respected Harvard Alumni Health Study[7, 8] support the contention that physical activity is closely associated with decreased risk of coronary heart disease. After monitoring Harvard alumni for nearly 20 years in a variety of epidemiological studies, researchers confirmed that sustained, vigorous physical activity produces the strongest reductions in CVD. Light and moderate physical activities such as golf, gardening, and walking are helpful in reducing CVD, but more vigorous activities (such as jogging, swimming, tennis, stair climbing, or aerobics) produce greater reductions in CVD.[7] Additionally, Harvard researchers found that physical activity produced reductions in CVD whether the daily activity comes in one long session or in two shorter sessions of activity.[8] The "bottom line" is this: To reduce your chances of experiencing CVD, you must engage in some form of regular, sustained, physical activity (see the box "Getting a Spiritual Lift through Physical Activity").

The American Heart Association began a new campaign called "Start" to encourage individuals and employers to "live longer, more heart-healthy lives through walking and other healthy habits." More information on this movement can be found on the American Heart Association website (www.americanheart.org/start).

If you are middle-aged or older and have been inactive, you should consult with a physician before starting an exercise program. Also, if you have any known health condition that could be aggravated by physical activity,

Getting a Spiritual Lift Through Physical Activity

Pick up almost any book on exercise, and you'll read about the "feel-good" effect. It's what happens when you start doing any type of aerobic activity, such as walking, running, or swimming. First you'll notice physical changes. You've got more energy. You're sleeping better. Maybe you're even a little less grouchy. In the long-term you will lower your risk for most chronic diseases, including coronary heart disease.

But something else is happening, too. Gradually, your outlook seems more positive. Things you couldn't even think about doing a few weeks ago seem possible. You find yourself thinking about starting to write poetry, figuring out what you want to do with your life, improving your grades, or making new friends. That's the feel-good effect spilling over into all areas of your life.

After a few weeks of starting your exercise program, you've dropped a few pounds and your clothes feel more comfortable. But how you think about yourself is changing, too. Maybe you're paying more attention to your appearance. Or you're eating in a healthier way—almost without thinking about it. What's happening is that your self-image is improving. The idea of taking care of yourself is starting to grow, so how you look, what you eat, and how you spend your time are becoming important.

Most health-related organizations (such as the American Heart Association) and government agencies concerned with health (such as the Centers for Disease Control and Prevention) have published recommendations for all individuals to be regularly active. Joining in physical activities with family or friends offers more than the obvious physical and social benefits. Canoeing, playing volleyball in the back yard, or backpacking builds connections. You see others in a new way, relate to them differently, gain new insights, and find ways to help others. People and experiences you may have taken for granted take on a new dimension, and you appreciate them more.

Some people get a spiritual lift from the great outdoors. Wilderness hiking, for example, transports you to a different setting. The quietness, beauty, and solitude can be soothing to the soul. You're looking at the sky, trees, and water. You're enjoying a very peaceful time. This feeling may seem to disappear as soon as you get back to your dorm, but it may make the things you need to deal with there a little easier.

To experience this type of spiritual lift, you don't have to become a marathon runner or climb a mountain. Start going for long walks—alone or with a friend. Start a group that plays games, such as basketball, tennis, or volleyball. Try going for an early morning swim. Get into bicycling. The spiritual effects may be hard to measure, but they'll surprise and reward you.

check with a physician first (see Chapter 4 for more information).

 TALKING POINTS You've started exercising many times by yourself, but you can't seem to stick to it. How would you convince a new friend that you can help each other get started on regular physical activity and keep it up?

Abnormal Blood Cholesterol Levels The third controllable risk factor for heart disease is high blood cholesterol level. Approximately 99.9 million American adults have a total cholesterol level of greater than 200 mg/dl, with 76.1 million having LDL ≥ 130 and 46 million having HDL < 40 mg/dl.[1] Generally speaking, the higher the levels of total and LDL cholesterol, the greater the risk for heart disease (Table 10.3). When high blood cholesterol levels are combined with other important risk factors, the risks become much greater.

Fortunately, blood cholesterol levels are relatively easy to measure. Many campus health and wellness centers provide cholesterol screenings for employees and students. These screenings help identify people whose cholesterol levels (or profiles) may be dangerous. Medical professionals have linked people's diets with their cholesterol levels. People with high blood cholesterol levels are encouraged

to consume a heart-healthy diet (see Chapter 5) and to become physically active. In recent years, researchers have developed a variety of drugs that are very effective at lowering cholesterol levels. In the section "Atherosclerosis," you will read more about cholesterol, particularly the cholesterol-carrying compounds—lipoproteins.

Table 10.3 Classification of Total Cholesterol, Triglycerides, LDL, and HDL Cholesterol

	Normal or Desirable	Borderline-High	High
Total cholesterol	< 200	200–239	≥ 240
Triglycerides	< 150	150–199	≥ 200
LDL cholesterol	< 130	130–159	≥ 160

	Low	Normal	High (Desirable)
HDL cholesterol	< 40	40–59	≥ 60

Source: National Cholesterol Education Program. *The Third Report of the Expert Panel on the Detection, Evaluation, and Treatment of High Blood Cholesterol in Adults.* NIH Publication No. 02-5215, September 2002.
Note: All values expressed in mg/dL.

High Blood Pressure The fourth of the six cardiovascular risk factors that can be changed is high blood pressure, or hypertension. Approximately 65 million Americans have hypertension, one-third of whom have not been diagnosed. High blood pressure can seriously damage a person's heart and blood vessels. High blood pressure causes the heart to work much harder, eventually causing the heart to enlarge and weaken. High blood pressure increases the risk of stroke, heart attack, congestive heart failure, and kidney disease.

When high blood pressure is seen with other risk factors, the risk for stroke or heart attack is increased tremendously. As you see in the section "Hypertension," this "silent killer" is easy to monitor and can be effectively controlled through a variety of approaches.

Diabetes Mellitus Diabetes mellitus (discussed in detail in Chapter 12) is a debilitating chronic disease that has a significant effect on the human body. Approximately 20.1 million Americans have diabetes, 30 percent of whom have not been diagnosed. In addition to increasing the risk of developing kidney disease, blindness, and nerve damage, diabetes increases the likelihood of developing heart and blood vessel diseases. More than 65 percent of people with diabetes die of some type of heart or blood vessel disease. The cardiovascular damage is thought to occur because of the abnormal levels of cholesterol and blood fat found in individuals with diabetes. With weight management, exercise, dietary changes, and drug therapy, diabetes can be relatively well controlled in most people. Despite careful management of this disease, diabetic patients remain quite susceptible to eventual heart and blood vessel damage.[9]

Obesity and Overweight According to the 2006 National Health and Nutrition Survey, 66.9 percent of American adults are overweight, and 34.1 percent are obese.[5] Even if they have no other risk factors, people who are obese are more likely than are people who are not obese to develop heart disease and stroke. Obesity, particularly if of the abdominal form, places considerable strain on the heart, and it tends to worsen both blood pressure and blood cholesterol levels. Men and women who are obese can expect a greater risk of heart disease, diabetes, gallbladder disease, osteoarthritis, respiratory problems, and certain cancers.[10] Maintaining body weight within a desirable range minimizes the chances of obesity ever happening. To accomplish this, you can elect to make a commitment to a reasonably sound diet and an active lifestyle.

 TALKING POINTS How could you tactfully bring up a friend's weight problem to show concern for his or her health?

Table 10.4 Criteria for Metabolic Syndrome

- Elevated waist circumference
  - Men: ≥ 40 inches
  - Women: ≥ 35 inches
- Elevated triglycerides
  - ≥ 150 mg/dL
- Reduced HDL cholesterol
  - Men: < 40 mg/dL
  - Women: < 50 mg/dL
- Elevated blood pressure
  - ≥ 130/85 mmHg
- Elevated fasting glucose
  - ≥ 100 mg/dL

Sources: The American Heart Association and the National Heart, Lung, and Blood Institute.

Metabolic Syndrome

Researchers and clinicians have recently observed that some risk factors seem to group together, most notably abdominal obesity, abnormal blood lipids, elevated blood pressure, and elevated fasting glucose. This grouping of risk factors has been called metabolic syndrome. A person is diagnosed with metabolic syndrome if she or he has three or more of the factors listed in Table 10.4. Individuals with metabolic syndrome (about 47 million Americans) are twice as likely to develop coronary heart disease, compared to those without this syndrome.

Another Risk Factor That Contributes to Heart Disease: Individual Response to Stress

The American Heart Association identifies one other risk factor that is associated with an increased risk of heart disease. This risk factor is one's *individual response to stress.*

Unresolved stress over a long period may be a contributing factor to the development of heart disease. Certainly, people who are unable to cope with stressful life experiences are more likely to develop negative dependence behaviors (for example, smoking, underactivity, poor dietary practices), which can then lead to cardiovascular problems through changes in blood fat profiles, blood pressure, and heart workload. (Chapter 3 covers ways of coping with stress.)

The news media frequently reports on new potential risk factors for heart disease; refer to the box "Making Sense of Medical Research News" for advice on evaluating medical news reports.

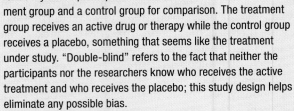

Have you ever been confused by a medical news report? Does it seem to you like the advice from medical research keeps changing? Some of this seeming confusion and conflict stems from the nature of scientific research—the results of many studies done over a long period may be needed to sort out confusing issues of cause and effect. However, some problems in deciphering medical news come from the way the news is presented by the mass media. News stories may sensationalize research findings by oversimplifying the results, leaving out important caveats, and failing to place the findings in the larger context of other research. To help make more sense out of medical news and determine which study results are most important for you, consider the following types and characteristics of medical research studies:

- *Results published in peer-reviewed scientific journals versus results presented at medical meetings.* Results published in journals have been reviewed by experts who can evaluate the study design and conclusions and help put the findings in context. Leading scientific journals tend to publish the most important studies. Results presented at medical meetings are typically preliminary findings from studies still in progress; they have not yet been reviewed and may never be published due to problems in study design or because hypotheses fail to pan out over the full course of the study.
- *Human studies versus animal or laboratory studies.* Results from animal or laboratory experiments provide important information, but further research is typically needed before the results of such experiments can be applied to humans. See Chapter 11 for more on animal research.
- *Retrospective (backward-looking) studies versus prospective (forward-looking) studies.* Studies that follow subjects going forward in time are generally more accurate and meaningful. Retrospective studies rely on people's memories and past medical records, which may be inaccurate or incomplete.
- *Observational (epidemiological) studies versus interventional studies.* An observational study looks at participants' lifestyle practices and health, comparing people who independently chose a particular health intervention against people who did not. Observational studies are good at showing associations between factors but cannot be used to prove cause-and-effect relationships because other lifestyle factors can influence the results.

  An interventional study, also known as a clinical trial, can be used to show causation. The most meaningful type of clinical trial is a *randomized, controlled, double-blind study.* In this type of study, researchers randomly divide participants into a treatment group and a control group for comparison. The treatment group receives an active drug or therapy while the control group receives a placebo, something that seems like the treatment under study. "Double-blind" refers to the fact that neither the participants nor the researchers know who receives the active treatment and who receives the placebo; this study design helps eliminate any possible bias.

- *Size and duration of the research study.* In general, studies that last longer and have more participants are likely to yield more meaningful results. Long study duration is key for research on chronic diseases; for example, a particular dietary change may reduce the risk of heart disease, but this reduction in risk may take 5 to 10 years to show up.
- *Participant characteristics.* Although this is not always the case, the results of a particular study are more likely to be relevant to you if you share key characteristics with the participants. For example, the results of a study on heart disease prevention in white men over age 65 may have limited relevance for a 25-year-old African American woman.
- *Relative risk versus absolute risk.* News media report on dramatic changes in relative risk—stating, for example, that a particular risk factor doubles your risk for a disease. When evaluating such statements, it is important to also consider your absolute risk of getting the disease. For example, if your absolute risk is only 1 in 100,000, then a doubling of risk would still mean that your overall risk of developing a disease is quite low.

Before you apply the findings from any research study to your own life, it is critical to put the findings into context. Find out what other experts recommend, especially major research associations and federal health agencies. A single study is rarely the final word on a health problem or treatment, and public health recommendations generally take into account all the available research into an issue. Also talk to your health care provider, who can help you make the choices most appropriate for your individual needs and situation.

Sources: Woloshin S, Schwartz LM. Media Reporting on Research Presented at Scientific Meetings: More Caution Needed, *Medical Journal of Australia,* 184(11), 576–580, 2006; Studying Research Studies: 10 Questions You Need to Ask, *Tufts University Health & Nutrition Letter,* June 2006; Making Sense of Medical News, *Consumer Reports on Health,* May 2005.

Forms of Cardiovascular Disease

The American Heart Association describes five major forms of CVD as coronary heart disease, hypertension, stroke, diseases of the arteries, and congestive heart failure. These five diseases account for over 87 percent of the deaths caused by CVD. Additionally, many other diseases influence the heart and blood vessels, such as congenital heart disease, rheumatic heart disease, and arrhythmias. (These CVDs are discussed later in this chapter.)

A person may have just one of these diseases or a combination of forms at the same time. Each form exists in varying degrees of severity. All forms are capable of causing secondary damage to other body organs and systems.

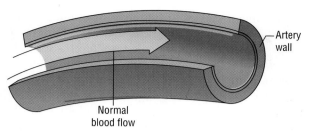

(A) Normal artery

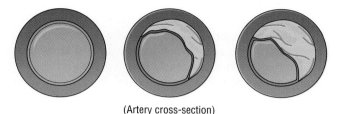

(Artery cross-section)

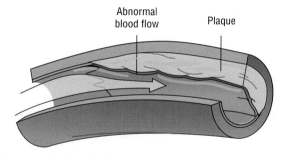

(B) Narrowing of artery due to plaque accumulation

Figure 10-3 Progression of Atherosclerosis This diagram shows how plaque deposits gradually accumulate to narrow the interior space of an artery. Shown enlarged here, coronary arteries are only as wide as a pencil lead.

Source: Adapted from National Heart, Lung, and Blood Institute, What Causes Coronary Artery Disease? www.nhlbi.nih.gov/health/dci/Diseases/Cad/CAD_Causes.html, May 15, 2007.

Coronary Heart Disease

This form of CVD, also known as *coronary artery disease*, involves damage to the vessels that supply blood to the heart muscle. The bulk of this blood is supplied by the coronary arteries. Any damage to these important vessels can cause a reduction of blood flow (with its vital oxygen and nutrients) to specific areas of heart muscle. The ultimate result of an inadequate blood supply is a heart attack. Approximately 330,000 deaths each year are from "sudden cardiac death," which occurs before a person can receive emergency medical treatment.

Atherosclerosis The principal cause of coronary heart disease (CHD) is **atherosclerosis** (Figure 10-3). Atherosclerosis produces a narrowing of the coronary arteries. This narrowing stems from the long-term buildup of fatty deposits, called *plaque,* on the inner walls of the

arteries. This buildup reduces the blood supply to specific portions of the heart. Often arteries of the heart can become totally blocked (occluded) owing to a clot so that all blood supply is stopped. Heart muscle tissue begins to die when it is deprived of oxygen and nutrients. This damage is known as **myocardial infarction.** In lay terms, this event is called a heart attack.

Biomarkers Within the past five years, researchers have found that a high blood level of the amino acid homocysteine may be related to an increased risk of CVD. It is thought that high concentrations of **homocysteine** may accelerate the atherosclerotic plaque formation process that clogs the artery passageways.[11] For persons who did not exhibit any of the traditional CHD risk factors (perhaps as many as 50 percent of the people who have heart attacks), the possibility that a blood test might identify this marker for heart disease was seen as good news.[11] If a person has a high homocysteine level, the theory is that he or she could probably lower the level by taking a multivitamin or by increasing the intake of certain B vitamins, especially B_6, B_{12}, and folic acid (folate). At the time of this writing, however, physicians and scientists are not fully convinced that this is a sound strategy.

While the jury remains undecided regarding the benefits of lowering homocysteine levels, a second possible marker for heart disease has emerged. This marker is a compound called **high sensitivity C-reactive protein (hsCRP).**[12] This protein is a by-product of the inflammation process. Persons who have elevated levels of hsCRP appear to be at greater risk of CHD than those with low levels. Research is presently under way to determine what causes hsCRP protein to reach high levels and for potential treatments. Some promising reports have emerged suggesting that statin medications (used to treat blood cholesterol abnormalities) may help reduce hsCRP protein levels.

> **Key Terms**
>
> **atherosclerosis** The buildup of plaque on the inner walls of arteries.
>
> **myocardial infarction** Heart attack; the death of part of the heart muscle as a result of a blockage in one or more of the coronary arteries.
>
> **homocysteine** An amino acid found in the bloodstream; high levels of homocysteine are thought to be related to an increased risk of coronary heart disease.
>
> **high sensitivity C-reactive protein (hsCRP)** A chemical compound found in the blood that is associated with inflammation; high levels are related to increased risk of coronary heart disease.

Cholesterol and Lipoproteins For many years, scientists have known that atherosclerosis is a complicated disease that has many causes. Some of these causes are not well understood, but others are clearly understood. Cholesterol, a soft, fatlike material, is manufactured in the liver and small intestine and is necessary in the formation of sex hormones, cell membranes, bile salts, and nerve fibers. Elevated levels of serum cholesterol (200 mg/dl or more for adults ages 20 and older, and 170 mg/dl or more for young people under age 20) are associated with an increased risk of developing atherosclerosis.[13]

The National Cholesterol Education Program has specific recommendations for improving your blood cholesterol concentration. The recommendations begin with what we call "therapeutic lifestyle changes," which include dietary modification, weight reduction for those overweight or obese, and regular physical activity.*

The three main dietary changes people can make to help lower their serum cholesterol level are lowering their intake of saturated fats, lowering their intake of dietary cholesterol, and lowering caloric intake to a level that does not exceed body requirements. The aim is to reduce excess fat, cholesterol, and calories in our diet while promoting sound nutrition. By adopting the therapeutic lifestyle changes, people with high serum cholesterol levels may be able to reduce their cholesterol levels by 30 to 55 mg/dl. However, these lifestyle changes do not affect people equally; some will experience greater reductions than others. Some will not respond at all to lifestyle changes and may need to take cholesterol-lowering medications.

Cholesterol is attached to structures called *lipoproteins*. Lipoproteins are particles that circulate in the blood and transport lipids (including cholesterol).[3]

*www.nhlbisupport.com/chd1/tlc_lifestyles.htm

> ### Key Terms
>
> **low-density lipoprotein (LDL)** The type of lipoprotein that transports the largest amount of cholesterol in the bloodstream; high levels of LDL are related to heart disease.
>
> **high-density lipoprotein (HDL)** The type of lipoprotein that transports cholesterol from the bloodstream to the liver, where it is eventually removed from the body; high levels of HDL are related to a reduction in heart disease.
>
> **calcium channel blockers** Drugs that prevent arterial spasms; used in the control of blood pressure and the long-term management of angina pectoris.
>
> **beta blockers** Drugs that reduce the workload of the heart, which reduces blood pressure and decreases the occurrence of angina pectoris.

The two major classes of lipoproteins are **low-density lipoproteins (LDLs)** and **high-density lipoproteins (HDLs).** A person's total cholesterol level is essentially determined by the amount of the LDLs and HDLs in a measured sample of blood. For example, a person's total cholesterol level of 200 mg/dl could be represented by an LDL level of 130 and an HDL level of 40, or an LDL level of 120 and an HDL level of 60. (Note that additional forms of lipoproteins do exist and carry some of the cholesterol in the blood; thus, the total cholesterol value is greater than the sum of LDL and HDL.)

After much study, researchers have determined that high levels of LDL are a significant cause of atherosclerosis. This makes sense, because LDLs carry the greatest percentage of cholesterol in the bloodstream. LDLs are more likely to deposit excess cholesterol into the artery walls. This contributes to plaque formation. For this reason, LDLs are often called the "bad cholesterol."[13] Borderline-high LDL levels (130–159 mg/dl) and high LDL levels (above 160 mg/dl) are determined partly by inheritance, but they are also clearly associated with smoking, poor dietary patterns, obesity, and lack of exercise.

In contrast, high levels of HDLs (60 mg/dl or higher) are related to a decrease in the development of atherosclerosis. HDLs are thought to transport cholesterol out of the bloodstream. Thus, HDLs have been called the "good cholesterol." Certain lifestyle alterations, such as quitting smoking, reducing obesity, regular aerobic-type exercise, and consumption of monounsaturated dietary fats, help many people increase their level of HDL.

Improving cholesterol levels is a significant step in reducing the risk of death from coronary heart disease. Since 1980 the percentage of American adults with high cholesterol has dropped from 27.8 percent to 18 percent. The main reason for this decrease was the introduction of the National Cholesterol Education Program in the mid-1980s. Before this program was instituted, measurement of blood cholesterol was not a routine part of health screenings. The recommendations from this program were updated in 1993 and then most recently in 2001.[13] Although identification and treatment of those with high total and LDL cholesterol levels remain important, the most recent report recommends more intensive therapy for individuals with multiple-risk factors for coronary artery disease. For people with elevated cholesterol levels, a 1 percent reduction in serum cholesterol level yields about a 2 percent reduction in the risk of death from heart disease.[13] If the therapeutic lifestyle changes are not completely effective or if the individual is at increased risk for coronary artery disease, then lipid-lowering medications are recommended. Among the most potent of these is a group of drugs called "statins." These medications have been shown to lower the risk of death from heart disease.

Angina Pectoris When coronary arteries become narrowed, chest pain, or angina pectoris, is sometimes felt.

This pain is caused by a reduced supply of oxygen to heart muscle tissue. Usually, a coronary artery disease patient feels angina when he or she becomes stressed or exercises too strenuously. Angina reportedly can range from a feeling of mild indigestion to a severe viselike pressure in the chest. The pain may extend from the center of the chest to the arms and even up to the jaw. Generally, the more severe the blockage, the more pain is felt. However, it is important to note that only 20 percent of heart attacks are preceded by long-standing angina.

Some cardiac patients relieve angina with the drug nitroglycerin, a powerful blood vessel dilator. This prescription drug, available in slow-release transdermal (through the skin) patches or small pills that are placed under the patient's tongue, causes a major reduction in the workload of the heart muscle. Other cardiac patients may be prescribed drugs such as **calcium channel blockers** or **beta blockers.**

Emergency Response to Heart Crises

Heart attacks need not be fatal. The consequences of any heart attack depend on the location of the damage to the heart, the extent to which heart muscle is damaged, and the speed with which adequate circulation is restored. Injury to the ventricles may very well prove fatal unless medical countermeasures are immediately undertaken. Recognizing a heart attack is critically important; see the box "Heart Attack Warning Signs."

Cardiopulmonary resuscitation (CPR) is one of the most important immediate countermeasures that trained people can use when confronted with a person having a heart attack. Public education programs sponsored by the American Red Cross and the American Heart Association teach people how to recognize, evaluate, and manage heart attack emergencies. CPR trainees are taught how to restore breathing (through mouth-to-mouth resuscitation) and circulation (through external chest compression) in people who require such emergency countermeasures. Frequently, colleges offer CPR classes through health science or physical education departments. We encourage each student to enroll in a CPR course. Additionally, automated external defibrillators (AEDs) are now located in many public buildings. Studies have reported that survival rates of those in cardiac arrest is greater than 90 percent when defibrillation is provided within the first minute.[14]

Diagnosis

A blood test, measuring cardiac muscle enzymes (markers of damage to the heart muscle), is usually performed initially. After a person's vital signs have stabilized, further diagnostic examinations can reveal the type and extent of damage to heart muscle. Initially an electrocardiogram (ECG) might be taken, which may be able to identify if areas of ischemia (insufficient blood flow) or damage has occurred to the heart muscle. Another test which may be used is echocardiography.

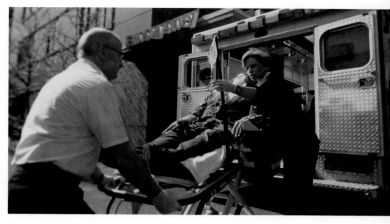

Emergency response teams help keep cardiac patients alive during transit to a medical facility.

This procedure can also detect ischemia. The diagnostic ability of both of these tests is improved if used in conjunction with exercise (that is, stress ECG or stress echocardiography). This test analyzes the electrical activity of the heart. Heart catheterization, also called *coronary arteriography,* is a minor surgical procedure that starts by placing a thin plastic tube into an arm or leg artery. This tube, called a *catheter,* is guided through the artery until it reaches the coronary circulation, where a radiopaque dye is then released. X-ray pictures called *angiograms* then record the progress of the dye through the coronary arteries. Areas of blockage are relatively easily identified.

Some newer techniques for noninvasive diagnosis of coronary artery disease are positron emission tomography (PET), electron beam computed tomography (EBCT),

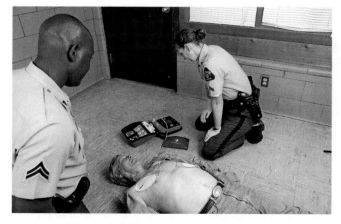

Automated external defibrillators (AEDs) are becoming more common in many places. With only a few hours of training, individuals can learn how to use an AED and become the first responders to an emergency situation. This action can be lifesaving for individuals experiencing a heart attack.

and magnetic resonance imaging (MRI). Now PET, EBCT, and MRI can be used to illustrate the anatomy of coronary arteries and the function of the heart, enabling physicians to evaluate such problems as valvular disease and cardiac shunts.

Nuclear medicine is another important tool in the diagnosis of cardiac disease. Nuclear medicine uses radiopharmaceuticals such as thallium-201 and technetium-99m sestamibi to evaluate perfusion of the heart muscle. Physicians use such tools to study the function of the heart and diagnose cardiac problems.

Treatment After the extent of damage has been determined, a physician or team of physicians can decide on a medical course of action. Treatments can be divided into two broad categories: surgical and nonsurgical.

Surgical Treatments Three types of surgical treatments for coronary heart disease are coronary artery bypass surgery, percutaneous coronary intervention, and heart transplants. More than a million of these surgical procedures are performed each year.

Currently popular is an extensive form of surgery called **coronary artery bypass surgery.** An estimated 253,000 patients had a total of 448,000 bypass procedures performed in 2006. The purpose of such surgery is to detour (bypass) areas of coronary artery obstruction by usually using a section of an artery from the patient's chest (the internal mammary artery) and grafting it from the aorta to a location just beyond the area of obstruction. Multiple areas of obstruction result in double, triple, or quadruple bypasses.

Surgeons have recently begun performing heart bypass surgery through a 3-inch incision in the rib cage, along with two to four small incisions in the patient's chest, rather than the traditional large, 12- to 15-inch incision. Physicians manipulate the coronary arteries through the small ports, and they view their work through a fiber-optic camera called a *thoracoscope.* This new technique results in much less pain and blood loss, a shorter

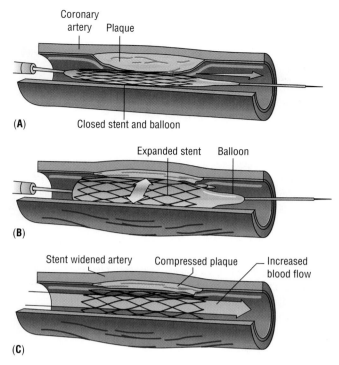

(A)
Coronary artery | Plaque
Closed stent and balloon

(B)
Expanded stent | Balloon

(C)
Stent widened artery | Compressed plaque | Increased blood flow

Figure 10-4 Percutaneous Coronary Intervention (A) A "balloon" is surgically inserted into the narrowed coronary artery. (B) The balloon is inflated, compressing plaque and fatty deposits against the artery walls. (C) A stent is left in place to prevent the artery from narrowing again at this site.

Source: Adapted from National Heart, Lung, and Blood Institute, What Is Coronary Angioplasty? www.nhlbi.nih.gov/health/dci/Diseases/Angioplasty/Angioplasty_WhatIs.html, May 15, 2007.

hospital stay, and a quicker recovery for the patient. This method has been nicknamed "keyhole" surgery and is still considered to be somewhat experimental.

A second type of surgery for coronary heart disease is **percutaneous coronary intervention (PCI),** often called angioplasty. In 2006, about 1,313,000 people with heart disease underwent PCI. PCI is an alternative to bypass surgery, involving the use of a coronary catheter (described earlier) to place a doughnut-shaped "balloon" directly into the narrowed coronary artery (Figure 10-4). When this balloon is inflated, plaque and fatty deposits are compressed against the artery walls, widening the space through which blood flows. These balloons usually remain within the artery for less than a minute. Renarrowing of the artery will occur in about one-quarter of PCI patients. Most patients are now having a **stent** (small mesh tube) inserted in the region where the coronary artery was enlarged by the balloon. Recently, these stents were being coated with drugs to prevent blood clotting at this site.

Balloon PCI can be used for blockages in the heart, kidneys, arms, and legs. The decision whether to have angioplasty or bypass surgery can be a difficult one to make.

In the past 10 years, a number of devices have been developed to remove the diseased material inside a coronary artery. These are called atherectomy devices. Inserted through a leg artery and held in place by a tiny inflated balloon, these motor-driven cutters shave off plaque deposits from inside the artery. A nose cone in the scraper unit stores the plaque until the device is removed.

The use of laser beams to dissolve plaque that blocks arteries has been slowly evolving. The FDA has approved three laser devices for use in clogged leg arteries. Other devices used to open coronary arteries are being researched. These techniques include thermal, photochemical, or acoustical energy to reduce the plaque.

A third and much less common type of surgery for heart disease is a heart transplant—replacing a diseased heart with a healthy heart from another person or with a mechanical device. For approximately 30 years, surgeons have been able to surgically replace a person's damaged heart with that of another human being. Although very risky, these transplant operations have added years to the lives of a number of patients who otherwise would have lived only a short time. In 2007, doctors performed 2,210 heart transplants in the United States.[1]

Artificial hearts have also been developed and implanted in humans. These mechanical devices have extended the lives of patients and have also served as temporary hearts while patients wait for a suitable donor heart. One of the important difficulties with artificial heart implantation has been the control of blood clots that may form, especially around the artificial valves. Blood clots can cause heart attacks or strokes that can be fatal.

Nonsurgical Treatments Nonsurgical treatments include various medications that can help reduce the risk of heart attacks, both in patients with existing heart disease

---

Key Terms

coronary artery bypass surgery A surgical procedure designed to improve blood flow to the heart by providing alternative routes for blood to take around points of blockage.

percutaneous coronary intervention (PCI) Any of a group of procedures used to treat patients suffering from an obstruction in an artery. Typically, a PCI involves inserting a slender balloon-tipped tube into an artery of the heart.

stent A device inserted inside a coronary artery during a percutaneous coronary intervention (PCI) to prevent the artery from narrowing at that site.

and in people with no history of heart attack. (For information on complementary and alternative approaches to treatment currently under study, see the box "Using Chelation Therapy to Treat Coronary Artery Disease.") Two commonly used medications are platelet inhibitors and aspirin.

Platelets are part of the physiological pathway that produces blood clots. Platelet inhibitors are a class of drugs that has been shown to prevent the formation of blood clots, a major cause of heart attacks, chest pain, and artery tightening after angioplasty. It is well established that platelet inhibitors reduce heart attacks in patients with unstable angina, or severe chest pain, by about half.[3] Observers say this new class of drugs will have a tremendous effect on the treatment of heart problems.

Studies released in the late 1980s highlighted the role of aspirin in reducing the risk of heart attack in men who had no history of previous attacks. Specifically, the studies concluded that for men with hypertension, elevated cholesterol levels, or both, taking one aspirin per day was a significant factor in reducing their risk of heart attack. Aspirin works by making the blood less able to clot, which reduces the likelihood of blood vessel blockages. Experts currently disagree about the age at which this preventive action should begin. The safest advice is to check with your physician before starting aspirin therapy.

Likewise, it now appears that women who take aspirin on a regular basis are less likely to have a heart attack than are women who do not take aspirin. However, women should first consult with their physicians about the correct dosage and the best way to use aspirin to protect their cardiovascular health.[15]

Hypertension

Just as your car's water pump recirculates water and maintains water pressure, your heart recirculates blood and maintains blood pressure. When the heart contracts, blood is forced through your arteries and veins. Your blood pressure is a measure of the force that your circulating blood exerts against the interior walls of your arteries and veins.

Measuring and Evaluating Blood Pressure Blood pressure is measured with a *sphygmomanometer*. A sphygmomanometer is attached to an arm-cuff device that can be inflated to stop the flow of blood temporarily in the brachial artery. This artery is a major supplier of blood to the lower arm. It is located on the inside of the upper arm, just above the elbow.

A health professional using a stethoscope listens for blood flow while the pressure in the cuff is released. Two pressure measurements are recorded: the **systolic pressure** is the highest blood pressure against the vessel walls during the heart contraction, and the **diastolic pressure** is the lowest blood pressure against the vessel walls when the heart relaxes (between heartbeats). Expressed in units of millimeters of mercury, blood pressure is recorded as the systolic pressure over the diastolic pressure, for example, 116/82.

Although a blood pressure of less than 120/80 is considered "normal" for adults, lower values do not necessarily indicate a medical problem. In fact, many young college women of average weight display blood pressures that seem to be relatively low (100/60, for example), yet these lowered blood pressures are quite "normal" for them.

What Is Hypertension?   Hypertension refers to a consistently elevated blood pressure. Generally, treatment for high blood pressure begins when a person has a systolic reading of 140 or above or a diastolic reading of 90 or above, although concern about health risks begins when a person reaches the prehypertensive range. Table 10.5 shows the classifications for blood pressure.

Based on data from 2005–2006, approximately 29 percent of adults have hypertension.[4] In the United States, more men have hypertension than women until age 45, when women surpass men. In terms of prevalence for U.S. adults age 20 and older, non-Hispanic black females have the highest rate (44 percent) of hypertension. Thirty-four percent of non-Hispanic white males and 31 percent of non-Hispanic white females have high blood pressure. Among Mexican American males in the United States, 27 percent have hypertension; 30 percent of Mexican American females have high blood pressure.[1]

Causes and Effects of Hypertension   The causes of 90 to 95 percent of the cases of hypertension are unknown, called essential hypertension. However, the health risks are real. Throughout the body, long-term hypertension makes arteries and arterioles become less elastic and thus incapable of dilating under a heavy workload. Brittle, calcified blood vessels can burst unexpectedly and produce serious strokes (brain accidents), kidney failure (renal accidents), or eye damage **(retinal hemorrhage).** Furthermore, it appears that blood clots are more easily formed and dislodged in a vascular system affected by hypertension. Thus hypertension can be a cause of heart attacks. Hypertension is a potential killer.

Hypertension is referred to as "the silent killer" because people with hypertension often are not aware that they have the condition. People with this disorder cannot feel the sensation of high blood pressure. The condition does not produce dizziness, headaches, or memory loss unless one is experiencing a medical crisis. Because it is a silent killer, it is estimated that 30 percent of the people who have hypertension do not realize they have it. Eleven percent know they have hypertension but are not taking any measures to reduce it. Twenty-six percent are on medication but do not keep their hypertension under control. Just 34 percent of people with hypertension are aware that they have high blood pressure *and* have it under control with medication.[16]

Prevention and Treatment   Hypertension is not thought of as a curable disease; rather, it is a controllable

Table 10.5	Blood Pressure Classification		
Blood Pressure (mm Hg)	**Normal**	**Prehypertension**	**Hypertension**
Systolic (top number)	less than 120	120–139	140 or higher
Diastolic (bottom number)	less than 80	80–89	90 or higher

High blood pressure, or hypertension, is defined in an adult as a systolic pressure of 140 mm Hg or higher and/or a diastolic pressure of 90 mm Hg or higher. Blood pressure is measured in millimeters of mercury (mm Hg).

Source: National Heart, Lung, and Blood Institute, *The Seventh Report of the Joint National Committee on Prevention, Detection, Evaluation, and Treatment of High Blood Pressure*, NIH Publication No. 03-5233, December 2003.

disease. When therapy is stopped, the condition returns. As a responsible adult, you should use every opportunity you can to measure your blood pressure regularly.

Weight reduction, physical activity, moderation in alcohol use, and as mentioned in Chapter 5, the dietary approaches to stop hypertension (DASH eating plan) are all recommended to reduce hypertension. These lifestyle modifications are now recommended therapy for individuals classified as prehypertensive. For overweight or obese people, a reduction in body weight may produce a significant drop in blood pressure. Physical activity helps lower blood pressure by expending calories (which may lead to weight loss in those who are overweight or obese) and through other physiological changes that affect the circulation. Moderation in alcohol consumption helps reduce blood pressure in some people (see the box "Can Alcohol Be Good for Your Heart?").

The restriction of sodium (salt) in the diet also helps some people reduce hypertension. Interestingly, this strategy is effective only for those who are **salt sensitive**—estimated to be about 25 percent of the population. Reducing salt intake would have little effect on the blood pressure of the rest of the population. Nevertheless,

Key Terms

systolic pressure   (sis **tol** ick) Blood pressure against blood vessel walls when the heart contracts.

diastolic pressure   (**dye** uh **stol** ick) Blood pressure against blood vessel walls when the heart relaxes.

retinal hemorrhage   Uncontrolled bleeding from arteries within the eye's retina.

salt sensitive   Term used to describe people whose bodies overreact to the presence of sodium by retaining fluid, thus increasing blood pressure.

Can Alcohol Be Good for Your Heart?

You have probably seen the controversial headlines over the past couple of years stating that moderate consumption of alcohol may reduce your risk of coronary heart disease. Such research is controversial because experts fear this may encourage problem drinkers or turn abstainers into problem drinkers.

Nevertheless, the evidence is strong that drinking alcohol in moderate amounts indeed reduces the risk of heart attack and death from coronary heart disease. The best evidence comes from population studies that show a reduction in coronary risk among moderate drinkers when compared with abstainers. The results are similar in both men and women, and among various ethnic groups. Moderate drinking is typically defined as one or two drinks a day for men and one a day for women.

Three possible explanations for the cardiovascular benefits are (1) that alcohol raises the level of protective high-density lipoprotein (HDL) cholesterol in the blood, making atherosclerosis less likely, (2) that alcohol inhibits blood clotting by helping to dissolve clots in blood vessels, and (3) that other substances in the alcoholic beverage may have antioxidant properties.

Researchers are looking at specific types of alcohol, such as red wine, but the results are not yet strong enough to justify recommending that people switch to wine from beer or liquor. It appears that the benefits come from any type of alcohol product.

The American Heart Association* makes the following recommendations:

- The beneficial effects of alcohol are limited to one to two drinks a day for men and one drink per day for women.

- Heavier consumption is related to many health problems, including alcoholism, high blood pressure, obesity, stroke, breast cancer, suicide, and accidents.

- Pregnant women should not use alcohol.

- Do not drink alcohol if you take aspirin on a regular basis. Check with your physician.

*American Heart Association, Alcohol, Wine, and Cardiovascular Disease, www.americanheart.org/presenter.jhtml?identifier=4422

---

because our daily intake of salt vastly exceeds our need for salt, the general recommendation to curb salt intake still makes good sense. The DASH eating plan also recommends foods that are rich in potassium and calcium.

Many of the stress reduction activities we discuss in Chapter 3 are receiving increased attention in the struggle to reduce hypertension. In recent years, behavioral scientists have reported the success of meditation, biofeedback, controlled breathing, and muscle relaxation exercises in reducing hypertension. Look for further research findings in these areas in the years to come.

Drugs used to lower high blood pressure are called *antihypertensives*. *Diuretic drugs* work by stimulating the kidneys to eliminate more fluid, thereby reducing blood volume. *Vasodilators* relax the smooth muscle in the walls of blood vessels (especially the arterioles), allowing the vessels to dilate (widen). Also used are calcium channel blockers, beta blockers, angiotensin converting enzyme (ACE) inhibitors, and other drugs that work in various ways to relax blood vessels. The most disturbing aspect of drug therapy for hypertension is that many patients refuse to take their medication on a consistent basis, probably because of the mistaken notion that "you must feel sick to be sick."

Some people taking these medications report uncomfortable side effects, including depression, reduced libido (sex drive), muscle weakness, impotence, dizziness, and fainting. Thus the medication's side effects may seem worse than the disease. This is all the more reason to emphasize the lifestyle modifications described earlier. Because of the poor record of patient compliance with hypertension drug therapy, many television and radio public service announcements are geared to the

hypertensive patient. Nutritional supplements, such as calcium, magnesium, potassium, and fish oil, have not proven to be effective and reliable in lowering blood pressure.

Stroke

A third major CVD is stroke. *Stroke* is a general term for a wide variety of crises (sometimes called *cerebrovascular accidents* [CVAs] or brain attacks) that result from blood vessel damage in the brain. African Americans have a 60 percent greater risk of stroke than White Americans do, probably because African Americans have a greater likelihood of having hypertension than do white Americans. About 795,000 (185,000 of which are recurrent events) people suffer a stroke in the United States each year, and of these, about a quarter die. A total of 143,574 Americans died of stroke in 2005.[1] Just as the heart muscle needs an adequate blood supply, so does the brain. Any disturbance in the proper supply of oxygen and nutrients to the brain can pose a threat.

Types of Strokes There are three main types of stroke, each affecting blood flow in the brain in a different way.

Cerebrovascular Occlusions Perhaps the most common form of stroke results from the blockage of a cerebral (brain) artery. Similar to coronary occlusions, **cerebrovascular occlusions** can be started by a clot that forms within an artery, called a *thrombus*, or by a clot that travels from another part of the body to the brain, called an *embolus* (Figure 10-5a and b). The resultant accidents (cerebral thrombosis or cerebral embolism) cause more

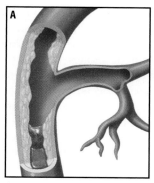

Thrombus
A clot that forms within a narrowed section of a blood vessel and remains at its place of origin.

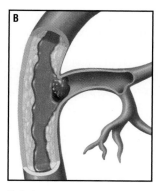

Embolus
A clot that moves through the circulatory system and becomes lodged at a narrowed point within a vessel.

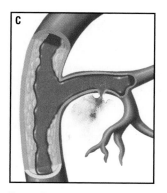

Hemorrhage
The sudden bursting of a blood vessel.

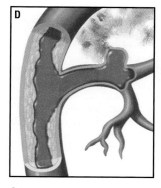

Aneurysm
A sac formed when a section of a blood vessel thins and balloons; the weakened wall of the sac can burst, or rupture, as shown here.

Figure 10-5 Causes of Stroke

than 88 percent of all strokes. The portion of the brain deprived of oxygen and nutrients can literally die.

Cerebral Hemorrhage A second type of stroke can result from an artery that bursts to produce a crisis called *cerebral hemorrhage* (Figure 10-5c). Damaged, brittle arteries can be especially susceptible to bursting when a person has hypertension.

Cerebral Aneurysm A third form of stroke is a *cerebral aneurysm*. An aneurysm is a ballooning or outpouching on a weakened area of an artery (Figure 10-5d). Aneurysms may occur in various locations of the body and are not always life threatening. The development of aneurysms is not fully understood, although there seems to be a relationship between aneurysms and hypertension. It is quite possible that many aneurysms are congenital defects. In any case, when a cerebral aneurysm bursts, a stroke results.

Diagnosis As for heart attacks, you should learn the symptoms of a stroke so you can act quickly to obtain help (Table 10.6). A person who reports any warning signs of stroke or periods of temporary lack of blood-flow to a region of the brain, called a **transient ischemic attack (TIA),** is given a battery of diagnostic tests, which could include a physical examination, a search for possible brain tumors, tests to identify areas of the brain affected, electroencephalogram, cerebral arteriography, and a **computerized axial tomography (CT)** or **magnetic resonance imaging (MRI) scan.** Many other tests can also be used.

Treatment Researchers recently made a breakthrough in the treatment of stroke, with the discovery that the clot-dissolving drug tissue plasminogen activators (TPA)

and the cell-rebuilding drug citicoline could reduce the severity of strokes.

In the past, physicians essentially waited for a stroke to end before assessing damage and beginning rehabilitation. Now, experts find that TPA can actually reduce the severity of a stroke as it is occurring. TPA was previously used to dissolve clots in the treatment of heart attacks. This same effect, applied during a stroke, can help prevent brain cells from "starving" to death because of a lack of blood supply. TPA is useful only for strokes caused by clots (embolism or thrombosis).

As a result, experts are reclassifying stroke as a medical emergency that must be treated as quickly as possible. To be effective, TPA must be administered in the first three hours of the stroke. After that time, brain cells have been damaged and TPA can worsen the damage. Because

---

Key Terms

cerebrovascular occlusions (ser ee bro **vas** kyou lar) Blockages to arteries supplying blood to the cerebral cortex of the brain; cause of the most common type of stroke.

transient ischemic attack (TIA) (**tran** see ent iss **key** mick) Strokelike symptoms caused by temporary spasm of cerebral blood vessels.

computerized axial tomography (CT) scan An X-ray procedure designed to illustrate structures within the body that would not normally be seen through conventional X-ray procedures.

magnetic resonance imaging (MRI) scan An imaging procedure that uses a powerful magnet to generate an image of body tissue.

Table 10.6 Risks Factors for and Warning Signs of Stroke

Risk Factors

- Over 60 years old
- Diabetes
- Smoking cigarettes
- Transient ischemic attack (TIA)—temporary lack of blood flow to a section of the brain—lasting longer than 10 minutes
- Localized body weakness or symptoms of speech impairment
- Atrial fibrillation—a form of irregular heartbeat

Warning Signs

- Sudden numbness or weakness of the face, arm, or leg, especially on one side of the body
- Sudden confusion, trouble speaking or understanding
- Sudden trouble seeing in one or both eyes
- Sudden trouble walking, dizziness, loss of balance or coordination
- Sudden, severe headache with no known cause

  If you or someone with you has one or more of these signs, don't delay! Immediately call 911 so an ambulance (ideally with advanced life support) can be sent for you.

Source: American Heart Association. Heart Attack, Stroke, and Cardiac Arrest Warning Signs, www.americanheart.org/presenter.jhtml?identifier=3053, August 15, 2007. Used with permission by The American Heart Association.

700,000 people suffer strokes and about one-quarter of them die each year, TPA has the potential to save thousands of lives a year.

Other treatment after a stroke depends on the nature and extent of the damage the patient has suffered. Some patients require surgery (to repair vessels and relieve pressure) and acute care in the hospital.

The advances made in the rehabilitation of stroke patients are amazing. Although some severely affected patients have little hope of improvement, our continuing advances in the application of computer technology to such disciplines as speech and physical therapy offer encouraging signs for stroke patients and their families.

Other Cardiovascular Diseases

A number of less common conditions can affect the functioning of the cardiovascular system. These include congenital heart disease, rheumatic heart disease, congestive heart failure, peripheral artery disease, and arrhythmias.

Congenital Heart Disease   A congenital defect is one that is present at birth. About 36,000 babies are born each year with one of at least 35 recognized congenital heart defects. In 2005, a total of 3,637 infants died from congenital heart disease.[1]

A variety of abnormalities may be produced by congenital heart disease, including valve damage, holes in the walls of the septum, blood vessel transposition, and an underdevelopment of the left side of the heart. All of these problems ultimately prevent a newborn baby from receiving adequate oxygenation of tissues throughout the body. A bluish skin color (cyanosis) is seen in some infants with such congenital heart defects.

The cause of congenital heart defects is not clearly understood, although one cause, rubella, has been identified. The fetuses of mothers who contract the rubella virus during the first three months of pregnancy are at great risk of developing congenital rubella syndrome (CRS), a catch-all term for a wide variety of congenital defects, including heart defects, deafness, cataracts, and mental retardation. Other hypotheses about the development of congenital heart disease implicate environmental pollutants, maternal use of drugs, including alcohol, during pregnancy, and unknown genetic factors.

Treatment of congenital defects usually requires surgery, although some conditions may respond well to drug therapy. Defective blood vessels and certain malformations of the heart can be surgically repaired. This surgery is so successful that many children respond quickly to the increased circulation and oxygenation. Many are able to lead normal, active lives.

Rheumatic Heart Disease   Rheumatic heart disease is the final stage in a series of complications started by a streptococcal infection of the throat (strep throat). Common symptoms of strep throat are

- Sudden onset of sore throat, particularly with pain when swallowing
- Fever
- Swollen, tender glands under the angle of the jaw
- Headache
- Nausea and vomiting
- Tonsils covered with a yellow or white pus or discharge

This bacterial infection, if untreated, can result in an inflammatory disease called *rheumatic fever* (and a related condition, *scarlet fever*). Rheumatic fever is a whole-body (systemic) reaction that can produce fever, joint pain, skin rashes, and possible brain and heart damage. A person who has had rheumatic fever is more susceptible to subsequent attacks. Rheumatic fever tends to run in families. About 1.8 million Americans suffer from various stages of rheumatic heart disease. In 2005, this disease killed 3,365 people.[1]

Damage from rheumatic fever centers on the heart's valves. For some reason the bacteria tend to proliferate in the heart valves. Defective heart valves may fail either to open fully (stenosis) or to close fully (insufficiency). A physician initially might diagnose valve damage when she hears a backwashing or backflow of blood (a **murmur**).

Further tests, including chest X-rays, cardiac catheterization, and echocardiography, can reveal the extent of valve damage. After it is identified, a faulty valve can be replaced surgically with a metal or plastic artificial valve or a valve taken from an animal's heart.

Congestive Heart Failure **Congestive heart failure** is a condition in which the heart lacks the strength to continue to circulate blood normally throughout the body. During congestive heart failure, the heart continues to work, but it cannot function well enough to maintain appropriate circulation. Venous blood flow starts to "back up." Swelling occurs, especially in the legs and ankles. Fluid can collect in the lungs and cause breathing difficulties and shortness of breath, and kidney function may be damaged. In 2005, congestive heart failure led to 58,933 deaths in the United States.[1]

Congestive heart failure can result from heart damage caused by congenital heart defects, lung disease, rheumatic fever, heart attack, atherosclerosis, or high blood pressure. Generally, congestive heart failure is treatable through a combined program of rest, proper diet, modified daily activities, and the use of appropriate drugs. Without medical care, congestive heart failure can be fatal.

Diseases of the Arteries **Peripheral artery disease (PAD),** also called *peripheral vascular disease (PVD),* is a blood vessel disease characterized by pathological changes to the arteries and arterioles in the extremities (primarily the legs and feet but sometimes the hands). PAD affects approximately 8 million Americans. These changes result from years of damage to the peripheral blood vessels. Important causes of PAD are cigarette smoking, a high-fat diet, obesity, and sedentary occupations. In some cases, PAD is aggravated by blood vessel changes resulting from diabetes.

PAD severely restricts blood flow to the extremities. The reduction in blood flow is responsible for leg pain or cramping during exercise, numbness, tingling, coldness, and loss of hair on the affected limb. The most serious consequence of PAD is the increased likelihood of developing ulcerations and tissue death. These conditions can lead to gangrene and may eventually necessitate amputation.

PAD is treated in multiple ways, including efforts to improve blood lipid levels (through diet, exercise, or drug therapy), to reduce hypertension, to reduce body weight, and to eliminate smoking. Blood vessel surgery may be a possibility.

Arrhythmias Arrhythmias are disorders of the heart's normal sequence of electrical activity that are experienced by more than 2 million Americans. They result in an irregular beating pattern of the heart. Arrhythmias can be so brief that they do not affect the overall heart rate. Some arrhythmias, however, can last for long periods of time and cause the heart to beat either too slowly or too rapidly. A slow beating pattern is called **bradycardia** (fewer than 60 beats per minute), and a fast beating pattern is called **tachycardia** (more than 100 beats per minute).

Hearts that beat too slowly may be unable to pump a sufficient amount of blood throughout the body. The body becomes starved of oxygen, and loss of consciousness and even death can occur. Hearts that beat too rapidly do not allow the ventricles to fill sufficiently. When this happens, the heart cannot pump enough blood throughout the body. The heart becomes, in effect, a very inefficient machine. It beats rapidly but cannot pump much blood from its ventricles. This pattern may lead to fibrillation, which is the life-threatening, rapid uncoordinated contractions of the heart. Interestingly, whether the heart pumps too slowly or too rapidly, the result is the same: inadequate blood flow throughout the body.

The person most prone to arrhythmia is the person with some form of heart disease, including atherosclerosis, hypertension, or inflammatory or degenerative conditions. The prevalence of arrhythmia tends to increase with age. Certain congenital defects may make a person more likely to have an arrhythmia. Some chemical agents, including high or low levels of minerals (potassium, magnesium, and calcium) in the blood, addictive substances (caffeine, tobacco, other drugs), and various cardiac medications, can all provoke arrhythmias.

Arrhythmias are most frequently diagnosed through an ECG (electrocardiogram), which records electrical activity of the heart. After diagnosis, a range of therapeutic approaches can be used, including simple monitoring (if the problem is relatively minor), drug therapy, use of a pacemaker, or the use of implantable defibrillators.

Key Terms

rheumatic heart disease Chronic damage to the heart (especially the heart valves) resulting from a streptococcal infection within the heart; a complication of rheumatic fever.

murmur An atypical heart sound that suggests a backflow of blood into a chamber of the heart from which it has just left.

congestive heart failure Inability of the heart to pump out all the blood that returns to it; can lead to dangerous fluid accumulations in veins, lungs, and kidneys.

peripheral artery disease (PAD) Atherosclerotic blockages that occur in arteries that supply blood to the legs and arms.

bradycardia Slowness of the heartbeat, as evidenced by a resting pulse rate of less than 60.

tachycardia Excessively rapid heartbeat, as evidenced by a resting pulse rate of greater than 100.

Related Cardiovascular Conditions Besides the cardiovascular diseases already discussed, the heart and blood vessels are subject to other pathological conditions. Tumors of the heart, although rare, occur. Infectious conditions involving the pericardial sac that surrounds the heart (*pericarditis*) and the innermost layer of the heart (*endocarditis*) are more commonly seen. Some people develop serious diseases of the heart valves. In addition, inflammation of the veins (*phlebitis*) is troublesome to some people.

Preventing Cardiovascular Disease

Although some factors that contribute to heart disease are beyond our control (nonmodifiable risk factors), there are many more things we can do to promote good heart health. The best news is that we are in control of a large part of our heart health. To exert this control in a positive manner, it is important to lead a heart-healthy lifestyle. Simply put, this means eating right, being regularly active, and controlling our body weight. The specifics related to dietary habits and physical activity recommendations were covered in detail in Chapters 4 and 5 and were also summarized in earlier sections of this chapter. However, it is also important to understand that some individuals have genetic factors that make them more susceptible to heart disease—so it is important to have regular medical checkups. If you are not able to control some of your risk factors, such as high blood pressure or high cholesterol, through lifestyle, then it is important to follow your doctor's advice in taking medications to treat these conditions before they lead to heart disease. Remember the old saying: an ounce of prevention is worth a pound of cure.

Taking Charge of Your Health

- Complete the Personal Assessment on pages 292–293 to determine your risk for heart attack and stroke.
- Review MyPyramid in Chapter 5 (page 127), and make changes to your diet so that it is more "heart healthy."
- Follow the surgeon general's recommendations and accumulate a moderate amount of physical activity daily or begin an aerobic exercise program that is appropriate for your current fitness level.
- If you are a smoker, resolve to quit smoking. Visit your physician to talk about safe and effective approaches. Begin putting your plan into action.
- Develop a plan to lower your dietary intake of saturated fat to keep your LDL cholesterol level low.
- Have your blood pressure checked, and review your weight, physical activity, alcohol intake, and salt intake to determine whether you can make changes in any of these areas.
- If you are overweight or obese, develop a plan to combine dietary changes and increased physical activity to lose weight gradually but steadily.

SUMMARY

- Cardiovascular diseases are responsible for more disabilities and deaths than any other disease.
- The vascular system refers to the body's blood vessels, including arteries, veins, arterioles, capillaries, and venules.
- A cardiovascular risk factor is an attribute that a person has or is exposed to that increases the likelihood of heart disease.
- The "big six" risk factors are tobacco smoke, physical inactivity, high blood cholesterol level, high blood pressure, diabetes mellitus, and abdominal obesity and overweight. These are risk factors that can be changed.
- Smokers have a heart attack risk that is more than twice that of nonsmokers. However, the risk of heart disease declines rapidly if the smoker quits.
- Regular aerobic exercise helps strengthen the heart muscle, maintain healthy blood vessels, and improve the vascular system's ability to transport blood and oxygen to the body.

- People with high blood cholesterol should eat a heart-healthy diet and become physically active.
- The five major forms of cardiovascular disease are coronary artery disease, hypertension, stroke, congestive heart failure, and diseases of the arteries.
- Each form of heart disease develops in a unique way and requires specialized treatment.
- Moderate alcohol consumption may be related to a lower risk of heart disease. However, heavy drinking increases cardiovascular disease risk.
- Weight reduction, physical activity, lowering alcohol use, sodium restriction, meditation, and antihypertensive drugs are often used to control hypertension.
- Other heart diseases include congenital heart disease, rheumatic heart disease, and heart arrhythmias.

REVIEW QUESTIONS

1. Identify the principal components of the cardiovascular system. Trace the path of blood through the heart and cardiovascular system.
2. How much blood does the average adult have? What are some of the important functions of blood?
3. Define cardiovascular risk factor. What relationship do risk factors have to cardiovascular disease?
4. Identify the risk factors for cardiovascular disease that cannot be changed. Identify the risk factors that can be changed. Identify the risk factor that is a contributing factor.
5. Describe the relationship between smoking and heart disease, including the role of environmental tobacco smoke. Explain the cardiovascular benefits of quitting smoking.
6. What is high sensitivity C-reactive protein (hsCRP)? What role might it play regarding cardiovascular disease?
7. What are the five major forms of cardiovascular disease? For each of these diseases, describe the disease, its cause (if known), and its treatment. Describe some additional CVDs.
8. Describe how high-density lipoproteins differ from low-density lipoproteins.
9. What problems does atherosclerosis produce?
10. Why is hypertension called the "silent killer"? What serious health problems can hypertension cause?
11. What are the warning signals of stroke? Identify and describe each of the four types of stroke.
12. What is a heart arrhythmia and what are its consequences? Identify the two main heart arrhythmia patterns.

ANSWERS TO THE "WHAT DO YOU KNOW?" QUIZ

1. True   2. True   3. False   4. False   5. False   6. True   7. True

Visit the Online Learning Center (**www.mhhe.com/payne11e**), where you will find tools to help you improve your grade including practice quizzes, key terms flashcards, audio chapter summaries for your MP3 player, and many other study aids.

SOURCE NOTES

1. American Heart Association. Heart Disease and Stroke: Statistical Update. *Circulation*, 119(3e), e21–e181, 2009.
2. Thibodeau GA, Patton KT. *Structure and Function of the Human Body* (11th ed.). St. Louis, MO: Mosby-Year Book, 2000.
3. Brubaker PH, Kaminsky LA, Whaley MH. *Coronary Artery Disease*. Champaign, IL: Human Kinetics, 2002.
4. Centers for Disease Control and Prevention. Facts on High Blood Pressure, www.cdc.gov/blood pressure/facts.htm.
5. National Center for Health Statistics. Health, United States, 2008, www.cdc.gov/nchs/data/hus/hus08.pdf#083
6. National Health Interview Survey (released), www.cdc.gov/nchs/data/nhis/earlyrelease/200903_07.pdf
7. Sesso HD, Paffenbarger RS, Lee I. Physical Activity and Coronary Heart Disease in Men: The Harvard Alumni Health Study. *Circulation*, 102, 975–980, 2000.
8. Lee I, Sesso HD, Paffenbarger RS. Physical Activity and Coronary Heart Disease in Men: Does the Duration of Exercise Episodes Predict Risk? *Circulation*, 102, 981–986, 2000.
9. American Diabetes Association. Standards of Medical Care in Diabetes. *Diabetes Care*, 30, S40–S41, 2007.
10. National Institutes of Health. *Clinical Guidelines on the Identification, Evaluation, and Treatment of Overweight and Obesity in Adults.* 1998.
11. American Heart Association. Homocyst(e)ine, Diet, and Cardiovascular Diseases. *Circulation*, 99, 178–182, 1999.
12. American Heart Association. Markers of Inflammation and Cardiovascular Disease. *Circulation*, 107, 499–511, 2003.
13. National Cholesterol Education Program. The Third Report of the Expert Panel on Detection, Evaluation, and Treatment of High Blood Cholesterol in Adults, NIH Publication No. 02-5215, 2002.
14. American Heart Association/American College of Sports Medicine. Automated External Defibrillators in Health/Fitness Facilities. *Circulation*, 105, 1147–1150, 2002.
15. American Heart Association. Aspirin as a Therapeutic Agent in Cardiovascular Disease. *Circulation*, 96, 2751–2753, 1997.
16. National Heart, Lung, and Blood Institute. *The Seventh Report of the Joint National Committee on Prevention, Detection, Evaluation, and Treatment of High Blood Pressure* (JNC 7). www.nhlbi.nih.gov/guidelines/hypertension/index.htm, July 21, 2003.

Personal Assessment

What is your risk for heart disease?

Coronary Disease Risk Prediction Score Sheet for Men Based on Total Cholesterol Level

For steps 1 through 6, determine the points for your characteristics and record these in the summary box (step 7). Using the point total, determine your risk score in step 8. Step 9 allows you to compare your risk level with that of the average person of your age. (If you are younger than 30 years old, use the 30–34 age group.) Ideally, you want your value to be at or below the "low risk" score.

Step 1

Age	
Years	Points
30–34	−1
35–39	0
40–44	1
45–49	2
50–54	3
55–59	4
60–64	5
65–69	6
70–74	7

Step 2

Total Cholesterol		
(mg/dl)	(mmol/L)	Points
<160	≤4.14	−3
160–199	4.15–5.17	0
200–239	5.18–6.21	1
240–279	6.22–7.24	2
≥280	≥7.25	3

Key	
Color	Risk
green	Very low
white	Low
yellow	Moderate
orange	High
red	Very high

Step 3

HDL Cholesterol		
(mg/dl)	(mmol/L)	Points
<35	≤0.90	2
35–44	0.91–1.16	1
45–49	1.17–1.29	0
50–59	1.30–1.55	0
≥60	≥1.56	−2

Step 4

Blood Pressure

Systolic (mm Hg)	Diastolic (mm Hg)				
	<80	80–84	85–89	90–99	≥100
<120	0				
120–129		0 pts			
130–139			1 pt		
140–159				2 pts	
≥160					3 pts

Note: When systolic and diastolic pressures provide different estimates for point scores, use the higher number.

Step 5

Diabetes	
	Points
No	0
Yes	2

Step 6

Smoker	
	Points
No	0
Yes	2

Risk estimates were derived from the experience of the NHLBI's Framingham Heart Study, a predominantly Caucasian population in Massachusetts, USA.

Step 7 (sum from steps 1–6)

Adding Up the Points	
Age	_____
Total Cholesterol	_____
HDL Cholesterol	_____
Blood Pressure	_____
Diabetes	_____
Smoker	_____
Point Total	_____

Step 8 (determine CHD risk from point total)

CHD Risk	
Point Total	10 Yr CHD Risk
≤−1	2%
0	3%
1	3%
2	4%
3	5%
4	7%
5	8%
6	10%
7	13%
8	16%
9	20%
10	25%
11	31%
12	37%
13	45%
≥14	≥53%

Step 9 (compare to man of the same age)

Comparative Risk		
Age (years)	Average 10 Yr CHD Risk	Low* 10 Yr CHD Risk
30–34	3%	2%
35–39	5%	3%
40–44	7%	4%
45–49	11%	4%
50–54	14%	6%
55–59	16%	7%
60–64	21%	9%
65–69	25%	11%
70–74	30%	14%

* Low risk was calculated for a man the same age, normal blood pressure, total cholesterol 160–199 mg/dl, HDL cholesterol 45 mg/dl, nonsmoker, no diabetes.

Source: www.nhlbi.nih.gov/about/framingham .risktmen.pdf.

Coronary Disease Risk Prediction Score Sheet for Women Based on Total Cholesterol Level

For steps 1 through 6, determine the points for your characteristics and record these in the summary box (step 7). Using the point total, determine your risk score in step 8. Step 9 allows you to compare your risk level with that of the average person of your age. (If you are younger than 30 years old, use the 30–34 age group.) Ideally, you want your value to be at or below the "low risk" score.

Step 1

Age	
Years	Points
30–34	−9
35–39	−4
40–44	0
45–49	3
50–54	6
55–59	7
60–64	8
65–69	8
70–74	8

Step 2

Total Cholesterol		
(mg/dl)	(mmol/L)	Points
<160	≤4.14	−2
160–199	4.15–5.17	0
200–239	5.18–6.21	1
240–279	6.22–7.24	1
≥280	≥7.25	3

Key	
Color	Risk
green	Very low
white	Low
yellow	Moderate
orange	High
red	Very high

Step 3

HDL Cholesterol		
(mg/dl)	(mmol/L)	Points
<35	≤0.90	5
35–44	0.91–1.16	2
45–49	1.17–1.29	1
50–59	1.30–1.55	0
≥60	≥1.56	−3

Step 4

Blood Pressure					
Systolic (mm Hg)	Diastolic (mm Hg)				
	<80	80–84	85–89	90–99	≥100
<120	−3 pts				
120–129		0 pts			
130–139			0 pts		
140–159				2 pts	
≥160					3 pts

Note: When systolic and diastolic pressures provide different estimates for point scores, use the higher number.

Step 5

Diabetes	
	Points
No	0
Yes	4

Step 6

Smoker	
	Points
No	0
Yes	2

Risk estimates were derived from the experience of the NHLBI's Framingham Heart Study, a predominantly Caucasian population in Massachusetts, USA.

TO CARRY THIS FURTHER . . .

Were you surprised with your score on this assessment? What were the factors that gave you the most points? See how changing those factors would lower your risk of heart disease.

Step 7 (sum from steps 1–6)

Adding Up the Points	
Age	_____
Total Cholesterol	_____
HDL Cholesterol	_____
Blood Pressure	_____
Diabetes	_____
Smoker	_____
Point Total	_____

Step 8 (determine CHD risk from point total)

CHD Risk	
Point Total	10 Yr CHD Risk
≤−2	1%
−1	2%
0	2%
1	2%
2	3%
3	3%
4	4%
5	4%
6	5%
7	6%
8	7%
9	8%
10	10%
11	11%
12	13%
13	15%
14	18%
15	20%
16	24%
≥17	≥27%

Comparative Risk		
Age (years)	Average 10 Yr CHD Risk	Low* 10 Yr CHD Risk
30–34	1%	<1%
35–39	1%	<1%
40–44	2%	2%
45–49	5%	3%
50–54	8%	5%
55–59	12%	7%
60–64	12%	8%
65–69	13%	8%
70–74	14%	8%

* Low risk was calculated for a woman the same age, normal blood pressure, total cholesterol 160–199 mg/dl, HDL cholesterol 55 mg/dl, nonsmoker, no diabetes.

Source: www.nhlbi.nih.gov/about/framingham.risktwom.pdf

11
chapter

Living with Cancer

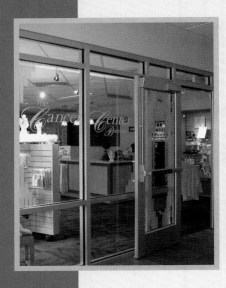

What Do You Know About Cancer?

1. Cancer involves conditions arising from the lack of cellular regulation. True or False?

2. The incidence of cancer is highest during childhood but declines with age. True or False?

3. Carcinogens are a class of recently developed cancer-fighting drugs. True or False?

4. Lung cancer is the leading cause of cancer deaths in both adult males and adult females. True or False?

5. Clear strategies, based on lifestyle changes, now exist to prevent all cancers. True or False?

6. No cancers are cured more easily today than a decade ago. True or False?

7. The "war on cancer" would be won if the use of tobacco products were completely eliminated. True or False?

Check your answers at the end of the chapter.

In spite of our understanding of its relationship to human health and our ceaseless attempts to prevent and cure it, progress in the "war on cancer" has been relatively limited. In this regard, cancer is clearly an "expensive" condition, in terms of both its human consequences and its monetary costs. However, concurrent with these costs are clear declines in the rate at which both breast and lung cancer are being diagnosed in the United States, and the survival rate for some types of cancer has significantly improved over the past several decades. Conversely, on the world stage, the picture is increasingly darker; in 2010, cancer became the leading cause of death, and cancer-related mortality is expected to double to 17 million by 2030.[1] It is estimated that 1,437,180 people developed cancer in 2008.* Once diagnosed, approximately 66 percent (adjusted for other causes of death) of this group will be alive 5 years later.[2] This 5-year period, called *relative survivability,* includes "persons who are living 5 years after diagnosis, whether disease free, in remission, or under treatment with evidence of another cancer."[2] The determination of survivability for particular forms of cancer, in time periods extending from 1 year, through 5, 10, and 15 years, is variable

*This figure does not include the majority of noninvasive cancers (carcinoma *in situ*), nor the million or more squamous cell and basal cell skin cancers.

because of a complexity of factors, including the substantial genetic variability within any one type of cancer, the differences in treatment protocols, the demands of data collection, and the nature of the population most likely to contract a particular form of cancer. Of course, predicting the length of survivability for a particular person upon diagnosis is virtually impossible. If one limits 2008's new cases to those forms of cancer for which early detection through screening is applicable (breast, colon, rectum, cervix, prostate, oral cavity, and skin), 86 percent will be alive after 5 years. Understandably, the term *cured* is used guardedly, since an initially diagnosed case of cancer can affect survivability beyond the end of the 5-year time period. Regardless of survivability, for those who develop cancer, the physical, emotional, and social costs will be substantial.

The financial cost of cancer to society is also troublesome. The National Institutes of Health (NIH) estimates that in 2007 alone cancer cost the American economy $214.2 billion, including $112.0 billion for loss of productivity due to death, $89.0 billion for direct medical costs, and $18.2 billion for indirect costs due to loss of productivity during treatment and recovery.[2] Not reflected in this total is the sizable amount of money spent on primary cancer prevention, such as school-based programs, public education efforts, and lobbying efforts intended to remove harmful products and pollutants from the environment. (See the box "Animal-Based Research on the Causes of Cancer" for more information on environmental carcinogens.)

Aside from the financial burdens of cancer, time burdens also come with receiving treatment. For example, during the initial year of treatment, the time spent on travel, waiting at appointments, receiving laboratory tests and imaging procedures, undergoing radiation procedures, and receiving chemotherapy infusions has been calculated at 360 hours for ovarian cancer, 272 hours for lung cancer, and 193 hours for kidney cancer.[3]

No single explanation can be given for why progress in eliminating cancer has been so limited. It is a combination of factors, including the aging of the population, continued use of tobacco, the high-fat American diet, the continuing urbanization and pollution of our environment, the lack of health insurance for an estimated 46 million Americans to pay for early diagnosis and proper treatment,[4] or simply our delayed recognition of cancer's true role in deaths once ascribed to other causes. Regardless, we continue to be challenged to control this array of abnormal conditions that we collectively call cancer. There is, however, increasing optimism that with a greater understanding of cancer genetics, real progress will finally be made. That said, however, the influences of the deep recession that has characterized the later years of the decade have not yet been assessed for our ability to maintain a productive response to the diagnosis, medical management, and prevention of cancer.

TALKING POINTS A close friend justifies her high-cancer-risk lifestyle by saying that "everyone will die of something." How would you counter this point?

Cancer: A Problem of Cell Regulation

Just as a corporation depends on individuals to staff its various departments, the body depends on its basic units of function, the cells. Cells band together as tissues, such as muscle tissue, to perform a prescribed function. Tissues in turn join to form organs, such as the heart, and organs are assembled into the body's several organ systems, such as the cardiovascular system. Such is the "corporate structure" of the body.

If individuals and cells are the basic units of function for their respective organizations, the failure of either to perform in a prescribed, dependable manner can erode the overall organization to the extent that it might not be able to continue. Cancer, the leading cause of death among adults under 80 years of age,[5] is a condition reflecting cell dysfunction in its most extreme form.

Cell Regulation

Most of the body's tissues lose cells over time. This continual loss requires that replacement cells come from areas of young and less specialized cells. The process of specialization required to turn the less specialized cells into mature cells is controlled by genes within the cells. On becoming specialized, these newest cells copy, or replicate, themselves. These two processes are carefully monitored by the cells' **regulatory genes.** Failure to regulate specialization and replication results in abnormal, or potentially cancerous, cells.

In addition to genes that regulate specialization and replication, cells also have genes designed to repair mistakes in the copying of genetic material (the basis of replication) and genes to suppress the growth of abnormal cells should it occur. Thus, repair genes and tumor

---

Key Terms

regulatory genes Genes that control cell specialization, replication, DNA repair, and tumor suppression.

oncogenes Faulty regulatory genes that are believed to activate the development of cancer.

proto-oncogenes (pro toe **on** co genes) Normal regulatory genes that may become oncogenes.

metastasis (muh **tas** ta sis) The spread of cancerous cells from their site of origin to other areas of the body.

---

suppressor genes, such as the *p53* gene (altered or missing in half of all cancers), can also be considered regulatory genes in place to prevent the development of abnormal cells. Should these genes fail to function properly, resulting in the development of malignant (cancerous) cells, the immune system (see Chapter 13) will ideally recognize their presence and remove them before a clinical (diagnosable) case of cancer can develop.

Because, when they are not working properly, specialization, replication, repair, and suppressor genes can become cancer-causing genes, or **oncogenes,** these four types of genes can also be referred to as **proto-oncogenes,** or potential oncogenes.[6] Beyond the involvement of the regulatory genes just discussed, nonregulatory genes also may have the potential to become oncogenic, resulting in an even wider array of cancer stimulators. Today nearly 200 different oncogenes have been identified. Further, multiple oncogenes may be involved in the development of a particular form of cancer.

Oncogene Formation

All cells have proto-oncogenes, so what events alter otherwise normal genes, including the critically important regulatory genes, causing them to become cancer-causing genes? Three mechanisms—genetic mutations, viral infections, and carcinogens—have received much attention.

Genetic mutations develop when dividing cells miscopy genetic information. If the gene that is miscopied is a gene that controls specialization, replication, repair, or tumor suppression (a proto-oncogene), the oncogene that results will allow the formation of cancerous cells. A variety of factors, including aging, free radical formation, and radiation, are associated with the miscopying of the complex genetic information that constitutes the genes found within the cell, including those intended to prevent cancer.

In both animals and humans, cancer-producing infectious agents, such as the feline leukemia virus in cats and the human immunodeficiency virus (HIV) and multiple forms of the human papillomavirus (HPV) in humans (see Chapter 13), have been identified. These viruses seek out cells of a particular type, such as cells of the immune system or the lining of the cervix, and substitute some of their genetic material for some of the cells' thus converting them into virus-producing cells. In so doing, they convert proto-oncogenes into oncogenes. Once converted into oncogenes, the altered genes are passed on through cell division.

A third possible explanation for the development of oncogenes involves the presence of environmental agents known as *carcinogens.* Over an extended period, carcinogens, such as chemicals found in tobacco smoke, polluted air and water, toxic wastes, and even high-fat foods, may convert proto-oncogenes into oncogenes. These carcinogens, such as those found in tobacco smoke, may work alone or in combination with co-carcinogenic promoters (see Chapter 9, Table 9.3) to alter the genetic material, including regulatory genes, within cells. Thus people might develop lung cancer only if they are exposed to the right combination of carcinogens over an extended period.

You may already see that some of the specific risk factors in each area—such as radiation in the development of mutations, sexually transmitted viruses in cancers of the reproductive tract, and smoking-introduced carcinogens in the development of lung cancer—can be moderated by adopting health-promoting behaviors.

Our understanding of the role of genes in the development of cancer is expanding rapidly. On occasion the public learns the identity of selected oncogenes. Very likely, many readers have heard of the *BRCA1* and *BRCA2* genes associated with breast and ovarian cancer, the *RAS* oncogene thought to influence 30 percent of all cancers, and the *p53* suppressor oncogene that may be involved in more cancers than is any other single oncogene. As geneticists continue to build on the base established by the Human Genome Project and in doing so discover additional genetic links to cancer, the possibility of some form of oncogene suppressor technology becomes a more realistic possibility in the war against cancer. That said, some within the scientific community believe that ultimately the etiology (cause) of cancer will prove to be so complex and multifaceted that the role of genetic causation will be more limited than it is currently anticipated to be.[7, 8] Rather, they feel that the ability to stop and then reverse cancerous changes at an early stage of development is more likely than is the prevention of this complex disease process. However, this text addresses the concepts of prevention in the belief that prevention-based practices reflect our personal contribution to the war on cancer.

The Cancerous Cell

Compared with noncancerous cells, cancer cells function in similar and dissimilar ways. It is the dissimilar aspects that often make them unpredictable and difficult to manage.

Perhaps the most unusual aspect of cancerous cells is their infinite life expectancy. Specifically, it appears that cancerous cells can produce an enzyme, *telomerase,* that blocks the cellular biological clock that informs normal cells that it is time to die. In spite of this ability to live forever, cancer cells do not necessarily divide more quickly than normal cells do. In fact, they can divide at the same rate or even on occasion at a slower rate.

In addition, cancerous cells do not possess the *contact inhibition* (a mechanism that influences the number of cells that can occupy a particular space at a particular time) of normal cells. In the absence of this property, cancer cells accumulate, altering the functional capacity of the tissue or organ they occupy. Further, the absence of *cellular cohesiveness* (a property seen in normal cells that "keeps them at home") allows cancer cells to spread

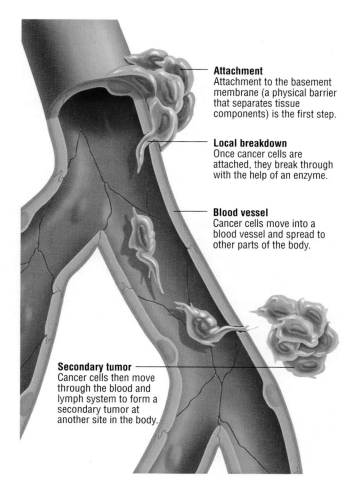

Attachment
Attachment to the basement membrane (a physical barrier that separates tissue components) is the first step.

Local breakdown
Once cancer cells are attached, they break through with the help of an enzyme.

Blood vessel
Cancer cells move into a blood vessel and spread to other parts of the body.

Secondary tumor
Cancer cells then move through the blood and lymph system to form a secondary tumor at another site in the body.

Figure 11-1 How Cancer Spreads   Locomotion (movement) is essential to the process of metastasis (spread of cancer). Scientists have identified a protein that causes cancer cells to grow arms, or pseudopodia, enabling them to move to other parts of the body.

Source: National Cancer Institute. *Horizons of Cancer Research,* NIH Pub. No. 89-3011 © 1989.

through the circulatory or lymphatic system to distant points via **metastasis** (Figure 11-1).[9] Interestingly, once migrating cancer cells arrive at a new area of the body, they "rediscover" their cellular cohesive capabilities. Adding to an understanding of cancer's spreading ability is a newly recognized role of pre-invasive lesions,[10] or disruptions in the basal layer of cells at the site of tumor formation, which allow for early outward migration of malignant cells. A final unique characteristic of cancerous cells is their ability to command the circulatory system to send them additional blood supply to meet their metabolic needs and to provide additional routes for metastasis. This *angiogenesis* capability of cancer cells makes them extremely hardy compared with noncancerous cells.[9]

Staging Cancer   In light of the interesting capabilities of malignant cells just described, it is critically important in the diagnosis and treatment of cancer that *oncologists* (physicians who have specialized in the care of cancer patients) know not only the type of cancer but also its extent. The latter determination is reflected in the concept of "staging" cancer.

For purposes of effective communication regarding the staging of cancer, the international medical community has adopted the *TNM* staging system.[2] This system first identifies the extent of a malignancy as to the extent of the primary tumor (T), whether it has or has not progressed to regional lymph node involvement (N), and the presence or absence of metastasis (M). On establishing a TNM profile of the tumor, a numerical stage (I, II, III, or IV) is determined. This categorization reflects: (I) *In situ* or "at the point of origin"; (II) *Local*—an invasive cancer confined to the organ of origin; (III) *Regional*—cancer extended into the immediately neighboring tissue or into regional lymph nodes; and (IV) *Distant*—cancer extended to distant parts of the body, either by discontinuous metastasis or through the lymphatic drainage to distant nodes.

On the basis of this system, important decisions regarding treatment, management, and prognosis (survivability) of the cancer are made—information important to all persons involved in the medical care to be received.

Benign Tumors

Noncancerous, or **benign,** tumors can also form in the body. These **tumors** are usually enclosed by a membrane and do not spread from their point of origin. Benign tumors can be dangerous when they crowd out normal tissue within a confined space.

Types of Cancer

Again, for the purposes of effective diagnosis and appropriate treatment, cancers can be named or labeled on the basis of their cell type of origin (such as hepatoma) and the organ in which they are located (such as the liver). To the medical community, the name of cancers, based on the cell type of origin, is most often used in making determination regarding diagnosis and treatment, whereas for the general public, the labeling of cancer on the basis of the organ of origin is more familiar and understandable. In this section the labeling based on the cell type of origin is given

brief consideration, while the body of the chapter describes cancer based on its organ of origin. In some cases labeling may also be extended back to embryonic germ layer of origin, but this is beyond the scope of this textbook.

For the majority of physicians and the patients with whom they must communicate, descriptions of cancer based on the organ of origin are technically adequate and, with explanation to patients, understandable. In the list that follows, several cell- or tissue-based cancers are discussed.

Carcinoma. Found most frequently in the skin, nose, mouth, throat, stomach, intestinal tract, glands, nerves, breasts, urinary and genital structures, lungs, kidneys, and liver; approximately 85 percent of all malignant tumors are classified as carcinomas.

Sarcoma. Formed in the connective tissues of the body; bone, cartilage, and tendons are the sites of sarcoma development; only 2 percent of all malignancies are of this type.

Melanoma. Arises from the melanin-containing cells of skin; found most often in people who have had extensive sun exposure, particularly a deep, penetrating sunburn; although once rare, the amount of this cancer has increased markedly in recent years; remains among the most deadly forms of cancer.

Neuroblastoma. Originates in the immature cells found within the central nervous system; neuroblastomas are rare; usually found in children.

Adenocarcinoma. Derived from cells of the endocrine glands.

Hepatoma. Originates in cells of the liver; although not thought to be directly caused by alcohol use, seen more frequently in people who have experienced **sclerotic changes** in the liver.

Leukemia. Found in cells of the blood and blood-forming tissues; characterized by abnormal, immature white blood cell formation; several forms are found in children and adults.

Lymphoma. Arises in cells of the lymphatic tissues or other immune system tissues; includes lymphosarcomas and Hodgkin's disease; characterized by abnormal white cell production and decreased resistance.

Figure 11-2 presents information about the estimated new cases of cancer and deaths from cancer at various sites in both men and women.[2] Table 11.1 on page 300 shows that cancer incidence and mortality rates vary among different racial and ethnic groups.

Cancer at Selected Sites in the Body

A second and more familiar way to describe cancer is on the basis of the organ site at which it occurs. The following discussion relates to some of these more familiar sites. A lack

---

> **Key Terms**
>
> **benign** Noncancerous localized nonmalignant tumors contained within a fibrous membrane.
>
> **tumor** Mass of cells; may be cancerous (malignant) or noncancerous (benign).
>
> **sclerotic changes** (skluh **rot** ick) Thickening or hardening of tissues.

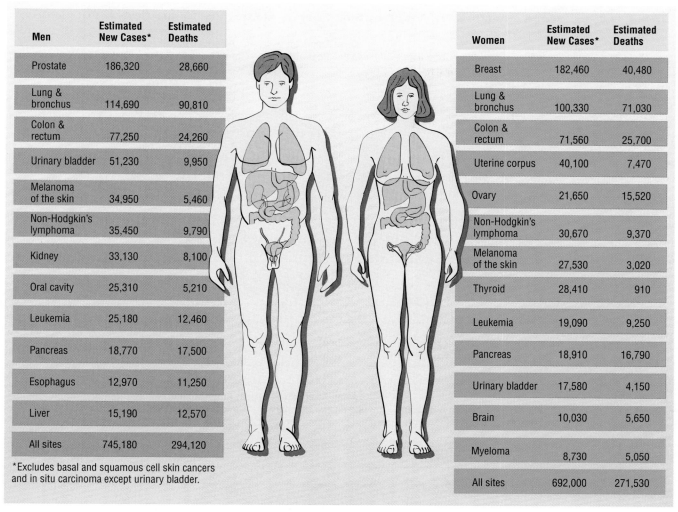

Men	Estimated New Cases*	Estimated Deaths
Prostate	186,320	28,660
Lung & bronchus	114,690	90,810
Colon & rectum	77,250	24,260
Urinary bladder	51,230	9,950
Melanoma of the skin	34,950	5,460
Non-Hodgkin's lymphoma	35,450	9,790
Kidney	33,130	8,100
Oral cavity	25,310	5,210
Leukemia	25,180	12,460
Pancreas	18,770	17,500
Esophagus	12,970	11,250
Liver	15,190	12,570
All sites	745,180	294,120

*Excludes basal and squamous cell skin cancers and in situ carcinoma except urinary bladder.

Women	Estimated New Cases*	Estimated Deaths
Breast	182,460	40,480
Lung & bronchus	100,330	71,030
Colon & rectum	71,560	25,700
Uterine corpus	40,100	7,470
Ovary	21,650	15,520
Non-Hodgkin's lymphoma	30,670	9,370
Melanoma of the skin	27,530	3,020
Thyroid	28,410	910
Leukemia	19,090	9,250
Pancreas	18,910	16,790
Urinary bladder	17,580	4,150
Brain	10,030	5,650
Myeloma	8,730	5,050
All sites	692,000	271,530

Figure 11-2 Cancer Cases and Deaths　These 2008 estimates of new cases of cancer and deaths from cancer reveal some significant similarities between men and women. Note that lung cancer is the leading cause of cancer deaths for both sexes.

Source: American Cancer Society. *Cancer Facts and Figures 2008*. Atlanta: American Cancer Society, Inc. Used with permission.

of space, in combination with the wide arrays of human cancers, limits the number of specific malignancies that can be described. Remember also that regular screening procedures can lead to early identification of cancer at these sites (see the box "Screening Guidelines for the Early Detection of Cancer in Asymptomatic People" on page 301).

Skin Cancer

In the footnote in Figure 11-2, you will see that the American Cancer Society (ACS) excludes two of the three forms of skin cancer and reports statistics only for melanoma, the least common form of skin cancer but the most serious of the three forms. However, when all three forms (melanoma, basal cell, and squamous cell) are taken into account, skin cancer is the most common kind of cancer, with an estimate of substantially more than 1 million new cases in 2008. On the basis of this prevalence, this textbook covers skin cancer first.

Thanks largely to our desire for a fashionable tan, many teens and adults have spent more time in the sun (and in tanning booths) than their skin can tolerate. As a result, skin cancer, once common only among people who had to work in the sun, is occurring with alarming frequency. In 2008, more than 1 million Americans developed basal or squamous cell skin cancer, and 63,360 cases of highly dangerous malignant melanoma were diagnosed.[2]

Deaths from skin cancer do occur, with 11,200 estimated in 2008. Approximately 75 percent of these deaths were the result of malignant melanoma.

Risk Factors　Severe sunburning during childhood and chronic sun exposure during adolescence and younger adulthood are largely responsible for the "epidemic" of skin cancer being reported. The current emphasis on screening for skin cancer may also be increasing the

Table 11.1 Incidence and Mortality Rates* by Site, Race, and Ethnicity, United States, 2000–2004

Incidence	White	African American	Asian American and Pacific Islander	American Indian and Alaska Native[†]	Hispanic/Latino[‡§]
All sites					
Males	556.7	663.7	359.5	321.2	421.3
Females	439.2	396.9	285.8	282.4	314.2
Breast (female)	132.5	118.3	89.0	69.8	89.3
Colon & rectum					
Males	60.4	72.6	49.7	42.1	47.5
Females	44.0	55.0	35.3	39.6	32.9
Kidney & renal pelvis					
Males	18.3	20.4	8.9	18.5	16.5
Females	9.1	9.7	4.3	11.5	9.1
Liver & bile duct					
Males	7.9	12.7	21.3	14.8	14.4
Females	2.9	3.8	7.9	5.5	5.7
Lung & bronchus					
Males	81.0	110.6	55.1	53.7	44.7
Females	54.6	53.7	27.7	36.7	25.2
Prostate	161.4	255.5	96.5	68.2	140.8
Stomach					
Males	16.2	17.5	18.9	16.3	16.0
Females	4.7	9.1	10.8	7.9	9.6
Uterine cervix	8.5	11.4	8.0	6.6	13.8

Mortality	White	African American	Asian American and Pacific Islander	American Indian and Alaska Native[†]	Hispanic/Latino[‡¶]
All sites					
Males	234.7	321.8	141.7	187.9	162.2
Females	161.4	189.3	96.7	141.2	106.7
Breast (female)	25.0	33.8	12.6	16.1	16.1
Colon & rectum					
Males	22.9	32.7	15.0	20.6	17.0
Females	15.9	22.9	10.3	14.3	11.1
Kidney & renal pelvis					
Males	6.2	6.1	2.4	9.3	5.4
Females	2.8	2.8	1.1	4.3	2.3
Liver & bile duct					
Males	6.5	10.0	15.5	10.7	10.8
Females	2.8	3.9	6.7	6.4	5.0
Lung & bronchus					
Males	72.6	95.8	38.3	49.6	36.0
Females	42.1	39.8	18.5	32.7	14.6
Prostate	25.6	62.3	11.3	21.5	21.2
Stomach					
Males	5.2	11.9	10.5	9.6	9.1
Females	2.6	5.8	6.2	5.5	5.1
Uterine cervix	2.3	4.9	2.4	4.0	3.3

*Per 100,000, age adjusted to the 2000 US standard population.
[†]Data based on Contract Health Service Delivery Areas (CHSDA), 624 counties comprising 54% of the US American Indian/Alaska Native population; for more information, please see Espey DK, Wu XC, Swan J, et al. Annual report to the nation on the status of cancer, 1975–2004, featuring cancer in American Indians and Alaska Natives.
[‡]Persons of Hispanic/Latino origin may be of any race.
[§]Data unavailable from the Alaska Native Registry and Kentucky.
[¶]Data unavailable from Minnesota, New Hampshire, and North Dakota.
Source: Ries LAG, Melbert D, Krapcho M, et al (Eds.). *SEER Cancer Statistics Review, 1975–2004*, National Cancer Institute, Bethesda, MD, www.seer.cancer.gov/csr/1975_2004/, 2007.

Screening Guidelines for the Early Detection of Cancer in Asymptomatic People

Site	Recommendation
Breast	• Yearly mammograms are recommended starting at age 40. The age at which screening should be stopped should be individualized by considering the potential risks and benefits of screening in the context of overall health status and longevity. • Clinical breast exams should be part of a periodic health exam about every 3 years for women in their 20s and 30s, and every year for women 40 and older. • Women should know how their breasts normally feel and report any breast change promptly to their health care providers. Breast self-exam is an option for women starting in their 20s. • Screening MRI is recommended for women with an approximately 20%–25% or greater lifetime risk of breast cancer, including women with a strong family history of breast or ovarian cancer and women who were treated for Hodgkin disease.
Colon and rectum	Beginning at age 50, men and women should begin screening with 1 of the examination schedules below: • A fecal occult blood test (FOBT) or fecal immunochemical test (FIT) every year • A flexible sigmoidoscopy (FSIG) every 5 years • Annual FOBT or FIT and flexible sigmoidoscopy every 5 years* • A double-contrast barium enema every 5 years • A colonoscopy every 10 years *Combined testing is preferred over either annual FOBT or FIT, or FSIG every 5 years, alone. People who are at moderate or high risk for colorectal cancer should talk with a doctor about a different testing schedule.
Prostate	The PSA test and the digital rectal examination should be offered annually, beginning at age 50, to men who have a life expectancy of at least 10 years. Men at high risk (African American men and men with a strong family history of 1 or more first-degree relatives diagnosed with prostate cancer at an early age) should begin testing at age 45. For both men at average risk and high risk, information should be provided about what is known and what is uncertain about the benefits and limitations of early detection and treatment of prostate cancer so that they can make an informed decision about testing.
Uterus	**Cervix:** Screening should begin approximately 3 years after a woman begins having vaginal intercourse, but no later than 21 years of age. Screening should be done every year with regular Pap tests or every 2 years using liquid-based tests. At or after age 30, women who have had 3 normal test results in a row may get screened every 2 to 3 years. Alternatively, cervical cancer screening with HPV DNA testing and conventional or liquid-based cytology could be performed every 3 years. However, doctors may suggest a woman get screened more often if she has certain risk factors, such as HIV infection or a weak immune system. Women ages 70 years and older who have had 3 or more consecutive normal Pap tests in the last 10 years may choose to stop cervical cancer screening. Screening after total hysterectomy (with removal of the cervix) is not necessary unless the surgery was done as a treatment for cervical cancer. **Endometrium:** The American Cancer Society recommends that at the time of menopause all women should be informed about the risks and symptoms of endometrial cancer, and strongly encouraged to report any unexpected bleeding or spotting to their physicians. Annual screening for endometrial cancer with endometrial biopsy beginning at age 35 should be offered to women with or at risk for hereditary nonpolyposis colon cancer (HNPCC).
Cancer-related checkup	For individuals undergoing periodic health examinations, a cancer-related checkup should include health counseling, and depending on a person's age and gender, might include examinations for cancers of the thyroid, oral cavity, skin, lymph nodes, testes, and ovaries, as well as for some nonmalignant diseases.

American Cancer Society guidelines for early cancer detection are assessed annually in order to identify whether there is new scientific evidence sufficient to warrant a reevaluation of current recommendations. If evidence is sufficiently compelling to consider a change or clarification in a current guideline or the development of a new guideline, a formal procedure is initiated. Guidelines are formally evaluated every 5 years regardless of whether new evidence suggests a change in the existing recommendations. There are 9 steps in this procedure, and these "guidelines for guideline development" were formally established to provide a specific methodology for science and expert judgment to form the underpinnings of specific statements and recommendations from the Society. These procedures constitute a deliberate process to ensure that all Society recommendations have the same methodological and evidence-based process at their core. This process also employs a system for rating strength and consistency of evidence that is similar to that employed by the Agency for Healthcare Research and Quality (AHRQ) and the U.S. Preventive Services Task Force (USPSTF).

Based on information in American Cancer Society. *Cancer Facts and Figures 2009.* Atlanta: American Cancer Society, Inc.

Table 11.2 Global Solar UV Index and Risk of Harm from Unprotected UV Exposure

UV Index	Risk Level	Recommended Protection
≥2	Low	Wear sunglasses on bright days. In winter, reflection off snow can nearly double UV strength. If you burn easily, cover up and use sunscreen.
3–5	Moderate	Take precautions, such as covering up, if you will be outside. Stay in shade near midday when the sun is strongest.
6–7	High	Reduce time in the sun between 10 a.m. and 4 p.m. Cover up, wear a wide-brim hat and sunglasses, and use sunscreen with an SPF of at least 15.
8–10	Very high	Take extra precautions; unprotected skin will be damaged and can burn quickly. Minimize sun exposure between 10 a.m. and 4 p.m. Otherwise, seek shade, cover up, wear a wide-brim hat and sunglasses, and use sunscreen with an SPF of at least 15.
11+	Extreme	Take all precautions; unprotected skin can burn in minutes. Avoid sun exposure from 10 a.m. to 4 p.m. Seek shade, cover up, wear a wide-brim hat and sunglasses, and apply sunscreen with an SPF of at least 15 liberally every 2 hours. Beachgoers should know that white sand and other bright surfaces reflect UV and will increase UV exposure.

Source: Environmental Protection Agency, Sunwise Program, UV Index Scale, www.epa.gov/sunwise1/uvindex2.html.

incidence of early-stage cancer being reported. Progress is being made in deterring people from pursuing the perfect tan. The American Academy of Dermatology reports that the incidence of deliberate tanning is down, and the use of sunscreens has increased. Occupational exposure to some hydrocarbon compounds can also cause skin cancer.

In spite of the progress reported by the American Academy of Dermatology, Americans continue to seek natural sources of sun or tanning salons for cosmetically related tanning, or they find that their exposure cannot be avoided owing to the nature of their jobs. In regard to "purposeful tanning" either outdoors or indoors, recent research has given some credibility to the contention that tanning is emotionally "addictive." Underlying this contention is a small but growing body of evidence that purposeful frequent tanning, using tanning beds, seems to elevate levels of beta-endorphins (a form of biological opiate) in the bloodstream. When frequent tanners have their ultraviolet (UV) stimulated opioid production blocked, they demonstrate withdrawal-like symptoms. Such is not the case in infrequent tanners and non-tanners.[11] In fact, people (most frequently younger women) who are so compulsive about tanning that they do so multiple times per week are now being described as "tanorexics." For all tanning salon users, and particularly the tanorexics, the UV radiation generated by tanning-bed bulbs was classified in August 2009 as a definitive carcinogenic agent, particularly for a person beginning tanning-bed use during the teen years.

For those who must or choose to seek extended periods of time in the sun, the most recently established UV Index, the Global Solar UV Index, can be found in Table 11.2. This daily index for your ZIP code (in the United States) can be accessed online at www.epa.gov/sunwise/uvindex.html. It is also often given on local television stations or in some local newspapers.

Prevention Prevention of skin cancer should be a high priority for people who enjoy the sun or must work outdoors. The use of sunscreen with a sun protection factor (SPF) of 15 or greater is very important. In addition, parents can help their children prevent skin cancer later in life by restricting their outdoor play from 11 a.m. to 2 p.m. Further, it should be noted that in response to concerns over tanning and sunburns during childhood, products intended to protect children from the sun, such as high-quality sunglasses, UV-blocking summer clothing and swim wear, stroller covers, and spray-on sunscreen with an SPF of 70 or higher, are now appearing in stores.

In fairness to readers, it must be mentioned that controversy abounds within the scientific community as to both the effectiveness of sunscreens and the form of sunscreen used (organic versus inorganic). That said, new technologies are under development and the current controversy may eventually be resolved. Regardless, practicing dermatologists continue to recommend their use. However, users are reminded that the level of protection provided is not doubled by simply doubling the SPF—for example, a sunscreen carrying an SPF of 30 does not provide twice the protection provided by a product with an SPF of 15.

A further rationale for preventing the development of skin cancer is the recently described relationship between skin cancer and the heightened probability of developing other forms of cancer later in life. Research suggests that people who have had skin cancer carry a 20 to 30 percent greater risk of developing other types of cancer than do people who have never developed skin cancer. (The Personal Assessment at the end of the chapter will help you determine your risk of developing this kind of cancer.)

Early Detection Although many doctors do not emphasize this point enough, the key to the successful treatment of skin cancer is early detection. For basal cell or squamous cell cancer, a pale, waxlike, pearly nodule or red, scaly patch may be the first symptom. Other types of skin cancer may be indicated by a gradual change in the appearance of an existing mole. A physician should be consulted if such a change is noted. Melanoma usually begins as a small, molelike growth that increases progressively in size, changes color, ulcerates, and bleeds easily. To help detect melanoma, the American Cancer Society recommends using the following guidelines: **A** for asymmetry, **B** for border irregularity, **C** for color (change), and **D** for a diameter greater than 6 mm.[2]

Figure 11-3 shows a mole that would be considered harmless and one that clearly demonstrates the ABCD characteristics just described. (See the box "Self-Examination for Melanoma" for a description of how to make a regular inspection of the skin.)

Treatment   When nonmelanoma skin cancer is found, an almost 100 percent cure rate can be expected. Treatment of these skin cancers can involve surgical removal by traditional excising or laser vaporization, destruction by burning or freezing, or destruction using X-ray therapy. When the more serious melanomas are found at an early stage, a high cure rate (99 percent) is accomplished using the same techniques. However, when malignant melanomas are more advanced, extensive surgery and chemotherapy are necessary. The 5-year survival rate for regionalized forms of the disease drops to 65 percent, and, unfortunately, long-term disease recovery is uncommon (15 percent).[2]

However, new treatments for malignant melanoma offer a ray of hope to people with the disease. Among the more promising of these is a combination therapy using interleukin-2, an immune system chemical that stimulates various "killer cells" within the immune system and a drug that activates phagocytic cells within the immune system. Additionally, a vaccine has been developed that stimulates the immune system to attack the melanoma cells more aggressively. This treatment-centered (rather than prevention-centered) vaccine uses components of the patient's own cancer cells to mobilize more white blood cells and produce more antibodies to fight the cancer.

Yet another new avenue of treatment of malignant melanoma is related to the melanoma cells' preference for a relatively low level of oxygenation in comparison with higher levels preferred by most cells. A new medication undergoing early trials enhances the melanoma cells' exposure to oxygen, thus rendering them less aggressive than is normally the case.

In addition to "regular" skin cancer and malignant melanoma, a second form of highly lethal skin cancer, *Merkel cell carcinoma,* is beginning to receive much needed attention.[12] This infrequently seen form of cancer first appears as a painless bump that can be mistaken for a cyst. If not excised at an early point, a biopsy performed, and then treated aggressively with radiation, this malignancy has a very high mortality rate.

Perhaps because nonmelanoma skin cancers are so common in adults (generally 40 years of age and older) and so successfully treated, we tend not to see these cancers as being a substantial problem. However, the medical management of the 1 million-plus cases diagnosed each

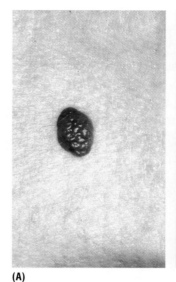 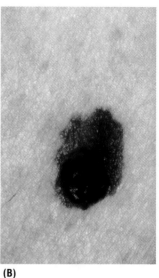

(A)   **(B)**

Figure 11-3 Normal Mole versus Malignant Melanoma   A: Normal mole. This type of lesion is often seen in large numbers on the skin of young adults and can affect any body site. Note its symmetrical shape, regular borders, uniform color, and relatively small size (actual size is about 6 millimeters). **B:** Malignant melanoma. Note its asymmetrical shape, irregular borders, uneven color, and relatively large size (actual size is about 2 centimeters).

year is a substantial cost to our heath care industry, and thus to us as individuals. When treated in a physician's office, the cost of removing a nonmelanoma skin cancer is approximately $500; when removed in an ambulatory (walk-in) clinic the cost increases to nearly $950; and when removed in the hospital the cost exceeds $4,300.[12]

Lung Cancer

Lung cancer is one of the most lethal and frequently diagnosed forms of cancer. Primarily because of the advanced stage of the disease at the time symptoms first appear, only 15 percent of all people with lung cancer (all stages) survive 5 years beyond diagnosis.[2] By the time a person is sufficiently concerned about having a persistent cough, blood-streaked sputum, and chest pain, it is often too late for treatment to be effective. This failure to be able to diagnose lung cancer in its earlier stages could, however, begin to change. Currently, the National Cancer Institute is studying the efficacy of *spiral CT scans* in detecting lung tumors earlier than can be done by conventional chest X-rays. At a current cost of $200 to $300, computerized axial tomography (CT) scanning technology is rapidly replacing the standard chest X-ray as the primary means of detecting lung cancer.[13]

Risk Factors   Today it is known that genetic predisposition is important in the development of lung cancer. Perhaps, in fact, the majority of people who develop this form

Through a routine physical exam, my brother found out he has melanoma. How should I check myself for this condition?

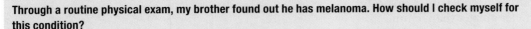

How to look for melanoma

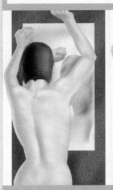 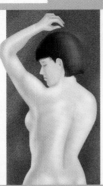 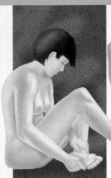 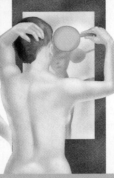 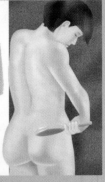

1. Examine your body front and back in the mirror, then right and left sides with arms raised.

2. Bend your elbows and carefully look at your palms, forearms, and under your upper arms.

3. Look at the backs of your legs and feet, the spaces between your toes, and the soles of your feet.

4. Examine the back of your neck and scalp with a hand mirror. Part your hair for a closer look.

5. Finally, check your back and buttocks with a mirror.

What to look for
Potential signs of malignancy in moles or pigmented spots:

Asymmetry

One half unlike the other half

Irregularity Border

Border irregular or poorly defined

Color

Color varies from one area to another; shades of tan, brown, or black

Diameter

Diameter larger than 6 mm, as a rule (diameter of a pencil eraser)

Source: Based on information from the American Academy of Dermatology.

of cancer have an inherited "head start." When people who are genetically at risk also smoke, their level of risk for developing lung cancer is significantly greater than it is for nonsmokers. Of particular interest at this time are multiple genes on chromosome 3. Damage to three tumor suppressors on this chromosome is found in virtually every case of small-cell lung cancer and 90 percent of nonsmall-cell lung cancer. Most of the remaining lung cancer cases appear in people who smoke but are not genetically predisposed.

Cigarette smoking is the single most important behavioral factor in the development of lung cancer. For men who smoke, the rate of lung cancer is 23 times higher than it is for men who do not smoke. For women who smoke, the rate is 13 times higher than for women who do not smoke. Smokers account for nearly 87 percent of all cases of lung cancer, and lung cancer itself produces at least 30 percent of all cancer-caused deaths.[2]

Since 1987, lung cancer has exceeded breast cancer as the leading cause of cancer death in women, although more new cases of breast cancer than lung cancer are diagnosed each year. The incidence of lung cancer in men has shown a gradual decline over the last several years that parallels their declining use of tobacco products. In contrast to men, in women the rate of lung cancer development has remained relatively constant over the last several years. Women tend to develop a different form of lung cancer than men, suggesting that they might absorb toxins more completely than men do.[14] Also, among nonsmokers, women are more likely to develop lung cancer, although recent studies have challenged this conclusion. (See the box "Lung Cancer in Nonsmokers" for more information on this group.) The tumor type found in women may also be estrogen-sensitive, as is true for forms of breast cancer, in comparison to the primary type developed by men.[14] One hopes that a decline in

Lung Cancer in Nonsmokers

The March 6, 2006, death of Dana Reeve, at the age of 44, from lung cancer shocked the nation and called to our attention the fact that even nonsmokers are susceptible to this highly lethal form of cancer. In August 2005, soon after the death of her husband, Christopher Reeve, Dana Reeve announced her illness and that she had begun a demanding course of treatment in an attempt to recover her health. As she battled, questions abounded as to why nonsmokers who reside with nonsmokers could be victims of lung cancer.

Dana Reeve's illness made us aware that women who are non-smokers are clearly more susceptible to developing lung cancer than are their male counterparts. Today it is recognized that nearly 20 percent of female lung cancer victims are nonsmokers. Experts speculate that females may be more susceptible than males to environmental carcinogenic agents, including secondhand smoke and radon gas. A second line of reasoning suggests that nonsmoking female lung cancer victims may have a genetic susceptibility to develop lung cancer through noncarcinogenic mechanisms, such as those described earlier in this chapter in the discussion of oncogene formation. Furthermore, the lung cancer that develops in nonsmoking women tends to be of a more aggressive type than that seen in males who are nonsmokers.

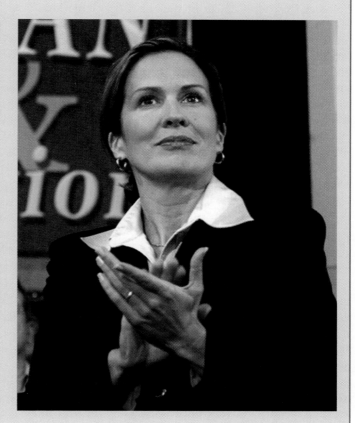

new cases of lung cancer will occur in women and reflect a continued decline in tobacco use.

Environmental agents, such as radon, asbestos, beryllium, uranium, and air pollutants, make a smaller contribution to the development of lung cancer. Radon alone may be the principal causative agent in most lung cancer found in nonsmokers.

Prevention The preceding information clearly suggests that not smoking or quitting smoking and avoidance of secondhand smoke (see Chapter 9) are the most important factors in the prevention of lung cancer. In addition, place of residence, particularly as it relates to air pollution, is a long-suspected risk factor for lung cancer. Nonsmokers who are considering living with a smoker or working in a confined area where secondhand smoke is prevalent should carefully consider the risk of developing lung cancer. A recent study does, however, lessen concern over moderate alcohol use and the risk of developing lung cancer.

Treatment The prognosis for surviving lung cancer remains extremely guarded. Depending on the type of lung cancer, its extent, and factors related to the patient's

overall health, various combinations of surgery, radiation, and chemotherapy remain the physicians' primary approach to treatment. Today, for persons with early-stage lung cancer, chemotherapy, following surgery, has increased survivability slightly. Additionally, experimental vaccines (LBLP25, TGF_beta2 antisense gene vaccine, GVAX) now in the early stages of testing have shown extremely encouraging results in patients with nonsmall-cell lung cancer, the most common form of the disease.[15] GVAX, in both patient-specific and nonspecific forms, is in Phase III clinical trials.[15] Also, a variety of new drugs now available or soon to be available for use in the treatment of non small-cell lung cancer (some for multiple types of cancer) include Iressa, Tarceva, Avastin, and Erbitux. The extent to which new agents are efficacious remains under study.

Despite the new vaccines and medication mentioned, in combination with older approaches to treating lung cancer, such as surgery, radiation, and chemotherapies, the level of improvement in survivability from lung cancer is nearly static (with some regional variability). In the opinion of experts, significant improvement cannot occur in the absence of even more aggressive reductions in smoking, particularly among women.[16]

Colorectal Cancer

Colorectal cancer—cancer of the colon (the large intestine) and the rectum (the terminal portion of the large intestine)—is the third most common kind of new cancer (excluding skin cancers) in both males and females, the second leading cause of cancer deaths in males (behind lung cancer), and the third leading cause of cancer deaths in females (behind lung and breast cancers) (see Figure 11-2).

Colorectal cancer, like many other forms of cancer, has a complex pathology, whose explanation lies beyond the scope of this book. However, classification as to the exact type of tumor and its location of origin within the colon or rectum will provide the oncologist with important information regarding the potential pattern of spread and the nature of treatment. Fortunately, when diagnosed in a localized state, colorectal cancer has a relatively high survival rate (90 percent when localized, and 68 percent for all stages).[2]

Risk Factors　Underlying the development of colorectal cancer are at least two potentially important areas of risk: genetic susceptibility and dietary patterns. Genes have recently been discovered that lead to familial colon cancer and familial polyposis (abnormal tissue growth that occurs before the formation of cancer) and are believed to be responsible for the tendency of colorectal cancer to run in families. Dietary risk factors include diets that are high in saturated fat from red meat and low in fruits and vegetables, which contain antioxidant vitamins and fiber. In regard to fiber's ability to prevent colorectal cancer, however, the ability of dietary fiber, when taken in supplement form, is in question.

In addition to familial and dietary links to an increased risk of colorectal cancer, alcohol use and smoking (alone or in combination) also appear related, particularly in terms of age of onset. In persons who regularly drink and/or smoke, colorectal cancer may appear five to seven years earlier than in those people who do not.[17] This pattern was particularly noted in males.

Prevention　Small outpouchings in the lower intestinal tract wall, called *polyps,* are frequently important in the eventual development of colorectal cancer. Prompt removal of polyps has been shown to lower the risk of colorectal cancer. Further, some evidence indicates that the development of colorectal cancer may be prevented or slowed through regular exercise, an increase in dietary calcium intake, and long-term folic acid supplementation. Additionally, oral contraceptive use may be protective for women. Recently, the belief that the consistent use of a low-dose (81 mg) aspirin could reduce polyp formation was strongly disputed, and is no longer recommended by the American Cancer Association for this purpose (although low-dose aspirin therapy is recommended in conjunction with cardiovascular disease prevention).

Little difference in polyp formation was noted between those taking daily aspirin therapy and those who did not.

Again, routine screening for colorectal cancer should be considered a form of prevention, much as prostate-specific autigen (PSA) testing is for prostate cancer and mammography is for breast cancer.

Early Detection　Listed below are the seven warning signs of cancer, which the acronym CAUTION will help you remember:

- **C**hange in bowel or bladder habits
- **A** sore that does not heal
- **U**nusual bleeding or discharge
- **T**hickening or lump in the breast or elsewhere
- **I**ndigestion or difficulty in swallowing
- **O**bvious change in a wart or mole
- **N**agging cough or hoarseness

In addition, a family history of inflammatory bowel disease, polyp formation, or colorectal cancer should make one more alert to symptoms.[2] In people over age 50, any sudden change in bowel habits that lasts 10 days or longer should be evaluated by a physician. The American Cancer Society's recommendations for colorectal cancer screening, beginning at age 50—including fecal occult blood tests, flexible sigmoidoscopy examinations, double-contrast barium enema examinations, and colonoscopy examinations—are detailed in the box "Screening Guidelines for the Early Detection of Cancer in Asymptomatic People" on page 301. However, in March 2005, the American College of Gastroenterology proposed that, because of the higher incidence of colorectal cancer in African Americans, routine colonoscopy should begin at age 45 for this group rather than at age 50. On the basis of information gleaned from the study just mentioned, smokers and regular users of alcohol could expect recommendations for earlier screening, beginning at age 45.

In 2008, additional colorectal cancer screening recommendations were introduced by other medical organizations that broadened the basic guidelines issued by the American Cancer Society (see page 301). Principal among these were recommendations by the U.S. Preventive Services Task Force regarding (1) discontinuation of *routine* colorectal screening for adults aged 76 to 85 years (although remaining responsive, via examination, to episodic signs of disease) and (2) discontinuance of all screening for persons over 85 years of age.[18]

Although not addressed as a recommendation, the value of "virtual colonoscopy" (in which a miniaturized camera is swallowed, thus allowing photography of the entire gastrointestinal tract) was substantiated for determining the identity of persons who did not require a traditional colonoscopy that would require the much-feared preparation and procedure of traditional scoping.

A second alternative technique for viewing the colon and rectum involves the use of CT scanning of the lower intestinal tract. Although adequately effective, this procedure also requires the preparation whose fear causes so many people to disregard the need for any colorectal screening. Additionally, some important limitations were recognized, as well as radiation exposure produced by the procedure.[19]

It should be noted that the digital stool-sample test (in which a finger, or "digit," is inserted into the rectum), which is the only stool-sample test used by many doctors and taken during physical examinations, as well as the newer test to find traces of cancer cell DNA in the stool, have both been found to be less effective than previously believed.

Treatment   When one or more of these screening procedures suggests the possibility of disease within the lower intestinal tract, a careful visual evaluation of the entire length of the colon will be undertaken. During colonoscopy, areas of concern can be biopsied and the presence of a malignancy confirmed. Upon diagnosis, a localized and noninvasive malignancy will be removed surgically. When an invasive tumor is identified, supportive treatment with radiation or chemotherapy is necessary. Metastatic cancer requires chemotherapy. New guidelines regarding screening for metastatic tumors arising from a primary colorectal cancer are being formulated. These guidelines are meant to remind physicians that metastatic tumors are unlikely to be found through use of colonoscopy.

Breast Cancer

Surpassed only by lung cancer, breast cancer is the second leading cause of death from cancer in women. It is the third leading cause of cancer deaths overall. Nearly one in eight women will develop breast cancer in her lifetime, resulting in an estimated 184,450 new invasive cases and 40,480 deaths in 2008. In men, an estimated 1,990 new cases and 450 deaths occurred in 2008 (see the box "Breast Cancer: A Rare Diagnosis in Men").[2] As women age, their risk of developing breast cancer increases. Regardless of age, however, waiting to learn whether a suspicious lump is benign or is a relatively harmless fluid-filled cyst is stressful. Today, 98 percent of women whose breast cancer is localized (confined to the breast) survive more than 5 years.

Most recently it has been reported that the actual rate of new cases of breast cancer has declined. According to data from 2004 (the last year for which actual versus estimated numbers of new cases of various forms of cancer are known), a 3.5 percent decline in new breast cancer cases was reported. Initial interpretation of this dramatic finding relates to a sharp decline in the use of menopause-related hormone replacement therapy and a disturbing decline in the use of mammograms.[20]

Risk Factors   Although all women and men are at some risk of developing breast cancer, the following groups of women have a higher risk:

- Women whose menstrual periods began at an early age, or whose menopause occurred late (although the former may be more important than the latter is)
- Women who had no children, had their first child later in life, or did not nurse
- Women who have used hormone replacement therapy (HRT)—particularly combined estrogen and progestin or combined estrogen and testosterone
- Women who have a high degree of breast density (high level of glandular tissues relative to fat) or biopsy-established hyperplasia
- Women whose diets are high in saturated fats, who are sedentary, or who are obese after menopause (particularly central body cavity obesity; see Chapter 6)
- Women who carry the *BRCA1* and/or *BRCA2* mutated tumor suppressor genes, or those with a strong family history of breast cancer

As mentioned, significant concern exists regarding the long-term use of hormone replacement therapy and the development of breast cancer in postmenopausal women. In fact, in a government-sponsored study (Women's Health Initiative Study) the link appeared so strongly and early that the study was terminated much earlier than had been planned. Researchers found that tumor development in women taking HRT versus those on a placebo was more common, that tumors were larger at diagnosis, and that tumors were more often invasive.[21] Many physicians are now advising that HRT be used only on a very short-term basis to relieve the symptoms of menopause, rather than the much longer period of time previously deemed appropriate.

While initial concerns about the risk of breast cancer in postmenopausal women was centered on the use of HRT medication combining estrogen and progesterone, recent attention is being directed to those using HRTs that combine estrogen and testosterone. These medications, often compounded (formulated) by pharmacists on the directions of a physician, may increase the risk of more invasive breast cancer.[22]

The effects of environmental pollutants and regional influences have also been investigated as causative factors in

---

Key Terms

sigmoidoscopy Examination of the sigmoid colon (lowest section of the large intestine), using a short, flexible fiber-optic scope.

colonoscopy (co lun **os** ko py) Examination of the entire length of the colon, using a flexible fiber-optic scope to inspect the structure's inner lining.

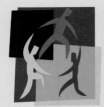

the development of breast cancer. Environmental pollutants vary from region to region and are influenced by a number of factors, including the type of industrial and agricultural activity in a particular area. A wide array of regional factors may be involved, including the genetic background of people in a given area and lifestyle differences involving diet, alcohol consumption, and exercise patterns.

The role of genetic predisposition in the development of breast cancer has also received considerable attention. For example, a small percentage (perhaps 5 to 10 percent) of women with breast cancer have inherited or developed mutations in one or both of two tumor suppressor genes (proto-oncogenes), *BRCA1* and *BRCA2*. Discovered in 1994 and 1995, respectively, and currently the focus of extensive research, more than 200 mutations in these genes have been identified. In a study involving 5,000 Ashkenazi Jews (Jews of Central and Eastern European descent) living in the Washington, D.C., area, mutation in the *BRCA1* gene resulted in a 56 percent greater chance of developing breast cancer by age 70 (versus a 13 percent greater risk for people without a mutated version of the gene).[23] In the years since these genes' identification, studies have been ongoing in an attempt to more accurately define the level of risk for developing breast cancer among women who carry one or both *BRCA1* or *BRCA2* mutations regardless of race or other aspects of ethnicity.[24,25] At this time, however, it cannot be definitively determined whether a given carrier of a mutated gene will actually develop cancer. Both of these genes are also associated with increased risk of developing ovarian cancer (see pages 316–317) and, perhaps, prostate cancer in men.

In addition to the much-studied *BRCA1* and *BRCA2* genes discussed earlier, other genetic mutations have

been implicated in the development of breast cancer, thus complicating further all aspects of screening, treatment, prevention, and public education. Among these additional mutations is one that influences a protein (MAP kinase) that functions as a "chemical switch" in controlling cell replication. In cancer patients with extra copies of the *HER-2* gene, cancerous cells are less likely to respond to chemotherapy. Yet another involves a portion of a gene (*CYP17*) that plays a role in the synthesis of estrogen, and a fourth mutation results in the malfunction of the important APC tumor suppressor gene.

The Personal Assessment at the end of the chapter may be helpful in determining your relative level of risk of developing breast cancer.

Prevention   As already discussed, a variety of risk factors are thought to be important in the development of most cases of breast cancer. Accordingly, some degree of prevention is possible when factors such as diet; alcohol use; physical activity level; decisions about contraception, pregnancy, and breast-feeding; occupational exposure to toxins; and even place of residence are considered.

For women who have a primary family history of breast cancer (sisters, mother, or grandmothers with the disease) and who have been found to carry one or both of the BRCA genes, an extreme form of prevention is also possible— **prophylactic mastectomy.** In this surgical procedure, both noncancerous breasts are removed, in an attempt to eliminate the possibility of future cancer development. When carefully planned, breast reconstruction surgery can be undertaken immediately, with satisfactory results (see the box "Drastic Measures to Prevent

Drastic Measures to Prevent and Treat Breast Cancer

When a combination of risk factors for breast cancer exists, including having a mother or sister who has developed breast cancer, having a high prevalence of breast cancer in family members over time, being a carrier of a breast cancer-related mutated gene, or having already had breast cancer, an increasing number of young women are electing to undergo prophylactic mastectomy. This decision was made in 2008 by television personality Christina Applegate.

In Ms. Applegate's case, a number of risk factors coalesced by an early age, including having a mother who had breast cancer, the identification of herself as a *BRAC1* carrier, an early-stage

malignancy in one breast, and suspicious masses removed from the other breast. Driven by these realities, she made the decision to have removed not only the breast in which cancer had already been diagnosed, but the other breast as well.

As mentioned in the textbook, the *BRAC1/2* genes also bear a heightened relationship to ovarian cancer and to prostate cancer in males. Perhaps after some time and based upon careful monitoring, including MRIs, women who have had a preventive mastectomy, such as Ms. Applegate, might also consider bilateral removal of the ovaries.

and Treat Breast Cancer"). Some physicians, however, recommend against the surgery, preferring to monitor susceptible women very carefully and frequently.

One important consideration related to this procedure is that not every person who carries a mutated tumor suppressor gene will develop cancer, making the surgery unnecessary.

At the present time, chemoprevention represents the newest approach to reducing the incidence of breast cancer. Intended for women with a high risk for the development of breast cancer (Gail Score higher than 1.66), two estrogen-related approaches are presently available.[26] The first involves the use of one of two medications (estrogen receptor modulators) that block the ability of estrogen to bind with potentially malignant breast cells whose future progression toward malignancy would be "fueled" by access to estrogen. The first of the two drugs is tamoxifen (Nolvadex) and the second is raloxifene (Evista). Both medications have relatively similar side effects, and both carry some risks for potentially serious conditions such as blood clots, endometrial (uterine wall) cancer, cataracts, and strokes. A woman considering chemoprevention will be carefully screened in terms of selecting the specific medication most compatible with her biomedical profile.

The third class of medications used in breast cancer chemoprevention are collectively known as aromatase inhibitors and function by decreasing the amount of estrogen produced in the body, rather than by blocking its availability to breast cells. Although not approved for use by premenopausal women, in postmenopausal women the aromatase inhibitors have been used in both treatment and chemoprevention of breast cancer. The principal risks in using this class of medication relate to fractures and the development of osteoporosis.

Early Detection: Breast Self-Examination
For several decades a fundamental component of early detection of breast cancer has been breast self-examination (BSE). Generally recommended for women 20 years of age and older, the procedure was to be performed during the

menstrual period or during the day immediately following the end of the menstrual period, when estrogen levels are at their lowest and cystic activity in breast tissue is minimal (or on the same day of each month by postmenopausal women). The box "Breast Self-Examination" illustrates the proper technique. Although breast self-examination is an easily learned technique, today its role as the primary method of detecting breast cancer in its earliest stage has been usurped by clinical breast examination (CBE) performed by a physician during scheduled checkups and by mammography and other imaging technologies. However, clinical breast examination also has been a source of some concern because of the inconsistencies among clinicians in performing the procedure. Steps have now been taken to correct this, and the American Cancer Society continues to strongly endorse its role in early breast cancer detection. Additionally, during physician visits in which CBE has been done, the ACS recommends that women review, with their clinicians, their own BSE techniques.

Early Detection: Mammography
Although researchers once disagreed about the age at which women should begin routine mammography and the extent to which mammography is effective in finding masses in dense breast tissue, today mammograms are physicians' best

---

Key Terms

prophylactic mastectomy Surgical removal of the breasts to prevent breast cancer in women who are at high risk of developing the disease.

Gail Score A numerical expression of the risk of developing invasive breast cancer, based on several variables such as age at first menstrual period, age at first live birth, results of previous biopsies, family history of breast cancer, and others. A score of 1.66% reflects a high level of risk.

Breast Self-Examination

I've never felt confident about doing a breast self-exam. What is the proper technique?

- Lie down and place your right arm behind your head. The exam is done while lying down, not standing up. This is because when you are lying down, your breast tissue spreads evenly over your chest wall and is as thin as possible, making it much easier to feel all the breast tissue.
- Use the finger pads of the three middle fingers on your left hand to feel for lumps in the right breast. Use overlapping, dime-size circular motions of the finger pads to feel the breast tissue.
- Use three different levels of pressure to feel all the breast tissue. Light pressure is needed to feel the tissue closest to the skin; medium pressure to feel a little deeper; and firm pressure to feel the tissue closest to the chest and ribs. A firm ridge in the lower curve of each breast is normal. If you're not sure how hard to press, talk with your doctor or nurse. Use each pressure level to feel the breast tissue before moving on to the next spot.
- Move around the breast in an up-and-down pattern starting at an imaginary line drawn straight down your side from the underarm and moving across the breast to the middle of the chest bone (sternum or breastbone). Be sure to check the entire breast area, moving downward until you feel only ribs and up to the neck or collarbone (clavicle).

- There is some evidence that the up-and-down pattern (sometimes called the vertical pattern) is the most effective pattern for covering the entire breast without missing any breast tissue.
- Repeat the exam on your left breast, using the finger pads of your right hand.
- While standing in front of a mirror with your hands pressing firmly down on your hips, look at your breasts for any changes of size, shape, contour, dimpling, pulling, or redness or scaliness of the nipple or breast skin. (Pressing your hands down on your hips contracts the chest wall muscles and enhances any breast changes.) Continue to look for changes with your arms down at your sides, and then with your arms raised up over your head with your palms pressed together.
- Examine each underarm while sitting up or standing and with your arm only slightly raised so you can easily feel in this area. Raising your arm straight up tightens the tissue in this area and makes it difficult to examine it.

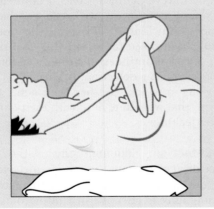
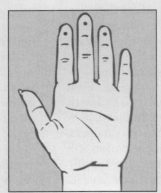
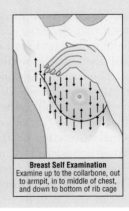

Breast Self Examination
Examine up to the collarbone, out to armpit, in to middle of chest, and down to bottom of rib cage

tool for the early detection of breast cancer. Accordingly, the American Cancer Society recommends that mammography begin at age 40.

Whether women begin routine mammography at 40, as advised by the ACS, or earlier particularly for women with previous breast cancer or a family history of breast disease, women should continue these examinations on an annual basis. Recommendations regarding mammography for older women (age 65 and older) are, however, a bit more individually determined and should be discussed annually with physicians. For older women, overall health status and expectations for reaching a normal life expectancy are weighed relative to the lessening cost-effectiveness of mammography.

Because of the important role routine mammography plays in the early identification of breast lesions, the Mammography Quality Standards Act (MQSA) is a valuable step toward ensuring that mammography is performed by experienced technicians, using correctly calibrated equipment, and interpreted by skilled radiologists. Every woman should be certain that her mammography is being performed in a MQSA-certified facility. However, even when interpreted by experienced radiologists, mammograms are at times difficult to interpret, leading to false-positive findings and the likelihood of additional (diagnostic versus screening) mammography, ultrasound, and/or biopsies. Although expensive and emotionally unsettling, the majority of these false-positive findings are eventually found to have been negative. The percentage of false-positive screenings varies with age, but overall, approximately 15 percent of women screened annually will on one occasion have a false-positive finding. Of course, there can also be false negatives (indicating no cancer, when in fact cancer is present).[27] These tragic occurrences can result in treatment being seriously delayed and are the basis for the highest percentage of medical malpractice lawsuits.

To secure the highest quality images for interpretation, the soft-tissue film-based mammography of the past is increasingly supplemented by newer technologies, including full-field digital mammography (FFDM), which replaces X-ray film with digital sensors capable of generating digitized images that can be viewed, stored, and electronically distributed in a secure fashion for interpretation at off-site locations, thus providing second and third opinions. Computer-aided detection (CAD)–based films, or digital mammography, is also finding its place in screening mammography. This technology feeds film-based or digitally produced images into a massive computerized library of normal breast images and "tags," in a visible manner, any portion of the breast that appears suspicious.

Many other technologies have been developed that could potentially aid in the screening or diagnosis of cancer, now or, most likely, in the future. Those with current applications include ultrasonography (ultrasound), which provides sound-wave-generated images, and magnetic resonance imaging, which produces an image by magnetically reorienting the molecular structure of human tissue. Both technologies are used, but not routinely, in breast cancer identification. Other technologies, including novel ultrasound, computer-aided detection with MRI, scintimammography, positron emission tomography (PET), and elastography, may be available for use in the future. At the current time they are not yet either FDA approved for general clinical use or FDA approved specifically for screening.

Ideally, these newer approaches will identify tumors in their earliest stages of development and reduce the percentage of false-positive and false-negative results associated with traditional mammography procedures.

Treatment The modern treatment of breast cancer involves a compliant interplay of the patient (and her family) with a variety of medical care professionals to deliver the most effective treatment available for the type and stage of the disease. Central to the team is, among others, the radiologist, general surgeon, pathologist, plastic-reconstructive surgeon, radiation oncologist, chemotherapy oncologists, a large array of technical support staff, and, of course, those providing continuous patient care. Not every position named above will be involved with every breast cancer patient, but all comprise the clinical resources available in a major cancer center.

If it can be assumed there is a "typical" case of breast cancer, it will most often involve a combination of major treatment modalities, including surgery, radiation therapy, chemotherapy, reconstructive surgery (if elected), and a period of rehabilitation, often using physical therapy or a tailored exercise program to maintain strength and flexibility in the shoulder girdle. In some cases, maintenance chemotherapy may continue well beyond the more familiar treatment period.

In the interest of brevity, only selected aspects of the postsurgical treatment protocol will be briefly described.[28]

Chemotherapy involves the use of drugs delivered intravenously or in pill form for the purpose of killing (in one or more manner) portions of a tumor that were incapable of being adequately addressed by surgery or cells that may have migrated to a location beyond the primary tumor site.

Radiation therapy, in a wide array of forms including brachytherapy, gamma knife therapy, and stereotactic radiosurgery, is intended to kill malignant cells during specific stages of cell division in which their genetic material is particularly vulnerable to the effects of radiation. The rapid replication rate of cancer cells makes radiation more effective in killing cancer cells than neighboring exposed cells above, below, and near the treatment field, such as those of skin, glandular tissue, vascular tissue, nervous tissue, and underlying musculature. Radiation physicists are routinely engaged in the planning of the type and extent of radiation to use.

Hormone therapy, similar in some ways to chemotherapy, is, as the name implies, directed at reducing the presence of a hormone, such as estrogen or, less commonly, progesterone, needed by the cancer cells, or by altering the ability of receptors on the surface of the cancer cells from interfacing with its needed hormone in spite of its normal level with the body.

Targeted therapy involves the formulation of drugs tailored to the uniqueness of the proteins manufactured by breast cancer patients' own cancer cells. The drugs Herceptin, Gleevec, and Avastin represent the current frontier of cancer therapy.

Prostate Cancer

If the names Bob Dole, General Norman Schwarzkopf, Jerry Lewis, and Colin Powell are familiar, then you know four older men who have been diagnosed with and treated for prostate cancer. In fact, prostate cancer is so common that in 2008 an estimated 186,320 new cases were diagnosed, and 28,660 men died of the disease.[2] Prostate cancer is a leading cause of cancer deaths in American men, exceeded only by lung cancer deaths.

The prostate gland is a walnut-size gland located near the base of the penis (see Figure 11-4). It surrounds the neck of the bladder and the urethra. The prostate secretes a number of components of semen, such as nutrients used to fuel sperm motility.

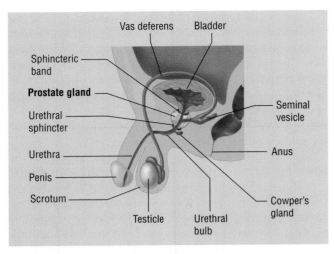

Figure 11-4 Location of the Prostate Gland within the Male Reproductive System

Risk Factors   Compared with other cancers, the risk factors for prostate cancer are less clearly defined. The most predictable risk factor is age. Currently, 65 percent of all prostate cancer cases are diagnosed in men over 65 years of age; however, cases in men under age 50 are not infrequent. African American men and men with a family history of prostate cancer are at greater risk of developing this form of cancer. This greater incidence of prostate cancer in African American males may be partially explained by the existence of an abnormal gene on chromosome 8 that is associated more commonly with prostate tumors in this racial group than in the general population.[29] A link between prostate cancer and dietary fat intake, including excessive red meat and dairy product consumption, has also been suggested. With the discovery of the *BRCA1* and *BRCA2* genes related to breast and ovarian cancer, a genetic link with prostate cancer was also established. Men with one of these genetic mutations have an increased risk of developing prostate cancer.

Prevention   Although the American Cancer Society does not specifically address prevention of prostate cancer, prevention is not an unrealistic goal. Clearly, moderation of dietary fat intake is a preventive step. Increased dietary intake levels of vitamin E and the micronutrient selenium have been shown to play a preventive role in prostate cancer. In addition, an ongoing assessment of the drug finasteride (Proscar), used in the treatment of benign prostatic hyperplasia (BPH) (enlargement of the prostate), has indicated that the drug can reduce the incidence of tumors of the prostate. In February 2008, results from the Prostate Cancer Prevention Trial provided sufficient evidence for the American Urological Association and the American Society of Clinical Oncology to conclude that maintenance use of finasteride was capable of lowering the risk of developing prostate cancer.[30]

Early Detection   Possible signs of prostate disease, including prostate cancer, often include difficulty urinating, frequent urination (particularly at night), continued wetness for a short time following urination, blood in the urine, low-back pain, and aching in the upper thighs. A physician should be consulted if any of these symptoms appear, particularly in men ages 50 or older. Screening for prostate cancer should begin by age 40. This screening consists of an annual rectal examination performed by a physician and a blood test, the **prostate-specific antigen (PSA) test,** administered every 2 years. Although the initial version of the PSA test was very successful in diagnosing prostate cancer, new, age-specific test values are now employed. These new interpretive standards allow increased specificity in determining risk. This said, however, the PSA test continues to deliver both false negative and false positive results. At this time there is considerable uncertainty as to whether screening for prostate cancer using the PSA test should be continued. Because of concern about the "overtreatment" of males who have elevated PSA levels, in combination with little apparent difference in the survival of men with prostate cancer based on whether they had or had not been screened, consensus is building that physicians should explain the limitations of the PSA test, and then allow their male patients to decide whether to be screened. For those males who have a history of PSA screenings, the velocity of a rise (over two consecutive tests) in the PSA levels could be more clinically significant than the absolute level of prostate-specific antigen, although this too is unresolved.[30]

Recommendations regarding whether use of PSA is no longer necessary after a certain age appear to have now been resolved. In 2008, the U.S. Preventive Services Task Force recommended that screening for men 75 years of age and older was no longer necessary.[31] Underlying this revision was the concern that in this age group the medical response to higher levels of PSA, such as biopsies, often produces undesirable consequences, such as erectile dysfunction, urinary incontinence, and bowel-related problems.

Another version of the PSA test has also been developed. This test can identify the "free" antigen most closely associated with the more aggressive forms of prostate cancer, thus cutting down on the false positives and extensive use of biopsies.[32] In addition, an ultrasound rectal examination is used in men whose PSA scores are abnormally high.

Treatment   Today prostate cancer is treated through surgical removal, cryotherapy (freezing), or the use of external radiation or the implantation of radioactive seeds (brachytherapy) into the gland, in combination with relatively short-term use of hormonal therapy, although the latter form of treatment is now seen as being of limited value, other than for older patients with more aggressive forms of the disease.[32] Now available for use in the treatment of prostate cancer is a new test to determine the probability of recurrence following initial treatment. This test uses seven biomarkers found in the blood that, at certain levels, can predict cancer recurrence with a high degree of accuracy.[33] In addition, an experimental vaccine has recently been tested on humans with promising results. Of course, each form of treatment carries the potential for side effects, including an 80 percent chance of impotence over a 10-year period; incontinence with surgery; diarrhea and tiredness with external radiation; some anal discomfort in association with the implantation of radioactive seeds into the prostate with internal radiation; and thinning of bones and some cardiovascular issues in conjunction with longer-term hormone therapy.

One form of prostate cancer grows so slowly that men whose cancer is of this type, whose tumors are very localized, and whose life expectancy is less than 10 years at the time of diagnosis, are not treated but are closely monitored for any progression of the cancer. The 5-year survival rate for men with localized prostate cancer is virtually 100 percent!

Testicular Cancer

Cancer of the testicle is among the least common forms of cancer; however, it is the most common solid tumor in men ages 15 to 34. Awareness of this type of cancer was raised in 1996 and 1997, when seven-time winner of the Tour de France Lance Armstrong and champion figure skater Scott Hamilton were diagnosed with testicular cancer. In both men, chronic fatigue and abdominal discomfort were the first symptoms of the disease. The American Cancer Society estimates that in 2008 testicular cancer was diagnosed in 8,090 men and caused the deaths of 380.[2]

Four forms of testicular cancer have been described: seminoma, teratoma, carcinoma, and choriocarcinoma. The most prevalent, seminoma, forms in the seminiferous tubules (where sperm originate) and is generally first observed during testicular self-examination as a small, hard mass on the side (or near the front) of the testicle. Fortunately, this form of testicular cancer is now highly curable.

Risk Factors Risk factors for testicular cancer are variable, ranging from family history to environmental factors. The disease is more frequently seen in white Americans and in men whose testicles were undescended during childhood. Additional risk factors, such as difficulty during the mother's pregnancy, elevated temperature in the groin, and mumps during childhood, have been reported. The incidence of this cancer has been increasing in recent decades, while a corresponding drop in sperm levels has also been observed. Although no single explanation can be given for these changes, environmental factors such as agricultural pesticide toxicity may be involved. Once pesticides are concentrated in the tissues of the human body, during pregnancy they mimic estrogen. This, in turn, may lead to testicular dysgenesis syndrome, or the failure of the testicles to develop normally. The suspicion that testicular cancer is linked to vasectomies appears to be unfounded.

Prevention Because risk factors for testicular cancer are so variable, prevention is limited to regular self-examination of the testicles. Symptoms such as fatigue, abdominal discomfort, and enlargement of the testicle should be reported to a physician, since these can be associated with other disease processes. A male infant with one or both testicles in the undescended position (resulting in an empty scrotum) should be seen promptly by a physician so that corrective procedures can be undertaken.

Early Detection In addition to the fatigue and abdominal distress reported by both Armstrong and Hamilton, symptoms of testicular cancer include a small, painless lump on the side or near the front of the testicle, a swollen or enlarged testicle, and a heaviness or dragging sensation in the groin or scrotum. The importance of testicular self-examination, as well as early diagnosis and prompt treatment, cannot be overemphasized for men in the at-risk age group of 15 to 34 years; see the box "Testicular Self-Examination."

Treatment Depending on the type, stage, and degree of localization of the tumor, surgical intervention generally includes removal of the testicle, spermatic cord, and regional lymph nodes. Chemotherapy and radiation might also be used. The highly publicized recovery of Lance Armstrong (and his subsequent accomplishments in professional biking) made the "Einhorn Regimen" (a combination of three chemotherapy agents) one of the chemotherapy protocols most widely recognized by the general public. Today, treatment is very effective, with 95.4 percent of all testicular cancer patients surviving 5 years and 99.3 percent surviving 5 years when the cancer was localized at the time of diagnosis.[2] It should be noted, however, that concern exists regarding the development of other forms of cancer, such as leukemia, later in life.

Cervical Cancer

In 2008, an estimated 11,070 new cases of cancer of the cervix (the anatomical neck of the uterus) occurred in the United States.[2] Fortunately, the death rate from cervical cancer has dropped greatly since 1950, largely because of the **Pap test.** This test screens for precancerous cellular changes (called *cervical intraepithelial neoplasia,* or *CIN*) and malignant cells. If malignant cells are found, it is

---

> **Key Terms**
>
> **prostate-specific antigen (PSA) test** A blood test used to identify prostate-specific antigen, an early indicator that the immune system has recognized and mounted a defense against prostate cancer.
>
> **Pap test** A cancer-screening procedure in which cells are removed from the cervix and examined for precancerous changes.

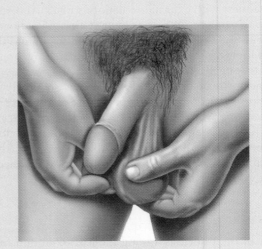
hoped that they represent only cancer in situ (at the site of origin), rather than a more advanced invasive stage of the disease. Unfortunately, this simple and relatively inexpensive screening test is still underused, particularly in women over age 60, the group in which cervical cancer is most frequently found.

Refinements in laboratory techniques and the incorporation of computerization have enhanced the diagnostic precision of the Pap test. ThinPrep represents the former, while PAPNET and FocalPoint have enhanced the technologist's ability to identify abnormal cells.

Risk Factors Because of the clear association between sexually transmitted infections and cervical cancer, risk factors for this form of cancer include early age of first intercourse, large number of sexual partners, history of infertility (which may indicate chronic pelvic inflammatory disease), and clinical evidence of *human papillomavirus* (*HPV*) infections (see pages 377–378 in Chapter 13). For patients with previous HPV infections or whose sexual history suggests a higher risk for HPV, a Pap-plus (a combination of the liquid pap and the HPV test) test has been shown effective in detecting the DNA from four HPVs that are known to be cancer causing, while being as easy to use as the traditionally used Pap test. Today the test is approved only for identifying HPV infection, but it is also capable of detecting both chlamydia and gonorrhea. In 2006 the first effective vaccine against the HPV variants associated

with cervical cancer became available. This vaccine and the forms of HPV against which it protects are described in greater detail in Chapter 13 on page 378. In 2008, the FDA extended the approved use of the Gardasil vaccine to include prevention against cancer of the vagina and the vulva (the external area adjacent to the vaginal opening).[34]

In addition to sexual history, cigarette smoking and socioeconomic factors are also risk factors for cervical cancer. The latter most likely relates to less frequent medical assessment, including infrequent Pap tests. (The Personal Assessment at the end of the chapter will help women evaluate their risk of developing cervical cancer.)

 TALKING POINTS Three risk factors are associated with HPV-induced cervical cancer: early age of first sexual intercourse, higher-than-average number of partners, and lack of protection against sexually transmitted diseases (for example, condoms). How would you introduce this topic to a teenage daughter, sister, or niece?

Prevention Sexual abstinence is the most effective way of reducing the risk of developing cervical cancer (for example, Catholic nuns have extremely low rates of cervical cancer). However, abstinence is unlikely to be the choice for most women; other alternatives include fewer sexual partners, more careful selection of partners to minimize contact with those at high risk, the use of condoms, and the use of spermicides. In addition, of course, regular medical assessment, including annual Pap tests (and the Pap-plus test), represents prevention through early detection. The HPV vaccine will further increase prevention.

Early Detection At this time, the importance of women having Pap tests for cervical cancer performed on a regular basis cannot be overemphasized. However, the specific scheduling of cervical screening is undergoing adjustment. For young sexually active women, initial screening using the Pap test (Pap-plus) should be undertaken within 3 years of first exposure. For young women not sexually at risk, or for women who have had a hysterectomy, the initial screening with the Pap test can be determined in consultation with health care providers. Once initiated, however, following three consecutive annual negative tests, the interval between tests may be increased upon discussion with health care providers. The American Cancer Society estimates that cervical cancer claimed the lives of 3,870 women in 2008.

The Pap test is not perfect, however. When tests are read in laboratories highly experienced in interpreting Pap slides, about 7 percent will be false negatives, resulting in a 93 percent accuracy rate. In less-experienced laboratories, false negatives may be as high as 20 percent. Unfortunately, not all women whose test results are accurately assessed as abnormal receive adequate follow-up care, nor do they have subsequent Pap tests regularly enough. For many women with an abnormal Pap test, visual assessment (colposcopy) of the cervix will be performed. Traditional technology generates some false negatives. However, a newer technology, the Luma Cervical Imaging System, has enhanced the ability of the clinician to visually identify signs of tissue change.

In addition to changes discovered by a Pap test, symptoms that suggest potential cervical cancer include abnormal vaginal bleeding between periods and frequent spotting.

Treatment Should precancerous cellular changes (CIN) be identified, treatment can include one of several alternatives. Physicians can destroy areas of abnormal cellular change using cryotherapy, electrocoagulation, laser destruction, or surgical removal of abnormal tissue. More advanced (invasive) cancer of the cervix can be treated with a hysterectomy combined with other established cancer therapies. A combination of radiation and chemotherapy is the most effective treatment for cervical cancer.

Uterine (Endometrial) Cancer

The American Cancer Society estimates that in 2008, 40,100 cases of uterine cancer (cancer within the inner wall of the body of the uterus, rather than within the cervix or neck of the uterus) were diagnosed in American women. In addition, 7,470 women died of the disease.[2] Although African Americans have a lower incidence of uterine cancer than White women do, their death rate is nearly twice as high.

Risk Factors Unlike cervical cancer, in which a strong viral link has been identified, the principal risk factor related to the development of endometrial cancer is a high estrogen level. Accordingly, the following factors are related to higher levels of estrogen and, thus, to the development of endometrial cancer:

- Early menarche (early onset of menstruation)
- Late menopause (prolonged exposure to estrogen)
- Lack of ovulation (infertility)
- Never having given birth
- Estrogen replacement therapy (ERT not moderated with progesterone)
- Obesity
- Use of tamoxifen (a drug used in breast cancer therapy)
- History of polycystic ovary syndrome
- Hereditary nonpolyposis colon cancer

To some degree, endometrial cancer is seen more frequently in people who are diabetic, are hypertensive, or have gallbladder disease.

Prevention The risk factors associated with high levels of estrogen are areas in which prevention might be targeted. In addition, the need for regular gynecological care that includes pelvic examination is a principal factor in minimizing the risk of uterine cancer. Pregnancy and the use of oral contraceptives both provide some protection from endometrial cancer.[2] Some degree of prevention may also be accomplished through a diet high in phytoestrogens that may provide an antiestrogenic effect. Most recently, however, an assessment of circulating enterolactone, the main form of dietary phytoestrogens in Westerns diets, failed to show a protective role against uterine cancer in ranges associated with normal dietary intake.[35]

Early Detection Compared with cervical cancer, which is routinely identified through Pap tests, endometrial cancer is much more likely to be suspected on the basis of symptoms (irregular or postmenopausal bleeding) and confirmed by biopsy. Although more invasive, biopsy is a more effective method than ultrasound to diagnose uterine cancer.

Treatment The treatment for early or localized endometrial cancer is generally surgical removal of the uterus (hysterectomy). Other therapies, such as radiation, chemotherapy, and hormonal therapy, may then be added to the treatment regimen. However, in terms of hormone replacement therapy (HRT), in which estrogen is combined with a synthetic progesterone, the FDA, The National Institute on Aging, and various medical associations now advise that no woman 65 or older with an intact uterus should take HRT owing to several concerns, including an increased risk for endometrial cancer. For women who are undergoing menopause and experiencing troublesome symptoms such as night sweats and hot flashes, HRT should be used in the smallest doses that provide relief and for the shortest duration possible.

Vaginal Cancer

Although rare, cancer of the vagina (the passage leading to the uterus) is of concern to a particular group of women: in the 1960s the daughters of more than 3 million mothers who were given the drug DES (diethylstilbestrol) to prevent miscarriages. Because of the effects of DES on the development of the fetal reproductive system, these daughters face the risk of developing a form of vaginal (and cervical) cancer called *clear cell cancer*. The medical community has been following large groups of daughters to better assess their level of risk. In a longitudinal study that followed such women and a control group of 1,374 unexposed age-mates, the risk of developing vaginal cancer was two to four times higher in the affected group than it was in women whose mothers were not given DES. A second study looking at the same population of women, who were exposed to DES during intrauterine development, demonstrated that they were now experiencing an earlier onset of menopause than was found in a group of age-mates who had not been exposed to DES.

Outside this unique group of women, vaginal cancer is relatively rare. The American Cancer Society estimates that in 2008, there were 2,210 new cases diagnosed, and 760 women died as the result of vaginal cancer.[2] Early detection can be accomplished using a Pap test when vaginal wall cell samples are taken. Treatment centers on surgical removal of the vagina and associated lymph nodes. Other supportive therapies may also be included in the treatment regimen.

Ovarian Cancer

Since the death in 1989 of actress Gilda Radner, a star in the early years of *Saturday Night Live,* public awareness of ovarian cancer has increased in the United States. The American Cancer Society estimates that in 2008, there were 21,650 new cases diagnosed, and 15,520 women died of the disease.[2] Most cases develop in women over age 40 who have not had children or began menstruation at an early age. The highest rate is in women over age 60. Today ovarian cancer causes more deaths than does any other form of female reproductive system cancer.

For a relatively small percentage of all women (10 percent), the inheritance of either the *BRCA1* or *BRCA2* suppressor gene mutation (see pages 297 and 308) significantly increases the risk of developing both breast and ovarian cancer. Today it is estimated that about 20 percent of all cases of ovarian cancer stem from these genetic mutations.

Beyond the 20 percent of cases attributed to genetic mutations, what might account for the majority of ovarian cancers? A number of studies, with varying degrees of assurance, suggest that decades of hormone replacement therapy (HRT) used to counter symptoms of menopause, maintain bone mass, and provide hormonal protection from heart disease could be responsible for the majority of ovarian cancers. As mentioned in conjunction with endometrial cancer, hormone replacement therapy is now used for only the briefest period of time.

Prevention   Methods of preventing or lowering the risk of developing ovarian cancer are very similar to those recommended for breast cancer. These include using oral contraceptives, giving birth and breast-feeding (for at least three months), reducing dietary fat intake, abstaining from alcohol use, and performing regular physical activity.

For the small group of women with a strong family history of ovarian cancer, a **prophylactic oophorectomy** should be seriously considered. In this surgical procedure, both ovaries are removed. Carefully monitored estrogen replacement therapy is then used to provide the protective advantages of estrogen in maintaining cardiovascular health and bone density.

Early Detection   Because of its vague symptoms, ovarian cancer has been referred to as a *silent cancer*. Women in whom ovarian cancer has been diagnosed often report that the only symptoms of their cancer's presence were digestive disturbances, gas, urinary incontinence, stomach distention, and crampy abdominal pain over a few short weeks. The last symptom should be medically evaluated immediately.

Three ovarian cancer tests are now available for use in early detection and progress monitoring of ovarian therapy. OvaSure is a new screening that the developer believes can identify a developing tumor in the ovary months or even a few years before it would have become invasive. Although approved by the FDA, OvaSure is undergoing evaluation based on the level of its ability to function as intended.

The two remaining tests, CA125 and HE4, are now used to monitor progress and effectiveness of therapies by determining the levels of antibodies against the ovarian cancer cells at various points in the treatment protocol and during follow-up, although they were used as screening tests as well.

For women with a strong family history of ovarian cancer (four primary family members who have had breast or ovarian cancer, with two or more cases occurring before age 50) or women of Ashkenazi Jewish descent (see page 308), genetic screening, newly available screening tests, and transvaginal ultrasound screening are likely to be recommended. These women may also be referred for participation in one of several prevention trials now under way.

Treatment At this time, treatment of ovarian cancer requires surgical removal of the ovary, followed by aggressive use of chemotherapy. Use of the chemotherapeutic drug paclitaxel (Taxol) initially results in a 50 percent survival rate 19 months after the completion of therapy. Recently, the use of an experimental three-drug combination—cyclophosphamide, paclitaxel, and cisplatin—has resulted in a 70 percent survival rate 22 months after chemotherapy. An even more recent advance in chemotherapy for ovarian cancer involves a two-drug therapy that, when delivered directly into the abdominal cavity, has extended survival rates beyond those associated with intravenous administration of the same agents—65.6 months versus 49.7 months.[36] The American Cancer Society reports survival rates at 5 years following diagnosis at 56 percent for younger women and 29 percent for those over age 65. Overall, the 1-year survival rate is 75 percent, with the 5-year rate at 45 percent. If diagnosed in its earliest stage of development, the 5-year survival rate is 92 percent.[2]

Pancreatic Cancer

Pancreatic cancer is one of the most lethal forms of cancer, with a survival rate of only 5 percent 5 years after diagnosis.[2] Because of this gland's important functions in both digestion and metabolic processes related to glucose utilization, its destruction by a malignancy leaves the body in a state incompatible with living.

In 2008 an estimated 37,680 new cases of pancreatic cancer were diagnosed, and 34,290 deaths occurred.[2]

Risk Factors Pancreatic cancer is more common in men than women, occurs more frequently with age, and develops most often in African American men. Smoking is clearly a risk factor for this form of cancer, with smokers more than twice as likely to develop the disease. Other risk factors have been tentatively suggested, such as chronic inflammation of the pancreas (pancreatitis), diabetes mellitus, alcohol-induced liver deterioration (cirrhosis), obesity, and high-fat diets.[2] Recently a meta-analysis (a restudy of earlier studies) assessed the long-term use of nonsteroidal anti-inflammatory drugs to see if they are a risk factor in the development of pancreatic cancer. No clear link was found between using these medications, including aspirin, and enhanced risk of pancreatic cancer.

Prevention Not smoking and abstaining from alcohol use are the most effective steps toward preventing this form of cancer. Further, reducing the risk of type 2 diabetes mellitus, through weight loss and exercise, would also make an important contribution to prevention. Annual medical examinations are, of course, associated with overall cancer prevention.

The role of dietary and supplemental vitamin D is currently being assessed. Preliminary findings from a group of studies that included nearly 120,000 men and women suggest a positive role for vitamin D in the prevention of pancreatic cancer.[37] A second study examined the relationship between UVB radiation (a form of UV radiation

Key Terms

prophylactic oophorectomy Surgical removal of the ovaries to prevent ovarian cancer in women at high risk of developing the disease.

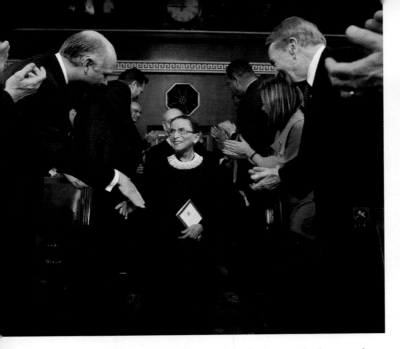

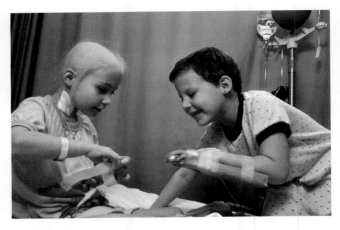

Chemotherapy involves the use of chemical agents given by mouth or injection to treat or control cancer. Chemotherapy typically affects rapidly dividing cells, which include cancer cells but also healthy cells in the blood, hair, and lining of the gastrointestinal tract. If healthy cells are damaged, side effects such as nausea and hair loss can occur.

Supreme Court Justice Ruth Bader Ginsburg, only the second woman to serve on the nation's highest court, was diagnosed with pancreatic cancer in 2009. Unfortunately, pancreatic cancer is among the most difficult forms of cancer from which to recover.

associated with exposure to solar energy) and several cancers and found an inverse relationship between the levels of solar radiation received and incidence of several cancers, including pancreatic cancer.[38] UV radiation is a facilitator of the production of vitamin D_3, so a speculative inference can be drawn regarding a protective role for this vitamin in minimizing the development of this form of cancer. At this time, however, there are no recommendations to increase vitamin D intake as a preventative for pancreatic cancer.

Early Detection   Early detection of this cancer is difficult because of the absence of symptoms until late in its course. Perhaps for people with a history of chronic pancreatitis, physicians might consider routine ultrasound assessment or CT scans. Once symptoms appear, a biopsy is performed.

Treatment   At this time there is no effective treatment for pancreatic cancer. Surgical removal of malignant sites within the gland, in addition to radiation and chemotherapy, is usually tried. Certainly, if a particular patient with pancreatic cancer qualifies, enrollment in a clinical trial would be worth consideration.

Lymphatic Cancer

An estimated 74,340 new cases of lymphoma (8,220 cases of Hodgkin's disease and 66,120 cases of non-Hodgkin's lymphoma) were diagnosed in 2008. The number of deaths from both forms of lymphoma was near 20,510.[2] The incidence of Hodgkin's disease has declined over the last 35 years, while the incidence of non-Hodgkin's disease has nearly doubled, but is now holding steady.[2]

Risk Factors   Risk factors for lymphoma are difficult to determine. Some possible factors are a general reduction in immune protection, exposure to toxic environmental chemicals such as pesticides and herbicides, the use of some biologics used in the treatment of autoimmune conditions (see Chapter 12), and viral infections. As you will learn in Chapter 13, the virus that causes AIDS (HIV) is a leukemia/lymphoma virus that was initially called HTLV-III (human T-cell leukemia/lymphoma virus-type III). A related leukemia/lymphoma virus, HTLV-I, is also suspected in the development of lymphatic cancer. The Epstein-Barr virus (EBV) may also play a role in lymphatic cancer development, as well as the hepatitis C virus.

Prevention   Beyond limiting exposure to toxic chemicals and sexually transmitted viruses, few recommendations can be made about prevention. Again, early detection and diagnosis can serve as a form of prevention, since early-stage cancer is more survivable than advanced disease.

Early Detection   Unlike other cancers, the early symptoms of lymphoma are diverse and similar to symptoms of other illnesses, most of which are not serious. These symptoms include enlarged lymph nodes (frequently a sign of any infection that the immune system is fighting), fever, itching, weight loss, and anemia.

Treatment   Although surgery (beyond a biopsy) is usually not associated with the treatment of lymphoma, a variety of other therapies are employed. Depending on the stage and type of lymphoma, therapy may involve only radiation treatment of localized lymph nodes, as is seen in non-Hodgkin's lymphoma. Radiation combined with chemotherapy is generally used in the treatment of late-stage non-Hodgkin's lymphoma. More recently, other therapies, including more aggressive chemotherapy, monoclonal antibody therapy, and bone marrow and stem cell transplantation, in combination with either high-dose or low-dose radiation have been employed with non-Hodgkin's lymphoma.

After completion of therapy, 1-year survival rates for Hodgkin's disease are near 92 percent and near 79 percent for non-Hodgkin's lymphoma. By the end of 5 years, these rates have dropped to 85 and 63 percent, respectively.[2] Lower rates of survival are seen at 10 years and beyond.

The Future of Cancer Prevention, Diagnosis, and Treatment

It has been decades since President Richard Nixon (1971) declared a national "war on cancer," and today the results are both encouraging and discouraging. On the positive side, impressive technological advances have been and continue to be made in the diagnosis and treatment of cancer. As mentioned throughout the chapter, new screening procedures as well as treatment protocols seem to appear at a consistent rate. Additionally, the death rates from a variety of cancers have fallen, including a 70 percent decrease in the rate for Hodgkin's disease and a 14 percent decline in the death rate for breast cancer. Death rates for cervical, stomach, uterine, colon, bladder, and thyroid cancers have also fallen. Today, the overall death rate for cancer is at its lowest point. Particularly important in this is a general increase in the public's awareness of cancer prevention and early detection.

On the negative side is the reality that cancer is not only a biological disease but also a disease (or more than 100 diseases) with strong sociopolitical implications. Central to this area are factors such as the inability of the majority of Americans to make needed changes in lifestyle in regard to smoking, alcohol use, exercise, weight management, and dietary practices. Also impeding progress is the absence of health care insurance for millions of Americans, which prevents early diagnosis and treatment of cancer. In fact, virtually every cancer in adults is negatively affected by one or more of these largely modifiable complicating factors.

In light of the 2008 presidential race, which led to the election of Democratic president accompanied by a Democratic house and a senate that is virtually equal in representation, the funding policies common to the first eight years of the decade many be slanted in different directions for the near future. Additionally, the deep recession that began mid-2007 and the continuing conflicts in the Middle East further cloud insights into the amount of money available for use in funding the war on cancer.

The 2009 fiscal year federal budget formulated by the outgoing Republican administration in 2008 allotted $4.81 billion to the National Cancer Institute. This amount had remained relatively level through the latter half of President George W. Bush's final term in office. With the change of administration, the National Cancer Institute submitted a budget for 2010 that requested an additional $2.19 billion. Given situations listed earlier, it would appear unlikely that this almost 50 percent increase is achievable. For those interested in the programs of the National Cancer Institute, the Online Learning Center (www.mhhe.com/payne11e) contains a link to a list of programs within the NCI and the amount of additional dollars each has requested.

In the final analysis, the "war" remains very challenging: progress is being made, setbacks occur, and the victory remains far from being in hand. The "Big C" remains.

Prevention Through Risk Reduction

Because cancer will probably continue to be the second most common cause of death among all adults, you should explore ways to reduce your risk of developing cancer. The following factors, which could make you vulnerable to cancer, can be controlled or at least recognized.

- *Know your family history.* You are the recipient of the genetic strengths and weaknesses of your biological parents and your more distant relatives. If you are able to determine that cancer is prevalent in your family medical history, you cannot afford to disregard this fact. It may be appropriate for you to be screened for certain types of cancer more often or at a young age. The importance of family history was clearly seen in our discussion of the *BRCA1/BRCA2* inheritance pattern and related decisions about prophylactic mastectomy and prophylactic oophorectomy.

- *Select and monitor your occupation carefully.* Because of recently discovered relationships between cancer and occupations that bring employees into contact with carcinogenic agents, you must be aware of the risks posed by certain job selections and assignments. Worksites where you will come into frequent contact with pesticides, strong solvents, volatile hydrocarbons, and airborne fibers could pay well but also shorten your life. The importance of this point is evident in reviewing the current list of environmental carcinogens studies funded by the National Cancer Institute. Included are studies that focus on indoor air pollution (tobacco smoke and cooking oils), dust (cotton, grain, plastic, and wood), organic solvents (benzene, carbon tetrachloride, toluene, xylene, and chlordane), organophosphates (diazinon, dichlorvos, malathion, triazines, and cyaniazine), polybrominated biphenyls, polychlorinated biphenyls, fumigants (ethylene), water pollution (chloride, phosphene, and fluoride), petroleum products (diesel fuel, gasoline, jet fuel), radiation (radon, neutron therapy, and reactor accidents), biological agents (chlamydia, HIV/HPV, helicobacter, hepatitis B and C), and radioisotopes (iodine and radium).

- *Do not use tobacco products.* You may want to review Chapter 9 on the overwhelming evidence linking all forms of tobacco use (including smokeless tobacco) to the development of cancer. Smoking is so detrimental to health that it is considered the number-one preventable cause of death along with obesity.

- *Monitor environmental exposure to carcinogens.* When one considers carcinogenic concerns related to types of employment, residential radon levels, ozone depletion leading to increased exposure to solar radiation, and environmental tobacco smoke (Chapter 9), one realizes that the environment holds great potential as a source of carcinogenic exposure. To the extent it is possible to select the environment in which you will reside, work, and recreate, you should add selecting a low-risk environment to your list of cancer-prevention activities.

- *Follow a sound diet.* As mentioned in conjunction with folic acid and colorectal cancer and high-fat diets and prostate cancer, dietary patterns are known to play both a causative and a preventive role in cancer. (Review Chapter 5 for information about dietary practices). In this chapter, emphasis was placed on the role of fruits and vegetables as excellent sources of nutrients, as well as important cancer-protective compounds known as phytochemicals. Consider these simple modifications to familiar food items that can be made in support of overall health:

  - For breakfast: Toast whole-grain bread and top with reduced-fat peanut butter and a sliced banana.
  - For lunch: Order salads, vegetable soups, or stir-fried vegetables when eating out.
  - For dinner: Add broccoli, green beans, corn, or peas to a casserole.
  - As a snack: Store cleaned, cut-up vegetables in the fridge at eye level and keep a low-fat or fat-free dip on hand.

  Should research demonstrate an even clearer role for nutrients, **chemoprevention** may become an even more widely practiced component of cancer prevention. Chemoprevention is not limited to food items and dietary supplements but can also involve pharmaceutical agents, such as aspirin and estrogen replacement therapy.

- *Control your body weight.* For women, obesity is related to a higher incidence of cancer of the uterus, ovary, and breast because obesity correlates with high estrogen levels. Maintaining a desirable body weight could improve overall health and lead to more

successful management of cancer should it develop. Examples of this point include the fact that obesity complicates the taking of biopsies and the mechanics of surgery, prolongs recovery time, and may alter the desired effect of some chemotherapy agents.

- *Exercise regularly.* Chapter 4 discusses in detail the importance of regular moderate exercise to all aspects of health, including reducing the risk of chronic illnesses. Moderate exercise increases the body's ability to deliver oxygen to its tissues and thus to reduce the formation of cancer-enhancing free radicals formed during incomplete oxidation of nutrients. Moderate exercise also stimulates the production of enzymes that remove free radicals.

- *Limit your exposure to the sun.* It is important to heed this message even if you enjoy many outdoor activities. Particularly for people with light complexions, the radiation received through chronic exposure to the sun may foster the development of skin cancer. Of course, the same advice applies to tanning beds, the use of which may lead to skin cancers, including melanoma.

- *Consume alcohol in moderation, if at all.* People who consume a lot of alcohol have an increased prevalence of several types of cancer, including cancer of the oral cavity, larynx, and esophagus. Whether this results directly from the presence of carcinogens in alcohol or is more closely related to the alcohol user's tendency to smoke has not yet been established.

Cancer and a Sense of Well-Being

Now that we have given ample consideration to several types of cancer, return to Chapter 1, page 15, and review Figure 1-2. In doing so, you can more fully appreciate the potentially negative impact that a chronic, demanding, and potentially life-shortening condition like cancer can have on a person's quest for a sense of well-being. Recall that ample resources from all dimensions of health are needed to engage in the activities that are required in fulfilling role responsibilities. Cancer diminishes the quantity and quality of these resources, sometimes requiring that roles be relinquished, such as a mother who can no longer adequately care for her children, or a student who can no longer attend classes.

As a person with cancer becomes less capable of meeting role fulfillment, this growing inability over time minimizes progress in fulfilling the even larger developmental expectation of his or her life cycle stage. As this occurs, the cancer victim's sense of well-being, normally fueled by the knowledge that progress can be sustained, is lessened. Further, because of the reciprocity that exists between all of the elements depicted in Figure 1-2, resource deterioration continues, often at an accelerated pace, and a sense of life satisfaction declines further. For cancer victims whose prognosis is poor, a sense of despair can develop to the extent that both death and dying may become the central focus of their remaining time.

> ### Key Terms
>
> **chemoprevention** Cancer prevention using food, food supplements, and medications thought to bolster the immune system or reduce the damage caused by carcinogens.

Taking Charge of Your Health

- Stay attuned to media reports about cancer so that you can make informed choices.
- Support agencies devoted to the prevention of cancer.
- Monitor your work, home, and recreational environments to determine whether they are placing you at risk for cancer.
- Perform regular self-examinations for forms of cancer that can be detected through these techniques.
- Undergo the recommended cancer screening procedures for your age and sex.
- If you have cancer, participate actively in your own treatment.

SUMMARY

- Cancer is a condition in which the body is unable to control the specialization, replication, and repair of cells or the suppression of abnormal cell formation.
- A variety of agents, including genetic mutations, viruses, and carcinogens, stimulate the conversion of regulatory genes (proto-oncogenes) into oncogenes.
- Skin cancer prevention requires protection from excessive ultraviolet ray exposure.
- Cigarette smoking and genetic predisposition are both related to the development of lung cancer.
- Mammograms are an important component of breast cancer identification. Drugs capable of preventing breast cancer are available; however, their use is being carefully studied.
- Regular use of Pap tests is related to the early detection of cervical cancer. Sexually transmitted viral infections are strongly suspected of causing cervical cancer.

- Uterine (endometrial) cancer is more common than cervical cancer. High levels of estrogen are strongly associated with this form of cancer.
- The PSA test improves the ability to diagnose prostate cancer. Age, high-fat diets, and inheritance of a mutated suppressor gene are known risk factors.
- Colorectal cancer has a strong familial link and is seen in populations that consume diets high in fat and low in fruits and vegetables. Polyp formation is associated with an increased risk of this form of cancer.
- Early detection based on self-examination and screening is the basis for the identification and successful treatment of many cancers.
- Risk reduction, through living a wellness lifestyle, remains at the heart of cancer prevention.

REVIEW QUESTIONS

1. What is the relationship between regulatory genes and tumor suppressor genes in the development of cancer? Why are regulatory genes called both proto-oncogenes and oncogenes?
2. What properties do cancer cells possess that are lacking in normal cells?
3. What are some of the major types of cancer, based on the tissue from which they originate? What are some of the more familiar cancers based on organ of origin?
4. What signs indicate the possibility that a skin lesion has become cancerous?
5. What are the principal factors that contribute to the development of lung cancer? Of breast cancer?
6. When should regular use of mammography begin, and which women should begin using it earliest?
7. What important information can be obtained with the use of Pap tests? What innovations are associated with the Pap-plus test?
8. How does the PSA test contribute to the early detection of prostate cancer?
9. What are the steps for effective self-examination of the breasts and testicles? What is the current status of breast self-examination?
10. What are the risk reduction activities identified in this chapter?

ANSWERS TO THE "WHAT DO YOU KNOW?" QUIZ

1. True   2. False   3. False   4. True   5. False   6. False   7. False

Visit the Online Learning Center (**www.mhhe.com/payne11e**), where you will find tools to help you improve your grade including practice quizzes, key terms flashcards, audio chapter summaries for your MP3 player, and many other study aids.

SOURCE NOTES

1. Boyle P. The globalization of cancer. *Lancet,* 368(9536), 629–630, 2006.
2. American Cancer Society. *Cancer Facts & Figures 2008.* Atlanta: American Cancer Society, 2008.
3. Yabroff KR, et al. Patient Time Costs Associated with Cancer Care. *Journal of the National Cancer Institute,* 99(1), 14–23, 2007.
4. DeHavas-Walt C, Proctor B, Smith J. *Income, Poverty, and Health Insurance Coverage in the United States: 2007.* U.S. Census Bureau. August 2008.
5. Jemal A, et al. Trends in the Leading Causes of Death in the United States, 1997–2002. *Journal of the American Medical Association,* 294(10), 1255–1259, 2005.
6. Saladin KS. *Anatomy and Physiology: The Unity of Form and Function* (5th ed.). New York: McGraw-Hill, 2010.
7. Barker SW, Kasprio J. Common Susceptibility Genes for Cancer: Search for the End of the Rainbow. *British Medical Journal,* 332(7550), 1150–1152, May 2006.
8. Orr N, Chanock S. Common Genetic Variation and Human Disease. *Advances in Genetics,* 62, 1–32, 2008.
9. Schwad M (Ed.). *Encyclopedia of Cancer* (Vols. 1–4), (2nd ed.). Springer, 2008.
10. Man Y, Gardner WA. Bad Seeds Produce Bad Crops: A Single Stage-Process of Prostate Tumor Invasion. *Journal of Biological Sciences,* 4, 246–258, 2008.
11. Kasur M, et al. Induction of withdrawal-like symptoms in a small randomized controlled trial of opioid blockage in frequent tanners. *J Am Acad Dermatol,* 54(4), 709–711, April 2006.
12. Louafi A, et al. Merkel Cell Carcinoma: Study of 24 Cases and Review of the Literature. *Annales de chirurgie plastique et esthétique,* February 13, 2009. [Epub ahead of print]
13. Henschke CI, et al. Survival of Patients with Stage 1 Lung Cancer Detected on CT Screening. 2006. *New England Journal of Medicine,* 355(17), 1763–1771, October 26, 2006.
14. Duby S, Siegried JM, Traynor AM. Nonsmall-Cell Lung Cancer and Breast Carcinoma: Chemotherapy and Beyond. *Lancet Oncology,* 7(5), 416–424, May 2008.
15. Nemunaitis J, Nemunaitis J. A Review of Vaccine Clinical Trials for Nonsmall Cell Lung Cancer. *Expert Opinion on Biological Therapy,* 7(1), 89–102, January 7, 2007.
16. Jemal A, et al. Annual Report to the Nation of the Status of Cancer, 1975–2005, Featuring Trends in Lung Cancer, Tobacco Use, and Tobacco Control. *Journal of the National Cancer Institute,* 100(23), 1672–1698, December 3, 2008.
17. Zisman AL, et al. Association Between the Age at Diagnosis and Location of Colorectal Cancer and Use of Alcohol and Tobacco: Implications for Screening. *Archives of Internal Medicine,* 166(6), 629–634, March 27, 2006.
18. Whitlock EP, et al. Screening for Colorectal Cancer: A Targeted, Updated Systematic Review for the U.S. Preventive Services Task Force. *Annals of Internal Medicine,* 149(9), 638–656, November 4, 2008.
19. Johnson CD, et al. Accuracy of CT Colonography for Detection of Large Adenomas and Cancers. *New England Journal of Medicine,* 359(12), 1207–1217, September 19, 2008.
20. Ravdin P, et al. *A Sharp Decrease in Breast Cancer Incidence in the United States in 2003.* Proceeding from the 2006 annual San Antonio Breast Cancer Symposium (SABCS). Oral Presentation, Dec. 14, 2006.
21. Chlebowski RT. Influence of Estrogen Plus Progestin on Breast Cancer and Mammography in Healthy Post-Menopausal Women: The Women's Health Initiative Randomized Trial. *Journal of the American Medical Association,* 289(24), 3243–3254, 2003.
22. Tamimi RM, et al. Combined Estrogen and Testosterone Use and Risk of Breast Cancer in Postmenopausal Women. *Archives of Internal Medicine,* 166(14), 1483–1489, July 24, 2006.
23. Krainer M, et al. Differential Contributions of BRAC1 and BRAC2 to Early-Onset Breast Cancer. *New England Journal of Medicine,* 336(20), 1416–1421, 1997.
24. Nanda R, et al. Genetic Testing in an Ethnically Diverse Cohort of High-Risk Women: A Comparative Analysis of BRAC1 and BRAC2 Mutations in American Families of European and African Ancestry. *Journal of the American Medical Association,* 294(15), 1925–1933, 2005.
25. Armstrong K, et al. Racial Differences in the Use of BRAC1/2 Testing Among Women with a Family History of Breast or Ovarian Cancer. *Journal of the American Medical Association,* 293(14), 1729–1736, 2005.
26. *Breast Cancer Chemoprevention: Medicines That Reduce Breast Cancer Risk.* 2009. MayoFoundation. www.mayoclinic.com/health/breast-cancer/WO00092
27. Mammography. Radiological Society of North America (RSNA). 2006. *RadiologyInfo.* August 15; 1–8; www.radiologyinfo.org/en/info.cfm?pg=mammo&bhcp=1.
28. *Breast Cancer Treatment.* 2009. Mayo Foundation. www.mayoclinic.org/breast-cancer/treatment.html
29. Amundadottir LT, et al. A Common Variant Associated with Prostate Cancer in European and African Populations. *Nature Genetics,* 38(6), 652–658, June 2006. Canby-Hagino E, et al. Looking Forward to New Paradigms in Prostate Cancer Screening and Prevention. *European Urology,* 51(1), 27–33, January 2007.
30. *ASCO/AUA guidelines recommends men and their doctors discuss using 5-ARIs to reduce prostate cancer risk.* News Release. American Society of Clinical Oncology, ASCO Annual Meeting, Chicago, IL, February 25, 2009.
31. U.S. Preventive Task Force. Screening for Prostate Cancer: U.S. Preventive Task Force Recommendation Statement. *Annals of Internal Medicine,* 149, 185–191, 2008.
32. Lu-Yao GL, et al. Survival Following Primary Androgen Deprivation Therapy Among Men with Localized Prostate Cancer. *Journal of the American Medical Association,* 300(2), 173–181, 2008.
33. Shariat SF, et al. Improved Prediction of Disease Relapse After Radical Prostatectomy Through a Panel of Preoperative Blood-Based Biomarkers. *Clinical Cancer Research,* 14(12), 3785–3791, 2008.
34. U.S. Food and Drug Administration. FDA News. FDA Approves Expanded Use of Gardasil to Include Preventing Certain Vulvar and Vaginal Cancers. Retrieved September 12, 2008, from www.fda.gov/bbs/topics/NEWS/2008/NEW01885.html
35. Zeleniuch-Jacquotte A, et al. Circulating Enterolactone and Risk of Endometrial Cancer. *International Journal of Cancer,* 119(10), 2376–2381, November 15, 2006.
36. Armstrong DK, et al. Intraperitoneal Cisplatin and Paclitaxel in Ovarian Cancer. *New England Journal of Medicine,* 354(1), 34–43, January 5, 2006.
37. Skinner HG, et al. Vitamin D Intake and the Risk of Pancreatic Cancer in Two Cohort Studies. *Cancer Epidemiology, Epidemiology Biomarkers and Prevention,* 15 (9), 1688–1695, September 2006.
38. Boscoe FP, Schymura MJ. Solar Ultraviolet-B Exposure and Cancer Incidence and Mortality in the United States, 1993–2002. *BMC Cancer,* 6, 264, 2006.

Personal Assessment

Are you at risk for skin, breast, or cervical cancer?

Some people may have a higher than average risk of developing particular types of cancer. These people can be identified by certain risk factors.

This simple self-testing method is adapted from one by the American Cancer Society to help you assess your risk factors for three common types of cancer. These are the major risk factors but by no means represent the only ones that might be involved.

Check your response to each risk factor. Add the numbers in the parentheses to arrive at a total score for each cancer type. Find out what your score means by reading the information in each "Interpretation" section. You are advised to discuss the information with your physician if you are at a higher risk.

Skin Cancer

1. Frequent work or play in the sun
   A. Yes (10)
   B. No (1)

2. Work in mines, around coal tars, or around radioactivity
   A. Yes (10)
   B. No (1)

3. Complexion—fair skin or light skin
   A. Yes (10)
   B. No (1)

YOUR TOTAL POINTS _____

Explanation

1. Excessive ultraviolet light causes skin cancer. Protect yourself with a sunscreen.
2. These materials can cause skin cancer.
3. Light complexions need more protection than others.

Interpretation

Numerical risks for skin cancer are difficult to state. For instance, a person with a dark complexion can work longer in the sun and be less likely to develop cancer than can a light-complected person. Furthermore, a person wearing a long-sleeved shirt and a wide-brimmed hat may work in the sun and be less at risk than is a person who wears a bathing suit and stays in the sun for only a short period. The risk increases greatly with age.

The key here is if you answered yes to any question, you need to realize that you have above-average risk.

Breast Cancer

1. Age group
   A. 20–34 (10)
   B. 35–49 (40)
   C. 50 and over (90)

2. Race/nationality
   A. Asian American (5)
   B. African American (20)
   C. White (25)
   D. Mexican American (10)

3. Family history of breast cancer
   A. Mother, sister, or grandmother (30)
   B. None or unknown (10)

4. Your history
   A. No breast disease (10)
   B. Previous noncancerous lumps or cysts (25)
   C. Previous breast cancer (100)

5. Maternity
   A. First pregnancy before age 25 (10)
   B. First pregnancy after age 25 (15)
   C. No pregnancies (20)

YOUR TOTAL POINTS _____

Interpretation

Under 100   Low-risk women should follow the 2008 ACS cancer screening guidelines. Note that the role of BSE has been redefined. Consult your physician's possible modifications to this protocol.

100–199   Moderate-risk women should consult their physicians to determine whether the ACS guidelines should be followed as stated or, possibly, be modified in terms of scheduling or procedures employed. Note that the role of BSE has been redefined.

200 or more   High-risk women should consult their physicians to determine whether the ACS guidelines should be followed as stated or, very likely, be modified in terms of scheduling or procedures employed. Note that the role of BSE has been redefined.

Personal Assessment—*continued*

Cervical Cancer*

1. Age group
   A. Under 25 (10)
   B. 25–39 (20)
   C. 40–54 (30)
   D. 55 and over (30)

2. Race/nationality
   A. Asian American (10)
   B. Puerto Rican (20)
   C. African American (20)
   D. White (10)
   E. Mexican American (20)

3. Number of pregnancies
   A. 0 (10)
   B. 1 to 3 (20)
   C. 4 and over (30)

4. Viral infections
   A. Herpes and other viral infections or ulcer formations on the vagina (10)
   B. Never (1)

5. Age at first intercourse
   A. Before 15 (40)
   B. 15–19 (30)
   C. 20–24 (20)
   D. 25 and over (10)

6. Bleeding between periods or after intercourse
   A. Yes (40)
   B. No (1)

YOUR TOTAL POINTS _____

Explanations

1. The highest occurrence is in the 40-and-over age group. The numbers represent the relative rates of cancer for different age groups. A 45-year-old woman has a risk three times higher than that of a 20-year-old.

2. Puerto Ricans, African Americans, and Mexican Americans have higher rates of cervical cancer.
3. Women who have delivered more children have a higher occurrence.
4. Viral infections of the cervix and vagina are associated with cervical cancer.
5. Women with earlier intercourse and with more sexual partners are at a higher risk.
6. Irregular bleeding may be a sign of uterine cancer.

Interpretation

40–69—This is a low-risk group. Ask your doctor for a Pap test. You will be advised how often you should be tested after your first test.

70–99—In this moderate-risk group, more frequent Pap tests may be required.

100 or higher—You are in a high-risk group and should have a Pap test (and pelvic examination) as advised by your doctor.

TO CARRY THIS FURTHER . . .

Regardless of score, you should discuss with your physician the desirability of the Pap-plus test (or one similar to it); it is designed to identify the presence of DNA from one or more of the HPV strains associated with cervical cancer.

___

*Lower portion of uterus. These questions would not apply to a woman who has had a complete hysterectomy.

Source: Adapted from the American Cancer Society.

Managing Chronic Conditions

What Do You Know About Chronic Diseases?

1. Chronic conditions most often develop slowly, but once in place they abruptly abate or resolve. True or False?

2. When an X-link recessive condition exists, the biological mother is defined as the carrier, while the male child is the afflicted recipient of that condition. True or False?

3. Congenital abnormalities, such as a cleft lip or cleft palate, develop shortly after birth. True or False?

4. Type 1 diabetes mellitus and type 2 diabetes mellitus are exactly the same condition, except that one form requires the use of insulin (from outside the body), while the other does not. True or False?

5. Irritable bowel syndrome becomes defined as irritable bowel disease if more than one year of treatment does not result in significant improvement. True or False?

6. Multiple sclerosis (MS) is a chronic condition of the nervous system, although its cause lies in the abnormal functioning of the immune system. True or False?

7. Parkinson's disease and Alzheimer's disease are both conditions reflecting changes to the brain's ability to use neurotransmitters in the normal manner. True or False?

Check your answers at the end of the chapter.

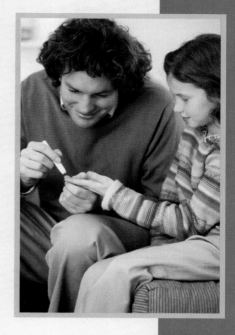

In clinical medicine, thousands of diseases, illnesses, and conditions can be diagnosed and treated. For ease of communication, these diseases and illnesses have been individually named and categorized. We have chosen a set of categories—*genetic/inherited, congenital, metabolic, autoimmune, degenerative,* and *infectious*—and a sample of conditions that we believe you will be interested in learning about. Knowledge of these conditions will increase your understanding of chronic disease processes and how they differ from infectious diseases. Where appropriate, you will also find useful information about risk factors and lifestyle changes you can make to reduce your risk of developing a chronic condition.*†

*Only a clinician can diagnose and treat these conditions. The information contained in this chapter is intended only to inform.
†We have placed each condition into its most appropriate category. However, the characteristics of a given condition may overlap with those in a second group. We will point this out when it occurs.

The young woman that we want you to meet was, not too many years ago, taking a personal health course much like you are now. She was bright, highly engaged, and eager for the world that awaited her beyond college. However, early in the semester in which she was in this class, absences due to illness began to accumulate, a brief period of hospitalization occurred, and by semester's end she had been diagnosed with Crohn's disease. Crohn's disease is characterized by episodes of diarrhea, rectal bleeding, malabsorption of nutrients, and frequent periods of generalized fatigue. Daily scheduled activities are often interrupted by periods of hospitalization and, on a near daily basis, the frequent need for restroom facilities.

The academic year following the diagnosis of Crohn's disease was even more disrupted when the young woman experienced initial episodes of cyclic vomiting syndrome, a condition characterized by the unanticipated onset of vomiting (as often as 15 to 20 times per day) shortly after the ingestion of food. Upon extensive evaluation at an internationally renowned medical institution, the label "idiopathic gastroparesis" was assigned to her newest problem. As the condition worsened, nutritional intake was accomplished by using a catheter surgically implanted into the small intestine through which nutritive-dense liquids were introduced—the delivery of 900 calories required up to 12 hours per day. Eventually, a gastric pacemaker was implanted into her abdominal cavity, thus increasing gastric emptying to a level adequate to abandon the use of tube feedings. This latter form of intervention allowed a window of improved health. Unfortunately, however, the effectiveness of the gastric pacemaker proved difficult to maintain, and the use of tube feeding was reinstated.

At this time, the young woman who was so recently in the same personal health course that you are, and still only in her late 20s, has been diagnosed with multiple sclerosis, a disease reflected in the loss of "insulation" around nerves necessary to conduct electrical impulses to skeletal muscles, impeding movement-related activities, including mobility.

In light of this multiplicity of illnesses, daily activities center around taking multiple drugs by mouth, feedings, and injections of an MS disease modifying medication, the use of a "walker" to navigate, and finding someone to drive her to doctor appointments. Her once wide circle of friends has been reduced to a loving spouse and family, home care providers, and a network of devoted cyberfriends—most of whom share some of the same medical conditions.

If this seems to be an unusually severe collection of illnesses for one young person to have, it certainly is. If you're considering that it was in any way "asked for," it wasn't. In fact, this young woman lived a "health-enhanced lifestyle" in all of the ways you will learn about in this textbook. Rather, it is yet another example of the unpredictable nature of life's journey. However, in spite of her own inability to ensure a high level of health through healthy living, she would nevertheless encourage you to take your health seriously because *"when it is gone, you'll miss it."* To see you do any less would be truly distressing to her.

The first five categories of conditions—genetic/inherited, congenital, metabolic, autoimmune, and **degenerative**—are discussed in the sections that follow. They have in common a slow, gradual course of development and remain a part of people's lives for long periods of time; thus they are said to be **chronic** conditions. Conversely, the infectious diseases are often quickly contracted and, once treatment has begun, stay active for a limited amount of time. These are referred to as the **acute** conditions (although HIV/AIDS is now defined as a chronic condition because of its extended duration). This sixth category, the infectious conditions, comprises illnesses caused by pathogenic organisms often transmitted from person to person. These conditions are discussed separately, in Chapter 13. The worldwide HIV/AIDS epidemic, the novel H1N1 pandemic, the increasing threat of infectious diseases such as methicillin-resistant *Staphylococcus aureus* (MRSA), and the comeback of familiar infections that are now resistant to antibiotics make this separate coverage necessary.

Three types of chronic conditions—obesity, cardiovascular disease, and cancer—are also addressed separately (in Chapters 6, 10, and 11, respectively) because of their importance to so many families and to the health of the nation. Many other chronic conditions are addressed in appropriate chapters throughout the book. For example, low-back pain is discussed in Chapter 4, osteoporosis in Chapter 4, and chronic obstructive lung disease in Chapter 9. Even though these conditions are not discussed in this chapter, they too fit into one or more of the categories described and are either chronic or acute in nature.

Chronic Disease Prevention

With the well-deserved emphasis placed on the prevention of heart disease and cancer, you might expect that virtually all diseases are preventable if you follow a wellness lifestyle. While it is true that many conditions are strongly linked to the lifestyle choices you make, we know little about how to prevent most of the chronic diseases described in this chapter (see the box "When It Is Gone, You'll Miss It!"). Learning about these conditions reminds us that even the most carefully tended human body is vulnerable to the effects of aging and the array of diseases that, in many cases, we do not yet understand. Accordingly, we are challenged to move beyond our perception of health as the absence of disease and illness. As we first discussed in Chapter 1 and as depicted

Chronic Illness—The End or a Turning Point?

Most people diagnosed with a chronic illness go through a period of serious adjustment. For college students, the necessary adaptations feel particularly burdensome because so few of their peers are faced with equal demands. Not only must self-care routines be changed, but the help of others may be necessary to carry out that care. The limitations imposed by a chronic illness can restrict the activities and behavior of the affected individual and his or her family and friends. Financial matters (including the ability to afford medications), the need to see physicians frequently, and insurance issues add to the person's stress. When their lives change so profoundly, young people can feel isolated and singled out in a negative way.

People respond to the diagnosis of a chronic illness in various ways. Frequently, their first reaction is denial. When this occurs, care may be delayed. At the same time, school and work performance and relationships begin to suffer from the internalized stress. Eventually, though, denial gives way to anger, which is often directed at others. Common targets of this anger are people close to the ill person, such as family and friends. Then anger broadens to include the world or God (for "letting these things happen"). Eventually, the demands of the illness, combined with a sense of futility, give way to acceptance. At this stage, the individual's resourcefulness surfaces as he or she looks within for untapped sources of strength. Gradually, the person becomes open to the assistance offered by others, begins to discover new interests and abilities, and realizes that life is not over—just different.

The decision to accept the chronic condition often brings a sense of inner peace and allows for a new approach to living. People who believe that they will not be given a burden too great for them to bear may rise to the challenge and find a level of strength that they—and others—didn't know they had. With acceptance comes new learning experiences. The person begins to understand the limitations of the body, to appreciate what true friendships are, and to recognize the importance of emotional resources once taken for granted. Even more significant is the realization that the spiritual dimension of health is bountiful. As the daily challenges of the illness continue, the person realizes that his or her personal beliefs and values have not only survived but are even stronger.

---

in Figure 1-2, on page 15, only then can we see that the value of health is not what it prevents, but rather what it makes possible—a life characterized by growth and development through each stage of the life cycle (see the box "Chronic Illness—The End or a Turning Point?").

Genetic/Inherited Conditions

Genetic or inherited conditions can occur in any of three ways: (1) abnormal genetic material (genes) are transmitted from one or both biological parents at conception; (2) abnormal genetic material is formed by mutation of normal genetic material at a very early stage of cellular replication and, subsequently, passed on with each cell doubling; or (3) an abnormal number of chromosomes—more or fewer than the normal number of 46—is inherited or formed. We will present brief descriptions of conditions from this broad category, including Klinefelter's syndrome, Turner's syndrome, cystic fibrosis, and color vision deficiency.

In discussing chronic diseases, other than the more prominent ones such as cardiovascular disease, cancer, and diabetes mellitus, we must note that few requirements for reporting the incidence of such diseases exist (unlike infectious diseases). For example, very few states keep records of autoimmune diseases such as lupus; fewer than 10 monitor developmental disabilities; and less than one-half of the states report on asthma. Because of these inadequacies it is likely that many chronic diseases are underestimated, so emerging trends are difficult to determine, and environmental factors associated with their development remain unrecognized.

Abnormal Number of Sex Chromosomes

At the time of conception (fertilization) an ovum (egg) from the biological mother containing 23 chromosomes is penetrated by a sperm from the biological father that also contains 23 chromosomes. This fusion of genetic material results in an initial human cell that contains 46 chromosomes, the number found in virtually every human cell. Of these 46 chromosomes, two are **sex chromosomes** (an X from the biological mother and an X or Y from the biological father). A normal male would thus possess a 44XY (44 nonsex chromosomes plus an X chromosome and a Y chromosome) chromosomal profile, and a normal female would be depicted as 44XX. Occasionally,

---

Key Terms

degenerative A slow but progressive deterioration of the body's structure or function.

chronic Develops slowly and persists for an extended period of time.

acute Having a sudden onset and a prompt resolution.

sex chromosomes The X and Y chromosomes that determine sex; chromosomes other than the autosomes.

---

people are born who possess more or fewer than the normal 46 chromosomes because they have more than or fewer than the normal 2 sex chromosomes.

Klinefelter's Syndrome
Klinefelter's syndrome is one condition in which an abnormal number of sex chromosomes is present. It occurs in males and is a relatively rare (1 in 1,000 male births) condition in which a Y sex chromosome from the biological father is combined with two X sex chromosomes.[1] Klinefelter's syndrome would be graphically depicted as 44XXY, for a total of 47 chromosomes.

Although they look normal at birth, male children with Klinefelter's syndrome gradually show signs of the condition by the time they reach puberty. Men with Klinefelter's syndrome are often tall, very thin, and have gynecomastia (breast enlargement). In addition, a small penis, small testicles, and underdeveloped secondary sexual characteristics are typical. Men with Klinefelter's syndrome are generally infertile and may have some impairment in learning ability and personality adjustment. The unique components of Klinefelter's syndrome are thought to reflect the feminizing influence of the additional X chromosome.

Turner's Syndrome
Another genetic condition caused by an altered sex chromosome number is Turner's syndrome. It occurs in females (1 in 5,000 female births) when one of the 2 X chromosomes is missing, resulting in a chromosomal number of 45.[1] This pattern is graphically depicted as 44X0, with 0 reflecting the absence of the second X chromosome. Women with Turner's syndrome have equivalent versions of many of the problems seen in men with Klinefelter's syndrome: infertility, a characteristic body type, and diminished secondary sex characteristics.

Inherited Genetic Mutations

Cystic Fibrosis
No inherited condition claims more children's and young adults' lives than does cystic fibrosis (CF). In the United States, in about 1 of every 2,000 live births is an infant born with this inherited condition. Early treatment is beneficial, and CF is one of 29 conditions for which the March of Dimes recommends testing in newborns; visit this book's Online Learning Center (www.mhhe.com/payne11e) for a list of neonatal screening requirements for your state. In past decades, life expectancy for children with cystic fibrosis was only about 8 years. Today, however, with a fuller understanding of the disease and with more effective forms of treatment, life expectancy has increased significantly, to about 30 years. Unfortunately, the disease is very demanding, and effective management requires daily intervention.

Cystic fibrosis causes a profound disruption in the function of the **exocrine glands** in several areas of the body. This impaired function is due to the body's inability to produce a protein that helps regulate chloride content within the secretory cells of various exocrine glands. In the absence of this protein, the glands cannot produce certain enzymes needed to carry out important bodily functions.

For example, CF impairs the ability of the pancreas, an exocrine gland, to produce digestive enzymes. CF is known to affect other exocrine glands as well. It reduces the ability of sweat glands to conserve electrolytes, the ability of mucous glands lining the airway to control mucus production, and the ability of secretory glands within the digestive tract to produce digestive enzymes. These impairments of normal function underlie significant problems in respiration and digestion.[2]

The management of CF has improved dramatically in recent years. Diets designed to maintain weight and support growth, respiratory therapy to maintain the health of the airways, a newly approved inhaled antibiotic, a vaccine effective against CF's principal pneumonia-causing bacterium, and new drugs have improved the quality of life and increased the life expectancy of people with CF. On a few occasions, **gene replacement therapy** through inhalation of virus-containing microscopic beads of genetic material has been attempted, but the existence of lung disease is a major obstacle to the effective delivery of the beads. Lung transplantation has, on a very limited basis, been undertaken as a last-resort treatment for cystic fibrosis. To date the results of these transplants have been so poor as to deem them inferior to the currently recommended treatment standards.[3] Accordingly, CF remains an incurable, life-shortening disease.

Like sickle-cell disease, which is described next, CF shows a **recessive inheritance pattern.** Genetic testing can determine whether a person who is apparently free from CF might, in fact, carry a copy of the recessive gene. In addition, if an at-risk pregnancy has occurred, chorionic villus sampling or amniocentesis can be performed, although this carries a risk of miscarriage.

Sickle-Cell Trait and Sickle-Cell Disease
Of all the chemical compounds found within the body, few occur in as many forms as hemoglobin, which helps bind oxygen to red blood cells. Two forms of hemoglobin are associated with *sickle-cell trait* and *sickle-cell disease*. With an occasional exception, it is African Americans who can possess either form of this abnormal hemoglobin. Those who inherit the trait form do not develop the disease but are capable of transmitting the gene for abnormal hemoglobin to their offspring. Those who inherit the disease form face a shortened life characterized by periods of pain and impairment called *crises*.

Approximately 8 percent of African Americans carry the recessive gene for sickle-cell trait; they experience little impairment, and they can transmit the gene to their children. For approximately 1.5 percent of African

Americans, however, sickle-cell disease is a painful, incapacitating, and life-shortening condition. Red blood cells are elongated, crescent-shaped (or sickled), and unable to pass through the body's minute capillaries (Figure 12-1). The body responds to the presence of these abnormal red blood cells by removing them very quickly. This sets the stage for anemia—thus the condition is often called *sickle-cell anemia*. In addition to anemia, this form of the condition is associated with many serious medical problems, including impaired lung function, congestive heart failure, gallbladder infections, bone changes, abnormalities of the eyes and skin, and, occasionally, extremely serious pulmonary hypertension, for which all patients should be screened and treated.[2] Until recently, living beyond early adulthood was not possible. Today, however, with effective screening and new medications, people with sickle-cell disease may live to reach 50 years of age.

In about 1 percent of people with sickle-cell disease, a bone-marrow or stem-cell transplant may be able to give the body the ability to produce a normal form of hemoglobin. Early results are promising and raise hope of a "cure" of sorts, although the number of patients who might be helped by this therapy is small. In addition, a newly introduced drug, hydroxyurea, has provided some relief from the pain caused by the clogging of vessels and the discomfort of acute chest congestion. The drug also reduces the number of blood transfusions normally needed to relieve pain.

Recently it was found that long-term transfusion can increase the risk of heart and liver damage, but its benefits outweigh this risk.

Screening to determine whether a woman or her partner carries the recessive gene may be the only key for preventing sickle-cell trait and disease. Genetic counseling can then help couples weigh the risk of passing on the gene to their children. Today, for couples at risk for passing on the gene, an ovum can be fertilized **in vitro,** the resulting embryo can then be tested, and if the ovum is found to be free of the condition it can be implanted in the uterus. This eliminates the need for any decision regarding a therapeutic abortion.

Sex-Chromosome-Linked Inherited Genetic Mutations

Color Vision Deficiency Recessive genetic mutations located on a maternal sex chromosome (which is always an X chromosome) present a unique problem for male offspring. The crux of the problem lies in the male's inability to "offset" or "override" the mutated gene's influence because he lacks a second X chromosome containing a normal version of the mutated gene. Females can carry the mutated gene but will not be affected by the abnormal trait because they have a normal second X chromosome. Color vision deficiency is such a condition.

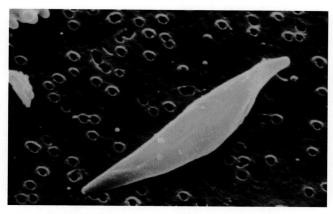

Figure 12-1 A Sickled (Crescent-Shaped) Red Blood Cell in a Person with Sickle-Cell Disease The red blood cells are elongated and thus cannot pass through the body's minute capillaries, causing periods of pain and impairment called *crises.*

Color vision deficiency, once called color blindness, occurs in approximately 1 in 8 white males, but it is slightly less prevalent in African American males and is rarely seen in females, as they would have to inherit two X chromosomes that both carry the recessive trait.

Virtually all persons with color vision deficiency are capable of seeing colors, although distinguishing shades of color is often difficult to very difficult. The extent to which this inherited condition is a problem for children and adults covers a wide continuum—from the condition's being almost unrecognizable, to interfering in learning colors as a young child, to difficulty in coordinating clothing selections, to being incapable of employment in occupations where color differentiation is a necessary skill.

Although color vision deficiency can be diagnosed easily by a physician or vision specialist, there is no treatment for or "outgrowing" of, the condition. Parents should have their children screened, particularly if they notice that a child has symptoms such as amblyopia (lazy

> ### Key Terms
>
> **exocrine glands** Glands whose secretions are released through tubes or ducts, such as sweat glands.
>
> **gene replacement therapy** An experimental therapy in which a healthy human gene is incorporated into a harmless virus to be delivered to cells that have an abnormal version of the gene.
>
> **recessive inheritance pattern** The inheritance of traits whose expression requires that they be carried by both biological parents.
>
> **in vitro** Outside the living body, in an artificial environment.

eye), nystagmus (rapid, small, jerking, or roving movement of the eye), or sensitivity to light.[4]

Fragile X Syndrome A second inherited genetic mutation linked to the sex chromosomes is fragile X syndrome, the condition most currently *known* to be associated with autism and an important player underlying mental retardation, most often in males. At the heart of fragile X syndrome is the mutation of a gene (FMR1) on the X chromosome. When functioning normally, this gene orchestrates the production of a protein that is important in communication between neurons (nerve cells) within the brain.[5] When this gene is "turned off," as occurs in fragile X syndrome, it can cause difficulties in cognitive function (both learning and memory) and movement, behavioral changes, connective tissue disorders, unique physical features of the face, and fertility issues in females.

Because females have a second X chromosome, fragile X syndrome is often more muted in females than in males. Young boys with fragile X syndrome commonly have symptoms of attention deficit hyperactivity disorders (ADHD), anxiety disorders, and difficulty sustaining eye contact or engaging in sustained verbal communication with others. Most males with this condition are defined as cognitively delayed, and a smaller percentage (10 to 15 percent), when tested for cognitive function, are defined as borderline or mildly mentally retarded.

As young males with fragile X syndrome grow older, physical features of their faces often change noticeably—the face of an adult male with fragile X syndrome is often very elongated and the ears are large and protruding. Hand flapping and hand biting are common behaviors in persons with fragile X syndrome.

Interventions relating to fragile X syndrome are multifaceted and involve a wide array of professionals in areas related to speech and language development, cognitive development, gross motor development, sensory integration, and behavioral management.[6] When their efforts are coordinated, these professionals can help persons with fragile X syndrome reach their full potential for self-sufficiency.

Congenital Abnormalities

The second group of conditions, congenital abnormalities, refers to abnormalities that are present at birth. These conditions are caused by inappropriate changes in tissues (and thus in organs and organ systems) during embryonic development. Although both inherited (genetic) and congenital conditions are present at birth, congenital abnormalities differ in that they do not involve an atypical number of chromosomes, or an inherited chromosomal abnormality.

During the first three months of pregnancy (the first trimester), the embryo is "constructed" within the protective confines of the uterus. Tissues, organs, and organ systems are formed and take their proper positions according to the complex genetic blueprint established at conception. The embryo will be fully formed by the end of this three-month period. Subsequent enlargement (growth) and refinement (maturation) will occur during the fetal period, which comprises the second and third trimesters.

A congenital abnormality is a condition caused by the inappropriate or incomplete development of a particular embryonic structure or the failure of a structure to function properly at birth. In the section that follows, we will describe selected types of congenital abnormalities. Some congenital abnormalities are so severe that they are incompatible with life, even within the uterus. Thus the embryo is spontaneously aborted by the body (this event is commonly known as a *miscarriage*). Some other congenital abnormalities are life threatening, but the pregnancy can be carried to full term. And in many other cases the abnormality is recognized early in the child's life and can be corrected, or may even be so minor that it is not problematic.

No single factor is responsible for causing congenital abnormalities. They generally form early in pregnancy, during the critical weeks when the embryo's organs are being formed. They may be the result of genetic mutation or environmental factors, such as infections and drugs. Most congenital abnormalities, however, are caused by a complex interplay of factors, some genetic and some environmental. Thus their cause is considered to be **multifactorial.**

Cleft Palate and Cleft Lip

In the early weeks of embryonic life, the structures of the face, including the lips and roof of the mouth, form as separate halves on each side of the midline. Failure of the upper lip to fuse results in a split or cleft lip. Failure of the roof of the mouth to fuse causes cleft palate. One of these conditions (or both) occurs in about 1 of every 800 live births.

Although a genetic predisposition may be a factor in some cases of cleft lip and palate, the cause of these conditions is unknown. Environmental factors, such as the use of certain medications during pregnancy, alcohol use, and smoking, may contribute to varying degrees.[7]

If a child's cleft lip or cleft palate is not corrected, he or she may have trouble eating or speaking clearly. In addition, cosmetic concerns may be at issue, an adequate bone foundation for tooth stability may not be established, and significant hearing loss may occur.[7] For these reasons, surgery is recommended to correct both conditions and prevent these difficulties. Figure 12-2 shows a child with cleft lip and cleft palate before surgery.

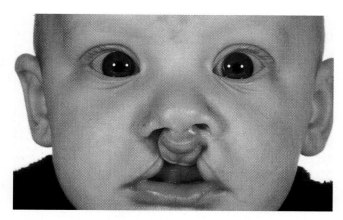

Figure 12-2 An Infant with Cleft Lip and Cleft Palate This common congenital abnormality is repaired before the child is two years old. Surgical correction is usually quite successful, both cosmetically and functionally.

Surgery to repair a cleft lip is usually performed when the infant is three to four months old, whereas surgery to repair a cleft palate is usually completed before the child reaches his or her second birthday. If the nasal passages and throat structures are involved, additional surgeries may be required to achieve the high level of success that characterizes today's medical care of these facial abnormalities.

Patent Foramen Ovale (PFO)

During intrauterine life, blood flow in the fetal heart bypasses the right ventricle, the chamber that normally pumps unoxygenated blood to the lungs for oxygenation (see Chapter 10). The lungs are bypassed because the fetus is in effect "under water" and, thus, cannot use its lungs. A hole (the foramen ovale) in the interatrial septum, the wall that divides the upper right chamber of the heart from the upper left chamber, provides the necessary passageway around the lungs. At the time of birth, however, when the fetus begins to breathe air, this hole is normally closed by a small flap of tissue. The blood is then redirected from the right atrium into the right ventricle to be sent to the lungs.[8]

In about one in five live births, the foramen ovale fails to close completely, without any apparent leakage of blood. In the absence of other cardiac abnormalities, this patent foramen ovale does not cause any problems, is rarely identified, and, thus, prompts no medical attention. In some infants or children, however, a patent foramen ovale may leak, allowing unoxygenated blood to flow into the left atrium and then into the left ventricle of the heart and out into the general circulation.[8] This leakage may result in some **cyanosis** and cause a heart murmur to develop.

Patent foramen ovale is usually diagnosed by the child's primary care physician. No treatment is needed unless other heart abnormalities exist or the volume of unoxygenated blood reaching the left side of the heart is too great.

The possible worsening of the leakage of PFO (both diagnosed and undiagnosed) in adults who regularly scuba dive has caused concern. Researchers speculate that inappropriate decompression techniques, resulting in dangerous ambient pressures and the formation of nitrogen bubbles, in combination with a small patent foramen ovale, may increase the risk of decompression illness as small nitrogen bubbles are distributed throughout the body by the arterial blood flow.[9] Experts disagree somewhat about whether scuba divers should undergo an echocardiogram to test for the presence of a patent foramen ovale. If you are concerned, discuss the issue with your physician.

The patent foramen ovale congenital abnormality is associated with a risk of stroke and migraine headache. Physicians are now more inclined to suggest undertaking surgical repair of these cardiovascular abnormalities years after their initial discovery as a preventive measure against midlife stroke.[10] In regard to migraine headaches, it has been established that a high percentage of persons with this abnormality also have debilitating migraine headaches, and that many found relief after surgical repair.[11]

Scoliosis

Most cases of scoliosis (abnormal lateral spinal curvatures) have no known cause and are thus classified as *idiopathic*. For a small percentage, particularly when present at birth, a genetic basis is thought to exist. In general, curvatures that are less than 10 degrees (or 20 degrees and nonprogressive) are considered postural malalignments and do not require treatment.

Most spinal curvatures begin as a lateral deviation of the spine (curvature to the side) in either the thoracic (upper back) or lumbar (lower back) region (Figure 12-3). The normally aligned spine above or below the initial curvature then begins to curve in the opposite direction to offset the original curvature. This eventually gives the spine an "S" shape. If it is not corrected, the increasing curvature of the spine causes the vertebrae that form the spinal column to rotate. As the vertebrae rotate forward, the ribs follow accordingly, eventually altering the entire

> **Key Terms**
>
> **multifactorial** Requiring the interplay of many factors; refers to the cause of a disease or condition.
>
> **cyanosis** Blue coloration of the lips, skin, and nail beds caused by inadequate oxygenation of the blood.

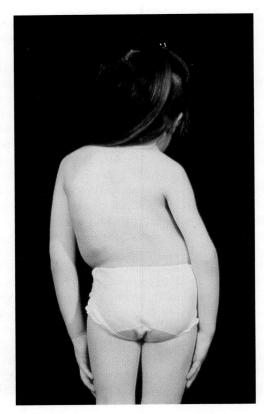

Figure 12-3 Scoliosis Evidence of scoliosis is commonly noted in late childhood or early adolescence.

architecture of the chest cavity. This causes noticeable postural problems, including uneven positioning of the shoulder blades and a "rib hump" deformity. In addition, the changing shape of the chest compresses the heart, lungs, and related structures that pass through the middle of the chest. Increasing disfiguration and discomfort accompany each degree of additional curvature and rotation.

For most people with scoliosis, the curvature that initially develops during the preteen years progressively worsens until the spine stops growing after puberty. Since treatment is the key to preventing these problems, most American elementary schools screen students between the 4th and 6th grades to identify children who need additional evaluation. Children should be screened every 6 to 9 months until growth of the spine slows and then stops. Curvatures of 20 degrees but less than 30 degrees when initially diagnosed may require treatment but will generally not progress after skeletal growth stops. Curvatures greater than 30 degrees will, however, usually continue to increase well after skeletal growth has stopped and into adulthood unless effective treatment is undertaken.

In this country, scoliosis is treated by orthopedic surgeons. Once the spine has been radiographically evaluated

and the precise nature of the condition determined, one of the following three treatment options is chosen:

- *Do nothing.* Depending on the patient's age and the degree of curvature, it may be appropriate to do nothing and simply monitor the condition to see whether further change occurs.

- *Use a brace.* In children and adolescents, a curve in the mild range (between 25 and 35 degrees) is most effectively treated by bracing the back with a specially fitted brace for 23 hours per day. This treatment continues until the spine has moved into acceptable alignment. Recently a procedure called anterior vertebral stapling has been used in treating curvatures of 30 degrees or less, thus eliminating the need for bracing.

- *Undergo surgery.* When a curvature in a preteen or adolescent is near or beyond 45 degrees, the treatment of choice may well be surgical realignment of several vertebrae within and beyond the curvature.

Only about 2 percent of females and 1 percent of males have scoliosis. For those who do, however, new options regarding treatment will be forthcoming, one hopes.

Metabolic Disorders

The third category of chronic conditions is metabolic. Metabolic disorders are caused by the body's inability to control chemical processes that regulate the building up (anabolism) and tearing down (catabolism) of tissue. Diabetes mellitus type 2 and diabetes mellitus type 1 are, perhaps, the most familiar of the metabolic disorders.

Congenital abnormalities, which you learned about in the last section, are caused by abnormal structure that leads to abnormal function. The metabolic disorders, on the other hand, are caused directly by abnormal function. The body is unable to normally utilize various nutrients in the growth and repair of tissues and in the regulation of body processes. The conditions described in this section have clear metabolic components. They may also have some characteristics that overlap with other categories of conditions. For example, a genetic predisposition is associated with type 2 diabetes mellitus and an autoimmune response with type 1 diabetes.

Diabetes Mellitus

News headlines tell us that American youth are at high risk for developing type 2 diabetes mellitus and its associated heart disease and other health problems. We used to believe that type 2 diabetes was a disease of middle age. The CDC launched SEARCH for Diabetes in Youth,[12] a campaign intended to find children and adolescents with a set of prediabetes markers, referred to as metabolic

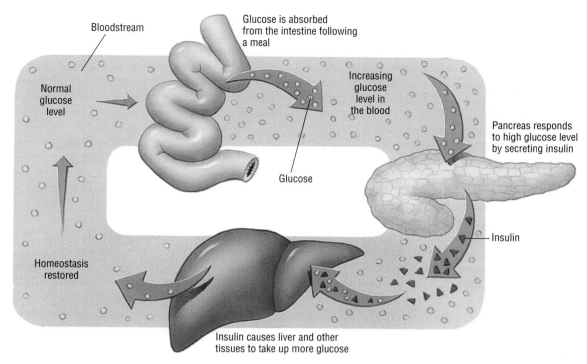

Figure 12-4 Normal Blood Glucose Regulation The secretion of insulin is regulated by a mechanism that tends to reverse any deviation from normal. Thus an increase in blood glucose level triggers secretion of insulin. Since insulin promotes glucose uptake by cells, blood glucose level is restored to its lower, normal level.

syndrome, likely resulting from a childhood of poor diet and gross inactivity, in combination with a genetic predisposition for diabetes (see Chapter 10 for more on metabolic syndrome). Those younger persons who had already progressed to clinical levels of insulin resistance were also sought out by this CDC-sponsored program.

Additionally, the American Diabetes Association issued new guidelines to hone the diagnostic criteria and the pharmacological treatment for children, adolescents, and young adults with previously unrecognized type 2 diabetes mellitus.[13]

Type 2 Diabetes In people who do not have diabetes mellitus, the body's need for energy is met through the "burning" of glucose (blood sugar) within the cells. Glucose is absorbed from the digestive tract and carried to the cells by the blood or stored in the liver as glycogen for later conversion back to glucose.[8] Glucose passes into the cell through a transport system that moves the glucose molecule across the cell's membrane. Activation of this glucose transport mechanism requires the hormone **insulin** (Figure 12-4). Specific receptor sites for insulin can be found on the cell membrane. Insulin is also required for the conversion of glucose into glycogen in the liver and for the formation of fatty acids in adipose cells. Insulin is produced in the islet cells of the pancreas. The release of insulin from the pancreas corresponds to the changing levels of glucose within the blood.[8]

In adults, and tragically in an increasing percentage of children and adolescents, with a genetic predisposition for developing type 2 diabetes, trigger mechanisms (most likely obesity and inactivity) begin a process through which the body cells become increasingly less sensitive to the presence of insulin. The growing ineffectiveness of insulin in moving glucose into cells causes the buildup of glucose in the blood. Elevated levels of glucose in the blood give rise to **hyperglycemia,** a hallmark symptom of type 2 diabetes mellitus.

In response to this buildup, the kidneys begin the process of filtering glucose from the blood. Excess glucose then spills over into the urine resulting in frequent urination. This removal of glucose in the urine is a second important symptom of type 2 diabetes. Increased thirst, a third symptom of developing diabetes, occurs in response to the movement of fluid from extracellular spaces into the circulatory system to maintain homeostasis.

Key Terms

insulin A hormone produced by the islet cells of the pancreas that is necessary for the normal utilization of glucose.

hyperglycemia The condition of having an abnormally high blood glucose level.

For many adults with type 2 diabetes or with a pre-diabetic status often referred to as "glucose intolerance" or "lowered insulin sensitivity," dietary modification (with an emphasis on monitoring total carbohydrate intake, not just sugar), weight loss, and regular exercise is the only treatment required to maintain an acceptable level of glucose. Weight loss improves the condition by "releasing" more insulin receptors, and exercise increases the actual number of receptor sites. With better insulin recognition, the person can return to a more normal state of functioning.

For people whose condition is more advanced, dietary modification, increased activity, and weight loss alone will not be effective in managing the condition, and oral drugs that stimulate insulin output, called hypoglycemic agents, will be required. Increasingly, very aggressive management, including both hypoglycemic agents and insulin, is successfully reducing risks associated with the disease. Many persons, however, have difficulty controlling blood sugar levels even with the use of insulin.

In addition to genetic predisposition and obesity as important factors in type 2 diabetes mellitus, unresolved stress appears to play a role in the development of hyperglycemic states (see the box "A Wellness Plan for Preventing Type 2 Diabetes Mellitus"). Although stress alone probably cannot produce a diabetic condition, it is likely that stress can induce a series of endocrine changes that can lead to a state of hyperglycemia. Depression too can elevate blood glucose levels and thus increase the risk of expressing type 2 diabetes.

Diabetes in both of its principal forms can cause serious damage to virtually all of the body's organ systems, but particularly the cardiovascular, nervous, and renal systems. Some common complications of diabetes are cataract formation, glaucoma, dental caries, kidney disease, gangrene, and impotence.

For the 23.6 million Americans with diagnosed diabetes, the estimated 5.7 million not yet diagnosed, as well as the 57 million who are afflicted with dimensions of metabolic syndrome,[14] their future health will be determined by prompt diagnosis and treatment, subsequent daily monitoring, and compliance with suggested lifestyle adjustments. Perhaps no single group of Americans is more susceptible for rapid decline in the direction of type 2 diabetes mellitus than Hispanic Americans of Mexican descent.

As mentioned previously, self-monitoring of glucose levels is a critical component of diabetes prevention. To this end, the American Diabetes Association has fine-tuned its recommendations regarding self-monitoring.[13] When using plasma glucose (finger prick) monitoring (glucometer), the following levels are applicable for the general adult population:

- 90 mg/dl to 130 mg/dl before meals and 110 mg/dl to 150 mg/dl at bedtime
- Less than 180 mg/dl one to two hours after meals

Modified values are assigned by the ADA for use in monitoring plasma glucose levels in children and in pregnant women. Modification levels for children are related to the nervous system's need for blood glucose during development; pregnant women need to monitor themselves for the development of a transitory form of diabetes known as gestational diabetes.

A second set of indices for monitoring diabetes involves the amount of glycated (think "sugar coated") hemoglobin (A1C or HbA1C) in the blood (hemoglobin is the oxygen-carrying pigment on the surface of red blood cells). Once taken, the results give a picture of the average glucose in the blood over a two- to three-month period. The American Association of Clinical Endocrinologists considers 6.5 mg/dl or less as the upper limit of normal, while the American Diabetes Association considers the upper limit as 7 mg/dl or less. A reading above 7 mg/dl is reflective of glucose intolerance or insulin insensitivity.

A third important biomedical index to maintain, in addition to hemoglobin faction and blood glucose, in the prevention of type 2 diabetes is that of blood pressure. Today, for persons of susceptibility, it is now advised that blood pressure readings be 135 or less over 80 or less.

Type 1 Diabetes A second type of diabetes mellitus is type 1 diabetes mellitus. The onset of this type of diabetes usually occurs before age 35, most often during childhood. In contrast to type 2 diabetes, in which insulin is produced but is ineffective because of insensitivity, in type 1 diabetes the body produces no insulin at all. Destruction of the insulin-producing cells of the pancreas by the immune system (possibly in search of a viral infection within the islet cells of the pancreas) accounts for this sudden and irreversible loss of insulin production.

In most ways the two forms of diabetes are similar, with the important exception that type 1 always requires the use of insulin from an outside source, whereas many people with type 2 diabetes mellitus will not require supplemental insulin, though some might need to take insulin to adequately overcome the insulin insensitivity that is the hallmark of type 2 diabetes. Today insulin is taken by injection (one to four times per day) or through the use of an insulin pump, which provides a constant supply of insulin. Delivery of insulin by inhalation has recently been introduced. Transdermal delivery of insulin (by a patch) is also an option. Development of the glucometer, a highly accurate device for measuring the amount of glucose in the blood, allows better management of this condition. Progress toward development of an immunization for type 1 diabetes mellitus and in vitro pancreas cell transplantation also has occurred.

An even more recently introduced variation of a transplant-based treatment (or cure) of type 1 diabetes is the use of cadaver islet cells. These cells are harvested from the pancreas of a nondiabetic deceased donor and

A Wellness Plan for Preventing Type 2 Diabetes Mellitus

I've recently been diagnosed with type 2 diabetes. How can I live well with this condition?

The rate at which Americans develop type 2 diabetes mellitus is on the rise, partly because the population is aging. The disease typically affects older people and thus is sometimes called *adult-onset diabetes*. African Americans, Hispanic Americans, and Native Americans are at greater risk than are members of other ethnic groups, but anyone can develop the disease. There is no foolproof way to prevent diabetes, but you can take steps to lower your risk.

- *Obesity and Overweight*
  Not all obese people become diabetic, but 90 percent of people with diabetes are overweight. In addition, body fat distribution is important—those who are heavy around the middle ("apple shaped") are more susceptible to the disease than those whose fat is stored in the buttocks and thighs ("pear shaped"). Evidence indicates that both men and women who gain weight in adulthood increase their risk of diabetes. A recent study conducted at Harvard University showed that women who had gained 11 to 17 pounds since age 18 doubled their risk of diabetes; those who had gained between 18 and 24 pounds tripled their risk.

  If diabetes runs in your family and you are overweight, you are four times as likely to become diabetic as a person with neither risk factor and twice as likely as a person with only one of these risk factors. Whatever your family history, staying within a healthy weight range and losing weight if you are overweight (see Chapter 6) will lower your risk of diabetes. If you tend to weight-cycle (repeatedly lose weight and then gain it back), keep trying. It is not true, as was once believed, that weight-cycling (yo-yo dieting) is in itself harmful to health.

- *Genetics*
  Some progress has been made in identifying the genes that predispose a person to become obese or develop diabetes, but many more years of research will undoubtedly be required before this knowledge is of any practical use. As already mentioned, a family history of diabetes puts you at increased risk. This does not mean that people with a family history are certain to develop diabetes. But if the disease runs in your family, you should try to reduce other risk factors.

- *Diet*
  Following a sound diet is a worthwhile step toward preventing diabetes. A semivegetarian diet (see Chapter 5) is known to lower the risk of heart disease and cancer and may also lower the risk of diabetes. It is low in fat, especially animal fat, and rich in fruits, grains, vegetables, and low-fat or non-fat dairy products. Such a diet is unlikely to promote weight gain and often promotes weight loss. It also provides the vitamins, minerals, and other nutrients you need to help prevent chronic diseases.

- *Exercise*
  Direct evidence shows that regular physical activity helps prevent diabetes. In one study, researchers from the University of California at Berkeley and Stanford University found that men who were very active—expending 3,500 calories in exercise per week—were only half as likely to develop diabetes as men who were sedentary, expending less than 500 calories per week in leisure-time activity. In fact, those who benefited most from exercise were those at highest risk for diabetes.

  Other strong evidence indicates that vigorous exercise has a protective effect against diabetes in both women and men. This is not just because exercise can promote weight loss—physical activity lowers blood sugar whether or not you lose weight.

- *Vitamin and Mineral Supplements*
  There is no evidence that any supplement can prevent diabetes, despite manufacturers' claims for chromium and other supplements. People with diabetes are often deficient in some vitamins and minerals, such as vitamin E, zinc, magnesium, and occasionally chromium. But these deficiencies may be caused in part by a reduced ability to absorb and utilize these nutrients. Thus they may be a result of the disease, not the cause.

- *Smoking*
  Smoking boosts your risk of diabetes and exacerbates the disease if you already have it. If you are a smoker, do whatever it takes to quit (see Chapter 9). Diabetes is just one of the many serious threats to your health that will be greatly reduced if you stop smoking now.

- *Stress*
  Stress negatively influences type 2 diabetes mellitus in two ways. First, with regard to physiological function, the body's natural response to stress (see Chapter 3) increases the level of glucose and free fatty acids in the blood, thus placing greater than normal demands on the diabetic's already compromised insulin response. Second, during periods of stress people with diabetes may not maintain the level of control over their condition that is normally in place. This can occur in different ways. For example, while stressed, they may be too occupied to monitor blood glucose levels on a regular basis, they may alter their dietary patterns in a less than healthful manner, or they may decrease their level of physical activity and thus lower their level of insulin sensitivity.

  When taken in combination, the detrimental influence of stress and the control of type 2 diabetes mellitus demand advanced coping capabilities on the part of the person with this form of diabetes. Chapter 3 discusses at length ways in which persons can increase their ability to prevent stress, moderate its intensity, or expend the high blood glucose levels found in association with the stress response.

Source: © Health Letter Associates, 1996, 1997, www.wellnessletter.com. Used with permission.

implanted into the pancreas of a person with type 1 diabetes. This experimental procedure is under refinement.

With both forms of diabetes mellitus, sound dietary practices, physical activity, and control of stress are important for keeping blood glucose levels within a normal range. When diabetes mellitus is not properly managed, several serious problems can result, including blindness, gangrene, kidney disease, and heart attack. It has also been recently found that people with diabetes have an increased risk for the development of cognitive decline, including Alzheimer's disease, before the age of 65, adding yet another significant health concern for the rapidly expanding diabetic population.[15] People who cannot establish good control of the disease are likely to die prematurely.

Double-Diabetes or Type 3 Diabetes Most recently a "third" form of diabetes mellitus has appeared in the medical literature. This form is seen in children with type 1 diabetes, who usually have normal insulin receptors but must take exogenous insulin. In these children, most likely because of their metabolic syndrome, their body loses the ability to recognize exogenous insulin, leading to the development of type 2 diabetes mellitus. When both forms of diabetes mellitus coexist in a person, that condition is called *double diabetes* or *type 3 diabetes mellitus*.[16]

Hypoglycemia

When people with type 1 diabetes do not eat enough, exercise too much, or take too much insulin, they may develop excessively low levels of blood sugar (blood glucose), resulting in a state of classic **hypoglycemia.** In nondiabetic people, difficulty maintaining high enough blood glucose levels may also be associated with drug use, liver damage, partial removal of the stomach, fasting, pancreatic tumors, and rare forms of adrenal and breast tumors, or as a prediabetic symptom.[17] People who have classic hypoglycemia experience headaches, mild confusion, low energy levels, anxiety, sweating, and tremors. They may look pale and behave somewhat abnormally. The form of hypoglycemia just described is the form seen routinely by medical personnel and on occasion by classroom teachers, coaches, and the parents of children with type 1 diabetes.

A rare form of hypoglycemia called *reactive hypoglycemia* is seen in people who are hypersensitive to the presence of sugar in the blood. In these people, a meal that is high in simple carbohydrates (sugars) stimulates excessive insulin production. This insulin removes blood sugar too quickly, leading to a state of hypoglycemia. People with reactive hypoglycemia have the same symptoms seen in hypoglycemia caused by other factors.

Before reactive hypoglycemia can be definitively diagnosed, the many other causes of low blood sugar (including diabetes mellitus) must first be ruled out. Treatment of reactive hypoglycemia involves dietary modification centered on the consumption of frequent, small meals that contain high levels of complex carbohydrates and few simple carbohydrates. These dietary modifications make the movement of glucose into the bloodstream more gradual, thus eliminating high glucose loads. This "spacing out" of glucose delivery to the blood reduces the body's tendency to overproduce insulin.

In the 1970s the diagnosis of hypoglycemia was made by some physicians to placate patients who complained of vague symptoms of anxiety, moodiness, fatigue, and a loss of interest in normal activities. Once clinical conditions such as depression were ruled out, patients were told that they "must be experiencing hypoglycemia." Patients were then put on a special diet and assured that they would begin to feel better "now that the problem was known." In many cases, patients reported dramatic improvement. Thus hypoglycemia was, for the better part of a decade, much more "common" than it is now believed to be. Today, this less frequently seen, yet still controversial, hypoglycemia is referred to as *idiopathic hypoglycemia,* or, perhaps to some degree yet, *functional hypoglycemia* by some. Central to its clear substantiation is a normal blood glucose reading at the time of symptoms (which can be difficult to obtain) and suggestions of emotional issues on a valid mental health inventory.

Autoimmune/Hypersensitivity Disorders

In Chapter 13 you'll learn more about the immune system. Until that time, the immune system can be described as an integrated collection of tissues, organs, and specific areas of endocrine (ductless) cells working to protect the body from foreign protein. On occasion, however, the immune system fails to recognize the body's own protein as being familiar (self) and mistakenly identifies its own protein as foreign (other) and begins attacking it in an attempt to "protect" the body. When this begins, an **autoimmune disorder** has begun. In this section of the chapter, examples of the autoimmune response will be described.

Fibromyalgia

Fibromyalgia syndrome (FMS) is a chronic condition with symptoms that are so complex an affected person might never be diagnosed and treated despite years of discomfort. For the 2 percent of the adult population believed to have FMS, intermittent periods of morning stiffness, muscle pain, fatigue, numbness and tingling, poor sleep, chronic headaches, jaw discomfort, and many other problems are often seen simply as signs of aging or stress. To trained physicians (often rheumatologists), however, these symptoms may indicate FMS. Accordingly, this syndrome can be diagnosed and effectively treated. Of course, other chronic conditions can coexist with FMS.

The cause of fibromyalgia is becoming more focused. Earlier theories focused on a wide array of causative factors ranging from emotional (depression), neurological (both peripheral and central nervous system), and hormonal, to environmental. Today, with the assistance of positron emission tomography (PET) scans and other diagnostic tools, focus is clearly more directed toward subtle differences in processing pain-related information within the central nervous system (CNS) and differences in neurotransmitter response to pain stimuli. This said, however, associations continue to be found between the existence of fibromyalgia and other events and conditions, including emotional and physical traumas, immune system hypersensitivity, and thyroid dysfunction.

The diagnosis of FMS is based on medical history and the assessment of discomfort in 18 so-called *tenderpoint locations* (see Figure 12-5). For research purposes, people who experience pain in at least 11 of the 18 tenderpoints are diagnosed with FMS. A lower number of "hits" is considered to be diagnostic in a nonresearch setting. Most people with chronic discomfort will be found to have several tenderpoints during the examination. People who lack tender points and morning stiffness, but, as in fibromyalgia, have chronic widespread pain, may have one or more comorbid conditions, including depression, anxiety, irritable bowel syndrome, chronic fatigue syndrome, systemic lupus erythematosus, or rheumatoid arthritis.[18]

The treatment of fibromyalgia centers on improving sleep and reducing pain. Physicians can prescribe medications to enhance the effectiveness of sleep-inducing neurotransmitters (such as serotonin and norepinephrine). Central to today's treatment of fibromyaliga is the medication pregabalin (Lyrica), a drug whose primary role is to enhance the quality of sleep. Although the medication is associated with adverse reaction in some patients, for most users improvement in scores on pain-measuring scales is routinely reported.[19] In addition to the use of pregabalin, nonsteroidal anti-inflammatory drugs (NSAIDs), such as ibuprofen, are used for pain relief. Mild sedatives and muscle relaxants are also employed. Other therapies include synthetic narcotics or transdermal patches for pain relief, acupuncture, and therapeutic massage. Treatments for fibromyalgia also include nonmedication-based approaches, such as acupuncture, cognitive-behavioral therapy, and relaxation therapy. Research on the effectiveness of these treatments is limited. However, there is some evidence that aerobic exercise may be efficacious.[19]

The prognosis for people with FMS is unclear, since few long-term studies have been carried out. For most patients, the condition will remain chronic, with periods of remission and active discomfort occurring intermittently. Whether daily functioning will be significantly impaired later in life remains to be seen.

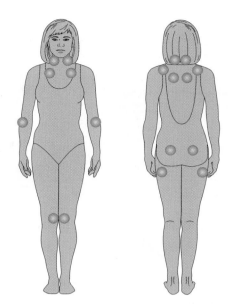

Figure 12-5 Tenderpoint Locations   Persons with fibromyalgia experience tenderness in at least 11 of the 18 tenderpoint locations.

Asthma

Bronchial asthma is a chronic respiratory disease characterized by acute attacks of breathlessness and wheezing caused by chronic airway inflammation with episodes of narrowing of the bronchioles. Although the mechanisms associated with asthmatic attacks are understood, the reason that some people develop a high level of immune system hypersensitivity is not fully known. The identification of a gene (which may be one of several) related to asthma suggests a genetic predisposition that is expressed during exposure to one or more triggering agents, or allergens.

Two main types of asthma have been identified: extrinsic and intrinsic. In extrinsic asthma, allergens such as pollen, urban air pollutants, dust mites, mold spores, animal fur or dander, and feathers produce sudden and severe bronchoconstriction that narrows the airways. Increased sputum production further narrows the bronchioles and restricts the passage of air. This narrowing fosters the development of chronic inflammation of the airways, which is the most damaging aspect of asthma. Wheezing is most pronounced when the person attempts to exhale air through the narrowed air passages.

Key Terms

hypoglycemia The condition of having an abnormally low blood glucose level.

autoimmune disorders Disorders caused by the immune system's failure to recognize the body as "self"; thus the body mounts an attack against its own cells and tissues.

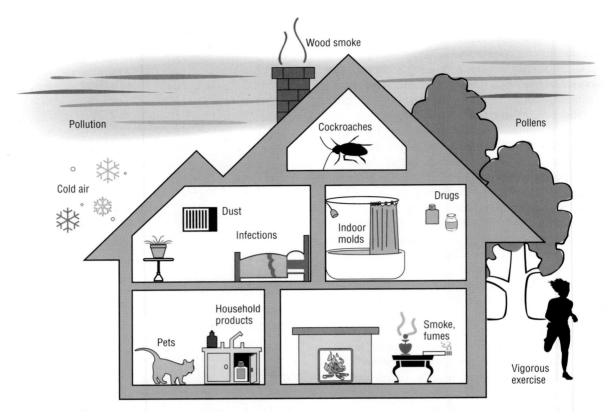

Figure 12-6 Common Asthma Triggers If you have asthma, do you know which triggers are troublesome for you?

For many people with asthma, exercise, cigarette smoke, and certain foods or drugs can cause an asthma attack (Figure 12-6). Physicians once suspected that immunizations (for measles, mumps, and rubella) predisposed people to extrinsic asthmatic attacks by hypersensitizing the immune system, but this view currently finds lessened support.

The incidence of extrinsic asthma increased within the general population and particularly among children during the 1980s and 1990s. Today that increase has leveled. That said, however, asthmatic attacks account for nearly one-fifth of the pediatric emergency room visits in this country. Minority children, in particular, are most at risk of developing asthma and dying from its complications. Underlying this increased risk for asthma among minority children is a combination of factors. Among the environmental factors potentially causing this increase are the diminished quality of both outdoor and indoor urban air quality (acidic particles), high levels of urban violence (stress), and overexposure to ozone in high-density traffic areas. However, genetic predisposition may also play an important role in this increase; studies comparing asthma levels among children of different races who share the same environment consistently find higher rates among minority children than their nonminority classmates. A final environmental factor that may account for some of the reported increase

is the more complete reporting of acute asthmatic attacks and deaths (by hospital ERs) without, unfortunately, the much-needed increase in initial diagnosis and medical management that would have prevented the acute attacks and death.

Intrinsic asthma, the less common form, has similar symptoms but is most closely related to obesity, stress, frequent respiratory tract infections, hormone replacement therapy (for perimenopausal and postmenopausal women),[20] or possibly by the aftereffects of maternal antibiotics taken during pregnancy. Allergens play a lesser role in this form of asthma, which may be more strongly influenced by genetic predisposition for a hypersensitive immune response to foreign protein (allergens).

Prevention or effective management of asthma is often possible using a combination of approaches. Most important, of course, is the maintenance of high-level wellness through a healthful lifestyle that includes a sound diet, regular exercise, and effective stress management. Each person who has asthma should work with his or her physician to develop a sound, individually tailored management plan. If you have asthma, complete the Personal Assessment at the end of the chapter to determine whether you are doing all you can to manage your condition effectively.

A number of components can be included in an asthma management plan. Exercises that are well tolerated, such as swimming, can help maintain a more normal level of respiratory function. Immunotherapy, in which the patient with extrinsic asthma is desensitized through injections of weakened allergens, is often attempted. In addition, the careful use of corticosteroid drugs several times per day by inhalation reduces inflammation. However, in early 2006 the FDA raised concerns about the use of other asthma-related medications, often in combination with these widely use corticosteroids. "Black box" warnings were added to the labels of these medications to call attention to the possibility of fatal interactions. As a point of interest, inhalers used in the treatment of asthma went "green" on January 1, 2009.

Additional drugs have recently been introduced. Among these are *antileukotrienes* that reduce the immune system's ability to foster inflammation,[21] a new class of engineered antibodies that bind to natural antibodies, thus preventing the activation of mast cells that trigger the asthmatic response, and others that reduce the effects of exercise and cold air that frequently trigger asthma attacks.

Bronchial thermoplasty is a newly developed surgical approach to the treatments of asthma. In this procedure, a transmitter-tipped catheter is passed through the trachea and into the main airway leading to each lung. Once the catheter is in place, high-frequency radio waves are sent through the catheter to destroy a portion of the smooth muscle layer of airway wall, thus reducing the amount of narrowing of the airway that can occur.[22] Each year in this country, several thousand people die as the result of asthma attacks. Some experts believe that this number could be reduced if physicians were more aggressive in their treatment of the bronchial inflammation component of the condition.

For the 1.5 million Americans (many of them children) with extreme hypersensitivity to peanut-based allergens, which can lead to potentially fatal asthmatic attacks (50 to 100 per year), the development of a peanut-allergy drug was much anticipated. However, development of the medication has been curtailed due to safety concerns that arose during early stages of human trials. In 2008, the American Academy of Pediatrics softened several of its earlier restrictive recommendations for women regarding prenatal and neonatal maternal dietary practices that were intended to help reduce subsequent food allergies in their children. However, early in prenatal care, women should aggressively call attention to family histories of food allergies.

Irritable Bowel Syndrome (IBS) and Inflammatory Bowel Disease (IBD)

Although these conditions have strikingly similar labels, they are different in several important ways. IBS is a *syndrome*—the presence of an array of symptoms in the absence of a single definable disease. IBD involves more definitive pathological processes that give rise to more discernible conditions. IBS and IBD both are significantly more common in females than in males, and both can coexist in the same person.

Irritable bowel syndrome (IBS) is characterized by highly uncomfortable episodes of spasticity-based pain, diarrhea, or constipation that are localized to the colon, or large intestine. Even for persons who are only occasionally afflicted with constipation or diarrhea, the mere thought of having to deal frequently with unpredictable pain, diarrhea, and constipation should elicit feelings of compassion for those with IBS. *Spastic colon* is also an antiquated term used frequently by the general public to describe this condition. For some diagnosed with IBS, the drug Zelnorm has proven effective in reducing the frequency and duration of symptoms by helping coordinate nerve and muscle activity of the colon, although currently the safety of this drug is in question. As distressing as this condition can be, it is important to remember that IBS is nonprogressive and localized to the colon, causes no damage to the colon, and, though painful, can be controlled with noninvasive measures, and is never fatal. Diet, stress management, and medication can help control the alienating and embarrassing issues associated with IBS.

In comparison to IBS, inflammatory bowel disease (IBD) is a more highly defined pathological progress that involves invasive, inflammatory changes to the gastrointestinal tract. Two recognizable diseases that fall under the label IBD are ulcerative colitis (UC) and Crohn's disease (CD).

Treatments for ulcerative colitis depend on the severity and duration of symptoms, but they focus on promptness of diagnosis and initiation of treatment, minimization of complications (such as anemia and malabsorption), maintenance of normal growth (when dealing with young children), and establishing remission, in which symptoms and disease progression are significantly minimized. Treatment options include dietary changes, enteral (tube) feeding, "gut rest," antidiarrheal medications, and the use of corticosteroids when symptoms have been present for a longer duration. Inflammation is identified through abnormal bloodwork results or visual changes seen through a colonoscopy. A class of nonsteroidal anti-inflammatory drugs, the aminosalicylates, may be used to sustain periods of remission. During very active periods of disease, immunomodulator drugs may be used to suppress inflammation, but these drugs compromise immune system function and their use must be carefully monitored.[23] Removal of the colon, known as a colectomy, may be the only "cure" for this condition. Patients with ulcerative colitis have a significantly elevated risk of colon cancer.

Unlike ulcerative colitis, Crohn's disease can occur anywhere along the course of the gastrointestinal tract ("from tip to tail"), from the mouth and lips to the anus. This condition involves clear pathological changes within the gastrointestinal tract and, unlike ulcerative colitis, is the only form of IBD that can penetrate the wall of the gastrointestinal tract. At times, persons with Crohn's disease can develop **fistulas,** open pathways between the gastrointestinal wall and neighboring structures, such as the vagina and urinary bladder.

Crohn's disease is increasingly treated with immunosuppressive drugs. These bioengineered antibodies, aimed principally against tumor necrosis factor (TNF), are intended to counter the immune system's inappropriate destruction of elements within the intestinal wall (see Chapter 13 for additional information on immune system function). Because they suppress the immune system, these biologics must be monitored carefully and patients should take extra caution to avoid exposure to colds, flu, and other opportunistic infections. Also of considerable concern is the possibility that persons taking tumor necrosis factor (TNF) drugs will develop fungal infections, including histoplasmosis, which if not treated could be fatal.[24] Most recently, concern about the use of biologics has arisen in relationship to the risk of future lymphatic cancers. Surgery is often needed to remove the colon and parts of the small intestine when inflammation does not respond to treatment with diet and drugs. Unfortunately, Crohn's disease often "reappears" near the site where the bowel was removed or in other areas of the GI tract. Therefore, many Crohn's patients develop "short-gut syndrome" and issues of gross malnutrition when they lose significant amounts of intestine in areas where nutrients are absorbed.

Along with the inflammatory changes that happen to the GI tract in a person with IBD, there are "extraintestinal manifestations," involving the eyes, skin, and joints. There might also be side effects related to the medications.

Though there is no known "cure," neither IBS nor IBD is generally considered to be fatal. One complication from IBD, known as toxic megacolon, is the most likely possible exception to that contention. Toxic megacolon, in which extensive inflammation of the colon wall occurs, must be addressed immediately and aggressively. It can arise from excessive inflammatory or bowel obstruction from either ulcerative colitis or Crohn's disease and can cause the colon to perforate. Usually treatment for this involves removal of the entire colon.

Key Terms

fistula A fissure, break, or hole in the wall of an organ.

self-antigens The cells and tissues that stimulate the immune system's autoimmune response.

systemic (sis **tem** ic) Distributed or occurring throughout the entire body system.

Although the etiology of IBD is not completely known, there are strong indications that genetic mutations underlie its development, leading to the establishment of an autoimmune reaction to proteins within the gastrointestinal wall. It has also been found that there are family patterns of both IBS and IBD, further suggesting that genetically based etiologies are in play.

Systemic Lupus Erythematosus (SLE)

Systemic lupus erythematosus, or simply *lupus,* is one of the most familiar autoimmune disorders or connective tissue disorders. These conditions are caused by an extensive and inappropriate attack by the body's immune system on its own tissues, which then serve as **self-antigens.** (See Chapter 13 for a discussion of the immune response.)

The word **systemic** refers to the widespread destruction of fibrous connective tissue and other tissues. *Erythematosus (erythema-* means "red") refers to the reddish rash that imparts a characteristic "mask" to the face of a person with SLE. The disease is seen in women 25 times more often than in men, and it first appears during young adulthood, although it is now known that auto-antibodies may first appear in the blood as much as a decade before the first observable symptoms of SLE appear (see the box "Lupus—Different in Women and Men?"). Subsequent studies have substantiated the appearance of auto-antibodies and other immune system indicators months before the appearance of the first clinically evident conditions related to SLE.[25] In a sizable portion of persons who will eventually be confirmed to have lupus, IgM-RF (rheumatoid factor) will be found upon assessment of its presence in the blood. Not surprisingly, the appearance of arthritic changes will be the first clinically observed changes in structure heralding the definitive diagnosis of SLE.[26]

Particularly interesting in most large studies is the gender inequity reported among African American women and women of Hispanic and Asian origin than among other women.

The course of systemic lupus erythematosus is gradual, with intermittent periods of inflammation, stiffness, fatigue, pleurisy (chest pain), and discomfort over wide areas of the body, including muscles, joints, and skin. Similar changes may take place in the tissues of the nervous system, kidneys, and heart.

Researchers do not know why the immune system attacks the body in such an extensive and aggressive way. It is likely, however, that a combination of genetic predisposition, hormones (estrogen), chronic emotional stress (see Chapter 3), ultraviolet radiation (including sunlight), and an earlier viral infection may be involved in its development.

A physician may suspect lupus based on the patient's description of her symptoms and make a diagnosis using a number of laboratory tests, including the identification of an SLE factor in the blood. A skin biopsy may be taken

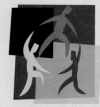

Learning from Our Diversity

Lupus—Different in Women and Men?

From a purely statistical point of view, systemic lupus erythematosis (SLE) is much more common in women. In fact, 90 percent of all cases are seen in women, with the age of onset generally in young adulthood. In light of the preponderance of SLE in younger (premenopausal) women, a high level of estrogen seems very likely to be a principal factor in the development of the condition in women who are genetically predisposed to the condition. Conversely, high levels of androgenic hormones (principally testosterone) provide a protective influence against the development of SLE in men. When SLE is seen in younger men, however, androgenic hormone levels are generally found to be lower than normal. Not surprisingly, SLE is more often initially diagnosed in older men, when testosterone levels have fallen with age. Understandably, after menopause, when estrogen levels have fallen drastically, women are only twice as likely as men to develop SLE.

As noted in the text discussion of SLE, a wide array of organ systems are negatively influenced by SLE. However, when the condition is found in younger men, the degree of kidney damage is greater than that seen in younger women. Because of this damage to the urinary system, younger male SLE victims are more vulnerable than are their female counterparts to life-shortening effects of renal failure. However, because pregnancy is unique to women, the pregnancy/childbirth complications brought about by SLE (increased incidence of miscarriages, premature births, and preeclampsia) distinguish women with SLE from those without SLE.

Beyond the gender-specific aspects of SLE just mentioned, the condition generally appears in a fairly similar fashion in both sexes. For each, prompt diagnosis and appropriate treatment are the keys to a longer and healthier life.

---

to confirm structural changes in the connective tissue layer below the skin.

Management of lupus generally involves the occasional or long-term use of NSAIDs, malarial drugs for the skin rash, and a low dose of prednisone (a corticosteroid) to reduce fever, treat episodes of pleurisy, and minimize certain neurological symptoms. The immune system itself may be medically suppressed as well. These treatments must be carefully monitored because they have serious side effects.

Management of lupus centers on the prevention of episodes of the disease called *flares*. These periods of active lupus are often triggered by exposure to the sun, periods of fatigue, or an infectious disease, all of which should be avoided as much as possible.

 TALKING POINTS You learn that two young women who are your coworkers have recently been diagnosed with lupus and Crohn's disease, respectively. How can you be supportive of them? What would you say to them about their conditions, particularly on days when it is obvious that they are not feeling well?

Multiple Sclerosis (MS)

For proper nerve conduction to occur within portions of the brain and the spinal cord, an insulating sheath of myelin must surround the neurons (nerve cells). In the progressive disease multiple sclerosis (MS), the cells that produce myelin are destroyed, myelin production ceases, and the underlying motor nerves are badly damaged. Neurological functioning eventually becomes so disrupted that vital functions are significantly impaired. The cause of MS is not known. Research continues to focus

on virus-induced autoimmune mechanisms in which T cells attack viral-infected myelin-producing cells. At this time a large number of viruses have been discovered in the cerebrospinal fluid (CSF) of persons with MS and other neurological disorders. These viruses generally are not found in persons who do not have these conditions. Among the most actively accessed viruses are herpes simplex virus 1 (HSV-1), herpes simplex virus 2 (HSV-2), Epstein-Barr virus (EBV), varicella zoster virus (VZV), human cytomegalovirus (HCMV), human herpes virus 6 (HHV-6), and the JC virus (JCV). Patients with different forms of MS will have different collections of viruses. However, the virus most commonly found in the spinal fluid of persons with MS (regardless of type) and others with neurological disorders is the VZV, making it a chief suspect in the etiology of multiple sclerosis.[27] Some immune system evidence of this virus can be found in about 90 percent of all Americans, but not at the levels associated with MS.

MS usually appears for the first time during the young adult years. It may take one of four forms, depending on the interplay of periods of stabilization (remitting), renewed deterioration (relapsing), continuous deterioration (progressive), and combinations of the above. The initial symptoms of the condition are often visual impairment, prickling and burning in the extremities, and an altered gait. In its most advanced stages, movement is greatly impaired, and mental deterioration may be present. It should be noted, however, that MS may be a "silent epidemic" among children, including those younger than 10 years of age. To facilitate a more timely diagnosis of MS, children showing mild tremors or reporting intermittent dimming of vision should be seen by a pediatric neurologist. It is currently estimated that over 20,000 American children may have early-onset MS.

The definitive diagnosis of MS is made through MRI scans for lesions (areas of myelin erosion) in the spinal nerves or the brain. Additionally, a newly developed blood test can assist physicians in determining at what point in time assertive medical management of patients should begin following the initial presentation of symptoms.

Treatment of MS is aimed at reducing the severity of symptoms and extending the periods of remission. Today a variety of therapies are used, including immune system–targeted biologics, steroid drugs, drugs to relieve muscle spasms, a medication to fight fatigue, injections of nerve blockers, and physical therapy.

At the heart of modern treatment of MS are several drugs, all of which were developed since 1993, some as recently as 2006. Among these are five *immunomodulating biologics*—Avonex, Betaseron, and Rebif (all versions of interferon alpha and beta and taken by injection), and Copaxon and Tysabri (which use different avenues to modify the activity of the immune system and are taken by injection and infusion, respectively); and an *immunosuppressant biologic*, Novantrone (initially developed for the treatment of cancer, taken four times per year by infusion). The goals of these therapies are to reduce the frequency of attacks, reduce the accumulation of lesions within the spinal cord and brain, and slow the accumulation of disabilities. Encouraging news was reported by researchers at Northwestern University who were able to reverse some MS deterioration by implanting bone marrow stem cells that were taken from patients before the chemotherapy-based suppression of their immune systems.[28]

Additional medications are available to address complications of MS, such as spasticity and the use of statins (cholesterol-lowering drugs) in MS-developing laboratory mice. To date, this represents the closest approximation of "prevention" that has been obtained in the field of MS treatment.

Psychotherapy is an important adjunct to the treatment of MS. Profound periods of depression often accompany the initial diagnosis of this condition. Emotional support is helpful in dealing with the progressive impairment associated with the condition; see the box "Support Is Just a Click Away" for more information.

Degenerative Diseases

A fifth category of chronic conditions is that of degenerative diseases. Conditions within this category are among the most debilitating of all chronic conditions in that they generally appear late in life, in conjunction with the overall frailty of advanced age, and thus put great demand on caregivers. Eventually, expensive institutional care is required when the level of debilitation prevents the afflicted persons from meeting the activities of daily living (ADL) or even maintaining a sense of self and of the world in which they live. Paramount among these degenerative conditions are Parkinson's disease and Alzheimer's disease.

For help on how to be a comfort to a person with a degenerative disease, see the box "Delivering the Very Best Medicine—No Prescription Required" on page 344.

Parkinson's Disease

Once called "shaking palsy," Parkinson's disease is now recognized as a specific neurological disorder belonging to a family of conditions called *motor system disorders*. Parkinson's disease involves the chronic progressive loss of dopamine production within specific areas of the brain. These areas, called the substantia nigra and striatum, transmit signals required to produce purposeful muscle activity that leads to more highly coordinated movement. The four primary signs of the disease reflect this loss of muscular coordination: (1) tremor or trembling in the hands, arms, legs, jaw, and face; (2) rigidity or stiffness of the limbs or trunk; (3) slowness of movement; and (4) postural instability and impaired balance. As these symptoms worsen, people with Parkinson's disease become progressively less able to talk, walk, and perform simple tasks associated with daily living.

As is true for Alzheimer's disease, Parkinson's disease can be staged using one or both of the following systems.[29] The most basic way to classify a person's progression in Parkinson's disease is in terms of early, moderate, or advanced stage. The advanced stage is characterized by loss of independence in terms of activities of daily living, limited efficacy of medications being used, significant changes in posture, limited speech, and frequent changes in movement.

The more complex system for staging uses Stage I through Stage V. In Stage V, persons are almost totally confined to bed or to a chair, whereas in Stage IV both sides of the body are affected, the person needs substantial help in standing or walking, and tasks of daily living are difficult to impossible to accomplish without assistance.

Parkinson's-like symptoms are associated with other conditions, such as head injury, tumors, prolonged use of tranquilizers, and manganese and carbon monoxide poisoning. The labels *Parkinson's syndrome* and *atypical Parkinson's* are used to describe these conditions. It is believed that as many as one in five elderly Americans shows some Parkinsonian signs.

About 500,000 Americans have been diagnosed with primary Parkinson's disease, and about 50,000 new cases are diagnosed annually. The exact number of people with this condition has always been difficult to establish with certainty, since some people assume that these changes are the result of aging and thus do not seek medical evaluation. The incidence of Parkinson's disease is the same in men and women. The condition is usually first seen in people over age 50, with 60 being the average age at first diagnosis. Compared with African Americans and Asian Americans, Whites are more likely to be diagnosed with Parkinson's disease. A relatively small percentage of people develop the disease as early as age 40. Slightly fewer cases of Parkinson's disease are seen among smokers than among nonsmokers (the risks of smoking, however, greatly outweigh the slightly lower risk of Parkinson's disease among smokers).

Three explanations of the cause of Parkinson's disease have been proposed. The first involves the formation of highly excited unstable chemical compounds known as *free radicals*. With aging, the formation of these highly unstable free radicals increases, and they accumulate within a large variety of body tissues. These free radicals seek stability by physically altering the chemical structure of tissues with which they have contact, including the cells of the substantia nigra. Once damaged, the cells of the substantia nigra and striatum die; thus their dopamine production is lost and the symptoms of Parkinson's appear.

The second possible explanation relates to environmental toxins that are suspected to produce Parkinson's-like symptoms in humans. However, no widely occurring environmental toxins of this nature have been discovered that could account for the large number of cases of Parkinson's disease in this country and around the world. This theory was, however, given support by a follow-up on responses from over 140,000 persons initially surveyed in 2001 as part of the Cancer Prevention Study II Nutrition Cohort. From this large study population, nearly 6 percent had substantial exposure to pesticides as farmers, ranchers, or fishermen. These individuals had a 70 percent higher incidence of Parkinson's disease than a matched group from within the population who had no substantial exposure to pesticides.[30] In two more recent studies, including one in California using GPS mapping to identify specific areas where pesticides were used and areas of non-use from which a control group was drawn,[31] and one in Texas using self-reporting of exposure to pesticides,[32] a direct relationship was demonstrated between exposure and elevated risk of Parkinson's disease.

The third theory about the cause of Parkinson's disease suggests an inherited predisposition associated with genetic material found within the mitochondria of cells. Mitochondria are cell structures in which energy is produced to fuel specific cellular tasks, such as the production of dopamine. Currently, however, a genetic basis for Parkinson's is thought most likely only in those cases of the disease that occur in persons considerably younger than typical victims and often with a substantial family history of the condition—perhaps 10 percent of all cases of Parkinson's disease.

Parkinson's disease is usually diagnosed by a neurologist after the patient is referred by a primary care physician. Although there is no single test for diagnosing Parkinson's disease, medical imaging, such as CT scans and MRI scans, may be helpful in ruling out conditions that mimic the disease.

Several medications are used to delay the progression of the disease. Each of these medications functions in one of two ways. The dopamine enhancers, best represented by levodopa, are chemically converted into dopamine, thus sustaining an adequate level of dopamine needed for coordinating motor control. Still a valuable contributor in the treatment of Parkinson's, the use of levodopa is now being delayed until the patient has undergone initial treatment with a second class of drugs, the dopamine agonists.

The dopamine agonist drugs, unlike levodopa, do not increase the amount of dopamine within selected brain areas; instead, they influence dopamine receptors in the brain to better recognize the diminished dopamine still being produced in the brain. Administering this second class of medications during the earliest stage of the disease makes it possible to delay the use of levodopa until later in the disease's progression, while avoiding certain problems associated with the early use of levodopa.

As helpful as these medications are, however, their influence is temporary and at best only slows the progress of the disease.

Although only in the earliest stage of human trials, a compound derived from glial cells, called GDNF, has shown a clear ability to increase dopamine production while at the same time reducing the limitations in the loss of motor control initially present. Considerable research and development remains to be done on this new treatment approach; currently, this research remains in tissue culture and animal stages.

Pharmacological treatment of Parkinson's disease can also be combined with the surgical implantation of a deep brain stimulation (DBS) unit. When implanted, this device delivers controlled electrical impulses, via electrodes, to targeted areas of the brain (principally the thalamus) in order to complete the electrical transportation of information once based on the availability of dopamine. This technology is most often used in later stages of the disease, but the procedure is not without potential downsides, including infections associated with surgical implantation of the device and a measure of cognitive decline that eventually resolves after six months for many patients.[33]

The use of stem cells to generate new dopamine-producing neurons has been a much anticipated "cure"

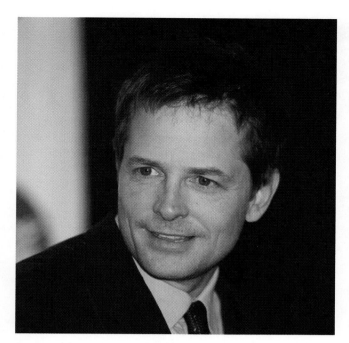

Actor Michael J. Fox has Parkinson's disease and actively supports research for a cure.

for Parkinson's disease. To date, the use of stem cells in the United States has been limited, partly due to the controversy surrounding their collection. Even farther into the future, it might become possible to implant entire neurons, thereby eliminating the time required for implanted stem cells to undergo the specialization and replication necessary to be effective therapies for Parkinson's.

At this time a radically different form of treatment for Parkinson's disease is under refinement. A **xenotransplant**-based technique has been developed through which fetal pig cells are transplanted into the brains of Parkinson's patients for the purpose of reestablishing functional dopamine-producing cells in the areas of the brain deprived of this ability by the disease. In the limited number of persons having had this procedure, levels of success are sufficiently high to encourage continued study, in spite of some ethical and safety (animal-to-human virus transmission) concerns regarding the use of animal tissues.

 TALKING POINTS Your grandmother seems increasingly frustrated by your grandfather's "clumsiness" and has complained that he is becoming increasingly unsteady and nervous. What might you say to her about his condition? What would you suggest she say to him?

Alzheimer's Disease (AD)

Although it affects only 1 to 2 percent of elderly people, organic brain syndrome, in either its acute or chronic form, is a collection of incapacitating, heart-rending, and costly afflictions. **Alzheimer's disease** is the best known of these conditions, affecting approximately 5 million adults in this country and perhaps as many as 12 million worldwide. Today, more than ever before, it is *the* disease associated with aging. Recently the concept of "predementia" changes was introduced, although only initial research has been completed. A very tentative estimate of 1 million newly afflicted middle-aged persons per year has been suggested.[34]

The initial signs of Alzheimer's disease are often subtle and may be confused with mild depression or frontotemporal dementia (FTD), a collection of degenerative brain disorders. At this stage of the disease process, however, the person might have some difficulty answering questions like these:

- Where are we now?
- What month is it?
- What is today's date?
- When is your birthday?
- Who is the president?

During the ensuing months, people with this condition experience greater memory loss, confusion, and **dementia.** In the most advanced stage, people with Alzheimer's disease are incontinent (unable to control bladder and bowel function), display infantile behavior, and finally become totally incapacitated as a result of the destruction of brain tissue. Patients with advanced Alzheimer's disease usually must be institutionalized.

Several theories have been advanced about the cause of Alzheimer's disease. Increasing evidence indicates that genetic mutations on chromosomes 1, 14, 19, or 21 may encourage the development of the disease.[35] Other theories suggest links between Alzheimer's disease and abnormal protein development, deficiencies in acetylcholine (a neurotransmitter) production, loss of nicotine receptors in specific areas of the brain, abnormal blood flow, or exposure to infectious agents or toxins.

Key Terms

xenotransplant A transplant of tissue from an animal, such as a pig, to a human recipient.

Alzheimer's disease Adult-onset form of dementia resulting from loss of acetylcholine production within specific areas of the brain.

dementia The loss of cognitive abilities, including memory and reason.

In the current classification system for AD, two principal categories are used, *early-onset AD* (before age 65) and *late-onset AD* (after age 65). Early-onset AD, encompassing types 1, 3, and 4, accounts for approximately 25 percent of all AD patients and is clearly an inherited form of the disease. Chromosomes 1 (*PSEN2* gene), 14 (*PSEN1* gene), and 21 (*APP* gene) have been identified as factors in this form of the disease. Late-onset AD, designated as type 2, the most prevalent form of the disease, is less clearly understood from a genetic point of view, although chromosome 19 (*APOE* gene) is believed to be involved. The *APOE* gene on chromosome 19 comes in three versions, E2, E3, and E4; the *E4* form is associated with heightened risk for Alzheimer's disease.

In addition to chromosomes 1, 14, 19, and 21, chromosomes 9, 10, and 12 are also of interest. It has been suggested that perhaps as many as 20 specific genes involved in the development of AD are located on these and other chromosomes. Of these genes, strong interest exists in the *SORL1* gene, which plays a role in amyloid beta protein production.[36]

The precise diagnosis of Alzheimer's disease and similar disorders is difficult to make before the patient dies. Only during an autopsy can the characteristic signs of the disease—*neurofibrillary tangles* (twisted strands of neuronal material) and *senile plaque* (compressed masses of cellular material, badly damaged nerve fibers, and a core composed of *amyloid beta protein*)—be identified to confirm the diagnosis. Before death, all other conditions capable of causing dementia must be individually ruled out. Thus, tentative or probable diagnosis of Alzheimer's disease is made by a process of elimination. Newer medical imaging technologies, such as MRIs and PET scans, have become so refined that it is now possible to confirm the diagnosis of Alzheimer's disease before death. Today these technologies have been combined with the application of selected memory tests allowing clinicians to clearly view subtle signs of diminished functional activity in specific areas of the brain. Using

this approach, the ability to predict the development of Alzheimer's disease, particularly in persons with a known genetic marker for the condition, is at hand.

Effective drugs to treat Alzheimer's disease have not yet been developed. That said, four drugs (Razadyne [galantamine], Exelon [rivastigmine], Aricept [donepezil], and Cognex [tacrine]) provide temporary improvement in intellectual function in mild to moderate AD by inhibiting the enzyme that breaks down the neurotransmitter *acetylcholine,* whose diminished availability is the basis of Alzheimer's disease.[37] The drug Cognex remains on the market, but its use has become minimal. A fifth medication, Namenda (menantine), used in moderate to severe AD, functions by blocking glutamate, a substance capable of damaging neurons. Many additional drugs are in various stages of development, including Flurizan, a slightly modified version of an NSAID initially developed for use in treating arthritis that is thought capable of preventing the actual formation of amyloid beta proteins.

At this time, a wide array of studies attempting to link behavioral patterns to the prevention of cognitive diseases that occur with aging and decline, including the development of AD, are under way. Among these are studies assessing the role of fatty acids (particularly n-3 omega fatty acid) in preventing cognitive decline, the role of exercise (particularly brisk walking) in improving cognitive capabilities in aging adults, and the contributions of regular light alcohol consumption in protecting against Alzheimer's-like conditions. Additional studies in the same vein include those related to the effectiveness of NSAIDs in preventing cognitive decline, as well as their interactions with other AD-approved medications, the ability of antioxidant vitamins (carotenes, vitamin C, and vitamin E) to prevent dementia, and the role of high-dose HRT in the cause or exacerbation of cognitive decline, including AD. Current studies in prevention-oriented research are investigating the role of the Mediterranean diet (see Chapter 5), reductions in dietary fats, and steps needed to reduce the growing incidence of metabolic syndrome (prediabetes) that is developing at alarming rates in this country and around the world. See the box "Busy Brains Don't Need Special Exercise" for information on how some companies are offering "brain-fitness" products that appeal to the fear of cognitive decline.

In addition to the speculative preventive approaches just described, vaccines for the prevention of Alzheimer's disease are now in clinical trials. These vaccines utilize a version of the beta-amyloid protein's DNA to stimulate an immune response against the beta-amyloid that occurs in conjunction with the disease. On the basis of the animal-based trials, immunizations appear safe, but their effectiveness requires continuing study.[38]

In addition to the vaccine research just mentioned, new delivery systems for Alzheimer's medications are under development. Among these new delivery techniques are skin patches, similar to those used in nicotine dependency and birth control, and implantable rods, similar to those used to deliver contraceptive medications.

Chronic Conditions and a Sense of Well-Being

Now that we have given ample consideration to several types of chronic conditions, return to Chapter 1, page 15, to review Figure 1-2. In doing so, you can more fully appreciate the potentially negative impact that a chronic, demanding, and potentially life-shortening chronic condition can have on a person's quest for a sense of well-being. Recall that ample resources from all dimensions of health are needed to engage in the activities required to fulfill role responsibilities. Chronic conditions diminish the quantity and quality of these resources, requiring that, in some cases, roles be relinquished. For example, the CEO of a company may be forced to take a reduced leadership role to deal with the effects and treatment of her condition, or a father may similarly be unable to meet all the demands placed on him by his children.

As a person with a chronic condition becomes less capable of meeting role fulfillment, over time the growing inability in meeting role expectations can minimize progress in fulfilling the even larger developmental expectation of his or her life-cycle stage. As this occurs, the chronically ill victim's sense of well-being, normally fueled by the knowledge that progress can be sustained, is lessened. Further, because of the reciprocity that exists between all of the elements depicted in Figure 1-1, resource deterioration continues, often at an accelerated pace, and a sense of life satisfaction declines further. For victims of chronic conditions whose prognosis is poor, a sense of despair can develop to the extent that both death and dying may become the central focus of their remaining time.

Taking Charge of Your Health

- Stay attuned to media reports about chronic conditions so that you can make informed choices.

- Support agencies devoted to the prevention of chronic health conditions.

- Monitor your work, home, and recreational environments to determine whether they are enhancing your risk for developing a chronic health condition.

- Undergo the recommended screening procedures and other preventive procedures

related to chronic conditions for your age and sex.

- If you have a chronic condition, participate actively in your own treatment.

SUMMARY

- Chronic conditions can be classified into several categories: genetic/inherited, congenital, metabolic, autoimmune, and degenerative.
- Klinefelter's syndrome and Turner's syndrome are conditions reflecting an abnormal number of sex chromosomes.
- Cystic fibrosis and sickle-cell trait and disease are conditions reflecting the inheritance of one or more recessive genetic traits.
- Color vision deficiency and fragile X syndrome are sex-linked inherited recessive conditions reflecting recessive traits carried on the X chromosome. Males exhibit the symptoms, while females are carriers.

- Cleft lip, cleft palate, and patent foramen ovale (PFO) are congenital abnormalities, reflecting developmental errors in the formation of the face and heart, respectively, that occur during the embryonic stage of intrauterine life. Scoliosis likely begins during intrauterine development, but may progress postnatally.
- Type 2 and type 1 diabetes mellitus are metabolic disorders reflecting insulin-based difficulties in the production of insulin or its recognition, thus depriving the body of its normal ability to utilize blood glucose. Type 3 diabetes reflects a combination of types 1 and 2 in the same individual.

- Fibromyalgia, systemic lupus erythematosus (SLE), and asthma are chronic conditions reflecting immune system dysfunction either by overresponding to allergens or by attempting to destroy the body's own proteins.
- Irritable bowel syndrome and inflammatory bowel disease reflect gastrointestinal system conditions, primarily seen in females, related to hypersensitivity or autoimmune responses. Multiple sclerosis (MS) is caused by an attack by the immune system on cells that produce myelin, the insulation critical to nervous system function in the brain and spinal cord.
- Parkinson's disease is characterized by loss of fine muscular control caused by the gradual cessation of dopamine production within the brain.
- Alzheimer's disease is a form of dementia (or loss of cognitive ability) caused by the gradual loss of the brain's ability to produce acetylcholine, a neurotransmitter essential for normal mental functioning.

REVIEW QUESTIONS

1. Identify and describe the five categories of chronic conditions presented in this chapter.
2. What is the genetic basis of Turner's syndrome? Klinefelter's syndrome? What physical features characterize persons with Turner's syndrome and Klinefelter's syndrome?
3. Cystic fibrosis is a *recessive genetic disorder;* explain this term. What functional difficulties are experienced by people with cystic fibrosis? What is the condition's long-term prognosis?
4. What complex protein structure is present in an abnormal form in people with sickle-cell disease? What shape are the red blood cells in people with this condition? Why are genetic screening and counseling considered important for sickle-cell disease and trait?
5. What is the function of the foramen ovale in the fetal heart? What recreational pursuit may be compromised by the presence of a patent foramen ovale?
6. What are the differences between type 2 diabetes and type 1 diabetes? How do the treatments for these conditions differ?
7. Identify three symptoms that characterize fibromyalgia. What role do tenderpoints play in the diagnosis of fibromyalgia?
8. How are intrinsic asthma and extrinsic asthma similar? In what important way are they different? In what population group is this increase most noticeable and distressful? What factors might account for this increase?
9. Systemic lupus erythematosus is an *autoimmune disorder;* explain this term. What environmental factors seem to trigger outbreaks or "flares" of SLE? In what gender is SLE most prevalent?
10. What neurotransmitters are inadequately produced in people with Parkinson's disease and Alzheimer's disease? In which specific areas of the brain are the production of these neurotransmitters lost? How do drugs used to manage the condition work?

ANSWERS TO THE "WHAT DO YOU KNOW?" QUIZ

1. False   2. True   3. False   4. False   5. False   6. True   7. True

Visit the Online Learning Center (**www.mhhe.com/payne11e**), where you will find tools to help you improve your grade including practice quizzes, key terms flashcards, audio chapter summaries for your MP3 player, and many other study aids.

SOURCE NOTES

1. Lewis R. *Human Genetics* (7th ed.). New York: McGraw-Hill, 2006.
2. McCance KL, Huether SE. *Pathophysiology: The Biologic Basis for Disease in Adults and Children* (5th ed.). St. Louis, MO: Mosby, 2005.
3. Liou TG, et al. Lung Transplantation and Survival in Children with Cystic Fibrosis. *New England Journal of Medicine,* 357(21), 2143–2152, November 22, 2008.
4. Subramanian M. (Reviewer). *Medical Encyclopedia.* Colorblindness. Medline Plus. U.S. National Library of Medicine. February 22, 2007. www.nlm.nih.gov/medlineplus/ency/article/001002.htm
5. *FMRI.* Genetics Home Reference. U.S. National Library of Medicine. January 2007. www.ghr.nlm.gov/gene=fmrl:jsessionid=E6116810908DB808BC79DB18A88FF47B.
6. The National Fragile X Foundation. *Intervention.* February 10, 2009. www.fragilex.org/html/home.shtml
7. Bartoshesky LE (Reviewer). *Cleft Lip and Palate.* The Nemours Foundation. October 2008. www.kidshealth.org/parent/medical/ear/cleft_lip_palate.html
8. Saladin KS. *Anatomy and Physiology: Unity of Form and Function* (5th ed.). New York: McGraw-Hill, 2010.
9. Honek T, et al. Paradoxical Embolization and Patent Foramen Ovale in Scuba Divers: Screening Possibilities. *Vnitmí Lékarství,* 53(2), 143–146, February 2007.
10. Kutty S, et al. Causes of Recurrent Focal Neurologic Events After Transcatheter Closure of Patent Foramen Ovale with the CarioSEAL Septal Occluder. *American Journal of Cardiology,* 101(10), 1487–1492, May 15, 2008.
11. Spies C, Schrader R. Transcatheter Closure of Patent Foramen Ovale in Patients with Migraine Headache. *Journal of Interventional Cardiology,* 19(6), 552–557, December 2006.
12. *Fact Sheet: Search for Diabetes in Youth.* Centers for Disease Control and Prevention. January 2007. www.searchfordiabetes.org.
13. Clinical Practice Recommendations 2008. Standards of Medical Care in Diabetes. American Diabetes Association. *Diabetes Care,* 31, Supplement 1, 2008.

14. *Total Prevalence of Diabetes & Pre-Diabetes.* American Diabetes Association. 2007. www.diabetes.org/diabetes-statistics/prevalence.jsp

15. Xu W, et al. Mid- and Late-Life Diabetes in Relation to the Risk of Dementia: A Population-Based Twin Study. *Diabetes,* 58(1), 71–77, January 2009.

16. Libman IM, Becker JD. Coexistence of Type 1 and Type 2 Diabetes Mellitus: "Double" diabetes? *Pediatric Diabetes,* 4(2), 110–113, June 2003.

17. National Diabetes Information Clearinghouse (NIDC). Hypoglycemia. 2008. www.diabetes.niddk.nih.gov/dm/pubs/hypoglycemia/index.htm

18. Weir PY, et al. The Incidence of Fibromyalgia and Its Associated Comorbidities: A Population-Based Retrospective Cohort Study Based on International Classification of Diseases, 9th Revision Codes. *Journal of Clinical Rheumatology,* 12(3), 124–128, June 2006.

19. Aumpron JE, Moulin DE. Fibromyalgia: Presentation and Management with a Focus on Pharmacological Treatment. *Pain Research & Management,* 13(6), 477–483, November–December 2008. Stephens S, et al. Feasibility and Effectiveness of an Aerobic Exercise Program in Children with Fibromyalgia: Results of a Randomized Controlled Pilot Trial. *Arthritis and Rheumatism,* 59(10), 1399–1406, October 15, 2008.

20. Gomez RF, et al. Hormone Replacement Therapy, Body Mass Index, and Asthma in Perimenopausal Women: A Cross Sectional Survey. *Thorax,* 61(1), 24–40, January 2006.

21. Fukui Y, et al. Efficacy of Leukotriene Receptor Antagonists in Asthma Treatment and Analysis of Background Factors Evaluated by a Questionnaire Survey Among Physicians. *Nihon Kokyuki Gakkai Zasshi,* 46(12), 972–980, December 2008.

22. Martin N, Pavord ID. Bronchial Thermoplasty for the Treatment of Asthma. *Current Allergy and Asthma Reports,* 9(1), 88–95, January 2009.

23. Nguyen GC, Harris ML, Dassopoulos T. Insights in Immunomodulatory Therapies for Ulcerative Colitis and Crohn's Disease. *Current Gastroenterology Reports,* 8(6), 499–505, December 2006.

24. Information for Healthcare Professionals: Cimzia (certolizumab pegol), Embrel (etanercept), Humira (adalimumab), and Remicade (infliximab). U.S. Food and Drug Administration. Center for Drug Evaluation and Research. September 4, 2008. www.fda.gov/CDER/drug/InfoSheets/HCP/TNF_blockersHCP.htm

25. McClain MT, et al. The Prevalence, Onset, and Clinical Significance of Antiphospholipid Antibodies Prior to Diagnosis of Systemic Lupus Erythematosus. 2004. *Arthritis and Rheumatism,* 50(4), 1226–1232, April 2004.

26. Heinien LD, et al. Clinical Criteria for Systemic Lupus Erythematosus Precede Diagnosis, and Associated Autoantibodies Are Present Before Clinical Symptoms. *Arthritis and Rheumatism,* 56(7), 2344–2351, July 2007.

27. Mancuso R, et al. Increased Prevalence of Varicella Zoster virus DNA in Cerebrospinal Fluid from Patients with Multiple Sclerosis. *Journal of Medical Virology,* 79(2), 192–199, February 2007.

28. Burt RK, et al. Autologous Non-Myeloablative Haemopoietic Stem Cell Transplantation in Relapsing-Remitting Multiple Sclerosis: A Phase I/II Study. *Lancet Neurology,* 8(3), 244–253, March 2009.

29. Classification of Parkinson's Disease: Stages of Parkinson's Disease. *A–Z Health Guide from WebMD,* April 2005. www.webmd.com/hw/health_guide_atoz/stp1229.asp?navbar=93188.

30. Ascherio A, et al. Pesticide Exposure and Risk for Parkinson's Disease. Annals of Neurology, 60(2), 197–203, August 2006.

31. Costello S, et al. Parkinson's Disease and Residential Exposure to Maneb and Paraquat from Agricultural Applications in the Central Valley of California. *American Journal of Epidemiology,* 169(8), 919–926, 2009.

32. Dhillon As, et al. Pesticide/Environmental Exposures and Parkinson's Disease in East Texas. *Journal of Agromedicine,* 13(1), 37–48, 2008.

33. Weaver FH, et al. Bilateral Deep Brain Stimulation vs Best Medical Therapy for Patients with Advanced Parkinson Disease: A Randomized Controlled Trial. *Journal of the American Medical Association,* 301(1), 63–73, January 7, 2009.

34. Mortimer JA, Petersen RC. Detection of Prodromal Alzheimer's Disease. *Annals of Neurology,* 64(5), 479–480, November 2008.

35. *Alzheimer's Disease Genetics Facts Sheet* (updated February 24, 2009). Alzheimer's Disease Education & Referral Center. National Institute on Aging. U.S. National Institutes of Health. www.nia.nih.gov/Alzheimers/Publications/geneticsfs.htm

36. Rogaeva E, et al. The Neuronal Sortilin-Related Receptor *SORL1* Is Genetically Associated with Alzheimer Disease. *Nature Genetics,* 39(2), 168–177, February 2007.

37. *Treatment* (updated February 24, 2009). Alzheimer's Disease Education & Referral Center. National Institute on Aging. U.S. National Institutes of Health. www.nia.nih.gov/Alzheimers/AlzheimersInformation/Treatment/.htm

38. Okura Y, Matsumoto Y. Recent Advance in Immunotherapies for Alzheimer's Disease: with Special References to DNA Vaccinations. *Human Vaccines,* 5(6), June 12, 2009.

Personal Assessment

Are you managing your asthma effectively?

Place a checkmark next to each statement that applies to you.

Reducing or Avoiding Asthma Triggers

_____ I have identified my asthma triggers.

_____ I do not smoke, and I avoid environmental tobacco smoke as much as possible.

_____ I use and properly maintain an air filter and an air conditioner to keep my home cleaner and more comfortable.

_____ I avoid vacuuming, or I use a dust mask.

_____ I avoid mowing the lawn, or I use a dust mask.

_____ I avoid wood stoves and fireplaces.

_____ I use dustproof encasings on my pillows, mattress, and box spring.

_____ I use a dehumidifier as necessary in my home to reduce indoor mold.

_____ I use window shades or curtains made of plastic or other washable material for easy cleaning.

_____ My closets contain only needed clothing; clothing I do not currently wear is stored in plastic garment bags.

_____ I do not sleep or lie down on upholstered furniture.

_____ If I have a pet, it does not sleep in or go into the bedroom.

_____ I avoid perfume and cologne, cleaning chemicals, paint, and talcum powder as much as possible.

Preventing and Managing Asthma Attacks

_____ I have learned everything I can about asthma.

_____ I take medications as prescribed by my physician whether or not I am having an attack.

_____ I carry my inhaler with me at all times.

_____ I have asked my physician to help me develop a crisis plan for managing a severe asthma attack.

_____ I keep emergency numbers by the phone.

_____ I have learned about my asthma medications and know how quickly they should work.

_____ I use a peak flow meter to anticipate and respond quickly to asthma attacks.

Interpretation

17 or more items checked: You are doing a great job avoiding asthma triggers and preventing and managing asthma attacks.

14 to 16 items checked: In many ways you are doing a good job of managing your asthma. However, you may be unnecessarily exposing yourself to common asthma triggers, or your plan for preventing and managing asthma attacks may need some work.

13 or fewer items checked: You could be managing your asthma much more effectively. Modify your home and activities as necessary to avoid common asthma triggers. Talk to your physician right away about establishing an asthma management plan and an emergency plan. Remember, asthma can be fatal, and poor preventive asthma management is an important contributing factor. Don't let it happen to you!

TO CARRY THIS FURTHER . . .

Discuss this assessment with other members of your family or your roommates. Secure their cooperation in helping you maintain a clean home free of dust, pet hair, smoke, and other asthma triggers. Make sure they know what to do to help you in case of a severe asthma attack.

Preventing Infectious Diseases

What Do You Know About Infectious Diseases?

1. Infectious diseases follow a predictable pathway as they move from an infected person to a soon-to-be infected person. True or False?

2. The immune system can be "armed" to fight a particular infectious disease by only one process—contracting the particular disease and then recovering from it. True or False?

3. Nosocomial infections are most often contracted in large public gatherings, such as an indoor sports arena. True or False?

4. On the college campus, the student group most susceptible to contracting bacterial meningitis is the graduate students. True or False?

5. Because of concerns over tampon misuse, health officials are strongly encouraging women to discontinue the use of internal sanitary protection products (tampons). True or False?

6. Today the American public seems less interested in the HIV/AIDS pandemic than it was in the past. True or False?

7. The most effective way to avoid contracting STDs is through abstaining from sexual activity. True or False?

Check your answers at the end of the chapter.

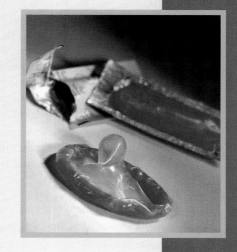

In the nineteenth century, infectious diseases were the leading cause of death. These deaths came after exposure to the organisms that produced such diseases as smallpox, tuberculosis (TB), influenza, whooping cough (pertussis), typhoid, diphtheria, and tetanus. However, since the early 1900s, improvements in public sanitation, the widespread use of antibiotic drugs, and vaccinations have considerably reduced the number of people who die from infectious diseases. People now die more often from chronic disease processes.

Today, however, we have a new respect for infectious diseases. By the end of 2008, it was estimated that 39.5 million people worldwide were living with HIV/AIDS, with long-range projections pointing to 70 million in the absence of effective prevention programs. We are witnessing a resurgence of TB. We recognize the role of pelvic infections in infertility. We also know that failure to fully immunize children has laid the groundwork for a return of whooping cough, polio, and other serious childhood diseases. In fact, some experts suggest that because of HIV/AIDS and the emergence and reemergence of infectious diseases, today's young adults may have a lower life expectancy than did the generation immediately ahead of them.

Several new types of infectious disease have appeared, and new concerns have been raised about the spread of familiar infectious diseases:

- The extremely virulent viruses, such as the Ebola virus in Zaire, which is fatal to 75 percent of those who contract it; a vaccine is only now under development. The danger of moving into clinical trials, however, seems daunting to researchers.

- The increasing resistance of bacteria such as *Staphylococcus aureus, Enterococcus,* and *Mycobacterium* (which causes tuberculosis) to antibiotics as the result of overuse and improper use, as well as the biological "redesign" of the organisms themselves (see the box "Are Americans Too Clean?").

- The now-completed cross-country march of the mosquito-borne West Nile virus, and, of course, the presence of avian influenza, could be knocking on the door of North America.

- The resurgence of cholera in Zimbabwe resulting from the deterioration of the water supply and sanitation in the face of ongoing political conflict and the displacement of large segments of the population. By the end of 2008, nearly 24,000 cases had been identified, with a fatality rate of 5 percent.

- The massive outbreak of EV-71 (enterovirus-71) resulting in hand, foot, and mouth disease. The infection afflicted thousands of children in China during the time of the Olympic Torch Relay in 2008. In one 24-hour period, the reported incidence jumped from 19,962 cases to 24,932. More than 25 children died from the results of the infection.

- The novel H1N1 (swine) influenza pandemic that first appeared in Mexico during the spring of 2009 and then spread to different areas in the World.

Infectious Disease Transmission

Infectious diseases can generally be transmitted from person to person, although the transfer is not always direct. Infectious diseases can be especially dangerous because they can spread to large numbers of people, producing **epidemics** or **pandemics.** The following sections explain the process of disease transmission and the stages of infection.

Pathogens

For a disease to be transferred, a person must come into contact with the disease-producing agent, or **pathogen,** such as a virus, bacterium, or fungus. When pathogens enter our bodies, the pathogens can sometimes resist body defense systems, flourish, and produce an illness. We commonly call this an *infection.* Because of their small size, pathogens are sometimes called *microorganisms,* or *microbes.*[1] Table 13.1 describes infectious disease agents and some of the illnesses they produce.

Chain of Infection

The movement of a pathogenic agent through the various links in the chain of infection (Figure 13-1) explains how diseases spread.[1] Not every pathogenic agent moves all the way through the *chain of infection,* because various links in the chain can be broken. Therefore, the presence of a pathogen creates only the potential for causing disease.

Agent The first link in the chain of infection is the disease-causing **agent.** Whereas some agents are very

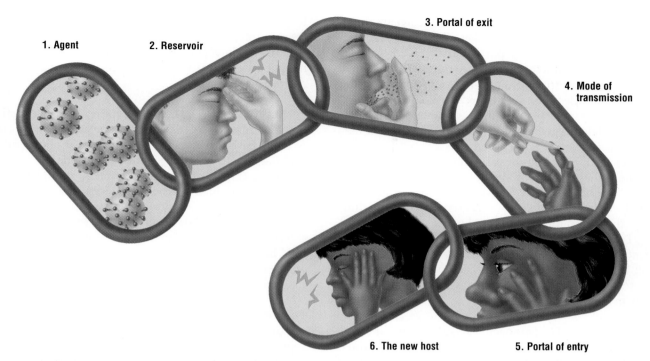

Figure 13-1 Chain of Infection The example above shows a rhinovirus, which causes the common cold, being passed from one person to another. 1. the *agent* (pathogen) is a rhinovirus; 2. the *reservoir* is the infected person; 3. the *portal of exit* is the respiratory system (coughing); 4. the *mode of transmission* is indirect hand contact; 5. the *portal of entry* is the mucous membranes of the uninfected person's eye; and 6. the virus now has a *new host*.

Table 13.1 Pathogens and Common Infectious Diseases

Pathogen	Description	Representative Disease Processes
Viruses	Smallest common pathogens; nonliving particles of genetic material (DNA) surrounded by a protein coat; require host cells for growth and replication	Rubeola, mumps, chicken pox, rubella, influenza, warts, colds, oral and genital herpes, shingles, AIDS, genital warts
Prion	Potentially self-replicating protein, lacking both DNA and RNA, virus-like in size	Creutzfeldt-Jakob disease, Gerstmann-Straussler-Scheinker syndrome, "mad cow" disease (bovine spongiform encephalopathy)
Bacteria	One-celled microorganisms with sturdy, well-defined cell walls; three distinctive forms: spherical (cocci), rod shaped (bacilli), and spiral shaped (spirilla)	Tetanus, strep throat, scarlet fever, gonorrhea, syphilis, chlamydia, toxic shock syndrome, Legionnaires' disease, bacterial pneumonia, meningitis, diphtheria, Lyme disease
Fungi	Plantlike microorganisms; molds and yeasts	Athlete's foot, ringworm, histoplasmosis, San Joaquin Valley fever, candidiasis
Protozoa	Single-cell, nucleated, primitive, parasitic animal-like organisms, capable of motility	Malaria, amebic dysentery, trichomoniasis, vaginitis
Rickettsia	A type of bacteria, with many virus-like characteristics, that requires host cells for growth and replication	Typhus, Rocky Mountain spotted fever, rickettsialpox
Parasitic worms	Many-celled, relatively simple animals; represented by tapeworms, leeches, and roundworms	Dirofilariasis (dog heartworm), elephantiasis, onchocerciasis

Source: From Barbara Hamann, *Disease: Identification, Prevention and Control*, 3/e, © 2007 The McGraw-Hill Companies, Inc. Used with permission.

virulent and lead to serious infectious illnesses such as HIV, which causes AIDS, others produce far less serious infections, such as the common cold. Through mutation, some pathogenic agents, particularly viruses, can become more virulent.

Reservoir Infectious agents require the support and protection of a favorable environment to survive. This environment forms the second link in the chain of infection and is called the *reservoir*. For many of the most common infectious diseases, the reservoirs are the bodies of people who are already infected. Here the agents thrive before being spread to others. These infected people are, accordingly, the hosts for particular disease agents. In some infectious illnesses, a person's reservoir status may be restored after treatment and apparent recovery from the original infection. This is because some pathogens, particularly viruses, can remain sequestered (hidden), emerging later to give rise to another infection. The herpes viruses are often sequestered.

For other infectious diseases, however, the reservoirs are the bodies of animals. Avian (bird) flu is a much discussed animal-reservoir disease. The infected birds are not always sick and do not always show symptoms similar to those seen in infected people.

The third type of reservoir in which disease-causing agents can live is in a nonliving environment, such as the soil. The spores of the tetanus bacterium, for example, can survive in soil for up to 50 years, entering the human body in a puncture wound.

Portal of Exit   For pathogenic agents to cause diseases and illnesses in others, they must leave their reservoirs. Thus the third link in the chain of infection is the *portal of exit,* or the point at which agents leave their reservoirs.

The principal portals of exit are familiar—the digestive system, urinary system, respiratory system, reproductive system, and the blood, especially with infectious diseases that infect humans.

Mode of Transmission   The fourth link in the chain of infection is the *mode of transmission,* or the way in which pathogens move from reservoirs to susceptible hosts. Two principal methods are direct transmission and indirect transmission.

We see three types of direct transmission in human-to-human transmission. These include contact between body surfaces (such as kissing, touching, and sexual intercourse), droplet spread (inhalation of contaminated air droplets), and fecal-oral spread (feces on the host's hands are brought into contact with the new host's mouth), as could occur when changing the diaper of an infected infant.

Indirect transmission between infected and uninfected people occurs when infectious agents travel by means of nonhuman materials. Vehicles of transmission include inanimate objects (known as *fomites*), such as water, food, soil, towels, clothing, and eating utensils.

Infectious agents can also be indirectly transmitted through vectors. The term *vector* describes living things, such as insects, birds, and other animals, that carry diseases from human to human. An example of a vector is the deer tick, which transmits Lyme disease.

Airborne indirect transmission includes the inhalation of infected particles that have been suspended in an air source for an extended time. Unlike droplet transmission, in which both infected and uninfected people must be in close physical proximity, noninfected people can become infected through airborne transmission by sharing air with infected people who were in the same room hours earlier. Viral infections such as German measles can be spread this way.

Portal of Entry   The fifth link in the chain of infection is the *portal of entry.* As with the portals of exit, portals of entry have three primary methods that allow pathogenic agents to enter the bodies of uninfected people. These are through the digestive system, respiratory system, and reproductive system. In addition, a break in the skin provides another portal of entry. In most infectious conditions, the portals of entry are the same systems that served as the portals of exit from the infected people. In HIV, however, we see cross-system transmission. Oral and anal sex allow infectious agents to pass between the warm, moist tissues of the reproductive and digestive systems.

The New Host   All people are, in theory, at risk for contracting infectious diseases and thus could be called susceptible hosts. In practice, however, factors such as overall health, acquired immunity, health care services, and health-related behavior can affect susceptibility to infectious diseases (see the box "Infectious Disease: A Challenge for Older Adults").

Stages of Infection

When a pathogenic agent assaults a new host, a reasonably predictable sequence of events begins. That is, the disease moves through five distinctive stages.[1] You may be able to recognize these stages of infection each time you catch a cold.

1. *The incubation stage.* This stage lasts from the time a pathogen enters the body until it multiplies enough to produce signs and symptoms of the disease. The duration of this stage can vary from a few hours to many months, depending on the virulence of the organisms, the concentration of organisms, the host's level of immune responsiveness, and other health problems. This stage has been called a *silent stage.* The pathogen can be transmitted to a new host during this stage, but this is not likely. A host may be infected during this stage but not be infectious. HIV infection is an exception to this rule.

2. *The prodromal stage.* After the incubation stage, the host may experience a variety of general signs and symptoms, including watery eyes, runny nose, slight fever, and overall tiredness for a brief time. These symptoms are nonspecific and may not be severe enough to force the host to rest. During this stage the pathogenic agent continues to multiply. Now the host is capable of transferring pathogens to a new host, but this is not yet the most infectious stage

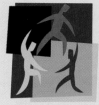

It's not always easy for young adults in excellent health to recover quickly and completely from some infectious diseases. Later in life the recovery often becomes much more difficult and in some cases impossible. For a variety of reasons, older adults do not recover from infectious conditions with the same resiliency as they once did.

Central to this issue is the gradual degradation of the immune system over time. For reasons not fully understood, the immune system loses both its ability to recognize the presence of pathogens that have entered the body and its ability to mount an effective response against them. Particularly important in this regard are the decreased prevalence of active immune system cells and the inability of existing immune cells to respond effectively. Whether this reduced level of immune protection is a "programmed" aspect of aging (all human life does end at some point in time) or whether it reflects a process that is preventable (perhaps through lifestyle modifications) remains hotly debated. Perhaps no group of older adults is at greater risk because of a compromised immune system than are those with AIDS. The nearly 80,000 persons over age 50 with this immune-system-destroying disease have a decreased ability to resist all infectious conditions, even when their HIV levels are suppressed through drug therapy.

In addition to the normal aging of their immune systems, older adults are generally afflicted with a variety of chronic conditions. The presence of multiple chronic illnesses (known as comorbidity) places the body under great stress, which also undermines the immune system. The combined effects of these conditions result in damage to different organ systems of the body—most importantly, the cardiovascular system, the respiratory system, and the renal system. Any time these systems are compromised by the effects of illness, either chronic or acute, the body becomes particularly vulnerable to infectious agents that routinely exist in our environment.

Compounding this situation is the inability of many older adults to understand the potential seriousness of infections at this stage of their lives. They may even have a false sense of confidence that their bodies are just as "good" at warding off infections as they once were. In addition, a lack of social support, isolation from health care facilities, and the inability to afford expensive prescription medication together make important medical care less available at a time when it could be effective.

When these factors are combined, as they are for many older adults, serious and even fatal infectious conditions become a reality. Therefore, anyone who is responsible for the health and well-being of older persons needs to understand their susceptibility to infectious conditions and recognize the fact that timely and competent care is of critical importance.

---

of an infectious disease. One should practice self-imposed isolation during this stage to protect others. Again, HIV infection is different in this stage.

3. *The clinical stage.* This stage, also called the *acme* or *acute stage,* is often the most unpleasant stage for the host. At this time the disease reaches its highest point of development. Laboratory tests can identify or analyze all of the clinical (observable) signs and symptoms of the particular disease. The likelihood of transmitting the disease to others is highest during this peak stage; all of our available defense mechanisms are in the process of resisting further damage from the pathogen.

4. *The decline stage.* The first signs of recovery appear during this stage. The infection is ending or, in some cases, falling to a subclinical level. People may suffer a relapse if they overextend themselves.

5. *The recovery stage.* Also called the *convalescence stage,* this stage is characterized by apparent recovery from the invading agent. The disease can be transmitted during this stage, but this is not probable. Until the host's overall health has been strengthened, he or she may be especially susceptible to another (perhaps different) disease pathogen. Fortunately, after the recovery stage, further susceptibility to the pathogenic agent is typically lower because the body has built up immunity. This buildup of immunity is not always permanent; for example, many sexually transmitted diseases can be contracted repeatedly.

We will discuss HIV/AIDS later in the chapter; for now, however, we need to note that this critically important pandemic infectious disease does not easily fit into the five-step model of infectious diseases just presented. In individuals infected with HIV there is an initial asymptomatic *incubation stage,* followed by a *prodromal stage* characterized by generalized signs of immune system inadequacy. However, once the level of specific protective cells of the immune system declines to the point that the body cannot be protected from opportunistic diseases, and the label AIDS is assigned, the five-stage model becomes less easily applied.

Body Defenses: Mechanical and Cellular-Chemical Immune Systems

Much as a series of defensive alignments protect a military installation, so too is the body protected by sets of defenses. These defenses can be classified as either mechanical or cellular-chemical (Figure 13-2). Mechanical defenses are first-line defenses, because they physically separate the internal body from the external environment. Examples include the skin, the mucous

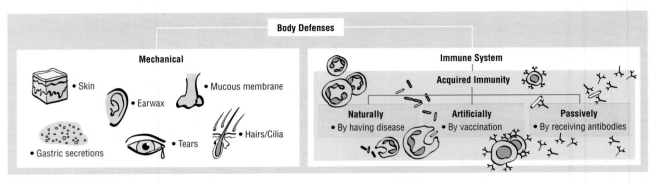

Figure 13-2 Body Defenses Against Invading Organisms   Mechanical defenses are the first line of protection, since they separate the internal body from the external environment. The immune system defenses include chemicals and specialized cells that provide protection from a vast array of antigens.

membranes of the respiratory and gastrointestinal tracts, earwax, the hairs and cilia that filter incoming air, and even tears. These defenses serve primarily as a shield against foreign materials that may contain pathogenic agents. These defenses can, however, be disarmed, such as when tobacco smoke kills the cilia that protect the airway, resulting in chronic bronchitis, or when contact lenses reduce tearing, leading to irritation and eye infection.

The second component of the body's protective defenses is the cellular-chemical system or, more commonly, the **immune system.** The immune system is far more specific than the mechanical defenses. Its primary mission is to eliminate microorganisms, foreign protein, and abnormal cells from the body. A wellness-oriented lifestyle, including sound nutrition, effective stress management, and regular exercise, supports this important division of the immune system. The microorganisms, foreign proteins, or abnormal cells that activate this cellular component are collectively called *antigens*.[2]

Divisions of the Immune System

Closer examination of the immune system, or cellular-chemical defenses, reveals two separate but highly cooperative groups of cells. One group of cells originates in the fetal thymus gland and has become known as *T cell–mediated immunity,* or simply **cell-mediated immunity** The second group of cells that makes up cellular immunity are the B cells (bursa of Fabricius), which are the working units of **humoral immunity.**[3] Cellular elements of both cell-mediated and humoral immunity are found within the bloodstream, the lymphatic tissues of the body (including that within the gastrointestinal system), and the fluid that surrounds body cells. In addition to the two major divisions of the immune system, a variety of antibodies, phagocytes (large white cells) such as natural killer (NK) cells, monocytes and macrophages; granulocytes (including neutrophils, eosinophils, and basophiles); important large protein complexes called *complement*

function in ways both independent of cell-mediated immunity and humoral immunity and in cooperation with these two major divisions of the immune system. When viewed collectively, these components directly eat antigens (phagocytosis), release caustic chemicals that degrade antigens, and send out chemical messengers that support cellular and humoral responses.

Although we are born with the structural elements of both cell-mediated and humoral immunity, developing an immune response requires that components of these cellular systems encounter and successfully defend against specific antigens. When the immune system has done this once, it is, in most cases, primed to respond quickly and effectively if the same antigens appear again. This confrontation produces a state of **acquired immunity (AI).**[1] Acquired immunity develops in different ways, as shown in Figure 13-2.

- **Naturally acquired immunity (NAI)** develops when the body is exposed to infectious agents. Thus when we catch an infectious disease, we fight the infection and in the process become immune (protected) from developing that illness if we encounter these agents again. For example, when a child catches chicken pox and recovers, it is unlikely that the child will develop a subsequent case of chicken pox. Before the advent of immunizations, this was the only way of developing immunity.

- **Artificially acquired immunity (AAI)** occurs when the body is exposed to weakened or killed infectious agents introduced through vaccination or immunization. As in NAI, the body fights the infectious agents and records the method of fighting the agents. Young children, older adults, and adults in high-risk occupations should consult their physicians about immunizations.

- **Passively acquired immunity (PAI),** a third form of immunity, results when antibodies are introduced into the body. These extrinsic antibodies are for a variety of specific infections, and they are produced

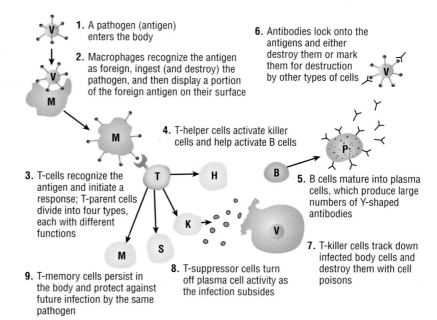

Figure 13-3 The Immune Response Cellular and chemical elements act together to destroy pathogens and guard against repeat infections such as the viral (V) infected cell shown.

1. A pathogen (antigen) enters the body

2. Macrophages recognize the antigen as foreign, ingest (and destroy) the pathogen, and then display a portion of the foreign antigen on their surface

3. T-cells recognize the antigen and initiate a response; T-parent cells divide into four types, each with different functions

4. T-helper cells activate killer cells and help activate B cells

5. B cells mature into plasma cells, which produce large numbers of Y-shaped antibodies

6. Antibodies lock onto the antigens and either destroy them or mark them for destruction by other types of cells

7. T-killer cells track down infected body cells and destroy them with cell poisons

8. T-suppressor cells turn off plasma cell activity as the infection subsides

9. T-memory cells persist in the body and protect against future infection by the same pathogen

outside the body (either in animals or by the genetic manipulation of microorganisms). When introduced into the human body, they provide immediate protection until the body can develop a more natural form of immunity. This form of short-term but immediate protection is provided when the emergency room staff administers a tetanus-toxoid "booster." Note that in PAI no actual pathogenic agents are introduced into the body—only the antibodies against various forms of disease-causing agents.

Regardless of how infectious agents are acquired, either through NAI or through AAI, the result is an "arming" of the body's own immune system. This process is frequently labeled as *active immunity*. This contrasts to PAI, in which the body "borrows" another's immune elements without actual involvement of the body's own immune system. The latter case is called *passive immunity*.[4]

In addition to the forms of immunity just described, unborn infants are also provided with a period of short-term immunity via the biological mother's immune system elements crossing the placental barrier (see Chapter 17) and then following birth via breast milk. This *maternal immunity*, however, gradually deteriorates but is concurrently being replaced by the child's own increasingly functional immune system.

Collectively, these forms of immunity can provide important protection against infectious disease.

The Immune Response

Fully understanding the function of the immune system requires a substantial understanding of human biology and is beyond the scope of this text. Figure 13-3 presents a simplified view of the immune response.

When antigens (whether microorganisms, foreign protein, or abnormal cells) are discovered within the body, various types of white blood cells confront and destroy some of these antigens. Principal among these

---

Key Terms

immune system The system of cellular and chemical elements that protects the body from pathogens, abnormal cells, and foreign protein.

cell-mediated immunity Immunity provided principally by the immune system's T cells, working both alone and in combination with highly specialized B cells; also called *T cell–mediated immunity.*

humoral immunity Immunity, also called *B cell–mediated immunity,* that is responsible for the production of critically important immune system elements known as *antibodies.*

acquired immunity (AI) A form of immunity resulting from exposure to foreign protein (most often wild, weakened, or killed pathogenic organisms).

naturally acquired immunity (NAI) A type of acquired immunity resulting from the body's response to naturally occurring pathogens.

artificially acquired immunity (AAI) A type of acquired immunity resulting from the body's response to pathogens introduced into the body through immunizations.

passively acquired immunity (PAI) A temporary immunity achieved by providing extrinsic antibodies to a person exposed to a particular pathogen.

blood cells are the *macrophages* (very large white blood cells) that begin ingesting antigens as they are encountered. In conjunction with this "eating" of antigens, macrophages display segments of the antigen's unique protein coat on their outer surface. Now in the form of macrophage/antigen complexes, macrophages transport their captured antigen identifiers to awaiting T cells, whose recognition of the antigen will initiate the full cell-mediated immune response. This involves the specialization of "basic" T cells into four forms: T-helper cells, T-killer cells, T-suppressor cells, and T-memory cells.

Once T-helper cells have been derived from T-"parent" cells by the presence of the macrophage/antigen complex, they notify a second component of cellular immunity, the T-killer cells. T-killer cells produce powerful chemical messengers that activate specific white blood cells that destroy antigens through the production of caustic chemicals called cytotoxins, or "cell poisons." In addition to the T-helper cells' activation of T-killer cells, T-helper cells also play a critical role in the activation of B cells, principal players in the expression of humoral immunity.

Activation of the humoral immunity component of the overall immune response involves the T-helper cells' ability to construct a working relationship among themselves, the macrophage/antigen complexes (mentioned earlier), and the small B cells. Once these three elements have been constituted into working units, the B cells are transformed into *plasma cells*. Plasma cells then utilize the information about the antigen's identity to produce massive numbers of **antibodies.** On release from the plasma cells, these antibodies then circulate throughout the body and capture free antigens in the form of *antigen/antibody complexes*.[4] The "captured" antigens are now highly susceptible to a variety of white blood cells that ingest or chemically destroy these infectious agents.

To ensure that the response to the presence of the antigen can be appropriately controlled, a third group of T cells, the T-suppressor cells, have been formed by the activation of T-parent cells. These T-suppressor cells monitor the outcome of the humoral response (antibody formation) and, when comfortable with the number of antibodies produced, turn off further plasma cell activity. The fourth group of specialized T cells, the T-memory cells, record this game plan for fighting the antigen invasion so that any subsequent similar invasion will be quickly fought.

An additional group of cells that operates independently from the T cell/B cell interplay just described are

the *natural killer (NK) cells*. These immune cells continuously patrol the blood and intracellular fluids looking for abnormal cells, including cancer cells and viral-infected cells. When these are found, the NK cells attack them with destructive cytotoxins in a process called *lysing*.[4] (Can you think of a popular household sanitizing product that uses a version of *lysing* in its brand name?)

Without a normal immune system employing both cellular and humoral elements, we would quickly fall victim to serious and life-shortening infections and malignancies. As you will see later, this is exactly what occurs in many people infected with HIV.

Emerging medical technology holds promise for repairing damaged immune systems. Perhaps in the not too distant future, *adult stem cells* can be harvested from other areas of the body of a person whose immune system has been compromised, or from the body of a carefully matched donor, and used to return a damaged immune system to a normal level of functioning. A second form of immune system repair involves harvesting *cord blood (stem) cells* taken from the umbilical cord blood collected and "banked" at birth.[5] After careful matching, these cells can be transplanted into a recipient in anticipation that they will specialize into the cell type needed by the damaged or diseased immune system. The virtual absence of any specialization in stem cells at the time of harvesting provides an opportunity for the highly generic stem cells to develop into immune system cells once they are transplanted into the recipient's body. Perhaps the most interesting use of this technology first occurred in October 2000, when a young cancer victim's immune system was restarted via a stem cell transplant obtained from the cord blood of her newborn brother, who was conceived for the purpose of being a stem cell donor. It should be noted, however, that this was a highly unusual procedure. Considerable controversy surrounded the use of stem cells obtained from embryonic or fetal tissue sources and the use of federal funds to create new stem cell lines was prohibited during the eight years of George W. Bush's presidency. However, very shortly after the inauguration of President Barack Obama in 2009, the restriction on the use of federal funds was lifted.[6] This action was welcomed by American stem cell researchers, who had to watch progress in other countries surpass that occurring in the United States during the Bush presidency. Even though these are considered to be the "best" stem cells, restrictions by the federal government (and several states) on their collection and use have forced clinicians to use stem cells from the sources mentioned earlier, as well as from cadavers.

Immunizations

Although the incidence of several childhood communicable diseases is at or near the lowest level ever, we are risking a resurgence of diseases such as measles, polio, diphtheria, and rubella. The possible increase in

---

Key Terms

antibodies Chemical compounds produced by the body's immune system to destroy antigens and their toxins.

childhood infectious illnesses is based on the disturbing finding that only 81 percent of American preschoolers are adequately immunized, which is principally due to the failure of many parents to complete their children's immunization programs. Today health professionals are attempting to raise the level of immunization to 90 percent of all children under the age of 2 years.

Vaccinations against several potentially serious infectious conditions are available and should be given. These include the following:

- *Diphtheria.* A potentially fatal illness that leads to inflammation of the membranes that line the throat, to swollen lymph nodes, and to heart and kidney failure
- *Whooping cough.* A bacterial infection of the airways and lungs that results in deep, noisy breathing and coughing
- *Hepatitis B.* A viral infection that can be transmitted sexually or through the exchange of blood or bodily fluids; seriously damages the liver
- *Hepatitis A.* A viral infection contracted from fecal contamination of food or water
- *Haemophilus influenzae type B.* A bacterial infection that can damage the heart and brain, resulting in meningitis, and can produce profound hearing loss
- *Tetanus.* A fatal infection that damages the central nervous system; caused by bacteria found in the soil
- *Rubella (German measles).* A viral infection of the upper respiratory tract that can cause damage to a developing fetus when the mother contracts the infection during the first trimester of pregnancy
- *Measles (red measles).* A highly contagious viral infection leading to a rash, high fever, and upper respiratory tract symptoms
- *Polio.* A viral infection capable of causing paralysis of the large muscles of the extremities
- *Mumps.* A viral infection of the salivary glands
- *Chicken pox.* A varicella zoster virus spread by airborne droplets, leading to a sore throat, rash, and fluid-filled blisters
- *Meningococcus.* A bacterial infection of the membranes covering the brain; symptoms are flulike
- *Pneumococcal infection.* A bacterium capable of causing infections, including pneumonia and heart, kidney, and middle-ear infections
- *Childhood diarrhea.* Caused by a rotavirus, this form of diarrhea is responsible for 55,000 to 70,000 hospitalizations, and 20 to 60 deaths, annually of infants and young children

Parents of newborns should take their infants to their family-care physicians, pediatricians, or well-baby clinics operated by county health departments to begin the immunization process. The immunization schedules for children 0 through 6 years of age and for persons aged 7 through 18 years of age posted on the Online Learning Center (www.mhhe.com/payne11e) are recommended by the American Academy of Pediatrics, the American Academy of Family Physicians, and the Centers for Disease Control and Prevention. As children quickly discover, and parents already know, most of today's immunizations are administered by injection. To improve compliance with the immunization schedule (some parents have a fear of "shots" resulting from early childhood experiences and thus avoid completing the schedule), researchers are attempting to develop a single immunization that would combine many individual vaccines. In addition, research is being conducted on new delivery systems, including a skin patch, nasal spray, and vaccine-enriched foods, such as potatoes.

In recent years, concern has arisen regarding the role of childhood immunizations in the development of other serious childhood physical and emotional health problems, such as type 1 diabetes mellitus, asthma, autism, and sudden infant death syndrome (SIDS). At this time, studies investigating the possible relationship between recommended immunizations and the conditions mentioned previously have found no demonstrable cause-and-effect relationships. For persons interested in more in-depth information regarding adverse affects and contraindications associated with immunizations, the Vaccine Adverse Events Reporting System (VAERS), administered by the Food and Drug Administration (FDA) and the CDC, is in the public domain. Like other reporting systems, the VAERS has limitations; however, information from a wide array of research studies can be readily obtained through the system.[7]

Although immunization is universally viewed as important for infants and children, adults have immunization needs that can be unmet. Accordingly, the CDC's National Immunization Program now provides an immunization schedule for adults. Figure 13-4 lists the immunizations that should be updated or initially received by adults (see the Online Learning Center for more information on the Adult Immunization Schedule). Adults are particularly underprotected in regard to diphtheria and tetanus.

On a final note, as mentioned above, some are concerned that a causative relationship exists between the MMRP childhood immunization and the development of autism.[7] Despite many studies in the United States and abroad, no substantial proof of this contention has been found. Still, the claim persists, most notably by actress Jenny McCarthy. However, in February 2009, the U.S. Court of Claims, a unique form of court used for adjudicating claims of this nature, pronounced that there is little if any evidence to support the immunization-autism claim, thus negating demands made by parents for compensation by the government's Vaccine Injury Compensation Program.

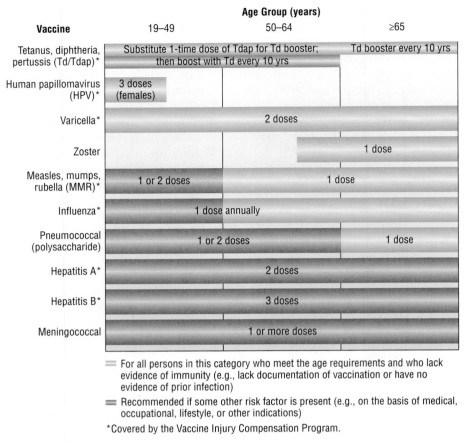

Vaccine	Age Group (years)		
	19–49	50–64	≥65
Tetanus, diphtheria, pertussis (Td/Tdap)*	Substitute 1-time dose of Tdap for Td booster; then boost with Td every 10 yrs		Td booster every 10 yrs
Human papillomavirus (HPV)*	3 doses (females)		
Varicella*	2 doses		
Zoster			1 dose
Measles, mumps, rubella (MMR)*	1 or 2 doses	1 dose	
Influenza*	1 dose annually		
Pneumococcal (polysaccharide)	1 or 2 doses		1 dose
Hepatitis A*	2 doses		
Hepatitis B*	3 doses		
Meningococcal	1 or more doses		

≡ For all persons in this category who meet the age requirements and who lack evidence of immunity (e.g., lack documentation of vaccination or have no evidence of prior infection)

≡ Recommended if some other risk factor is present (e.g., on the basis of medical, occupational, lifestyle, or other indications)

*Covered by the Vaccine Injury Compensation Program.

Figure 13-4 Immunizations Recommended for Adults   For additional information, visit www.cdc.gov/nip.

Source: Centers for Disease Control and Prevention. Recommended Adult Immunization Schedule—United States, October 2008–September 2009. *MMWR* 2008:57:Q1–Q4.

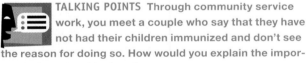 **TALKING POINTS** Through community service work, you meet a couple who say that they have not had their children immunized and don't see the reason for doing so. How would you explain the importance of having this done?

Causes and Management of Selected Infectious Diseases

This section focuses on some of the common infectious diseases and some diseases that are less common but serious. You can use this information as a basis for judging your own disease susceptibility.

Nosocomial Infections

Although the classroom, residence hall, home, work-site, and virtually any place where people gather in large numbers and in close proximity would seem "ideal" places to contract an infectious disease, a better place might come as a surprise—any place where nosocomial infectious agents call "home." Nosocomial infections are infections spread in conjunction with the delivery of health care services—most often from providers to patients or from patients to other patients. Persons who are hospitalized are particularly vulnerable to the development of a potentially fatal nosocomial infection. Recent examples of these infectious agents include *Clostridium difficile (C-diff)*, most often contracted by hospitalized persons who are on antibiotics; methicillin-resistant *Staphylococcus aureus*, generally referred to as MRSA, or even "flesh-eating bacterium"; and a collection of infectious agents (HIV, hepatitis C, and syphilis) transplanted in conjunction with the use of untested "stolen" human tissues supplied to hospitals by unethical tissue banks. Also considered nosocomial would be the fungal agent isolated from contaminated contact lens solution that resulted in *Fusarium keratitis* leading to temporary blindness.

Each year approximately 2.2 million persons develop an infection directly linked to the health care system, including 780,000 in association with operations. Contact with infectious agents occurs in a variety of ways, including the failure of personnel to wash or glove their hands properly prior to conducting examinations, the use of contaminated medical equipment such as endoscopes

Table 13.2 Is It a Cold or the Flu?

Symptoms	Cold	Flu
Fever	Rare	Usual; high (100 degrees F to 102 degrees F); occasionally higher, especially in young children); lasts 3–4 days
Headache	Rare	Common
General aches, pains	Slight	Usual; often severe
Fatigue, weakness	Sometimes	Usual; can last up to 2–3 weeks
Extreme exhaustion	Never	Usual; at the beginning of the illness
Stuffy nose	Common	Sometimes
Sneezing	Usual	Sometimes
Sore throat	Common	Sometimes
Chest discomfort, cough	Mild to moderate; hacking cough	Common; can become severe
Complications	Sinus congestion, middle ear infection, asthma	Pneumonia, bronchitis; can be life threatening
Prevention	Wash your hands often; avoid close contact with anyone with a cold	Annual vaccination; antiviral drugs—see your physician
Treatment	Antihistamines, decongestants, nonsteroidal anti-inflammatory medicines	Antiviral medicines—see your physician

Note: The need to consult a physician as the result of complications that might arise during the course of a cold or flu is not unknown. During the course of a cold, any of the following should be called to the attention of a physician: (1) when a cold fails to resolve within 5 to 7 days, (2) when an elevated temperature develops (above 103 degrees F), or (3) when a "deep chest" cough develops that produces either a brownish-tinged sputum or does not respond to OTC cough medication. Similar complications can occur in conjunction with the flu and require consultation with a physician. In addition, prolonged vomiting and diarrhea also should be called to the attention of a physician. Upon contracting the flu, children, older adults, pregnant women, and all persons with chronic conditions such as diabetes mellitus, cardiovascular diseases, and malignancies should be carefully monitored and complications should be promptly reported to a physician.

Source: National Institute of Allergy and Infectious Diseases, "Is it a cold or the flu?" 2008.

and catheters, failure to maintain sterile operating areas during surgery, the widespread use of central-lines (catheters implanted directly into a large artery near the collarbone), receiving intravenous medications contaminated during their manufacture, contact with visitors who are infectious, sharing a semiprivate room with an infectious roommate, and even from the clothing of physicians and other staff members.

Two factors make today's nosocomial infections particularly serious. The first, of course, is that these infections strike people who by virtue of being institutionalized are less than healthy. Second is the fact that the organisms most frequently associated with these infections are among the most pathogenic with which we have contact.

Today, disease control officials debate the generally stated mortality attributed to nosocomial infections (ranges from 32,000 to 100,000 deaths). MRSA infections alone are thought to be responsible for 20,000 deaths. Some experts suggest that a relatively large percentage of the hospital and nursing home infections are in patients who are already terminal or so frail that infection was only an exacerbating factor in their demise. Accordingly, they believe that these deaths should not be included in the mortality statistics associated with nosocomial infections.

Because of the potential seriousness of nosocomial infections, persons entering the health care arena should discuss infection control with their physician, including the proper procedures for self-care, the possible need for greater isolation while an inpatient, and the desirability of restricting visitation.

The Common Cold

The *common cold,* an acute upper-respiratory-tract infection, must reign as humankind's supreme infectious disease. Also known as **acute rhinitis,** this highly contagious viral infection can be caused by an array of viruses, including rhinoviruses (the most common cause of colds), respiratory syncytial viruses, para-influenza viruses, human metapneumoviruses, and adenoviruses. Colds are particularly common when people spend time in crowded indoor environments, such as classrooms. Colds are so common that over 1 billion cases occur each year in this country. The average American adult has 2 to 4 colds per year; children have 6 to 10.

The signs and symptoms of a cold are fairly predictable. Runny nose, watery eyes, general aches and pains, a listless feeling, and a slight fever all may accompany a cold in its early stages. Eventually the nasal passages swell, and the inflammation may spread to the throat. Stuffy nose, sore throat, and coughing may follow (Table 13.2). The senses of taste and smell are blocked, and appetite declines.

> **Key Terms**
>
> **acute rhinitis** The common cold; the sudden onset of nasal inflammation.

Fighting the Common Cold

Everyone, at one time or another, thinks about how to prevent a cold or how to recover from one. For many people the use of herbal or homeopathic products seems worthy of consideration. Four such products are routinely suggested as being effective in the prevention and/or recovery from colds (and in some cases the flu).

Remember, however, that neither dietary supplements nor homeopathic medications must undergo the rigorous clinical trials required by the FDA for prescription medications. Nor do they need to meet the standards for safety and effectiveness required by the FDA for OTC products. Anecdotal information and studies conducted in other countries are the primary basis for the claims made for these products.

Echinacea, a dietary supplement derived from the roots of the purple coneflower (*Echinacea purpurea*), is purported to be effective in strengthening the immune system and in so doing reducing the number of colds typically contracted during the course of a year. However, in an article appearing in the *New England Journal of Medicine* (July 2005), researchers at the University of Virginia reported that echinacea was ineffective in the prevention of colds.

Elderberry, in extract form, represents a second herbal product whose ability to prevent the development of colds and influenza has been reported. Additionally, elderberry extract has been reported to be effective in reducing the duration of flu-related symptoms from the usual six days to as few as two days. Mild gastrointestinal complications have also been reported in conjunction with elderberry extract use if taken without food in the stomach.

Goldenseal, an herbal product, is generally taken in combination with echinacea. It is believed that goldenseal has some antibacterial efficacy, as well as the ability to stimulate the production of mucus within the respiratory track. To date no antiviral capabilities have been demonstrated with goldenseal, so a direct influence on cold and flu agents seems unlikely. Herbalists suggest that goldenseal detoxifies the body in some fashion.

Oscillococcinum, a nonherbal homeopathic flu medication popular in Europe, contains small quantities of duck liver (see the discussion of homeopathic medication in Chapter 18). Underlying the purported effectiveness of oscillococcinum is its vaccinelike protection resulting from a heightened immune system response to the minuscule amount of flu virus contained in the infected duck liver.

When you notice the onset of symptoms, you should begin managing the cold promptly. After a few days, most of the cold's symptoms subside. In the meantime, you should isolate yourself from others, drink plenty of fluids, eat moderately, and rest.

In addition to the unpleasantness of the symptoms associated with colds, these nearly universal respiratory infections are also expensive. Collectively, colds cost the American economy $40 billion annually, owing to lost work and out-of-pocket expenditures on cold medications.

Some of the many OTC cold remedies can help you manage a cold. These remedies will not cure your cold but may lessen the discomfort associated with it. Nasal decongestants, expectorants, cough syrups, and aspirin or acetaminophen can give some temporary relief. Follow label directions carefully. (For information on herbal and homeopathic remedies, see the box "Fighting the Common Cold.")

In light of the information regarding the treatment of colds given in Table 13.2 and discussed earlier, it is critically important to know that the FDA has determined that the use of OTC cold medication is inappropriate (and potentially fatal[9]) for children under 2 years of age.[8] Recommendations for older children are currently under review. Particularly when using cold medication you should follow these important points:[8]

- Check the "active ingredients" section of the DRUG FACTS label.

- Be very careful if you are giving more than one OTC cough and cold medication to a child.

- Carefully follow the directions in the DRUG FACTS part of the label.

- Only use the measuring spoons or cups that come with the medicine or those made for measuring drugs.

- Choose childproof safety caps and store medications out of the reach of children.

- Never use a cough or cold medication to sedate a child or make him or her sleepy.

Giving young children fluids, the passage of time, and TLC is a safer alternative and will reduce the likelihood of a visit to a hospital's emergency department.

If a cold persists, as evidenced by prolonged chills, fever above 103 degrees F, chest heaviness or aches, shortness of breath, coughing up rust-colored mucus, or persistent sore throat or hoarseness, you should contact a physician. Because we now consider colds to be transmitted most readily by hand contact, you should wash your hands frequently.

Two factors seem predictable in terms of "preventing" colds. The first involves the less than average number of colds seen in children between 6 and 11 years of age who had attended larger preschool programs (more than six other children).[10] The second factor involved a lower than average number of colds in adults who exercised at vigorous levels of intensity.[11]

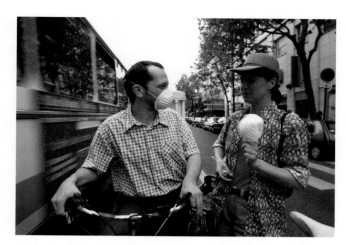

With the 2009 occurrence of the swine flu pandemic, the value of wearing masks as a means of minimizing disease transmission was debated. The couple shown above reflect the uncertainity of the extent to which masks are effective in preventing the spread of the flu virus.

Seasonal Influenza

Influenza is also an acute contagious disease caused by viruses. Some influenza outbreaks have killed thousands and even millions of people, such as the influenza pandemics of 1889–1890, 1918–1919, 1957, and 2003–2004. The viral strains that produce this infectious disease have the potential for more severe complications than the viral strains that produce the common cold. The viral strain for a particular form of influenza enters the body through the respiratory tract. After brief incubation and prodromal stages, the host develops signs and symptoms not just in the upper respiratory tract but throughout the entire body. These symptoms include fever, chills, cough, sore throat, headache, gastrointestinal disturbances, and muscular pain (see Table 13.2).

Antibiotics are generally not prescribed for people with influenza, except when the patient has a possible secondary bacterial infection. Physicians may recommend only aspirin, fluids, and rest. Parents are reminded not to give aspirin to children because of the danger of Reye's syndrome. Reye's syndrome is an aspirin-enhanced complication of influenza in which central nervous system changes can occur, including brain swelling. For a person hoping to avoid the debilitating symptoms of flu, four antiviral prescription medications are currently approved by the FDA: Tamiflu, Relenza, Symmetrel, and Flumadine. Unfortunately, the 2008–2009 flu season, although mild by past standards, revealed that the A H1N1 virus was rapidly becoming resistant to Tamiflu. Relenza (available only for nasal inhalation) was an effective substitute for Tamiflu, except for persons unable to use an inhalant because of respiratory problems and asthma. For these persons, use of the two remaining medications was their only option. On an encouraging note, new antiviral medications are in clinical trials. The influenza vaccine is formulated one year in advance of the flu season in which it will be used, so its composition will be based on the types of flu viruses seen in Asia during the prior year.

Most young adults can cope with the milder strains of seasonal influenza that appear each winter or spring. However, pregnant women and older people—especially older people with additional health complications, such as heart disease, kidney disease, emphysema, and chronic bronchitis—are not as capable of handling this viral attack. People who regularly come into contact with the general public, such as teachers, should also consider annual flu shots.

Today a possible 105 million Americans could receive annual "flu shots." In past years, these annual immunizations, tailored to work against the flu viruses anticipated for the coming flu season, were principally received by adults over 50 years of age and others with special needs. During the flu epidemic of 2003–2004, younger adults moved into the recipient population. The nation's supply of 115 million doses of vaccine for the 2006–2007 flu season proved to be adequate, as, again, thousands of people from within the eligible pool chose not to be immunized.

Today the pool of eligible recipients of seasonal influenza vaccine has become almost inclusive. Revised recommended guidelines issued in June 2006 now approve the influenza vaccine for people 6 months of age and older. Receipt of the vaccine is deemed particularly important for people at risk of complications should they experience an episode of the flu and for a variety of persons who "simply can't afford to have the flu." This latter and sizable group includes people over 65, people with muscle and nerve disorders, women who will be pregnant during the flu season (November–February), all children between 16 and 59 months of age, people with chronic health problems such as cardiovascular disease and metabolic disorders such as diabetes, people with compromised immune systems such as HIV/AIDS and transplant recipients, those in people-centered occupations (medical personnel, teachers, and child care providers), people who provide essential community services (law enforcement, fire protection, and military personnel), people who live in communal residences (college residence halls or prisons), and people planning on traveling to the Southern Hemisphere between April and September.

In the near future, the term *flu shot* may be less frequently heard. In June 2003, the FDA approved the sale of Flumist, a nasal spray inhalation delivery system for influenza vaccine. Its use is approved for people ages 2 to 49. Its use is not, at this time, recommended for persons most in need of the highest level of protection.

The flu season generally runs from November through February, with nearly 115,000 persons developing clear symptoms of influenza, and 36,000 dying from its complications.

Avian (Bird) Influenza and Novel-H1N1 (Swine) Influenza

In 2003, the World Health Organization (WHO) became aware of the presence of a virus that was not among the predictable viral strains that make up the seasonal human flu viruses. An apparently modified version of a virus that was formerly limited to avian species (principally in Near Eastern countries) was now beginning to spread to humans via contact with the excrement of chickens and ducks. In an attempt to stem transmission of the A-H5NI virus, millions of chicken and ducks were destroyed, principally in China, Korea, Japan, Vietnam, and Indonesia.

As the Avian Flu virus began migrating into other areas of the world, reports surfaced of cases in the Near East, Middle East, Asia, Europe, Africa, and to a very limited extent in North America. By August 2009, 438 cases had been reported and 262 deaths had occurred. Although some isolated cases of A-H5N1 influenza in humans suggest that the virus has developed some potential for human-to-human transmission, that capability seems limited. Nonetheless, the world health community remains vigilant in monitoring the virus because more aggressive mutations could still occur, creating the potential for an Avian Flu pandemic. Visit the Online Learning Center (www.mhhe.com/payne11e) to view a timeline of Avian influenza.

Today, however, the concern regarding an Avian Flu pandemic has been significantly replaced with the existence of a Stage 6 pandemic of novel-H1N1 (Swine) Influenza that began in Mexico in March 2009. Although the H1N1 virus is routinely found in pigs in North America, this virus is distinctly different, having incorporated genetic material from other viruses, including a swine virus common to European and Asian swine, the Avian virus (H5N1), and one or more human flu viruses, and is thus known as novel H1N1.

The novel-H1N1 virus is easily spread from an infected person to other people (new hosts) via respiratory inhalation (coughing and sneezing), or by handling a contaminated object such as a towel and then touching the nose or mouth. The novel-H1N1 infection presents with a variety of symptoms, including cough, fever, sore throat, runny nose, chills, body aches, and lethargy. Symptoms range from minimal to severe. Fortunately, it appears that the majority of infected persons recover, although as with seasonal flu, deaths have occurred. Current antiviral medications shorten the period of symptoms and reduce their discomfort, but will not prevent infection.[12]

Given the virulence of the novel-H1N1 virus, and the rapidity with which it spread within North America and throughout the world in conjunction with global interconnectedness, the world health community began immediate formulation and production of preventative vaccines, guidelines for immunizing various segments of the population (for which school facilities were pressed into use), and periods of home isolation for those infected. By August 2009, more than 180,000 cases of Swine Flu had been reported and 1,799 deaths had occurred, although the WHO acknowledges that these numbers are likely understated because of its backlog of information. Additionally, some countries either lack efficient reporting systems or have curtailed reporting into their own reporting centers because of lack of resources or logistical difficulties associated with rural area reporting. For students wanting to follow the unfolding of the pandemic, weekly updates are available at http://www.who.int/csr/don/en.

Tuberculosis

Experts considered *tuberculosis (TB)*, a bacterial infection of the lungs resulting in chronic coughing, weight loss, and sometimes death, to be under control in the United States until the mid-1980s. The number of cases surged then, however, with a peak of 26,283 cases in 1992. The number has declined since then, with 12,898 cases reported in 2008, a 49 percent decline from 1992.[13] However, public health officials must continually monitor this infectious disease, because people visit or immigrate to the United States from areas of the world in which TB is considerably more common and because drug-resistant strains of the bacterium continue to develop.

Today, three forms of drug-resistant TB have emerged, including monodrug-resistant TB, multiple-drug-resistant (MDR) TB from which only 50 percent recover, and most recently, extensively drug-resistant (XDR) TB. Mortality from XDR TB is virtually 100 percent. In a recent assessment of reports from wide areas of the world, the CDC reported that in the industrialized nations of the world, 6 to 7 percent of the multiple-drug-resistant TB cases are of the XDR TB form. The rate of XDR TB infection remains relatively low (although increasing) in the United States—with 49 cases reported between 1993 and 2006.[14] However, in Africa, the former Soviet Union, and areas of Asia, there could be a total of around 180,000 cases of XDR TB. Globally, tuberculosis, in all of its forms, is estimated to number 9 million cases, claiming 2 million lives annually.

Tuberculosis thrives in crowded places where infected people are in constant contact with others, since TB is spread by coughing. This includes prisons, hospitals, public housing units, and even college residence halls. In such settings, a single infected person can spread the TB agents to many others.

When healthy people are exposed to TB agents, their immune systems can usually suppress the bacteria well enough to prevent symptoms from developing and to reduce the likelihood of infecting others. When the immune system is damaged, however, such as in some older adults, malnourished people, and those who are infected with HIV, the disease can become established and eventually be transmitted to other people at risk.

Underlying the global tuberculosis problem is a multitude of factors, including those already mentioned. Additional factors, found even in the United States, include antiquated treatment protocols, time delays associated with traditional testing for TB, and failure of patients to be compliant in taking medications. Global efforts are under way to address as many of these factors as possible—including educational programs through WHO and other international agencies, multinational research efforts in the development of new antibiotics, and a more prompt and sensitive diagnostic test. The CDC has recommended adoption of the QuantiFERON-TB Gold test (QFT Gold). Although this test is more expensive than the traditional tuberculin-based skin test for detecting active TB in persons once vaccinated with Bacillus Calmette-Guerin (BCG),[15] it requires only a single blood draw and no return trip to a clinic for assessment, and will give more accurate results (fewer false positives).

Pneumonia

Pneumonia is a general term that describes a variety of infectious respiratory conditions. There are bacterial, viral, fungal, rickettsial, mycoplasmal, and parasitic forms of pneumonia. However, bacterial pneumonia, with more than 90 serotypes, is the most common form and is often seen with other illnesses that weaken the body's immune system. In fact, pneumonia is so common in the frail older adult that it is often the specific condition causing death.

Older adults with a history of chronic obstructive lung disease, cardiovascular disease, diabetes, or alcoholism often encounter a potentially serious midwinter form of pneumonia known as *acute (severe) community-acquired pneumonia*. Characteristics of this condition are the sudden onset of chills, chest pain, and a cough that produces sputum. In addition, a symptom-free form of pneumonia known as *walking pneumonia* is also commonly seen in adults and can become serious without warning.

As the number of older Americans grows, recommendations regarding immunization against pneumococcal pneumonia have been established and vaccination programs undertaken. Today, the recommendation for an adult initial pneumonia vaccination is age 65, with starting ages as early as 19 years for people with specific health conditions or those who work in high-risk settings.

The cost effectiveness of pneumonia immunizations for older adults, and particularly for minority older adults, is well established. The first known drug-resistant strains of pneumonia have been identified in this country. As a result, some experts are calling for an even more comprehensive vaccination plan for older adults.

In children under the age of 5 years, pneumococcal disease is annually responsible for an array of infectious conditions, including 4.9 million cases of otitis media (middle ear infection), 700 cases of meningitis, 17,000 cases of bacterial blood infections, and 200 deaths.[16] In spite of the prevalence and potential severity of pneumococcal disease in young children, the incidence of this infectious condition is beginning to recede as a larger percentage of children gain the protection provided by the polyvalent immunization now included in the recommended immunization schedule.

Mononucleosis

College students who contract **mononucleosis ("mono")** can be forced into a long period of bed rest during a semester when they can least afford it. Other common diseases can be managed with minimal disruption, but the overall weakness and fatigue seen in many people with mono sometimes require a month or two of rest and recuperation.

Mono is a viral infection in which the body produces an excess of mononuclear leukocytes (a type of white blood cell). After uncertain, perhaps long, incubation and prodromal stages, the acute symptoms of mono can appear, including weakness, headache, low-grade fever, swollen lymph glands (especially in the neck), and sore throat. Mental fatigue and depression are sometimes reported as side effects of mononucleosis. After the acute symptoms disappear, the weakness and fatigue usually persist—perhaps for a few months.

Mono is diagnosed by its characteristic symptoms. The Monospot blood smear can also be used to identify the prevalence of abnormal white blood cells. In addition, an antibody test can detect activity of the immune system that is characteristic of the illness.

This disease is most often caused by an Epstein-Barr virus (EBV), so antibiotic therapy is not recommended. Treatment usually includes bed rest and the use of OTC remedies for fever (aspirin or acetaminophen) and lozenges for sore throat. Corticosteroid drugs can be used in

---

Key Terms

mononucleosis ("mono") A viral infection characterized by weakness, fatigue, swollen glands, sore throat, and low-grade fever.

extreme cases. Rupture of the spleen is an occasional, but serious, consequence of the condition, particularly in persons who are too physically active during their recovery. Adequate fluid intake and a well-balanced diet are also important in the recovery stages of mono. Fortunately, the body tends to develop NAI to the mono virus, so repeat infections of mono are unusual. However, persons on immunosuppressant drugs, such as Remicade for Crohn's disease, are somewhat likely to experience a recurrence of mononucleosis or other EBV-related infections.

For years, mono has been labeled the "kissing disease"; however, mono is not highly contagious and is known to be spread by direct transmission in ways other than kissing. No vaccine has been developed for mononucleosis. The best preventive measures are the steps that you can take to increase your resistance to most infectious diseases: (1) eat a well-balanced diet, (2) exercise regularly, (3) sleep sufficiently, (4) use health care services appropriately, (5) live in a reasonably healthful environment, and (6) avoid direct contact with infected people.

Chronic Fatigue Syndrome

Chronic fatigue syndrome (CFS) may be the most perplexing "infectious" condition physicians see. First identified in 1985, this mononucleosis-like condition is most often seen in women in their 40s and 50s. People with CFS, often busy professional people, report flulike symptoms, including severe exhaustion, fatigue, headaches, muscle aches, fever, inability to concentrate, allergies, intolerance to exercise, and depression. Examinations of the first people with CFS revealed antibodies to the Epstein-Barr virus. Thus observers assumed CFS to be an infectious viral disease (and initially called it *chronic Epstein-Barr syndrome*).

In the years since its first appearance, the condition has received great attention that has produced considerable confusion over its exact nature. In fact, several theories have been advanced to identify the cause (or causes) of CFS. As suggested earlier, some experts believe an infectious agent may be partially responsible, possibly a virus such as EBV, cytomegalovirus, enteroviruses, human T-cell lymphotrophic virus, or human herpes virus 6. To date, no specific virus has been consistently isolated. A second explanation involves an extended challenge to the immune system, possibly activated by an initial viral infection and resulting in the overproduction of immune system chemicals that produce flulike symptoms. Perhaps the most creditable explanation involves a more complex causation for CFS. This model suggests involvement of emotional, environmental, and infectious factors, all influencing the stress response (see Chapter 3), in association with a possible genetic predisposition.

Since there is no definitive diagnosis (or treatment) for CFS, a probable diagnosis will be based on a medical history featuring exercise-induced malaise, nonrefreshing sleep, impairment of memory, muscle pain, multiple joint pain, unusual headaches, sore throat, and tenderness in the neck or swollen lymph nodes in the armpits. In combination, these characteristic markers of CFS will be chronic in nature and clearly disabling (see the box "Living with a Chronic Infectious Disease—Life Is Not Over, Just Different").

Bacterial Meningitis

Since approximately 1995, a formerly infrequently seen but potentially fatal infectious disease, *meningococcal meningitis*, has appeared on college campuses, suggesting that college students are currently at greater risk of contracting the disease than are their noncollege peers. Particularly interesting is the fact that among college students, the risk of contracting this infection on campus is highest for those students living in residence halls, suggesting that close living quarters, as well as sharing cigarettes and beverages, kissing (exchanging infectious oral fluids), and contact with students from other areas of the world favor transmission of the bacteria. Since many colleges and universities require that first-year students reside in residence halls, it is in this group that the incidence of meningococcal meningitis is highest. Additionally, this group of students is most likely to be in large-section lecture classes and take meals in large dining facilities. Annually, about 150 cases of meningococcal meningitis occur on American college campuses, resulting in 15 deaths per year. Understandably, more and more colleges and universities are requiring, as a condition of admission, documentation of immunization against bacterial meningitis. Additionally, a growing number of states are requiring that health care providers provide clearly stated information regarding the value of meningococcal meningitis immunization. Some people, however, have questioned the cost-effectiveness of immunizing all entering college students. Skepticism about cost-effectiveness aside, today's late childhood-adolescent immunization schedule suggests vaccine against meningococcal meningitis be given at age 11 to 12 years. By doing so, when this population moves on to the college campus where group living is common, the "herd immunity" provided by an immunized majority will protect those non-immunized classmates who "slipped through the cracks."

> **Key Terms**
>
> **chronic fatigue syndrome (CFS)** An illness that causes severe exhaustion, fatigue, aches, and depression; mostly affects women in their 40s and 50s.
>
> **Lyme disease** A bacterial infection transmitted by deer ticks.

Living with a Chronic Infectious Disease—Life Is Not Over, Just Different

A chronic infectious disease can wear down your body and your spirit. First, you've got to deal with the pain, fatigue, and medicinal side effects associated with the condition. But you also need to learn to adapt everything—your routine, your relationships, and your work—to the illness. As the quality of your life changes dramatically, you may feel depressed, frustrated, and alone. What is the best way to handle the different aspects of your life as you learn to cope with a long-term illness such as chronic fatigue syndrome, hepatitis, or HIV? Will it ever be possible to enjoy a full life again?

Certainly your intimate relationships may also be strained. Your partner may not understand the new limits your illness places on your activities, especially if you were very active before. The best approach is open and honest communication. Try to dispel (or come to terms with) any fears your partner may have about your illness. Take all necessary precautions to avoid infecting your partner if the disease is transmissible. Also, reassure your partner that you're taking these precautions so that he or she won't become ill. Make a point of including your partner in your daily routines. Keep him or her informed of all doctor's appointments, procedures you must undergo, and any news of progress or setbacks. Share your feelings as a way of reducing anxiety for both of you. Create adaptations so that you can still enjoy a romantic relationship. Make the most of your time together, and find new ways to enjoy each other's company.

If you have children, they will also be affected by your illness. Young children may not understand why you can't take them for a sled ride when you feel sick or why you can't go to a school play because of a doctor's appointment. It's best to let children know that their fears and anxieties are valid and that you want them to share them with you. Tell them about your prognosis, taking care not to make any false promises of recovery if that is not expected. Spend time with each child—helping with homework, reading a story, or doing light chores around the house. Always allow the child to ask questions.

From your home to your workplace, your life will change along with your condition. As you adapt to your new situation, it is important to:

- *Be your own best friend.* Eat well, exercise as much as you can, rest when you need to, and follow the treatments prescribed by your physician.

- *Know and understand your limits.* Don't feel guilty about not doing things you used to do before you got sick. Instead, set goals and handle responsibilities as your condition allows.

- *Find new things to do for fun.* This is a good time to start a new hobby that's relaxing. You can also make adaptations so that you can continue activities you've always enjoyed. Maybe you can't run three miles a day, but an after-dinner walk might be a pleasant substitute.

- *Communicate openly with others.* Share your feelings respectfully, and allow others around you to share theirs. Together, you can calm your fears, instill hope in each other, and foster a sense of belonging.

- *Remain positive.* Remember, life is not over—just different. Look forward to the good days, when you feel well, and take advantage of them. Create new ways to fulfill your needs and desires. Remain positive about the future and your treatment. New discoveries do occur, and treatments are always evolving. However, be realistic about your situation. Joining a support group may be one of the best things you can do for yourself.

What you learn about yourself throughout your illness may surprise you. You may discover a strength of spirit you never knew you had. Some days may be very hard, but somehow you get through them. You may see life in a new way—slowing down and taking pleasure in a job well done, enjoying friendships more, listening to your inner voice, spending time with your children, taking a second look at nature, and being thankful for today and tomorrow.

Meningococcal meningitis is a bacterial infection of the thin membranous coverings of the brain. In its earliest stages, this disease can easily be confused with the flu. Symptoms usually include a high fever, severe headache, stiff neck, nausea with vomiting, extreme tiredness, and the formation of a progressive rash. For about 10 percent of people who develop this condition, the infection is fatal, often within 24 hours. Therefore the mere presence of the symptoms just described signals the need for immediate medical evaluation. If done promptly, treatment is highly effective.

Lyme Disease

Lyme disease is an infectious disease that has become a significant health problem in eastern, southeastern,

upper midwestern, and West Coast states, with 27,444 cases in 2007 (23,305 in 2006). The significant increase in the number of cases of Lyme disease since 1992 (when 9,909 cases were reported) most likely reflects widening geographical distribution of the disease, a greater awareness of its symptoms by the general public, and more consistent reporting by physicians. This bacterial disease results when infected blacklegged ticks (also called deer ticks), usually in the nymph (immature) stage, attach to the skin and inject the infectious agent as they feed on a host's blood. The deer ticks become infected by feeding, as larvae, on infected white-footed mice.

The symptoms of Lyme disease vary but typically appear within 30 days as small red bumps surrounded by a circular red rash at the site of bites. The red rash has been described as being like a "bull's eye" in appearance—a pale center surrounded by a reddish margin. However, in some persons this characteristic rash does not appear, thus other symptoms must be recognized so that diagnosis is not delayed. Flu like symptoms, including chills, headaches, muscle and joint aches, and low-grade fever, may accompany this acute phase. A chronic phase develops in about 20 percent of untreated infected persons. This phase may produce disorders of the nervous system, heart, or joints. Fortunately, Lyme disease can be treated with antibiotics. Unfortunately, however, no immunity develops, so infection can recur. Some physicians order tests and begin antibiotic therapy too quickly. The basis of treatment should be the appearance of clinical symptoms, not simply the reporting of a tick bite. Lyme disease may be more difficult to diagnose in children than in adults.

Chronic Lyme disease is today at the center of controversy regarding its treatment and, even, to an extent, its actual existence[17]—akin in this regard to CFS. This form of Lyme disease is determined to exist if symptoms are still present at 6 months following the completion of the standard treatment protocol. In many cases, physicians place their late-Lyme-disease patients on prophylactic antibiotics based solely on the information provided by patients, and often without explaining the negative consequences of doing so.

In contrast to that approach, other physicians will first order blood tests to determine the presence and level of antibodies for the causative agent (*B. burgdorferi*) in the blood before beginning antibiotic treatment. If the antibody titers are very low or nonexistent, treatment will be restricted to symptomatic protocols, with reassurance that patients no longer have Lyme disease. For both acute and chronic Lyme disease, the ideal is never to have become the new host for an infected deer tick. Lyme disease prevention is thus described.

People who live in tick-prone areas, including near small urban/suburban woodlots, and participate in outdoor activities can encounter the nearly invisible tick nymphs. These people should check themselves frequently to be sure that they are tick-free. They should tuck shirts into pants, tuck pants into socks, and wear gloves and hat when possible. They should shower after coming inside from outdoors and check clothing for evidence of ticks. Pets, particularly dogs who enjoy outdoor play and then return indoors, can carry infected ticks into the house. If you find ticks, carefully remove them from the skin with tweezers and wash the affected area. There is no vaccine available for humans, so prevention is very important. Repellants containing DEET or permethrin are effective in repelling ticks; they should be used according to directions on the label. A form of "natural" prevention seems to occur in conjunction with frequent noninfected tick exposure in the past, but this should not discourage persons from using preventive measures.

As a final aside on Lyme disease, in July 2006 the FDA issued a news release to inform the public of adverse reactions, including a death, to Lyme disease medication bismacine, or chromacine.[18] This untested and thus unapproved compound contains bismuth, a heavy metal that can seriously damage the cardiovascular and renal systems. Bismacine is compounded as an injection by some local druggists, under the auspices of "alternative" practitioners.

Hantavirus Pulmonary Syndrome

Since 1993 a small but rapidly growing number of people have been dying of extreme pulmonary distress caused by the leakage of plasma into the lungs. In the initial cases, the people lived in the Southwest, had been well until they began developing flulike symptoms over one or two days, then quickly experienced difficulty breathing, and died only hours later. Epidemiologists quickly suspected a viral agent such as the *hantavirus,* known to exist in Asia and, to a lesser degree, in Europe. Exhaustive laboratory work led to the culturing of the virus and confirmed that all of these patients had been infected with an American version of the hantavirus. Researchers identified this latest infectious condition as *hantavirus pulmonary syndrome.*

Today hantavirus pulmonary syndrome has been reported in areas beyond the Southwest, including most of the western states and some of the eastern states. The common denominator in all these areas is the presence of deer mice. It is now known that this common rodent serves as the reservoir for the virus. In fact, so common is the mouse that in 2000 the National Park Service began warning hikers, campers, and off-road bikers that hantavirus probably existed in every national park and that caution should be taken to avoid high-risk sites. As recently as 2006, nine new cases were reported in five southwestern states, resulting in five deaths.[19]

The virus moves from deer mice to humans when people inhale dust contaminated with dried virus-rich rodent urine or saliva-contaminated materials, such as nests. If you must remove rodent nests from a house, barn, or shed, wear rubber gloves, pour a disinfectant or bleach on the nests and soak them thoroughly, and finally, pick up the nests with a shovel and burn them or bury them in holes that are several feet deep. This said, prevention is a better alternative to removing nests and can be accomplished by sealing up holes in structures, trapping and disposing of deer mice in an effective manner, and cleaning up sources of food that would otherwise attract mice.

Because there is no vaccine for hantavirus pulmonary syndrome, people who likely have been exposed to the infected excrement of deer mice should seek early evaluation of flulike symptoms.

West Nile Virus

First detected in New York City in 1999, *West Nile virus* was, by the summer of 2000, identified in 6 eastern states.

By the end of 2002, the West Nile virus had spread westward to include 34 states. By the end of 2003, the West Nile virus had been found in all but 2 of the 48 contiguous U.S. states. By the end of 2006, the virus had been identified in all of the contiguous states, with human cases reported in all but 5 states. In 2007, the CDC reported a total of 3,630 cases of West Nile virus (WNV), of which 1,227 involved neurological involvement (WNND), and 2,350 reported principally fever (WNF) as their primary symptom. There were 117 deaths from West Nile virus infections, principally in older adults and the chronically ill, and in all cases from the WNND form of the disease.[20] In 2008, 1,370 cases were initially reported, a substantial drop from the 2007 total. A number of variables were determined to have caused this decline including drier weather conditions, better screening of homes, improved mosquito control, and more consistent use of mosquito repellents by the general public. Unfortunately, it was learned in early 2009 that the 2008 figures were underreported because of defects in widely used testing kits. A revision of the 2008 data is forthcoming.

This vector-borne infectious virus is transmitted from a reservoir, most often birds, by mosquitoes that in turn infect humans.[1] Human-to-human transmission (via mosquitoes) apparently does not occur, although the CDC has reported at least four cases of virus transmission in conjunction with infected transplanted tissue. West Nile virus infection involves flulike symptoms, including fever, headache, muscle ache, fatigue, and joint pain. In young children, persons with immune systems weakened by HIV, and older adults, West Nile virus infection may involve encephalitis (WNND), a potentially fatal inflammation of the brain. Physicians recommend that any unusual neurological symptoms be considered as a possible West Nile infection. The West Nile virus deaths that have occurred since the infection's initial appearance in 1999 have been the result of encephalitis.

In an attempt to determine the extent of the West Nile virus range, public health officials throughout the United States have tested mosquitoes, sentinel chickens, crows, other birds, cows, and other animals, including humans. Additionally, mosquito habitats are being treated in an attempt to reduce the vector population. Public service announcements focusing on protection against mosquito bites are routinely made in high-risk areas. Additionally, a newly developed immunization that protects birds is being field tested; a horse vaccine is available. There is currently no human vaccine approved for use, although development is ongoing.

Additional aspects of the disease have been reported to the CDC, including the presence of the virus in blood transfusions. (Today, clinically recovered patients cannot give blood for 60 days following release from the hospital.) The West Nile virus has also been isolated from breast milk, and cases of prenatal transmission have been confirmed. Also, a new test to accurately screen for infected blood has been developed, as has a new diagnostic test that significantly reduces the time needed to obtain confirmation of the West Nile virus.

Tampon-Related Toxic Shock Syndrome

Toxic shock syndrome (TSS) made front-page headlines in 1980, when the CDC reported a connection between TSS and the presence of a specific bacterial agent (*Staphylococcus aureus*) in the vagina associated with the use of tampons.

Superabsorbent tampons can irritate the vaginal lining three times more quickly than regular tampons do. This vaginal irritation is aggravated when the tampon remains in the vagina for a long time (more than five hours). When this irritation begins, the staphylococcal bacteria (which are usually present in the vagina) have relatively easy access to the bloodstream. When these bacteria proliferate in the circulatory system, their resultant toxins produce a massive T-cell response (see pages 356–358). These immune system products exacerbate the effects of the bacterial toxin on body tissues, leading to symptoms including fever (102° F or above), headache, vomiting, sore throat, muscle aches, a sunburn-like rash, bloodshot eyes, reduced urination, and peeling of the skin on the hands and soles of the feet. A woman with TSS can die, usually as a result of cardiovascular failure, if left untreated. Fortunately, less than 10 percent of women diagnosed as having TSS die.

To minimize the risk of TSS, all premenopausal women, particularly those new to use of tampons, should consider these recommendations for safe tampon use: (1) tampons should not be the sole form of sanitary protection used, and (2) tampons should not remain in place for too long. Women should change tampons every few hours and intermittently use sanitary napkins. Tampons should not be used during sleep. Some physicians recommend that tampons not be used at all if a woman wants to be extraordinarily safe from TSS.

Hepatitis

Hepatitis is an inflammatory process in the liver that can be caused by several viruses. Types A, B, C (once called non-A and non-B), D, and E have been recognized. Hepatitis can also be caused indirectly from abuse of alcohol and other drugs. General symptoms of hepatitis include

---

Key Terms

toxic shock syndrome (TSS) A potentially fatal condition caused by the proliferation of certain bacteria in the vagina whose toxins enter the general blood circulation.

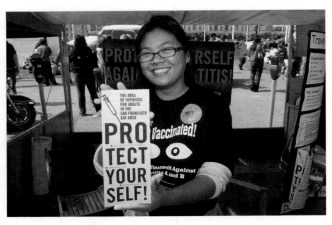

Effective vaccines are available for both hepatitis A and hepatitis B.

fever, nausea, loss of appetite, abdominal pain, fatigue, and jaundice (yellowing of the skin and eyes).[1]

Type A hepatitis is often associated with consuming fecal-contaminated food, such as raw shellfish raised in fecal-contaminated water, raw vegetables field-washed in contaminated water, or contaminated drinking water. As an example, in November 2003, 520 patrons of a Chi-Chi's Mexican restaurant near Pittsburgh became ill and 3 died as a result of eating contaminated green onions. Poor sanitation, particularly in the handling of food and diaper-changing activities, has produced outbreaks in child care centers. Experts estimate that up to 200,000 people per year experience this viral infection. This number far exceeds the reported 26,000 to 27,000 cases per year, suggesting that a very large reservoir exists among children who are routinely asymptomatic before 6 years of age. In 2005 it was recommended that all children between 1 and 2 years of age be immunized against hepatitis A. Today that recommendation is in place, with the first immunization given at 12 months and the second by 18 months of age. Persons who contract hepatitis A generally develop acquired immunity, thus preventing a recurrence.[21]

Type B hepatitis (HBV) is spread in various ways, including sexual contact, intravenous drug use, tattooing, body piercing, and even sharing electric razors. On the basis of these modes of transmission, college students should be aware of their potential risk for HBV infection. Beyond the risk factors just identified, medical and dental procedures are also a potential means of transmitting the virus, including patient to practitioner and practitioner to patient transmission. Chronic HBV infection has been associated with liver cirrhosis and is the principal cause of liver cancer. An effective immunization for hepatitis B is now available; thus, the incidence of HBV in children and adolescents has dropped by one-fifth since 1999. However, an increase has been noted in people over 19 years of age. Although it is given during childhood, it should be seriously considered for older unvaccinated people and college students. In 2002 the American Academy of Pediatrics recommended that all newborns be immunized before leaving the hospital. Adults should seriously consider being immunized against hepatitis B, particularly if they are likely to have multiple sex partners, have sex partners from high-risk groups, or are a caregiver to an infected person. For those who are infected, several medications are now available for use in treating hepatitis B.

Hepatitis C is contracted in ways similar to hepatitis B (sexual contact, tainted blood, in association with tattooing and piercings, and shared needles). In the absence of immunization, the pool of infected people is in excess of 4.1 million, and the death rate is expected to climb. Currently a dual-drug therapy for HCV involving multiple forms of interferon in combination with the drug ribavirin is the treatment of choice. Many infected persons remain asymptomatic for decades, and many persons infected with HCV recover from this liver-threatening infection. People in the latter group appear to have a genetically based ability to stimulate a high level of natural killer (NK) cells within the immune system.[22] In a recent study, a two-drug combination treatment resulted in a virus-free state for nearly 60 percent of a large group of infected persons treated for 1 year. In spite of encouraging news such as this, recovery from HCV infection seems less likely the case for infected African Americans, a phenomenon that cannot currently be explained.

The newly identified type D (delta) hepatitis is very difficult to treat and is found almost exclusively in people already suffering from type B hepatitis, since the hepatitis D virus requires the presence of the hepatitis B virus in order to gain full pathogenicity. This virus, like type B hepatitis and HIV, makes unprotected sexual contact, including anal and oral sex, very risky. Hepatitis E, associated with water contamination, is rarely seen in this country other than in people returning from hepatitis E virus–endemic areas of the world.

AIDS

Acquired immunodeficiency syndrome (AIDS) has become the most devastating infectious disease in recent history, and it is virtually certain to be among the most devastating diseases in history unless a cure is forthcoming. Setting aside for the present the international scope of the HIV/AIDS epidemic, statistics for the United States alone paint a distressing picture. On the basis of data reported through 2007, a total of 1,051,875 Americans have been diagnosed with AIDS, and 583,298 have died from its effects (or 55.4 percent of all cases).[23, 24] Table 13.3 shows the estimated number of persons living with HIV/AIDS at the end of 2007, by race/ethnicity, sex, and transmission

Table 13.3 Estimated Numbers of Persons Living with HIV/AIDS at the End of 2007, by Race/Ethnicity, Sex, and Transmission Category—34 States with Confidential Name-Based HIV Infection Reporting

Transmission category	White, not Hispanic		Black, not Hispanic		Hispanic		Asian/ Pacific Islander		American Indian/Alaska Native		Total	
	No.	%	No.	%	No.	%	No.	%	No.	%	No.	%
Male adult or adolescent												
Male-to-male sexual contact	121,702	79	84,965	51	41,866	60	1,883	77	1,052	64	253,804	64
Injection drug use	11,769	8	35,946	21	15,754	23	157	6	221	13	64,335	16
Male-to-male sexual contact and injection drug use	12,205	8	11,220	7	4,062	6	72	3	231	14	28,081	7
High-risk heterosexual contact	5,957	4	34,093	20	7,649	11	306	12	127	8	48,515	12
Other	1,604	1	1,188	1	434	1	38	2	13	1	3,322	1
Subtotal	153,236	100	167,412	100	69,765	100	2,455	100	1,644	100	398,057	100
Female adult or adolescent												
Injection drug use	9,033	33	22,561	24	6,030	28	72	11	198	32	38,266	26
High-risk heterosexual contact	17,566	65	71,100	75	15,501	71	547	82	404	66	106,139	72
Other	545	2	1,306	1	335	2	50	8	12	2	2,287	2
Subtotal	27,144	100	94,966	100	21,865	100	669	100	614	100	146,692	100
Child (<13 yrs at diagnosis)												
Perinatal	842	84	4,344	92	1,209	92	28	78	21	91	6,506	91
Other	158	16	393	8	104	8	8	22	2	9	676	9
Subtotal	1,000	100	4,737	100	1,313	100	36	100	23	100	7,181	100
Total	**181,380**	**100**	**267,116**	**100**	**92,943**	**100**	**3,160**	**100**	**2,281**	**100**	**551,932**	**100**

Note. These numbers do not represent reported case counts. Rather, these numbers are point estimates, which result from adjustments of reported case counts. The reported case counts have been adjusted for reporting delays and for redistribution of cases in persons initially reported without an identified risk factor, but not for incomplete reporting.
Source: Centers for Disease Control and Prevention. *HIV/AIDS Surveillance Report, 2009.* Vol. 19, Table 10.

category in 34 states with confidential name-based reporting. Note that for adolescents and adults, male-to-male homosexual contact, female heterosexual contact, and male injection drug use are the leading means of transmission. When HIV/AIDS data are viewed in terms of race and ethnicity, it will be noticed that there is a disproportionate distribution of cases for African Americans and Latinos, in comparison to other groups. Based on data from the American Community Survey (2007),[25] the Hispanic Origin Population Survey (2008),[26] the U.S. Census Bureau study of persons of Hispanic origin, combined with the CDC's HIV/AIDS data through 2007, Whites compose 74.1 percent of the American population but were 33.8 percent of the U.S. persons living with HIV/AIDS at the end of 2007. Hispanics constitute 15.1 percent of the U.S. population but 16.9 percent of the HIV/AIDS cases, while African Americans constitute 12.4 percent of the population but 47.3 percent of the HIV/AIDS cases. As reported for 2007, Asian Americans, at 4.4 percent of the population, have only 0.6 percent of the cases, while Native Americans and Alaska Natives compose 0.8 percent of the population and 0.4 percent of the HIV/AIDS cases. There is no easy explanation for the discrepancies seen in these data.

In addition to the human tragedy suggested by these statistics, the financial cost of treating the HIV/AIDS epidemic is sizable. Today, with the array of medications for use in sustained treatment for individuals with HIV/AIDS, life expectancy can exceed 20 years. Accompanying this extended survival period is a huge financial outlay. A single year of treatment in 2003 could range from $21,900 for persons with a CD4 count above 500 cells/mm^3 to as much as $57,600 for persons with a CD4 count below 50 cells/mm^3.[27] In most cases, these costs are paid for through a combination of federal, state, and private programs. These programs include Medicaid, Medicare, the Ryan White CARE Act, private health insurance, the Department of Veterans Affairs, and various community health centers and other safety net providers.[28]

Cause of AIDS   AIDS is the disease caused by HIV, a virus that attacks the CD4 T-helper cells of the immune system (see pages 357–358). When HIV attacks CD4 T-helper cells, people lose the ability to fight off a variety of infections that would normally be easily controlled. Because these infections develop while people are vulnerable, they are collectively called *opportunistic infections.* HIV-infected (HIV-positive) patients become increasingly vulnerable to infection by bacteria, protozoa, fungi, and several viruses. A variety of malignancies also develop during this period of immune-system vulnerability.

HIV positive with AIDS was originally diagnosed based on the presence of specific conditions. Among these were *Pneumocystis carinii* pneumonia and Kaposi's sarcoma, a rare but deadly form of skin cancer. Gradually, experts recognized that additional conditions were associated with advancing deterioration of the immune system and thus added them to the list of AIDS conditions. This list now includes almost 30 definitive conditions, with more conditions being added as they become apparent. Among the conditions found on the current version of the list are toxoplasmosis within the brain, cytomegalovirus retinitis with loss of vision, lymphoma involving the brain, recurrent salmonella blood infections, and a wasting syndrome that includes invasive cervical cancer in women, recurrent pneumonia, and recurrent tuberculosis. Today, however, experts tend to assign the label of HIV positive with AIDS to HIV-infected people when their level of CD4 T-helper cells drops below 200 cells per cubic microliter of blood, regardless of whether specific conditions are present. (CD4 cells are the type of cells most often infected and destroyed by HIV.)

Spread of HIV   HIV cannot be contracted easily in comparison to other infectious conditions such as colds, flu, and some childhood infections that can spread quickly within a classroom or office complex. The chances of contracting HIV through casual contact with HIV-infected people at work, school, or home are extremely low or nonexistent. HIV is known to be spread only by direct sexual contact involving the exchange of bodily fluids (including blood, semen, and vaginal secretions), the sharing of hypodermic needles, transfusion of infected blood or blood products, and perinatal transmission (from an infected mother to a fetus or newborn baby). For HIV to be transmitted, it must enter the bloodstream of the noninfected person, such as through needles or tears in body tissues lining the rectum, mouth, or reproductive system. Current research also indicates that HIV is not transmitted by sweat, saliva, tears, or urine, although the virus may be found in very low concentrations in these fluids. The virus cannot enter the body through the gastrointestinal system because digestive enzymes destroy the virus. An exception to this generalization, however, might exist, as studies conducted in Africa indicate that transmission can occur in conjunction with breast-feeding infants. A second exception involves the transmission of HIV between infected persons and their uninfected sexual partners during episodes of unprotected oral sex when the uninfected persons have evident gingivitis and bleeding gums.

Women are at much greater risk than men are of contracting HIV through heterosexual activity because of the higher concentration of lymphocytes in semen (± 10 million lymphocytes/tsp) than in vaginal secretions ($\pm 1,200$ thousand lymphocytes/tsp). This susceptibility is evidenced in part by the increasing percentage of women with AIDS who were infected through heterosexual contact—from 8 percent in 1981, to 19 percent in 1993, and 72 percent in 2007.[29] Women under age 25 contract the virus principally through heterosexual contact.

Diagnosis of HIV Infection   HIV infection is diagnosed through a clinical examination, laboratory tests for accompanying infections, and an initial screening test. Should the initial screening test produce a negative result, persons at risk for infection should be rescreened in three to six months. For persons reluctant to present themselves for screening in a clinical setting, home screening tests are also available. Regardless, once initial screening has been undertaken, to eliminate the small chance of a false positive having occurred, more sensitive tests can be administered, including the enzyme-linked immunosorbent assay (ELISA) and Western blot test. Although expensive and not completely reliable, even more recently developed tests are now available. One of these tests identifies the existence of viral mutations known to be drug resistant, while another helps determine whether a particular drug will function in suppressing the contracted viral strain. This information helps physicians structure treatment protocols.

The Course of HIV Infection   Some newly infected people experience flulike symptoms within a month or two after exposure to HIV. The symptoms usually disappear within a few weeks and are typically mistaken for another illness. During this period, people carry high levels of HIV in their blood and genital fluids and are very infectious. The immune system fights back, which reduces the HIV level in the body; this immune response also produces the antibodies that can be detected through testing. Unlike with most other infections, however, the immune system is unable to clear HIV from the body, despite a strong immune response.

The next stage of HIV infection—an asymptomatic stage—may last from a few months to more than 12 years. In Western countries, the average time between infection and the appearance of symptoms is about 10 to 12 years in untreated individuals. The length of the asymptomatic stage may be influenced by such factors as age, gender, overall health status, access to health care, and the particular strain of HIV causing the infection. During this period, the virus is actively multiplying and killing cells of the immune system, and the HIV-positive individual can transmit the infection. This long incubation period is one of the key reasons why widespread testing is recommended; if people know they are infected, they can take steps to avoid transmitting HIV to others. To counter the reality of such a lengthy incubation period, the American College of Physicians now strongly encourages that all patients 13 years of age and older should be screened for HIV, with re-screening to be determined on a case-by case basis.[30]

As the status of the immune system worsens, symptoms begin to appear, including enlarged lymph nodes, loss of energy, frequent fevers and sweats, and persistent infections. As described earlier, a diagnosis of AIDS is made when a person develops one of the AIDS-defining conditions or the level of CD4 T helper cells drops below 200 (healthy adults typically have CD4 counts over 1,000 per mm^3). People with AIDS are vulnerable to many opportunistic infections and may become very ill.

Treatment of HIV Infection   Although no treatment currently exists to cure HIV infection, drugs are available to help reduce the level of HIV in the body, prevent opportunistic infections, and improve chances for survival. Decisions about treatment are usually made on the basis of blood tests and symptoms. CDC guidelines recommend treatment when a person has an AIDS-defining condition or when CD4 cell counts are low and viral counts are high. Currently, it appears that considerable discussion is occurring regarding initial antiviral medications when the CD4 T-helper cell count reaches a level of 350 mm^3, or even at 500 mm^3; earlier recommendations delayed initiation of treatment at levels as low as 250 mm^3 and even 200 mm^3. Today initial or modified antiviral treatments can be altered relative to CD4 T-helper cell counts depending on the viral load and its relative rate of increase.[31]

Currently, there are different classes of drugs used to treat HIV-infected persons. One major class prevents the virus from duplicating itself inside infected CD4 T-helper cells. A second major class blocks HIV virus entry into the cells. Combinations of drugs are taken, a treatment approach referred to as highly active antiretroviral therapy, or HAART. Since the introduction of HAART, death rates from AIDS have declined for patients who can stick to treatment regimens and tolerate the side effects of the drugs (see the box "From Fear to Hope, and Now Benign Neglect—AIDS in the News").

Drug Resistance in HIV Infection   Consistent with other pathogenic agents, both bacterial and viral, HIV has the ability to develop drug resistance during the course of HIV/AIDS treatment and might already be drug resistant at the time of transmission. This possibility first reached national attention in 2005 when a male in New York contracted an HIV infection that almost immediately was found to be resistant to each of the three drug protocols first tried. The person then progressed rapidly to AIDS. A similar situation developed in San Francisco shortly afterward.

In comparison to these apparently "wild" drug-resistant viruses, it is now recognized that in 10 to 20 percent of the persons under treatment, a resistant-related mutation will develop within a portion of the virus pool infecting their body. These drug-resistant viruses diminish the antiretroviral therapy's ability to sustain manageable levels of CD4 cells and to keep the viral load at the lowest levels possible. Unfortunately, the percentage of people who will develop an antiretroviral-resistant status is rising.

Today, trials are under way, using newly developed technology, to develop a test that would be much faster than previous tests in detecting the mutated viruses. When such a test becomes available, it will be possible to adjust drug cocktails early in the course of treatment, leading to a more therapeutically effective approach to HIV/AIDS treatment. In fact, a newly approved test that measures the levels of antiviral drugs in hair can be used to accurately predict the long-term success of the antiviral treatment being used.[32]

HIV/AIDS on the World Stage   In comparison to one and a half decades of media attention directed primarily to HIV/AIDS in the United States, attention through the late 1990s and thus far into the current decade is increasingly drawn toward the "AIDS Crisis" that is occurring in other areas of the world. Principal among these are Africa, the Indian subcontinent, and areas of Asia and Latin America. Figure 13-5 on page 375 depicts the strikingly disproportionate number of cases in sub-Saharan Africa compared to other areas of the world, and thus the urgency being expressed on the part of the international community, including the industrialized nations, world relief agencies, the pharmaceutical industry, as well as philanthropic foundations and celebrities.

The extent to which the international scope of the HIV/AIDS crisis can be ameliorated seems highly uncertain, at best. In the absence of a vaccine to immunize against HIV, and given the limited availability of effective prevention programs and the prohibitive cost of the antiretroviral medication required to manage declining health, time may be running out for those now infected and those likely to soon join them. On a somewhat brighter side, international pharmaceutical corporations have loosened their originally restrictive policies on the manufacturing and sale of antiretroviral agents, and are now allowing generic versions of some antiretroviral medications to be manufactured in the homelands of people in need.

On AIDS Day 2008, a small debate occurred challenging two aspects of the global AIDS epidemic (see Figure 13-5). The first challenge was directed toward concerns that data supporting the extent of the global scope of the epidemic have been overstated in recent years, given treatment and prevention efforts. The dire reality of Africa's HIV/AIDS epidemic status, however, remains undisputable. The second concern expressed was related to the $200 million spent annually by UNAIDS

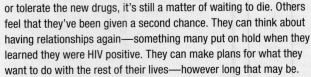
(the umbrella WHO organization) being misdirected by disregarding the treatment and prevention of pneumonia, a condition that kills more children annually than AIDS, measles, and malaria combined. Whether one or both of these challenges to the "hogging" of treatment and prevention resources are valid remains unclear but interesting to consider.

Prevention of HIV Infection   Can HIV infection be prevented? The answer is a definite yes. HIV infection rates on college campuses are considered low (approximately 0.2 percent), but students can be at risk. Every

person can take several steps to reduce the risk of contracting and transmitting HIV. All these steps require understanding one's behavior and the methods by which HIV can be transmitted. Some appropriate steps for college-aged people are abstinence, safer sex, sobriety, and communication with potential sexual partners. To ensure the greatest protection from HIV, one should abstain from sexual activity.

The box "Reducing Your Risk of Contracting HIV" lists recommendations for safer sex, sobriety, and the exchange of honest, accurate information about sexual histories.

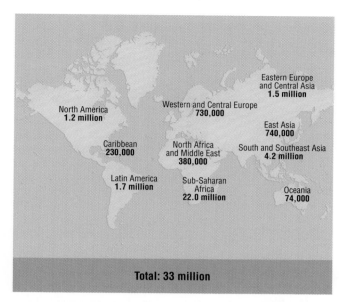

Figure 13-5 Estimated Number of Adults and Children Living with HIV at the End of 2007 For every person counted in these statistics, there is a face and a story. What are you doing to protect yourself from HIV/AIDS?

Source: Joint United Nations Programme on HIV/AIDS (UNAIDS) and World Health Organization (WHO). *2008 Report on the Global AIDS Epidemic.* Geneva: UNAIDS, www.unaids.org.

However, it is increasingly apparent that it is difficult (or nearly impossible) for people to remember and then apply these guidelines. Accordingly, the CDC is beginning a gradual "reversal of course" away from an emphasis on prevention toward a medical model based on testing, contact identification, and individual counsel. Initial testing, the beginning point of this model, will initially occur in homeless shelters, drug treatment

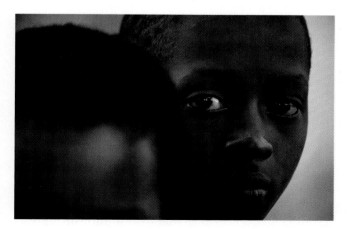

These children are among the thousands of orphaned children in Africa fending for themselves following the death of their parents from AIDS.

centers, jails, and in conjunction with prenatal care. A 2005 recommendation by the CDC added a new dimension to possible adoption of a medical model for HIV/AIDS prevention. This recommendation suggests that all persons potentially exposed to possible HIV infection through rape, accident (needle pricks or blood splatter to the eyes), occasional drug use, or unprotected intercourse be immediately started on a drug cocktail within 72 hours and continued for 28 days in hopes of preventing infection. At this point, the effectiveness of this prophylactic approach is based on positive results using primates and the monkey form of HIV.

 TALKING POINTS In a job interview with a representative from a large pharmaceutical company, you are asked about your feelings regarding the affordability of HIV/AIDS medications in third world countries. What would your response be?

Sexually Transmitted Diseases

Sexually transmitted diseases (STDs) were once called venereal diseases (for Venus, the Roman goddess of love). Today the term *venereal disease* has been superseded by the broader terms *sexually transmitted disease* or *sexually transmitted infections*. Despite preference some instructors might have for the new term (STI), your text will retain the older designation (STD), as it is the term used by the CDC (the terms are interchangeable). Experts currently emphasize the successful prevention and treatment of STDs rather than the ethics of sexuality. Thus one should consider the following points: (1) By age 25 years, approximately one-third of all adults will have contracted a sexually transmitted disease—most often chlamydia, herpes simplex, or human papillomavirus infection; (2) a person can have more than one STD at a time; (3) the symptoms of STDs can vary over time and from person to person; (4) the body develops little immunity for STDs; and (5) STDs can predispose people to additional health problems, including infertility, birth defects in their children, cancer, and long-term disability. In addition, the risk of HIV infection is higher when sexual partners are also infected with STDs. Most STDs are treated with an array of antibacterial, antiviral, and antifungal prescription medications. For more information on specific treatments, visit the Online Learning Center. The latest treatment guidelines, published by the CDC in 2006, serve as the basis of this online information. Updates are available at www.cdc.gov/std/treatment.

This section focuses on the STDs most frequently diagnosed among college students (chlamydia, gonorrhea, human papillomavirus infection, herpes simplex, syphilis, and pubic lice). Complete the Personal Assessment at the end of this chapter to determine your risk of contracting an STD.

Chlamydia (Nonspecific Urethritis)

Chlamydia is thought to be one of the most prevalent STDs in the United States today. Chlamydia infections occur an estimated 3 times more frequently than does gonorrhea and up to 10 times more frequently than syphilis. In 2007, 1,108,374 cases were reported by the CDC.[33] Because of its high prevalence in sexually active persons between 15 and 24 years of age (782,013 cases in 2007), they should be screened for chlamydia twice a year, even in the absence of symptoms. Because chlamydia frequently accompanies gonorrheal infections, a dual therapy is often appropriate when gonorrhea is found. Sexually active people in this age range should also be considered for routine screening, particularly if they have a history of multiple sex partners and have not practiced a form of barrier contraception (see Figure 13-6).

Chlamydia trachomatis is the bacterial agent that causes the chlamydia infection. Chlamydia is the most

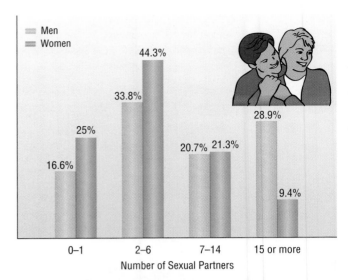

Figure 13-6 Number of Lifetime Sexual Partners among Adults Age 20–59 Years The fewer the number of partners you've had, the lower your risk of contracting HIV or an STD. How many partners have you had, and how accurate is your count? People may be less than truthful when answering sensitive questions. In addition, researchers have found that the methods used by men and women to calculate or estimate their number of sexual partners tend to lead to underestimation by women and overestimation by men.

Source: National Center for Health Statistics. 2007. Drug use and sexual behaviors reported by adults: United States, 1999–2002. *Advance Data from Vital and Health Statistics* No. 384. Lovers and liars: How many sex partners have you really had? University of Michigan News Service, February 13, 2006, www.umich.edu/news/index.html?Releases/2006/Feb06/r021306d.

common cause of nonspecific urethritis (NSU). NSU describes infections of the **urethra** and surrounding tissues that are not caused by the bacterium responsible for gonorrhea. About 80 percent of men with chlamydia display gonorrhea-like signs and symptoms, including painful urination and a whitish pus discharge from the penis. As in gonorrheal infections and many other STDs, most women report no overt signs or symptoms. A few women might exhibit a mild urethral discharge, painful urination, and swelling of vulval tissues. The recommended treatment for chlamydia is treatment with antibiotics (see the Online Learning Center for specifics). The infected person should carefully comply with instructions to abstain from sexual intercourse.

Both sexual partners should receive treatment to avoid the ping-pong effect—the back-and-forth reinfection that occurs among couples when only one partner receives treatment. Furthermore, as with other STDs, having chlamydia once does not effectively confer immunity.

Unresolved chlamydia can lead to the same negative health consequences that result from untreated gonorrheal infections. In men the pathogens can invade and damage the deeper reproductive structures (the prostate gland, seminal vesicles, and Cowper's glands). Sterility can result. The pathogens can spread further and produce joint problems (arthritis) and heart complications (damaged heart valves, blood vessels, and heart muscle tissue).

In women the pathogens enter the body through the urethra or the cervical area. If the invasion is not properly treated, it can reach the deeper pelvic structures, producing a syndrome called **pelvic inflammatory disease (PID).** The infection may attack the inner uterine wall (endometrium), the fallopian tubes, and any surrounding structures to produce this painful syndrome. A variety of further complications can result, including sterility, ectopic (tubal) pregnancies, and **peritonitis.** Infected women can transmit a chlamydia infection to the eyes and lungs of newborns during a vaginal birth. Detecting chlamydia and other NSUs early is of paramount concern for both men and women.

In 2003 and 2004 the Netherlands reported the first appearance of a particularly virulent form of chlamydia—*Lymphogranuloma venereum* (LGV)—which had been contracted by gay men. In comparison to the more commonly seen chlamydia, LGV presents with enlargement of lymph nodes in the groin area, genital or rectal ulceration, and anal spasms. Although cases are now being seen in this country, the prevalence of LGV is still speculative.

Human Papillomavirus

The appearance of another STD, **human papillomavirus (HPV),** is unwanted news. Because HPV infections are generally asymptomatic, the exact extent of the disease is unknown. A study of a group of sexually active college women found HPV infection in approximately 20 percent of the women. HPV-related changes to the cells of the cervix are found in nearly 5 percent of the Pap tests taken from women under age 30. Researchers currently believe that risk factors for HPV infection in women include (1) sexual activity before age 20, (2) intercourse with three or more partners before age 35, and (3) intercourse with a partner who has three or more partners. By 50 years of age, 80 percent of sexually active women will have contracted an HPV infection. The extent of HPV infection in men is even less clearly known, but it is probably widespread. It has even been suggested that virtually all sexually active persons will have acquired some form of HPV during their lifetime.

HPV infection is alarming because some of the nearly 100 strains of the virus are strongly associated with precancerous changes to cells lining the cervix, illustrating the importance of the new viral Pap-plus test (see Chapter 11). Additionally, visible genital warts (cauliflowerlike, raised, pinkish-white lesions) are associated with viral forms 6 and 11, while viral forms 16, 18, 31, 33, and 35 foster changes in other areas (Figure 13-7). Found most commonly on the penis, scrotum, labia,

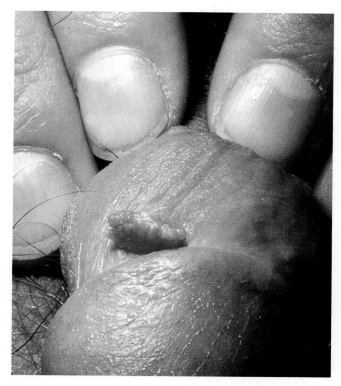

Figure 13-7 A Human Papillomavirus Infection (Genital Warts)

cervix, and around the anus, these lesions represent the most common symptomatic viral STD in this country. Although most genital wart colonies are small, they may become very large and block the anus or birth canal during pregnancy.

> ### Key Terms
>
> **sexually transmitted diseases (STDs)** Infectious diseases that are spread primarily through intimate sexual contact.
>
> **chlamydia** The most prevalent sexually transmitted disease; caused by a nongonococcal bacterium.
>
> **urethra** (yoo **ree** thra) The passageway through which urine leaves the urinary bladder.
>
> **pelvic inflammatory disease (PID)** An acute or chronic infection of the peritoneum or lining of the abdominopelvic cavity and fallopian tubes; associated with a variety of symptoms or none at all and a potential cause of sterility.
>
> **peritonitis** (pare it ton **eye** tis) Inflammation of the peritoneum, or lining of the abdominopelvic cavity.
>
> **human papillomavirus (HPV)** Sexually transmitted viruses, some of which are capable of causing precancerous changes in the cervix; causative agent for genital warts.

Treatment for HPV, including genital warts, may include patient-applied gels or creams or physician-administered cryotherapy, topical medication, or surgery. Regardless of treatment, however, the viral colonies will probably return. One should use condoms to attempt to prevent transmission of HPV.

As noted in Chapter 11, in conjunction with cervical cancer, a vaccine effective for HPV 6 and 11 (genital warts) and 16 and 18 (cervical cancer) has been approved for use by the FDA (Gardasil). The current recommendation calling for the inoculation of young women between the ages of 9 and 26 years, and older if just beginning sexual activity, is strongly encouraged by the health care community. The CDC recommends that the preferred (or most reasonable) age for receiving the initial vaccination is between ages 11 and 12. In states that are considering mandatory inoculation as a part of required school-based immunizations, controversy abounds. With approximately 7 percent of children sexually active by age 13, and nearly 25 percent by age 15, when is young too young? Some experts suggest that when young women clearly display signs of sexual maturation, including the onset of menstruation, then the inoculation is appropriate. The need for an eventual booster has not yet been determined, but current recommendations suggest a booster might be needed in about 10 years following initial vaccination to sustain an effective level of protection. By mid 2009, about 30 percent of young women aged 13 to 17 years had received the Gardasil vaccine (3 million out of 10 million girls in that age range).

Additional vaccines are under development, some intended for use in newly infected patients, some for long-established infections but before clear changes in the cervical-lining cells occur, and others for more advanced cervical cancer. Most of the last two classes of vaccines are for treatment rather than prevention of HPV infections.

Gonorrhea

Another extremely common (355,991 cases reported in 2007) STD, *gonorrhea* is caused by a bacterium (*N. gonorrhoea*).[33] The incidence of gonorrhea rose 18 percent between 1997 and 2001, perhaps, in part, because of decreasing fear of HIV/AIDS brought about by the effectiveness of the protease inhibitors being widely reported at that time. However, since 2001 the reported cases of gonorrhea have declined; but in 2005 a marked upturn was reported over the 2004 level, and by 2007 the level had increased by 4.9 percent over the 2005 level.[33,34]

In men this bacterial agent can produce a milky-white discharge from the penis, accompanied by painful urination. About 80 percent of men who contract gonorrhea report varying degrees of these symptoms. This figure is approximately reversed for women: only about 20 percent of women are symptomatic and thus report varying degrees of frequent, painful urination, with a slimy yellow-green discharge from the vagina or urethra. Oral sex with an infected partner can produce a gonorrheal infection of the throat (pharyngeal gonorrhea). Gonorrhea can also be transmitted to the rectal areas of both men and women.

An interesting finding relative to gonorrhea in adolescents suggests that the incidence of gonorrhea within the adolescent population correlated closely with the consumption of beer, suggesting that alcohol consumption fosters a higher level of high-risk sexual behavior, including earlier onset of sexual activity, an increased number of partners, and less selectivity in choosing those partners. With heavy consumption of beer on many college campuses, this finding does not bode well for the highly asymptomatic female population.

Physicians diagnose gonorrhea by culturing the bacteria. The only class of drugs recommended by the CDC for treatment of gonorrhea is the cephalosporins. Although prevalent in other areas of the world, drug-resistant strains are not extensive in the United States. However, a clear increase in drug-resistant strains has been reported along the West Coast, in various Pacific areas, such as Hawaii, other Pacific Islands, and Asia. Infected persons who might have contracted the disease while in these areas should report this information to their physicians. An alternative treatment plan for persons with drug-resistant strains of gonorrhea appears in the Online Learning Center. For the latest updates on treatments for gonorrhea, see the CDC website, www.cdc.gov/std.

Testing for gonorrhea is included as a part of prenatal care so that infections in mothers can be treated before they give birth. If the birth canal is infected, newborns can easily contract the infection in the mucous membranes of the eye.

Herpes Simplex

Public health officials think that the sexually transmitted genital herpes virus infection rivals chlamydia as the most prevalent STD. To date, about 45 million Americans have been diagnosed, although the asymptomatic (thus undiagnosed) population could increase this figure substantially. *Herpes* is really a family of more than 50 viruses, some of which produce recognized diseases in humans (chicken pox, shingles, mononucleosis, and others). One subgroup, called herpes simplex 1 virus (HSV-1), produces an infection called *labial herpes* (oral or lip herpes). Labial herpes produces common fever blisters or cold sores around the lips and oral cavity. Herpes simplex 2 virus (HSV-2) is a different strain that produces similar clumps of blisterlike lesions in the genital region (Figure 13-8). Laypeople call this second type of herpes the STD type, but both types produce

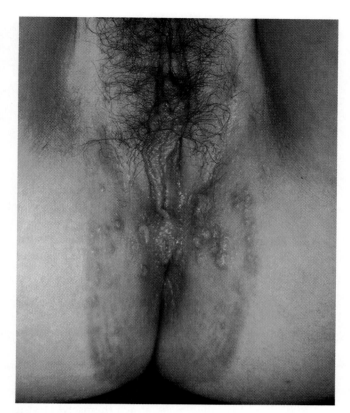

Figure 13-8 A Severe Herpes Infection

identical clinical pictures. About 5 to 30 percent of cases are caused by HSV-1. Oral-genital sexual practices most likely account for this crossover infection.

Herpes appears as a single sore or as a small cluster of blisterlike sores. These sores burn, itch, and (for some) become very painful. The infected person might also report swollen lymph glands, muscular aches and pains, and fever. Some patients feel weak and sleepy when they have blisters. The lesions may last from a few days to a few weeks. Viral shedding lasts a week on average; then the blisters begin scabbing, and new skin is formed. Even when the patient has become asymptomatic, viral transmission is still possible.

Herpes is an interesting virus for several reasons. It can lie dormant for long periods. For reasons not well understood but perhaps related to stress, diet, or overall health, the viral particles can be stimulated to travel along the nerve pathways to the skin and then create an active infection. Thus herpes can be considered a recurrent infection. Fortunately for most people, recurrent infections are less severe than the initial episode and do not last as long. Because herpes may occur at intervals following initial treatment with antivirals, two choices exist. One is to treat each recurrence as it arises (episodic recurrent treatment), and the second is to attempt to suppress recurrence through continuous use of medication (daily suppressive therapy). Additionally, physicians

may recommend other medications for relief of various symptoms. Visit the Online Learning Center for more information about treatment. Genital herpes is almost always diagnosed through a clinical examination.

At this time a much anticipated Phase III trial is under way testing new vaccines manufactured by GlaxoSmithKline Biologicals. Earlier, but in much smaller trials, it was found that the vaccine was effective in providing protection for about 70 percent of the female subjects but was almost completely ineffective for males. The current trial, still ongoing, involves two versions of the vaccine, one version intended to be a prophylactic (preventive) vaccine and the other a therapeutic (treatment) vaccine. Most likely the vaccine technology will employ genetically altered viruses in which genes controlling replication will have been removed or altered in a manner preventing viral replication.

Currently, the best method of preventing herpes infection is to avoid all direct contact with a person who has an active infection. Do not kiss someone with a fever blister—or let them kiss you (or your children) if they have an active lesion. Do not share drinking glasses or eating utensils. Check your partner's genitals. Do not have intimate sexual contact with someone who displays the blisterlike clusters or rash. Condoms are only marginally helpful and cannot protect against lesions on the female vulva or the lower abdominal area of men. Be careful not to infect yourself by touching a blister and then touching any other part of your body.

Although there is currently no cure for HSV-2, antiviral medication can be effectively employed. Intended as prophylactic medications (to be taken daily), these antiviral medications do reduce the number and duration of viral shedding episodes. Certainly, the sexual partners of persons infected with HSV-2 need to be fully aware and involved in the management of this sexually transmitted infection. Infected persons can best accomplish this communication by becoming educated about their condition, determining the appropriate point in the relationship to introduce this important information, answering in an honest manner questions asked by the new partner, and finally, by building a mutually agreed-upon plan regarding all aspects of sexual intimacy during periods of potential disease transmission.

Newborn babies are especially susceptible to the virus if they come into contact with an active lesion during birth. Newborns have not developed the defense capabilities to resist the invasion. They can quickly develop

---

Key Terms

shingles Painful fluid-filled skin eruptions along underlying sensory nerve pathways—caused by reactivation of once-sequestered herpes zoster (chicken pox) virus.

a systemic (general) infection (neonatal herpes) that is often fatal or local infections that produce permanent brain damage or blindness. Fortunately, most of these problems can be prevented through proper prenatal care. A cesarean delivery can be performed if viral particles might be present at birth, although this is done less often today than in the past.

Syphilis

Syphilis is a serious disease that, left untreated, can cause death. The chance of contracting syphilis during a single sexual encounter with an infected partner is about 30 percent. Syphilis takes a well-established course after it is contracted. The syphilis bacterium, *Treponema pallidum,* is a spirochete. It is transmitted from an infected person to a new host through intimate contact. Moist, warm tissue, such as that lining the reproductive, urinary, and digestive tracts, offers an ideal environment for the agent.

If contracted during an episode of unprotected coitus, syphilis incubates without symptoms for 10 to 90 days, followed by the characteristic primary stage of the disease, which lasts 1 to 5 weeks. A small, raised, painless sore called a chancre forms. This highly infectious lesion is not easily identified in 90 percent of women and 50 percent of men; thus these people generally do not seek treatment. The chancre heals in 4 to 8 weeks.

The extremely contagious secondary stage of the disease occurs 6 to 12 weeks after initial infection. The infectious agents are now systemic, so symptoms may include a generalized body rash, a sore throat, or a patchy loss of hair. A blood test (VDRL) will be positive, and treatment can be effectively administered. If untreated, the second stage subsides within 2 to 6 weeks. A pregnant woman can easily transmit syphilis to her fetus during this stage. Congenital syphilis often results in stillbirth or an infant born with a variety of life-threatening complications. Early treatment of infected pregnant women can prevent congenital syphilis.

After the secondary stage subsides, an extended period of noninfectiousness occurs. The infectious agents remain dormant within the body cells, and the infected person displays few clinical signs during this state. This latent stage of 15 to 30 years was, in the past, often unrecognized, thus masking the relationship between contraction of disease and the earlier clinical stage, and the latter terminal manifestation of the untreated disease was difficult to connect. During late-stage syphilis, tissue damage is profound and irreversible. The person suffers damage to the cardiovascular system, central nervous system, eyes, and skin, and death from the effects of the disease is likely.

In 1950, a record 217,558 cases of syphilis were reported in this country. The number of cases then fell steadily to fewer than 80,000 cases in 1980. From 1980 through 1990 the incidence climbed, reaching nearly 140,000 cases in 1990. Another decline then began, and in 1993 the number of cases dropped to 101,259. In 2000 the CDC reported that syphilis had fallen to the lowest level (5,972) in 42 years. By 2005, however, reported cases of primary syphilis had risen to 8,724. In 2007, the CDC reported 10,768 new cases of syphilis.[34]

Whether the upward trend in the number of reported cases of primary syphilis continues remains to be seen. As has been true for most of the last few decades, a high percentage of cases have been associated with HIV infections, largely among gay men in several larger cities. Observers have noted an alarming increase in infant syphilis in children born to mothers who use drugs and support their habit through sexual activity. For specific information on the antibiotics used in the treatment of syphilis, visit the Online Learning Center.

Pubic Lice

Three types of lice infect humans: the head louse, the body louse, and the pubic louse all feed on the blood of the host. Except for the relatively uncommon body louse, these tiny insects do not carry diseases. They are, however, very annoying.

Pubic lice, also called *crabs,* attach themselves to the base of the pubic hairs, where they live and lay their eggs (nits). These eggs move into a larval stage after one week; after two more weeks, they develop into mature adult crab lice. People usually notice they have a pubic lice infestation when they suffer intense itching in the genital region. Prescription and OTC creams, lotions, and shampoos are usually effective in killing both the lice and their eggs, although some reports suggest that lice are becoming resistant to OTC treatments.

Lice are not transmitted exclusively through sexual contact but also by contact with contaminated bedsheets and clothes. If you develop a pubic lice infestation, you must thoroughly treat yourself, your clothes, your sheets, and your furniture. Listed following are specific steps to be taken to eradicate pubic lice:[35]

- Wash the infested area; towel dry.

- Follow label directions in using lice medications. Dry with clean towel.

- Following application of lice medications, remove nits from hair shaft with fingernails.

- Put on clean underwear and clothing after treatment.

- Machine wash all clothing and bedding used by the infected person during the 2–3 days before treatment (use the hot wash cycle for at least 20 minutes).

- Dry-clean clothing that is not washable. Store in plastic bags for two weeks

- Inform sexual partners that they are at risk of infestation, and should be examined and treated.

- Do not have sex until treatment is completed.
- Repeat treatment in 9–10 days if lice are still found.

Vaginal Infections

Three common pathogens produce uncomfortable *vaginal infections*. The first is the yeast or fungus pathogen *Candida (Monilia) albicans,* which produces the yeast infection often called *thrush*. These organisms, commonly found in the vagina, seem to multiply rapidly when some unusual stressor (pregnancy, use of birth control pills or antibiotics, diabetes) affects a woman's body. This infection, now called *vulvovaginal candidiasis (VVC),* is signaled by a white- or cream-colored vaginal discharge that resembles cottage cheese. Vaginal itching and vulvar swelling are also commonly reported. Current treatment is based on the use of one of several prescription and OTC azole drugs. For women who have recurrent VVC, some degree of prophylactic suppression of candidiasis seems possible. As has been recommended for all STDs discussed here, the Online Learning Center provides an extensive listing of recommended and alternative prescription-based medications now used in the treatment of STDs. When OTC medications exist for use in treating sexually transmitted infections, such as those used with vaginal infections, they too are listed.

Men rarely report this monilial infection, although some may report mildly painful urination or a barely noticeable discharge at the urethral opening or beneath the foreskin of the penis.

A second type of sexually transmitted vaginal infection is somewhat less easily described in terms of a clearly defined pathogenic agent. Rather, *bacterial vaginosis (BV)* reflects an imbalance in the normal relationships among all vaginal flora, leading to some bacterial forms gaining a level of pathogenicity sufficient to allow the formation of abnormal symptoms. Included among these signs of microbial imbalance are abnormal vaginal discharge, a strong fishlike odor (most often following intercourse), burning during urination, and clinical indicators that can be ascertained by visual inspection by a physician and laboratory test results.[36]

BV has been labeled an STD because it is rarely seen in women who are celibate or who have had a very limited number of sexual partners. Increased risk is associated with having a new sexual partner, having had multiple sexual partners, having used an intrauterine device (IUD), and frequent douching. Directly or indirectly, having BV seems to increase the risk of contracting HIV, contracting other STDs, and developing pelvic inflammatory disease (PID). Bacterial vaginosis is usually treated with antibiotics (see the Online Learning Center). In some cases, the condition resolves itself with changes in sexual practices.

The protozoan *Trichomonas vaginalis,* a third STD-related pathogenic agent, also produces a vaginal infection. This parasite can be transmitted through sexual intercourse or by contact with contaminated (often damp) objects, such as towels, clothing, or toilet seats, that may contain some vaginal discharge. In women, this infection, called *trichomoniasis,* or "trich," produces a foamy, yellow-green, foul-smelling discharge that may be accompanied by itching, swelling, and painful urination. Although topically applied treatments with limited effectiveness for trichomoniasis are available, only one highly effective oral medication is currently on the market. Men infrequently contract trichomoniasis but may harbor the organisms without realizing it. They also should be treated to minimize reinfection of partners.

The vagina is warm, dark, and moist, an ideal breeding environment for a variety of organisms. Unfortunately, some highly promoted commercial products seem to increase the incidence of vaginal infections. Among these are tight panty hose (without cotton panels), which tend to increase the vaginal temperature, and commercial vaginal douches, which can alter the acidic level of the vagina. Both of these products might promote infections. Avoiding public bathrooms when possible is also a good practice. Of course, if you notice any unusual discharge from the vagina, you should report this to your physician.

Cystitis and Urethritis

Cystitis, an infection of the urinary bladder, and urethritis, an infection of the urethra, occasionally can be caused by a sexually transmitted organism. Such infections can also be caused by the organisms that cause vaginitis and organisms found in the intestinal tract. A culture is required to identify the specific pathogen associated with a particular case of cystitis or urethritis. The symptoms are pain when urinating, the need to urinate frequently, a dull aching pain above the pubic bone, and the passing of blood-streaked urine.

Physicians can easily treat cystitis and urethritis with antibiotics when the specific organism has been identified. The drug Monurol, which requires only a single dose, has proved effective. Few complications result from infections that are treated promptly. If cystitis or urethritis is left untreated, the infectious agent could move upward in the urinary system and infect the ureters and kidneys. These upper-urinary-tract infections are more serious and require more extensive evaluation and aggressive treatment. Therefore one should obtain medical care immediately upon noticing symptoms.

Urinary tract infections in men, not related to the gonorrhea bacterium, are extremely common. These cases of nongonococcal urethritis (NGU) are sexually transmitted in predictable ways, with a discharge from the penis and pain on urination being the symptoms that bring men into treatment. Recently it was established that NGU is also transmitted in conjunction with oral sex, when the recipient's penis is exposed to infectious agents from his partner.[37]

A study involving urinary tract infections in mice, whose urinary tract infections are virtually identical to those in humans, demonstrated that the bacteria involved often avoid complete antibiotic elimination. This occurs when the bacteria clump into pods that are then covered by a "bio-film" produced by the organisms. The film retards further antibody effectiveness, allowing the infection to be re-established when antibiotics have been cleared from the body.

Preventing cystitis and urethritis depends to some degree on the source of the infectious agent. One can generally reduce the incidence of infection by urinating completely (to fully empty the urinary bladder), particularly following intercourse, and by drinking ample fluids to flush the urinary tract. Drinking cranberry juice has been found to reduce urinary tract infections. Prevention of urinary tract infections cannot be disregarded, from both medical and cost perspectives. As noted, untreated cystitis and urethritis can be the basis of serious damage to the kidneys. These two infections combined are the second greatest cause of antibiotic use—which is both costly and increasingly losing effectiveness.

Sexually Transmitted Diseases, Health, Role Fulfillment, and a Sense of Well-Being

In recalling Figure 1-2 on page 15 in which a more broadly based perception of health was depicted, it should be easy to understand that a sexually transmitted disease (both acute and chronic) can interfere with the competent fulfillment of role expectations. Particularly for those who "push the sexual envelope" in terms of the number and types of partners, various types and degrees of impairment may become hindrances to undertaking the daily tasks that are demanded by various roles and may eventually compromise the degree to which self-identity, emotional independence, social interconnectivity, and the assumption of responsibility for the well-being of self and others can be accomplished. If health is, as your text contends, a reflection of your resourcefulness for living life well, then STDs contribute nothing that is positive to that list.

Taking Charge of Your Health

- Since microorganisms develop resistance to antibiotics, continue taking all such medications until gone, even when the symptoms of the infection have subsided.

- Check your current immunization status to make sure you are protected against preventable infectious diseases.

- If you are a parent, take your children to receive their recommended immunizations as necessary.

- Because of the possibility of contracting HIV/AIDS and sexually transmitted diseases, incorporate disease prevention into all of your sexual activities.

- Use the Personal Assessment at the end of this chapter to determine your risk of contracting a sexually transmitted disease.

- If you have ever engaged in high-risk sexual behavior, get tested for HIV.

SUMMARY

- A variety of pathogenic agents are responsible for infectious conditions.
- A chain of infection with six potential links characterizes every infectious condition.
- One can acquire immunity for some diseases through both natural and artificial means. Children and adults should be immunized according to a schedule.
- The immune system's response to infection relies on cellular, chemical, and humoral elements.
- Nosocomial infections are infections that develop in conjunction with the delivery of health care services, most often in hospitals and nursing homes.
- The common cold and influenza produce many similar symptoms but differ in their infectious agents, incubation period, prevention, and treatment. Avian (bird) flu may be the basis of the next influenza pandemic and novel H1N1 influenza has already reached a pandemic level.
- Tuberculosis and pneumonia are potentially fatal infections of the respiratory system.
- Bacterial meningitis, a potentially fatal infection of the linings that cover the brain, is of increasing concern on college campuses.
- Hantavirus pulmonary syndrome is caused by a virus carried by ticks; human-to-human transmission has also been reported.
- Hepatitis B (serum hepatitis) is a viral infectious condition that produces serious liver damage. Other varieties are hepatitis A, C, D, and E.

- HIV/AIDS is a widespread, incurable viral disease transmitted through sexual activity, through intravenous drug use, in infected blood products, or across the placenta during pregnancy.

- There are a variety of sexually transmitted diseases, many of which do not produce symptoms in most infected women and many infected men.

REVIEW QUESTIONS

1. Describe the six links in the chain of infection.
2. What are the two principal cellular/chemical components of the immune system, and how do they cooperate to protect the body from infectious agents, foreign protein, and abnormal cells?
3. What is a nosocomial infection, and in what settings are nosocomial infections most likely to develop?
4. How are the common cold and influenza similar? How do they differ in their causative agents, incubation period, prevention, and treatment?
5. Why is bacterial meningitis of greater concern on the college campus than elsewhere?
6. Why is outdoor activity a risk factor for contracting Lyme disease?

7. What role do birds play in the transmission of the West Nile virus? What insect is the vector?
8. How is hepatitis B transmitted, and which occupational group is at greatest risk of contracting this infection? How do forms A, C, D, and E compare with hepatitis B?
9. How is HIV transmitted? How are HIV/AIDS currently treated, and how effective is the treatment? In what areas of the world does the HIV/AIDS epidemic seem virtually unchecked?
10. Why are women more often asymptomatic for STDs than men?

ANSWERS TO THE "WHAT DO YOU KNOW?" QUIZ

1. True   2. False   3. False   4. False   5. False   6. True   7. True

Visit the Online Learning Center (**www.mhhe.com/payne11e**), where you will find tools to help you improve your grade including practice quizzes, key terms flashcards, audio chapter summaries for your MP3 player, and many other study aids.

SOURCE NOTES

1. Hamann B. *Disease Identification, Prevention, and Control* (3rd ed.). New York: McGraw-Hill, 2007.
2. Salidin KS. *Anatomy and Physiology: Unity of Form and Function.* (5th ed.). New York: McGraw-Hill, 2010.
3. *Understanding the Immune System: How It Works.* National Institute of Allergy and Infectious Disease, National Cancer Institute. NIH Publication No. 03-5423. September 2003. www.niaid.nih.gov/publications/immune/the_immune_system.pdf.
4. Vander A, Sherman J, Luciano D. *Human Physiology: The Mechanisms of Body Function* (11th ed.). New York: McGraw-Hill, 2008.
5. Thornley I, et al. Private Cord Blood Banking: Experiences and Views of Pediatric Hematopoietic Cell Transplantation Physicians. *Pediatrics,* 123(3), 1011–1017, March 2009.
6. Tanne JH. Obama Reverses US Federal Funding on Stem Cell Research. *BMJ,* 338, b1011, doi: 10.1136/bmj.b1011, March 2009.
7. Vaccine Adverse Event Reporting System (VAERS). 2008. Department of Health and Human Services. Food and Drug Administration. Centers for Disease Control and Prevention. www.vaers.hhs.gov
8. *FDA Recommends the Over-the-Counter Cough and Cold Products Not Be Used for Infants and Children Under 2 Years of Age.* Public Health Advisory. U.S. Food and Drug Administration. Department of Health and Human Services. January 17, 2008 (updated October 10).
9. Vernacchio L, et al. Pseudoephedrine Use Among US Children, 1999–2006: Results from the Slone Survey. *Pediatrics,* 122(6), 1299–1304, December 2008.
10. Ball TM, et al. Influence of Attendance at Day Care on the Common Cold from Birth Through 13 Years of Age. *Archives of Pediatrics & Adolescent Medicine,* 156(2), 121–126, 2002.
11. Mattews CE, et al. Moderate to Vigorous Physical Activity and Risk of Upper-Respiratory-Tract Infections. 2002. *Clinical Journal of Sport Medicine,* 34(8), 1242–1248, 2002.
12. Centers for Disease Control and Prevention. Novel H1N1 Flu (Swine Flu) and You. August 5, 2009. www.cdc.gov/h1n1flu/ga.htm
13. Trends in Tuberculosis: United States: 2008. *Morbidity and Mortality Weekly Report,* 58(10), March 20, 2009.
14. Extensively Drug-Resistant Tuberculosis—United States, 1993–2006. *Morbidity and Mortality Weekly Report,* 56(11), 250–253, March 23, 2007.
15. Kariminia A, et al. Comparison of QuantiFERON TB-G to TST for Detecting Latent Tuberculosis Infection in a High-Incidence Area Containing BCG-Vaccinated Population. *Journal of Evaluation in Clinical Practice,* 15(1), 148–151, February 2009.
16. *Streptococcus pneumoniae disease.* Division of Bacterial and Myocotic Diseases. CDC. August 11, 2005. www.cdc.gov.sjlibrary .org/ncidod/dbmd/diseaseinfo/streppneum_t.htm.
17. Feder HM, et al. A Critical Appraisal of "Chronic-Lyme Disease." *New England Journal of Medicine,* 357, 1422–1430, October 4, 2007.
18. FDA News. *FDA Warns Consumers and Health Care Providers Not to Use Bismacine, Also Known as Chromacine.* July 21, 2006. www.fda .gov/bbs/topics/NEWS/2006/NEW01415.html.
19. Brillman J, et al. Update on Emerging Infections from the Centers for Disease Control and Prevention. *Annals of Emergency Medicine,* 48(5), 594–595, November 2006.
20. West Nile Virus Activity—United States, 2007. *Morbidity and Mortality Weekly Report,* 57(26), 720–723, July 4, 2008.
21. CDC. *Hepatitis: A Fact Sheet,* October 4, 2006. www.cdc.gov/hepatitis.

22. Irshad M, et al. Hepatitis C Virus (HCV): A Review of Immunological Aspects. *International Reviews of Immunology,* 27(6), 497–517, 2008.
23. Centers for Disease Control and Prevention. Estimated Numbers of AIDS Cases, by Year of Diagnosis and Selected Characteristics, 2003–2007 and Cumulative—United States and Dependent Areas. (Table 4.) *HIV/AIDS Surveillance Report.* (Last Revised February 18, 2009). www.cdc.gov/hiv/topics/surveillance/resources/reports/2007report/table4.htm
24. Centers for Disease Control and Prevention. Estimated Numbers of Deaths of Persons with AIDS by Year of Death and Selected Characteristics, 2003–2007 and Cumulative—United States and Dependent Areas. (Table 8.) *HIV/AIDS Surveillance Report.* (Last Revised February 18, 2009). www.cdc.gov/hiv/topics/surveillance/resources/reports/2007report/table8.htm
25. United States—Race and Ethnicity. American Fact Finder. 2007. U.S. Census Bureau. www.factfinder.census.gov/servlet/ACSSAFFPeople?_submenuId_10&_see=on
26. *U.S. Hispanic Population Surpasses 45 Million Now 15 Percent of Total.* U.S. Census Bureau News. US Department of Commerce. May 1, 2008. www.census.gov/Press-Release/www/releses/archives/population/011910.html
27. Gebo K, et al Contemporary Costs of HIV Health Care in the HAART era. Program and abstracts of the 13 Conference on retroviruses and opportunistic infections. February 5–8, 2006, Denver, Abstract 537.
28. Financing HIV/AIDS Care: A Quilt with Many Holes. *HIV/AIDS Policy Issue Brief.* The Henry Kaiser Family Foundation. May 2008, p. 8. www.kff.org
29. Centers for Disease Control and Prevention. *Estimated Numbers of Persons Living with HIV/AIDS at the End of 2007, by Race/Ethnicity and Transmission Category—34 States with Confidential Name-Based HIV Infection Reporting* (Table 10). *HIV/AIDS Surveillance Report.* (Last Revised February 18, 2009).
30. Qaseem A, et al. Screening for HIV in Health Care Settings: A Guidance Statement from the American College of Physicians. *Annals of Internal Medicine,* 150(2), 1256, January 20, 2009.
31. CDC Department of Health and Human Services. *Summary: CDC Expert Consultation on the Effect of Antiretroviral Therapy on Risk of Sexual Transmission and HIV Infection and Superinfection.* January 9, 2009. www.cdc.gov/hiv/topics/resources/other/arv-therapy-risk.htm
32. Gandhi M, et al. Protease Inhibitor Levels in Hair Strongly Predict Virologic Response in Treatment. *AIDS,* 23(4), 471–478, February 20, 2009.
33. Centers for Disease Control and Prevention. Cases of Sexually Transmitted Diseases Reported by State Health Departments and Rates per 100,000 Population: 1941–2007 (Table 1). *STD Surveillance 2007.* January 13, 2009.
34. Centers for Disease Control and Prevention. Cases of Sexually Transmitted Diseases Reported by State Health Departments and Rates per 100,000 Population: 1941–2007 (Table 10). *STD Surveillance 2007.* January 13, 2009.
35. Centers for Desease Control and Prevention. *Fact Sheet: Lice.* Division of Parasitic Diseases. May 2008. www.cdc.gov/lice.html
36. *Fact Sheet: Bacterial Vaginosis.* Division of STD Prevention. Centers for Disease Control and Prevention. 2007. www.cdc.gov/std/healthcomm/fact_sheets.htm
37. Handsfield H. Nongonococcal Urethritis: A Few Answers but Mostly Questions. *Journal of Infectious Diseases,* 193 (3), 333–335, February 1, 2006.

Personal Assessment

What is your risk of contracting a sexually transmitted disease?

A variety of factors interact to determine your risk of contracting a sexually transmitted disease (STD). This inventory is intended to provide you with an estimate of your level of risk.

Circle the number in each row that best characterizes you. Enter that number on the line at the end of the row (points). After assigning yourself a number in each row, total the numbers appearing in the points column. Your total points will allow you to interpret your risk for contracting an STD.

Age

						Points
1	3	4	5	3	2	_____
0–9	10–14	15–19	20–29	30–34	35+	

Sexual Practices

0	1	2	4	6	8	_____
Never engage in sex	One sex partner	One sex partner but that person has had other partners	Two to five sex partners	Five to ten sex partners	Ten or more sex partners	

Sexual Attitudes

0	1	8	1	7	8	_____
Will not engage in nonmarital sex	Premarital sex is okay if it is with future spouse	Any kind of premarital sex is okay	Extramarital sex is not for me	Extramarital sex is okay	Believe in complete sexual freedom	

Attitudes toward Contraception

1	1	6	5	4	8	_____
Would use condom to prevent pregnancy	Would use condom to prevent STDs	Would never use a condom	Would use the birth control pill	Would use other contraceptive measure	Would not use anything	

Attitudes toward STD

3	3	4	6	6	6	_____
Am not sexually active so I do not worry	Would be able to talk about STD with my partner	Would check out an infection to be sure	Would be afraid to check out an infection	Can't even talk about an infection	STDs are no problem—easily cured	

YOUR TOTAL POINTS _____

Interpretation

5–8—Your risk is well below average
9–13—Your risk is below average
14–17—Your risk is at or near average
18–21—Your risk is moderately high
22+—Your risk is high

TO CARRY THIS FURTHER . . .

Having taken this Personal Assessment, were you surprised at your level of risk? What is the primary reason for this level? How concerned are you and your classmates and friends about contracting an STD?

Source: Centers for Disease Control and Prevention.

part five

Sexuality and Reproduction

Sexuality is an important part of our being. It colors the way we interact with the world around us and affects our goals, relationships, and roles in society.

1. **Physical Dimension**
   Sexuality is closely related to the physical dimension of health. For example, our bodies mature at puberty, we respond to sexual arousal, we make choices about contraception and pregnancy, and we adjust our sexual behavior as we age. Sexual experiences and relationships can be very complex and demanding because they are fueled by energy and time. They are enhanced when the body is well maintained, rested, and relatively free from illness.

2. **Emotional Dimension**
   One of the most stressful aspects of life is sexual intimacy. Feelings about your own sexual behavior can range from exhilaration to ambivalence to depression. Being comfortable with your sexuality comes from being guided by your core values, knowing how to express your sexual feelings openly, being able to set limits when appropriate, and understanding how to communicate effectively with your partner.

3. **Social Dimension**
   Because sexuality often involves interaction with others, the development of social skills in this area is imperative. For many, dating is an excellent arena in which to establish specific social skills. As a relationship becomes more serious, communication skills will grow. These skills are important factors in the process of mate selection and marriage for those who choose this path.

4. **Intellectual Dimension**
   As a relationship matures, opportunities abound for contemplation, analysis, and reflection. You may have to sort through your feelings, examine your values, and use lessons from past experiences as you take part in this process of introspection. You will also draw on your intellectual resources as you learn about reproductive anatomy, fertility, sexual response, contraception, and birth.

5. **Spiritual Dimension**
   As an intimate relationship progresses, you may have to explore your feelings about your sense of morality, the appropriateness of premarital sex, or the value of fidelity in a marriage or other long-term committed relationship. Dating, courtship, and particularly marriage offer opportunities to enhance your spirituality by extending sympathy, support, and love to another person. Some people even find the sexual act itself to be a way of expressing their spirituality.

6. **Occupational Dimension**
   Decisions about reproduction can have a significant effect on your occupational dimension of health. Women who are pregnant may have to work even when they are not feeling well. Then they must decide how much time to take off work after the child is born. They and their partners must also make difficult choices about long-term child care arrangements. The decisions they make will affect their occupational satisfaction and sense of fulfillment.

Exploring the Origins of Sexuality

What Do You Know About the Origins of Sexuality?

1. A fertilized ovum with the sex chromosomes XX is a biological male. True or False?

2. One's sexuality is based upon both biological and psychosocial factors. True or False?

3. Both women and men have seminal vesicles. True or False?

4. Most women experience very similar menstrual cycles. True or False?

5. The release of luteinizing hormone (LH) causes ovulation to take place. True or False?

6. Hormone replacement therapy (HRT) reduces cardiovascular risks. True or False?

7. PMS tends to occur in women in the days just before menstruation. True or False?

Check your answers at the end of the chapter.

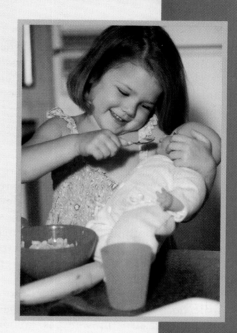

Early in this new millennium, we have reached a better understanding of both the biological and psychosocial factors that contribute to the complex expression of our sexuality. As a society, we are now inclined to view human behavior in terms of a complex script written on the basis of both biology and conditioning.

Reflecting this understanding is the way in which we use the words *male* and *female* to refer to the biological roots of our sexuality and the words *man* and *woman* to refer to the psychosocial roots of our sexuality. In this chapter, we explore human sexuality as it relates to the dynamic interplay of the biological and psychosocial bases that form our masculinity or femininity.

Biological Bases of Human Sexuality

Within a few seconds after the birth of a baby, someone (a doctor, nurse, or parent) emphatically labels the child: "It's a boy," or "It's a girl." For the parents and society as a whole, the child's biological sexuality is being displayed and identified. Another female or male enters the world.

Genetic Basis

At the moment of conception, a Y-bearing or an X-bearing sperm cell joins with the X-bearing ovum to establish the true basis of biological sexuality.[1] A fertilized ovum with sex chromosomes XX is biologically female, whereas a fertilized ovum bearing the XY sex chromosomes is biologically male. Genetics forms the most basic level of an individual's biological sexuality.

Gonadal Basis

The gonadal basis for biological sexuality refers to the growing embryo's development of *gonads*.[2] Male embryos develop testes about the 7th week after conception, and female embryos develop ovaries about the 12th week after conception.

Structural Development

The development of male or female reproductive structures is initially determined by the presence or absence of hormones produced by the developing testes— androgens and müllerian inhibiting substance (MIS). With these hormones present, the male embryo starts to develop male reproductive structures (penis, scrotum, vasa deferens, seminal vesicles, prostate gland, and Cowper's glands).

Because the female embryo is not exposed to these male hormones, it develops the characteristic female reproductive structures: uterus, fallopian tubes, vagina, labia, and clitoris.

Key Terms

nocturnal emission Ejaculation that occurs during sleep; "wet dream."

menopause Decline and eventual cessation of hormone production by the female reproductive system.

spermatogenesis (sper **mat** oh **jen** uh sis) The process of sperm production.

psychosocial sexuality Masculine and feminine aspects of sexuality.

gender General term reflecting a biological basis of sexuality; the male gender or the female gender.

gender identity Recognition of one's gender.

gender preference Emotional and intellectual acceptance of one's own gender.

Biological Sexuality and the Childhood Years

The growth and the development of the child in terms of reproductive organs and physiological processes have traditionally been thought to be "latent" during the childhood years. However, a gradual degree of growth occurs in both girls and boys. The reproductive organs, however, undergo faster growth at the onset of puberty and achieve their adult size and capabilities shortly thereafter.

Puberty

The entry into puberty is a gradual maturing process for young girls and boys. For young girls, the onset of menstruation, called *menarche,* occurs at about age 12 or 13 but may come somewhat earlier or later.[3] Early menstrual cycles tend to be anovulatory (ovulation does not occur). Menarche is usually preceded by a growth spurt that includes the budding of breasts and the growth of pubic and underarm hair.[4]

Young males follow a similar pattern of maturation, including a growth spurt followed by a gradual sexual maturity. However, this process takes place about 2 years later than it does in young females. Genital enlargement, underarm and pubic hair growth, and a lowering of the voice commonly occur. The male's first ejaculation is generally experienced by the age of 14, most commonly through **nocturnal emission** or masturbation. For many young boys, fully mature sperm do not develop until about age 15.

Reproductive capability declines only gradually over the course of the adult years. In the woman, however, the onset of **menopause** signals a more direct turning off of the reproductive system than is the case for the male adult. By the early to mid-50s, virtually all women have entered a postmenopausal period, but for men, relatively high-level **spermatogenesis** may continue for a decade or two.[4]

The story of sexual maturation and reproductive maturity cannot, however, be solely focused on the changes that take place in the body. Now we will discuss the psychosocial processes that accompany the biological changes.

 TALKING POINTS Your 12-year-old son comes to you and says that all of his male friends are starting to grow facial hair. He is worried that his own beard will never begin. What could you say to him that could ease his fears?

Psychosocial Bases of Human Sexuality

If you visualized growth and development of sexuality as a ladder (Figure 14-1), one vertical rail of the ladder would represent our biological sexuality. Arising at various points

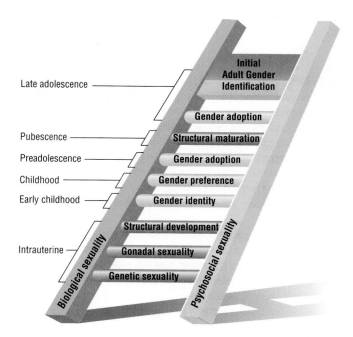

Figure 14-1 Growth and Development of Sexuality Our sexuality develops through biological and psychosocial stages.

Late adolescence — Initial Adult Gender Identification

Gender adoption

Pubescence — Structural maturation

Preadolescence — Gender adoption

Childhood — Gender preference

Early childhood — Gender identity

Structural development

Gonadal sexuality

Intrauterine — Genetic sexuality

Biological sexuality / Psychosocial sexuality

---

along this rail would be rungs representing the sequential unfolding of the genetic, gonadal, and structural components. These biological bases of our sexuality can be considered the "hardwired" parts of our sexuality. They are rooted in the linkages of our parents' genetic backgrounds. These are the parts of our sexuality over which we have little control.

Because humans, more so than any other life form, can rise above a life centered on reproduction, we have a second dimension or rail to our sexuality—our **psychosocial sexuality.** The reason we possess the ability to be more than reproductive beings is a question for the theologian or the philosopher. We are considerably more complex than the hardwired functions determined by biology. The process that transforms a male into a man and a female into a woman begins at birth and continues to influence us throughout the course of our lives.

It is during this transformation into a man or woman that we humans have some ability to influence our gender development. Here is where we occasionally are able to make decisions that influence both the way we view ourselves as men or women and the way we are viewed as men or women by others. This is the part of our sexuality that is not completely hardwired by our genetic background.

Gender Identity

Although expectant parents may prefer to have a child of a particular **gender,** they frequently must wait until the birth of the baby to have their question answered.

External genitals "cast the die," and femininity or masculinity begins to receive its traditional reinforcement by the parents and society in general. By the eighteenth month, typical children have both the language and the insight to correctly identify their gender. They have established a **gender identity.**[4] The first rung rising from the psychosocial rail of the ladder has been climbed.

Gender Preference

During the preschool years, children receive the second component of the scripting required for the full development of psychosocial sexuality—**gender preference.** Gender preference refers to the emotional and intellectual acceptance of one's birth gender. Reaching this rung on the psychosocial rail of the ladder takes place during the preschool years, when nearly every boy prefers being a boy and nearly every girl prefers being a girl.

During the preschool years, parents typically begin to control the child's exposure to experiences traditionally reserved for children of the opposite gender. This is particularly true for boys; parents often stop a boy's play activities if they perceive them as being too feminine. (Note: The concept of gender preference is not to be confused with sexual preference. Sexual preference refers to a sexual and/or emotional attraction to sexual partners. Sexual preference is discussed in Chapter 15 in a section titled "Sexual Orientation.")

Attitudes toward gender roles have become more flexible in recent years. Many parents now allow their children to pursue the activities they enjoy, regardless of whether the activities were once considered strictly masculine, such as playing baseball or building a model airplane, or feminine, such as growing flowers or cooking.

Parents should not become alarmed if their children or teenagers experiment with their gender identity through their appearance or activities. Such experimentation is natural and a part of finding the gender identity that best fits them. Such children often become very secure in their gender identity as adults.

With the recent acceleration in the importance of competitive sports for women, many of the skills and experiences once reserved for boys are now being fostered in young girls. What effect, if any, this movement will have on the speed at which gender preference is reached will be a topic for further research.

Gender Adoption

The process of reaching an initial adult gender identification requires a considerable period of time. The specific knowledge, attitudes, and behavior characteristic of adults must be observed, analyzed, and practiced. The process of acquiring and personalizing these "insights" about how men and women think, feel, and

Music Video Portrayals of Men and Women

Back in the 1950s, many American adults were shocked to see the early rock-and-roll performers (like Elvis Presley) shaking their hips as they gyrated to a strange new music form. Half a century later, song writers and music performers continue to shock today's adults. Just ask for a middle-aged adult's comments after watching music videos on TV for 30 minutes.

Not surprisingly, today's young adults seem less concerned than their parents and mentors about the impact that music lyrics and music videos might have. College students we talk to seem to pass them off as "mere entertainment"—a temporary escape from their classes and busy lives. Just fun. Harmless.

But have you stopped to think how these lyrics and videos tend to portray men and women? Have you thought about how they might show a skewed look at the gender roles of men and women? Aren't the men in music videos generally the ones in control of everything? And aren't women generally seen as less in control and more manipulative? Many women in music videos must use their beauty and their sexuality (not their brains) to "trap" the powerful man.

Some would argue that the lyrics in many of the songs don't help portray how a healthy relationship between two people might take place. Lyrics in some songs speak openly about sexual manipulation, lies and deceit, sexual prowess, revenge, power, dominance, and physical and emotional pain. Critics of today's music and videos are especially concerned that young children and adolescents will learn inappropriate ways to deal with interpersonal relationships.

What do you think about this? Are the critics just complaining about something that should be viewed simply as an "escape"? In other words, are people making a mountain out of the proverbial molehill?

And what about you personally? Do you think much about the messages in the music you listen to or the videos you watch? Do you believe that music lyrics and videos have influenced the way you see yourself as a man or woman? Have you tried to apply something you learned in a song or saw in a music video to your personal life? Do you believe that the relationships depicted in music videos generally reflect "reality" or a world of fiction? If you see these media products as forms of escapism, should they even try to portray reality? How do you think your friends would answer these questions?

One thing is for sure: this controversy won't end anytime soon.

---

act is reflected by the term **gender adoption,** the first and third rungs below the initial adult gender identification rail of the ladder in Figure 14-1. This process is influenced by many cultural and social factors; see the box "Music Video Portrayals of Men and Women."

In addition to constructing a personalized version of an adult sexual identity, the child and particularly the adolescent must construct a gender schema for a member of the opposite gender. The world of adulthood, with its involvement with intimacy, parenting, and employment, requires that men know women and women know men. Gender adoption provides an opportunity to begin constructing the equally valuable "pictures" of what the genders are like.

Initial Adult Gender Identification

By the time young people have climbed all of the rungs of the sexuality ladder, they have arrived at the chronological point in the life cycle when they need to construct an initial adult **gender identification.** You might notice that this label seems remarkably similar to the terminology used to describe one of the developmental tasks being used in this textbook. In fact, the task of forming an initial adult identity is closely related to developing an initial adult image of oneself as a man or a woman. Although most of us currently support the concept of "person" in many gender-neutral contexts (for some very valid reasons), we still must identify ourselves as either a man or a woman.

Androgyny: Sharing the Pluses

Our society has increasingly accepted an image of a person who possesses both masculine and feminine qualities. This accepted image has taken decades to develop because our society traditionally has reinforced rigid masculine roles for men and rigid feminine roles for women.

For a variety of reasons, the traditional picture has changed. **Androgyny,** or the blending of both feminine and masculine qualities, is more clearly evident in our society now than ever before. Today it is quite common to see men involved in raising children (including changing diapers) and doing routine housework. It is also quite common to see women entering the workplace in jobs traditionally managed by men and participating in sports traditionally played by men. Men are not scoffed at when they are seen crying after a touching movie. Women are not laughed at when they choose to assert themselves. The disposal of many sexual stereotypes has benefited our society immensely by relieving people of the pressure to be 100 percent "womanly" or 100 percent "macho."

Research data suggest that androgynous people are more flexible and independent, have greater self-esteem, have more positive attitudes toward sexuality, and show more social skills and motivation to achieve.[4] (Complete the Personal Assessment at the end of this chapter to explore your own attitudes about sexuality and sex roles.)

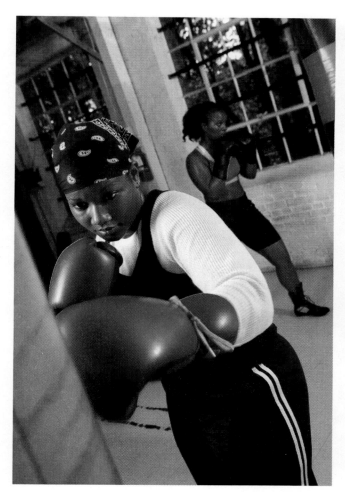
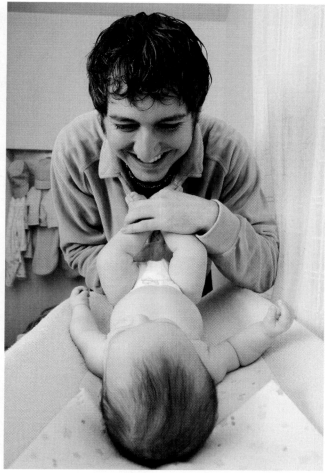

Just as women have broken into traditionally male careers and activities, many men have taken on jobs and tasks that were once considered women's exclusive domain.

 TALKING POINTS How could you demonstrate to your grandmother that the blending of gender roles is a positive development?

Reproductive Systems

The most familiar aspects of biological sexuality are the structures that comprise the reproductive systems. Each structure contributes in unique ways to the reproductive process. Thus, with these structures, males have the ability to impregnate. Females have the ability to become pregnant, give birth, and nourish infants through breast-feeding. In addition, many of these structures are associated with nonreproductive sexual behavior.

Male Reproductive System

The male reproductive system consists of external structures of genitals (the penis and scrotum) and internal structures (the testes, various passageways or ducts,

seminal vesicles, the prostate gland, and the Cowper's glands) (Figure 14-2A).

The Testes   The *testes* (also called *gonads* or *testicles*) are two egg-shaped bodies that lie within a saclike structure called the *scrotum*. During most of fetal development, the testes lie within the abdominal cavity. They descend into the scrotum during the last two months of fetal life.

Key Terms
gender adoption The long process of learning the behavior that is traditional for one's gender.
gender identification Achievement of a personally satisfying interpretation of one's masculinity or femininity.
androgyny (an **droj** en ee) The blending of both masculine and feminine qualities.

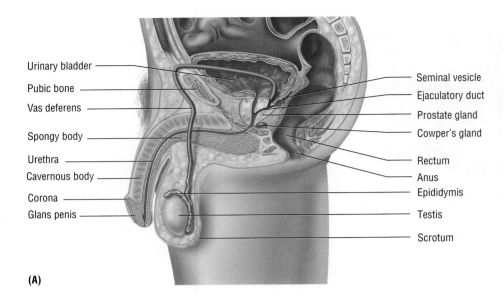

Figure 14-2 The Male Reproductive System **A:** Side view, **B:** Front view.

Urinary bladder

Pubic bone

Vas deferens

Spongy body

Urethra

Cavernous body

Corona

Glans penis

Seminal vesicle

Ejaculatory duct

Prostate gland

Cowper's gland

Rectum

Anus

Epididymis

Testis

Scrotum

(A)

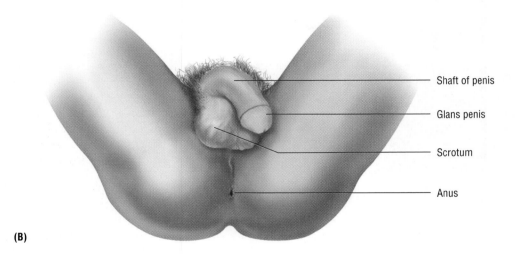

Shaft of penis

Glans penis

Scrotum

Anus

(B)

The testes are housed in the scrotum because a temperature lower than the body core temperature is required for adequate sperm development. The walls of the scrotum are composed of contractile tissue and can draw the testes closer to the body during cold temperatures (and sexual arousal) and relax during warm temperatures. Scrotal contraction and relaxation allow a constant, productive temperature to be maintained in the testes (Figure 14-2B).

A cross-sectional view of a single testis reveals an intricate network of structures called *seminiferous tubules.* Within these 300 or so seminiferous tubules, the process of sperm production (spermatogenesis) takes place. Sperm cell development starts at about age 11 in boys and is influenced by the release of the hormone **interstitial cell-stimulating hormone (ICSH)** from the pituitary gland. ICSH does primarily what its name suggests: it stimulates specific cells (called *interstitial cells*) within the testes to begin producing the male sex hormone

testosterone. Testosterone in turn is primarily responsible for the gradual development of the male secondary sex characteristics at the onset of puberty. By the time a boy is approximately 15 years old, sufficient levels of testosterone exist so that the testes become capable of full spermatogenesis.

Before the age of about 15, most of the sperm cells produced in the testes are incapable of fertilization. The production of fully mature sperm (*spermatozoa*) is triggered by another hormone secreted by the brain's pituitary gland—**follicle-stimulating hormone (FSH).** FSH influences the seminiferous tubules to begin producing spermatozoa capable of fertilization.

Ducts Spermatogenesis takes place around the clock, with hundreds of millions of sperm cells produced daily. The sperm cells do not stay in the seminiferous tubules but rather are transferred through a system of *ducts* that lead into the *epididymis.* The epididymis is a tubular coil that attaches to the back side of each testicle. These collecting structures house the maturing sperm cells for two to three weeks. During this period the sperm finally become capable of motion, but they remain inactive until they mix with the secretions from the accessory glands (the seminal vesicles, prostate gland, and Cowper's glands).

Each epididymis leads into an 18-inch passageway known as the *vas deferens*. Sperm, moved along by the action of hairlike projections called *cilia*, can also remain in the vas deferens for an extended time without losing their ability to fertilize an egg.

Seminal Vesicles

The two vasa deferens extend into the abdominal cavity, where each meets with a *seminal vesicle*—the first of the three accessory structures or glands. Each seminal vesicle contributes a clear, alkaline fluid that nourishes the sperm cells with fructose and permits the sperm cells to be suspended in a movable medium. The fusion of a vas deferens with the seminal vesicle results in the formation of a passageway called the *ejaculatory duct*. Each ejaculatory duct is only about one inch long and empties into the final passageway for the sperm—the urethra.

Prostate Gland

The ejaculatory duct is located within the second accessory gland—the *prostate gland* (see Figure 14-2A). The prostate gland secretes a milky fluid containing a variety of substances, including proteins, cholesterol, citric acid, calcium, buffering salts, and various enzymes. The prostate secretions further nourish the sperm cells and also raise the pH level, making the mixture quite alkaline. The alkalinity permits the sperm to have greater longevity as they are transported during ejaculation through the urethra, out of the penis, and into the highly acidic vagina.

Cowper's Glands

The third accessory gland, the *Cowper's glands*, serves primarily to lubricate the urethra with a clear, viscous mucus. These paired glands empty their small amounts of preejaculatory fluid during the arousal stage of the sexual response cycle. Alkaline in nature, this fluid also neutralizes the acidic level of the urethra. Viable sperm cells can be suspended in this fluid and can enter the female reproductive tract before full ejaculation by the male.[5] This may account for many of the failures of the "withdrawal" method of contraception.

The sperm cells, when combined with secretions from the seminal vesicles and the prostate gland, form a sticky substance called **semen.**[6] Interestingly, the microscopic sperm actually makes up less than 5 percent of the seminal fluid discharged at ejaculation. Contrary to popular belief, the paired seminal vesicles contribute about 60 percent of the semen volume, and the prostate gland adds about 30 percent.[1] Thus the fear of some men that a **vasectomy** will destroy their ability to ejaculate is completely unfounded (see Chapter 16).

During *emission* (the gathering of semen in the upper part of the urethra), a sphincter muscle at the base of the bladder contracts and inhibits semen from being pushed into the bladder and urine from being deposited into the urethra.[7] Thus semen and urine rarely intermingle, even though they leave the body through the same passageway.

Penis

Ejaculation takes place when the semen is forced out of the *penis* through the urethral opening. The involuntary, rhythmic muscle contractions that control ejaculation result in a series of pleasurable sensations known as *orgasm*.

The urethra lies on the underside of the penis and extends through the three cylindrical chambers of erectile tissue (two *cavernous bodies* and one *spongy body*). Each of these three chambers provides the vascular space required for sufficient erection of the penis. When a male becomes sexually aroused, the areas become congested with blood (*vasocongestion*). After ejaculation or when a male is no longer sexually stimulated, these chambers release the blood into the general circulation and the penis returns to a **flaccid** state.

The *shaft* of the penis is covered by a thin layer of skin that is an extension of the skin that covers the scrotum. This loose layer of skin is sensitive to sexual stimulation and extends over the head of the penis, except in males who have been circumcised. The *glans* (or head) of the penis is the most sexually sensitive (to tactile stimulation) part of the male body. Nerve receptor sites are especially prominent along the *corona* (the ridge of the glans) and the *frenulum* (the thin tissue at the base of the glans).

Age-Related Hormone Changes

Later in life, men begin to experience some changes in their reproductive system. The level of androgens, or male hormones,

---

Key Terms

interstitial cell-stimulating hormone (ICSH) (in ter **stish** ul) A gonadotropic hormone of the male required for the production of testosterone.

follicle-stimulating hormone (FSH) A gonadotropic hormone required for the initial development of ova (in the female) and sperm (in the male).

semen A secretion containing sperm and nutrients discharged from the urethra at ejaculation.

vasectomy A surgical procedure in which the vasa deferens are cut to prevent the passage of sperm from the testicles; the most common form of male sterilization.

flaccid (**fla** sid) Nonerect; the state of erectile tissue when vasocongestion is not occurring.

Chapter Fourteen Exploring the Origins of Sexuality

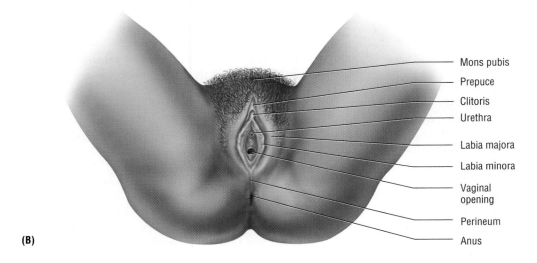

Fallopian (uterine) tube

Uterus

Urinary bladder

Pubic bone

Mons pubis

Urethra

Clitoris

Prepuce

Labia minora

Labia majora

(A)

Fimbriae

Ovary

Cervix

Cervical os (opening)

Rectum

Anus

Vagina

Bartholin's gland

Vaginal opening

(B)

Mons pubis

Prepuce

Clitoris

Urethra

Labia majora

Labia minora

Vaginal opening

Perineum

Anus

decreases with age, and the size of the prostate gland often increases. A deficiency of androgens has been found to cause health concerns in older men, including a lack of strength and energy, changes in mood, lower interest in sex, decreased bone density, and a decrease in muscle mass. Some are calling this the male menopause, or **andropause.** [8]

As a result, researchers are studying the benefits and risks of androgen replacement therapy in older men, similar to the hormone replacement therapy given to women. The benefits are an increase in bone and muscle mass, improved muscular and cardiovascular function, improved sexual function, and an overall better sense of well-being. The possible risks include an increased incidence of prostate disease, cardiovascular problems, and sleep apnea.[9] Androgen replacement therapy is available through prescription injections and implants, transdermal patches, oral pills, and a gel applied daily to the skin surface.[9]

Female Reproductive System

The external structures (genitals) of the female reproductive system consist of the mons pubis, labia majora, labia minora, clitoris, and vestibule (Figure 14-3). Collectively these structures form the *vulva* or vulval area.

Mons Pubis The *mons pubis* is the fatty covering over the pubic bone. The mons pubis (or mons veneris, "mound of Venus") is covered by pubic hair and is quite sensitive to sexual stimulation.

Labia Majora and Labia Minora The *labia majora* are large longitudinal skin folds that cover the entrance to the vagina, whereas the *labia minora* are the smaller longitudinal skin folds that lie within the labia majora. These hairless skin folds of the labia minora join at the top to form the *prepuce.* The prepuce covers the glans of the *clitoris,* which is the most sexually sensitive part of the female body.

Clitoris   In terms of its tactile sensitivity, the *clitoris* is the most sensitive part of the female genitals. It contains a glans and a shaft, although the shaft is below the skin surface. It is composed of erectile tissue that can become engorged with blood. It is covered by skin folds (the clitoral prepuce) and can collect **smegma** beneath these tissue folds.[4]

Vestibule   The *vestibule* is the region enclosed by the labia minora. Evident here are the urethral opening and the entrance to the vagina (vaginal orifice). Also located at the vaginal opening are the *Bartholin's glands,* which secrete a minute amount of lubricating fluid during sexual excitement.

The *hymen* is a thin layer of tissue that stretches across the opening of the vagina. Once thought to be the only indication of virginity, the intact hymen rarely covers the vaginal opening entirely. Openings in the hymen are necessary for the discharge of menstrual fluid and vaginal secretions. Many hymens are stretched or torn to full opening by adolescent physical activity or by the insertion of tampons. In women whose hymens are not fully ruptured, the first act of sexual intercourse will generally accomplish this. Pain may accompany first intercourse in females with relatively intact hymens.

The internal reproductive structures of the female include the vagina, uterus, fallopian tubes, and ovaries. Among some cultural groups, the vulvas of young girls are subject to the practice of female genital mutilation (see the "Female Genital Mutilation" box).

Vagina   The *vagina* is the structure that forms a canal from the orifice, through the vestibule, to the uterine cervix. Normally the walls of the vagina are collapsed, except during sexual stimulation, when the vaginal walls widen and elongate to accommodate the erect penis. Only the outer third of the vagina is especially sensitive to sexual stimulation. In this location, vaginal tissues swell considerably to form the **orgasmic platform.**[6] This platform constricts the vaginal opening and in effect "grips" the penis (or other inserted object)—regardless of its size. Thus the belief that a woman receives considerably more sexual pleasure from men with large penises is not supported from an anatomical standpoint.

Uterus   The *uterus* (or *womb*) is approximately the size and shape of a small pear. This highly muscular organ is capable of undergoing a wide range of physical changes, as evidenced by its enlargement during pregnancy, its contraction during menstruation and labor, and its movement during the orgasmic phase of the female sexual response cycle. The primary function of the uterus is to provide a suitable environment for the possible implantation of a fertilized ovum, or egg. This implantation, should it occur, takes place in the innermost lining of the uterus—the *endometrium*. In the mature female,

the endometrium undergoes cyclic changes as it prepares a new lining on a near-monthly basis.

The lower third of the uterus is called the *cervix*. The cervix extends slightly into the vagina. Sperm can enter the uterus through the cervical opening, or *cervical os*. Mucous glands in the cervix secrete a fluid that is thin and watery near the time of ovulation. Mucus of this consistency apparently facilitates sperm passage into the uterus and deeper structures. However, cervical mucus is much thicker during portions of the menstrual cycle when pregnancy is improbable, and during pregnancy, to protect against bacterial agents and other substances that are especially dangerous to the developing fetus.

The upper two-thirds of the uterus is called the *corpus* or *body*. This is where the fertilized ovum generally implants into the uterus.

Fallopian Tubes   The upper portion of the uterus opens into *two fallopian tubes,* sometimes called *oviducts* or *uterine tubes,* each about four inches long. The fallopian tubes are each directed toward an ovary. They serve as a passageway for the ovum in its weeklong voyage toward the uterus. In most cases, conception takes place in the upper third of the fallopian tubes.

Ovaries   The *ovaries* are analogous to the testes in the male. Their function is to produce the ovum, or egg. Usually, one ovary produces and releases just one egg each month. Approximately the size and shape of an unshelled almond, an ovary produces viable ova in the process known as *oogenesis*.

The ovaries also produce the female sex hormones through the efforts of specific structures within the ovaries. These hormones play multiple roles in the development of female secondary sex characteristics, but their primary function is to prepare the endometrium of the uterus for possible implantation of a fertilized ovum. In the average healthy female, this preparation takes place about 13 times a year for a period of about 35 years. At menopause, the ovaries shrink considerably and stop nearly all hormonal production.

Menstrual Cycle   Each month or so, the inner wall of the uterus prepares for a possible pregnancy. When

---

Key Terms

andropause   Significant decrease in androgenic hormone production in aging men; also called male menopause.

smegma   Cellular discharge that can accumulate beneath the clitoral hood or the foreskin of an uncircumcised penis.

orgasmic platform   Expanded outer third of the vagina, which grips the penis during sexual intercourse.

Female Genital Mutilation

Although sometimes referred to as female circumcision, the practice of surgically altering a young girl's vulva is more appropriately called female genital cutting (FGC) or female genital mutilation (FGM). This procedure is practiced in 28 African countries, several countries in the Middle East, and among some Muslims in Indonesia and Malaysia.* And even in the United States. In November 2006 in Lawrenceville, Georgia, an Ethiopian immigrant was convicted of aggravated battery and cruelty to children in a trial in which he was accused of using scissors to remove his 2-year-old daughter's clitoris in 2001. He was sentenced to 10 years in prison. This was thought to be the first criminal case in the United States that involved FGM.[†]

Typically, the procedure takes one of three forms: the removal of the clitoral hood (circumcision), the removal of the clitoris and perhaps the labia minora (clitoridectomy), and the drastic removal of the clitoris, inner lips, and part of the outer lips (infibulation).

For people from Western cultures, these practices may seem barbaric. Indeed, numerous international treaties, conventions, and relief organizations (World Health Organization, United Nations, CARE, United Nations Children's Fund) have developed policy statements that condemn these practices.[‡ §] Often performed by native women with crude instruments in unsanitary conditions, FGM takes place without the use of anesthetics. Female infants or young girls are subjected to this ritualistic cutting. Obvious dangers include severe bleeding, infection, and the formation of scar tissue.

Infibulation is sometimes extended to incorporate the sewing together of the remaining parts of the labia majora. This is thought to ensure virginity in a woman, but poses major risks when a newlywed husband tries to force his penis through the sewn area. Sometimes a midwife must first cut through the scar tissue to open the entrance to the vagina. Years after FGC, women face the possibility of serious complications with childbirth.

It is estimated that FGC and FGM have been performed on over 130 million women worldwide.[§] At face value, these procedures may seem gruesome to us in the West, yet we must pause to consider imposing our values on other cultures . . . cultures that readily accept these acts as important to the foundations of their belief systems. To many of us, these procedures represent a sexist devaluation of women. Yet this is normative behavior for groups of people who believe in carrying traditional values for their society. FGC and FGM pose real ethical dilemmas for those of us in Western cultures. What are your thoughts on this?

* Hyde JS, DeLamater JD. *Understanding Human Sexuality* (10th ed.). New York: McGraw-Hill, 2007.
† *Jury Convicts Father in Genital Mutilation of Girl*, MSNBC.com., November 1, 2006, www.msnbc.msn.com/id/15515179/.
‡ *Female Genital Mutilation*, World Health Organization, www.who.int/mediacentre/factsheets/fs241.
§ *Female Genital Mutilation/Cutting*, United Nations Children's Fund, www.unicef.org.

a pregnancy does not occur (as is the case throughout most months of a woman's fertile years), this lining must be released and a new one prepared. The breakdown of this endometrial wall and the resultant discharge of blood and endometrial tissue is known as *menstruation* (or *menses*) (Figure 14-4). The cyclic timing of this is controlled by a woman's hormones.

Girls generally have their first menstrual cycle, the onset of which is called *menarche,* around age 12 or 13. However, menarche ranges widely, from about age 9 to 17 years.[4] Over the past few decades, the age of menarche has been dropping gradually. This drop appears to be related to heredity, improved overall health, better childhood nutrition, and increased caloric intake. These factors in combination produce the increased body weight evident today in many young adolescent girls that seems to trigger an earlier menarche.

After a girl first menstruates, her cycles may be anovulatory for a year or longer before a viable ovum is released during her cycle. She will then continue this cyclic activity until age 45 to 55.

This text refers to a menstrual cycle that lasts 28 days. Be assured that few women display absolutely perfect 28-day cycles. Most women fluctuate by a few days to a week or more around this 28-day pattern.

It is not uncommon for some women to experience irregular cycles (cycles that differ in length) and even occasional mid-cycle spotting (small amounts of reddish discharge). These events are most likely to occur in young women who are just establishing their cycles, women who are approaching or moving through menopause, and women who are just starting to use hormone-based contraceptive methods. Major life changes, certain illnesses and medications, and unresolved stress can also affect the length of a woman's cycle. Any woman who experiences a significant, dramatic change from her usual pattern should contact her physician or health care practitioner.[4]

Your knowledge about the menstrual cycle is critical for your understanding of pregnancy, contraception, menopause, and issues related to the overall health and comfort of women; see the box "Endometriosis." Although seemingly complicated, each segment of the cycle can be studied separately for better understanding.

The menstrual cycle can be thought of as occurring in three segments or phases: the menstrual phase (lasting about one week), the preovulation phase (also lasting about one week), and the postovulation phase (lasting about two weeks). Day 1 of this cycle starts with the first day of bleeding, or menstrual flow.

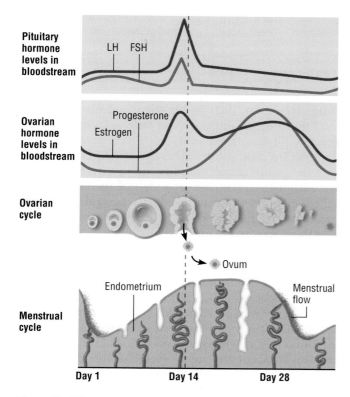

Pituitary hormone levels in bloodstream

LH FSH

Ovarian hormone levels in bloodstream

Progesterone

Estrogen

Ovarian cycle

Ovum

Menstrual cycle

Endometrium

Menstrual flow

Day 1   Day 14   Day 28

Figure 14-4 Menstrual Cycle The menstrual cycle involves the development and release of an ovum, supported by hormones from the pituitary gland, and the buildup of the endometrium, supported by hormones from the ovaries, for the purpose of establishing a pregnancy.

Menstrual Phase The *menstrual phase* signals the woman that a pregnancy has not taken place and that her uterine lining is being sloughed off. During a five- to seven-day period, a woman will discharge about one-fourth to one-half cup of blood and tissue. (Only about one ounce of the menstrual flow is blood.) The menstrual flow is heaviest during the first days of this phase. Because the muscular uterus must contract to accomplish this tissue removal, some women have uncomfortable cramping during menstruation. Most women, however, report more pain and discomfort during the few days before the first day of menstrual flow.

Today's methods of absorbing menstrual flow include the use of internal tampons and external pads. Caution must be exercised by the user of tampons to prevent the possibility of toxic shock syndrome (TSS) (see Chapter 13). Because menstrual flow is a positive sign of good health, women are encouraged to be normally active during menstruation.

Preovulation Phase The *preovulation phase* of the menstrual cycle starts about the time menstruation stops. Lasting about one week, this phase is first influenced by the release of follicle-stimulating hormone (FSH) from

Endometriosis

Endometriosis is a condition in which endometrial tissue that normally lines the uterus is found growing within the pelvic cavity. Because the tissue remains sensitive to circulating hormones, it is the source of pain and discomfort during the latter half of the menstrual cycle. Endometriosis is most commonly found in younger women and is sometimes related to infertility in women with severe cases.

In addition to painful cramping before and during menstruation, the symptoms of endometriosis include low-back pain, pain during intercourse, painful bowel movements, heavy menstrual flow, and difficulty becoming pregnant. Many women with endometriosis, however, experience no symptoms.*

Treatment of endometriosis largely depends on its extent. Drugs to suppress ovulation, including birth control pills, may be helpful in mild cases. For more severe cases, surgical removal of the tissue or a hysterectomy may be necessary. For some women, endometriosis is suppressed during pregnancy and does not return after pregnancy.

*WebMd.com. Endometriosis Health Center: Sexual Health: Your Guide to Endometriosis. www.women.webmd.com/endometriosis/endometriosis, January 11, 2009.

the pituitary gland. FSH circulates in the bloodstream and directs the ovaries to start the process of maturing approximately 20 primary ovarian *follicles*. Thousands of primary egg follicles are present in each ovary at birth. These follicles resemble shells that house immature ova. As these follicles ripen under FSH influence, they release the hormone *estrogen*. Estrogen's primary function is to direct the endometrium to start the development of a thick, highly vascular wall. As FSH secretions are reduced, the pituitary gland prepares for the surge of the **luteinizing hormone (LH)** required to accomplish ovulation.[10]

In the days immediately before ovulation, one of the primary follicles (called the *graafian follicle*) matures fully. The other primary follicles degenerate and are absorbed by the body. The graafian follicle moves toward the surface of the ovary. When LH is released in massive quantities on about day 14, the graafian follicle bursts to release the fully mature ovum. The release of the ovum is called ovulation. Regardless of the overall length of a

Key Terms

luteinizing hormone (LH) (loo ten eye zing) A gonadotropic hormone of the female required for fullest development and release of ova; ovulating hormone.

woman's cycle, **ovulation** occurs 14 days before her first day of menstrual flow.

The ovum is quickly captured by the fingerlike projections (*fimbriae*) of the fallopian tubes. In the upper third of the fallopian tubes, the ovum is capable of being fertilized in a 24- to 36-hour period. If the ovum is not fertilized by a sperm cell, it will begin to degenerate and eventually be absorbed by the body.

Postovulation Phase   After ovulation, the *postovulation phase* of the menstrual cycle starts when the remnants of the graafian follicle restructure themselves into a **corpus luteum.** The corpus luteum remains inside the ovary, secreting estrogen and a fourth hormone called *progesterone*. Progesterone, which literally means "for pregnancy," continues to direct the endometrial buildup. If pregnancy occurs, the corpus luteum monitors progesterone and estrogen levels throughout the pregnancy. If pregnancy does not occur, high levels of progesterone signal the pituitary to stop the release of LH and the corpus luteum starts to disintegrate on about day 24. When estrogen and progesterone levels diminish significantly by day 28, the endometrium is discharged from the uterus and out the vagina. The postovulation phase ends, and the cycle is complete.

Related Conditions

Premenstrual Syndrome (PMS)   PMS is a collection of physical and psychological symptoms that occur in the days just before menstruation in many women of childbearing age. The physical symptoms may include weight gain, breast tenderness, fatigue, headaches, backaches, and abdominal cramps (**dysmenorrhea**). The psychological symptoms can include irritability, tension, anxiety, mood swings, depression, difficulty concentrating, and aggressiveness. These symptoms vary from woman to woman and from one menstrual cycle to the next. It has been estimated that 85 percent of women experience at least some of these symptoms on a regular basis.[11]

The specific cause of PMS is unknown, but it is likely related to the changing levels of estrogen and progesterone as a woman's body prepares for menstruation. Treating the symptoms of PMS often starts with a healthy diet—reducing one's intake of caffeine, salt, and simple sugar, and increasing one's intake of complex carbohydrates by eating more fresh fruits and vegetables. A simple, daily vitamin/mineral combination pill might also be helpful. Physical exercise is highly recommended to reduce PMS symptoms and elevate one's mood.

For some women, taking a warm bath or placing a heating pad on the abdomen eases menstrual cramping. The following exercise routine can also help target menstrual cramping:

- Lie face up with the knees and legs bent; perform abdominal breathing about 10 times. Feel the abdomen slowly inflate and then slowly fall.

- Stand and hold the back of a chair; lift one heel off the floor, then the other. Repeat 20 times.

- Lie on your back; lift and bring your knees to your chin; repeat 10 times.

Over-the-counter nonsteroidal anti-inflammatory drugs (NSAIDs), such as ibuprofen and naproxen, and over-the-counter diuretics can help alleviate uncomfortable physical symptoms. For severe cases of PMS, a physician can prescribe medications. These might include certain antidepressants and prescription diuretics. Although in the past progesterone therapy or combined estrogen-progesterone birth control pills were prescribed for relief from PMS, recent research indicates that these approaches are generally ineffective.[12]

Premenstrual Dysphoric Disorder (PMDD)   Premenstrual dysphoric disorder (PMDD) is a severe form of PMS and occurs in about 2 to 10 percent of menstruating women.[13] As with PMS, PMDD expresses itself in the latter half of the menstrual cycle in the days before menstruation begins. The symptoms of PMDD are similar to those of PMS, but they are so severe that they cause major disruptions in a woman's personal relationships, social activities, and employment. With PMDD, the mood swings, tension, irritability, depression, anger, appetite changes, sleep problems, loss of control, difficulties concentrating, and physical symptoms are magnified far beyond that seen in women with PMS.

To make a diagnosis of PMDD, a physician will likely give a woman a thorough medical examination, including a review and analysis of her symptoms and medical history. He or she will want to rule out emotional problems (such as depression) as possible causes of the symptoms, as well as medical or gynecological concerns (such as endometriosis, menopause, or fibroid tumors) that could also account for the symptoms.

The cause of PMDD appears to be a connection between hormonal fluctuations and a lowered level of serotonin, a neurotransmitter that helps transmit nerve signals. Methods of treatment of PMDD focus on many of the same strategies used to manage PMS: good nutrition, regular aerobic exercise, psychological counseling (to develop coping strategies), and the use of over-the-counter pain relievers and diuretics. Additionally, the FDA has approved the use of three prescription antidepressants to help relieve the symptoms of PMDD. Some physicians prescribe common birth control pills or other hormonal drugs to women coping with PMDD, although their effectiveness remains uncertain.[13]

Recently the U.S. Food and Drug Administration (FDA) approved a newer type of birth control pill, marketed as Yasmin and YAZ. These pills both contain estrogen and a progestin called drospirenone. Yasmin is a low-estrogen variety, and YAZ is a very low estrogen pill. The drospirenone seems to have a unique hormone action and also functions as a diuretic to relieve bloating and breast tenderness. YAZ has been approved by the FDA to treat PMDD symptoms.[12]

Fibrocystic Breast Condition In some women, particularly those who have never been pregnant, stimulation of the breast tissues by estrogen and progesterone during the menstrual cycle results in an unusually high degree of secretory activity by the cells lining the ducts. The fluid released by the secretory lining finds its way into the fibrous connective tissue areas in the lower half of the breast, where in pocketlike cysts the fluid presses against neighboring tissues. Excessive secretory activity produces in many women a benign fibrocystic breast condition characterized by swollen, firm, or hardened tender breast tissue before menstruation.

Researchers have begun to describe the importance of a healthy diet in preventing fibrocystic breast condition, in particular a low-fat, low-salt, low-red-meat diet that is rich in whole grains, fish, and chicken. The reduction or elimination of caffeine found in coffee, tea, soft drinks, and chocolate might also help reduce these benign breast changes. In some cases, vitamin E and vitamin B-complex supplementation have helped.[4] Women with more extensive fibrocystic conditions can be treated with drugs that have a "calming" effect on progesterone production. Occasional draining of cysts can bring relief.

Amenorrhea **Amenorrhea** is a condition characterized by the absence of menstruation. The lack of menstruation, if not caused by aging or pregnancy, is categorized as either primary or secondary amenorrhea.[7] *Primary amenorrhea* occurs when girls have passed the age of 16 and have never menstruated. Perhaps these girls have not yet reached a critical body weight (with the increased ratio of body fat) to trigger the menstrual cycle to begin. Additionally, some girls may have inherited a familial tendency to mature later than most of their peers. At an appropriate time for their bodies, these girls will start to menstruate. However, in cases where the primary amenorrhea is determined to be caused by hormonal deficiencies or abnormal body structure, hormone therapy can be quite useful.

Secondary amenorrhea occurs when a previously menstruating woman ceases to menstruate. Likely reasons for secondary amenorrhea include pregnancy, breast-feeding, or the use of hormonal contraceptives. Less common reasons could be linked to unresolved stress, a reduction in body fat, hormonal irregularities, or serious athletic training. Other causes could be anorexia (see Chapter 6) or the female athlete syndrome (see Chapter 4). If a woman has not menstruated in six months and is not pregnant, not breast-feeding, and not using hormonal contraceptives, she should consult with her physician or medical care professional.[7]

Menopause For the vast majority of women in their late 40s through their mid-50s, a gradual decline in reproductive system function, called *menopause,* occurs. Menopause is a normal physiological process, not a disease process. It can, however, become a health concern for some middle-aged women who have unpleasant side effects resulting from this natural ending of ovum production and menstruation.

As ovarian function and hormone production diminish, the hypothalamus, ovaries, uterus, and other estrogen-sensitive tissues must adjust. The extent of menopause as a health problem is determined by the degree to which **hot flashes,** night sweats, insomnia, vaginal wall dryness, depression and melancholy, breast changes, and the uncertainty of fertility are seen as problems.

Many of today's midlife women are likely to find menopause to be a relatively positive experience. The end of fertility, combined with children leaving home, makes the middle years a period of personal rediscovery for many women; see the box "No Fear of 50."

For women who are troubled by the changes brought about by menopause, physicians may prescribe **hormone replacement therapy (HRT).** This can relieve many symptoms and offer benefits to help reduce the incidence of osteoporosis (see Chapters 4 and 5). However, HRT has recently been found to increase the risk of breast cancer and cardiovascular problems.[14, 15] These concerns have caused many women to reconsider their use of HRT. See the box "Women and Heart Disease" in Chapter 10.

There are alternative approaches to HRT that women can try to ease the symptoms of menopausal changes. Reducing the intake of spicy foods, caffeine, and alcohol may help with hot flashes and night sweats. Vitamin E and soy products help some women, and the use of certain herbs (especially black cohosh) is being studied. The use of a prescription antidepressant (such as Prozac or Paxil) may reduce hot flashes in some women.

Key Terms

ovulation The release of a mature egg from the ovary.

corpus luteum (kore pus **loo** tee um) Cellular remnant of the graafian follicle after the release of an ovum.

dysmenorrhea Abdominal pain caused by muscular cramping during the menstrual cycle.

amenorrhea The absence of menstruation.

hot flashes Unpleasant, temporary feelings of warmth experienced by women during and after menopause, caused by blood vessel dilation.

hormone replacement therapy (HRT) Medically administered hormones to replace hormones lost as the result of menopause.

Chapter Fourteen Exploring the Origins of Sexuality

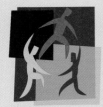

Learning from Our Diversity

No Fear of 50: The New Model for Menopause

Just a generation ago, menopause was regarded almost as a dreaded disease by many women—not to mention the men who were married to them. It was seen not just as the end of fertility but as the loss of youth, attractiveness, femininity, sex appeal, and sexual enjoyment. Both women and their husbands dreaded the onset of hot flashes, mood swings, depression, and loss of sex drive that were commonly believed to be every woman's fate during premenopause. In the minds not just of middle-aged women but also of men and young people, the definition of menopause was "old."

That was then; this is now. With the first women of the baby boom generation dealing with menopause, it's a whole new story. The generation that said it would never get old is not taking menopause on the chin—instead, today's women are fighting back, with every weapon at their command. Regular exercise and stress reducers like meditation and yoga go a long way toward easing the emotional swings associated with menopause—and a balanced diet, rich in healthful sources of calcium, helps stabilize mood and prevent osteoporosis. For some women, hormone replacement therapy (HRT) is helpful in alleviating unpleasant symptoms of menopause and in reducing bone loss. However, recent concerns over HRT have caused other women to opt not to use HRT and instead pursue treatments offered by alternative medicine, or simply let nature take its course.

Many of the "new" 50-plus women are treating menopause as a natural process instead of a disease. Rather than using menopause as an excuse to stop exercising and eating healthfully, these women and thousands of others see it as a compelling reason to stay fit.

With their children grown and gone, midlife women who have spent decades raising a family now find that they have time to themselves—and for themselves. Career women, whether they're mothers or not, have usually achieved their major goals or are in sight of them, and they no longer need to make an all-out push to scale the corporate or professional ladder. There's more time for friendships, for hobbies and interests, for travel, and for contemplating instead of competing. There's more time for the healthful, self-nuturing pursuits that help ease the transition into menopause. And there's more life to be lived than at any time in the past. No longer considered the figurative end of a woman's life, menopause now is increasingly regarded as a passage into the next stage, with all the challenges and rewards it offers.

Increasingly, physicians are rejecting the "menopause as disease" model in favor of a more positive approach that empowers women to manage this stage of their lives proactively instead of being overwhelmed or overmedicated by it. Women of the baby boom generation may be aging—but they're not doing it passively.

Vaginal dryness can be helped by the use of over-the-counter lubricants and moisturizers, vaginal estrogen creams, and regular sexual activity. Insomnia can be countered with the use of good sleeping patterns (consistent bedtime hour, a small glass of warm milk, and reduced caffeine, alcohol, and food intake before bed).

Interestingly, physical activity cuts across most of the issues related to menopause. Physical activity has been

Discovering Your Spirituality

Sexuality as a Means of Spiritual Discovery

Few would argue that many of our expressions of sexuality are truly wonderful. For example, the enjoyment we can receive from a warm caress or an intimate kiss can be stimulating beyond imagination. The fact that our biological anatomy can function in ways that make us feel pleasure can be viewed as one of life's most rewarding gifts.

However, expressions of sexuality can extend beyond merely "feeling good." One's sexuality is an experience that encompasses the whole individual. It is much more than a biological act, a means of procreation, or an orgasmic release. While sexuality is all of these things, it also is a means of conveying intimacy to another person. Ultimately, sexuality is a form of intimate communication between two people. Through sexual expressions, one can convey feelings of love, devotion, caring, individuality, and openness. Of course, these feelings can also be communicated in nonsexual ways, but the depth of feelings that comes with sexual intimacy is especially powerful, and it is perhaps driven and enhanced by strong biological forces.

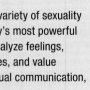

When sexuality is considered from this broader perspective, it can be viewed as a journey into personal understanding. This can evolve into a lifelong spiritual journey that constantly challenges one's values and stances on a variety of sexuality issues. In this spiritual journey, the brain, the body's most powerful sex organ, plays key roles. The brain helps one analyze feelings, moral and religious issues, relationship possibilities, and value stances. The brain also helps one learn about sexual communication, sexual technique, and sexual pleasure.

As you read the sexuality material in this unit, you will see that sexuality encompasses the whole person, in a variety of ways and in a variety of circumstances. Sexual expression is much more than just "doing it." For those who think otherwise, remember that "people who are only interested in sex are probably not very interesting people." Look for the ways in which your sexuality is connected to other aspects of your life.

demonstrated to help sleep patterns, provide emotional balance, encourage mental acuity, and bolster cardiovascular function. Physical activity also makes people feel better about their bodies and, thus, become potentially more interested in sexual activity that in turn can help maintain vaginal lubrication.

Taking Charge of Your Health

- Take the Personal Assessment at the end of this chapter to determine how traditional or nontraditional your attitudes are toward sexuality.
- If you wish to become more flexible and expand your social skills, identify ways in which you can increase your androgynous behavior. For example, learn to cook, expand your assertiveness skills, do volunteer work with children, join a club sports team, or learn how to invest in the stock market.

- Most college sexuality textbooks encourage readers to become familiar with their external reproductive "body parts." If you believe that this is important, study the illustrations in this chapter, find a handheld mirror, undress, and identify these structures as best you can.
- If you are a woman who has a significant amount of menstrual pain, try some of the treatment suggestions in this chapter.
- If you are a man who is essentially "clueless" about the menstrual cycle and would

like to understand it much better, study the information in this chapter. If you have a very close female friend and you wish to validate some of this information, ask her (diplomatically, of course) if you could get her "impressions" of this natural phenomenon.
- Read the *Discovering Your Spirituality* box and see if you agree that sexuality can be a means of spiritual discovery.

SUMMARY

- The biological basis of human sexuality includes genetic, gonadal, and structural components.
- The structural basis of sexuality begins as the male and female reproductive structures develop in the growing embryo and fetus. Structural sexuality changes as one moves through adolescence and later life.
- The psychosocial basis of human sexuality includes gender identity, gender preference, gender adoption, and initial adult gender identification.
- Androgyny is the blending of feminine and masculine qualities.
- The male and female reproductive structures are external and internal. The complex functioning of these structures is controlled by hormones.

- The menstrual cycle's primary functions are to produce ova and to develop a supportive environment for the fetus in the uterus.
- Endometriosis is a condition in which endometrial tissue that normally lines the uterus grows within the pelvic cavity, causing pain before and during menstruation and can lead to infertility.
- Fibrocystic breast condition is characterized by swollen, firm, or hardened tender breast tissue before menstruation.
- Postmenopausal hormone therapy has benefits in treating the symptoms of menopause but may carry risks for some women.

REVIEW QUESTIONS

1. Describe the following foundations of our biological sexuality: the genetic basis, the gonadal basis, and structural development.
2. Define and explain the following psychosocial sexuality terms: gender identity, gender preference, gender adoption, and initial adult gender identification.
3. Define androgyny and explain its advantages.
4. Identify the major components of the male reproductive system. Trace the passageway for sperm.
5. Identify the major components of the female reproductive system. Trace the passageway for ova.

6. Identify and describe the four main hormones that control the menstrual cycle.
7. What are some of the nondrug techniques for reducing the symptoms of PMS?
8. What are the symptoms of fibrocystic breast condition and endometriosis?
9. Describe the difference between primary and secondary amenorrhea.
10. Name two circumstances in which postmenopausal hormone therapy might be prescribed for women.

ANSWERS TO THE "WHAT DO YOU KNOW?" QUIZ

1. False   2. True   3.   False   4. False   5. True   6. False   7. True

Visit the Online Learning Center (**www.mhhe.com/payne11e**), where you will find tools to help you improve your grade including practice quizzes, key terms flashcards, audio chapter summaries for your MP3 player, and many other study aids.

SOURCE NOTES

1. Thibodeau GA, Patton KT. *Anatomy and Physiology* (6th ed.). St. Louis, MO: Mosby, 2006.
2. Sherwood L. *Human Physiology: From Cells to Systems* (6th ed.). Belmont, CA: Cengage, 2007.
3. Hyde JS, DeLamater JD. *Understanding Human Sexuality* (10th ed.). New York: McGraw-Hill, 2009.
4. Crooks R, Baur K. *Our Sexuality* (10th ed.). Belmont, CA: Wadsworth, 2008.
5. Kelly GF. *Sexuality Today: The Human Perspective* (8th ed.). New York: McGraw-Hill, 2006.
6. Carroll JL. *Sexuality Now: Embracing Diversity* (2nd ed.). Belmont, CA: Cengage, 2007.
7. Strong B, Yarber WL, Sayad BW, DeVault C. *Human Sexuality: Diversity in Contemporary America* (6th ed.). New York: McGraw-Hill, 2008.
8. Schieszer J. Male Menopause Out of the Closet. MSNBC Interactive, October 1, 2006. www.msnbc.com/id/3543479/.
9. WebMd.com. Testosterone Replacement Therapy: Is it Right for You?, January 10, 2009. http://men.webmd.com/testosterone-replacement-therapy.
10. Hatcher RA, et al. *Contraceptive Technology* (19th ed.). New York: Ardent Media, 2007.
11. Shuman T. *Sexual Health: Your Guide to Premenstrual Syndrome.* WebMD Content Article, February 2006, www.webmd.com/content/Article/10/2953_497.htm.
12. WebMD.com Premenstrual Syndrome (PMS): Medications, January 10, 2009, www.women.webmd.com/pms/premenstrual-syndrome-pms-medications.
13. Shuman T. Sexual Health: Your Guide to Premenstrual Dysphoric Disorder. WebMD Content Article, February 2006, www.webmd.com/content/Article/10/2953_498.htm.
14. Writing Group for the Women's Health Initiative Investigation. Risks and benefits of estrogen plus progestin in healthy postmenopausal women: Principal results from the Women's Health Initiative Randomized Controlled Trial. *Journal of the American Medical Association,* 288(3), 321–333, July 17, 2002.
15. Hormone Therapy Is No Heart Helper. *Harvard Heart Letter,* 13(2), 2–4, October 2004.

Personal Assessment

Sexual Attitudes: A Matter of Feelings

Respond to each of the following statements by selecting a numbered response (1– 5) that most accurately reflects your feelings. Circle the number of your selection. At the end of the questionnaire, total these numbers for use in interpreting your responses.

1. Agree strongly
2. Agree moderately
3. Uncertain
4. Disagree moderately
5. Disagree strongly

Men and women have greater differences than they have similarities.	1	2	3	4	5
Homosexuality and bisexuality are immoral and unnatural.	1	2	3	4	5
Our society is too sexually oriented.	1	2	3	4	5
Pornography encourages sexual promiscuity.	1	2	3	4	5
Children know far too much about sex.	1	2	3	4	5
Education about sexuality is solely the responsibility of the family.	1	2	3	4	5
Dating begins far too early in our society.	1	2	3	4	5
Sexual intimacy before marriage leads to emotional stress and damage to one's reputation.	1	2	3	4	5
Sexual availability is far too frequently the reason that people marry.	1	2	3	4	5
Reproduction is the most important reason for sexual intimacy during marriage.	1	2	3	4	5
Modern families are too small.	1	2	3	4	5
Family planning clinics should not receive public funds.	1	2	3	4	5
Contraception is the woman's responsibility.	1	2	3	4	5
Abortion is the murder of an innocent child.	1	2	3	4	5
Marriage has been weakened by the changing role of women in society.	1	2	3	4	5
Divorce is an unacceptable means of resolving marital difficulties.	1	2	3	4	5
Extramarital sexual intimacy will destroy a marriage.	1	2	3	4	5
Sexual abuse of a child does not generally occur unless the child encourages the adult.	1	2	3	4	5
Provocative behavior by the woman is a factor in almost every case of rape.	1	2	3	4	5
Reproduction is not a right but a privilege.	1	2	3	4	5

YOUR TOTAL POINTS _____

Interpretation

20–34 points—A very traditional attitude toward sexuality

35–54 points—A moderately traditional attitude toward sexuality

55–65 points—A rather ambivalent attitude toward sexuality

66–85 points—A moderately nontraditional attitude toward sexuality

86–100 points—A very nontraditional attitude toward sexuality

TO CARRY THIS FURTHER . . .

Were you surprised at your results? Compare your results with those of a roommate or close friend. How do you think your parents would score on this Personal Assessment?

Understanding Sexual Behavior and Relationships

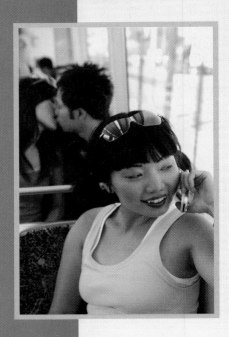

What Do You Know About Sexual Behavior and Relationships?

1. Transgendered persons differ from transsexuals. True or False?

2. Most males are multiorgasmic. True or False?

3. In the sexual response pattern, the plateau stage follows the orgasmic stage. True or False?

4. Children raised in lesbian or gay families overwhelmingly grow up with a heterosexual orientation. True or False?

5. Fellatio can be performed on female partners. True or False?

6. After orgasm, the length of the resolution phase is usually longer in older men. True or False?

7. In comparison to mutual monogamy, serial monogamy increases the likelihood of exposure to infectious diseases. True or False?

Check your answers at the end of the chapter.

As we move through a new millennium, we have reached a greater understanding of the psychosocial factors that contribute to the complex expression of our sexuality. In this chapter, we explore human sexuality as it relates to the dynamic interplay of the psychosocial bases of sexual behavior and relationships. We begin by examining the human sexual response pattern.

The Human Sexual Response Pattern

Although history has many written and visual accounts of the human's ability to be sexually aroused, it was not until the pioneering work of Masters and Johnson that the events associated with arousal were clinically documented.[1] These researchers posed the following five questions, which gave direction to a series of studies involving the scientific evaluation of human sexual response.

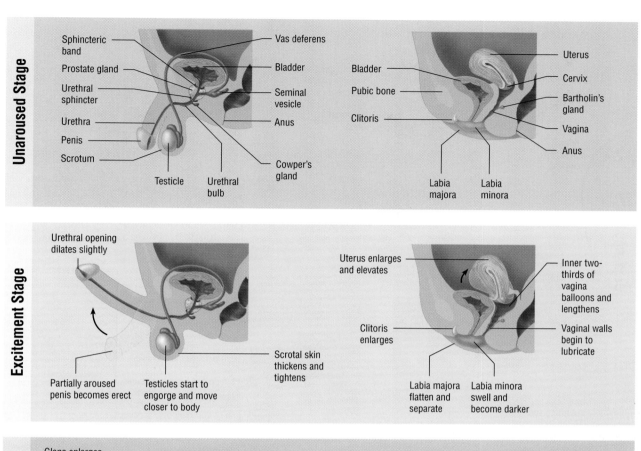

Figure 15-1 The Sexual Response Pattern in Men and Women

(Continued on next page)

Do the Sexual Responses of Men and Women Have a Predictable Pattern?

The answer to the first question posed by the researchers was an emphatic *yes.* A predictable sexual response pattern was identified;[1] it consists of an initial **excitement stage,** a **plateau stage,** an **orgasmic stage,** and a **resolution stage.** Each stage involves predictable changes in the structural characteristics and physiological function of reproductive and nonreproductive organs in both the male and female. These changes are shown in Figure 15-1.

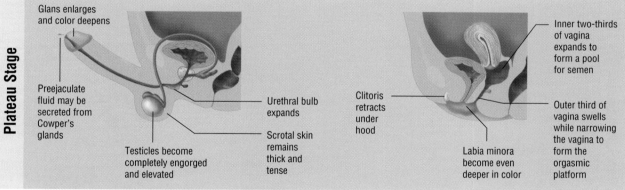

Key Terms

excitement stage Initial arousal stage of the sexual response pattern.

plateau stage Second stage of the sexual response pattern; a leveling off of arousal immediately before orgasm.

orgasmic stage Third stage of the sexual response pattern; the stage during which neuromuscular tension is released.

resolution stage Fourth stage of the sexual response pattern; the return of the body to a preexcitement state.

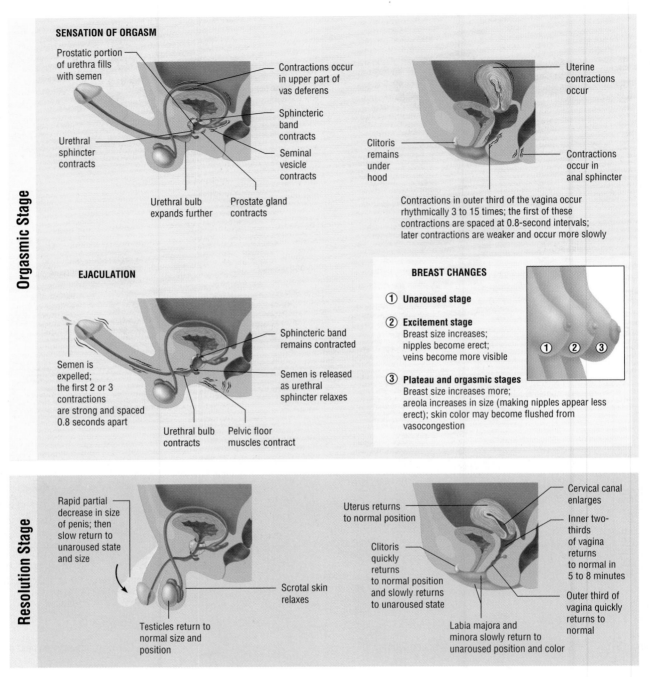

Figure 15-1 *Continued*

Is the Sexual Response Pattern Stimuli-Specific?

The research of Masters and Johnson[1] clearly established a *no* answer to the second question concerning stimuli specificity. Their findings demonstrated that several senses can supply the stimuli necessary for initiating the sexual response pattern. Although touching activities might initiate arousal in most people and maximize it

for the vast majority of people, in both men and women, sight, smell, sound, and *vicariously formed stimuli* can also stimulate the same sexual arousal patterns.

What Differences Occur in the Sexual Response Pattern?

Differences between Men and Women   In response to the third question, several differences are observable when comparing the sexual response patterns of men and women:

- With the exception of some late adolescent males, the vast majority of men are not multiorgasmic. The **refractory phase** of the resolution stage prevents most men from experiencing more than one orgasm in a short time, even when sufficient stimulation is available.

- Women possess a **multiorgasmic capacity.** Masters and Johnson found that as many as 10 to 30 percent of all female adults routinely experience multiple orgasms.

- Although they possess multiorgasmic potential, some 10 percent of all women are *anorgasmic*—that is, they never experience an orgasm through **coitus.** [1] For many of these women, orgasms can be experienced when masturbation provides the stimulation.

- When measured during coitus, men reach orgasm far more quickly than do women. However, when masturbation is the source of stimulation, women reach orgasm as quickly as men.

More important than any of the differences pointed out is the finding that the sexual response patterns of men and women are far more alike than they are different. Not only do men and women experience the four basic stages of the response pattern, but they also have similar responses in specific areas, including the **erection** and *tumescence* of sexual structures; the appearance of a **sex flush;** the increase in cardiac output, blood pressure, and respiratory rate; and the occurrence of *rhythmic pelvic thrusting.* [1]

Differences Among Subjects Within a Same-Gender Group   When a group of subjects of the same gender was studied in an attempt to answer questions about similarities and differences in the sexual response pattern, Masters and Johnson noted considerable variation. Even when variables such as age, race, education, and general health were held constant, the extent and duration of virtually every stage of the response pattern varied.

Differences Within the Same Individual   For a given person the nature of the sexual response pattern does not remain constant, even when observed over a relatively short period. A variety of internal and external factors can alter this pattern. The aging process, changes in general health status, levels of stress, altered environmental settings, use of alcohol and other drugs, and behavioral changes in a sexual partner can cause one's own sexual response pattern to change from one sexual experience to another. See the boxes "Sexual Performance Difficulties and Therapies" and "The Ultimate Aphrodisiac?" for additional information about other factors affecting the sexual response pattern.

What Are the Basic Physiological Mechanisms Underlying the Sexual Response Pattern?

The basic mechanisms in the fourth question posed by Masters and Johnson are now well recognized. One factor, *vasocongestion,* or the retention of blood or fluid within a particular tissue, is critically important in the development of physiological changes that promote the sexual response pattern. [1] The presence of erectile tissue underlies the changes that can be noted in the penis, breasts, and scrotum of the male and the clitoris, breasts, and labia minora of the female.

A second mechanism now recognized as necessary for the development of the sexual response pattern is that of *myotonia,* or the buildup of neuromuscular tension within a variety of body structures. [2] At the end of the plateau stage of the response pattern, a sudden release of the accumulated neuromuscular tension gives rise to the rhythmic muscular contractions and pleasurable muscular spasms that constitute orgasm, as well as ejaculation in the male. [3]

What Role Is Played by Specific Organs and Organ Systems in the Sexual Response Pattern?

The fifth question posed by Masters and Johnson, which concerns the role played by specific organs and organ systems during each stage of the response pattern, can be readily answered by referring to the material presented in Figure 15-1. As you study this figure, remember that direct stimulation of the penis and either direct or indirect stimulation of the clitoris are the principal avenues toward orgasm. Also, intercourse represents only one activity that can lead to orgasmic pleasure. [4]

Key Terms

refractory phase That portion of the male's resolution stage during which sexual arousal cannot occur.

multiorgasmic capacity Potential to have several orgasms within a single period of sexual arousal.

coitus (**co** ih tus) Penile-vaginal intercourse.

erection The engorgement of erectile tissue with blood; characteristic of the penis, clitoris, nipples, labia minora, and scrotum.

sex flush The reddish skin response that results from increasing sexual arousal.

Sexual Performance Difficulties and Therapies

For all of the predictability of the human sexual response pattern, many people find that at some point in their lives, they are no longer capable of responding sexually. The inability of a person to perform adequately is identified as a sexual difficulty or dysfunction. Sexual difficulties can have a negative influence on a person's sense of sexual satisfaction and on a partner's satisfaction. Fortunately, most sexual difficulties can be resolved through strategies that use individual, couple, or group counseling. Most sexual performance difficulties stem from psychogenic factors.

Difficulty	Possible Causes	Therapeutic Approaches
Women		
Orgasmic Difficulties Inability to have orgasm	Lack of knowledge about female responsiveness; inadequate sexual arousal; interpersonal problems with partner; anxiety, fear, guilt, anger, poor self-concept	Counseling to improve a couple's communication; educating a woman and her partner about female responsiveness; teaching a woman how to experience orgasm through masturbation
Vaginismus Painful, involuntary contractions of the vaginal muscles	Previous traumatic experiences with intercourse (rape, incest, uncaring partners); fear of pregnancy; religious prohibitions; anxiety about vaginal penetration of any kind (including tampons)	Counseling to alleviate psychogenic causes; gradual dilation of the vagina with woman's fingers or dilators; systematic desensitization exercises; relaxation training
Dyspareunia Painful intercourse	Insufficient sexual arousal; communication problems with partner; infections, inflammation; structural abnormalities; insufficient lubrication	Individual and couple counseling with a focus on relaxation and communication; medical strategies to reduce infections and structural abnormalities; additional lubrication
Men		
Erectile Dysfunction Inability to achieve an erection (impotence)	Chronic diseases (including diabetes, vascular problems, and chemical dependencies); trauma; numerous psychogenic factors (including anxiety, guilt, fear, poor self-concept)	Medical intervention (including possible vascular surgery, drugs, or the use of penile implants or pumps); couple counseling using sensate focusing, pleasuring, and relaxation strategies
Rapid Ejaculation Ejaculating too quickly after penile penetration; premature ejaculation	Predominantly psychogenic in origin; a man's need to prove his sexual prowess; anxiety associated with previous sexual experiences	Counseling to free the man from the anxiety associated with rapid ejaculation; altering coital position, masturbation before intimacy, use of the squeeze technique as orgasm approaches
Dyspareunia Painful intercourse	Primarily physical in origin; inability of the penile foreskin to retract fully; urogenital tract infections; scar tissue in seminal passageways; insufficient lubrication	Medical care to reduce infection or repair damaged or abnormal tissue; additional lubrication

Sexual Orientation

Sexual orientation refers to the direction in which people focus their sexual interests. People can be attracted to opposite-gender partners, same-gender partners, or partners of both genders.

Heterosexuality

Heterosexuality (or heterosexual orientation) refers to an attraction to opposite-gender partners. (*Heteros* is a Greek word that means "the other.") A heterosexual person is sometimes called *straight*. Throughout the world, this is the most common sexual orientation. For reasons related to species survival, heterosexuality has its most basic roots in the biological dimension of human sexuality. Beyond its biological roots, heterosexuality has significant cultural and religious support in virtually every country in the world. Worldwide, laws related to marriage, living arrangements, health benefits, child rearing, financial matters, sexual behavior, and inheritance generally support relationships that are heterosexual in nature. However, this may soon be changing. (See page 420 for information regarding same-sex marriage.)

Homosexuality

Homosexuality (or homosexual orientation) refers to an attraction to same-gender partners. The term *homosexuality* comes from the Greek word *homos,* meaning "the same." The term *gay* can refer to males or females, whereas the word *lesbian* is used only in reference to females.[5]

The distinctions among the categories of sexual orientation are much less clear than their definitions might suggest. Most people probably fall somewhere along a continuum between exclusive heterosexuality and exclusive homosexuality. Kinsey in 1948 presented just such a continuum.[6]

Students often wonder, "What makes a person gay?" This question has no simple answer. (College sexuality textbooks devote entire chapters to this topic.) Some research has pointed to differences in the sizes of certain brain structures as a possible biological or anatomical basis for homosexuality.[7] Other research proposes possible genetic, environmental, hormonal, or other foundations.

Two studies published in 2006 in the *Proceedings of the National Academy of Sciences* support the biological basis for sexual orientation. One study identified different neural pathways that lesbians and nonlesbians use to process pheromone-like stimuli in the hypothalamic region of the brain.[8] The other study examined four groups of Canadian men (944 subjects) and discovered that men with at least several older brothers were more

likely to be gay than were men without older brothers or with just one or two older brothers. This effect was seen only in those men whose older brothers had the same biological mother. The effect was not seen in men whose older brothers were stepbrothers or adopted brothers. The lead researcher theorized that there was some unknown prenatal mechanism (perhaps a mother's increasing immune response to male fetuses, a "maternal memory" for male gestations) that caused her to develop anti-male antibodies that altered the brain chemistry and development of her subsequent male fetuses.[9]

However, for sexual orientation in general, no single theory has emerged that fully explains this complex developmental process. The consensus of scientific opinion is that people do not choose their sexual orientation. Thus, being straight or being gay is something that "just happens." Most gays and lesbians report that no specific event "triggered" them into being gay. Many also indicate that they knew that their orientations were different from those of other children as far back as their prepuberty years.

Given the many challenges of being gay in a straight world, it would seem logical that gays and lesbians do not make conscious efforts to become gay. It is also highly unlikely that heterosexual persons actually choose to be straight. Sexual orientation is something that just unfolds. (See the box "Coming Out—Then What?" on page 410 for insight into some of the issues that gays and lesbians need to face.)

Although operational definitions of sexual orientation may vary from researcher to researcher, Kinsey estimated that about 2 percent of American females and 4 percent of American males were exclusively homosexual.[6, 10] More recent estimates place the overall combined figure at about 10 percent of the population. The expression of same-gender attraction is not uncommon.

TALKING POINTS How would you react if a close family member told you that he or she was gay? Could you be supportive or at least communicate your feelings without anger or criticism?

Bisexuality

People who have the ability to be attracted to either gender are referred to as *bisexuals*. Bisexuals may fall into one of several groups: those who are (1) genuinely attracted to both genders, (2) gay but also feel the need to behave heterosexually, (3) aroused physically by the same gender but attracted emotionally to the opposite gender, (4) aroused physically by the opposite gender, but attracted emotionally to the same gender. Some people participate in a bisexual lifestyle for extended periods, whereas others move quickly to a more exclusive orientation. The size of the bisexual population is not accurately known. (See the box "Challenges for Bisexuals" for more information on bisexual men and women.)

Gender Identity Issues

Gender identity refers to the recognition of oneself as a male or female. As noted in Chapter 14, this recognition initially takes place within about 18 months after birth.

Most people then move through their lives, adopting many or all of the traditional gender roles for their biological sex. Most feel reasonably comfortable with who they are as a man or a woman.

However, this typical pattern does not occur for everyone: (a) Some individuals are not comfortable with their biological sex. They struggle with the issue of transsexualism. (b) Transgendered people prefer not conforming to society's traditional expectations for their sex. (c) Other individuals are comfortable with their gender identity but find sexual pleasure from dressing in clothes that are more culturally "appropriate" for the opposite gender. These persons engage in transvestism.

Transsexualism

Transsexualism is an uncommon sexual variation in which a person rejects his or her biological sexuality. The male transsexual believes that he truly is a "woman trapped in a man's body." He desires to be the woman who he knows he is. Likewise, the female transsexual believes that she is a male existing in a woman's body. She desires to be the man who she knows she is. (Note that sex therapists and psychiatrists do not view transsexuals as homosexual in their sexual orientation.)

For transsexuals, the periods of gender preference and gender adoption (see Chapter 14) are perplexing as they attempt, often with little success, to resolve the conflict between what their mind tells them is true and

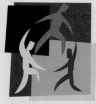
People whose sexual orientation is toward both men and women are termed *bisexuals.* This can be a confusing label, however. For example, if a man has had one sexual experience with a man, but all of his other sexual experiences are with women, does this mean he is a bisexual? And what about the woman who has sequential relationships with men, followed by an occasional relationship with a woman? Is she bisexual? What about people who are sexually attracted to one gender, but are emotionally more attracted to the other gender? The labels can get confusing and can make one wonder about the value of any label describing sexual orientation. This is just one of the many challenges facing bisexual people.

Some experts suggest that bisexuals (those who have had at least one sexual experience with a man and one with a woman) probably outnumber exclusive homosexuals (those who have had sexual experience *only* with persons of their own gender).* One might think that this larger group would be better understood by society, but that seems not to be the case. Bisexuals may have a larger field of potential partners, but this benefit may be offset by the difficulty of "fitting" into society.

Heterosexual people, gay males, and lesbians may not view bisexuality as acceptable, believing that the bisexual person is just incapable of making the decision to go one way or the other.† They may accuse the bisexual person of wanting the best of both worlds, as if "having it all" (in terms of sexual possibilities and experiences) is an inappropriate, bad thing. Then there is the issue of telling a new dating partner that you are attracted to both men and women. Some new partners may find this reality a distinct "turnoff."

For these reasons, numerous college and university counseling centers are expanding their outreach programs to include programs for bisexual students. If you are interested, you might check into the offerings of your campus counseling center to see if they provide educational information, support groups, or specialized counseling for bisexual students. Many campuses also have student groups that focus on gay, lesbian, bisexual, and transgendered students.

Interestingly, it appears that more and more bisexual students are "coming out" despite the challenges they may face. In the near future, we may find more public acceptance for people who are bisexual. Would you consider increased public acceptance of bisexuality to be a good or bad thing?

*Hyde JS, DeLamater JD. *Understanding Human Sexuality* (10th ed.). New York: McGraw-Hill, 2009.
†Kelly GF. *Sexuality Today: The Human Perspective* (8th ed.). New York: McGraw-Hill, 2006.

what their body displays. Adolescent and young adult transsexuals may cross-dress, undertake gay or lesbian relationships (which they view as heterosexual relationships), and experiment with hormone replacement therapy. Sometimes, transsexuals actively pursue a sex reassignment operation. Thousands of these surgeries have been performed at some of the leading medical centers in the United States. For more detailed information about transsexualism, including theories about the origins of transsexualism, you could consult a textbook used in college human sexuality courses or search the Internet for pertinent websites.

Transgenderism

People who are **transgendered** present appearances and personas that do not conform to the gender role expectations that society has established for their sex. Thus, transgendered persons tend to be nonconformists to traditional sex roles.[11] Transgendered women take on characteristics and mannerisms of men, and transgendered men take on characteristics and mannerisms of women. They might cross-dress on a full- or part-time basis, although they usually do not do this for sexual arousal purposes (as transvestites typically do).

Do transgendered persons differ from transsexuals? Yes, they are two different categories, according to

Some people do not conform to the gender-role expectations that society has established for their sex.

Key Terms

transsexualism A sexual variation in which a person rejects his or her biological sexuality.

transgendered Refers to persons whose appearance and behaviors do not conform to society's traditional gender role expectations.

sexuality experts.[11] The main distinction is that transgendered persons do not feel the need to surgically change their bodies to achieve the physical structures of the other sex. Transsexuals feel trapped in an opposite-sex body, and many would like to have their genitals and body appearance be consistent with the "sex they know themselves to be." However, transgendered individuals know and accept the sex to which they were born; yet they prefer to take on and display mannerisms of the other sex.

Transvestism

Public figures such as Dennis Rodman, Eddie Izzard, Harvey Fierstein, and RuPaul have turned a spotlight on cross-dressing, or transvestism. The term **transvestism** is typically used to describe a heterosexual male who, from time to time, dresses as a woman. (Some gay men and women enjoy cross-dressing on occasion.) The practice of transvestism can range from simple sexual gratification from the wearing of feminine clothing, to the expression of the feminine side of the individual's personality. Although many transvestites wish to express the feminine aspects of their personality, most are satisfied with their gender role and their biological gender. Many are married and may or may not have shared this aspect of their personality with their partner.

One large study found that typical cross-dressers are virtually indistinguishable from non-cross-dressing men in their personality traits, sexuality, and measures of psychological wellness.[12]

Years ago, psychologists attempted to cure cross-dressers, but today most have recognized that cross-dressing is lifelong and that they can obtain better results by teaching the cross-dresser to accept his feminine side.

It is rare for a female to be a transvestite, perhaps because the norms for women's clothing are far less restrictive than those for men. For example, while it might be quite normal to see your grandmother wearing a flannel shirt and blue jeans around the house, it would be surprising for you to see your grandfather watching NFL football wearing a frilly negligee.

Patterns of Sexual Behavior

Although sex researchers may see sexual behavior in terms of the human sexual response pattern described earlier, most people are more interested in the observable dimensions of sexual behavior.

Celibacy

Celibacy can be defined as the self-imposed avoidance of sexual intimacy. Celibacy is synonymous with sexual abstinence. People could choose not to have a sexually intimate relationship for many reasons. For some,

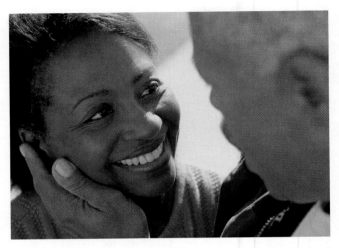

Any sensual contact can be a form of communication and sexual expression between partners.

celibacy is part of a religious doctrine. Others might be afraid of contracting a sexually transmitted disease. For most, however, celibacy is preferred simply because it seems appropriate for them. Celibate people can certainly have deep, intimate relationships with other people—just not sexual relationships. Celibacy may be short term or last a lifetime, and no identified physical or psychological complications appear to result from a celibate lifestyle.

Masturbation

Throughout recorded history, **masturbation** has been a primary method of achieving sexual pleasure. Through masturbation, people can explore their sexual response patterns. Traditionally, some societies and religious groups have condemned this behavior based on the belief that intercourse is the only "right" sexual behavior. With sufficient lubrication, masturbation cannot do physical harm. Today masturbation is considered by most sex therapists and researchers to be a normal source of self-pleasure.

Fantasy and Erotic Dreams

The brain is the most sensual organ in the body. In fact, many sexuality experts classify **sexual fantasies** and **erotic dreams** as forms of sexual behavior. Particularly for people whose verbal ability is highly developed, the ability to create imaginary scenes enriches other forms of sexual behavior.

Sexual fantasies are generally found in association with some second type of sexual behavior. When occurring before intercourse or masturbation, fantasies prepare a person for the behavior that will follow. As an example, fantasies experienced while reading a book may focus your attention on sexual activity that will occur later in the day.

When fantasies occur with another form of sexual behavior, the second behavior may be greatly enhanced by the supportive fantasy. Both women and men fantasize during foreplay and intercourse. Masturbation and fantasizing are inseparable activities.

Erotic dreams occur during sleep in both men and women. The association between these dreams and ejaculation resulting in a nocturnal emission (wet dream) is readily recognized in men. In women, erotic dreams can lead not only to vaginal lubrication but to orgasm as well.

Shared Touching

Virtually the entire body can be an erogenous zone when sensual contact between partners is involved. A soft, light touch, a slight application of pressure, the brushing back of a partner's hair, and gentle massage are all forms of communication that heighten sexual arousal.

Genital Contact

Two important purposes can be identified for the practice of stimulating a partner's genitals. The first is the tactile component of **foreplay.** Genital contact, in the form of holding, rubbing, or caressing, heightens arousal to a level that allows for progression into intercourse.

The second role of genital contact is that of *mutual masturbation to orgasm.* Stimulation of the genitals so that both partners have orgasm is a form of sexual behavior practiced by many people, as well as by couples during the late stage of a pregnancy. For couples not desiring pregnancy, the risk of conception is virtually eliminated when this becomes the form of sexual intimacy practiced.

As is the case in other aspects of intimacy, genital stimulation is best enhanced when partners can talk about their needs, expectations, and reservations. Practice and communication can shape this form of contact into a pleasure-giving approach to sexual intimacy.

Oral-Genital Stimulation

Oral-genital stimulation brings together two of the body's most erogenous areas: the genitalia and the mouth. Couples who engage in oral sex consistently report that this form of intimacy is highly satisfactory. Some people have experimented with oral sex and found it unacceptable, and some have never experienced this form of sexual intimacy. Some couples prefer not to participate in oral sex because they consider it immoral (according to religious doctrine), illegal (which it is in some states), or unhygienic (because of a partner's unclean genitals). Some couples may refrain because of the mistaken belief that oral sex is only for gays and lesbians. Regardless of the reason, a person who does not consider oral sex to be pleasurable should not be coerced into this behavior.

Because oral-genital stimulation can involve an exchange of body fluids, the risk of disease transmission is real. Small tears in mouth or genital tissue may allow transmission of disease-causing pathogens. Only couples who are absolutely certain that they are free from all sexually transmitted diseases (including HIV infection) can practice unprotected oral sex. Couples in doubt should refrain from oral-genital sex or carefully use a condom (on the male) or a latex square to cover the female's vulval area. Increasingly, latex squares (dental dams) can be obtained from drugstores or pharmacies. (Dentists may also provide you with dental dams, or you can make your own latex square by cutting a condom into an appropriate shape.)

Three basic forms of oral-genital stimulation are practiced by both heterosexual and homosexual couples.[11] **Fellatio,** in which the penis is kissed, licked, or sucked by the partner, is the most common of the three. **Cunnilingus,** in which the vulva of the female is kissed, licked, or penetrated by the partner's tongue, is only slightly less frequently practiced.

Mutual oral-genital stimulation, the third form of oral-genital stimulation, combines both fellatio and cunnilingus. When practiced by a heterosexual couple, the female partner performs fellatio on her partner while her male partner performs cunnilingus on her. Gay couples can practice mutual fellatio or cunnilingus.

Intercourse

Sexual intercourse (coitus) refers to the act of inserting the penis into the vagina. Intercourse is the sexual behavior that is most directly associated with **procreation.** For some, intercourse is the only natural and appropriate form of sexual intimacy.

Key Terms

transvestism Atypical behavior in which a person derives sexual pleasure from dressing in the clothes of the opposite gender.

masturbation Self-stimulation of the genitals.

sexual fantasies Fantasies with sexual themes; sexual daydreams or imaginary events.

erotic dreams Dreams whose contents elicit a sexual response.

foreplay Activities, often involving touching and caressing, that prepare individuals for sexual intercourse.

fellatio (feh **lay** she oh) Oral stimulation of the penis.

cunnilingus (cun uh **ling** gus) Oral stimulation of the vulva or clitoris.

procreation Reproduction.

The incidence and frequency of sexual intercourse is a much-studied topic. Information concerning the percentages of people who have engaged in intercourse is readily available in textbooks used in sexuality courses. Data concerning sexual intercourse among college students may be changing somewhat because of concerns about HIV infection and other STDs, but a reasonable estimate of the percentage of college students who have engaged in sexual intercourse is 60 to 75 percent.

These percentages reflect two important concepts about the sexual activity of college students. The first is that most college students are having intercourse. The second concept is that a large percentage (25–40 percent) of students are choosing to refrain from intercourse. Indeed, the belief that "everyone is doing it" may be a bit shortsighted. From a public health standpoint, we believe it is important to provide accurate health information to protect those who choose to have intercourse and to actively support a person's right to choose not to have intercourse.

Sexually active couples need to share their expectations concerning techniques and the desired frequency of intercourse. Even the "performance" factors, such as depth of penetration, nature of body movements, tempo of activity, and timing of orgasm, are increasingly important to many couples. Issues concerning sexually transmitted diseases (including HIV infection) are also critically important for couples who are contemplating intercourse. These factors also need to be explored through open communication.

A variety of books (including textbooks) provide written and visually explicit information on intercourse positions. Four basic positions for intercourse—*man above, woman above, side by side,* and *rear entry*—each offers relative advantages and disadvantages.

Anal Sexual Activity

Some couples practice **anal intercourse,** in which the penis is inserted into the rectum of a partner. Anal intercourse can be performed by both heterosexual couples and gay men. According to a report in the journal *Archives of Sexual Behavior,* about 20 to 25 percent of college students have experienced anal intercourse.[13] The anal sphincter muscles contract tightly and tend to resist entry. Thus, couples who engage in anal intercourse must do so slowly, gently, and with adequate amounts of water-based lubricants. Because of the danger of tearing tissues in the rectal area, HIV transmission risk is increased if the inserting male is infected.[3] Unless it is absolutely certain that both partners are uninfected, the inserting male should always wear a condom. Even with a condom, disease transmission is possible, since during anal intercourse, condoms are more likely to tear than during penis-vaginal intercourse. Couples practicing anal sex must not follow anal insertion with insertion into the mouth or vagina because of the likelihood of transmitting infectious agents.

For many people, anal intercourse is not only unpleasant, but simply unnatural for humans. For others, the anal area is just another part of the human body that is especially sensitive to stimulation, and they enjoy the pleasurable sensations that come from intercourse or the insertion of a well-lubricated finger or sex toy. Some people enjoy kissing ("rimming") or touching in the anal area, but this should occur only when the anal area has been fully cleansed or covered with a sheet of protective plastic wrap. As with all sexual behavior, couples need to communicate clearly their feelings about any activity. If one partner is uncomfortable about an activity and wants to stop, his or her feelings must be supported by the other person. A desire for a particular sexual activity must not turn into sexual coercion or a sexual assault.

Secondary Virginity

Some individuals who have previously engaged in sexual intercourse have chosen to refrain from further sexual intercourse. They are said to be practicing **secondary virginity.** The practice of secondary virginity reflects a conscious choice for persons to wait until a time when they feel it's all right to resume intercourse.

The decision to be a secondary virgin can be made for a number of reasons. Some prefer to return to abstinence for moral or religious reasons, while others wish to wait until there is more commitment in the relationship. Some come to the realization that they are not yet physically or emotionally ready for intercourse. Others do not want to risk pregnancy or the possibility of contracting a sexually transmitted disease. Some do not have the time or energy needed to become involved in a sexual relationship.

Those who choose secondary virginity are quick to point out its advantages. They no longer worry about certain risks, such as pregnancy or contracting an STD. They no longer have to worry about the expense of contraception or the side effects from certain forms of birth control. Some feel great relief knowing that they are successfully following their own moral compass or religious beliefs. By pursuing secondary virginity, they can focus a great deal more time and energy on other important aspects of their relationship.

Sexuality and Aging

Students are often curious about how aging affects sexuality. This is understandable because we live in a society that idolizes youth and demands performance. Many younger people become anxious about growing older because of what they think will happen to their ability to express their sexuality. Interestingly, young adults are willing to accept other physical changes of aging (such as the slowing down of basal metabolism, reduced lung capacity, and even wrinkles) but not those changes related to sexuality.

Research shows that, although sexual activity does decline with age, the capacity to enjoy sex is not altered, and a significant proportion of older adults remain sexually active.[4]

As with other aspects of aging, certain anatomical and physiological changes will be evident, but these changes do not necessarily reduce the ability to enjoy sexual activity. Most experts in sexuality report that many older people remain interested in sexual activity. Furthermore, those who are exposed to regular sexual activity throughout a lifetime report being most satisfied with their sex lives as older adults.[11]

As people age, the likelihood of alterations in the male and female sexual response patterns increases. In the postmenopausal woman, vaginal lubrication commonly begins more slowly, and the amount of lubrication usually diminishes. However, clitoral sensitivity and nipple erection remain the same as in earlier years. The female capacity for multiple orgasms remains the same, although the number of contractions that occur at orgasm typically is reduced.

In the older man, physical changes are also evident. This is thought to be caused by the decrease in the production of testosterone between the ages of 20 and 60 years. After age 60 or so, testosterone levels remain relatively steady. Thus many men, despite a decrease in sperm production, remain fertile into their 80s.[11] Older men typically take longer to achieve an erection (however, they are able to maintain their erection longer before ejaculation), have fewer muscular contractions at orgasm, and ejaculate less forcefully than they once did. The volume of seminal fluid ejaculated is typically less than in earlier years, and its consistency is somewhat thinner. The resolution phase is usually longer in older men. In spite of these gradual changes, some elderly men engage in sexual intercourse with the same frequency as do much younger men.

Bonds Between People

As people develop their relationships, they often form bonds that start with friendship and dating activities and then move toward intimacy and love. Let's explore these stepping-stones.

Friendship

One of the exciting aspects of college life is that you will probably meet many new people, some of whom will become your best friends. Because of your common experiences, it is likely that you will keep in contact with a few of these friends for a lifetime. Close attachments to other people can have an important influence on all of the dimensions of your health.

What is it that draws friends together? With the exception of physical intimacy, many of the same growth experiences seen in dating and mate selection are also seen in the development of friendships. Think about how you and your best friend developed the relationship you now have. You probably became friends when you shared similar interests and experiences. Your friendship progressed (and even faltered at times) through personal gains or losses. In all likelihood, you cared about each other and learned to share your deepest beliefs and feelings. You cemented your bond by turning your beliefs into behaviors. You resolved conflicts (see the box "Resolving Conflict Through Better Communication").

Throughout the development of a deep friendship, the qualities of trust, tolerance, empathy, and support must be demonstrated. Otherwise, the friendship can fall apart. You will soon note that the qualities seen in a friendship are very similar to the qualities noted in the upcoming description of companionate love (page 417). In both cases, people develop deep attachments through extensive familiarity and understanding.

Dating

A half-century ago, the events involved in a dating relationship were somewhat predictable. People met each other through their daily activities or groups of friends, and a formal request for a date was made. Ninety-nine times out of a hundred, the requestor was male and the invitee was female. After a period of formal and informal dates, the two made a commitment to steady dating or decided to "date around." If the relationship progressed, further commitments were made (for example, letter jackets, class rings, or other jewelry items were exchanged). After months or years of a committed relationship, the couple decided to get married. The man invariably asked for the woman's "hand" (after first receiving permission from her parents), and plans for a wedding ceremony were made.

Does this form of dating and mate selection exist now in the new millennium? For some couples, yes. The traditional way of dating and selecting a life partner works well for them. However, many young and midlife adults prefer a more flexible, less predictable format for

---

Key Terms

anal intercourse A sexual act in which the erect penis is inserted into the rectum of a partner.

secondary virginity The discontinuation of sexual intercourse after initial exploration.

Resolving Conflict Through Better Communication

Every relationship presents challenges to the individuals involved. Therapists would argue that couples who can learn to resolve conflict effectively have the best chance of maintaining long-term relationships. The hallmark of effective conflict resolution is that each person ends up feeling respected by his or her partner. Not surprisingly, this process is built on effective communication.

Here are some successful ways to communicate better to manage conflict:

- Show mutual respect. Remain calm.
- Identify and resolve the real issue.
- Be a good listener.
- Seek areas of agreement.
- Do not interrupt.
- Mutually participate in decision making.
- Be cooperative and specific.
- Focus on the present and future—not the past.
- Don't try to assign blame.
- Say what you are thinking and feeling.
- When talking, use sentences that begin with "I."
- Avoid using sentences that start with "You" or "Why."
- Set a time limit for discussing problems.
- Accept responsibility.
- Do something fun together.

dating and finding a person they might choose to marry. For example, more than ever, women are playing a more assertive role when it comes to initiating and establishing the ground rules for a relationship.

Interestingly, a large number of our students do not even like to use the word *dating* because it connotes a formalized pattern of behavior followed by their parents and grandparents. Many college students today seem to prefer "hanging out" with a group of 5 to 10 friends, instead of pairing off with a partner and doing only "couple activities."

When students do start to pair off and become exclusive in their dating, they tend to pursue a pattern called **serial monogamy.** In serial monogamy, a person dates one person exclusively until the relationship ends. Then another partner is found, and that couple dates exclusively for a period of time until that relationship eventually ends. In this pattern of dating, individuals do not date multiple people simultaneously. They go through mutually exclusive relationships, one after the other.

Students can fool themselves into believing that their dating patterns reflect **mutual monogamy.** Some couples believe that going out with another person as long as six months or a year reflects mutual monogamy. (Technically, for the six months or the year of going out, it can be called mutual monogamy.) When that relationship ends and a new one begins, however, the persons involved must understand that their dating pattern is developing into a serial pattern.

One critical health issue involved with serial monogamy is the increased possibility of exposure to infectious diseases, including all of the sexually transmitted diseases and HIV. While less risky than having indiscriminate sexual activities with multiple partners at the same time, serial monogamy still exposes a person to a new partner who may or may not be harboring a disease pathogen. Individuals who have a series of intimate relationships with multiple persons need to be especially vigilant in their safe sex practices. They need to understand clearly that their new partner could be exposing them to a rich pool of infectious diseases.

Online Dating

In the last decade, online dating services have become well-established on the Internet. Now, two people can meet each other in a truly virtual way. You probably know people who have used these services. Some have found them helpful, and some have found them frustrating. Regardless, television ads for the most popular Internet dating sites tell us it is easy to find the "person of your dreams" online.

Users of online dating services should keep things in perspective and remain generally skeptical. Remember that the people you are meeting online can portray themselves in any way they wish to. It is very possible that people you meet online don't look like the photo you see, don't have the finances or job they claim to have, and might not even be "childless and single." They may write romantic prose but be interested only in finding someone for sex. Someone who claims to be 23 years old could be any age—53 years old or 13 years old. You never really know.

For these reasons, you should keep up your defenses. Never reveal personal data about yourself that could be used against you—for instance, never give out your full name, your birthday, your ID numbers, your address, your phone numbers, or any specific work information. If your virtual relationship progresses to the point that you want to meet the person face-to-face, you must again be very careful. It is possible that the person could be a predator of some kind. Only agree to meet in a very public place with other people around, so that you can safely remove yourself from the situation, if necessary. Perhaps go with a friend to meet this new person.

During this first, brief meeting, watch for any particular clues that make you feel uneasy. If you discover any such distraction, think twice about having a second meeting. If things go well, who knows? Maybe you've found a real possibility. However, it could (and should) take a long time to determine if this person's initial positive presentation can stand the test of time, as you learn more and more about the reality of this person's life.

Intimacy

When most people hear the word **intimacy,** they immediately think about physical, sexual intimacy. However, sexuality experts and family therapists prefer to view intimacy more broadly, as any close, mutual, verbal or nonverbal behavior within a relationship. In this sense, intimate behavior can range from sharing deep feelings and experiences with a partner to sharing profound physical pleasures with a partner.

Intimacy is present in both love and friendship. You have likely shared intimate feelings with your closest friends, as well as with those you love. Intimacy helps us feel connected to others and allows us to feel the full measure of our own self-worth.

 TALKING POINTS Your teenage son equates intimacy with sex. How would you explain the emotional intimacy involved in marriage?

Love

Love may be one of the most elusive yet widely recognized concepts that describe some level of emotional attachment to another. Various forms of love include friendship and erotic, devotional, parental, and altruistic love. Other behavioral scientists[11] have focused primarily on two types of love most closely associated with dating and mate selection: *passionate love* and *companionate love.*

Passionate love, also described as romantic love or **infatuation,** is a state of extreme absorption in another. It is characterized by intense feelings of tenderness, elation, anxiety, sexual desire, and ecstasy. Often appearing early in a relationship, passionate love typically does not last very long. Passionate love is driven by the excitement of being closely involved with a person whose character is not fully known.

If a relationship progresses, passionate love is gradually replaced by companionate love. This type of love is a less intense emotion than passionate love. It is characterized by friendly affection and a deep attachment that is based on extensive familiarity with the loved one.[11] This love is enduring and capable of sustaining long-term mutual growth. Central to companionate love are feelings of empathy for, support of, and tolerance of the partner. Complete the Personal Assessment at the end of this chapter to determine whether you and your partner are truly compatible.

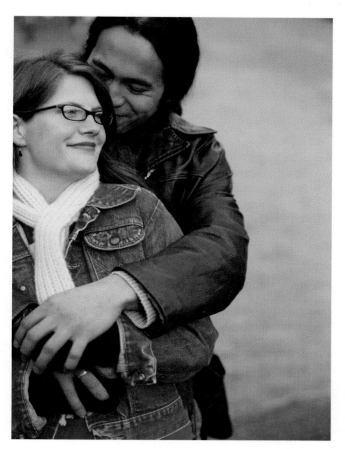

Companionate love is capable of sustaining mutual long-term growth.

Qualities of a Healthy Relationship

Perhaps the best thing a person could have is a truly fantastic relationship with someone. Such a relationship might be better than getting straight A's, better than looking like a movie star, and better than winning the lottery. But how do you know if what you have is a great relationship? Said in another way, what are the qualities that reflect a healthy relationship?

> **Key Terms**
>
> **serial monogamy** A pattern of dating in which a person is involved in a series of exclusive relationships, one after the other.
>
> **mutual monogamy** A pattern of dating in which a person is involved exclusively with one partner.
>
> **intimacy** Any close, mutual, verbal or nonverbal behavior within a relationship.
>
> **infatuation** A relatively temporary, intensely romantic attraction to another person.

Although bookstore shelves are filled with hundreds of books that try to pinpoint the answer to this question, here are some basic qualities that reflect a healthy relationship. In a healthy relationship, partners should feel safe and treat each other with respect. Partners should enjoy spending time with each other, yet they still feel good about having some personal, private time. In a healthy relationship, partners trust each other and openly communicate their needs, concerns, and feelings. Partners in a good relationship are interested in each other's lives, including their families, work activities, and recreational needs. If the relationship is sexually intimate, partners are honest and open about their past and current sexual activity. There also should be no sexual coercion in a healthy relationship.[14]

Even great relationships have their ups and downs (see the box "How 'Real' Are the Relationships Seen on TV Dramas and Soaps?"). For the long run, partners need to have some healthy optimism, a measure of flexibility, and a willingness to compromise during the tough times. Perhaps the simplest sign of a healthy relationship is that it has a lot more positive aspects to it than negative ones.

Communication in Relationships

As you read this chapter, you might notice that one of the recurring messages is the importance of effective communication between partners in a relationship. Furthermore, the sections on friendship, dating, intimacy, love, and marriage become meaningless unless you realize that true satisfaction in these areas is grounded in effective communication. When you think about it, effective communication is the basis for *all healthy relationships.*

For this reason, we encourage all readers to take advantage of every available opportunity to learn effective communication skills. You might find these opportunities in college courses. Most speech and communication departments have courses that teach personal communication skills. Look for pertinent courses in psychology and counseling psychology departments. Most colleges and universities also offer one or more human sexuality courses in their biology, psychology, sociology, consumer sciences, or health science departments. The counseling center on your campus may offer programs that can improve your communication skills. Finally, your campus library or bookstore will have popular books that may be very useful.

Recognizing Unhealthy Relationships

Sadly, sometimes people do not recognize or heed the warning signs of an unstable relationship, so they stay involved long after the risks outweigh the benefits of the relationship. These warning signs include abusive behavior, whether it is emotional or physical abuse (see Chapter 19). Another red flag is excessive jealousy about a partner's interactions with others. Sometimes excessive jealousy evolves into controlling behavior, as one partner attempts to manage the daily activities of the other partner. By definition, controlling behavior limits your creativity and freedom.

Other warning signs are dishonesty, irresponsibility, lack of patience, and any kind of drug abuse. We certainly do not want to see these qualities in those we have initially judged to be "nice people," even though these unappealing characteristics may be obvious to others. If you suspect that any of these problems may be undermining your relationship, talk about your concerns with one or two trusted friends, and then seek the advice of a professional counselor at your college or university. Life is too short to spend it with people who are making your life miserable.

Ending a Relationship

One of life's real challenges is dealing with the breakup of a relationship. Generally speaking, the longer the relationship has lasted, the more difficult it is to end it. While a bad first date can halt a potential relationship quickly, a partnership that has gone on for a few weeks, months, or years can be much more complicated. However, it is best to act quickly after making the firm judgment that the relationship is over. This allows you both not to waste time on a relationship that just isn't working out.

Each breakup situation is different, but there are some common threads to keep in mind. Unless you have been treated poorly (by a partner who cheated, lied, abused, manipulated, or disrespected you), try to show some personal *respect* and *courtesy* to the other person. Whether it is in a face-to-face meeting, a phone call, a text message, or an email, try also to keep the message *clear and simple.* You can state that you just don't think the relationship is working and that you want to move on. Don't feel that you have to identify a specific event that caused you to want to break up, and don't place blame on the other person. Don't feel that you have to justify yourself or explain your reasons, either. Keep the message *short.*[15]

One hopes the ending of a relationship will be emotionally beneficial for both of you. If not, and you have lingering concerns over the breakup, you should seek help from your college's counseling center or a trusted friend or professor. If your former partner becomes abusive or threatening in some way (perhaps by harassing you through stalking, constant e-mailing, or incessant phoning), you should contact your campus security department or local police. (See Chapter 19 about protecting your safety.)

Relationships and Lifestyles

A variety of formal and informal relationships and lifestyles exist in our society. Here are a few of the most common ones.

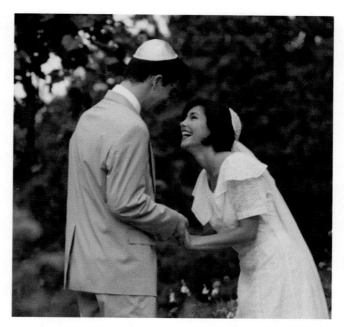

Recent statistics show that both men and women are waiting longer to get married.

Marriage

Just as there is no single best way for two people to move through dating and mate selection, marriage is an equally variable undertaking. In marriage, two people join their lives in a way that affirms each as an individual and both as a legal pair. They are able to resolve issues constructively (see the box "Improving Marriage"). However, for a large percentage of couples, the demands of marriage are too rigorous, confining, and demanding. They will find resolution for their dissatisfaction through divorce or extramarital affairs. For most, though, marriage will be an experience that alternates periods of happiness, productivity, and admiration with periods of frustration, unhappiness, and disillusionment with the partner. Each marriage is unique. Each marriage provides an opportunity for the partners to share a lifetime of experiences.

As we move through the early years of this new century, we see certain trends in marriage. The most obvious of these is the age at first marriage. Today men are waiting longer than ever to marry. Now the median age at first marriage for men is 27.5 years.[16] In addition, these new husbands are better educated than in the past and are more likely to be established in their careers. Women are also waiting longer to get married and tend to be more educated and career oriented. Recent statistics indicate that the median age at first marriage for women is 25.9 years.[16]

Marriage still appeals to most adults. Currently, 75 percent of adults age 18 and older are married, widowed, or divorced.[17] Thus one-quarter of today's adults have never married.

Gay and Lesbian Partnerships

To believe that adult partnerships are reserved only for heterosexual couples is to avoid reality. In the United States and in many parts of the world, gays and lesbians are forming partnerships that, in many ways, mimic those of heterosexuals. It no longer is unusual to see same-sex men and women openly living together in one household. Gay and lesbian couples buy houses together and share property rights. As businesses restructure their employee benefits packages, gays and lesbians are covering their partners on health care plans and making them beneficiaries on their insurance policies and retirement plans.

A search of the literature will indicate that gay and lesbian partnerships have many of the same characteristics and problems as heterosexual couples.[3] Like straight couples, they struggle with interpersonal issues related to their relationship and their lifestyle. They work to decide how best to juggle their financial resources, their leisure time, and their friends and extended families. If they live together in an apartment or house, they must decide how to divide the household tasks.

If children are present in the household, they must be cared for and nurtured. These children could have come from an adoption, a previous heterosexual relationship, or, in the case of a lesbian couple, from artificial insemination. Research indicates that children raised in gay or lesbian families overwhelmingly grow up with a heterosexual orientation, and are like other children from heterosexual families in terms of their adjustment, mental health, social skills, and peer acceptance.[3]

Same-Sex Marriage

One area in which gay and lesbian couples differ from heterosexual couples is in their ability to obtain a legal

marriage. In the last few years, this inequity has been the focus of an intense national debate over same-sex marriage. The issues are complex, primarily because of the differences in state laws and the various courts' interpretations of those laws. At this point in the debate, here is where same-sex marriage stands.

If enacted, same-sex marriages would grant gay couples a legal marriage document that allows for an array of legal and economic benefits, including joint parental custody, insurance and health benefits, joint tax returns, alimony and child support, inheritance of property, hospital visitation rights, family leave, and a spouse's retirement benefits. (Social Security benefits come from a federal program and are not influenced by state laws.)

Currently, the states of Massachusetts, Connecticut, Iowa, Vermont, and New Hampshire are the only states

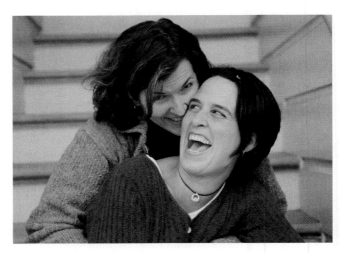

Legalization of same-sex marriage would grant gay and lesbian couples a wide range of legal and economic rights.

that have legalized same-sex marriage. (California once allowed same-sex marriage, but in November 2008, voters passed a constitutional amendment, Proposition 8, limiting marriage "to one man and one woman." In 2009, an appeal of Proposition 8 was unsuccessful. However, same-sex marriages performed before Proposition 8 were permitted to remain valid in California.) Most states do not recognize same-sex marriages formed in other jurisdictions.[18]

In 2000, the Vermont legislature passed the nation's first "civil union" law, which granted legal status to gay and lesbian couples. Vermont's law conferred on same-sex couples all the benefits that the state allowed for heterosexual married couples. Since then, Connecticut, New Jersey, and New Hampshire have also passed civil union legislation. However, these civil unions are not generally recognized in other states.

In an attempt to counter movements toward same-sex marriage, 41 states have established state constitutional amendments or state laws that restrict marriage to one man and one woman. A handful of states have established laws that grant "domestic partner" benefits (but not marriage) to committed gay and lesbian couples who register with the state government. Among these are California, Oregon, Hawaii, Maine, the District of Columbia, and Washington.[18]

It is conceivable that the debate over same-sex marriages could push more states to adopt domestic partnership legislation, with the hopes of preserving bans on actual gay and lesbian marriages. Some members of the U.S. Congress have attempted to rally support for a federal constitutional amendment that would ban gay marriage, but at the present time there appears to be insufficient political energy to push this legislation forward. Many observers believe that ultimately the U.S. Supreme Court will have to rule on the constitutionality of same-sex marriage.

Divorce

Marriages, like many other kinds of interpersonal relationships, can end. Today, marriages—relationships begun with the intent of permanence "until death do us part"—end through divorce nearly as frequently as not.

Why should approximately half of marital relationships end? Unfortunately, marriage experts cannot provide one clear answer to this question. Rather, they suggest that divorce is a reflection of unfulfilled expectations for marriage on the part of one or both partners, including the following:

- The belief that marriage will ease your need to deal with your own faults and that your failures can be shared by your partner
- The belief that marriage will change faults that you know exist in your partner

- The belief that the high level of romance of your dating and courtship period will be continued through marriage
- The belief that marriage can provide you with an arena for the development of your personal power, and that once married, you will not need to compromise with your partner
- The belief that your marital partner will be successful in meeting all of your needs

If these expectations seem to be ones you anticipate through marriage, then you may find that disappointments will abound. To varying degrees, marriage is a partnership that requires much cooperation and compromise. Marriage can be complicated. Because of the high expectations that many people hold for marriage, the termination of marriage can be an emotionally difficult process to undertake.

The American attitude toward divorce swung like a pendulum during the last century. Divorce has gone from being an embarrassing, painful ordeal, to a common, relatively simple legal procedure. More recently, some observers have begun to question the wisdom of no-fault divorce.

Our society is concerned about the well-being of children whose parents divorce. Different factors, however, influence the extent to which divorce affects children. Included among these factors are the gender and age of the children, custody arrangements, financial support, and the remarriage of one or both parents. Many children must adjust to accept their new status as a member of a blended family.

Singlehood

For many people, being single is a lifestyle that affords the potential for pursuing intimacy, if desired, and provides an uncluttered path for independence and self-directedness. Other people, however, are single because of divorce, separation, death, or the absence of an opportunity to establish a partnership. The U.S. Census Bureau indicates that 43 percent of women and 40 percent of men over the age of 18 are currently single.[17]

Single people can have many different living arrangements. Some single people live alone and choose not to share a household. Other arrangements for singles include cohabitation, periodic cohabitation, singlehood during the week and cohabitation on the weekends or during vacations, or the platonic sharing of a household with others. For young adults, large percentages of single men and women live with their parents.

Like living arrangements, the sexual intimacy patterns of singles are individually tailored. Some singles practice celibacy, others pursue intimate relationships in a **monogamous** pattern, and others have multiple partners. As in all interpersonal relationships, including marriage, the levels of commitment are as variable as the people involved.

Cohabitation

Cohabitation, or the sharing of living quarters by unmarried people, represents yet another alternative to marriage. According to the U.S. Census Bureau, the number of unmarried, opposite-gender couples living together totals over 5.2 million couples.[17] The number of reported same-gender couples totaled nearly 800,000 in the year 2005.

Although cohabitation may seem to imply a vision of sexual intimacy between male and female roommates, several forms of shared living arrangements can be viewed as cohabitation. For some couples, cohabitation is only a part-time arrangement for weekends, during summer vacation, or on a variable schedule. In addition, **platonic** cohabitation can exist when a couple shares living quarters but does so without establishing an intimate relationship. Close friends, people of retirement age, and gay couples might all be included in a group called cohabitants.

How well do cohabitation arrangements fare against marriage partnerships in terms of long-term stability? A report prepared by the CDC's National Center for Health Statistics[19] indicated that unmarried cohabitations are generally less stable than marriages. The probability of a first marriage ending in separation or divorce within 5 years was found to be 20 percent, but the probability of a premarital cohabitation breaking up within 5 years was 49 percent. After 10 years, the probability of a first marriage ending was 33 percent, compared with 62 percent for cohabitations.

Single Parenthood

Unmarried young women continue to become pregnant and then become single parents in this country. In 2005, unmarried mothers accounted for 37 percent of all newborn births in the United States.[17] There is also a significantly different form of single parenthood: the planned entry into single parenthood by older, better-educated people, the vast majority of whom are women.

In contrast to the teenaged girl who becomes a single parent through an unwed pregnancy, the more mature woman who desires single parenting has usually planned carefully for the experience. She has explored several important concerns, including questions regarding how she will become pregnant (with or without the knowledge of a male partner or through artificial insemination), the need for a father figure for the child, the effect of single parenting on her social life, and, of course, its effect on her career development. When these questions have been resolved, no legal barriers stand in the way of her becoming a single parent.

A very large number of women and a growing number of men are actively participating in single parenthood as a result of a divorce settlement or separation agreement involving sole or joint custody of children. Increasing numbers of single persons are now adopting children. In 2006, single women headed up 8.4 million households with children under the age of 18. In contrast, single men headed up 2.1 million households in the year 2006 with children under the age of 18.[17]

Key Terms

monogamous (mo **nog** a mus) Paired relationship with one partner.

cohabitation Sharing of a residence by unrelated, unmarried people; living together.

platonic Close association between two people that does not include a sexual relationship.

Taking Charge of Your Health

- Take the Personal Assessment at the end of this chapter to learn how compatible you and your partner are.

- If being around someone whose sexual orientation is different from yours makes you feel uncomfortable, focus on getting to know that person better as an individual.

- If you are in an unhealthy relationship, take the first step toward getting out of it through professional counseling or group support.

- If you are in a sexual relationship, communicate your sexual needs to your partner clearly. Encourage him or her to do the same so that you can have a satisfying sex life.

- Consider whether your lifetime plan will include singlehood, marriage, cohabitation, single parenthood, or a gay partnership. Evaluate your current plan in relation to that plan.

SUMMARY

- Men and women share the four stages of sexual response: excitement, plateau, orgasmic, and resolution.
- Direct stimulation of the penis and direct or indirect stimulation of the clitoris are the principal avenues toward orgasm.
- The three sexual orientations are heterosexuality, homosexuality, and bisexuality.
- Most sex therapists and researchers consider masturbation to be a normal source of self-pleasure.
- Shared touching, genital contact, oral-genital stimulation, and intercourse are common forms of sexual intimacy.
- Physiological changes may alter the way in which some older people perform sexually.

- Passionate love is gradually replaced by companionate love, which is characterized by deep affection and attachment.
- Although the legality of gay and lesbian marriages continues to be debated, committed relationships between members of the same sex often mimic the dynamics of heterosexual marriages.
- Although most people marry at some time in their lives, other relationships and lifestyles exist, including singlehood, cohabitation, and single parenthood.
- Most relationships can be improved through better communication.

REVIEW QUESTIONS

1. What similarities and differences exist between the sexual response patterns of males and females? Do both women and men experience vasocongestion and myotonia?
2. Explain the differences between heterosexuality, homosexuality, and bisexuality. How common is each of these sexual orientations in our society?
3. What is the general distinction between a transsexual person and a transgendered person?
4. Define celibacy, masturbation, sexual fantasies, erotic dreams, shared touching, genital contact, oral-genital stimulation, and sexual intercourse.
5. What precautions must be considered if a couple decides to engage in anal sexual activity?

6. Identify the physiological changes that occur in men and women as they get older.
7. Identify five warning signs of an unhealthy relationship. What are some successful ways to end a relationship?
8. What is meant by serial monogamy? What is meant by secondary virginity?
9. What are some differences between passionate love and companionate love?
10. In what ways do gay and lesbian partnerships differ from heterosexual partnerships?

ANSWERS TO THE "WHAT DO YOU KNOW?" QUIZ

1. True   2. False   3. False   4. True   5. False   6. True   7. True

Visit the Online Learning Center (**www.mhhe.com/payne11e**), where you will find tools to help you improve your grade including practice quizzes, key terms flashcards, audio chapter summaries for your MP3 player, and many other study aids.

SOURCE NOTES

1. Masters WH, Johnson VE. *Human Sexual Response*. Philadelphia: Lippincott, Williams and Wilkins, 1966.
2. Strong B, Yarber WL, Sayad BW, DeVault C. *Human Sexuality: Diversity in Contemporary America* (6th ed.), New York: McGraw-Hill, 2008.
3. Hyde JS, DeLamater JD. *Understanding Human Sexuality* (10th ed.). New York: McGraw-Hill, 2009.
4. Carroll JL. *Sexuality Now: Embracing Diversity* (2nd ed.). Belmont, CA: Cengage Learning, 2007.
5. Kelly GF. *Sexuality Today: The Human Perspective* (8th ed.). New York: McGraw-Hill, 2006.
6. Kinsey AC, Pomeroy WB, Martin CE. *Sexual Behavior in the Human Male* (reprint ed.). Bloomington: Indiana University Press, 1998.
7. Allen LS, Gorski RA. Sexual Orientation and the Size of the Anterior Commissure in the Human Brain. *Proceedings of the National Academy of Sciences*, 89(15), 7199–7202, 1992.
8. Berglund H, Lindstrom P, Savic I. Brain Response to Putative Pheromones in Lesbian Women. *Proceedings of the National Academy of Sciences*, 103(21), 8269–8274, 2006.
9. Bogaert AF. Biological Versus Nonbiological Older Brothers and Men's Sexual Orientation. *Proceedings of the National Academy of Sciences*, 103(28), 10771–10774, 2006.
10. Kinsey AC, et al. *Sexual Behavior in the Human Female* (reprint ed.). Bloomington: Indiana University Press, 1998.
11. Crooks RL, Baur K. *Our Sexuality* (10th ed.). Belmont, CA: Wadsworth, 2008.
12. Brown GR, et al. Personality Characteristics and Sexual Functioning of 188 Crossdressing Men. *J Nervous Mental Dis* 185(5), 265–273, 1996.
13. Baldwin JI, Baldwin JD. Heterosexual Anal Intercourse: An Understudied, High-Risk Sexual Behavior. *Archives of Sexual Behavior*, 29(4), 357–373, 2000.
14. Health Services at Columbia University. Healthy vs. Unhealthy Relationships. www.goaskalice.columbia.edu.
15. Health Services at Columbia University. Breaking Up Can Be Hard to Do. www.goaskalice.columbia.edu.
16. U.S. Census Bureau. *Median Age at First Marriage: 2006*. 2006 American Community Survey. www.census.gov.
17. U.S. Census Bureau. *Statistical Abstract of the United States: 2008* (127th ed.). Washington, DC: U.S. Department of Commerce, 2007.
18. National Conference of State Legislatures. *Same Sex Marriage, Civil Unions and Domestic Partnerships: June 2009*. www.ncsl.org.
19. Bramlett MD, Mosher WD. *Cohabitation, Marriage, Divorce, and Remarriage in the United States*. U.S. Centers for Disease Control and Prevention, National Center for Health Statistics, Vital Health Statistics, 23(22), 2002.

Personal Assessment

How compatible are you?

This quiz will help test how compatible you and your partner's personalities are. You should each rate the truth of these 20 statements based on the following scale. Circle the number that reflects your feelings. Total your scores and check the interpretation following the quiz.

1 Never true
2 Sometimes true
3 Frequently true
4 Always true

We can communicate our innermost thoughts effectively.	1	2	3	4
We trust each other.	1	2	3	4
We agree on whose needs come first.	1	2	3	4
We have realistic expectations of each other and of ourselves.	1	2	3	4
Individual growth is important within our relationship.	1	2	3	4
We will go on as a couple even if our partner doesn't change.	1	2	3	4
Our personal problems are discussed with each other first.	1	2	3	4
We both do our best to compromise.	1	2	3	4
We usually fight fairly.	1	2	3	4
We try not to be rigid or unyielding.	1	2	3	4
We keep any needs to be "perfect" in proper perspective.	1	2	3	4
We can balance desires to be sociable and the need to be alone.	1	2	3	4
We both make friends and keep them.	1	2	3	4
Neither of us stays down or up for long periods.	1	2	3	4
We can tolerate the other's mood without being affected by it.	1	2	3	4
We can deal with disappointment and disillusionment.	1	2	3	4
Both of us can tolerate failure.	1	2	3	4
We can both express anger appropriately.	1	2	3	4
We are both assertive when necessary.	1	2	3	4
We agree on how our personal surroundings are kept.	1	2	3	4

YOUR TOTAL POINTS _____

Interpretation

20–35 points—You and your partner seem quite incompatible. Professional help may open your lines of communication.

36–55 points—You probably need more awareness and compromise.

56–70 points—You are highly compatible. However, be aware of the areas where you can improve.

71–80 points—Your relationship is very fulfilling.

TO CARRY THIS FURTHER . . .

Ask your partner to take this test too. You may have a one-sided view of a "perfect" relationship. Even if you scored high on this assessment, be aware of areas where you can still improve.

Managing Your Fertility

What Do You Know About Birth Control?

1. Birth control and contraception mean the same thing. True or False?

2. The periodic abstinence approach is similar to "natural family planning." True or False?

3. In the United States, condoms are available in one size only. True or False?

4. Emergency contraception (Plan B) produces a medication abortion. True or False?

5. Intrauterine devices (IUDs) are safe and effective for most women. True or False?

6. Women who take "the pill" for many years are likely to get breast cancer. True or False?

7. Many states have enacted laws that prohibit "partial-birth abortions." True or False?

Check your answers at the end of the chapter.

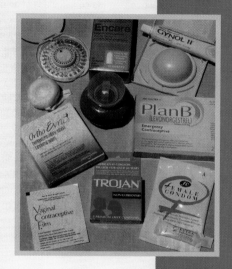

How you decide to control your fertility will have an important effect on your future. Your understanding of information and issues related to fertility control will help you make responsible decisions in this complex area.

Basic Concepts of Fertility Control

This chapter begins with some basic concepts related to fertility control. After reading the material in the next four short subsections, you should be better prepared to examine closely the many birth control methods available today. We start with a terminology distinction.

There's More to Sex Than You Thought

Are you ready for sex? If you're not sure, take time to think it over. If you start having sex before you're ready, you might feel guilty. You might feel bad because you realize this step isn't right for you now. Or your religious upbringing may make you feel as though you're doing something wrong. You also may not be ready for the emotional aspects of a sexual relationship. Most important, you will probably have difficulty handling the complexities of an unplanned pregnancy or a sexually transmitted disease.

If you do feel ready for sex, you still have a choice. Sex may be okay for you now. It may be personally fulfilling, something that enhances your self-esteem. Alternatively, you can choose to abstain from sex until later—another way of enhancing your self-esteem. You'll feel empowered by making the decision for yourself, rather than doing what is expected. Being strong enough to say "no" can also make you feel good about yourself. For some, making this decison may reflect a renewed commitment to spiritual or religious concerns.

If you're married, sex is a good way of connecting as a couple. It's something that the two of you alone share. It's a time to give special attention to each other—taking a break from the kids, your jobs, and your other responsibilities. It's a way of saying: "This relationship is important—it's something I value."

Going through a pregnancy together is another opportunity for closeness. From the moment you know that you're going to be parents, you're connected in a new way. Your focus becomes the expected child. You'll watch the fetus grow on ultrasound, go to parenting and Lamaze classes together, visit the doctor together, mark the various milestones, and share new emotions. When your child is born, you'll be connected as never before.

Whether you're thinking about starting to have sex, making the decision to wait, or examining the sexual life you have now, you can't ignore the possibilities and the consequences. Is the time right for you? Are you doing this for yourself or for someone else? What do you think you will gain from waiting? Do you expect your future partner to also have made the decision to wait? What do you expect to get from a sexual relationship—pleasure, intimacy, love? What do you expect to give? Do you want an emotional commitment? Do you view sex and love as inseparable? Do you understand how sex can enhance your spirituality? Taking time to consider these questions can make you feel good about yourself—no matter what you decide.

Birth Control Versus Contraception

Any discussion about the control of your **fertility** should start with an explanation of the subtle differences between the terms **birth control** and **contraception.** These terms reflect different perspectives about fertility control. *Birth control* is an umbrella term that refers to all the procedures you might use to prevent the birth of a child. Birth control includes all available contraceptive measures, as well as sterilization and abortion procedures.

Contraception is a much more specific term for any procedure used to prevent the fertilization of an ovum. Contraceptive measures vary widely in the mechanisms they use to accomplish this task. They also vary considerably in their method of use and their rate of success in preventing conception. A few examples of contraceptives are condoms, hormonal contraceptives, spermicides, and diaphragms.

Beyond the methods mentioned, certain forms of sexual behavior not involving intercourse could be considered forms of contraception. For example, mutual masturbation by couples virtually eliminates the possibility of pregnancy. This practice, as well as additional forms of sexual expression other than intercourse (such as kissing, touching, and massage), has been given the generic term **outercourse.** Outercourse protects against unplanned pregnancy and may also significantly reduce the transmission of sexually transmitted diseases,

including HIV infection (see the box "There's More to Sex Than You Thought").

Reasons for Choosing to Use Birth Control

People use birth control for many reasons. Many career-minded individuals carefully plan the timing and spacing of children to best provide for their children's financial support without sacrificing their job status. Others choose methods of birth control to ensure that they will never have children. Some use birth control methods to permit safe participation in a wide variety of sexual behaviors. Fear of contracting a sexually transmitted disease prompts some people to use particular forms of birth control (see the box "Discussing Birth Control with Your Partner").

Financial and legal considerations can be significant factors in the choice of certain birth control methods. Many people must of necessity take the cost of a method into account when selecting appropriate birth control. The cost of sterilization and abortion can prohibit some low-income people from choosing these alternatives, especially because federal funds do not support such procedures. A number of states have established statutes and policies that make contraceptive information and medical services relatively difficult to obtain.

I have a new girlfriend and I think we are moving closer and closer to having sex. I know we should talk about birth control and disease prevention, but I don't know how to start. What should I do?

If you believe there is even a chance you will engage in any kind of sex, or if you think your partner may pursue sex with you, you should be prepared and discuss the possibility before being swept along by the heat of an encounter. In addition, you and your partner will feel more comfortable about your relationship and your sexual activity if you first discuss your feelings about contraception, disease prevention, and pregnancy. Consider the following topics:

- First, the fact that you are discussing contraception together does not necessarily mean that you will engage in sex. In addition, you can discuss abstinence as a very effective form of contraception.
- Discussing contraception and disease prevention with your partner is not rude. It is simply common sense.
- Talking about contraception is a way of sharing responsibility and intimacy. It can bring you closer.
- Which type(s) of contraception will you use? See the section "Selecting Your Contraceptive Method" for help in making your choices.

- If you feel unsure about how to broach the subject or are undecided about any of the issues, consider discussing the subject with a counselor or physician before you talk with your partner.
- Sort out your own feelings and understand all the alternatives, including their advantages and disadvantages, before you open the discussion.
- Pick the right occasion. Don't wait until you have begun sexual activity.
- Both partners have dignity and worth, and should be treated with dignity. If you and your boyfriend or girlfriend are discussing contraception and you have different views, you each have the right to your opinions. If necessary, you can agree to disagree.
- Listen carefully and ask questions. Speak honestly about your own feelings and beliefs.
- Who will pay for the contraceptive method? Will both partners share the cost?
- What will both of you do if the female partner becomes pregnant?

Have you discussed these issues in the past before initiating sex with a partner? Do you plan to discuss these issues in the future?

Another important consideration in the use of birth control methods is the availability of professional services. An example of the effect of this factor may be the selection of birth control methods by college students. Some colleges and universities provide contraceptive services through their student health centers. Students enrolled in these schools have easy access to low-cost, comprehensive contraceptive services. Students enrolled in colleges that do not provide such complete services may find that access to accurate information and clinical services is difficult to obtain and that private professional services are expensive.

For many people, religious doctrine will be a factor in their selection of a birth control method. One example is the opposition of the Roman Catholic Church and other religious groups to the use of contraception other than periodic abstinence.

Theoretical Effectiveness Versus Use Effectiveness

People considering the use of a contraceptive method need to understand the difference between the two effectiveness rates given for each form of contraception. *Theoretical effectiveness* is a measure of a contraceptive method's ability to prevent a pregnancy when the method is used precisely as directed during every act of intercourse. *Use effectiveness,* however, refers to the effectiveness of a method in preventing conception when used by the general public. Use effectiveness rates take into account factors that lower effectiveness below that based on "perfect" use. Failure to follow proper instructions, illness of the user, forgetfulness, physician (or pharmacist) error, and a subconscious desire to experience risk or even pregnancy are a few of the factors that can lower the effectiveness of even the most theoretically effective contraceptive technique.

Effectiveness rates are often expressed as the percentage of women users of childbearing age who do not become pregnant while using the method for one year. For some methods the theoretical-effectiveness and

Key Terms

fertility The ability to reproduce.

birth control All the methods and procedures that can prevent the birth of a child.

contraception Any method or procedure that prevents fertilization.

outercourse Sexual activity that does not involve intercourse.

Table 16.1 Effectiveness Rates of Birth Control for 100 Women During the First Year of Use

| Method | Estimated Effectiveness | | Advantages | Disadvantages |
	Theoretical	Use		
No method (chance)	15%	15%	Inexpensive	Totally ineffective
Withdrawal	96%	73%	No supplies or advance preparation needed; no side effects; men share responsibility for family planning	Interferes with coitus; very difficult to use effectively; women must trust men to withdraw as orgasm approaches
Periodic abstinence	91%–99%	75%	No supplies needed; no side effects; men share responsibility for family planning; women learn about their bodies	Difficult to use, especially if menstrual cycles are irregular, as is common in women; abstinence may be necessary for long periods; lengthy instruction and ongoing counseling may be needed
Spermicide (gel, foam, suppository, film)	82%	71%	No health risks; can be used with condoms to increase effectiveness considerably	Must be inserted 5 to 30 minutes before coitus; effective for only 30 to 60 minutes; some concern about nonoxynol-9
Diaphragm	94%	84%	No major health risks, easily carried in purse, can be used during breast-feeding, no impact on a woman's hormones, usually cannot be felt by either partner	Cannot be used during menstruation; must be left in place for at least 6 hours after coitus; must be fitted by clinician; some women may find it awkward or embarrassing to use; some concern about nonoxynol-9
FemCap (no previous births) (previous births)	? ?	86% 71%	No major health risks, easily carried in purse, can be used during breast-feeding, no impact on a woman's hormones, usually cannot be felt by either partner	Similar to diaphragm disadvantages above
Lea's Shield	?	85%	No major health risks, easily carried in purse, can be used during breast-feeding, no impact on a woman's hormones, usually cannot be felt by either partner	Similar to diaphragm disadvantages above; must be left in place at least 8 hours after last intercourse
Sponge (no previous births) (previous births)	91% 80%	84% 68%	Easy to use; not messy; protection is good for 24 hours and multiple acts of intercourse; no prescription required	Not reusable; contraceptive protection is reduced for women with previous births; some concern about nonoxynol-9
Male condom Male condom with spermicide	98% 99%	85% 95%	Easy to use; inexpensive and easy to obtain; no health risks; very effective protection against some STDs; men share responsibility for family planning	Must be put on just before coitus; some men and women complain of decreased sensation; some concern about nonoxynol-9
Female condom	95%	79%	Relatively easy to use; no prescription required; polyurethane is stronger than latex; provides some STD protection; silicone-based lubrication provided; useful when male will not use a condom	Contraceptive effectiveness is not as high as with male condom; couples may be unfamiliar with a device that extends outside the vagina; more expensive than male condoms

continued

use-effectiveness rates are vastly different; the theoretical rate is always higher than the use rate. Table 16.1 presents data concerning estimated effectiveness rates, advantages, and disadvantages of many birth control methods.

Selecting Your Contraceptive Method

In this section, we discuss some of the many factors that should be important to you as you consider selecting a contraceptive method. Completing the Personal Assessment at the end of this chapter will help you to make this decision.

Those who wish to exercise a large measure of control over their fertility can consider the following:

- It should be safe.
- It should be effective.
- It should be reliable.
- It should be reversible.
- It should be affordable.
- It should be easy to use.
- It should not interfere with sexual expression.

Table 16.1 Continued

Method	Estimated Effectiveness		Advantages	Disadvantages
	Theoretical	Use		
IUD			Easy to use; highly effective in preventing pregnancy; does not interfere with coitus; repeated action not needed	May increase risk of pelvic infection and infertility in a very small percentage of women; not usually recommended for women who have never had a child; must be inserted by health care personnel; may cause heavy bleeding and pain in some women
ParaGard (copper T)	99%+	99%+		
Mirena (progestin)	99%+	99%+		
Combined pill (estrogen + progestin)	99%+	92%	Easy to use; highly effective in preventing pregnancy; does not interfere with coitus; regulates menstrual cycle; reduces heavy bleeding and menstrual pain; helps protect against ovarian and endometrial cancer	Must be taken every day; requires medical examination and prescription; minor side effects such as nausea or menstrual spotting; possibility of cardiovascular problems in a small percentage of users
Minipill (progestin only)	99%+	92%		
Contraceptive ring (estrogen + progestin)	99%+	92%	Easy to use after learning how to insert; remains in place 3 weeks	Like other hormonal methods, does not protect against STDs; requires physician prescription; possibility of cardiovascular problems in a small percentage of users
Contraceptive patch (estrogen + progestin)	99%+	92%	Easy to apply; must change weekly for 3 weeks	No STD protection; requires physician prescription; possibility of cardiovascular problems in a small percentage of users
Depo-Provera	99%+	97%	Easy to use; highly effective for 3-month period; continued use prevents menstruation	Requires supervision by a physician; administered by injection; some women experience irregular menstrual spotting in early months of use
Contraceptive implant	99%+	99%+	Easy to use; protection is good for 3 years; progestin only; can be used while breast-feeding; no medicine to take daily	No STD protection; requires physician to insert or remove; may cause temporary irregular bleeding; possibility of cardiovascular problems in a small percentage of users
Tubal ligation	99%+	99%+	Permanent; removes fear of pregnancy	Surgery-related risks; generally considered irreversible
Vasectomy	99%+	99%+	Permanent; removes fear of pregnancy	Generally considered irreversible

Source: Adapted from Hatcher RA, et al. *Contraceptive Technology*, 19th ed. New York: Ardent Media, 2007; and Planned Parenthood Federation of America. *Birth Control.* www.plannedparenthood.org.

Behavioral Contraceptive Methods

The first contraceptives we'll discuss are those that are based on the sexual behavior of a couple. As with all approaches to contraception, a clear understanding of each method can help you make decisions about sexual activity and birth control that are right for you. For guidelines on locating accurate information on the Web, see the box "Information Online—Birth Control and Sexuality."

Abstinence

Abstinence as a form of birth control has gained attention recently on college campuses. This method is as close to 100 percent effective as possible. There have

been isolated reports in medical literature of pregnancy without sexual intercourse, usually involving ejaculation by the male near the woman's vagina. Avoiding this situation should raise the effectiveness of abstinence to 100 percent.

Abstinence as a form of birth control has additional advantages in that it gives nearly 100 percent protection from sexually transmitted diseases, it is free, and it does not require a visit to a physician.

However, significant concerns exist about the effectiveness of educational programs that encourage abstinence. A large five-year study published in the January 2009 issue of the journal *Pediatrics* supported earlier studies that found that teens who "pledged virginity until marriage" were just as likely to have sex as nonpledgers, were less likely to use contraceptives when they had sex, had similar rates of oral and anal sex, and had similar rates of sexually transmitted diseases as nonpledgers. Also, pledgers did not differ in lifetime number of sexual partners and age at time of first sex.[1]

Abstinence works effectively only when it is broadly defined (to include many sexual behaviors) and used correctly and consistently. Abstinence is a challenging proposition for many adolescents and young adults.

Withdrawal

Withdrawal, or **coitus interruptus,** is the contraceptive practice in which the erect penis is removed from the vagina just before ejaculation of semen. Theoretically, this procedure prevents sperm from entering the deeper structures of the female reproductive system. The use effectiveness of this method, however, reflects how unsuccessful the method is in practice (see Table 16.1).

Strong evidence suggests that the clear preejaculate fluid that helps neutralize and lubricate the male urethra can contain *viable* (capable of fertilization) sperm.[2] This sperm can be deposited near the cervical opening before withdrawal, which explains the relatively low effectiveness of this method. Furthermore, withdrawal does not protect users from the transmission of sexually transmitted diseases (STDs). It should never be considered a reliable contraceptive approach.

Periodic Abstinence

Five approaches are included in the birth control strategy called **periodic abstinence:** (1) the calendar method, (2) the temperature method, (3) the cervical mucus method, (4) the symptothermal method, and (5) the standard days method.[3] All five methods attempt to determine the time a woman ovulates. Figure 16-1 shows a day-to-day fertility calendar that reflects a woman's fertile period. Most research indicates that an ovum is viable for only about 24 to 36 hours after its release from the ovary. (After they are inside the female reproductive tract, some sperm can survive up to a week.) When a woman can accurately determine when she ovulates, she must refrain from intercourse long enough for the ovum to begin to disintegrate. Fertility awareness, rhythm, natural birth control, and natural family planning are other terms for periodic abstinence. Remember that periodic abstinence methods *do not* provide protection against the spread of STDs, including HIV infection.[2]

Periodic abstinence is the only contraceptive method endorsed by the Roman Catholic Church. For some

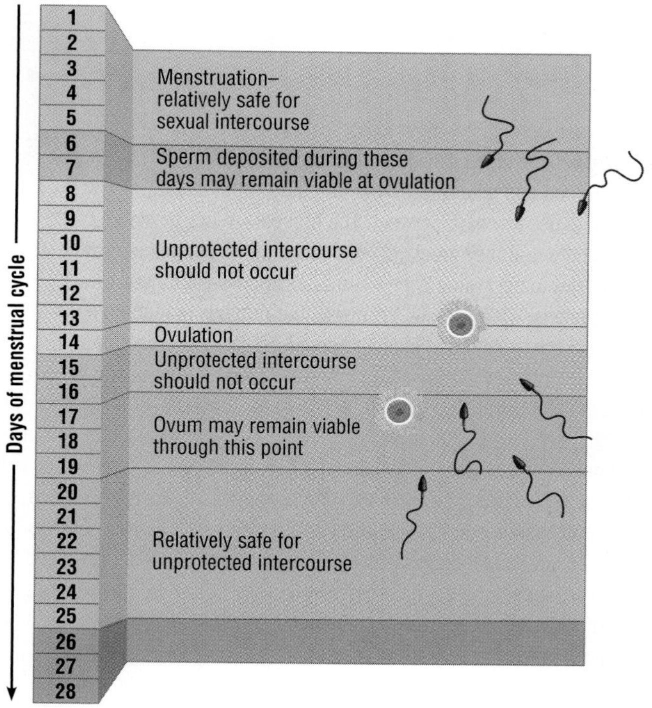
Days of menstrual cycle
1
2
3
4
5
6
7
8
9
10
11
12
13
14
15
16
17
18
19
20
21
22
23
24
25
26
27
28
Menstruation–
relatively safe for
sexual intercourse
Sperm deposited during these
days may remain viable at ovulation
Unprotected intercourse
should not occur
Ovulation
Unprotected intercourse
should not occur
Ovum may remain viable
through this point
Relatively safe for
unprotected intercourse

Figure 16-1 Periodic Abstinence These methods try to pinpoint when a woman is most likely to ovulate. Remember that most women's cycles are not consistently perfect 28-day cycles like those shown in most illustrations.

people who have deep concerns for the spiritual dimension of their health, selecting a method other than periodic abstinence may entail a serious compromise of beliefs.

The **calendar method** requires close examination of a woman's menstrual cycle for the last 6 to 12 cycles. Records are kept of the length (in days) of each cycle. A *cycle* is defined as the number of days from the first day of bleeding of one cycle to the first day of bleeding of the next cycle.

To determine the days she should abstain from intercourse, a woman should subtract 18 from her shortest cycle; this is the first day she should abstain from intercourse. Then she should subtract 11 from her longest cycle; this is the last day she must abstain from intercourse.[4]

The *temperature method* requires a woman (for about three or four successive months) to take her body temperature every morning before she rises from bed. A finely calibrated thermometer, available in many drugstores, is used for this purpose. The theory behind this method is that there is a distinct correlation between body temperature and the process of ovulation. Around the time of ovulation, the body temperature rises at least 0.4 degree F and remains elevated until the start of menstruation. The woman is instructed to refrain from intercourse during the interval when the temperature change takes place.

Drawbacks of this procedure include the need for consistent, accurate temperature readings and the realization that all women's bodies are different. Some women may not fit the temperature pattern projection because of biochemical differences in their bodies. In addition, body temperature can fluctuate. Temperature kits cost about $10 to $12 in drugstores.[5]

The *cervical mucus method* is another periodic abstinence technique. Generally used with other periodic abstinence techniques, this method requires a woman to evaluate the daily mucus discharge from her cervix. Users of this method become familiar with the changes in both appearance (from clear to cloudy) and consistency (from watery to thick) of their cervical mucus throughout their cycles. Women are taught that the unsafe days are when the mucus becomes clear and is the consistency of raw egg whites. Such a technique of ovulation determination must be learned from a physician or family planning professional.

The *symptothermal method* of periodic abstinence combines the use of the calendar, temperature, and cervical mucus methods. Family planning professionals consider the symptothermal method preferable to a single periodic abstinence approach.

The newest periodic abstinence approach is called the *standard days method*. This method is appropriate only for women who have menstrual cycles that are consistently between 26 and 32 days long. It is not to be used by women who have variable cycles that are shorter than 26 days or longer than 32 days. Having had just one cycle in the past year shorter than 26 days or longer than 32 days should encourage a woman NOT to use the standard days method. She should meet with her health care provider and discuss an alternative method.

To use this method, women must count the days of their menstrual cycle, with day 1 as the first day of menstrual bleeding. Women can have intercourse on days 1 to 7. On days 8 to 19, women should refrain from penis/

Key Terms

withdrawal (coitus interruptus) (co ih tus in ter **rup** tus) A contraceptive practice in which the erect penis is removed from the vagina before ejaculation.

periodic abstinence Birth control methods that rely on a couple's avoidance of intercourse during the ovulatory phase of a woman's menstrual cycle; also called *fertility awareness* or *natural family planning.*

calendar method A form of periodic abstinence in which the variable lengths of a woman's menstrual cycle are used to calculate her fertile period.

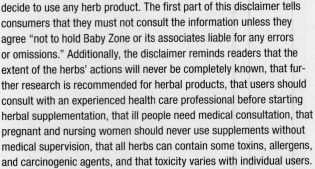
vaginal intercourse or use a barrier method of contraception. Days 8 to 19 are the fertile days. From day 20 until the end of the cycle, unprotected intercourse can take place.[4] Keep in mind that the standard days method does not protect against the transmission of STDs.

Those who wish to practice one of these periodic abstinence methods should consult a professional to learn how to chart their menstrual cycle and detect the physical signs that help predict the "unsafe" days. Besides the lack of protection against STDs, the periodic abstinence methods have the following potential problems:

- Partner may be uncooperative.
- Couple may take risks during "unsafe" days.
- Record-keeping may be poor.
- Illness and lack of sleep can affect body temperature.
- Vaginal infections and douches change mucus.
- Method cannot be used if the woman has irregular periods or temperature patterns.

Over-the-Counter Contraceptive Methods

OTC methods are ones that couples can choose easily because they do not require a physician's prescription, they are readily available in supermarkets or drugstores,

and they are approved by the U.S. Food and Drug Administration (FDA). They all work by providing some kind of obstacle or mechanism that prevents the sperm from joining with an ovum.

Some OTC herbal products are available for couples who are trying to conceive a baby. (See the box "Herbal Answers for Fertility Questions.") However, it is important to note that OTC herbal products are not evaluated or approved by the Food and Drug Administration.

Spermicides

Spermicides are agents that are capable of killing sperm. When used alone, they offer a moderately effective form of contraception for the woman who is sexually active on an infrequent basis. Modern spermicides are generally safe (but see the following precaution), reversible forms of contraception that can be obtained without a physician's prescription in most drugstores and supermarkets. They are available in foams, creams, jellies, film, or suppositories. Spermicides are relatively inexpensive. Applicator kits cost about $8, and refills cost around $4 to $8 (see Figure 16-2). Suppositories and film are also priced in this range.[5]

Spermicides are made of water-soluble bases with a sperm-killing agent in the base. Frequently, spermicides are used with other contraceptives, such as diaphragms, shields, caps, and condoms. Spermicides do not protect

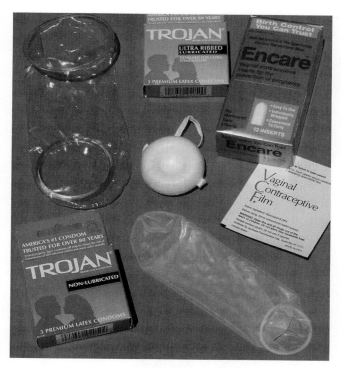

Over-the-counter methods of contraception are widely available in drugstores and supermarkets. They include male and female condoms, spermicides, and the contraceptive sponge.

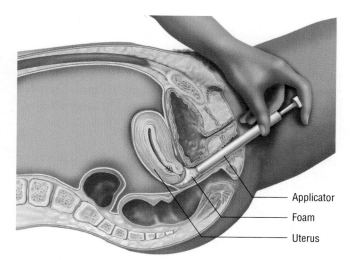

Applicator
Foam
Uterus

Figure 16-2 Use of Spermicide Spermicidal foams and suppositories are placed deep into the vagina in the region of the cervix no longer than 30 minutes before intercourse.

users from contracting pathogens that cause various STDs. In fact, people who use nonoxynol-9 many times each day are more likely to transmit infections, including HIV.[5] This is due to an increase in skin irritations and abrasions, which provide the avenue for passage of pathogens into the bloodstream.

Couples should realize that condoms, when used consistently and correctly, provide much better disease protection and contraceptive effect than spermicides used alone. However, the small amount of nonoxynol-9 that is added to the lubricant with some condoms is not sufficient to serve as an effective backup contraceptive if the condom breaks. Thus, some health centers and family planning agencies have stopped distributing condoms coated with a spermicide.[6] If you and/or your partner have concerns about your use of spermicides, you should seek advice from your health care provider.

Condoms

Colored or natural, smooth or textured, straight or shaped, plain or reservoir-tipped, dry or lubricated—the latex condom is approaching an art form. Nevertheless, the familiar **condom** remains a safe, effective, reversible contraceptive device. All condoms manufactured in the United States must be approved by the FDA.

For couples who are highly motivated in their desire to prevent a pregnancy, the effectiveness of a condom can approach that of an oral contraceptive. A condom can be nearly 100 percent effective when used with contraceptive foam. For couples who are less motivated, the condom can be considerably less effective. Condoms cost from 50¢ to $2.50 each, but are often free in college health centers or local health departments or clinics.

The condom offers a measure of protection against sexually transmitted diseases. For both the man and the woman, chlamydial infections, gonorrhea, HIV infection, and other STDs are less likely to be acquired when the condom is used correctly (see the box "Maximizing the Effectiveness of Condoms"). Some lubricated condoms also contain a spermicide, yet the small amount of spermicide present in the condom's lubricant is not enough to consistently prevent conception if the condom should break. Current recommendations are to use dry condoms or lubricated condoms without spermicide. Also, any additional lubricants used should be water-based lubricants.

The FDA has approved two types of nonlatex condoms. The polyurethane male condom and the polyurethane female condom are available as one-time-use condoms. These condoms are good alternatives for people who have an allergic sensitivity to latex, estimated to be up to 7 percent of the population.[7] Also, they are thinner and stronger than latex condoms and can be

> **Key Terms**
>
> **spermicides** Chemicals capable of killing sperm.
>
> **condom** A shield designed to cover the erect penis and retain semen upon ejaculation; "rubber."

Maximizing the Effectiveness of Condoms

I have used condoms a few times, but I was always in a hurry and never read the small print instructions. My current partner asked me if "I knew what I was doing" the last time we had intercourse. What do I need to know to use condoms more effectively?

These simple directions for using condoms correctly, in combination with your motivation and commitment to regular use, should provide you with reasonable protection:

- *Keep a supply of condoms at hand.* Condoms should be stored in a cool, dry place so that they are readily available at the time of intercourse. Condoms that are stored in wallets or automobile glove compartments may not be in satisfactory condition when they are used. Temperature extremes are to be avoided. Check the condom package for the expiration date.

- *Do not test a condom by inflating or stretching it.* Handle it gently and keep it away from sharp fingernails.

- *For maximum effectiveness, put the condom on before genital contact.* Either the man or the woman can put the condom in place. Early application is particularly important in the prevention of STDs. Early application also lessens the possibility of the release of preejaculate fluid into the vagina.

- *Unroll the condom on the erect penis.* For those using a condom without a reservoir tip, a half-inch space should be left to catch the ejaculate. To leave this space, pinch the tip of the condom as you roll it on the erect penis: do not leave any air in the tip.

- *Lubricate the condom if this has not already been done by the manufacturer.* When doing this, be certain to use a water-soluble lubricant and not a petroleum-based product such as petroleum jelly. Petroleum can deteriorate the latex material. Other oil-based lubricants, such as mineral oil, baby oil, vegetable oil, shortening, and certain hand lotions, can quickly damage a latex condom. Use water-based lubricants only!

- *After ejaculation, be certain that the condom does not become dislodged from the penis.* Hold the rim of the condom firmly against the base of the penis during withdrawal. Do not allow the penis to become flaccid (soft) while still in the vagina.

- *Inspect the condom for tears before throwing it away.* If the condom is damaged in some way, immediately insert a spermicidal agent into the vagina or consider using emergency contraception (see page 440).

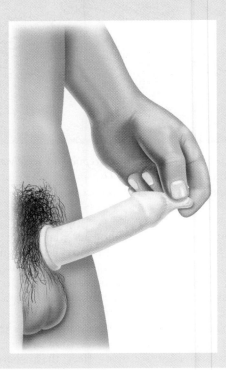

used with oil-based lubricants. Currently, these condoms are believed to provide a level of protection against STDs that is close to that of latex condoms. The contraceptive effectiveness of the polyurethane condoms remains somewhat less than that of the male latex condom.[8]

Contraceptive Sponge

The **contraceptive sponge** is a small, pillow-shaped polyurethane device containing nonoxynol-9 spermicide. The sponge is dampened with tap water and inserted deep into the vagina to cover the cervical opening. This device provides contraceptive protection for up to 24 hours, regardless of the number of times intercourse occurs. After the last act of intercourse, the device must be left in place for at least 6 hours. Once removed, the sponge must be discarded. The sponge must not be left in place for longer than 24 or 30 hours because of the risk of toxic shock syndrome.[4]

Used alone, the sponge does not provide reliable protection against STDs and HIV infection. Consult your physician if you are concerned about the use of

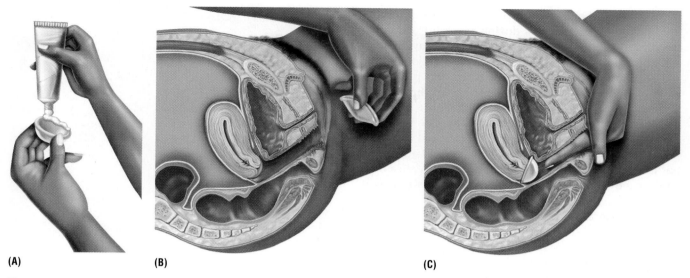

(A)   **(B)**   **(C)**

Figure 16-3 Use of a Diaphragm   **A:** Spermicidal cream or jelly is placed into the diaphragm. **B:** The diaphragm is folded lengthwise and inserted into the vagina. **C:** The diaphragm is then placed against the cervix so that the cup portion with the spermicide is facing the cervix. The outline of the cervix should be felt through the central part of the diaphragm.

nonoxynol-9 spermicide. In women who have not given birth, the contraceptive effectiveness of the sponge is similar to that of the diaphragm. The sponge is less effective in women who have given birth.[4] A package of three sponges costs between $9 and $15.[5]

Prescription Contraceptive Methods

Many approaches to contraception require a physician's prescription. Generally, these methods have higher effectiveness rates, but they also come with possible risks and side effects to the user. Some devices require careful fitting or placement. Some prescription methods use devices that require the user to follow careful instructions. Some approaches use hormones that can have dangerous consequences for a very small percentage of users. It is for these reasons that these products or approaches are not available on an over-the-counter basis.

Diaphragm

The **diaphragm** is a soft rubber cup with a springlike metal rim that rests in the top of the vagina. The diaphragm covers the cervical opening (Figure 16-3). During intercourse the diaphragm stays in place quite well and cannot usually be felt by either partner.

The diaphragm is always used with a spermicidal cream or jelly placed inside the cup and around the rim. When used properly with a spermicide, the diaphragm is a relatively effective contraceptive, and when combined with the man's use of a condom, its effectiveness is even greater. The diaphragm must be inserted before

intercourse. It should provide effective protection for 6 hours. If this time interval extends beyond 6 hours, some clinicians recommend that additional spermicide be placed in the vagina.

Use of additional spermicide with multiple acts of intercourse is optional. After intercourse, the diaphragm must be left in place for at least 6 hours before it is removed. Because of the risk of toxic shock syndrome (TSS), the diaphragm must not remain in the vagina

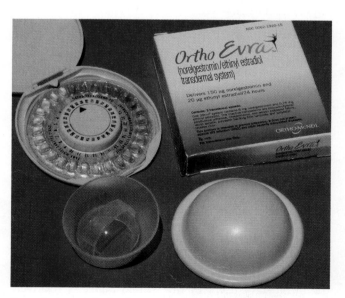

Prescription methods of contraception are those that include hormones, such as combined oral contraceptives and the contraceptive patch, and those that require expert fitting, such as the diaphragm and FemCap.

longer than 24 hours.[4] Women should avoid using diaphragms, caps, and shields during any kind of vaginal bleeding, including menstruation.[5] It is always best to ask a health care provider for specific instructions.

Diaphragms must always be fitted and prescribed by a physician.[9] The cost of obtaining a diaphragm and keeping a supply of spermicide may be higher than that of other methods. Typically, it costs $15 to $75 for a diaphragm and $8 to $17 for the spermicidal cream or jelly. An examination may cost between $50 and $200, but it will be less at family planning clinics. Also, a high level of motivation to follow the instructions *exactly* is important.

Diaphragms and other vaginal barrier methods (caps and shields) do not provide reliable protection against STDs and HIV infection. Recent concerns about the spermicide nonoxynol-9 should prompt users to ask their physicians to recommend which spermicidal cream or jelly to use with diaphragms. If you are concerned about possible HIV infection, either avoid sexual activity or use a latex condom.

Lea's Shield and FemCap

The two newest barrier methods for women were approved by the FDA in 2002. Both methods are used with a spermicide. *Lea's Shield* is a reusable oval device made of silicone rubber that fits closely over the cervix. An attached loop helps in the removal from the vagina. The Lea's Shield works much like a diaphragm, but it has a central air valve that permits air to move out from beneath the shield and permit a closer fit. This device comes in only one size and must be prescribed by a physician. The first-year use effectiveness of this device (85 percent) is about the same as that for diaphragms (84 percent).

The *FemCap* is a reusable hat-shaped silicone rubber cap that completely covers the cervix. Coated with spermicide, the FemCap's brim fits snugly against the deep vaginal walls. An attached strap helps in the removal of this device. The FemCap must be prescribed by a physician and comes in three sizes. Among women who have never been pregnant or given birth vaginally, the first-year use effectiveness of this device is 86 percent. Costs for these new devices are similar to those for diaphragms.[5]

Intrauterine Device (IUD)

The **intrauterine device (IUD)** is the most popular reversible contraceptive method in the world, although the number of users in the United States is relatively small. It can be an excellent choice for women who desire a long-term, hassle-free, reversible, highly effective method of contraception. The IUD is especially advantageous to women who have already had at least one child,

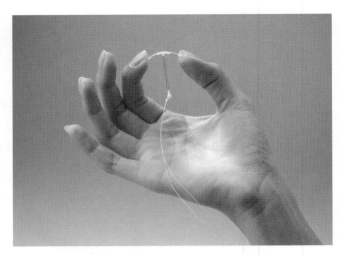

The T-shaped ParaGard IUD works by releasing copper ions that impair sperm function and prevent fertilization.

are in a stable, monogamous relationship, and perhaps are unable to take daily birth control pills.

Two types of IUDs are available in the United States: a T-shaped one containing the hormone progestin (Mirena) and a T-shaped one wrapped with copper wire (ParaGard). The Mirena IUD works by thickening cervical mucus, inhibiting sperm survival, and producing a thin endometrial lining that will not support a fertilized ovum. In some women, the Mirena inhibits ovulation. The ParaGard works by releasing copper ions that impair sperm function and prevent fertilization.[4] The Mirena IUD substantially reduces menstrual flow, but the ParaGard may increase menstrual flow. About 20 percent of women who use the Mirena IUD stop having their periods altogether.[10]

The Mirena provides highly effective contraceptive protection for 5 years and the ParaGard for 12 years. Only a skilled physician can prescribe and insert an IUD. As with many other forms of contraception, IUDs do not offer protection against STDs, including the AIDS virus.[9]

For many years, the public has been concerned about two potentially serious side effects: *uterine perforation* (in which the IUD embeds itself into the uterine wall) and pelvic inflammatory disease (PID, a widespread infection of the abdominal cavity). Recent research, however, indicates that these events rarely happen, especially when the IUD is inserted by a skilled clinician. Between 2 and 10 percent of IUD users experience *expulsion* (muscular contractions which force the IUD out of the uterus) within the first year of use.[4]

As Table 16.1 indicates, IUDs are highly effective birth control devices. The cost for an IUD ranges from $175 to $500, which includes an exam, insertion, and a follow-up visit.[5]

Oral Contraceptives

First introduced in the United States in 1960, today's **oral contraceptive pill** provides one of the highest effectiveness rates of any of the reversible contraceptive methods. Only the IUD, the implant, and the injection provide higher effectiveness rates. Worldwide, more than 75 million women are currently using oral contraceptives.[4]

Use of the pill requires a physician's examination and prescription. Because oral contraceptives are available in a wide range of formulas, follow-up examinations are important to ensure that a woman is receiving an effective dosage with as few side effects as possible. Matching the right prescription with the woman may require a few consultations.

Combined Pills   All oral contraceptives contain synthetic (laboratory-made) hormones. The typical *combined pill* uses both synthetic estrogen and synthetic progesterone in each of 21 pills. With *triphasic pills,* the level of estrogen remains constant, but the level of progestin varies every 7 days.

The FDA has approved two *extended-cycle oral contraceptives* (Seasonale and Seasonique) that contain active hormones for 84 days (12 weeks) followed by 1 week of pills containing inactive ingredients.[3] Women using Seasonale or Seasonique have only four menstrual periods each year. In early 2007, the FDA approved the newest extended-cycle pill, called Lybrel. This contraceptive pill contains low-dose hormones that are taken each day for a full year. Despite having no menstrual periods for 365 days, most women using Lybrel report having some breakthrough bleeding or spotting during the early months of use.[11]

The contraceptive effect of the pill can be compromised in women who are also taking certain medicines or supplements. The antibiotic rifampin reduces the pill's effectiveness. Interestingly, other antibiotics do not make the pill less effective. But certain antifungal drugs taken orally for yeast infections, certain anti-HIV protease inhibitors, some anti-seizure medications, and the over-the-counter plant supplement St. John's Wort (sometimes used for mild depression) all have the ability to make the pill less effective. Thus it is very important for a woman to talk with her clinician about the medicines she is taking before she is given any prescription method of birth control.[5]

Oral contraceptives function in several ways. The estrogen in the pill tends to reduce ova development. The progesterone in the pill helps reduce the likelihood of ovulation (by lowering the release of luteinizing hormone). The progesterone in the pill also causes the uterine wall to develop inadequately and helps thicken cervical mucus, thus making it difficult for sperm to enter the uterus. As with many forms of contraception, *oral contraceptives do not protect against the transmission of STDs, including HIV infection.*

The physical changes produced by the oral contraceptive provide some beneficial side effects in women. Because the synthetic hormones are taken for 21 days and then are followed by **placebo pills** or no pills for 7 days, the menstrual cycle becomes regulated. Even women who have irregular cycles immediately become "regular." Because the uterine lining is not developed to the extent seen in a non-pill-taking woman, the uterus is not forced to contract with the same amount of vigor. Thus menstrual cramping is reduced, and the resultant menstrual flow is diminished. Research indicates that oral contraceptive use can provide protection against anemia, PID, noncancerous breast tumors, acne, recurrent ovarian cysts, ectopic pregnancy, endometrial cancer, endometriosis, and ovarian cancer.[4]

The negative side effects of the oral contraceptive pill can be divided into two general categories: (1) unpleasant and (2) potentially dangerous. The unpleasant side effects generally subside within two or three months for most women. A number of women report some or many of the following symptoms:

- Tenderness in breast tissue
- Nausea
- Mild headaches
- Slight, irregular spotting
- Weight gain
- Fluctuations in sex drive
- Mild depression
- More frequent vaginal infections

The potentially dangerous side effects of the oral contraceptive pill are most often seen in the cardiovascular system. Blood clots, strokes, hypertension, and heart attack seem to be associated with the estrogen component of the combined pill. However, when compared with nonusers, the risk of dying from cardiovascular complications is only slightly increased among healthy young oral contraceptive users. Additionally, multiple scientific studies have determined that oral contraceptive use has little, if any, effect on the development of breast cancer,

---

Key Terms

intrauterine device (IUD)   A small, plastic, medicated or unmedicated contraceptive device that prevents pregnancy when inserted in the uterus.

oral contraceptive pill   A pill taken orally, composed of synthetic female hormones that prevent ovulation or implantation; "the pill."

placebo pills (pla **see** bo)   Pills that contain no active ingredients.

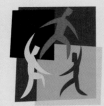
even among women with a family history of breast cancer. This is especially true for women who started taking the pill after 1978, when lower dose formulations began.[4]

Most health professionals agree that the risks related to pregnancy and childbirth are much greater than those associated with oral contraceptive use. Certainly, a woman who is contemplating the use of the pill must discuss all of the risks and benefits with her physician.

There are some **contraindications** for the use of oral contraceptives. If you have a history of blood clots, migraine headaches, liver disease, a heart condition, high blood pressure, obesity, diabetes, hepatitis, cirrhosis, breast or uterine cancer, or if you are too young to have started consistent menstrual cycles, the pill probably should not be your contraceptive choice. Providing a physician with a complete and accurate health history is important before a woman starts to take the pill.

Two additional contraindications continue to draw considerable attention by the medical community. Cigarette smoking and advancing age are highly associated with an increased risk of potentially serious side effects. Increasing numbers of physicians are not prescribing oral contraceptives for their patients who smoke. The risk of cardiovascular-related deaths is greatly enhanced in women over age 35. The risk is even higher in female smokers over 35. The data are quite convincing.[4]

For the vast majority of women, however, the pill, when properly prescribed, is safe and effective. Careful scrutiny of one's health history and careful follow-up examinations when a problem is suspected are essential elements that can provide a good margin of safety. Monthly pill packs cost $15 to $50 at drugstores and less at clinics. An exam may cost $35 to $250.[5]

What about an oral contraceptive for men? See the box "The Male Contraceptive Pill" for information on the medical and social challenges of developing a pill for men.

Minipills   Some women prefer not to use the combined oral contraceptive pill. Thus, to avoid some of the potentially serious side effects of the combined pill, some physicians are prescribing **minipills.** These oral contraceptives contain no estrogen—only low-dose progesterone in all pills in the 28-day pill pack. The minipill seems to work by thickening cervical mucus, preventing ovulation, and producing a thin endometrial lining.[4] The effectiveness of a minipill is slightly lower than that of the combined pill. *Breakthrough bleeding* and **ectopic pregnancy** are more common in minipill users than in combined-pill users. The cost of minipills is similar to that of combined pills.

Injectable Contraceptive

Depo-Provera is a highly effective (99 percent+) injectable progestin contraceptive that provides protection for 3 months. This hormone shot works primarily by preventing ovulation and thickening the cervical mucus to keep the sperm from joining with the egg.

The most common side effects of Depo-Provera are irregular bleeding and spotting followed by *amenorrhea* (the absence of periods).[4] In particular, new users of Depo-Provera report occasional breakthrough bleeding as the most common unpleasant side effect.[4] When the woman's body adjusts to the presence of this drug, breakthrough bleeding diminishes, and the most common side effect is amenorrhea. This is understandable, because the drug inhibits ovulation. Many women consider amenorrhea to be a desirable effect of Depo-Provera use. Women who stop using Depo-Provera may experience infertility for a period of up to one year.[4] The cost of Depo-Provera ranges from $35 to $75 per injection. The initial exam could cost $35 to $250.[5]

Contraceptive Implant

In July 2006, the FDA approved the use of a progestin-based contraceptive implant called Implanon. This thin, flexible plastic device is about the size of a matchstick and is inserted just under the skin of the upper arm. Implanon works by slowly releasing progestin for up to three years. The progestin inhibits ovulation and also thickens the cervical mucus to prevent the sperm from joining with an egg. Studies indicate that this contraceptive implant is nearly as effective as sterilization.[4]

Many of the health concerns that apply to other hormone-based contraceptives (including drug interactions that can lower its effectiveness) apply to the implant as well. The costs of the device and its insertion range from $400 to $800. Removal of the implant costs $75 to $150.[5]

Contraceptive Ring

One of the newest contraceptives on the market is the vaginal **contraceptive ring** (NuvaRing). Available by prescription, NuvaRing is a thin polymer ring (2⅛ inches in diameter and ⅛ inch thick) that contains synthetic estrogen and progestin. Users insert this device deep into the vagina where it remains for 3 weeks. At the end of the third week, the device is removed for a week and the woman has her period. The NuvaRing provides effective contraception (99 percent+ effective when used perfectly) for the entire 4-week time frame.

The ring functions in a manner similar to the oral contraceptive pill: It reduces the chances of ovulation and thickens cervical mucus. Women who use the ring cannot at the same time use shields, caps, or diaphragms as a backup method. The contraceptive ring does not protect against sexually transmitted diseases, including the virus that causes HIV/AIDS. As with all prescribed forms of contraception, women should discuss all the benefits, risks, and possible side effects with their health

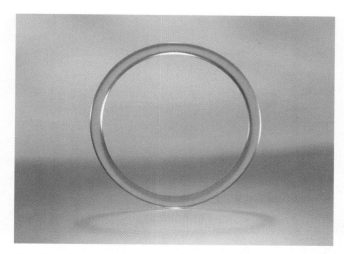

The NuvaRing contraceptive ring is a flexible ring about 2⅛ inches in diameter. When inserted into the vagina, it delivers a low dose of hormones similar to those found in oral contraceptives.

care provider. The costs of the contraceptive ring are about $15 to $50 per month for the device and $35 to $250 for the exam.[5]

Contraceptive Patch

In 2002 the Ortho Evra **contraceptive patch** became available to women. This patch contains continuous levels of estrogen and progestin delivered from a 1¾-inch square patch that is applied weekly to one of four areas on the woman's body: the buttocks, abdomen, upper chest (front and back, excluding the breasts), or upper outer arm.[12] The patch remains attached even while a woman

---

Key Terms

contraindications Factors that make the use of a drug inappropriate or dangerous for a particular person.

minipills Low-dose progesterone (progestin) oral contraceptives.

ectopic pregnancy A pregnancy in which the fertilized ovum implants at a site other than the uterus, typically in the fallopian tubes.

contraceptive ring Thin, polymer contraceptive device containing estrogen and progestin; placed deep within the vagina for a three-week period.

contraceptive patch Contraceptive skin patch containing estrogen and progestin; replaced each week for a three-week period.

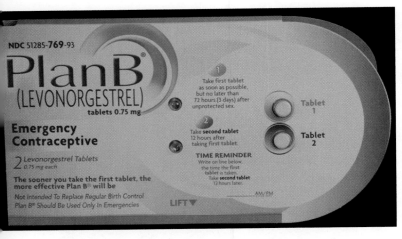

Plan B emergency contraception consists of two doses of hormones taken about 12 hours apart. Nonprescription behind-the-counter access to Plan B has been approved for women age 17 and older.

bathes, swims, or exercises. After 3 weeks of patches, the woman uses no patch for the fourth week, during which time she has her period. The patch functions in a manner similar to the oral contraceptive pill. Like all hormonal methods of contraception, the patch does not protect against sexually transmitted diseases, including the virus that causes HIV/AIDS. The patch costs about $15 to $50 per month. The exam may cost $35 to $250.[5]

Many women have used the patch successfully, but some concerns have arisen over possible increased cardiovascular risks (blood clots, strokes, heart attacks) due to the way the hormones are delivered to the user. On the home page of the Ortho Evra website, the manufacturer clearly states that patch users will be exposed to about 60 percent more estrogen than if they were taking a typical oral birth control pill that contains 35 μg of estrogen.[12] For this reason, it is especially important that potential users discuss with their health care provider whether this is a good contraceptive choice for them. This precaution is even more important for women who are smokers and women over the age of 35.

Emergency Contraception

Emergency contraception is designed to prevent pregnancy after unprotected vaginal intercourse such as when a condom breaks, when a couple uses no method of contraception, or when someone forces another to have intercourse. This method is also called postcoital or "morning after" contraception. (Emergency contraception is not the "abortion pill" or RU-486.) Emergency contraception is available in two forms: emergency hormonal contraception and the insertion of an IUD.

Currently, the FDA has approved one oral contraceptive (Plan B) for use specifically as emergency contraception, although physicians may prescribe other oral contraceptives for this purpose. Plan B consists of 2 progestin-only pills, the first dose of which should be taken as soon as possible (but not later than 120 hours or 5 days) after unprotected intercourse. Typically, a second dose follows 12 hours after the first pill. The sooner the first dose is taken after intercourse, the better the contraceptive protection. (Alternatively, a woman can choose to take both pills at once.) Plan B reportedly reduces the risk of pregnancy by 89 percent, if started within three days of unprotected intercourse.[5]

Emergency contraception works by preventing ovulation or fertilization. If a woman is already pregnant, Plan B will not cause an abortion or affect the pregnancy. In 2006 the FDA decided to allow Plan B to be sold as an over-the-counter product, similar to the way nicotine-replacement medications are made available to the public. Thus, Plan B is available behind the pharmacy counter (not on aisle shelves) to women and men age 17 and older. Some pharmacists may ask for identification to verify a young person's age. People under age 17 will need a physician's prescription to get Plan B.[5]

The most commonly reported side effects of emergency hormonal contraception are nausea and vomiting. Less than 25 percent of users of progestin-only pills experience nausea.[5] The use of antinausea medication can help offset the nausea and vomiting. Some women also report fatigue, breast tenderness, abdominal pain, headaches, and dizziness. These side effects subside within a day or two after treatment. Costs for Plan B range from $10 to $45.[5]

A copper IUD is a less commonly used, but highly effective, form of emergency contraception. To function as an emergency contraceptive, however, the ParaGard IUD must be inserted by a clinician within 5 days of unprotected intercourse.

Permanent Contraceptive Methods

All the contraceptive mechanisms or methods already discussed have one quality in common: They are reversible. Although microsurgical techniques are providing medical breakthroughs, **sterilization** should still be considered an irreversible procedure.[13] When you decide to use sterilization, you no longer control your own fertility because you will no longer be able to produce offspring. Attempts to reverse sterilization are quite difficult and very expensive.

Therefore, couples considering sterilization procedures usually must undergo extensive discussions with a physician or family planning counselor to identify their true feelings about this finality. People must be aware of the possible changes in self-concept they might have after

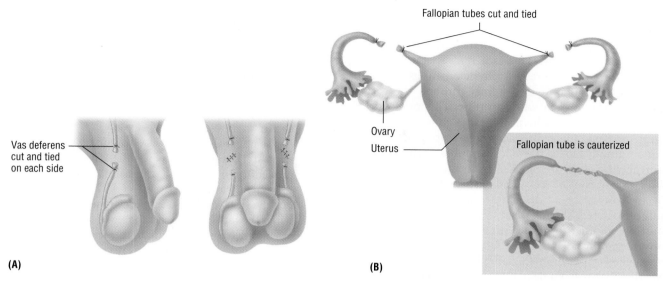

Figure 16-4 The Most Frequently Used Forms of Male and Female Sterilization   A: Vasectomy. B: Tubal ligation.

Labels in figure:
- Vas deferens cut and tied on each side
- (A)
- Fallopian tubes cut and tied
- Ovary
- Uterus
- Fallopian tube is cauterized
- (B)

sterilization. If you are a man who equates fertility with masculinity, you may have trouble accepting your new status as a sterile man. If you are a woman who equates motherhood with femininity, you might have adjustment problems after sterilization. Some people later regret not being able to have children. Sterilization does not protect one against STDs, including HIV infection.

Male Sterilization

The male sterilization procedure is called a *vasectomy*. Accomplished with a local anesthetic in a physician's office, this 20- to 30-minute procedure consists of the surgical removal of a section of each vas deferens. After a small incision is made through the scrotum, the vas deferens is located and a small section removed. The remaining ends are either tied or *cauterized* (Figure 16-4A).

Immediately after a vasectomy, sperm may still be present in the vas deferens. A backup contraceptive is recommended until a physician microscopically examines a semen specimen. This examination usually occurs about six weeks after the surgery. After a vasectomy, men can still produce male sex hormones, get erections, have orgasms, and ejaculate. (Recall that sperm account for only a small portion of the semen.) Some men even report increased interest in sexual activity because their chances of impregnating a woman have been virtually eliminated.

What happens to the process of spermatogenesis within each testicle? Sperm cells are still being produced, but they are destroyed by specialized white blood cells called *phagocytic leukocytes*.

The future may hold a reversible form of vasectomy, as researchers experiment with injecting a plug-forming material into the vas deferens, with the intention that the plug could be removed at a later date if desired. The cost of a vasectomy ranges from $350 to $1,000.[5]

Female Sterilization

The most common method of female sterilization is called *tubal ligation*. During this procedure, the fallopian tubes are cut and the ends tied back. Some physicians cauterize the tube ends to ensure complete sealing (Figure 16-4B). The fallopian tubes are usually reached through the abdominal wall. In a *minilaparotomy*, a small incision is made through the abdominal wall just below the navel. The resultant scar is small and is the basis for the term *band-aid surgery*.

Female sterilization requires about 20 to 30 minutes, with the patient under a local or general anesthetic. The use of a laparoscope has made female sterilization much simpler than in the past. The laparoscope is a small tube equipped with mirrors and lights. Inserted through a single incision, the laparoscope locates the fallopian tubes before they are cut, tied, or cauterized. When

Key Terms

emergency contraception Contraceptive measures used to prevent pregnancy within five days after unprotected intercourse; also called *postcoital* or *morning-after* contraception.

sterilization Generally permanent birth control techniques that surgically disrupt the normal passage of ova or sperm.

a laparoscope is used through an abdominal incision, the procedure is called a *laparoscopy*.

In 2002, a new method of female sterilization was approved by the FDA. This is a nonincision approach (the Essure coil), whereby a physician inserts a small, soft metallic coil into the vagina, through the cervix, and directly into each fallopian tube. This procedure is done under local anesthetic and takes about a half-hour. Once inserted, the coils encourage scar tissue growth that eventually blocks the fallopian tubes. If the tubes are obstructed, sperm are blocked from meeting the ovum. After three months, a woman returns to her physician for an X-ray test that determines whether the tubes are fully obstructed. During these first three months, couples must use another form of birth control. Cramping is the most common side effect. In rare cases, Essure coils can be expelled or perforate the fallopian tube.[3] Reports indicate that Essure has a near 100 percent effectiveness rate.[4]

Women who are sterilized still produce female hormones, ovulate, and menstruate. However, the ovum cannot move down the fallopian tube. Within a day of its release, the ovum will start to disintegrate and be absorbed by the body. Freed of the possibility of becoming pregnant, many sterilized women report an increase in sex drive and activity.

Female sterilization is very effective, with failure rates of only 1 to 2 per 1,000 procedures. The complications tend to be few and minor, and there appear to be no serious long-term side effects. Tubal ligation costs $1,500 to $6,000.[5]

Two other procedures produce sterilization in women. *Ovariectomy* (the surgical removal of the ovaries) and *hysterectomy* (the surgical removal of the uterus) accomplish sterilization. However, these procedures are used to remove diseased (cancerous, cystic, or hemorrhaging) organs and are not primarily considered sterilization techniques.

 TALKING POINTS You and your husband have children. And you'd like to stop taking the pill for health reasons. Your husband says you're pressuring him to have a vasectomy. How can you keep the dialogue going in a cooperative way?

Abortion

Regardless of the circumstances under which pregnancy occurs, women may now choose to terminate their pregnancies. No longer must women who do not want to be pregnant seek potentially dangerous, illegal abortions. On the basis of current technology and legality, women need never experience childbirth. The decision will be theirs to make.

Abortion is a highly controversial, personal decision—one that needs serious consideration by each woman. On the basis of the landmark 1973 U.S. Supreme Court case *Roe v. Wade*, the United States joined many of the world's most populated countries in legalizing abortion within the following guidelines:

1. For the first three months of pregnancy (first trimester), the decision to abort lies with the woman and her doctor. Most abortions are performed in the first trimester.
2. For the next three months of pregnancy (second trimester), state law may regulate the abortion procedure in ways that are reasonably related to maternal health.
3. For the last weeks of pregnancy (third trimester) when the fetus is judged capable of surviving if born, any state may regulate or even prohibit abortion except where abortion is necessary to preserve the life or health of the mother.

In 2005, 1.21 million women made the decision to terminate a pregnancy in the United States.[14] Thousands of additional women probably considered abortion but elected to continue their pregnancies.

See the box "New President, New Policy" for an update on American policy regarding international family planning agencies that deal with abortion.

First-Trimester Abortion Procedures

The first trimester consists of the first 13 weeks (91 days) of pregnancy. During the first 49 days after a woman's last menstrual period, a woman has two options for terminating a pregnancy: *vacuum aspiration* or *medication abortion*. Once 63 days have passed, only vacuum aspiration is an abortion option. Eighty-eight percent of all abortions are performed during the first trimester.[4]

Vacuum Aspiration There are two common methods of performing vacuum aspiration abortions. Both procedures can be performed in a physician's office or in a hospital. Both procedures require **dilation** of the cervix. The method used depends on how long the woman has been pregnant. Together, these methods represent the most widely used abortion procedures in the United States.

The **manual vacuum aspiration (MVA)** procedure can be performed in the earliest part of the first trimester, from the time a woman knows she is pregnant up to 10 weeks after her last period. After a physician injects a local anesthetic into the cervix, dilators can be used to enlarge the cervical opening. The physician then inserts a small tube into the uterus and applies suction with a handheld instrument. By rotating and moving this small tube across the uterine wall, the physician can empty the uterus. A return visit to the physician is an important follow-up procedure.[4]

After the first month of pregnancy and throughout the first trimester, physicians typically select **dilation and suction curettage (D&C)** (frequently called *vacuum aspiration*) as the abortion procedure of choice. D&C is similar to MVA, but the clinician uses a vacuum machine rather than a manually operated suction instrument. The clinician tends to use more sedation for the woman, in addition to the local cervical anesthetic. The cervix is stretched open with dilators that gradually enlarge the opening to permit the insertion of a tube into the cervix. This tube is attached to a vacuum machine that empties the uterus with gentle suction. If the physician believes that additional endometrial tissue remains in the uterus, he or she can use a **curette** to scrape the wall of the uterus. A subsequent visit to the clinician is an important follow-up procedure. Costs range from $350 to $900.[5]

Medication Abortion Mifepristone (formerly called RU-486) and methotrexate are drugs that can be used to induce a **medication abortion** during the first trimester of pregnancy. After years of testing in the United States, the FDA gave approval to the so-called "abortion pill" in 2000. The pill is marketed under the name Mifeprex and is available only through physicians. The cost of using mifepristone is about the same as the cost of first-term surgical procedures, or about $350 to $650.[5]

Under the FDA's regimen, women must use mifepristone within 49 days of their last menstrual period. Mifepristone blocks the action of progesterone and causes the lining of the uterus to break down. Women take three pills at the first doctor visit and then return 48 hours later to take a second drug, misoprostol, which causes menstruation to occur, usually within about 5 hours.

A third visit to a physician is necessary to ensure that the woman is recovering well from the procedure.

Physicians will want to make certain that there is no infection or excessive bleeding and that the uterus is fully emptied. Over a decade of research studies have indicated that the use of mifepristone is around 95 percent effective, when used during the first 7 weeks of pregnancy.[15]

Methotrexate is a drug used since the 1950s for cancer treatment. Physicians have found that it is effective in inducing an early-term medication abortion. However, in comparison to mifepristone, methotrexate is rarely used. If medication abortions continue to gain favor with women and their physicians, it is likely that more women will use physicians' offices, rather than abortion clinics, for abortion services. In 2005, 13 percent of all abortions were medication abortions.[14]

Second-Trimester Abortion Procedures

When a woman's pregnancy continues beyond the 13th week of gestation, termination becomes a more difficult matter. The procedures at this stage become more complicated, take longer to be completed, and generally cost more than first-trimester abortions.

Dilation and Evacuation Between 13 and 16 weeks of pregnancy, the abortion method of choice is **dilation and evacuation (D&E).** Some physicians use this method up through 24 weeks or more of pregnancy.[4] The D&E is a more involved surgical procedure than is a D&C and generally requires greater dilation of the cervix, larger medical instruments (including forceps), suction, and

Key Terms

abortion Induced premature termination of a pregnancy.

dilation Gradual expansion of an opening or passageway, such as the cervix.

manual vacuum aspiration (MVA) The abortion procedure performed in the earliest weeks after a pregnancy is established.

dilation and suction curettage (D&C) (kyoo re **taage**) A surgical procedure in which the cervical canal is dilated to allow the uterine wall to be scraped; vacuum aspiration.

curette A metal scraping instrument that resembles a spoon, with a cup-shaped cutting surface on its end.

medication abortion An abortion caused by the use of prescribed drugs.

dilation and evacuation (D&E) Second-trimester abortion procedure that requires greater dilation, suction, and curettage than first-trimester vacuum aspiration procedures.

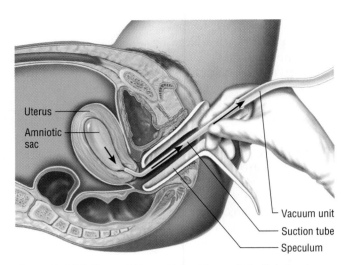

Figure 16-5 Dilation and Evacuation The cervix is dilated and the contents of the uterus are aspirated (removed by suction). This procedure is used to perform abortions during the second trimester.

curettage (see Figure 16-5). Some women may be given a general anesthetic during D&E procedures. After D&E, a return visit to the clinician is an important follow-up procedure. *Note:* Procedures that once used drugs or salt solutions to induce a second-trimester abortion are so rarely used today that we have chosen not to describe them.

Partial-Birth Abortion Since the late 1990s, *partial birth abortion* (technically called *intact dilation and extraction*) has been a contentious legal issue because many legislators believed it was too gruesome a procedure to be permitted. In the April 2007 *Gonzales v. Carhart* decision, the U.S. Supreme Court upheld the federal Partial-Birth Abortion Ban of 2003. This Supreme Court ruling paved the way for individual states to enact bans on this rarely used, middle-to-late second-semester abortion procedure. Within three months of the April 2007 ruling, Louisiana became the first state to pass a partial-birth abortion ban.

At the time of this writing, 31 states had enacted bans on partial-birth abortions. All 31 states have a provision that allows some type of exception to the ban in cases when a woman's life or health is in danger.[16] (For the current status of laws pertaining to partial-birth abortion, go to www.guttmacher.org.)

Third-Trimester Abortion Procedures

If an abortion is required in the latter weeks of the gestational period, a surgical procedure in which the fetus will be removed (*hysterotomy*) or a procedure in which the entire uterus is removed (*hysterectomy*) can be undertaken. As you can imagine, these procedures are more complicated and involve longer hospitalization, major abdominal surgery, and an extended period of recovery.

A Final Word

In the heat of passion, people often fail to think rationally about the potential outcomes of unprotected sex. Therefore, the time to prepare for the romantic moment is *before* you are in a position where you don't want to think about the possibility of an unintended result. If you choose to be sexually active, find a form of protection that works well for you and use it consistently. If you choose not to be sexually active, realize that this is a viable choice that can be 100 percent effective.

Taking Charge of Your Health

- Use the Personal Assessment at the end of this chapter to help you determine which birth control method is best for you.

- If you have a partner, discuss your personal preferences with him or her.

- Talk to your doctor about the health aspects of different types of birth control before making your decision.

- Find out as much as you can about the newest types of contraception (Seasonale, NuvaRing, Mirena, FemCap, Lea's Shield, Implanon, Essure, and Ortho Evra).

- Think about your likelihood of becoming pregnant or contracting an STD, and discuss with your partner how you might handle these possibilities if they should occur.

SUMMARY

- Each birth control method has both a theoretical-effectiveness rate and a use-effectiveness rate.
- Many factors should be considered when deciding which contraceptive is best for you.
- Sterilization is usually considered an irreversible procedure.
- The birth control pill is safe and effective for the vast majority of women, but it does not protect against sexually transmitted diseases.
- Among the newest hormonal contraceptives are the ring, the patch, the implant, and extended-cycle oral contraceptives.

- The contraceptive sponge is more effective with women who have not given birth to children.
- Two types of IUDs are available: a hormone-containing IUD and a copper-wrapped IUD.
- Emergency contraception is safe and effective in preventing pregnancy when used within 5 days of unprotected intercourse.
- The FDA has approved the drug mifepristone (formerly called RU-486) to induce a medication abortion during the first trimester of pregnancy.
- Abortion procedures vary according to the stage of the pregnancy.

REVIEW QUESTIONS

1. Explain the difference between the terms *birth control* and *contraception*. Give examples of each.
2. Identify some of the factors that should be given careful consideration when selecting a contraceptive method. Explain each factor.
3. What is periodic abstinence? Identify and describe each of the five approaches to this birth control strategy.
4. What are the current concerns over the use of the spermicide nonoxynol-9?
5. How do minipills differ from the combined oral contraceptive pills?
6. What is emergency contraception? For what circumstances might this be used?
7. In what form is Depo-Provera delivered to a woman?
8. Describe the various sterilization procedures.
9. Identify and describe the different abortion procedures that are used during each trimester of pregnancy.
10. What is a medication abortion?

ANSWERS TO THE "WHAT DO YOU KNOW?" QUIZ

1. False   2. True   3. False   4. False   5. True   6. False   7. True

Visit the Online Learning Center (**www.mhhe.com/payne11e**), where you will find tools to help you improve your grade including practice quizzes, key terms flashcards, audio chapter summaries for your MP3 player, and many other study aids.

SOURCE NOTES

1. Rosenbaum JE. Patient Teenagers? A Comparison of the Sexual Behaviors of Virginity Pledgers and Matched Nonpledgers. *Pediatrics* (online), 131(1), e110–e120, January 2009.
2. Hyde JS, DeLamater JD. *Understanding Human Sexuality* (10th ed.). New York: McGraw-Hill, 2009.
3. Crooks RL, Baur K. *Our Sexuality* (10th ed.). Belmont, CA: Wadsworth, 2008.
4. Hatcher RA, et al. *Contraceptive Technology* (19th ed.). New York: Ardent Media, 2007.
5. Planned Parenthood Federation of America. *Birth Control.* www.plannedparenthood.org/health-topics/birth-control, accessed January 20, 2009.
6. Carroll JL. *Sexuality Now: Embracing Diversity* (2nd ed.). Belmont, CA: Cengage Learning, 2007.
7. DeNoon D. Best Condoms Still Latex, WebMd Health. March 21, 2003. www.mywebmd.com.
8. Steiner MJ, et al. Contraceptive Effectiveness of a Polyurethane Condom and a Latex Condom: A Randomized Controlled Trial. *Obstetrics and Gynecology*, 101(3), 539–547, 2003.
9. Strong B, Yarber WL, Sayad BW, DeVault C. *Human Sexuality: Diversity in Contemporary America* (6th ed.), New York: McGraw-Hill, 2008.
10. Bayer Pharmaceuticals website. What Is Mirena? www.mirena-us.com, accessed January 23, 2009.
11. Wyeth Pharmaceuticals website. Is Lybrel Right for You? www.lybrel.com, accessed January 24, 2009.
12. Ortho-McNeil-Janssen Pharmaceuticals website. About ORTHO EVRA. www.orthoevra.com, accessed January 23, 2009.
13. Kelly GF. *Sexuality Today: The Human Perspective* (8th ed.). New York: McGraw-Hill, 2006.
14. Guttmacher Institute. Facts on Induced Abortion in the United States. www.guttmacher.org, accessed January 23, 2009.
15. Creinin MD, et al. Mifepristone and Misoprostol and Methotrexate/Misoprostol in Clinical Practice for Abortion. *American Journal of Obstetrics and Gynecology*, 188 (3), 664–669, 2003.
16. Guttmacher Institute. State Policies in Brief: Bans on "Partial-Birth" Abortion as of January 1, 2009. www.guttmacher.org, accessed January 24, 2009.

Personal Assessment

Which birth control method is best for you?

To assess which birth control method would be best for you, answer the following questions, and check the interpretation section.

Do I: Yes   No

1. Need a contraceptive right away?   ____   ____
2. Want a contraceptive that can be   ____   ____
   used completely independent of
   sexual relations?
3. Need a contraceptive only once in   ____   ____
   a great while?
4. Want something with no harm-   ____   ____
   ful side effects?
5. Want to avoid going to the   ____   ____
   doctor?
6. Want something that will   ____   ____
   help protect against sexually
   transmitted diseases?
7. Have to be concerned about   ____   ____
   affordability?
8. Need to be virtually certain that   ____   ____
   pregnancy will not result?
9. Want to avoid pregnancy now but   ____   ____
   want to have a child sometime in
   the future?
10. Have any medical condition or   ____   ____
    lifestyle that may rule out some
    form of contraception?

Interpretation

If you have checked **Yes** to number:

1. Condoms, spermicides, and sponges may be easily purchased without prescription in any pharmacy.
2. Sterilization, oral contraceptives, hormone rings, patches, or injections, implants, and periodic abstinence techniques do not require that anything be done just before sexual relations.
3. Diaphragms, condoms, sponges, or spermicides can be used by people who have coitus only once in a while. Periodic abstinence techniques may also be appropriate but require a high degree of skill and motivation.
4. IUD use should be carefully discussed with your physician. For most women, IUDs are quite safe. Sometimes the use of oral contraceptives or hormone products results in some minor discomfort and, on rare occasions, may have harmful side effects.

5. Condoms, spermicides, and sponges do not require a prescription from a physician.
6. Condoms help protect against sexually transmitted diseases. Nonoxynol-9 may increase STD transmission in some users. No method (except abstinence) can guarantee complete protection.
7. Be a wise consumer: Check prices, ask pharmacists and physicians. The cost of sterilization is high, but there is no additional expense for a lifetime.
8. Sterilization provides near certainty. Hormone-based contraceptives, IUDs, or a diaphragm-condom-spermicide combination also give a high measure of reliable contraceptive protection. Periodic abstinence, withdrawal, and douche methods should be avoided. Outercourse may be a good alternative.
9. Although it is sometimes possible to reverse sterilization, it requires surgery and is more complex than simply stopping use of any of the other methods.
10. Smokers and people with a history of blood clots should probably not use oral contraceptives or other hormone approaches. Some people have allergic reactions to a specific spermicide or latex material. Some women cannot be fitted with a diaphragm, shield, or cap. The woman and her health care provider will then need to select another suitable means of contraception.

TO CARRY THIS FURTHER . . .

There may be more than one method of birth control suitable for you. Always consider whether a method you select can also help you avoid an STD. Study the methods suggested here, and consult Table 16.1 to determine what method may be most appropriate.

Source: Adapted from K. Haas and A. Haas, *Understanding Sexuality* (3rd ed.). St. Louis: Mosby, 1993. Used with permission by Adelaide Haas.

Becoming a Parent

What Do You Know About Pregnancy and Parenting?

1. If a fetus has a heartbeat above 140, then it's a boy. True or False?

2. The acidic level in the vagina is destructive to sperm. True or False?

3. In each human pregnancy, there are four trimesters. True or False?

4. Typically, the longest stage of labor is the third stage. True or False?

5. Amniocentesis helps to identify chromosomal abnormalities. True or False?

6. Women's health issues are responsible for more cases of infertility than men's health issues. True or False?

7. IVF-ET is the most frequently used assisted reproductive technology. True or False?

Check your answers at the end of the chapter.

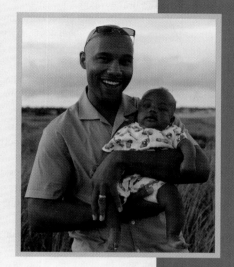

Although birth control is especially important for many young couples, most couples eventually want to have children and raise a family. In the past, couples had their children very soon after either high school or college. Now the trend seems to be to wait longer before having children. Most likely, educational, economic, contraceptive, and occupational factors have laid the groundwork for this trend. To the relief of many people, medical research indicates that women over the age of 30 or 35 are quite able to have healthy babies.

Parenting Issues for Couples

Before deciding to have children, couples should frankly discuss the effects that pregnancy and a newborn child will have on their lives (see the box "Parenthood Expands Personal Growth"). In addition, couples who are sexually active should consider these same issues, because very few contraceptive methods are

Parenthood Expands Personal Growth

Becoming a parent is almost always an exciting experience. Through nine months of pregnancy, anticipation of the baby increases on a daily basis. What sex will the baby be? How much hair will he or she have? How large will the baby be? Will the baby be a healthy child? Will the labor and delivery go smoothly? How will the household be changed as a result of the baby? How will the parents interact with each other after the baby enters the picture?

All these parental thoughts are centered on the baby and its presence. This is natural. Carrying a pregnancy to term and adjusting to the new baby are exciting, challenging, and exhausting experiences for the parents. There are times when new parents wonder how they ever got themselves into this situation. But there are many more times when parents are likely to be immensely thankful and proud to be parents of a newborn child.

Sometimes as we watch the growth and development of a newborn baby, we fail to think about the opportunities parenthood provides for the parents themselves to grow and develop. Parenthood presents an extra dimension to the lives of most parents. Although one can see this extra dimension in a number of ways, perhaps the most noticeable change is in the depth and quality of human relationships.

Perhaps most easily seen is the connection between mother and child. Living together, sharing nutrients (ideally only good ones), and protecting each other for nine months forges a spiritual bond between mother and child that remains for a lifetime. They experience labor and delivery in a way unique to themselves. Although fathers may be able to sense how strong this bond is, they never can fully understand or feel how close this mother-child connection is and how strong it tends to remain. *Parenthood is a life-altering experience for a woman.*

After becoming parents, fathers also tend to forge close, intimate bonds with their children, but these bonds are more likely related to the interactions they experience with the children as they grow and develop. Sometimes to their surprise, fathers find out that they have marvelous capabilities to adjust to the new demands a baby presents. Many fathers develop unexpected talents at nurturing their children. Perhaps because of this, more and more fathers are choosing to stay at home and raise their children, while their spouse works to support the family financially. This arrangement was virtually unheard of just three decades ago. *Indeed, parenthood is also a life-altering experience for a man.*

Parenthood encourages men and women to expand their focus from themselves (and their careers, their interests, their friends) to a broader spectrum of other people. This spectrum will certainly include the child, but also health care providers, teachers, school officials, their child's friends, the friends' parents and perhaps religious leaders, law enforcement personnel, and sports coaches. Parents will be required to expand their communication skills, their patience, and their insights as they try to raise their children the best way they can. Through this struggle comes added personal growth for the parents.

A final area in which parenthood offers a new dimension for the parents concerns the intimate bond between the parents themselves. Although it doesn't always happen (and the divorce statistics tell a compelling story), the process of conceiving a child, birthing a child, and raising a child to adulthood can make two people grow together in a way unmatched by any other experience. Older adult couples will often say that their most significant shared experience was raising their children. Many agree that it was through this experience that they gained a depth of understanding about each other that enriched their lives and established their most intimate connection. *In this sense, parenthood is a spiritual, life-altering experience for the parents.*

---

100 percent effective all the time, and pregnancy can result from nearly any act of intercourse. For students contemplating single parenthood, we ask that you consider these issues as they relate to your particular situation and to excuse our consistent use of plural pronouns.

Deciding to Become Parents

Here are some questions to consider before deciding to become parents:

- What effect will pregnancy have on us individually and collectively?

- Why do we want to have a child?

- What effect will a child have on the images we have constructed for ourselves as adults?

- Can we afford to have a child and provide for its needs?

- How will the responsibilities related to raising a child be divided?

- How will a child affect our professional careers?

- Are we ready now to accept the extended responsibilities that can come with a new child?

- How will we rear our child in terms of religious training, discipline, and participation in activities?

- Are we ready to part with much of the freedom associated with late adolescence and the early young-adult years?

- How will we handle the possibility of being awakened at six o'clock or earlier each morning for the next few years?

- What plans have we made in the event that our baby (or fetus) has a serious birth defect?

- Are we capable of handling the additional responsibilities associated with having a disabled child?

- Are we comfortable with the thought of bringing another child into an already overcrowded, violent, bigoted, and polluted world?

If these questions seem strikingly negative in tone, there is indeed a reason for this. We believe that all too frequently the "nuts and bolts" issues related to child-bearing and parenting are ignored or at least are placed on the back burner. Of course, future parents will consider how cute and cuddly a new baby will be, how holidays will be enhanced with a new child, and how pleased the grandparents will be; however, we consider these issues to be secondary to the serious realities of having a child enter your lives. Complete the Personal Assessment at the end of this chapter to explore your feelings about parenting.

 TALKING POINTS If you think you would like to have children someday, would you feel comfortable discussing these issues with your partner? How would you start the conversation?

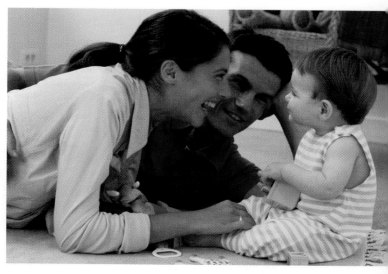

For many young couples, the rewards of raising a family outweigh the stress that inevitably accompanies parenthood.

Becoming a Parent Through a Stepfamily

Some people will become parents through a marriage in which one or both adult partners bring children from a previous relationship.[1] This newly constituted household is called a stepfamily.

Although some people call this a *blended family,* the National Stepfamily Resource Center (NSRC) believes the preferred term is a *stepfamily*. Children in stepfamilies do not lose their individual identities and instantly "blend" into a new family while losing attachments to the parent who is not a part of the new marriage. Things are rarely that smooth. If both parents remarry, a child may become a member of two stepfamilies and, perhaps, face even more obstacles concerning family loyalty. It is natural for children to wonder where they fit in or where they belong. Calling a newly constituted family a blended family may set up too many unrealistic expectations for children and adults and make adjustments more difficult. For example, children may balk when told that they are to consider their new family to be the family that deserves all their attention and loyalty.[1]

It is beyond the scope of this chapter to outline the challenges (and joys) that come with becoming a parent through a stepfamily arrangement. The NSRC, a clearinghouse for research-based information about stepfamily relationships, indicates that for stepfamilies to be successful, parents should

- Nurture and enrich the couple relationship.
- Reveal and understand emotions.
- Have realistic expectations.

- Develop new roles.
- Seek support and see the positive.

Throughout the merging of families into stepfamilies, clear communication, honest feelings, and a positive attitude about one's new role can help the process run more smoothly. It is quite possible that new family relationships can be wonderful experiences for all involved.

Parenting Across Cultures

In their recent text *Transcultural Health Care,* Purnell and Paulanka describe the various ways ethnic groups in America tend to view babies and young children.[2] In the Amish culture, children are seen as gifts from God and are enthusiastically welcomed into families. Amish families have an average of seven children per family and, unlike in other ethnic groups in America, this fertility pattern has not changed for the past century. Large families prize children because they are not only gifts from God, but they are also valuable resources on low-tech, labor-intensive family farms.

Children are considered a blessing to Jewish families. Children are to be afforded an education that prepares them for progress in society as well as increased understanding of their Jewish heritage. To that end, many Jewish children attend public school but also attend Hebrew school a couple of afternoons each week during the school year. Jewish children play important roles in most of the holiday celebrations and religious services. Parents are expected to treat their children fairly and to be flexible, caring, and attentive to discipline.[2]

Although there is much change taking place as Chinese increase their assimilation into the United States,

Which Personal Media Should You Trust for Information on Pregnancy?

Some sources of communication and information are the "personal media" to which we are exposed on a daily basis. These media include our immediate family members, our relatives, our friends and peer groups, and people we respect in our communities. Frequently, these personal media have had a wealth of experiences that, at least to us, give them a measure of credibility. They have "walked the walk" and, in a strange way, we now feel obligated to hear them "talk the talk."

And perhaps that's all we should do with our personal media sources—just listen. Here are some of the "pearls of wisdom" we might hear:

- If the baby's heart rate is above 140, then it's a boy.
- Mixing a common cleaning solution with a mother's urine will show you the sex of her forthcoming child.
- If the Mom craves sweets, it will be a girl. If she craves salty foods, it will be a boy.
- Pregnant women should drink plenty of water, or the amniotic fluid will get dirty.
- Pregnant women should not take baths.
- Having sex on even days of the month will produce boy babies.
- If you sleep on your right side while pregnant, you will have a girl.
- If you hold your hands above your head while pregnant, you could strangle the fetus.
- Eating spicy food near the baby's due date will cause early contractions.

If you check the Internet, you will find many sources of pregnancy folklore through advertised books, websites, and publications. Some of these sources of folklore are indeed fascinating, especially ones coming from non-Western cultures far away from the United States.

Because pregnancy and childbirth are such beautiful, complex, and mysterious events, they lend themselves easily to folklore. And "gems of wisdom" coming from folklore are easily passed on to couples having their first child. These couples are so new to pregnancy that they don't know what to believe. They may believe the most ridiculous information because they trust their personal media sources—friends, family, and older relatives.

What would be good advice for a pregnant woman who feels a bit overwhelmed with traditional "pearls of wisdom" and folklore recommendations about how to handle her pregnancy? We would encourage her to simply listen, nod her head, and smile. Then, if she has a question or feels uncomfortable about a pregnancy question or topic, make certain she asks her physician, nurse, or health care provider during her next visit. Undoubtedly, they have heard all of the urban legends, latest medical breakthroughs, or bits of folklore before and are willing to set the record straight.

For instance, regarding those "pearls of wisdom" listed previously—they are all—*False.*

---

many Chinese American families still hold on to Chinese traditions. Children are highly valued, but the number of children in a family tends to be small, perhaps because of China's one-child rule. Independence is usually not fostered, and parents make many decisions for the children even into young adulthood. Teens are expected to work hard in school, score well on exams, and help with chores around the home.[2]

In discussing Arab Americans' views of children, Purnell and Paulanka write that high fertility rates tend to be favored because of the belief that "God decides family size" and because families follow Islamic dictates regarding birth control, treatment of infertility, and abortion. Procreation is considered the primary reason for a marriage, since it enhances family strength. As with a number of cultures around the world, pregnancy tends to occur early in the marriage, and there is a preference for boys over girls. The sex of a child can be a great concern for the pregnant woman, and observers will often note the way in which the mother "carries" her baby during the pregnancy (girls are thought to be carried high and boys to be carried low).[2] See the box "Which Personal Media Should You Trust for Information on Pregnancy?" for more on folklore related to pregnancy.

Pregnancy: An Extension of the Partnership

Pregnancy is a condition that requires a series of complex yet coordinated changes to occur in the female body. This chapter follows pregnancy from its beginning, at fertilization, to its conclusion, with labor and childbirth. Fathers-to-be share many of the joys and worries of pregnancy and childbirth.

Physiological Obstacles and Aids to Fertilization

Many sexually active young people believe that they will become pregnant (or impregnate someone) only when they want to, despite their haphazard contraceptive practices. Because of this mistaken belief, many young people do not consistently use contraceptives. Young adults must remember that, to ensure the survival of our species, our bodies were designed to promote pregnancy. It is estimated that about 85 percent of sexually active women of childbearing age will become pregnant within one year if they do not use some form of contraception.[3]

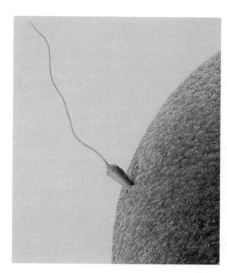

The surface of an ovum is penetrated by sperm at fertilization.

With regard to pregnancy, each act of intercourse can be considered a game of physiological odds. Obstacles exist that may reduce a couple's chance of pregnancy, including the following.

Obstacles to Fertilization

1. *The acidic level of the vagina is destructive to sperm.* The low pH of the vagina kills sperm that fail to enter the uterus quickly.
2. *The cervical mucus is thick during most of the menstrual cycle.* Sperm movement into the uterus is more difficult, except during the few days surrounding ovulation.
3. *The sperm must locate the cervical opening.* The cervical opening is small and may not be located by most sperm.
4. *Half of the sperm travel through the wrong fallopian tube.* Most commonly, only one ovum is released at ovulation. The two ovaries generally "take turns" each month. The sperm have no way of "knowing" which tube they should enter. Thus it is probable that half will travel through the wrong tube.
5. *The distance sperm must travel is relatively long compared with the tiny size of the sperm cells.* Microscopic sperm must travel about seven or eight inches after they are inside the female.
6. *The sperm's travel is relatively "upstream."* The anatomical positioning of the female reproductive structures necessitates an "uphill" movement by the sperm.
7. *The contoured folds of the tubal walls trap many sperm.* These folds make it difficult for sperm to locate the egg. Many sperm are trapped in this maze.

There are also a variety of aids that tend to help sperm and egg cells join. Some of these are listed next.

Aids to Fertilization

1. *An astounding number of sperm are deposited during ejaculation.* Each ejaculation contains about a teaspoon of semen.[4] Within this quantity are between 200 and 500 million sperm cells. Even with large numbers of sperm killed in the vagina, millions are able to move to the deeper structures.
2. *Sperm are deposited near the cervical opening.* Ejaculation into the vagina by the penis places the sperm near the cervical opening.
3. *The male accessory glands help make the semen nonacidic.* The seminal vesicles, prostate gland, and Cowper's glands secrete fluids that provide an alkaline environment for the sperm. This environment helps sperm be better protected in the vagina until they can move into the deeper, more alkaline uterus and fallopian tubes.[5]
4. *Uterine contractions aid sperm movement.* The rhythmic muscular contractions of the uterus tend to cause the sperm to move in the direction of the fallopian tubes.
5. *Sperm cells move rather quickly.* Despite their tiny size, sperm cells can move about one inch per hour. Powered by sugar solutions from the male accessory glands and the whiplike movements of their tails, sperm can reach the distant third of the fallopian tubes in less than 8 hours as they swim in the direction of the descending ovum.
6. *After they are inside the fallopian tubes, sperm can live for days.* Some sperm may be viable for up to a week after reaching the comfortable, nonacidic environment of the fallopian tubes. Most sperm, however, will survive an average of 48 to 72 hours. Thus they can "wait in the wings" for the moment an ovum is released from the ovary.
7. *The cervical mucus is thin and watery at the time of ovulation.* This mucus allows for better passage of sperm through the cervical opening when the ovum is most capable of being fertilized.

Signs of Pregnancy

Aside from pregnancy tests done in a professional laboratory, a woman can sometimes recognize early signs and symptoms. The signs of pregnancy have been divided into three categories.

Presumptive Signs of Pregnancy

Missed period after unprotected intercourse the previous month

Nausea on awakening (morning sickness)

Increase in size and tenderness of breasts

Darkening of the areolar tissue surrounding the nipples

Probable Signs of Pregnancy

Increase in the frequency of urination (the growing uterus presses against the bladder)

Increase in the size of the abdomen

Cervix becomes softer by the sixth week (detected by a pelvic examination by a clinician)

Positive pregnancy test

Positive Signs of Pregnancy

Determination of a fetal heartbeat

Feeling of the fetus moving (*quickening*)

Observation of the fetus by ultrasound or optical viewers

Home Pregnancy Tests Using a woman's urine, home pregnancy tests detect the presence of human chorionic gonadotropin (hCG), a hormone produced during pregnancy by the woman's placenta.[6] These tests contain monoclonal antibodies, which are molecules coated with a substance that bonds to the hCG hormone. If hCG is present, a colored stripe, dot, or other symbol appears in the test windows. Improved technology has made these home test kits highly accurate.

Although the makers of today's tests say their products can detect hCG as soon as the very day a missed period was supposed to begin, they also advise taking the test again a few days later to help confirm the result. If the result is positive, one should see a doctor as soon as possible.

Agents That Can Damage a Fetus

A large number of agents that come into contact with a pregnant woman can affect fetal development. Many of these (rubella and herpes viruses, tobacco smoke, alcohol,

---

> **Key Terms**
>
> **trimester** A three-month period; human pregnancies encompass three trimesters.
>
> **zygote** A fertilized ovum.
>
> **blastocyst** Early stage of the developing life form that embeds itself into the endometrial lining of the uterus.
>
> **embryo** Developmental stage from the end of the second week after conception until the end of the eighth week.
>
> **fetus** Developmental stage from the beginning of the ninth week after conception until birth.
>
> **spontaneous abortion** Any cessation of pregnancy resulting from natural causes; also called a *miscarriage*.

---

and virtually all other drugs) are discussed in other chapters of this text. The best advice for a pregnant woman is to maintain close contact with her obstetrician during pregnancy and to consider carefully the ingestion of any over-the-counter (OTC) drug (including aspirin, caffeine, and antacids) that could possibly harm the fetus.

Pregnant women should also avoid exposure to radiation. Such exposure, most commonly through excessive X-rays or radiation fallout from nuclear testing, can irreversibly damage fetal genetic structures. In addition, pregnant women should avoid Accutane, a drug prescribed for the treatment of cystic acne that can severely damage the fetus.[7]

Intrauterine Development

Intrauterine development takes place over the course of three **trimesters.** Most pregnancies last from 38 to 42 weeks. For purposes of illustration, we will consider each trimester to be 13 weeks. The growth and development during these trimesters occurs in a typical pattern for most pregnancies.

First Trimester The first 13-week trimester starts at conception, when the egg and sperm unite to form a structure called the **zygote** (Figure 17-1). The zygote, or fertilized egg, undergoes a series of cellular changes as it grows and makes its weeklong journey down the fallopian tube to the uterus. About the 10th day after conception, the zygote, now called a **blastocyst,** embeds itself into the endometrial lining of the uterus. From the end of 2 weeks after conception until the end of the eighth week, the growing structure is called an **embryo.** After 8 weeks and until the birth, it is called a **fetus.**

The first trimester is characterized by rapid cellular growth. By the end of the first trimester, the fetus weighs only about one ounce, yet most body organs are formed and the fetus can move.[8] It is currently thought that about half of all pregnancies end in **spontaneous abortion** during the early weeks of the first trimester, usually before the woman realizes she is pregnant. These miscarriages usually result from a genetic defect or a serious developmental problem.

Second Trimester The second trimester is characterized by continued growth and maturation. During this time, the organs continue to grow and physicians can hear the fetal heartbeat with a stethoscope. The bone structures are fully evident during the second trimester. The fetus starts to look more and more like an infant.

Additionally, the mother's breast weight increases by about 30 percent because of the deposition of 2 to 4 pounds of fat. This fat serves as a reserve energy source for the mother should she decide to nurse her baby. For this reason, good maternal nutrition is essential during the second trimester.[8]

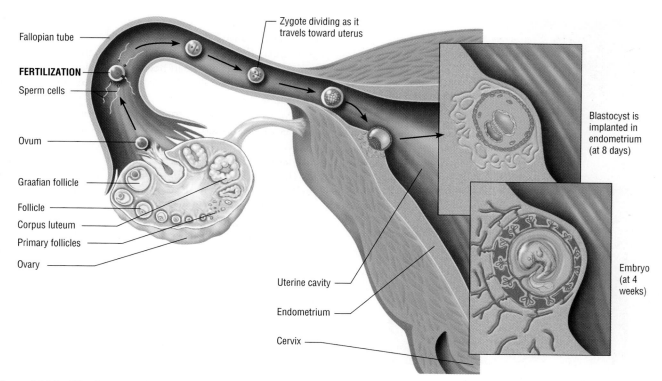

Figure 17-1 Fertilization and Implantation　After its release from the follicle, the ovum begins its weeklong journey down the fallopian tube. Fertilization generally occurs in the outermost third of the tube. Now fertilized, the ovum progresses toward the uterus, where it embeds itself in the endometrium. A pregnancy is established.

Third Trimester　The third trimester is another critical time for the developing fetus. At the beginning of this trimester, the fetus generally weighs 2 to 3 pounds. Over the final 13 weeks of gestation, the fetus will double in length and multiply its weight by up to five times.

This is also the time when the fetus absorbs considerable amounts of the minerals iron and calcium from the mother. For this reason, the mother must maintain

The fetus at 16 weeks' gestation within the amniotic sac.

sound eating patterns and avoid her body's depletion of mineral stores, perhaps by taking a vitamin and mineral supplement containing iron, which would reduce her risk of developing anemia during the final trimester.[8]

Maintaining a Healthy Pregnancy　Having a healthy pregnancy and delivering a healthy child actually should begin in the months before conception. During these pre-conception months, obstetricians advise women to stop smoking, stop drinking alcoholic beverages, eat well, get physical exercise, avoid or treat infections, avoid unnecessary exposure to toxic chemicals, and ask a physician before consuming any drug (prescription or over-the-counter).

Why the early start? Many women do not know that they are pregnant until after they miss a menstrual period. If they wait to alter their lifestyle until after they are certain of the pregnancy, they could inadvertently put the child's health at risk. Tremendous embryonic and fetal growth and development take place in the earliest weeks after conception. So it's best to plan ahead—before conception.

Once the pregnancy is established, it is important to follow additional guidelines:

- Arrange for prenatal care.
- Consume a well-balanced diet.

Chapter Seventeen　Becoming a Parent

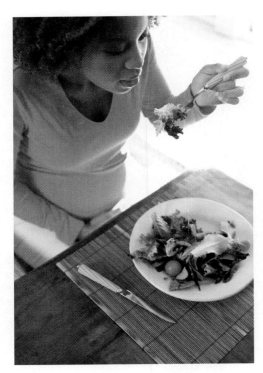

Strategies for maintaining a healthy pregnancy include consuming a well-balanced diet, engaging in appropriate physical activity, and avoiding tobacco, alcohol, and other drugs.

- Take a vitamin supplement that contains folic acid.
- Exercise according to your physician's recommendation.
- Avoid and treat infections.
- Avoid alcohol, tobacco, and other drugs.
- Limit your caffeine intake.
- Stay away from X-rays, hot tubs, and saunas.
- Stay away from toxic chemicals.

An expectant dad can also participate in this healthy approach by matching the woman's lifestyle changes. This provides sound emotional support for the pregnancy and, as an added bonus, improves the overall health of the dad.

Childbirth: The Labor of Delivery

Childbirth, or *parturition*, is one of the true peak life experiences for both men and women. Most of the time, childbirth is a wonderfully exciting venture into the unknown. For the parents, this intriguing experience can provide a stage for personal growth, maturity, and insight into a dynamic, complex world.

During the last few weeks of the third trimester, most fetuses move deeper into the pelvic cavity in a process called *lightening*. During this movement, the fetus's body rotates and the head begins to engage more deeply into the mother's pelvic girdle. Many women report that their babies have "dropped."

Another indication that parturition may be relatively near is the increased reporting of *Braxton Hicks contractions*.[9] These uterine contractions, which are of mild intensity and often occur at irregular intervals, may be felt throughout a pregnancy. During the last few weeks of pregnancy (*gestation*), these mild contractions can occur more frequently and cause a woman to feel as if she is going into labor (false labor).

Labor begins when uterine contractions become more intense and occur at regular intervals. The birth of a child can be divided into three stages: (1) effacement and dilation of the cervix, (2) delivery of the fetus, and (3) expulsion of the placenta (Figure 17-2). For a woman having her first child, the birth process lasts an average of 12 to 16 hours. The average length of labor for subsequent births is much shorter—from 4 to 10 hours on the average. Labor is very unpredictable. Labors that last from 1 to 24 hours occur daily at most hospitals.

Stage One: Effacement and Dilation of the Cervix

In the first stage of labor the uterine contractions attempt to thin (*efface*) the normally thick cervical walls and to enlarge (*dilate*) the cervical opening.[4] These contractions are directed by the release of prostaglandins and the hormone oxytocin into the circulating bloodstream. In women delivering their first babies, effacement will occur before dilation. In subsequent deliveries, effacement and dilation usually occur at the same time.

The first stage of labor is often the longest. The cervical opening must thin and dilate to a diameter of 10 cm before the first stage of labor is considered complete.[5] Often this stage begins with the dislodging of the cervical mucus plug. The subsequent *bloody show* (a mucus plug and a small amount of blood) at the vaginal opening may indicate that effacement and dilation have begun. Another indication of labor's onset may be the bursting or tearing of the fetal amniotic sac. "Breaking the bag of waters" refers to this phenomenon, which happens in various measures in expectant women.

The pain of the uterine contractions becomes more intense as the woman moves through this first stage of labor. As the cervical opening effaces and dilates 0 to 3 cm, many women report feeling happy, exhilarated, and confident. In the early phase of the first stage of labor, the contractions are relatively short (lasting 15–60 seconds) and the intervals between contractions range from 20 minutes to 5 minutes as labor progresses. However,

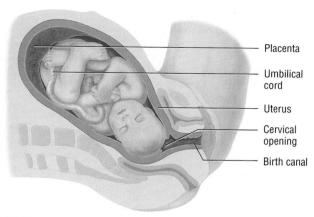

(A) First stage: Effacement and dilation. Uterine contractions thin the cervix and enlarge the cervical opening.

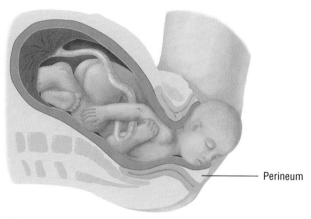

(B) Second stage: Delivery of the fetus. Uterine contractions are aided by mother's voluntary contractions of abdominal muscles. The fetus moves through dilated cervical opening and birth canal.

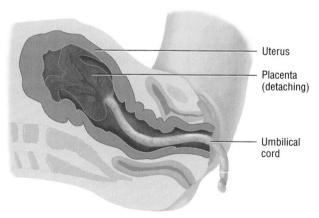

(C) Third stage: Delivery of the placenta. Placenta detaches from uterine wall and is delivered through the birth canal.

Figure 17-2 Labor and Delivery

these rest intervals will become shorter and the contractions more forceful when the woman's uterus contracts to dilate 4 to 7 cm.

In this second phase of the first stage of labor, the contractions usually last about 1 minute each, and the rest intervals drop from about 5 minutes to 1 minute over a period of 5 to 9 hours.

The third phase of the first stage of labor is called *transition*. During transition, the uterus contracts to dilate the cervical opening to the full 10 cm required for safe passage of the fetus out of the uterus and into the vagina (birth canal).[7] This period of labor is often the most painful part of the entire birth process. Fortunately, it is also the shortest phase of most labors. Lasting 15 to 30 minutes, transition contractions often last 60 to 90 seconds each. The rest intervals between contractions are short and vary from 30 to 60 seconds.

An examination of the cervix by a nurse, midwife, or physician will reveal whether full dilation of 10 cm has occurred (see the box "Midwifery on the Rise" for more on the role of midwives). Until the full 10 cm dilation, women are cautioned not to "push" the fetus during the contractions. Special breathing and concentration techniques help many women cope with the first stage of labor.

Stage Two: Delivery of the Fetus

When the mother's cervix is fully dilated, she enters the second stage of labor, the delivery of the fetus through the birth canal. Now the mother is encouraged to help push the baby out (with her abdominal muscles) during each contraction. In this second stage the uterine contractions are less forceful than during the transition phase of the first stage and may last 60 seconds each, with a 1- to 3-minute rest interval.

This second stage may last up to 2 hours in first births.[4] For subsequent births, this stage will usually be much shorter. When the baby's head is first seen at the vaginal opening, *crowning* is said to have taken place. Generally, the back of the baby's head appears first. (Infants whose feet or buttocks are presented first are said to be delivered in a *breech position.*) After the head is delivered, the baby's body rotates upward to let the shoulders come through. The rest of the body follows quite quickly. The second stage of labor ends when the fetus is fully expelled from the vagina. In the past, deliveries were often performed with an *episiotomy,* a surgical incision of the **perineum** intended to prevent lacerations (tearing) during delivery.

> ### Key Terms
>
> **false labor** Conditions that resemble the start of true labor; may include irregular uterine contractions, pressure, and discomfort in the lower abdomen.
>
> **perineum** In the female, the region between the vulva and the anus.

Midwifery on the Rise

For the past century, most of the women in the United States who went into labor followed a fairly standard procedure. This included a trip to the hospital and a lengthy wait in a labor room. The actual birth then took place in a delivery room, which was a surgical room equipped to handle most medical emergencies. Doctors and nurses were always close by to watch the expectant mother and to track the high-tech monitors.

This scenario is rapidly changing with the increased use of midwives, many of whom help deliver babies within hospital settings, at free-standing birthing centers, or in the homes of the pregnant women. Two types of nurse-midwives are certified by the American College of Nurse-Midwives (ACNM). A certified nurse-midwife (CNM) is trained and certified in the two disciplines of nursing and midwifery, while the certified midwife (CM) has training and certification in midwifery. All certified nurse-midwives have baccalaureate degrees and 85 percent also have master's or doctoral degrees. By 2010, all graduates of midwifery education programs will be required to have a master's degree to be eligible to take the certification exam of the American Midwifery Certification Board. Two percent of CNMs are men.*

Both CNMs and CMs operate within a framework of a health care system that provides for consultation, collaborative management, or referral to additional medical care according to the health needs and condition of the pregnant woman. If the woman needs specialized help during the pregnancy or emergency care during labor, certified midwives do not hesitate to access the traditional medical system. Since 97 percent of midwife deliveries take place within hospitals, this care is usually easily attainable. Presently, less than 3 percent of midwife-assisted births occur at free-standing birthing centers or in private homes.

Today, over 10 percent of all vaginal births in the United States are attended by midwives. In the year 2005, certified midwives attended more than 305,000 births. With 39 ACNM-certified midwifery training programs in place at some of the most prestigious universities in the country (for example, Vanderbilt University, Baylor College of Medicine, the University of Michigan, and Yale University), this trend will likely continue.

Note: "Doulas" are assistants in the labor process who are trained to provide physical, emotional, and informational support to mothers before, during, and after childbirth. They are not trained or certified as midwives. Certified doulas attend a three-day course and then meet other certification requirements. Unlike CNMs and CMs, doulas are not academically trained to provide professional clinical care. A college degree is not required for becoming a doula.

*American College of Nurse-Midwives. *Fact Sheets and QuickInfo,* www.midwife.org.

Immediately after the birth, and again 5 minutes later, the newborn's physical health frequently is evaluated by obstetrical assistants using the Apgar score system. The baby will be judged (rated either 0, 1, or 2) on five criteria including appearance (color), pulse, response to foot stimulation, muscle tone, and respiration. After 5 minutes, 98 percent of infants score 7 or above. An Apgar score of less than 5 after 5 minutes indicates the possibility of a serious defect.

Newly delivered babies often look "unusual." Their heads are often cone-shaped as a result of the compression of cranial bones that occurs during the delivery through the birth canal. Within a few days after birth, the newborn's head assumes a much more normal shape. Most babies (of all races) appear bluish at first until they begin regular breathing. All babies are covered with a coating of *vernix,* a white, cheeselike substance that protects the skin.

Stage Three: Delivery of the Placenta

Usually within 30 minutes after the fetus is delivered, the uterus again initiates a series of contractions to expel the placenta (or *afterbirth*). The placenta is examined by the attending physician to ensure that it was completely expelled. Torn remnants of the placenta could lead to dangerous hemorrhaging by the mother. Often the physician manually examines the uterus after the placenta has been delivered.

After the placenta has been delivered, the uterus continues with mild contractions to help control bleeding and start the gradual reduction of the uterus to its normal, nonpregnant size. This final aspect of the birth process is called **postpartum.** External abdominal massage

---

> **Key Terms**
>
> **postpartum** The period after the birth of a baby during which the uterus returns to its prepregnancy size.
>
> **cesarean delivery** (si **zare** ee an) Surgical removal of a fetus through the abdominal wall.
>
> **bonding** Important initial recognition established between the newborn and those adults on whom the newborn will depend.
>
> **teratogenic agent** Any substance that is capable of causing birth defects.

of the lower abdomen seems to help the uterus contract, as does an infant's nursing at the mother's breast (see the box "Benefits of Successful Breast-Feeding").

Cesarean Deliveries

A **cesarean delivery** (cesarean birth, C-section) is a procedure in which the fetus is surgically removed from the mother's uterus through the abdominal wall. This type of delivery, which is completed in up to an hour, can be performed with the mother having a regional or a general anesthetic.

In 2006, the percentage of deliveries by cesarean section reached an all-time high of 31.1 percent.[10] The increasing use of cesarean deliveries is questioned by some medical experts, although others point to the need for this kind of delivery when one or more of the following factors are present:

- The fetus is improperly positioned.
- The mother's pelvis is too small.
- The fetus is especially large.
- The fetus shows signs of distress.
- The umbilical cord is compressed.
- The placenta is being delivered before the fetus.
- The mother's health is at risk.

Although a cesarean delivery is considered major surgery, most mothers cope well with the delivery and postsurgical and postpartum discomfort. The hospital stay is usually a few days longer than for a vaginal delivery. The mother can still nurse her child and may still be able to have vaginal deliveries with later children. More and more hospitals are allowing the father to be in the operating room during cesarean deliveries. Fortunately, research indicates that early **bonding** between child, mother, and father can still occur with cesarean deliveries. Cesarean deliveries are much more expensive than vaginal deliveries.

Problems in Fetal Development and Pregnancy

Most women progress through their three trimesters of pregnancy without any major complications for either their own health or the health of the baby. Sometimes there are difficulties, but fortunately, many of these problems can be identified and successfully managed. Genetic and prenatal counseling can be especially helpful.

Genetic and Prenatal Counseling

Genetic and prenatal (before birth) counseling are two of the most beneficial advances in medical technology. Genetic counselors can provide timely, accurate, and complete information to patients, while maintaining the attitude that the patient's values should guide the decisions.

The March of Dimes is the nation's preeminent organization with the mission to "improve the health of babies by preventing birth defects, premature birth, and infant mortality."[11] The March of Dimes indicates that people who should be especially interested in genetic counseling include the following:

- Women who plan to be pregnant after age 35 (see the box "Pregnancy and Parenting After 40").
- Couples who already have a child with an inherited disorder, birth defect, or mental retardation.
- Women who have had three or more miscarriages or had babies who died in infancy.
- Men or women who think that their job, lifestyle, or medical history might pose a risk to a current or future pregnancy. Such concerns might be exposure to certain medications, chemicals, radiation, drugs, or infections. These substances are frequently called **teratogenic agents.**
- Couples who understand that certain genetic defects occur in their ethnic group. Examples are Tay-Sachs disease, a fatal nervous system disease that can occur in people of Eastern European Jewish ancestry, and sickle-cell disease, a blood disorder that can occur in African Americans.

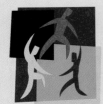

Learning from Our Diversity

Pregnancy and Parenting After 40

Women who become pregnant in their 40s are not a new phenomenon. What is new is women becoming pregnant (or adopting or using surrogate mothers) at a time when many women begin menopause.* For example, Susan Sarandon delivered a child when she was in her mid-40s, and presidential hopeful John Edwards's wife, Elizabeth, delivered a child in her late 40s and another in her early 50s. Other examples are Sharon Stone (adopted a child in her late 40s), Diane Keaton (adopted two children in her 50s), and Cheryl Tiegs (had twins in her 50s using the services of a surrogate mother).

The reasons for births after age 40 are several. Some couples may have tried to conceive for years and only succeeded when in their 40s. Other women and couples delayed pregnancy in order to build their careers, travel, or become more financially secure. In addition, fertility technology, microsurgery, and the use of donor eggs or sperm have finally given many couples the baby they long wanted.

It is not unusual to see men becoming fathers in their later 50s or 60s. Well-known people like Rod Stewart, Larry King, Michael Douglas, and Paul McCartney became new fathers in later middle age. Indeed, there is plenty of evidence that sperm function in older men does not diminish much from that seen in younger men.[†]

However, women experience a decline in fertility as they age. Traditionally, women have been discouraged from becoming pregnant for the first time in their 40s because of the health risks to the mother and the risk of birth defects for the baby. The risk of having a child with a birth defect also increases as the mother's age increases. For example, about 1 out of 1,400 babies born to women in their 20s has Down syndrome, while 1 out of 100 babies born to women in their 40s has Down syndrome.[‡]

Older women suffer more complications than younger women during pregnancy and childbirth. The risk of miscarriage is 12 to 15 percent for women in their 20s but rises to 25 percent in women at age 40. Older women are more likely than younger women to develop gestational diabetes or high blood pressure during a pregnancy. Older moms also are more likely to have low-birth-weight babies (under 5.5 pounds) or stillbirths (births of a baby who has died). The incidence of cesarean births is slightly higher for older moms as well.[‡]

If this sounds discouraging, remember that women who want to have a baby in their 40s should use this information to *prevent problems* rather than let it discourage them from having a baby. Revisit the recommendations in the section "Maintaining a Healthy Pregnancy." These guidelines are important for all pregnant women to follow. Women in their 40s who want to start their families should consider the following additional points:

- To identify all of your options, consult with your obstetrician/gynecologist before trying to become pregnant.
- Make sure you have early prenatal (before birth) care. The first 8 weeks of development are especially important for the baby.
- Don't skip any doctor appointments. Your health must be carefully monitored.
- Get appropriate prenatal screening tests, including ones that test for genetic disorders. Your doctor will advise you on these tests.

Following these strategies will help a woman minimize the chances of having complications for herself and her baby. The odds for success are still in her favor.

*Hesse, M. Famous Older Moms. AARP Online. www.aarpmagazine.org/lifestyle/famous_older.html.
[†]Crooks RL, Baur K. *Our Sexuality* (10th ed.). Belmont, CA: Wadsworth, 2008.
[‡]WebMD. Pregnancy: Having a Baby After Age 35. www.webmd.com/content/Article/51/40823.htm.

- Couples who are first cousins or other close blood relatives.
- Pregnant women who have had screening tests that indicate that their pregnancy may be at increased risks for complications or birth defects.[12]

The genetic counselor might use a variety of methods to gather information about the couple, including DNA testing, other medical tests, medical records, family histories, and autopsy reports. When a couple receive genetic counseling before conception and learn that they have a high risk of conceiving a child with a birth defect, then they have a variety of options still open to them, such as artificial insemination by a donor, ovum donation, and adoption.

If you have already become pregnant, you should still work with your physician to identify risk factors in your first prenatal visit. This allows time for tests to be conducted and medical records to be reviewed. (These tests are explained in the next section of this chapter.) In general, couples may want to consider receiving genetic counseling and testing while they still have the legal option to terminate the pregnancy.

Testing for Fetal Abnormalities

Many women undergo tests during pregnancy to check for birth defects, genetic disorders, and other problems. A few of the most common tests are ultrasound scans, the quad marker screen, amniocentesis, and chorionic villus sampling (CVS). Each of these tests can be helpful in diagnosing problems, but the tests are not necessary for every pregnancy. Women should check with their doctor about which, if any, are appropriate.

Ultrasound Ultrasound technology uses high-frequency sound waves to form pictures of the fetus on a computer screen. The test can verify a due date; determine multiple

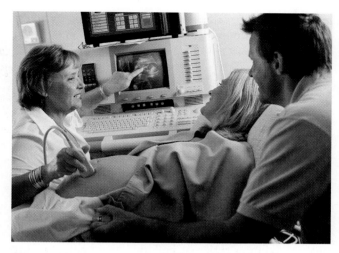

Ultrasound scans are used to check the growing fetus for possible abnormalities, as well as size, development, position, and many other factors.

fetuses or major abnormalities; check the overall health, development, sex, and position of the baby; measure the amniotic fluid; and check the position of the placenta. There are no known risks from the tests. Ultrasound tests are painless and take about 30 minutes to complete.[13]

Quad Marker Screen The quad marker screen is a simple blood test that predicts the likelihood of a certain problem occurring with the pregnancy or the fetus. The quad marker screen does not diagnose the problem, however.[14] The test is used only during the 15th and 20th weeks of pregnancy. It analyzes the mother's blood sample for levels of four substances (two proteins produced by the baby's liver and two hormones produced by the placenta). The quad marker screen results can indicate a variety of possible problems, including brain and spinal cord defects and genetic disorders like Down syndrome. The results provide additional information about the possibility of twins and the age of the fetus.

In over 98 percent of pregnancies, normal test results predict healthy babies and uncomplicated births. Abnormal results from a quad marker screen do not necessarily mean that a problem exists. A small percentage of women with elevated, abnormal results will be carrying a fetus with a birth defect. Follow-up tests, such as amniocentesis, may be used to make a more definitive diagnosis.

Amniocentesis This test examines skin cells shed by the fetus into the surrounding amniotic fluid. Performed between the 15th and 18th weeks of pregnancy, the test involves inserting a long, thin needle through the mother's abdomen to extract less than an ounce of fluid from the womb. A local anesthetic reduces any discomfort. The cells must be cultured in a laboratory, and it may take two or three weeks for test results to be ready. The test is a reliable indicator of chromosomal abnormalities such as Down syndrome or genetic disorders such as Tay-Sachs disease, Hunter's syndrome, and sickle-cell disease. Amniocentesis can also identify neural tube defects. The accuracy of test results is 99.4 percent.[15]

While usually quite safe, amniocentesis can trigger cramping, leakage of amniotic fluid, and vaginal bleeding, and it may increase the risk of miscarriage by less than 1 percent. The test is done only on women at increased risk of having babies with genetic disorders or to assess the maturity of the baby's lungs in the last trimester.

Chorionic Villus Sampling Performed between 10 and 12 weeks of pregnancy, CVS can detect the same genetic abnormalities as amniocentesis, with the exception of neural tube defects. CVS is undertaken earlier in a pregnancy than amniocentesis. The results are usually available within 10 days. The test involves inserting a needle or catheter into the womb and extracting some of the chorionic villi (cells from the placenta that originate from the fertilized egg). These villi have the same genes as the fetus.

The test is quite safe, but CVS has a slightly greater risk of causing miscarriage than amniocentesis, since it takes place earlier in the pregnancy. Rare cases of babies born with finger and toe defects after CVS have been reported, but these seem to have been in tests undertaken before the ninth week. The accuracy of CVS results is 98 percent.[16]

 TALKING POINTS Are there people in your life who you can comfortably ask, "What was it like to go through labor and delivery?" Will you feel open enough to express any personal concerns you might have about your own fears of this process?

Infertility

Most traditional-age college students are interested in preventing pregnancy. However, other people are trying to do just the opposite: they are trying to become pregnant. It is estimated that about 10 percent of the U.S. population has a problem with *infertility*. These couples wish to become pregnant but are unsuccessful.

Causes of Infertility

What causes infertility? About 40 percent of infertility problems are attributed to male factors and about 40 percent are explained by female factors. Approximately 10 percent of the problems stem from a combination of female and male factors, while the remaining 10 percent come from unknown origins.[17]

Problems of infertility that may come from males include low sperm count, inability of the sperm to move properly, or structural abnormalities of the sperm. Female factors related to infertility center on lack of ovulation and obstructions in the fallopian tubes.

Preventing Infertility

Can you do anything to prevent infertility? There are many ways you can increase your chances of remaining fertile. Avoiding sexually transmitted diseases is one crucial factor. (See the guidelines for safe sex in Chapter 13.) The risk from multiple partners should encourage responsible sexual activity. Men and women should avoid working around hazardous chemicals or using psychoactive drugs. Being overweight or underweight, smoking, and heavy alcohol consumption are risk factors that reduce one's fertility.[18] Maintaining overall good health and having regular medical (and, for women, gynecological) checkups are excellent ideas. Because infertility is directly linked with advancing age, couples may not want to indefinitely delay having children.

Enhancing a Couple's Fertility

A number of approaches can be used to increase sperm counts. Among the simple approaches are the application of periodic cold packs on the scrotum and the replacement of tight underwear with boxer shorts. When a structural problem reduces sperm production, surgery can be helpful. Most experts (reproductive endocrinologists) suggest that couples have intercourse at least a couple of times in the week preceding ovulation. Frequent intercourse tends to lower sperm counts, so couples should not have sex more than often every 36 hours.[19]

Treatments for Infertility

A variety of approaches can be used with couples who are having fertility problems. These include artificial insemination, surgery, fertility drugs, and assisted reproductive technologies (ARTs).

Artificial Insemination Men can collect (through masturbation) and save samples of their sperm to use in a procedure called *artificial insemination by partner.* Near the time of ovulation, the collected samples of sperm are deposited near the woman's cervical opening. In a related procedure called *artificial insemination by donor,* the sperm of a donor are used. Donor semen is screened for the presence of pathogens, including the AIDS virus.

Surgery Causes of infertility in women center mostly on obstructions in the reproductive tract and the inability to ovulate. The obstructions frequently result from tissue damage (scarring) caused by infections. Chlamydial and gonorrheal infections often produce fertility problems. Other possible causes of structural abnormalities include scar tissue from previous surgery, fibroid tumors, polyps, and endometriosis. A variety of microsurgical techniques may correct some of these complications.

One of the most recent innovative procedures involves the use of **transcervical balloon tuboplasty.** In this procedure a series of balloon-tipped catheters are inserted through the uterus into the blocked fallopian tubes. After they are inflated, these balloon catheters help open the scarred passageways.

Fertility Drugs When a woman has ovulation difficulties, pinpointing the specific cause can be very difficult. Increasing age produces hormone fluctuations associated with lack of ovulation. Being significantly overweight or underweight also has a serious effect on fertility. However, in women of normal weight who are not approaching menopause, it appears that ovulation difficulties are caused by failure of synchronization between the hormones governing the menstrual cycle. Fertility drugs can help alter the menstrual cycle to produce ovulation. Clomiphene citrate (Clomid), in oral pill form, or injections of a mixture of luteinizing hormone (LH) and follicle-stimulating hormone (FSH) taken from the urine of menopausal women (Pergonal) are the most common fertility drugs available. Both are capable of producing multiple ova at ovulation.

Assisted Reproductive Technology (ART) For couples who are unable to conceive after drug therapy, surgery, and artificial insemination, the use of one of four assisted reproductive technologies (ARTs) can be helpful. One option is *in vitro fertilization and embryo transfer (IVF-ET).* This method is sometimes referred to as the "test tube" procedure. Costing over $10,000 per attempt, IVF-ET consists of surgically retrieving fertilizable ova from the woman and combining them in a glass dish with sperm. After several days, the fertilized ova are transferred into the uterus. IVF-ET accounts for 98 percent of all ART procedures.[20]

A second test tube procedure is called *gamete intrafallopian transfer (GIFT).* Similar to IVF-ET, this procedure deposits a mixture of retrieved eggs and sperm directly into the fallopian tubes.

Fertilized ova (zygotes) can also be transferred from a laboratory dish into the fallopian tubes in a procedure called *zygote intrafallopian transfer (ZIFT).* One

---

Key Terms

transcervical balloon tuboplasty The use of inflatable balloon catheters to open blocked fallopian tubes; a procedure used for some women with fertility problems.

advantage of this procedure is that the clinicians are certain that ova have been fertilized before the transfer to the fallopian tubes. GIFT and ZIFT combined account for less than 2 percent of ART procedures.[20]

The fourth (and newest) procedure is *intracytoplasmic sperm injection (ICSI)*. This is a laboratory procedure in which a single sperm cell is injected into a woman's retrieved egg. The fertilized egg is then transplanted into the woman's uterus. The cost and technical expertise involved in ICSI make it a seldom-used procedure for infertile couples.

Ethical Questions Remain   The January 2009 births of eight babies to a California woman (who already had six children through IVF-ET procedures) raised the eyebrows of many who struggle with the ethical issues surrounding high-tech infertility treatments. This was the second set of octuplets ever recorded in the United States.[21] The biggest challenge with extreme multiple births is the overall health of the babies and the mother. The risks to the infants include bleeding in the brain, intestinal problems, developmental delays, and learning disabilities that last a lifetime. (At the time of this writing, however, all eight babies and the mother appeared to be in good physical health.)

The general consensus among medical ethicists seems to be that the decision to implant such a large number of embryos into the woman was irresponsible. European countries limit the number of embryos to be implanted at one to three. In the California woman's case, she was apparently offered "selective reduction" to lower the number of implanted embryos, but she declined. A representative of the American Society for Reproductive Medicine indicated that the organization's guidelines suggest that no more than two embryos be implanted in a woman under the age of 35.[21] Where do you stand on this issue?

Options for Infertile Couples

The process of coping with infertility problems can be an emotionally stressful experience for a couple. Hours of waiting in physicians' offices, undergoing many examinations, scheduling intercourse, producing sperm samples, and undergoing surgical or drug treatments place multiple burdens on a couple. Knowing that other couples are able to conceive so effortlessly adds to the mental strain. Fortunately, support groups have been established to assist couples with infertility problems. (Some of these groups are listed in the box "Where to Find Help for Infertility and Adoption.")

Surrogate Parenting   Surrogate parenting is an option that has been explored, although the legal and ethical issues surrounding this method of conception have not been fully resolved. Surrogate parenting can take several

Where to Find Help for Infertility and Adoption

These agencies can provide you with information about infertility and give referrals to specialists in your area:

American Society for Reproductive Medicine
(205) 978-5000
www.asrm.org

Planned Parenthood Federation of America
(800) 230-7526
www.plannedparenthood.org

RESOLVE
(703) 556-7172
www.resolve.org

These agencies can provide help to prospective adoptive parents:

National Adoption Center
1-800-TO-ADOPT
www.adopt.org

National Council for Adoption
(703) 299-6633
www.adoptioncouncil.org

North American Council on Adoptable Children
(651) 644-3036
www.nacac.org

forms. Typically, an infertile couple makes a contract with a woman (the surrogate parent), who will then be artificially inseminated with semen from the expectant father. In some instances the surrogate receives an embryo from the donor parents. The surrogate carries the fetus to term and returns the newborn to the parents. In some cases, women have served as surrogates for their close relatives. Because of the concerns about true "ownership" of the baby, surrogate parenting may not be a particularly viable or legal option for many couples.

Adoption   For couples who have determined that biological childbirth is impossible, adoption offers an alternative. Adopted children currently represent about 2.5 percent of all children in the United States.

As the supply of adoptable infants has decreased, young women considering putting their babies up for adoption have gained new leverage. Couples determined to adopt a healthy infant have increasingly turned to independent adoptions arranged by a lawyer, or they may negotiate directly with the birth mother. Independent adoptions now surpass those arranged by social service agencies.

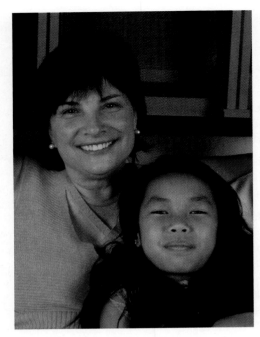

Adoption is an alternative for couples who cannot have or choose not to have a biological child. About 2.5 percent of children in the United States have been adopted.

Adoption is now a viable option for most adults. In the past, many states permitted only wealthy, heterosexual, young or midlife married couples to adopt children or become foster parents. Now, in many states, single persons can legally adopt children. Single gay and lesbian persons also can adopt. Same-sex couples may also adopt in many areas of the country. (Visit the nonprofit organization www.familieslikeours.org website for more information.)

The most important factors in adoption seem to be the ability of the adopting person or couple to be able to provide a stable, safe, and positive environment with sufficient space for the child. Adequate income is important, but being wealthy is not a requirement. (To find out more about adoption, visit www.naic.acf.hhs.gov, www.adopt.org, and www.davethomasfoundation.org.)

> ### Key Terms
>
> **human cloning** The replication of a human being.
>
> **enucleated egg** An ovum with the nucleus removed.
>
> **therapeutic cloning** The use of certain human replication techniques to reproduce body tissues and organs.
>
> **stem cells** Premature (pluripotent) cells that have the potential to turn into any kind of body cell.

Foster Parenting The number of children in foster care who are waiting to be reunited with their biological parents or awaiting adoption has risen steadily since the mid-1980s. Experts attribute the rise to family problems caused by parental drug abuse, unemployment, alcoholism, and other difficulties. Currently about one-half million children a year spend time in foster homes.

Like adoption, foster parenting has presented a variety of ethical and legal issues, especially the debate between "the best interests of the child" and parental rights.

 TALKING POINTS You have tried for a couple of years to get pregnant, and now you are ready to consider some of the newest options to increase the chances of conception. Your partner seems unwilling to spend much money for these high-tech procedures. You are ready to spend some of your retirement savings in this effort. How can you and your partner best come to an agreement on this issue?

What About Human Cloning?

Today's most controversial issue related to parenting is reproduction through **human cloning.** With the 1997 breakthrough cloning of the Scottish sheep Dolly, the possibility of human cloning emerged within the scientific community.

Cloning Techniques

To clone a human, the procedure would involve the following steps:[22]

- Doctors would surgically retrieve an egg from the female donor.
- The nucleus of this egg would be removed.
- A cell is taken from a cloning subject (a male or female).
- Through an electrical jolt, the cloning subject's cell is fused with the **enucleated egg.** This creates a clonal zygote. Shortly after, this clonal zygote divides over and over and develops into a clonal embryo.
- The clonal embryo is implanted in the womb of a surrogate mother.
- After nine months, a genetically matched reproduction of the cloning subject is born.

Reproductive Cloning

Although this step-by-step process may seem simple, it has never been accomplished with human subjects. In fact, it took scientists 277 attempts to produce Dolly, the cloned sheep.[22] The technical expertise to clone humans has not been fully developed, although some scientists believe it could be on the near horizon, if public policy would fully support this area of research.

However, public policy currently does not support human cloning. Several countries and a few states have passed laws banning human cloning.[22] The U.S. Food and Drug Administration (FDA) has warned researchers that any attempts at human cloning must first get FDA approval, which the FDA claims will not be forthcoming. Both the American Society for Reproductive Medicine and the National Academy of Sciences have voiced their opposition to human cloning.[23] Many public opinion polls have indicated that Americans are overwhelmingly against the use of cloning to produce babies.

Therapeutic Cloning

However, the potential use of a particular type of cloning has received much more popular public support in America. This is the use of cloning to reproduce body parts, tissues, and specific organs for use in medical transplant procedures. A baby is never reproduced in this cloning procedure.[23] In organ and tissue cloning, sometimes called **therapeutic cloning,** the clonal embryo is not implanted into a surrogate mother, but allowed to grow (divide) into a number of premature cells called **stem cells.** These stem cells have the potential to grow into any kind of body cell.

Theoretically, scientists could develop techniques that would cause these stem cells to grow into tissues or organs that would match the tissues or organs in the person who donated the genetic material. Because of this genetic match, these cloned organs would not be rejected after the transplant surgery. In essence, this technology permits a person's own body to be a human repair kit. Some predict that, in the not too distant future, scientists will be able to grow replacement organs like hearts, livers, and skin and replacement neurons for persons who suffer from Parkinson's or Alzheimer's disease.

When stem cells are removed from four-to-five-day-old embryos, the embryos die. For this reason, research involving embryonic stem cells has been a "political hot potato" in America for more than a decade. In 2001, political pressure encouraged President George W. Bush to prohibit federal research funds to be used for embryonic stem cell research, except for research using already existing stem cell lines. This policy effectively stifled human embryonic stem cell research in the United States.

However, shortly after the Bush administration left office in early 2009, the FDA approved the first human trials of embryonic stem cells. The FDA gave approval to the Geron Corporation to study whether specialized precursor nerve cells made from embryonic stem cells were safe to inject into patients with complete spinal cord injuries. The project was expected to involve 8 to 10 patients who are completely paralyzed below the 3rd to 10th vertebrae.[24] At the time of this writing, political pundits anticipate that the administration of President Barack Obama will further loosen restrictions on stem cell research and therapeutic cloning.

There are those who wonder if cloning represents "science gone mad." Some believe that any kind of cloning is unethical because it interferes with nature. Altering a woman's eggs, reprogramming cells, and tampering with embryos is something that is *simply wrong*. Regardless of the position you take on this issue, you can expect to see more scientific advances regarding cloning, especially therapeutic cloning.

Taking Charge of Your Health

- Use the Personal Assessment at the end of this chapter to help you think about your feelings about parenting.

- Talk to your partner (or roommate) about any ethical concerns that you think might be involved in human cloning.

- If you don't want a child at this time, make sure that you are managing your fertility accordingly, whether by abstinence or a highly effective form of contraception.

- If you are pregnant or think you might be pregnant, challenge yourself to avoid any agents that might damage your fetus.

- If you plan to become a parent one day, choose lifestyle behaviors that will enhance (not reduce) your fertility.

SUMMARY

- Couples have many important issues to discuss before deciding to have children.
- Several physiological factors can be either aids or obstacles to fertilization.

- Women can often recognize the presumptive and probable signs of pregnancy; a physician can determine positive signs of pregnancy.

- Pregnant women, and women attempting to become pregnant, should avoid agents that can damage the fetus, including all drugs (prescription, over the counter, and illicit), tobacco smoke, and alcohol.
- The nine months of pregnancy can be divided into three trimesters. The fetal growth and development during each trimester is unique.
- Childbirth takes place in three distinct stages: effacement and dilation of the cervix, delivery of the fetus, and delivery of the placenta.

- Certified nurse-midwives help deliver babies in a variety of hospital, birthing, and home settings.
- Genetic and prenatal counseling can provide much information to prospective parents.
- For couples with fertility problems, numerous strategies can be used to help conception take place.
- Having children through human cloning raises many ethical issues.

REVIEW QUESTIONS

1. How would you define the term *stepfamily*?
2. What are some obstacles and aids to fertilization presented in this chapter? Can you think of others?
3. What are the presumptive, probable, and positive signs of pregnancy?
4. Briefly describe the changes in intrauterine development during each trimester.
5. Identify and describe the events that occur during each of the three stages of childbirth. Approximately how long is each stage?

6. Who should seek genetic counseling? How can the counselor assess the couple's risk of having a child with birth defects?
7. Describe the level of training that certified nurse-midwives have. In what setting do most midwife deliveries take place?
8. What can be done to reduce chances of infertility?
9. Explain the IVF-ET, GIFT, ZIFT, and ICSI procedures.
10. What is the difference between human cloning and therapeutic cloning?

ANSWERS TO THE "WHAT DO YOU KNOW?" QUIZ

1. False   2. True   3. False   4. False   5. True   6. False   7. True

Visit the Online Learning Center (**www.mhhe.com/payne11e**), where you will find tools to help you improve your grade including practice quizzes, key terms flashcards, audio chapter summaries for your MP3 player, and many other study aids.

SOURCE NOTES

1. National Stepfamily Resource Center. *Frequently Asked Questions*, www.stepfamilies.info/, accessed February 1, 2009.
2. Purnell LD, Paulanka BJ. *Transcultural Health Care: A Culturally Competent Approach* (3rd ed.). Philadelphia: F. A. Davis, 2008.
3. Hatcher RA, et al. *Contraceptive Technology* (19th ed.). New York: Ardent Media, 2007.
4. Hyde JS, DeLamater JD. *Understanding Human Sexuality* (10th ed.). New York: McGraw-Hill, 2009.
5. Crooks RL, Baur K. *Our Sexuality* (10th ed.). Belmont, CA: Wadsworth, 2008.
6. WebMD. Your Guide to Pregnancy Tests. www.webmd.com/baby/guide/pregnancy-tests, accessed February 1, 2009.
7. Strong B, Yarber WL, Sayad BW, DeVault C. *Human Sexuality: Diversity in Contemporary America* (6th ed.). New York: McGraw-Hill, 2008.
8. Wardlaw GM, Hampl JS. *Perspectives in Nutrition* (7th ed.). New York: McGraw-Hill, 2006.
9. Carroll JL. *Sexuality Now: Embracing Diversity* (2nd ed.). Belmont, CA: Cengage Learning, 2007.
10. Martin JA, et al. Births: Final Data for 2006. *National Vital Statistics Reports*, 57(7), January 2009.
11. March of Dimes Foundation. *About Us*, www.marchofdimes.com/aboutus, accessed February 1, 2009.
12. March of Dimes Foundation. *Genetics and Pregnancy: The Genetics Revolution*, www.marchofdimes.com/printableArticles/4439_1126.asp, accessed February 1, 2009.
13. WebMD. *Prenatal Ultrasound*, www.webmd.com/baby/guide/ultrasound, accessed February 2, 2009.
14. WebMD. *Pregnancy: Quad Marker Screen*, www.webmd.com/baby/guide/quad-marker-screen, accessed February 2, 2009.
15. WebMD. *Pregnancy: Amniocentesis*, www.webmd.com/baby/guide/amniocentesis, accessed February 2, 2009.
16. WebMD. *Pregnancy: Chorionic Villus Sampling*, www.webmd.com/baby/guide/chorionic-villus-sampling, accessed February 2, 2009.
17. McAnulty RD, Burnette MM. *Exploring Human Sexuality: Making Healthy Decisions* (2nd ed.). Boston: Allyn & Bacon, 2004.
18. RESOLVE: The National Infertility Association. *Risk Factors*, www.resolve.org, accessed February 2, 2009.
19. WebMD. *Health Guide A–Z: Infertility—Home Treatment*, www.mywebmd.com/content/healthwise130/32439, accessed October 2, 2003.
20. WebMD. *A Couple's Guide: Trying to Conceive*, www.my.webmd.com/content/article/73/87996, accessed October 3, 2003.
21. Landau E. *Octuplets: Eight Times the Ethical Questions*, www.cnn.com/2009/HEALTH/01/30/embryos.ethics/index (January 30, 2009), accessed January 31, 2009.
22. Bonsor K. *How Human Cloning Will Work*, www.science.howstuffworks.com/human-cloning1.htm, accessed February 2, 2007.
23. DeNoon D. *Cloning FAQs and Fiction*, www.my.webmd.com/content/article/57/66221.htm, accessed September 24, 2003.
24. Falco M. *FDA Approves Human Embryo Stem Cell Study*, www.cnn.com/2009/HEALTH/01/23/stem.cell/index (January 23, 2009), accessed January 31, 2009.

Personal Assessment

How do you feel about parenting?

Respond to each of the following items based on your own opinions about parenting. Circle the letters that best match your response.

SA   **Strongly agree**
A   **Agree**
U   **Undecided**
D   **Disagree**
SD   **Strongly disagree**

1. One cannot parent successfully without, at the same time, being a generally successful adult member of the community.	SA	A	U	D	SD
2. It is inappropriate to view parenting as a method of achieving immortality.	SA	A	U	D	SD
3. Parenting requires that one be willing to make major personal sacrifices for the benefit of the child.	SA	A	U	D	SD
4. Parenting adds a large measure of vitality to an adult's life.	SA	A	U	D	SD
5. Parenting demands greater creativity than any other adult pursuit.	SA	A	U	D	SD
6. A person who cannot comfortably make decisions for others should not consider parenting.	SA	A	U	D	SD
7. A family cannot exist in the absence of children.	SA	A	U	D	SD

TO CARRY THIS FURTHER . . .

After completing this personal assessment, join three of your classmates in comparing and discussing your responses. What suggestions were made to help increase your awareness of all that parenting involves?

part six

Consumer and Safety Issues

Part Six includes chapters on consumer health and safety. The decisions you make in each of these areas can have a profound effect on your well-being in each dimension of your health.

1. Physical Dimension
The physical dimension of health is directly influenced by consumer decisions, such as the physician you choose. And, of course, it is crucial to learn how to protect yourself from physical harm caused by intentional or unintentional injury.

2. Emotional Dimension
The effect of an overcrowded, highly industrialized society on your emotional health is often evident. Yet an even more powerful influence is the potential for violence or unintentional injury. Many people who are rape survivors or victims of other crimes feel fearful or angry for years afterward. Those who have behaved violently themselves may find that the knowledge of their actions erodes their emotional health.

3. Social Dimension
Good health care consumers are made, not born. The decisions you make about your health are shaped by many people. Your doctor, for example, may give you information about behavior change, or your insurance agent may offer you several managed care options from which to choose. Effective interaction with these professionals and many other people can help you meet your health care needs.

4. Intellectual Dimension
Understanding violence-related issues and consumer options requires critical thinking skills. Isolating causes of safety-related problems and devising workable solutions are complex tasks. In addition, you must be able to analyze a number of variables to make difficult decisions about your health.

5. Spiritual Dimension
Nurturing our spirituality and caring for the well-being of others are inextricably intertwined. As we search for solutions to complex social and health-related issues, we must often make difficult decisions: For example, will we someday deny health insurance coverage to persons based on the existence of high-risk health behaviors such as tobacco use and a sedentary lifestyle? Or, might we someday legally define smoking by parents as a form of child abuse? To build a better world for future generations may be the most serious challenge to our spiritual commitment to serve others.

6. Occupational Dimension
Your occupational health can be enhanced by making sound decisions about your health care and personal safety. For example, choosing a health care provider who emphasizes prevention and positive behavior change will promote your overall well-being and minimize the number of days you are unable to work because of illness. In addition, avoiding intentional and unintentional injuries will allow you to perform at your peak.

Becoming an Informed Health Care Consumer

What Do You Know About Health Care?

1. In terms of assessing the honesty of health-related advertising, testimonials represent the highest level of trustworthiness. True or False?

2. On the basis of current educational standards and state licensing examinations, a doctoral degree in allopathic medicine (MD) and a doctoral degree in osteopathic medicine (DO) are essentially interchangeable. True or False?

3. Nurse practitioners are primary care providers who are permitted to diagnose and treat patients, doing so under the supervision of physicians. True or False?

4. To be permitted to practice in the United States, practitioners in all fields of complementary and alternative medicine (CAM) must pass licensing examinations supervised by the U.S. Department of Health and Human Services. True or False?

5. The sale of a generic version of a prescription medication is permitted upon the expiration of the patent protection period of the brand name medication. True or False?

6. You must have a prescription to purchase over-the-counter (OTC) medications in any state other than the state where you obtained your driver's license. True or False?

7. The safety and effectiveness of dietary supplements is established and carefully monitored by the Food and Drug Administration (FDA). True or False?

Check your answers at the end of the chapter.

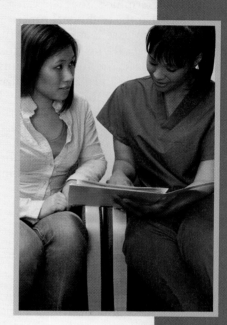

Health care providers often evaluate you by criteria from their areas of expertise. The nutritionist knows you by the food you eat. The physical fitness professional knows you by your body type and activity level. In the eyes of the expert in health consumerism, you are the product of the health information you believe, the health-influencing services you use, and the products you consume. When you make your decisions about health information, services, and products after careful study and consideration, your health will probably be improved. However, when your decisions lack insight, your health, as well as your pocketbook, may suffer.

That said, at this point an additional thought about health consumerism needs inclusion. The delivery of health care services (principally in the forms of medical care) could be undergoing changes in availability, method of delivery, and affordability that will make aspects of this chapter in need of changes that are not at this point determined. Your text can only sensitize you to the reality that the traditional American fee-for-services form of health care is no long serving us as well as it should and that calls for change are growing increasingly louder. Certainly, the current administration in Washington is listening and plans for change are being formulated. At the time of this writing, the United States and South Africa are the only highly industrialized countries yet to adopt a more nationalized or regionalized form of medical care services. Check the Online Learning Center (www.mhhe.com/payne11e) for the latest updates on government progress on reforming the health care system.

Health Information

The Informed Consumer

The Pew Charitable Trust's ongoing study of Internet use (Internet & American Life Project) provides current information on health-related Internet use.[1] The breadth of this interest is informative. Of the 95 million Americans who in 2004 conducted health-related searches, 66 percent of the searchers sought information pertaining to specific conditions and problems, 51 percent to treatment and management of conditions, 51 percent to nutrition and diet, 42 percent to exercise and fitness, 40 percent to prescription medications and over-the-counter (OTC) products, and 30 percent to alternative treatments. Further, 31 percent sought information regarding health insurance, 18 percent investigated environmental health issues, and 11 percent pursued sexual health information. Among the 16 areas searched, only 8 percent sought information pertaining to drug and alcohol use, whereas 7 percent investigated information pertaining to smoking cessation, the area least visited.

A more recent study (2008) by the same project suggests 75 to 80 percent of all Internet users do search the Web for health-related information.[2] A preponderance of this population are persons with disabilities or persons with recently identified health conditions. Internet users with broadband access are more likely to search than are those using a dial-up service.

In light of the breadth of these health interest areas, it is very likely that most people also turn to a variety of other sources for the information and access that they seek. Some of these sources are easily accessed, while others are more difficult to find but perhaps contain more appropriate information. In the section that follows, you will be introduced to several sources of health-related information. Complete the Personal Assessment at the end of this chapter to rate your own skills as a consumer of health-related information, products, and services.

Sources of Information

Your sources of information on health topics are as diverse as the number of people you know, the number of publications you read, and the number of experts you see or hear. No single agency or profession regulates the quantity or quality of the health-related information you receive. Readers will quickly recognize that all are familiar sources and that some provide more accurate and honest information than others.

Family and Friends The accuracy of information you get from a friend or family member may be questionable. Too often the information your family and friends offer is based on "common knowledge" that is wrong. In addition, family members or friends may provide information they believe is in your best interest rather than facts that may have a more negative effect on you.

Advertisements and Commercials Many people spend much of every day watching television, listening to the radio, and reading newspapers or magazines. Because many advertisements are health oriented, these are significant sources of information. The primary purpose of advertising, however, is to sell products or services. One newer example of this intertwining of health information with marketing is the "infomercial," in which a compensated studio audience watches a skillfully produced program that trumpets the benefits of a particular product or service. In spite of the convincing nature of these infomercials, however, the validity of their information is often questionable.

In contrast to advertisements and commercials, the mass media routinely offer public service messages, as mandated by the FCC, that give valuable health-related information. For example, the FCC ordered antismoking public-service announcements on television following the release of the first Surgeon General's Report on Smoking and Health (1964). These ads were powerful players in fostering a significant drop in smoking during the late 1960s and the 1970s.

Labels and Directions Federal law requires that many consumer product labels, including all medications and many kinds of food (see Chapter 5), contain specific information. For example, when a pharmacist dispenses a prescription medication, he or she must give a detailed information sheet describing the medication.

Many health care providers and agencies give consumers helpful information about their health problems or printed directions for preparing for screening procedures. Generally, information from these sources is accurate and current and is given with the health of the consumer foremost in mind.

Folklore Because it is passed down from generation to generation, folklore about health is the primary source of health-related information for some people.

The accuracy of health-related information obtained from family members, neighbors, and coworkers is difficult to evaluate. As a general rule, however, one should exercise caution relying on its scientific soundness. A blanket dismissal is not warranted, however, because folk wisdom is occasionally supported by scientific evidence. In addition, the emotional support provided by the suppliers of this information could be the best medicine some people could receive. In fact, for some ethnic groups, indigenous health care is central to overall health care. For example, within the Chinese American community, practitioners of traditional healing arts represent primary health care. Even though many Americans would consider this form of care "folk medicine," it is highly valued and trusted by those who find it familiar.

Testimonials People eagerly want to share information that has benefited them. Others may base their decisions on such testimonials. However, the exaggerated testimonials that accompany the sales pitches of the medical quack or the "satisfied" customers appearing in advertisements and on commercials and infomercials should never be interpreted as valid endorsements.

Mass Media Health programming on cable television stations, stories in lifestyle sections of newspapers, health care correspondents appearing on national network news shows, and the growing number of health-oriented magazines are sources of health information in the mass media.

In terms of the public's priority for specific media sources of health information, a gradual evolution is occurring. As recently as 1999, television, followed by magazines and newspapers, were the three principal sources of health-related news for American adults. Now, with more than 216 million Americans having cable or phone access,[3] these traditional sources of information are gradually losing popularity to the Internet. Most likely this trend will continue until a new information-sharing technology moves into the mainstream of American life.

Health-related information in the mass media is generally accurate, but it is sometimes presented so quickly or superficially that its usefulness is limited. The consumer who wants more complete coverage of a

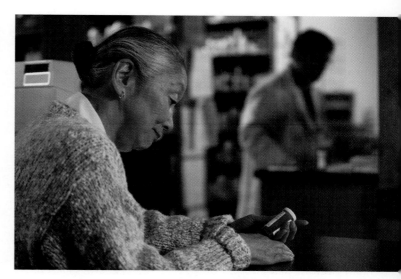

Labels and directions that accompany prescription medications are a good source of information for consumers.

health topic might acquire it by subscribing to a cable channel devoted partly or entirely to health-related programming, such as the Discovery Health Channel or The Learning Channel.

Practitioners The health care consumer also receives much information from individual health practitioners and their professional associations. In fact, today's health care practitioner so clearly emphasizes patient education that finding one who does not offer some information to a patient would be difficult. Education improves patient **compliance** with health care directives, which is important to the practitioner and the consumer.

Another important development in the trend toward health-related education is the evolution of the hospital as an educational institution. Moving beyond traditional educational activities, such as physician/staff in-house education and patient education, hospitals are extending their educational activities into the communities in a variety of ways, including newspapers, online websites, and public speaking bureaus. Wellness centers and larger multispecialty group practices are also engaged in informational outreach.

Online Computer Services We have already discussed the rapidly growing utilization of the Internet as a primary source of health-related information. We have even,

---

Key Terms

compliance Willingness to follow the directions provided by another person.

Table 18.1 Consumer Protection Agencies and Organizations

These agencies and organizations can be found in a variety of forms. Many are located within the organizational makeup of various federal agencies, while others, taking the form of free-standing organizations, are sustained in part by the validity of products, services, and corporate "good citizenship" of companies engaged in retail sales. Yet a third arena of operation for consumer protective services is within the confines of a highly creditable professional organization, such as the American Medical Association. Several consumer protective agencies and organizations are listed below.

Federal Agencies

Office of Consumer Affairs, Food and Drug Administration
(301) 827-5006
www.fda.gov/oca/aboutoca.htm

Federal Trade Commission
www.ftc.gov

Fraud Division, U.S. Postal Inspection Service
(202) 268-4299
www.usps.gov

Consumer Information Center
(719) 948-3334
www.pueblo.gsa.gov

U.S. Consumer Product Safety Commission Hotline
(800) 638-CPSC

Consumer Organizations

Consumers Union of the U.S., Inc.
(914) 378-2000
www.consumerreports.org

Professional Organizations

American Medical Association
(312) 464-5000
www.ama-assn.org

American Hospital Association
(312) 422-3000
www.aha.org

American Pharmaceutical Association
(202) 628-4410
www.aphanet.org

---

in a sense, concluded that you are or would be one of those users. This assumption may not, however, be as predictable as we believe.

In spite of the fact that today's health care system depends on computer technology to diagnose and treat illness and injury, medical professionals are perhaps the professionals least likely to use the Internet to correspond with their clients. In a study of medical practitioners across a wide range of medical specialties, only 16 percent had ever used e-mail to correspond with patients, and less than 3 percent had done so with any frequency.[4] It is not clear why physicians seem reluctant to correspond in this manner, but the medical establishment states concerns over privacy and issues of liability.

Another reason underlying this limited use of the Internet to communicate with patients is that only 4 percent of physicians have a completely computerized medical records system and only 13 percent have some degree of computerized records,[5] thus complicating all forms of clinician/patient exchange not associated with face-to-face contact.

 TALKING POINTS A family member considers herself good at diagnosing health problems. Since she hasn't been wrong in years, she no longer relies on physicians. What questions could you ask her to point out the dangers associated with her approach?

Health Reference Publications A substantial portion of all households own or subscribe to a health reference publication, such as the *Encyclopedia of Complementary*

Health Practices, the *Physicians' Desk Reference (PDR),* or a newsletter such as *The Harvard Medical School Health Letter* or *The Johns Hopkins Medical Letter: Health After 50.* Some consumers also use personal computer programs and DVDs or CDs featuring health-related information.

Reference Libraries Public and university libraries continue to be popular sources of health-related information. One can consult with reference librarians and check out audiovisual collections and printed materials. More and more of these holdings can be accessed through the home computer.

Consumer Advocacy Groups A variety of nonprofit consumer advocacy groups patrol the health care marketplace (Table 18.1). These groups produce and distribute information designed to help the consumer recognize questionable services and products. Large, well-organized groups, such as the National Consumers' League and Consumers Union, and smaller groups at the state and local levels champion the right of the consumer to receive valid and reliable information about health care products and services.

Voluntary Health Agencies Volunteerism and the traditional approach to health care and health promotion are virtually inseparable. Few countries besides the United States can boast so many national voluntary organizations, with state and local affiliates, dedicated to improving health through research, service, and public education. The American Cancer Society, the American

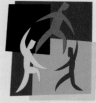

Learning from Our Diversity

Americans with Disabilities Act—New Places to Go

Although federal laws designed to end discrimination on the basis of gender and race were enacted in the United States decades ago, a law designed to address discrimination on the basis of physical and mental disabilities was not enacted until 1990. This law, the *Americans with Disabilities Act* (1990), has done a great deal to level the playing field for the disabled, both on the college campus and in the larger community. On campuses today, it's common to see students whose obvious disabilities would have prevented them from attending college before this law was enacted. Students with cerebral palsy, spina bifida, spinal cord injuries, sensory impairments, and orthopedic disabilities share living quarters, lecture hall seats, and recreational facilities with their nondisabled classmates.

Before the passage of ADA, colleges and universities were under little obligation to make their campuses barrier-free or even admit students with disabilities. Accordingly, generation after generation of highly qualified, but disabled students either remained undereducated or when admitted, continually struggled to move across campus, gain entry to buildings, access classrooms above those on the first floor, and, particularly, to reside on campus and to receive the personal care assistance associated with their particular forms of disability. Today compliance is so complete, it is estimated that between 11 and 15 percent of all college students meet the definition of "disabled."

Equally important are those students whose disabilities are largely unobservable. Students with learning disabilities, mental disabilities, and subtle but disabling chronic health conditions such as Crohn's disease, lupus, and fibromyalgia may pass unnoticed, yet their lives are equally challenged.

The Americans with Disabilities Act does not suggest that preferential treatment be given to students with disabilities, nor does it allow students to be unaccountable for their behavior. Instead, it seeks to create an environment—on the college campus and beyond—where people, regardless of disability, can learn new things, form meaningful relationships, and develop independence.

This law has the power to remove the physical and emotional barriers that can hinder a person with a disability from succeeding. For the first time, it allows students with disabilities to go where everyone else can—and beyond.

Red Cross, the National Multiple Sclerosis Society, and the American Heart Association all are voluntary (not-for-profit) health agencies. Consumers can, in fact, expect to find a voluntary health agency for virtually every health problem. College students should also note that volunteerism on their part, perhaps with a health agency like the Red Cross or the AHA, is both a personally satisfying experience and an activity viewed favorably by potential employers.

Government Agencies   Government agencies are also effective sources of information to the public. Through meetings and the release of information to the media, agencies such as the Food and Drug Administration, Department of Agriculture, Federal Trade Commission, U.S. Postal Service, and Environmental Protection Agency publicize health issues. Government agencies also control the quality of information sent out to the buying public, particularly through labeling, advertising, and the distribution of information through the mail. The various divisions of the National Institutes of Health regularly release research findings and recommendations to clinical practices, which in turn reach the consumer through clinical practitioners.

Despite their best intentions, federal health agencies are often less effective than the public deserves. A variety of factors, including inadequate staff, poor administration, lobbying by special interest groups, and political pressures, prevent these federal agencies from enforcing consumer-protection legislation. As a result, the public is left with a sense of false confidence in the consumer protection provided by the federal government.

State governments also distribute health-related information to the public. State agencies are primary sources of information, particularly in the areas of public health and environmental protection. (For an example of health care activism at work, see the box "Americans with Disabilities Act—New Places to Go.")

Qualified Health Educators   Health educators work in a variety of settings and offer their services to diverse groups. Community health educators work with virtually all of the agencies mentioned in this section; patient educators function in primary care settings; and school health educators are found at all educational levels. Health educators are increasingly being employed in a wide range of wellness-based programs in community, hospital, corporate, and school settings.

Health Care Providers

The sources of health information just discussed can greatly help us make decisions as informed consumers. The choices we make about physicians, health services, and medical payment plans reflect our commitment to remaining healthy and our trust in specific people who are trained in keeping us healthy. See the box "Choosing a Physician and a Hospital" for guidelines to help you make choices about health care providers that are right for you.

We're moving to a new town at the beginning of the summer. What will my parents and I need to know about choosing a new doctor and a hospital?

Choosing a Physician

- Get recommendations from local residents or people in the health care field, or call local hospitals for recommendations.
- Next, call the doctor's office and find out the following:
  - What are the office hours (when is the doctor available, and when can you speak to office staff)?
  - Does the doctor or someone else in the office speak the language you are most comfortable speaking?
  - How many other doctors "cover" for the doctor when he or she is not available? Who are they?
  - How long does it usually take to get a routine appointment?
  - Does the office send reminders about routine prevention tests?
  - What do you do if you need urgent care?
  - Does the doctor (or a nurse or physician assistant) give advice over the phone for common medical problems?
- After your initial visit, ask yourself, Did the doctor . . .
  - Give me a chance to ask questions?
  - Really listen to my questions?
  - Answer in terms I understood?
  - Show respect for me?
  - Ask me questions?
  - Make me feel comfortable?
  - Address the health problem(s) I came with?
  - Spend enough time with me?

Trust your own reactions when deciding whether this doctor is the right one for you. But you also may want to give the relationship some time to develop. It takes more than one visit for you and your doctor to get to know each other.

Choosing a Hospital

Keep the following questions in mind when choosing a hospital:

- Does the hospital meet national quality standards? Hospitals can choose to be surveyed by the Joint Commission on Accreditation of Healthcare Organizations (JCAHO) to make sure they meet certain quality standards; check for information at www.jcaho.org.
- How does the hospital compare with others in your area? State and consumer groups may study hospitals and issue reports and rankings. Call your state department of health, health care council, or hospital association to find out more; also, ask your doctor what she or he thinks about the hospital.
- Does your doctor have privileges (permission to admit patients) at the hospital? If not, you would need to be under the care of another doctor while at the hospital.
- Does your health plan cover care at the hospital?
- Does the hospital have experience with your condition? "General" hospitals handle a wide range of routine conditions, whereas "specialty" hospitals have a lot of experience with certain conditions (such as cancer or heart disease) or certain groups (such as children).
- How well does the hospital check and improve on its own quality of care? Ask the hospital quality management department how it monitors and improves the hospital's quality of care. Also, ask for any patient satisfaction surveys the hospital has done, as these will tell you how other patients have rated the quality of their care.

Source: U.S. Department of Health and Human Services, Agency for Healthcare Research and Quality. *Your Guide to Choosing Quality Health Care.* AHCPR Pub. No. 99-0012. Updated July 2001.

Why We Consult Health Care Providers

Most of us seek care and advice from medical and health practitioners when we have a specific problem (see Figure 18-1). A bad cold, a broken arm, or a newly discovered lump can motivate us to consult a health care professional. Yet *diagnosis* and *treatment* are only two reasons that we might require the services of health care providers.

We also might encounter health practitioners when we undergo *screening*. Screening most often involves a cursory (or noninvasive) collection of information that can quickly be compared to established standards often based on gender, age, race, or the presence of preexisting conditions. Your earliest experience with screening may have been in elementary school, where physicians, nurses, audiologists, and dentists sometimes examine children for normal growth and development patterns. As an adult,

your screening is more likely to be done on an individual basis by a physician's staff as a routine portion of every office visit when they collect baseline information such as height, weight, and blood pressure measurements. You may also encounter community-based screening when you stop at your local shopping mall's health fair and have your blood pressure taken or cholesterol checked. In both settings, the extent to which your data become incorporated into a larger data pool determines whether this screening is community-based or simply personally informing. Although screening should be considered much less precise than actual diagnosis, screening serves to identify people who should seek further medical examination.

Consultation is a fourth reason that knowledgeable consumers seek health care providers. A consultation is the use of two or more professionals to deliberate a person's

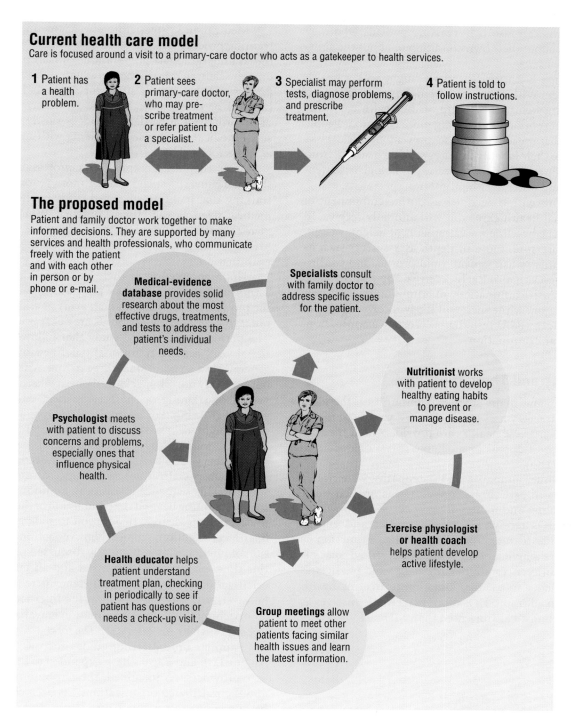

Current health care model

Care is focused around a visit to a primary-care doctor who acts as a gatekeeper to health services.

1 Patient has a health problem.

2 Patient sees primary-care doctor, who may pre-scribe treatment or refer patient to a specialist.

3 Specialist may perform tests, diagnose problems, and prescribe treatment.

4 Patient is told to follow instructions.

The proposed model

Patient and family doctor work together to make informed decisions. They are supported by many services and health professionals, who communicate freely with the patient and with each other in person or by phone or e-mail.

Medical-evidence database provides solid research about the most effective drugs, treatments, and tests to address the patient's individual needs.

Specialists consult with family doctor to address specific issues for the patient.

Nutritionist works with patient to develop healthy eating habits to prevent or manage disease.

Psychologist meets with patient to discuss concerns and problems, especially ones that influence physical health.

Exercise physiologist or health coach helps patient develop active lifestyle.

Health educator helps patient understand treatment plan, checking in periodically to see if patient has questions or needs a check-up visit.

Group meetings allow patient to meet other patients facing similar health issues and learn the latest information.

Figure 18-1 Current Versus Proposed Health Care Model   Compare the current health care model in the United States to selected aspects of a proposed model of health care.

Source: Adapted from Barr M, Ginsburg J. *The Advanced Medical Home: A Patient-Centered, Physician-Guided Model of Health Care.* A Policy Monograph of the American College of Physicians, January 2006. © Copyright 2006 American College of Physicians. All rights reserved.

specific health problem or condition. Consultations are especially helpful when **primary care health providers,** such as family practice physicians, gynecologists, pediatricians, internists, and general practice dentists, require the opinion of specialists. Using additional practitioners

> **Key Terms**
>
> **primary care health providers** Health care providers who generally see patients on a routine basis, particularly for preventive health care.

as consultants can also help reassure patients who may have doubts about their own condition or about the abilities of their physician.

Prevention is a fifth reason we might seek a health care provider. With the current emphasis on trying to stop problems before they begin, using health care providers for prevention is becoming more common. People want information about how to prevent needless risks and promote their health, and they seek such advice from physicians, nurses, dentists, exercise physiologists, patient educators, and other health promotion specialists.

When prevention becomes a routine component of your personal health care, you will annually receive, in addition to the baseline measurements of height, weight, and blood pressure, more in-depth assessments such as a blood chemistry assessment, lipid profile, and cardiogram. Women will also likely receive a Pap test (in some version), breast examination, mammography, and pelvic examination, while men will likely receive a prostate specific antigen (PSA) test, digital prostate examination, and testicular examination.

Physicians and Their Training

In every city and many smaller communities, the local telephone directory lists physicians in a variety of medical specialties. These health care providers hold the academic degree of doctor of medicine (MD) or doctor of osteopathy (DO).

At one time, allopathy and osteopathy were clearly different health care professions in terms of their healing philosophies and modes of practice. Today, however, MDs and DOs receive similar educations and engage in very similar forms of practice. Both can function as primary care physicians or as board-certified specialists. Their differences are in the osteopathic physician's greater tendency to use manipulation in treating health problems. In addition, DOs often perceive themselves as being more holistically oriented than MDs are.

Key Terms

allopathy (ah **lop** ah thee) A system of medical practice in which specific remedies (often pharmaceutical agents) are used to produce effects different from those produced by a disease or injury.

osteopathy (os tee **op** ah thee) A system of medical practice in which allopathic principles are combined with specific attention to postural mechanics of the body.

chiropractic Manipulation of the vertebral column to relieve misalignments and cure illness.

Medical and osteopathic physicians undergo a long training process. They usually take three to four years of initial undergraduate preparation with a heavy emphasis on the sciences. Most undergraduate schools have preprofessional courses of study for students interested in medical or osteopathic schools. However, this pattern of preprofessional academic work is slowly changing as some medical schools seek students with more of a liberal arts focused background.

After they are accepted into professional schools, students generally spend four or more years in intensive training that includes advanced study in the preclinical medical sciences and clinical practice. When they complete this phase of training, the students are awarded the MD or DO degree and then take the state medical license examination.

Upon completion of their basic medical education, a *transitional year* residency program follows in which the physician moves through an array of clinical areas in order to better define her or his area of specialized study. The period of specialized study that follows the transitional year, a more traditionally defined *residency,* will generally last an additional three to four years. For many, but certainly not all, specialized physicians, an additional period of training, a *subspecialization,* will add more years of training. For example, a newly graduated physician might next take a surgery-based transition-year program, followed by a specialization in cardiopulmonary surgery, eventually leading to a second full residency (subspecialization) in pediatric cardiopulmonary surgery. This sequence involves an additional decade or more of training beyond the completion of the premedical undergraduate degree. In addition to state and specialty board certification, comprehensive national certification of physicians is a frequently discussed possibility. At this time, no nationally required and all-encompassing certification of physician competency is required. Note, however, that with the advent of the Internet, something approaching this type of information is available through websites such as *America's Top Doctors.*[6]

Familiar online rating guides such as Craig's List, Angie's List, and Zagat's have expanded to include health care providers. As imagined, the response of physicians and their affiliated organizations has been characterized by condemnation, patient dismissals, and even threats of legal action against patients for defamation of character. One company, Medical Justice, initially an antimalpractice suit legal action group, now markets waiver forms for physicians to give their patients to sign in which patients promise not to engage in "Internet defamation."[7] Patients refusing to sign a waiver may risk losing the services of their care provider.

Whether the demands made on physicians and the currently much-discussed shortage of physicians that now exists in this country are influenced by issues of malpractice-litigation and defamation of character, this text cannot answer. What is known, however, is that unless current medical schools increase enrollments, new medical schools are built, and the recruiting of foreign physicians is not accelerated, our shortage of physicians will continue to increase. According to the Association of American Medical Colleges, at today's rate of physician production, we will have 750,000 physicians in this country by 2025, while our needs would be for an additional 159,000 physicians. Although more applications are being accepted, class sizes are expanding, and additional schools being constructed, it is doubtful that the shortage problem will soon be resolved.

Communication Between Patients and Their Health Care Providers

In the complex world of modern health care, it is of critical importance that patients communicate important information to their health care providers and, in turn, that they understand as fully as possible the information they receive from their providers. Following are 10 valuable suggestions from the Joint Commission on Accreditation of Healthcare Organizations and the U.S. Government's Agency for Healthcare Research and Quality.

- Take part in every decision about your health care.

- If you are not prepared to ask questions on your behalf, ask a family member or friend to fill this role for you.

- Tell your physician and pharmacist about every drug you are taking, including prescription drugs, OTC drugs, vitamins, supplements, and herbal products—bring them with you.

- Make certain that you get the results of every test, and understand what they mean.

- If you do not hear about test results, never assume that everything is all right. Call your doctor and ask.

- Whenever possible, choose a hospital where many patients receive the same procedure that you are to receive. Ask your physician or the hospital for the numbers of procedures performed.

- Ask hospital personnel if they have washed their hands before they begin touching you.

- If you are having surgery, make sure that you, your physician, and your surgeon all agree on what will be done during the operation.

- Insist that your surgeon write his or her initials or words such as *yes* or *this side* on the part of the body to be operated on. Put *no* on the opposite body part.

- When you are discharged, ask your doctor to explain your treatment plan, including changes in medications, restrictions on activity, and additional therapies you will need.

In many situations involving medical care, carefully communicated comments and questions between providers and patients can be the basis of the successful resolution of a health problem, as opposed to unnecessary delay, pain, discomfort, or even death.

Complementary, Alternative, and Integrative Care Practitioners

In addition to medical and osteopathic physicians, several other forms of health care offer alternatives within the large health care market. Included within this group of complementary or alternative forms of practice are chiropractic, acupuncture, homeopathy, naturopathy, herbalism, therapeutic touch, and ayurveda. Although the traditional medical community has long scoffed at these fields of practice as ineffective and unscientific, many people use these forms of health care and believe strongly that they are as effective as (or more effective than) allopathic and osteopathic medicine. As a result of this belief, today many physicians are better informed about complementary care methods and more comfortable discussing them with patients. Following are brief descriptions of some of the more popular of these complementary care fields and the practitioners that function within them. (Also reread the box "What Is Complementary Medicine?" in Chapter 1, which discusses the controversial nature of various fields of complementary or alternative care.)

Chiropractic Historically (and, to varying degrees, today) the underlying premise of **chiropractic** is that misalignment or subluxation of the spinal (vertebral) column is the primary cause of illness, and, thus, its realignment is the appropriate treatment for illness. Accordingly, chiropractic medical practice is primarily limited to vertebral adjustments, where manual manipulation of the spine is used to correct misalignments. With about 50,000 practitioners in the United States, chiropractic is the third-largest health profession, used by 15 to 20 million people. Some chiropractors use only spinal manipulation, whereas others use additional medical technologies, including dietary supplementation and various noninvasive technologies similar to those used by physical therapists and athletic trainers, including massage.

In spite of the fact that chiropractors undergo nearly the same number of years of initial medical school training (undergraduate plus four years to MD) as do primary care physicians and take courses closely aligned with those taken by physicians, current laws restrict the scope of chiropractic practice to noninvasive techniques initially consistent with the original theoretical basis of their discipline, "one cause—one cure of all illnesses and diseases." In 1998 the National Center for

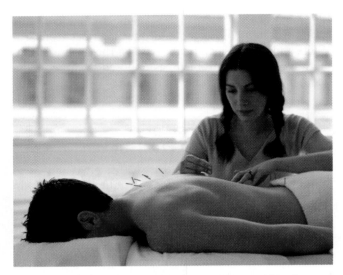

Acupuncture has received increasing acceptance within the Western medical community.

Complementary and Alternative Medicine[8] established a Comprehensive Center for Chiropractic Research (the 11th alternative medical field to receive such a center) to establish scientific standards for the study of chiropractic effectiveness.

Should careful study of chiropractic demonstrate limited effectiveness, then chiropractic medicine is likely to remain a user-friendly, highly popular but highly limited approach to health care. There is, however, a current trend of including chiropractic physicians within allopathic (conventional) medical groups, principally to treat those conditions clearly associated with postural conditions.

Acupuncture **Acupuncture** is, for Americans, the most familiar component of the 3,000-year-old Chinese medical system. This system is based on balancing the active and passive forces within the patient's body to strengthen the *qi* ("chee"), or life force. The system also employs herbs, food, massage, and exercise.

Key Terms

acupuncture Insertion of fine needles into the body to alter electroenergy fields and cure disease.

homeopathy (hoe mee **op** ah thee) The use of minute doses of herbs, minerals, or other substances to stimulate healing.

naturopathy (na chur **op** ah thee) A system of treatment that avoids drugs and surgery and emphasizes the use of natural agents, such as sunshine, to correct underlying imbalances.

herbalism An ancient form of healing in which herbal preparations are used to treat illness and disease.

Acupuncturists place hair-thin needles at certain points in the body to stimulate the patient's qi. These points are said to correspond to different organs and bodily functions and, when stimulated, help the body's own defenses fight illness.

Of all the Chinese therapies, acupuncture is the most widely accepted in the West. Researchers have produced persuasive evidence of acupuncture's effectiveness with treating low-back pain, adult postoperative pain, nausea and vomiting associated with chemotherapy, and pain following dental surgery. Acupuncture may also be effective in other areas such as addiction, headache, menstrual pain, fibromyalgia, osteoarthritis, and tennis elbow. However, because of the difficulty of conducting double-blind research that involves the insertion of needles, acupuncture research is challenging to design, thus its use may remain largely complementary. This limitation could soon change as pseudo-acupuncture needles, whose tips retract once the skin is initially punctured, have just become available, thus allowing double-blind studies to be conducted.

For information on the medical system originating in India, see the box "Ayurveda."

Manipulative Practices Although chiropractic medicine, osteopathic medicine, and physical therapy all fall under the heading of manipulative practices, this section addresses less widely used practices, including massage therapy, reflexology, rolfing, the Bowman technique, Trager bodywork, and a host of other practices that include pressing on muscles, bones, joints, soft tissue, and underlying blood and lymphatic vessels.[9] So varied are the techniques, including location of pressure, depth of pressure, and interval between applications of pressure, that it is difficult to compare one with another. That said, all techniques are based on the common agreement that the body is self-regulating and can heal itself, and that its parts are interdependent.

Although chiropractic, osteopathic, and physical therapy programs do sponsor research that appears in the medical literature (as identified by National Library of Medicine searches), the majority of the other techniques mentioned here have produced relatively little research, or research limited largely to patient observations and self-reporting. As a result, these practices remain "highly alternative" and are not covered by health insurance. On the positive side, relatively little risk is reported, particularly when practitioners are experienced.

Homeopathy Widely accepted in Europe, **homeopathy** is the leading alternative therapy in France. Homeopathy uses infinitesimal doses of herbs, minerals, or even poisons to stimulate the body's curative powers. The theory on which homeopathy is based, the *law of similars,* contends that if large doses of a substance can cause a problem, tiny doses can trigger healing. A few small studies

Considering Complementary Care

Ayurveda

Even older than Chinese medicine, India's ayurveda takes a preventive approach to health care, through focusing on the interplay of body, mind, and spirit—and is, perhaps, the most holistic of the world's principal approaches to health care. In the Indian subcontinent, this is the medical care for the masses.

The central principle of ayurveda is the integration and balance of the individual's body, mind, and spirit, both within the person, and between the individual and the environment. The individual and the environment must be in balance, for the ultimate well-being of both, as both contain elements of each other.

Important to ayurvedic medicine is the balanced nature of the constitution (or *prakriti*) appropriate to each individual. This constitution plays a critical role in how the individual expresses physiological processes, and thus maintains the internal and external balance needed for well-being. The prakriti, itself, is composed of three *dosha* (or qualities), each of which reflects combinations of the five basic elements of life—space, air, fire, water, and earth. Balance within each dosha, and between the three dosha, influences the balanced nature of the constitution or prakriti itself. The idea is that when balance exists, disease processes unique to each dosha will not develop. Dosha imbalances can result from lifestyle patterns, emotional factors such as stress, and environmental factors such as weather or the ambient germ pool.

Ayurvedic practitioners direct treatment toward the *elimination of impurities* from the body through dietary changes, fasting, and colonic cleansing of the gastrointestinal tract, and cleansing of the respiratory tract with nasal sprays and inhalations; *reducing symptoms* of imbalance through activities such as yoga, meditation, exercises, and relaxing in the sun, and through dietary changes; and *reducing worry and increasing harmony in life* by practicing peaceful thinking during exercising, yoga, and meditation. A fourth aspect of ayurvedic medical practice is the *elimination of existing physical and psychological discomfort* through massage directed at the body's 107 points where life's energy is stored within the body.

To date, no more than 1 percent of Americans have utilized the services of ayurvedic practitioners, and only a fraction of those using this form of health care have done so on a regular basis. For an American-trained physician to learn necessary aspects of ayurvedic medicine in order to combine both conventional (allopathic) and ayurvedic medicine, more than 200 hours of training would be required. Despite the limited awareness that most readers might initially have had about ayurveda, this ancient but increasingly available form of complementary care could seem very attractive from a philosophical perspective and because of a virtual absence of invasive procedures. However, it is important to understand that ayurvedic medical preparations tend to include heavy metals, such as lead, iron, and sulfur, which can lead to potentially serious levels of toxicity and reduce the effectiveness of medications important to allopathic medical practice.

Sources: *BackGround: What Is Ayurvedic Medicine?* National Center for Complementary and Alternative Medicine. National Institutes of Health. Department of Health and Human Services. October 2005. www.nccam.nih.gov/health/ayurveda/; Perspective: Ayurveda and Conventional Medicine. *CAM at the NIH* 12 (4): Fall 2005/Winter 2006. www.nccam.nih.gov/news/newsletter/2006_winter/perspective.htm.

---

showed homeopathy to be at least somewhat effective in treating hay fever, diarrhea, and flu symptoms, but members of the scientific community call the studies flawed or preliminary and suggest that the placebo effect was occurring. It was further concluded that on the basis of these studies there was no strong evidence in favor of homeopathy over conventional treatment methods. The Center recommended that larger, more carefully controlled studies be conducted.[10]

An interesting dimension to the marketing of homeopathy as an effective alternative to conventional medical care relates to the contention of some homeopathy physicians that the "molecular essence" of their homeopathic medicines can be sent via the Internet, thus allowing treatment to occur through cyberspace.

Naturopathy The core of naturopathic medicine is what Hippocrates called *medicatrix naturae,* or the healing power of nature. Proponents of **naturopathy** believe that when the mind and the body are in balance and receiving proper care, with a healthy diet, adequate rest, and minimal stress, the body's own vital forces are sufficient to fight off disease. Getting rid of an ailment is only the first step toward correcting the underlying imbalance that allowed the ailment to take hold, naturists believe. Correcting the imbalance might be as simple as rectifying a shortage of a particular nutrient, or as complex as reducing overlong work hours, strengthening a weakened immune system, and identifying an inability to digest certain foods.

Herbalism **Herbalism,** also known as herbology, phytotherapy, and herbal medicine, is without a doubt the most ancient form of medical treatment. As long ago as the Neandertal period (60,000 years ago), evidence indicates the use of plants for both food and medicine. Today herbalism is the principal form of medical treatment in developing areas of the world and is strongly supported in many developed areas as well. In the United States, botanicals provide the molecular models for many prescription medications and are principal players in the field of dietary supplementation. If prayer is excluded, herbal medicine is the most popular form of complementary and alternative medicine used in America.

Because plants contain active biochemical systems, they are known to produce a wide array of chemical compounds and bioactive metabolites. An experienced herbalist will know how to prepare such plants for human use. However, as with any bioactive material, there is a risk of toxic reaction rather than therapeutic response.[11]

Herbal medications and supplements can be dispensed in a variety of forms, including teas, coffees, tinctures, fluid and solid extracts, poultices (plasters), ointments, oils, pills, capsules, and powders. Even though many prescription medications are botanically based, the FDA classifies herbal preparations as dietary supplements because their safety and effectiveness have not been subjected to rigorous testing. Consumers use these preparations knowing relatively little about their safety and effectiveness, processing, formulation, and packaging/labeling. These risks must be taken seriously, particularly by anyone who uses herbal supplements in large quantities or in combination with prescription medications.

Today mainstream American and European pharmaceutical companies are gradually moving into the herbal supplement market. This may improve herbal safety and effectiveness, but the more sophisticated research/testing, manufacturing, marketing, and distribution could raise prices.

For readers interested in a quick tutorial regarding over forty of the more commonly used herbs, the NCCAM offers *Herbs at a Glance,* accessible through the Center's home page.[12] For those with a more serious intent, numerous books of the pharmacologically active components of botanicals are available in virtually every public and university library.

Therapeutic Touch (Biofield Therapy)   The *biofield* (or energy field) is believed by therapeutic touch practitioners to dwell within and immediately surround the body. For thousands of years, practitioners of biofield therapy, as exemplified by therapeutic touch, have attempted to identify irregularities or contractions in this electrical field and through appropriate touching (or near-touching of the body) restore its appropriate configuration. Once the biofield is aligned appropriately, the negative forces that have been disruptive to the physical and emotional balance required for healthful living are released. A second perception of biofield therapies is that through manipulation of the biofield a pathway or entry point is established that allows other health modalities, such as medications, to influence the restoration of the holistic balance needed for good health.

Nurses are the most likely practitioners of therapeutic touch and related therapies in the hospital setting. When therapeutic touch is used in a wellness-oriented manner, it is most often delivered by a certified practitioner. This is often a nurse practicing in a fee-for-service manner, a chiropractor, a naturopathic physician, or a psychologist.

The scientific literature regarding the effectiveness of therapeutic touch is very difficult to interpret. This is largely because of the difficulty of establishing double-blind experiments to study a therapeutic approach (that is, experiments in which neither practitioner nor patient knows whether the actual therapy versus a sham therapy is being delivered). A second difficulty is the problem of quantifying the outcome of the therapy. At this point it appears that therapeutic touch is somewhat effective in reducing anxiety, enhancing mood, improving sleep, and producing a higher level of relaxation among patients experiencing various emotionally traumatic medical treatments, such as breast cancer surgery, but this effectiveness is based largely on self-reported improvement and various inventories designed to assess feeling states.

If you would like to consult a practitioner in one of the alternative disciplines but you don't know where to start, see the box "Researching and Evaluating CAM Practitioners" for advice.

National Center for Complementary and Alternative Medicine   At the urging of many people in both the medical and complementary health care fields, the National Institutes of Health requested federal funding to establish a scientific center for the study of alternative medical care. Today the National Center for Complementary and Alternative Medicine assembles information about alternative approaches to medical care and provides a framework for well-controlled research into the effectiveness of each approach. Double-blind studies, so called because neither the participants nor the researchers know which treatment each participant is receiving, are being conducted. The first substantial recommendation regarding an alternative form of care, acupuncture, was released in 1998.

It will be interesting to note whether all the branches of complementary medical care will want their theories of treatment and prevention tested under the rigorous criteria used by the National Center for Complementary and Alternative Medicine and to see how they respond if the results are not favorable.

Restricted-Practice Health Care Providers

We receive much of our health care from medical physicians. However, most of us also use the services of various health care specialists, some of whom also have advanced graduate-level training.

Nurse Professionals   Nurses constitute a large group of health professionals who practice in a variety of settings. Their responsibilities usually depend on their academic preparation. Registered nurses (RNs) are academically

Building Media Literacy Skills

Researching and Evaluating CAM Practitioners

A campus flyer promotes acupuncture to relieve allergy symptoms. A close friend swears that the magnets built into her shoes relieve leg pain. A website for a local massage therapist advertises a specific type of massage to prevent migraines. What should you make of all these messages about complementary and alternative medicine (CAM)?

Information about CAM treatments and practitioners comes from many forms of media and can be difficult to evaluate. Compared to more traditional forms of medical care, there is often less scientific information available about CAM—and less regulation of CAM products and practitioners. It is important for you as a health care consumer to take an active role when you are considering CAM therapies. Don't rely on advertisements and testimonials as primary sources of information. The National Center for Complementary and Alternative Medicine (NCCAM) suggests the following strategies to assist you in your decision making about CAM.

Gathering Information

- If you are seeking a CAM practitioner, speak with your primary health care provider regarding the therapy you are interested in. Your doctor may know about the therapy and be able to advise you on its safety, use, and effectiveness, or possible interactions with any of your current medications. Ask if she or he can recommend a practitioner for the type of CAM you are seeking.
- Make a list of CAM practitioners and gather information about each before making your first visit. Ask basic questions about their credentials and practice. Where did they receive their training? What licenses or certifications do they have? Contact a professional organization for the type of practitioner you are seeking; the National Library of Medicine's Directory of Information Resources (dirline.nlm.nih.gov) includes many relevant associations. Many states also have regulatory agencies or licensing boards for certain types of practitioners.
- Ask how much the treatment will cost. Check with your insurer to see if the cost of therapy will be covered. If it is covered, check with local practitioners to see if they accept your insurance.
- After you select a practitioner, make a list of questions to ask at your first visit (see the following suggested list of questions).

Come to the first visit prepared to answer questions about your health history, including injuries, surgeries, and major illnesses, as well as prescription medicines, vitamins, and other supplements you take.

Having a Successful First Visit

Here are some questions you might want to ask during your first visit:

- What benefits can I expect from this therapy?
- What are the risks associated with this therapy?
- Do the benefits outweigh the risks for my disease or condition?
- What side effects can be expected?
- Will the therapy interfere with any of my daily activities?
- How long will treatment last? How often will my progress or plan of treatment be assessed?
- Will I need to buy any equipment or supplies?
- How much will the therapy cost?
- Do you have scientific articles or references about using the treatment for my condition?
- Could the therapy interact with conventional treatments?
- Are there any conditions for which this treatment should not be used?

Making Decisions

Assess your first visit and decide if the practitioner is right for you:

- Did you feel comfortable? Was the practitioner easy to talk with? Were you comfortable asking questions, and did the practitioner answer your questions satisfactorily?
- Was the practitioner open to how both CAM therapy and conventional medicine might work together for your benefit?
- Do the treatment plan and its associated costs seem reasonable and acceptable to you? Are you clear about the time and costs associated with treatment?

Source: National Center for Complementary and Alternative Medicine, Selecting a CAM Practitioner, NCCAM Publication No. D346 (February 2007), http://nccam.nih.gov/health/practitioner/index.htm.

---

prepared at two levels: (1) the technical nurse and (2) the professional nurse. The technical nurse is educated in a two-year associate degree program. The professional nurse receives four years of education and earns a bachelor's degree. Both technical and professional nurses must successfully complete state licensing examinations before they can practice as RNs.

In light of the important role that nurse professionals play in today's health care system, it is worrisome that a significant shortage of nurses exists. On the basis of enrollment data for nursing programs in this country,

and the number of nurses who have apparently left the workforce for various reasons, the current shortage of registered nurses is estimated to be 110,000. Projecting through 2012, it is estimated that 1.1 million new and replacement openings for nurses will exist in the United States, a need that will most likely not be met.[13]

Many professional nurses continue their education and earn master's and doctoral degrees in nursing or other health-related fields. Some professional nurses specialize in a clinical area (such as pediatrics, gerontology, public health, or school health) and become certified as *advanced practice nurses* (APNs). Currently four APN fields, including nurse midwives, nurse anesthetists, nurse practitioners, and nurse case managers, can be found in larger communities. Working in close association with physicians, APNs perform an array of diagnositic, treatment, and administrative activities once limited to physicians. The ability of these highly trained nurses to function at this level gives communities additional primary care providers and frees physicians to deal with more complex cases.

Licensed practical nurses (LPNs) are trained in hospital-based programs that last 12 to 18 months. Because of their brief training, LPNs' scope of practice is limited. Most LPN training programs are gradually being phased out. Additionally, some hospitals are financially assisting LPNs to transition into associate degree programs leading to the RN degree, or to be redefined as a nursing care technologist, at a lower rate of pay, if they do not receive the RN degree.

Allied Health Care Professionals   Our primary health care providers are supported by a large group of allied health care professionals, who are often responsible for highly technical services and procedures. These professionals include respiratory and inhalation therapists, radiographic technologists, nuclear medicine technologists, pathology technicians, general medical technologists, operating room technicians, emergency medical technicians, physical therapists, occupational therapists, cardiac rehabilitation therapists, dental technicians, physician assistants, and dental hygienists. Depending on the particular field, the training for these specialty support areas can take from one to five years of postsecondary school study. Programs include hospital-based training leading to a diploma through associate, bachelor's, and master's degrees. Most allied health care professionals must also pass state or national licensing examinations.

Self-Care/Home Care

The emergence of the **self-care movement** suggests that many people are becoming more responsible for maintaining their health. They are developing the expertise to prevent or manage many types of illness, injuries, and conditions. They are learning to assess their health status and treat, monitor, and rehabilitate themselves in a manner that was once thought possible only through a physician or some other health care specialist.

> **Key Terms**
>
> **self-care movement** The trend toward individuals taking increased responsibility for prevention or management of certain health conditions.

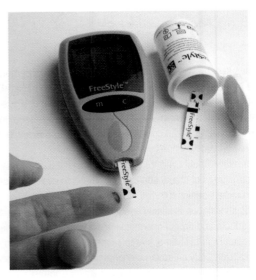

Self-care is appropriate in the management of certain chronic conditions, including diabetes. People with diabetes can monitor their blood sugar at home and make appropriate adjustments to their diet and medication schedule.

The benefits of this movement are that self-care can (1) reduce health care costs, (2) provide effective care for particular conditions, (3) free physicians and other health care specialists to spend time with other patients, and (4) increase interest in health-related activities.

Appropriate Self-Care   Self-care is an appropriate alternative to professional care in three areas. First, self-care may be appropriate for certain acute conditions that have familiar symptoms and are limited in their duration and seriousness. Common colds and flu, many home injuries, sore throats, and nonallergic insect bites are often easily managed with self-care. That said, there are some symptoms that might seem somewhat familiar that should not be responded to through self-care, but rather by seeing a physician promptly. These include a feeling of pressure or squeezing in the chest, a sudden severe headache, markedly blurred vision, difficulty talking or walking, dizziness and confusion, blood in urine or stool, unrelieved depression, and a cough with a yellow-green discharge. Self-care might be useful at some point, but not until the symptoms have been evaluated by a physician.

A second area in which self-care might be appropriate is therapy. For example, many people administer injections for diabetes mellitus, multiple sclerosis, allergies, and migraine headaches and continue physical therapy programs in their homes. Asthma and hypertension are also conditions that can be managed or monitored with self-care.

A third area in which self-care has appropriate application is health promotion. Weight loss programs, physical conditioning activities, smoking cessation, and

Good Health—What's It Worth, Now and Later?

The average life expectancy for women in the United States today is 80 years. For men, it's 76 years. That's a dramatic change from just a few generations ago. Thanks to tremendous advances in medical science and technology, many people are enjoying healthy, happy, and spiritually fulfilling lives well into their final years.

But this longevity comes with a price tag. It means that making healthful choices every day—including eating a balanced diet, getting exercise and adequate rest, and making opportunities for emotional and spiritual expression—takes on new importance. If you're going to live 10 "extra" years, what do you want to do with that time? Probably many of the things you're doing now, plus some different ones. Are you going to be able to meet the challenge—healthwise?

Taking charge of your health right now, when you're young and healthy, can be one of the most empowering things you do. By consciously choosing a healthy lifestyle—limiting your intake of alcohol, avoiding drugs and cigarette smoking, and limiting your sexual partners—you are building the foundation for good health in your later years.

If you should ever have a serious health problem, you'll be better equipped to handle it if you're used to taking care of yourself. You'll feel comfortable being involved in your treatment decisions and doing whatever you can to control the quality of your life. You'll see your health crisis as a challenge you need to deal with, instead of viewing yourself as a helpless victim.

Taking charge of your own health—by being an informed health care consumer, by choosing a healthy lifestyle, and by fostering a positive attitude—brings a sense of peace. It's knowing that you're doing everything you can to take care of yourself. It's enhancing the quality of your life today and preparing for an active and rewarding tomorrow.

---

stress-reduction programs are particularly well suited to self-care (see the box "Good Health—What's It Worth, Now and Later?").

A potential fourth area in home care, self-diagnosis, is emerging, and not without some concern. Perhaps beginning with the thermometer, progressing to the home pregnancy test and the mail-in HIV diagnostic kit, today in-home genetic testing is available. These genetic screening tests are readily available and consist of a swab that is used to obtain a scraping of cells from the inner cheek and a mail-in envelope. Upon processing cells for their DNA, persons can obtain a genetic profile as it relates to specific disease predispositions. Principal concerns associated with the use of these tests are the shortcutting of primary care physicians (although some brands require physician consent) and the absence of genetic counselors to work with clients after they receive the results of their tests. Currently, in-home genetic screening tests cost $200 to $400 and are readily available over the Internet.

Over a thousand diseases can now be tested for using genetic screening. However, test results based on self-collected samples of genetic material are not necessarily reliable. For example, laboratories processing such materials do not consistently demonstrate analytical validity (getting the right technological outcome from the tissue sample submitted) and clinical validity (verifying that the DNA results are related to a medically recognized condition). When samples submitted to online genetic testing services (by the U.S. Genetics and Public Policies Center) were retested, it was found that many of the initial test results did not meet acceptable criteria for validity. Furthermore, companies that were marketing dietary and exercise prescriptions based on genetic findings (nutrigenomic testing) were often advice inconsistent with genetic findings.[14] Today there is little governmental supervision over this growing form of self-care.

Home Health Care As the U.S. population ages, it is becoming increasingly common for family members to provide home care to older relatives. As the number of frail older people increases, home care can significantly reduce the need for institutional care. Home care also can be delivered by home health care specialists. In fact, this form of care is proving so cost-effective that some insurance programs, including *Medicare* and *Medicaid*, cover portions of the cost of home health care for older adults. (See the sections on Medicare and Medicaid on pages 485–487.)

A decision to provide family-based home care, particularly for older adults, is often made for admirable and understandable reasons, including love for the relative who needs care and the high cost of professional home care and institutional care. For the millions of families who have made this decision, providing home health care can be highly rewarding. It also can be very demanding, however, because of the needs and limitations of the person who requires care and the compromises the caregivers must make. Particularly when a spouse or family decides to provide care without the assistance of professional caregivers, they can jeopardize their own health long before the recovery or death of the person for whom they are caring. Even when their physical stamina seems unaffected, factors such as fatigue, emotional strain, postponement of personal and family goals, loss of social contact, and even physical abuse of caregivers by those receiving care can be substantial.

Although this portrays caregiving as an intense responsibility with the potential for detrimental influences on the well-being of those who give care, the process of providing care to a spouse, child, relative, or neighbor is generally more gradual. In this regard, a six-stage model of caregiving is often observed:[14] (1) I may help a relative, (2) I am beginning to help, (3) I am helping, (4) I am still helping, (5) my role is changing, and (6) my caregiving has ended. Whether stage 6 is the result of the arrival of professional home health caregivers, institutionalization of the relative, death of the relative, or the deterioration of the caregiver, the process is generally static in nature.

Health Care Facilities

Most of us have a general idea of what a hospital is. However, all hospitals are not alike. They usually fall into one of three categories—private, publicly owned, or voluntary. *Private hospitals* (or proprietary hospitals) function as profit-making hospitals. They are not supported by tax monies and usually accept only clients who can pay all their expenses. Although there are some exceptions, these hospitals are generally smaller than tax-supported public hospitals. Commonly owned by a group of business investors, a large hospital corporation, or a group of physicians, these hospitals sometimes limit their services to a few specific types of illnesses.

Publicly owned hospitals are supported primarily by tax dollars. They can be operated by government agencies at the state level (such as state mental hospitals) or at the federal level (such as the Veterans Administration Hospitals and various military service hospitals such as Walter Reed Army Medical Center in Washington, D.C., about which so much has been written in regard to conditions surrounding the care of wounded soldiers from Iraq and Afghanistan). Large county or city hospitals are frequently public hospitals. These hospitals routinely serve indigent segments of the population. They also function as *teaching hospitals.*

The most commonly recognized type of hospital is the *voluntary hospital.* Voluntary hospitals are maintained as nonprofit public institutions. Often supported by religious orders, fraternal groups, or charitable organizations, these hospitals usually offer a wider range of comprehensive services than do private hospitals or clinics. Voluntary hospitals are supported by patient fees (covered by health insurance), Medicare reimbursement, and Medicaid and public assistance reimbursement. To maintain this not-for-profit status, these hospitals must reinvest a significant portion of earned income into maintenance and improvement in their facilities.

In the last decade, hospitals, particularly private and voluntary hospitals, have expanded their scope of services. Today hospitals often operate *wellness centers,* stress centers, cardiac rehabilitation centers, chemical dependence programs, health education centers, and satellite centers for well-baby care and care for the homeless. During the 1990s two trends were observed in terms of hospital organization and ownership: the acquisition of small hospitals (such as county hospitals and smaller community hospitals) by larger regional hospitals and the reorganization of voluntary hospitals as for-profit hospitals. Both trends reflected the rapid movement of medical care in the direction of *managed care,* the term referring to the more profit-focused, cost-efficient, and third-party-controlled care reflective of the application of corporate strategies to the delivery of health care services.

The roots of the trend toward consolidation of the past decade, based on the cost effectiveness of managed care, the increased income for newer, larger hospitals, and the costs of new technology, have been increasingly replaced by hospitals' *desire to survive* as an institution. Today this trend to consolidate is more closely aligned with the financial difficulties surrounding the end-of-decade recession, the growing number of people who are uninsured or underinsured, the public demand for more affordable health care, and the growing focus on the "health care crisis" at all levels of government. Whether some of the innovated forms of health care delivery described later can be maintained during the current financial downturn remains to be seen, as these new delivery options face the same challenges faced by the more traditional hospitals.

Other health care facilities include clinics (both private and tax-supported), nursing homes (most of which are private enterprises), and rehabilitation centers. Rehabilitation centers are often supported by charitable organizations devoted to the care of chronically ill or handicapped people, orthopedically injured people, or burn victims. Increasingly, hospitals are decentralizing services into suburban areas, including the establishing of freestanding rehabilitation centers where patients receive some of their in-patient treatment, including physical and occupational therapy.

In recent years, many private, 24-hour drop-in medical emergency and surgical centers have appeared. These clinics have their own professional staffs of physicians, nurses, and allied health professionals. They compete directly with larger hospital-based facilities. Some clinics specialize in women's health needs, including gynecological care, prenatal care, and childbirth services.

Regardless of the type of health care institutions in which you seek services, both you and the institutions have legally binding rights that structure your relationship. Table 18.2 details both your rights as a patient and their rights as a licensed health care facility.

Table 18.2 Patients' Institutional Rights

Regardless of the type of institution in which you are a patient, you have a variety of rights. These are intended to protect you from unnecessary harm and financial loss. The hospital too can expect your cooperation as a patient.

As a patient, you can expect all of the following from the institution:

- To be treated with respect and dignity
- To be afforded privacy and confidentiality consistent with federal and state laws, institutional policies, and the requirements of your insurance carrier
- To be provided services on request, as long as they are reasonable and consistent with appropriate care
- To be fully informed of the identity of the physicians and staff providing care
- To be kept fully updated about your condition, including its management and your prognosis for recovery
- To be informed of any experimental or other research/educational projects that may be utilized in your treatment and to refuse such treatment
- To have the opportunity to specify advance directives (a living will, a life-prolonging statement, or the appointment of a health care representative) in order to facilitate health care decisions
- To receive an explanation of your bill for services regardless of the source of payment
- To present a complaint and receive a response about any aspect of your care or treatment and to have your complaint taken seriously
- To be involved in ethical considerations that arise during the course of your care

The institution can expect you, as a patient:

- To keep all appointments
- To provide all background information pertinent to your condition
- To treat hospital personnel with respect
- To ask questions and seek clarification about matters that affect you
- To follow the treatment prescribed by your physician
- To be considerate and respectful of other patients and to ensure that your visitors are considerate and respectful as well
- To satisfy your financial obligation to health care providers through the provision of insurance information and by arranging credit where applicable

As a patient, you may at any time:

- Refuse treatment
- Seek a second opinion
- Discharge yourself from the institution

Beyond the "universal" patient/institutional rights listed above, a wide array of more specialized rights exists regarding care issues related to language-based needs, sensory perception deficiencies (including access to communication-based technologies), and availability of companionship for selected hospitalized patients. Information pertaining to these needs can be found in *Hospitals and Effective Communication,* Office for Civil Rights, U.S. Department of Health and Human Services, March 7, 2007, www.hhs.gov/ocr/hospitalcommunication.html.

Health Care Costs and Reimbursement

There are many avenues for receiving health care. However, being able to pay for quality care is one of the greatest concerns of the American public. In 2007 (the most recent year for which statistics are available), nearly 43.3 million Americans were without health insurance for the entire year.[15] Some believe that adding those people who lacked coverage for a portion of the year to the preceding figure would result in a total number of 75 million people with less than full health care. Again using the most recent figures available, approximately 9 percent of persons under the age of 18 were uninsured;[16] however, if full-time students (covered by their parents' policies) were excluded, the remaining 18 to 24 years of age population would have 28 percent of their membership without any health insurance. Using 2004 data, when race and ethnicity were viewed, 33 percent of Hispanics, 30 percent of Native Americans and Native Alaskans, 20 percent of African Americans, and 15 percent of whites lacked health insurance coverage. Household income also reflects the same unevenness of health insurance coverage, as nearly a quarter of households with incomes below $25,000 lack coverage, in comparison to only 8.5 percent of households earning over $75,000.[17] Employed persons, regardless of age or race, who work in the service sector and lack benefits, such as food workers, and the self-employed often find access to individual health insurance policies too expensive. Approximately 11.5 percent of all American children lack access to the fullest range of health services owing to a lack of health insurance.[18]

Today, the use of data from 2004 and 2007 seems tenuous, if not useless, in painting a picture of the availability of health insurance for larger and larger segments of the American public as unemployment rates soar,

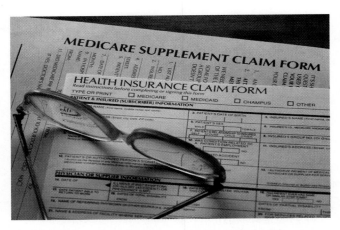

Health insurance helps consumers access quality health care, but millions of Americans have no insurance or have inadequate coverage.

employers begin to shop for cheaper and less comprehensive policies for their employees, and retirees lose their employer-provided benefits. Americans are less and less optimistic today about their ability to maintain adequate health insurance coverage, find reasonably priced health care, and afford long-term home-based or nursing home care than ever before. Unfortunately, the word *crisis* is appropriate to use when talking about our ability to afford high-quality health care today.

For reasons related to the current economic crisis already mentioned and the yet determined changes and types of control that will be needed to ensure any new approach to the delivery of health (medical) care services to the American population is adequate, it also becomes difficult to predict what the annual outlay of health care dollars will be. Certainly, the $2.6 trillion cost estimates made for 2009 (over $6,000 per person) will most likely continue to increase.

Stemming from the recession that is yet to be substantially reversed and significant changes in the political makeup in Washington, confusion over health care reform, in every form, is bombarding the American public, as well as drawing wide international interest. Until some agreements are reached, the status quo remains—overly expensive, highly impersonal, at times inaccessible, and too controlled by third-party interests. That said, although no widely accepted definitive plan has been advanced, one influential organization, the Institute of Medicine of the National Academy of Sciences, has defined important characteristics of an efficacious plan. Should such a plan be developed, it would include the following characteristics:[19]

- Health care coverage would be universal.
- Health care coverage would be continuous.
- Health care coverage would be affordable to individuals and families.
- Health care coverage would be affordable for society.

- Health care coverage would enhance health and well-being by providing access to high-quality care that is effective, safe, timely, patient-centered, and equitable.

Whether such a plan could be formulated and found acceptable by the many parties with highly vested interests in our current health care system remains far from certain. Regardless, the current system is badly damaged, if not broken. In the United States today, health care looks less like a right than like a privilege.

On a current ranking of countries by infant mortality data (deaths per 1,000 births), a salient measure of the availability of health care, the United States is thirty-sixth (6.33 deaths per 1,000 live births) in the world. And many Americans are traveling to Europe, India, Japan, and China for necessary surgeries that can be done for significantly less money abroad than in this country—in modern hospitals, by physicians who have been highly trained (often at U.S. medical schools). Without question, American medical education and sophisticated medical technology are reputed to be the best in the world, but they are accessible only to those Americans who can afford it.

Health Insurance

Given the turmoil just described, it is possible that health insurance policies, currently written and sold to employers and individuals by insurance companies, may change in significant ways, particularly if the federal government becomes a principal payee for tomorrow's insurance policies. If, however, the structure of health insurance policies remains largely intact, then the description of health insurance that follows will be applicable.

Health insurance is a financial agreement between an insurance company and an individual or group for the payment of health care costs. After paying a premium to an insurance company, the policyholder is covered for specific benefits. Each policy is different in its coverage of illnesses and injuries. Merely having an insurance policy does not mean that all health care expenses will be covered. Most health insurance policies require various forms of payments by the policyholder, which includes cost-sharing of the premium with your employer, deductible amounts, fixed indemnity benefits, coinsurance, and exclusions.

A *deductible* amount is an established amount that the insuree must pay before the insurer reimburses for services. For example, a person or family may have to pay the first $1,000 of the year's medical expenses before insurance begins providing any coverage.

A policy with *fixed indemnity* benefits will pay only a specified amount for a particular procedure or service. If the policy pays only $1,000 for an appendectomy and the actual cost of the appendectomy was $1,500, then the policy owner will owe the health care provider $500. A policy with full-service benefits, which pays the entire cost of a particular procedure or service, may be worth the extra cost.

Policies that have *coinsurance* features require that the policy owner and the insurance company share the costs of certain covered services, usually on a percentage basis. One standard coinsurance plan requires that the policyholder pay 20 percent of the costs above a deductible amount, and the company pays the remaining 80 percent.

An *exclusion* is a service or expense that is not covered by the policy. Elective or cosmetic surgery procedures, unusual treatment protocols, biologics and not-yet approved prescription medications, and certain kinds of consultations are common exclusions. Illness and injuries that already exist at the time of purchase (preexisting conditions) are often excluded. In today's turbulent health care climate, with looming governmental intervention, the insurance industry is "seeing the value" in curtailing the once-powerful preexisting-condition restrictions that characterized individual health insurance plans. In addition, injuries incurred during high-risk activities (ice hockey, hang gliding, mountain climbing, intramural sports) might not be covered by a policy.

Group Versus Individual Plans Health insurance can be obtained through individual policies or group plans. Group health insurance plans usually offer the widest range of coverage at the lowest price and are often purchased cooperatively by companies and their employees. In 2006, companies with health insurance benefits spent on average $11,480 for each employee's family health insurance plan—with the employer covering $8,508 of the $11,480 price, and the individual employee paying the remaining $2,973; a nonfamily policy (for a single employee) will cost the employer $3,615 and the employee $627, for total cost of $4,242.[20] In addition to family plans and individual (single member) plans, an individual + one plan is now available, allowing for more flexibility (and lower costs) when only a couple needs coverage. Fortunately, no employee is refused entry into a group insurance program. However, when employees leave the company, their previous group coverage can follow them for a prescribed period of time only, usually 18 to 24 months. Today, as many large American companies continue to lay off employees, the eventual loss of health insurance becomes a serious personal and family crisis. Fortunately, for persons who were employed by companies with 20 or more employees at the time of their job loss, the federal government allows them to carry their group health insurance for 18 months into the future. COBRA (Continuation of Health Coverage) costs, however, are paid entirely by the former employee, up to 102 percent of the plan's full cost.[21]

Individual policies (non-employer provided) can be purchased by one person (or a family) from an insurance company. These policies are often much more expensive than group plans and may provide much less coverage. Still, people who do not have access to a group plan should attempt to secure individual policies, because the financial burdens resulting from a severe accident or illness that is not covered by some form of health insurance can be devastating. Many colleges and universities offer annually renewable health insurance policies that students can purchase. Some questions to consider before purchasing an individual health insurance policy are these.

- Is the insurance company I'm considering rated favorably by *Best's Insurance Reports* or my state insurance department?
- Have I compared health insurance policies from at least two other companies?
- Can I afford this insurance policy?
- Do I understand the factors that might raise the cost of this policy?
- Do I clearly understand which health conditions are covered and which are not?
- Do I clearly understand the deductible amounts of this policy?
- Do I clearly understand all information in this policy that refers to exclusions and preexisting conditions?

High-Deductible Health Plans with Health Savings Accounts In HDHP/HSA accounts, pretax income is set aside in a "health savings account" (HSA) to be used exclusively for the payment of health care–related expenses, including enrollment in your employer's health insurance plan and expenses not covered by that plan. The HDHP component requires deductibles considerably higher than those normally required by health insurance plans—generally no lower than $1,000 for an individual plan and $2,000 for a family plan, but not to exceed $5,259 for an individual plan or $10,500 for a family plan.[22] On the positive side, the money set aside on a monthly basis is not taxed, the cost of the insurance is less because of the high deductible, and the account can be transferred with changes in employment. These plans also emphasize coverage of preventive care, a feature not generally covered by more traditional health insurance plans. The less attractive aspects of HDHP/HSA plans are the high deductible and unavailability of the pretax money for other uses.

Medicare

Since it was established in 1965, *Medicare* has been a key provider of health coverage for the nation's elderly. Medicare is a federally funded health insurance program for persons 65 years of age and older, as well as for persons of any age who have particular disabilities or permanent kidney failure. Funding for Medicare comes primarily from federal payroll taxes (FICA) and is administered by the Health Care Financing Administration, within the U.S. Department of Health and Human Services.

In its current configuration, Medicare is divided into two portions. Part A helps pay for care while in hospitals, as well as for care in skilled nursing facilities and hospice care, and for some home health care. Persons become eligible for Part A coverage on turning 65, on the condition of having paid Medicare taxes while working. Medicare Part A does require an annual deductible of $1,068 (historically deemed to be the equivalent of the first three days of hospital care).[23] Additionally, beginning in 2007, Part A–related deductions from Social Security monthly payments will be increased progressively for individuals with a total retirement income above $80,000 and for couples with a combined income above $160,000.[23] This Medicare Modernization Act legislation is intended to more equitably share the burden of the "universal" Part A portion of Medicare.

Part B is an optional portion of Medicare that can be chosen at the time of becoming eligible for Part A, or at selected times following initial eligibility. Unlike Part A, there is a monthly charge for Part B coverage. Currently, that charge is $96.40 per month for individuals making $85,000 or less or a couple making $170,000 or less but is subject to annual adjustment.[23] Part B helps pay for doctor's services, outpatient hospital care, and some other medical services not covered under Part A, including physical and occupational therapy, medical devices, and some home health care. Routine dental and vision care are not included. Like Part A, Medicare Part B also has a deductible, currently $135.[23]

Because of the universal nature of Medicare Part A and the affordable monthly charge for Part B, group health insurance plans to which many retirees belong require that Medicare be the "first payer" for services, thus allowing the group plan to be responsible for only that portion of health-related charges not covered by Medicare.

The Medicare Prescription Drug Improvement and Modernization Act of 2003 (now referred to as Part D) provides new prescription coverage options for Medicare recipients. Beginning in 2010, it provides prescription coverage through third-party providers for a premium of $31.94 per month. In 2010, after meeting an annual deductible of $310 Medicare covers 75 percent of the costs of prescription drugs, up to $2,830 per year; there is then a gap (the "donut hole") in coverage until out-of-pocket expenses reach $4,550 in a single year, at which point Medicare kicks in again and covers 95 percent of further costs for the remainder of the year.[23] The Medicare prescription drug program is expected to cost the Medicare system $724 billion during the first decade of its existence.

After its initial implementation in 2006, Medicare Part D remains confusing for many older persons, largely due to the large number of Part D coverage plans available in the marketplace, "windows" during which coverage can be changed, in combination with the array of medications that are frequently added or subtracted from the lists of medications covered, thus making some plans a "better fit" than other plans. That said, at this point acceptance of Part D has been strong, and first-year costs were slightly lower than initially anticipated. Further refinements in Medicare-based drug coverage will likely occur with time.

Medigap and Advantage Medicare Plans Because Medicare Parts A and B have deductibles and co-pays, along with areas that are not covered, most Medicare recipients select additional insurance coverage to assist them in addressing the out-of-pocket expenses associated with Medicare Parts A and B. These programs, featuring multiple levels of coverage and approved for sale by private-sector insurance companies, are often referred to as Medigap policies. The cost of individual policies vary widely, depending on the limitations found in less expensive policies and on the more comprehensive coverage of therefore more expensive versions.

A second form of supplemental coverage for Medicare recipients is the Advantage programs. These programs also come in a variety of forms and at differing costs, but have in common aspects of both drug coverage (Medicare Part D) and Medigap or supplemental coverage related to Part A and Part B deductibles and uncovered services.

Medicaid

Unlike Medicare, a program that is almost exclusively for persons 65 and older, as well as persons on disability and those with specific conditions such as end-stage renal failure,[23] *Medicaid* is a program designed to assist in meeting the health care needs of qualified persons regardless of age. Also unlike Medicare, which is a federal program entirely funded through Medicare tax withholdings (Part A), user-paid elected enrollment fees (Part B), and the new Part D, Medicaid is a federal- and state-funded program administered by each of the individual states.

Qualification for receiving Medicaid assistance can be perplexing. Federal Medicaid law sets mandatory eligibility standards, while optional eligibility standards allow each state to tailor many aspects of the program to fit its unique needs. Central to the majority of the federally mandated eligibility standards is the current Federal Poverty Level (FPL), as well as the standards related to the Aid to Families with Dependent Children (AFDC) program and the Temporary Assistance to Needy Families (TANF) program. Optional eligibility standards allow states to define some aspects of eligibility for pregnant women, disabled children, certain working disabled persons, and those designated as medically needy.

Federally mandated Medicaid services are wide ranging and include hospital services, physician services, laboratory/X-ray procedures, immunizations, family planning services, home health care services, transportation for medical care services, and nursing home services. This final service is of critical importance to older adults in that it pays for the majority of nursing home care required by this age group. Optional services, which are under state control, include prescription drugs, rehabilitation and physical therapy services, prosthetic devices, vision services, hearing services, and dental services, to include a few.

Health Maintenance Organizations

Health maintenance organizations (HMOs) are health care delivery plans under which health care providers agree to meet the covered medical needs of subscribers for a prepaid amount of money. For a fixed monthly fee, enrollees are given comprehensive health care with an emphasis on preventive health care. Enrollees receive their care from physicians, specialists, allied health professionals, and educators who are hired (group model) or contractually retained (network model) by the HMO.

Managed care, and HMOs in particular, was a reaction to the sharply climbing costs of health care that began in the 1980s. Businesses, which paid a large portion of health care costs through employee-benefit plans, complained that no one in the health care loop had an incentive to control costs. Employers complained that consumers paid only a deductible and a small copayment, giving them little cause to question prices; doctors faced little financial oversight; and insurance companies merely rubber-stamped the bills.

When HMOs presented an alternative, employers began offering their workers incentives to select HMOs over traditional fee-for-service coverage and thus attempted to rein in the runaway costs of health care. HMOs now cover nearly 74 million Americans. Membership is rising again following a gradual decline during mid-2005 when HMOs discontinued serving Medicare recipients (as a Medicare carve-out program) due to the cost of their prescription medication needs. However, in spite of growing enrollment, HMO premiums continue to rise at rates commensurate with other forms of health care coverage.[24]

HMOs are usually the least expensive but most restrictive type of managed care. The premiums are 8 to 10 percent lower than those for traditional plans, they charge no deductibles or coinsurance payments, and copayments are $15 to $20 per visit. However, you are limited to using the doctors and hospitals in the HMO's network, and you must get approval for treatments and referrals.

In theory, HMOs were to be the ideal blend of medical care and health promotion. Today, however, many observers are concerned that too many HMOs are being too tightly controlled by a profit motive in which physicians are being paid large bonuses to *not* refer patients to specialists or are prevented by "gag rules" from discussing certain treatment options with patients because of their costs to the HMOs.

Concerns, in addition to the "gag rules" mentioned, have also arisen over the years. Among these have been concerns related to the right of members to sue their HMOs for medical negligence, the provision of better ob-gyn coverage, and the development of a more efficient mechanism to appeal denial of services. However, in the last regard, in 2004 the Supreme Court ruled that HMO patients could not use more permissive state laws to sue HMOs for damages resulting from their refusal to approve particular medical services.

In spite of the problems just mentioned, HMOs remain, in theory, more cost-efficient than the traditional fee-for-service health care model. Cost containment is achieved, in part, because most of the medical services within a group model HMO are centralized, and there is little duplication of facilities, equipment, or support staff.

Other new approaches to reducing health costs are independent practice associations (IPAs) and preferred provider organizations (PPOs). An IPA is a modified form of an HMO that uses a group of doctors who offer prepaid services out of their own offices and not in a central HMO facility. IPAs are viewed as "HMOs without walls." A PPO is a group of private practitioners who sell their services at reduced rates to insurance companies. When a policyholder chooses a physician who is in that company's PPO network, the insurance company pays the entire physician's fee less the deductible and copay amounts. When a policyholder selects a non-PPO physician, the insurance company pays a smaller portion of that physician's fee. Today, more than 80 percent of Americans with health benefits are enrolled in a managed care plan (HMO, IPA, or PPO).

Extended or Long-Term Care Insurance

With the aging of the population and the greater likelihood that nursing home care will be required (at nearly $66,795 per year in 2006 for a semiprivate room), insurers have developed extended care policies.[25] When purchased at an early age (by one's mid-50s), these policies are much more affordable than if purchased when a spouse or family member will soon require institutional care. However, not all older adults will need extensive nursing home care, so an extended or long-term care policy could be an unnecessary expenditure.

Access to Health Care

With nearly 46 million (or perhaps more) Americans lacking any health insurance and with nearly a quarter of those with insurance being underinsured, Americans are finding it increasingly difficult to access their country's highly sophisticated health care system. The unemployed poor, working poor, and minorities have the most difficulty accessing health care. African Americans, Hispanic Americans, and Native Americans have the worst health status of all Americans, yet they receive the fewest health care services. Even for older Americans with Medicare, gaping holes exist in the types of care covered (for example, glasses and hearing aids are not covered) and the prices of prescription medications far exceed the coverage provided. Currently, the United States and South Africa are the only two major industrialized nations lacking a comprehensive and unified approach to meeting the health care needs of their populations.

Before proceeding to the conclusion of the chapter, allow your text to remind you of its contention that health is far more than the absence of illness and the reduction of risk for future illness, but rather a much more comprehensive view of resourcefulness as a person's resources are directed to role fulfillment and growth through each life-cycle stage. With this in mind, you should feel increasingly comfortable that your textbook sees the current "health care system crisis" as being more accurately defined as being a "medical care crisis."

Health-Related Products

As you might imagine, prescription and over-the-counter (OTC) drugs constitute an important part of any discussion of health-related products.

Prescription Drugs

Caution: Federal law prohibits dispensing without prescription. This FDA warning appears on the labels of approximately three-fourths of all medications. Prescription drugs must be ordered for patients by a licensed practitioner. Because these compounds are legally controlled and may require special skills in their administration, the public's access to these drugs is limited.

Although the *Physicians' Desk Reference* lists more than 2,500 compounds that can be prescribed by a physician, only 260 drugs made up the bulk of the nearly 3,435 million new prescriptions and refills, in the top 15 prescription classes, dispensed by online, mail-order, supermarket, mass-market, corporate, and independent pharmacies in 2008.[26] Total retail prescription sales of $291 billion for 2008 represent a 1.3 percent increase over 2007 sales.[27] Pharmaceutical sales growth in this range is far below the reliable 6 to 9 percent annual increases enjoyed for many consecutive years and suggests a downturn for the coming years. This reversal of fortunes for the pharmaceutical industry reflects a number of factors, including a decreasing number of new drugs coming into the market in 2007 and 2008, a significant number of brand name drugs moving out of patent protection and into generic sales, and the negative influences of the financial climate on the industry.

Research and Development of New Drugs

As consumers of prescription drugs, you may be curious about the process by which drugs gain FDA approval. The rigor of this process may be the reason that only about 16 new drugs were approved in 2008, the lowest number approved in several years, although 2007 saw 19 approved, and 2006 had 17 new approvals. This reduction from the former average of between 20 and 30 new drugs per year is believed to reflect the newer FDA stance (Quality First) that arose following the removal of medications after longer-term use found them to be less safe than initially believed.

The nation's pharmaceutical companies constantly explore the molecular structure of various chemical compounds in an attempt to discover important new compounds with desired types and levels of biological activity. Once these new compounds are identified, companies begin extensive in-house research with computer simulations and animal testing to determine whether clinical trials with humans are warranted. Of the 125,000 or more compounds under study each year, only a few thousand receive such extensive preclinical evaluation. Even fewer of these are then taken to the FDA to begin the evaluation process necessary to gain approval for further research with humans. When the FDA approves a drug for clinical trials, a pharmaceutical company can obtain a patent, which prevents the drug from being manufactured by other companies for the next 17 years.

If the 7 years of work needed to bring a new drug into the marketplace go well, a pharmaceutical company enjoys the remaining 10 years of legally protected retail sales. Today new "fast-track" approval procedures at the FDA are progressively reducing the development period, particularly for desperately needed breakthrough drugs such as those used to treat AIDS. Concern was expressed in 2000 that this "rush to approval" forced the FDA to utilize the services of independent evaluators, many of whom had ties to the pharmaceutical industry that could have influenced their assessments of a drug's readiness for marketing.

Figure 18-2 maps the long, arduous, and expensive process whereby a scant few of the tens of thousands of compounds, often derived from botanical sources, are, after nearly 7 years of testing and review, approved for market as the newest prescription medications. During these carefully monitored stages, pharmaceutical companies take biologically active molecules through computer modeling, synthesizing, testing in vitro, testing

Figure 18-2 New Drug Development and Approval

Only about 5 of 5,000 investigated compounds make it to human testing (clinical trials), and only about 1 in 5 drugs tested in people is eventually approved. The FDA is involved in two stages of drug development: A company files an Investigational New Drug Application (IND) to request approval to test a new drug in humans. If clinical trials indicate that the drug is safe and effective, the drug developer will then file a New Drug Application (NDA) seeking FDA approval to make the drug available for physicians to prescribe to patients. Additional testing and surveillance may be required after drug approval in order to evaluate long-term effects.

Source: Used with permission by Pharmaceutical Research and Manufacturers of America.

	Preclinical Testing		Clinical Trials				FDA		Phase IV
			Phase I	Phase II	Phase III				
Years	3.5		1	2	3		2.5	12 Total	
Test Population	Laboratory and animal studies	File IND at FDA	20 to 80 healthy volunteers	100 to 300 patient volunteers	1,000 to 3,000 patient volunteers	File NDA at FDA	Review process/ approval		Additional post-marketing testing required by FDA
Purpose	Assess safety and biological activity		Determine safety and dosage	Evaluate effectiveness, look for side effects	Verify effectiveness, monitor adverse reactions from long-term use				
Success Rate	5,000 compounds evaluated		5 enter trials				1 approved		

in animals, and human trials, and eventually some are approved for marketing. Note that in this example, of the 5,000 compounds initially introduced into the process, only 1 successfully completes the approval process to become a marketable prescription medication. For more information on the drug approval process, visit the website for the FDA Center for Drug Evaluation and Research (www.fda.gov/cder/handbook).

For decades the process of testing and reviewing new prescription medications involved human testing only on adult males (such as medical students, prisoners, patients). In the latter decades of the twentieth century, concerns were raised about the absence of women, and then children and older adults, in the testing process, and most recently testing using pregnant women. Today, when deemed appropriate for the best use of a new medication, these groups are included in the human testing protocol. Now, when a new medication comes onto the market, it is no longer necessary to extrapolate from adult male dosages in order to determine safe and effective use with women, children, or older adults.

An additional area of concern related to the research and development of prescription medications includes the extent to which the pharmaceutical industry will continue to voluntarily use children (and pregnant women) in reassessment of drug dosages initially determined for adult men and nonpregnant women.

Despite the importance that modern drugs and biologics play in today's practice of medicine, the American public is far from pleased with our pharmaceutical manufacturing industry. According to a joint survey by the Harvard School of Public Health, the Kaiser Family Foundation, and *USA Today,* 79 percent of those surveyed believed that the costs of prescriptions were unreasonable, 79 percent thought that unacceptably high costs were principally the fault of the drug companies, 74 percent felt that these companies were making excessive profits, and 51 percent and 60 percent felt that too

much was being spent on marketing to doctors and on public advertisements.[28] The final two issues, under the strong urging of Congress, will be sharply curtailed over the coming years, thus ending for doctors the free pens and note pads, paid trips to professional meetings held on tropical islands, free computer bags emblazoned with drug company logos, and industry-underwritten grand rounds where medical students see respected clinicians using the drugs of a particular company.

Generic Drugs

When a new drug comes into the marketplace, it carries three names: its **chemical name,** its **generic name,** and its **brand name.** While the 17-year patent is in effect, no other drug with the same chemical formulation can be sold. When the patent expires, other companies can manufacture a drug of equivalent chemical composition and market it under the brand-name drug's original generic name. Because extensive research and development are unnecessary at this point, producing generic drugs is far less costly than is developing the original brand-name drug. Nearly all states allow pharmacists to substitute generic drugs for brand-name drugs, as long as the prescribing physician approves. For those interested in viewing all of the current approved generics, the FDA updates each month its Generic Drug Approvals list.[29]

Key Terms

chemical name Name used to describe the molecular structure of a drug.

generic name Common or nonproprietary name of a drug.

brand name Specific patented name assigned to a drug by its manufacturer.

In recent years the pharmaceutical industry has actively attempted to extend the patent protection on several of the most profitable drugs on the market because their period of protected sales is expiring. In some cases the manufacturers have appealed directly to Congress for waivers to the current patent law, contending that they need the additional time to recoup research and development costs. This reason seems highly questionable to some people in light of the $4.35 billion spent by the drug industry in 2004 for advertising, most of which was directed to consumers through skillfully crafted television commercials (such as those for erectile dysfunction drugs), and to physicians in the wide variety of ways as previously discussed. In addition to direct appeals to Congress, other manufacturers have quietly "layered" additional patents onto their products to prevent manufacturers of generic versions from using the same shape or color used in brand name versions, even though the chemical formulations are no longer protected. In another approach, manufacturers of highly profitable brand name drugs have offered to pay manufacturers of generic drugs to not make generic versions of their products once the patent protection has expired.

Today a variety of reference books are available to inform consumers about the availability of generic drugs and the prescription drugs that they can legally be substituted for. *Mosby's Drug Reference for Health Professionals* series is a widely used reference focusing on both brand name drugs and generic equivalents. Updated annually, this publication is currently available in the 2010 edition.[30]

Over-the-Counter Drugs

When people are asked when they last took some form of medication, for many the answer might be, "I took aspirin (or a cold pill, or a laxative) this morning." In making this decision, people engaged in self-diagnosis, determined a course for their own treatment, self-administered their treatment, and freed a physician to serve people whose illnesses are more serious than theirs. None of this would have been possible without readily available, inexpensive, and effective OTC drugs.

Although 2,500 prescription drugs are available in this country, there are easily as many as 100,000 different OTC products, now classified as belonging to one or more of 80 different categories[31]—such as acne medications, laxatives, skin-bleaching agents, cold and cough suppressants, diaper rash ointments, and wart removal compounds. Incorporated into these thousands of products are 1 or more of the 800 FDA-approved (as safe and effective) active ingredients. Like prescription drugs, nonprescription drugs are regulated by the FDA. However, for OTC drugs, the marketplace is a more powerful determinant of success.

The regulation of OTC drugs is based on a provision in a 1972 amendment to the 1938 Food, Drug, and Cosmetic Act. As a result of that action, OTC drugs were placed in three categories (I, II, and III) based on the safety and effectiveness of their active ingredient(s). Today, only category I OTC drugs that are safe, effective, and truthfully labeled are to be sold without prescription. The FDA's drug-classification process also allows some OTC drugs to be made stronger and some prescription drugs to become nonprescription drugs by reducing their strength through reformulation. Whether the reformulation of a prescription drug into an OTC formulation is always to the consumer's advantage is questionable. For example, in 2003 Prilosec, a drug for reducing esophageal reflux disease, became available over the counter. Although Prilosec as an OTC drug is less expensive than it was as a prescription product, it is now no longer covered by health insurance. The loss of insurance coverage (usually 80 percent of the price once deductibles are met) makes the medication as expensive as, if not more expensive than, it was initially, at least for patients who have prescription coverage. Of course, because it is an OTC drug, a doctor appointment and resultant prescription are not required, but even this savings will soon be offset by the lack of insurance coverage if the medication is used over a long period of time.

Like the label shown in Figure 18-3, current labels for OTC products reflect FDA requirements. The labels must clearly state the type and quantity of active ingredients, alcohol content, side effects, instructions for appropriate use, warning against inappropriate use, and risks of using the product with other drugs (polydrug use). Unsubstantiated claims must be carefully avoided in advertisements of these products. In addition, under new labeling laws, the use of "black boxes" will be required when it is known that OTC medications hold risks, particularly when used in combination with other medications. An example of this occurred in 2008 when the use of OTC cough remedies was found ineffective and in fact dangerous when used by young children. In response to the concerns of the pediatric community, the OTC manufacturers agreed to "black box" the use of these popular products for children four years of age and younger. When used on a routine basis, OTC medications should be carefully discussed with a physician or a pharmacist.

As described in Chapter 5, dietary supplements are not regulated in the same way as OTC drugs; see the box "Dietary Supplements and the Self-Care Movement" on page 492 for more information.

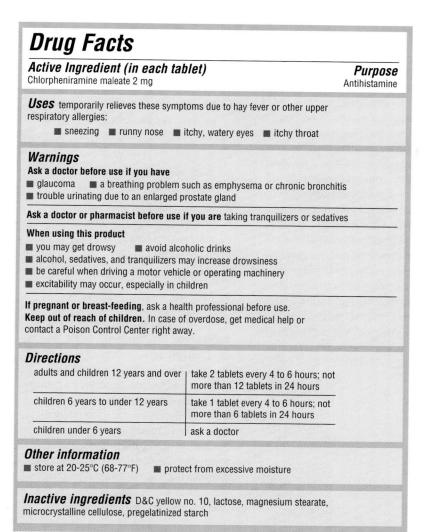

Drug Facts

Active Ingredient (in each tablet)	**Purpose**
Chlorpheniramine maleate 2 mg	Antihistamine

Uses temporarily relieves these symptoms due to hay fever or other upper respiratory allergies:

■ sneezing ■ runny nose ■ itchy, watery eyes ■ itchy throat

Warnings

Ask a doctor before use if you have

■ glaucoma ■ a breathing problem such as emphysema or chronic bronchitis
■ trouble urinating due to an enlarged prostate gland

Ask a doctor or pharmacist before use if you are taking tranquilizers or sedatives

When using this product

■ you may get drowsy ■ avoid alcoholic drinks
■ alcohol, sedatives, and tranquilizers may increase drowsiness
■ be careful when driving a motor vehicle or operating machinery
■ excitability may occur, especially in children

If pregnant or breast-feeding, ask a health professional before use.
Keep out of reach of children. In case of overdose, get medical help or contact a Poison Control Center right away.

Directions

adults and children 12 years and over	take 2 tablets every 4 to 6 hours; not more than 12 tablets in 24 hours
children 6 years to under 12 years	take 1 tablet every 4 to 6 hours; not more than 6 tablets in 24 hours
children under 6 years	ask a doctor

Other information

■ store at 20-25°C (68-77°F) ■ protect from excessive moisture

Inactive ingredients D&C yellow no. 10, lactose, magnesium stearate, microcrystalline cellulose, pregelatinized starch

Figure 18-3 Over-the-Counter Drug Label The FDA now requires over-the-counter drugs to carry standardized labels, such as the one at the left.

Health Care Consumer Fraud

A person who earns money by marketing inaccurate health information, unreliable health care, or ineffective health products is called a fraud, a **quack,** or a charlatan. **Consumer fraud** flourished with the old-fashioned medicine shows of the late 1880s. Unfortunately, consumer fraud still flourishes. You need look no further than large city newspapers to see questionable advertisements for disease cures and weight loss products. Quacks have found in health and illness the perfect avenues to indulge in **quackery**—to make maximum gain with minimum effort. Fraud can even occur after death; see the box "Modern 'Grave Robbing'" on page 493.

When people are in poor health, they may be afraid of becoming disabled or dying. So powerful are their desires to live and avoid suffering that people are vulnerable to promises of health improvement or a cure. Even though many people have great faith in their physicians, they also want access to experimental treatments or products touted as being superior to currently available therapies. When tempted by the promise of help, people sometimes abandon traditional medical care. Of course, quacks recognize this vulnerability and present a variety of "reasons" to seek their help. Gullibility, blind faith, impatience, superstition, ignorance, or hostility toward professional expertise eventually carries the day. In spite of the best efforts of agencies at all levels, no branch of government can protect

Key Terms

quack A person who earns money by purposely marketing inaccurate health information, unreliable health care, or ineffective health products.

consumer fraud Marketing of unreliable and ineffective services, products, or information under the guise of curing disease or improving health; quackery.

quackery The practice of disseminating or supplying inaccurate health information, unreliable health care, or ineffective health products for the purposes of defrauding another person.

Dietary Supplements and the Self-Care Movement

Currently, more than 50 percent of American adults are using an array of vitamins, minerals, herbal products, hormones, amino acids, and glandular extracts in their quest for improved health. People turn to dietary supplements rather than the dietary recommendations discussed in Chapter 5 for many reasons, including concern over their own morbidity and mortality, dissatisfaction with today's impersonal health care system, distrust in the safety of the food supply, and people's increasing inability to control other aspects of life. As a result, we are now spending an estimated $20 billion annually on dietary supplements—many of which appear unnecessary and some of which may be unsafe and ineffective. Recall that dietary supplement makers are not required to submit evidence of safety or effectiveness to the Food and Drug Administration, as is the case with prescription medications and, to a lesser degree, the OTC products.

In spite of the lack of available data on safety and effectiveness, the traditional medical community is showing increasing interest in the potential benefits of dietary supplements. A growing number of teaching hospitals are establishing departments of complementary medicine, and medical students are learning about the documented role (to the extent that it is known) that these supplements can play in promoting health. Additionally, major international pharmaceutical companies are beginning to market dietary

supplements. The reputation and resources of these companies are likely to generate more carefully controlled research into the safety and efficacy of these products. However, the extent to which the National Center for Complementary and Alternative Medicine (within the National Institutes of Health) will undertake carefully controlled studies of dietary supplements remains uncertain.

In the 1994 Dietary Supplement Health and Education Act, some degree of "clarity" was brought to the largely self-regulated dietary supplement industry. For the FDA little was gained in terms of having increased supervision over the safety and effectiveness of supplements or their production and packaging, as they remained "foods" by definition. The regulation of advertising of dietary supplements was retained by the Federal Trade Commission (FTC). Critics of this division of labor have contended that the FTC's regulation of dietary supplement advertising is less focused than it needs to be. The FTC has issued some guidelines regarding questionable claims in this advertising and urges concerned consumers to contact the FTC. The following are examples of advertising claims that would be the basis of such reporting:*

- A claim that the product is an effective cure-all for a wide variety of diseases, or can function as a diagnostic tool for identifying a health problem

- A claim that the product can treat or cure a specific disease or condition

- Phrasing such as "scientific breakthrough," "miraculous cure," or "ancient remedy"

- Technologically unfamiliar words such as *thermogenesis, hypothalamic appetite center,* or *metabolic substrates*

- Undocumented personal testimonials from patients or practitioners claiming spectacular results

- A claim that availability is limited or that a "holding deposit" is needed

- A promise of a no-risk guarantee

If you find such claims or wording in advertisements for a particular dietary supplement in a pamphlet, an infomercial, or other media, contact the FTC at www.ftc.gov. Similar claims or wording on a supplement's packaging should be reported to the FDA.

For readers seeking accurate information on dietary supplements, your textbook recommends *IBIDS,* the database on dietary supplements, from the Office of Dietary Supplements of the National Institutes of Health (NIH), which can be found at http://grande.nal.usda.gov/ibids/index.php.[32]

"Miracle" Health Claims: Add a Dose of Skepticism. Federal Trade Commission. Sept. 2001. www.ftc.gov/bcp/conline/pubs/health/frdheal.htm.

---

consumers from their own errors of judgment that so easily play into the hands of quacks and charlatans.

Regardless of the motivation that leads people into consumer fraud, the outcome is frequently the same. First, the consumer loses money. The services or products are grossly overpriced, and the consumers have little recourse to help them recover their money. Second, the consumers often feel disappointed, guilty, and angered by their own carelessness as consumers. Far too frequently, consumer fraud may lead to unnecessary suffering.

Becoming a Skilled Health Care Consumer

After reading this discussion of health information, services, and products, you should be a wiser, more prepared consumer. However, information alone is not enough.

Consider these six suggestions to help you become a more skilled, assertive consumer:

1. *Prepare yourself for consumerism.* In addition to offering this personal health course, your university may offer a course on consumerism. Libraries and bookstores offer trade books on a variety of consumer topics. Consumer protection agencies can guide you in some subjects. Government agencies also may help you in your choices. Unfortunately, most Americans have, at best, an intermediate level of health literacy, and many, particularly those for whom English is a second language, have even less. This is true in spite of attempts to add "plain language" to communications between health professionals and the general public.[33] Consumers must insist on receiving understandable explanations of information related to health issues.

Modern "Grave Robbing"

Perhaps one of the most distressing examples of health-related consumer fraud reached headline status in 2006 when it was discovered that a body-parts procurement business was working in conjunction with a mortuary (or individual mortuary employees) to harvest marketable human body parts for sale to medical schools for medical research or to hospitals for transplantation into living recipients. Modern "grave robbing" is, of course, illegal. All organ donations must have been legally authorized by the donor, or by the immediate family of the deceased. In addition to stealing and selling body parts, the mortuary deceived the survivors of the deceased into believing that the body had been handled properly in preparation for viewing before burial or cremation. This scandal reached public attention when investigators released X-rays showing that the mortuary had inserted PVC pipes and other "filler" to normalize the appearance of the body in areas where parts had been illegally removed.

Concurrent with the previous case, it was reported that a University of California, Los Angeles, employee assigned to the intake and preparation of donated (willed) bodies had earned over $1 million between 2000 and 2004 by selling body parts and tissues to a second party who in turn sold the material to over 20 hospitals and research institutions. News of this event led to a sharp decline in the number of bodies donated to the state's anatomical board in the year following.

In light of the high demand for, and limited supply of, human body parts for use in modern medical education, medical research, and medical practice, a cadaver is worth thousands of dollars, as virtually every type of tissue, individual body part, anatomical region (pelvis, intact leg, head, and so on), and, of course, the intact body, can be used. This said, how can a family be assured that no illegal harvesting has occurred? The answer, beyond only using the services of a "trusted" mortuary in the local community, is to request viewing of the prepared body before dressing and placement in the casket or in the retort prior to cremation—something many a grieving family member would be uncomfortable doing.

2. *Comparison shop.* In our free-enterprise system, virtually every service or product can be duplicated on the open market. Very few items or services are one-of-a-kind. Take the time to study your choices before you purchase a product or service.

3. *Insist on formal contracts and dated receipts.* Under the consumer laws in most states, you have a limited time in which to void a contract. Formal documentation of your actions as a consumer will give you the maximum protection available.

4. *Obtain written instructions and warranties.* Be certain of the appropriate use of any product you purchase. If you use a product inappropriately, you might void its warranty. Be familiar with what you can reasonably anticipate from the products and services you buy. In addition, be aware that a written warranty supersedes any verbal assurances a salesperson might make.

5. *Put your complaints in writing.* A carefully constructed record of your complaints is vital. Accurate records of the names and addresses of all companies and people with whom you have done business will enable you to document your actions as a consumer.

6. *Press for resolution of your complaints.* As a consumer, you are entitled to effective products and services. If your consumer complaints are not resolved, you have legal recourse through the courts. You should not hesitate to assert your rights, not only for your own sake, but for consumers who might later become victims.

Consumerism is an active relationship between you and a provider. If the provider is competent and honest and you are an informed and active consumer, both of you will profit from the relationship. However, if the provider is not competent or honest, you can protect yourself by employing the preceding six suggestions.

Taking Charge of Your Health

- Keep yourself well informed about current health issues and new developments in health care.

- Analyze the credibility of the health information you receive before putting it into practice.

- Select your health care providers by using a balanced set of criteria (see pages 472 and 479).

- Explore alternative forms of health care, and consider using them as a complement to traditional health care.

- In selecting a health insurance policy, compare various plans on the basis of several key factors, not simply cost (see page 485).

- Assemble a complete personal/family health history as soon as possible. Be sure to include information from older family members.

- Comply with all directions regarding the appropriate use of prescription and OTC medications.

SUMMARY

- Physicians can be either doctors of medicine (MDs) or doctors of osteopathy (DOs). They receive similar training and engage in similar forms of practice.
- Although alternative health care providers, including chiropractors, naturopaths, herbalists, and acupuncturists, meet the health care needs of many people, systematic study of these forms of health care is only now under way.
- Nursing at all levels is a critical health care profession. Advanced practice nurses represent the highest level of training within nursing.
- Self-care is often a viable approach to preventing illness and reducing the use of health care providers.
- Our growing inability to afford health care services has reached crisis proportions in the United States.

- Health insurance is critical to our ability to afford modern health care services.
- Medicare and Medicaid are governmental plans for paying for health care services.
- The development of prescription medication is a long and expensive process for pharmaceutical manufacturers. The cost of prescription medication is the most rapidly increasing aspect of health care affordability.
- OTC products have a role to play in the treatment of illness, but their safe use is based on following label directions.
- Critical health consumerism, including avoiding health quackery, requires careful selection of health-related information, products, and services.

REVIEW QUESTIONS

1. Identify and describe some sources of health-related information presented in this chapter. What factors should you consider when using these sources?
2. Describe the similarities between allopathic and osteopathic physicians. What is an alternative health care practitioner? Give examples of the types of alternative practitioners.
3. What are the theories underlying acupuncture and ayurveda?
4. In what ways is the trend toward self-care evident? What are some reasons for the popularity of this movement?
5. How do private, publicly owned, and voluntary (proprietary) hospitals differ?

6. Explain the following terms relating to health insurance: *deductible amount, fixed indemnity benefits, full-service benefits, coinsurance, exclusion,* and *preexisting condition.*
7. What is a health maintenance organization? How do HMO plans reduce the costs of health care? What are IPAs and PPOs?
8. What role do Medicare and Medicaid play in meeting the health care needs of the American public? Which portion of Medicare is universal? What elective options does Medicare offer?
9. What are the three criteria that must be met by an OTC drug?
10. What can a consumer do to avoid consumer fraud?

ANSWERS TO THE "WHAT DO YOU KNOW?" QUIZ

1. False   2. True   3. True   4. False   5. True   6. False   7. False

Visit the Online Learning Center (**www.mhhe.com/payne11e**), where you will find tools to help you improve your grade including practice quizzes, key terms flashcards, audio chapter summaries for your MP3 player, and many other study aids.

SOURCE NOTES

1. *Health Information Online.* Pew Internet & American Life Project. May 17, 2005. www.pewinternet.org/PPF/r/156/report display.asp.
2. *The Engaged E-Patient Population.* Pew Internet & American Life Project. August 26, 2008. www.ihealthbeat/org/.
3. China Tops US for Internet Population Lead. *PC World.* April 25, 2008. www.pcworld.com/businesscenter/article/145108/china
4. Physicians' Use of Email with Patients: Factors Influencing Electronic Communication and Adherence to Best Practices. *Journal of Medical Internet Research,* 8(1), e2, 2006. www.jmir.org/2006/1/e2.
5. DesRoches CM, et al. Electronic Health Records in Ambulatory Care—A National Survey of Physicians. *New England Journal of Medicine,* 359(1), 50–60, July 3, 2008.
6. America's Top Doctors. Castle Connolly Medical LTD. 2007. www.castleconnolly.com.
7. Medical Justice. Greensboro, NC. 2009. www.medicaljustice.com/medical-malpractice-crisis-det.asp.

8. National Center for Complementary and Alternative Medicine (NCCAM), National Institutes of Health. Health and Human Services. April 4, 2009. www.info@nccam.nih.gov.
9. *BackGround: Manipulative and Body-Based Practices: An Overview.* National Center for Complementary and Alternative Medicine. National Institutes of Health. U.S. Department of Health and Human Services. January 23, 2007. www.nccam.nih.gov/health/backgrounds/manipulative.htm.
10. National Center for Complementary and Alternative Medicine. *Questions and Answers About Homeopathy.* 2003. www.nih.gov/health/homeopathy/index.htm#al.
11. Lee JS. Medicinal Plants: A Powerful Health Aid? *Science Creative Quarterly,* 2(1), 7, 2007. www.scq.ubs.ca/?p=49.
12. *Herbs at a Glance.* National Center for Complementary and Alternative Medicine (NCCAM). National Institutes of Health. Health and Human Services. April 9, 2009.

13. Department for Professional Employees. Nurse: Vital signs. AFL-CIO. 2004. www.dpeaflcio.org/policy/factsheets/fs2004nurses.htm.

14. *Stages of Caregiving.* (Adapted from *The Caregiving Years* by Denise Brown.) National Family Caregivers Association and the National Alliance for Caregiving. 2004.

15. *Early Release of Selected Estimates Based on Data from the 2007 National Health Interview Survey.* June 25, 2008. Table 1.1a Number of persons without health insurance coverage, by age group, United States, 1997–2007. National Center for Health Statistics.

16. *Early Release of Selected Estimates Based on Data from the 2007 National Health Interview Survey.* June 25, 2008. Table 1.1 Percentage of persons without health insurance coverage, by age group, United States, 1997–2007. National Center for Health Statistics.

17. Health insurance coverage: 2004. U.S. Census Bureau. U.S. Department of Commerce. April 12, 2006. www.census.gov/hhes/www/hlth04asc.jtml.

18. Health & Nutrition (Table 120). *The 2007 Statistical Abstract.* U.S. Census Bureau. Department of Commerce. December 22, 2006. www.census.gov/compendia/statab/health nutrition.

19. Insuring America's Health: Principals and Recommendations. Institute of Medicine. National Academy of Science. January 12, 2004. www.iom.edu/?id=19175.

20. Rowland D. (January 31, 2007, testimony before the House Ways and Means Committee.) *Health Care Squeezing the Middle Class with More Cost and Less Coverage.* Kaiser Commission on Medicaid and the Uninsured. www.kff.org/uninsured/upload/7612.pdf.

21. *Continuation of Health Coverage–COBRA.* U.S. Department of Labor. April 10, 2009. www.dol.gov/dol/topic/health-plans/cobra.htm.

22. High Deductible Health Plans (HDHP) with Health Savings Accounts (HSA). Federal Employee Health Benefits 2007. U.S. Office of Personnel Management. www.opm.gov/hsa/index.asp.

23. *Medicare & You 2010.* Centers for Medicare & Medicaid Services CMS Publication No. 10050-53. 2009.

24. Managed care fact sheet. Managed Care National Care National Statistics. Health Care Web Summit. March 2007. www.mcareol.com/factshts/factnati.htm.

25. Houser A. *Nursing Home Research Report.* American Association of Retired Persons (AARP). October 2007. www.aarp,org/research/longtermcare/nursinghomes/fs10r_homes.html.

26. Top therapeutic classes by U.S. dispensed prescriptions. 2008 U.S. sales and prescription information. IMS Health Incorporated. 2009. www.imshealth.com/portal/site/imshealth.

27. *Top New Drugs and Pharmaceutical Trends of 2008.* USP News. University of the Sciences in Philadelphia. February 2, 2009. www.usp.edu/newsEvents,newsDetails.aspx?.

28. USA Today/Kaiser Family Foundation/Harvard School of Public Health. *The Public on Prescription Drugs and Pharmaceutical Companies.* (Conducted January 3–23, 2008.) March 4, 2008. www.kff.org/kaiserpolls/pomr030408pkg.cfm.

29. *Approved Drug Products with Therapeutic Equivalence Evaluations: Orange Book.* Center for Drug Evaluation and Research. Food and Drug Administration. U.S. Department of Health and Human Services. 2007. www.accessdata.fda.gov/scripts/cder/ob/default.cfm. Accessed April 3, 2009.

30. *Mosby's Drug Reference for Health Professionals* (2nd ed.). St. Louis: Mosby, 2010.

31. Rulemaking history of nonprescription products: Drug category list. Center for Drug Evaluation and Research. Food and Drug Administration. U.S. Department of Health and Human Services. Updated March 20, 2007. www.fda.gov/cder/octmonographs/rulemaking index.htm.

32. International Bibliographic Information on Dietary Supplements (IBIDS) Database. Office of Dietary Supplements. National Institutes of Health. 2009. www.ods.od.nih/gov/Health_Information/IBIDS.aspx.

33. Stableford S, Mettger W. Plain Language: A Strategic Response to the Health Literacy Challenge. *Journal of Public Health Policy,* 28(1), 71–93, 2007.

Personal Assessment

Are you a skilled health care consumer?

Circle the selection that best describes your practice. Then total your points for an interpretation of your health consumer skills.

1 Never
2 Occasionally
3 Most of the time
4 All of the time

1. I read all warranties and then file them for safekeeping.   1   2   3   4
2. I read labels for information pertaining to the nutritional quality of food.   1   2   3   4
3. I practice comparative shopping and use unit pricing, when available.   1   2   3   4
4. I read health-related advertisements in a critical and careful manner.   1   2   3   4
5. I challenge all claims pertaining to secret cures or revolutionary new health devices.   1   2   3   4
6. I engage in appropriate medical self-care screening procedures.   1   2   3   4
7. I maintain a patient-provider relationship with a variety of health care providers.   1   2   3   4
8. I inquire about the fees charged before using a health care provider's services.   1   2   3   4
9. I maintain adequate health insurance coverage.   1   2   3   4
10. I consult reputable medical self-care books before seeing a physician.   1   2   3   4
11. I ask pertinent questions of health care providers when I am uncertain about the information I have received.   1   2   3   4
12. I seek second opinions when the diagnosis of a condition or the recommended treatment seems questionable.   1   2   3   4
13. I follow directions pertaining to the use of prescription drugs, including continuing their use for the entire period prescribed.   1   2   3   4
14. I buy generic drugs when they are available.   1   2   3   4
15. I follow directions pertaining to the use of OTC drugs.   1   2   3   4
16. I maintain a well-supplied medicine cabinet.   1   2   3   4

TOTAL POINTS _____

Interpretation

16–24 points	A very poorly skilled health consumer
25–40 points	An inadequately skilled health consumer
41–56 points	An adequately skilled health consumer
57–64 points	A highly skilled health consumer

TO CARRY THIS FURTHER . . .

Could you ever have been the victim of consumer fraud? What will you need to do to be a skilled consumer?

Protecting Your Safety

What Do You Know About Safety?

1. Unintentional injuries harm more people than intentional injuries. True or False?

2. Suicides (self-directed violence) take more lives than homicides (interpersonal violence). True or False?

3. The rate of criminal victimization in the United States is at an all-time high. True or False?

4. The incidence of family violence, including intimate partner violence, maltreatment of children, and maltreatment of elders, has declined in recent years. True or False?

5. Children are safer from interpersonal violence after school than while in school. True or False?

6. More injuries occur at home than at any other location. True or False?

7. Motor vehicle crashes take more lives than any other type of injury. True or False?

Check your answers at the end of the chapter.

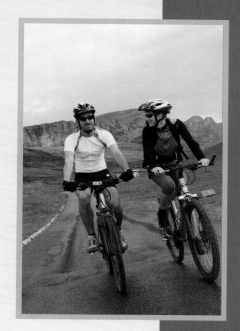

I t is nearly impossible to read a newspaper or watch the television news without seeing evidence of violence in our world. In addition to international terrorist incidents, which seem to be occurring with increasing regularity, there are reports of robberies, assaults, sexual offenses, and homicides. The newsroom adage "If it bleeds, it leads" seems to determine which items will receive top billing on the evening news. Is there that much violence in our communities, or are the news media just providing us with the kind of news we demand? After all, programs such as *Dexter, Law and Order,* and *CSI: Crime Scene Investigation* are among the most popular on television.

We can all think of examples of interpersonal violence in our communities, such as family violence, including intimate partner violence and child and elder maltreatment or school violence. There is violence on college campuses, where the binge-drinking rate is 40 percent, and there is violence in our streets as well, where youth gangs compete for territory. Needless to say, everyone is at some risk for becoming a victim of violence. For tips on ways to reduce your risk for becoming a victim of interpersonal violence, see the box "Don't Be a Victim of Violent Crime."

While it is true that interpersonal violence and the resulting injuries are serious problems in our society, it is important to keep the threat of interpersonal violence in perspective. The fact is, unintentional injuries injure and kill many more people than interpersonal violence does. For example, you are more than twice as likely to die from a motor-vehicle-related injury as from an intentional injury. Each year thousands of people die from motor vehicle crashes, unintentional poisonings, falls, fires, drowning, and firearms accidents, and millions more are injured. Even though the most serious unintentional injuries and injury deaths are reported in the media, they do not seem to carry the same "shock value" as intentional violence. Perhaps

we assume that these were chance occurrences— "accidents." However, many of these unintentional injuries and injury deaths could have been prevented with proper precautions.

In the first part of this chapter we discuss intentional injuries, injuries that result from interpersonal violence, and ways you can keep yourself safe. In the second part of this chapter, we examine unintentional injuries and suggest ways to prevent and control them. Our goal is to help you, the student, protect your health, by reducing your risk of becoming an injury victim. Complete the Personal Assessment at the end of this chapter to see whether you are adequately protecting your own safety.

Intentional and Unintentional Injuries

In 2007, in the United States there were 34.3 million injuries and poisonings for which individuals sought or received medical care.[1] Injuries are the fifth leading cause of death in this country, and they cause significant pain and suffering to people and families while placing a heavy financial burden on individuals and on the economy.[2]

Intentional and unintentional injuries are part of living in an imperfect world, and we cannot expect to eliminate these injuries completely. But we can take steps together, and as individuals, to reduce the number and seriousness of injuries. Many federal, state, and local agencies are involved in the prevention and control of injuries. These agencies include the National Center for Injury Prevention and Control, the National Center for Occupational Safety and Health, the National Highway Traffic Safety Administration, the Federal Trade Commission, the U.S. Coast Guard, numerous law enforcement agencies, and a large number of nongovernmental agencies.

You, too, can take steps to prevent and control injuries. In this chapter you will learn about types of injuries, their prevalence, and ways you can lower your risk of becoming the victim of an intentional or unintentional injury.

Intentional Injuries

Intentional injuries are injuries purposely inflicted either by the victim or by another person. Each year in the United States, intentional acts of violence, including suicides, result in approximately 50,000 deaths and another 2 million nonfatal injuries.[3] Included in these 50,000 fatal intentional injuries are approximately 30,000 suicides, the leading cause of intentional injury deaths, and 20,000 fatalities resulting from *interpersonal violence*. (See Chapter 2 for more information about suicide and suicide prevention.) In this chapter we discuss only those intentional injuries that result from interpersonal violence.

Interpersonal Violence

Interpersonal violence occurs in our homes and communities, including our schools, places of work, and college campuses. Interpersonal violence can be perpetrated by family members, friends, colleagues, acquaintances, strangers, or gang members. Motivations for these acts include material gain, power, anger, jealousy, and religious, racial, or ethnic hatred.

In 2006, an estimated 6.1 million violent crimes were committed against U.S. residents 12 years of age and older. This is equivalent to 26 violent crime victims for every 1,000 people living in the United States. While this rate may seem high, it remains at about half the 1994 rate.[4] An estimated 1.8 million persons were treated for nonfatal physical-assault-related injuries in emergency departments in 2006.[5] Although the physical assault rate is higher for males, the rate of assault-related visits to emergency departments is higher for females. The highest intentional injury rates for both genders were for the 20- to 24-year-old age group.[4]

Homicide The spectrum of interpersonal violence includes homicide, robbery, rape and other sexual assault, and simple and aggravated assault (assaults with a weapon). Homicide, or murder, is the intentional taking of one person's life by another person. Sadly, the United States leads the industrialized world in homicide rates. The homicide rate for 2005 was 5.6 per 100,000.[6] Homicide ranked as the 15th leading cause of death in the United States in 2005, accounting for 18,124 deaths.[3] Among 15- to 24-year-olds, of whom 5,466 were murdered, homicide was the second leading cause of death in 2005.[3] Seventy-nine percent of all homicide victims are male.[4]

While the U.S. homicide rate is higher than that of any European country, it has steadily declined since 1991, when it was 9.8 per 100,000 population.[6] The higher homicide rates in the early 1990s have been attributed to illegal drug trafficking in large cities.[7] The lower homicide rates of more recent years have been attributed to better community policing, tougher state laws regulating hand guns, and mandatory prison sentences. No other country has such a large proportion of its population in prison. It is estimated that 1 in every 15 people (6.6 percent) of the entire U.S. population will spend time in a state or federal prison. The chances of going to prison are higher for men (9.1 percent) than for women (1.8 percent).[8] From 2000 through 2007, the number of sentenced prisoners grew 15 percent while the general population grew 6.4 percent.[9]

Other Types of Interpersonal Violence Homicide is just one type of interpersonal violence. There are also robberies, rapes and other sexual assaults, and aggravated and simple assaults. Since 1993 the rate of violent victimization has fallen from 50 to 25 violent victimizations per 1,000 persons in 2006.[4] Victims of violent crimes tend to be male, black, under 25 years of age, and in the lower income brackets.[4, 10] Except for rape and other sexual assault, every violent crime victimization

---

Key Terms

intentional injuries Injuries that are purposely inflicted either by the victim or by another person.

homicide The intentional taking of one person's life by another person.

Table 19.1 Rape: Myth Versus Fact

Myth	Fact
Only women are raped.	Nearly 10 percent of rape victims (19,670) in 2003 were males.
Most rapists are strangers.	Seventy-four percent of male victims and 70 percent of female victims describe the offender as a nonstranger (intimate, other relative, or friend/acquaintance).
Most rapes occur in streets, alleys, and deserted places.	Ninety percent of rapes occur in living quarters—60 percent in the victim's residence.
Rapists are easily identified by their demeanor or psychological profile.	Most experts indicate that rapists do not differ significantly from nonrapists.
Rape is an overreported crime.	Only one in five rapes is reported.
Rape happens only to people in low socioeconomic classes.	Rape occurs in all socioeconomic classes. Each person, male or female, young or old, is a potential victim.
There is a standard way to avoid rape.	Each rape situation is different. No single method to avoid rape can work in every potential rape situation. Because of this, we encourage personal health classes to invite speakers from a local rape prevention services bureau to discuss approaches to rape prevention.

rate is higher for males than for females. Females were more likely to be victimized by someone they knew, while males were more often victimized by a stranger. The rate of violent victimization for Blacks was 41 percent higher than that for Whites, and the victimization rate for 16- to 24-year-olds was more than twice that for the overall population.[4, 10] While violent crimes against females (55 percent) were more likely to be reported than those against males (42 percent), it is estimated that only 38 percent of rapes and other sexual assaults were reported. Less than half of all violent crimes committed in 2005 were reported to police.[10]

Stalking In recent years the crime of **stalking** has received considerable attention. Stalking is "behavior directed at a specific individual involving repeated visual or physical proximity; nonconsensual communication; explicit or implied threats; or a combination thereof that would cause fear in a reasonable person."[11] Most stalkers are male. (One notable exception was the convicted female stalker of talk-show host David Letterman.) Many of these stalkers are excessively possessive or jealous and pursue people with whom they formerly had a relationship. Some stalkers pursue people with whom they have had only an imaginary relationship.

Some stalkers have served time in prison and have waited for years to "get back" at their victims. In some cases, stalkers go to great lengths to locate their intended victims and frequently know their daily whereabouts. Although not all stalkers plan to batter or kill their victims, their presence and potential for violence are enough to create an extremely frightening environment for the intended victim and family.

Fortunately, since 1990 virtually all states have enacted or tightened their laws related to stalking and have created stiff penalties for stalkers. In many areas the criminal justice system is proactive in letting possible victims of stalking know, for example, when a particular prison inmate is going to be released. In other areas, citizens are banding together to provide support and protection for people who may be victims of stalkers.

It has been reported that about 13 percent of college women are stalked in a given year.[12] If you think you are or someone you know is being stalked, contact the police (or a local crisis intervention hot line number) to report your case.

Rape and Other Sexual Assault As violence in our society increases, the incidence of *rape* and other *sexual assault* correspondingly rises. The victims of these crimes fall into no single category. Survivors of rape and other sexual assault include young and old, male and female. They can be people with mental retardation, prisoners, hospital patients, college students. We are all potential victims, and self-protection is critical. Table 19.1 deals with the myths surrounding rape.

Sometimes a personal assault begins as a physical assault that may turn into a rape. Rape is generally considered a crime of sexual aggression in which the victim is forced to have sexual intercourse. Current thought concerning rape characterizes this behavior as a violent act that happens to be carried out through sexual contact.

Key Terms

stalking Repeated visual or physical proximity, nonconsensual communication, or threats that would cause fear in a reasonable person.

Acquaintance rape refers to forced sexual intercourse between individuals who know each other. *Date rape* is a form of acquaintance rape that involves forced sexual intercourse by a dating partner. Studies on a number of campuses suggest that about 20 percent of college women report having experienced date rape; a recent report from the Bureau of Justice Statistics puts the figure at about 3 percent per year. This figure includes completed and attempted rapes.[12] A higher percentage of women report being kissed and touched against their will. Alcohol is frequently a significant contributing factor in these rape situations. (See Chapter 8 concerning alcohol's role in campus crime.) Some men have reported being psychologically coerced into intercourse by their female dating partners. In many cases the aggressive partner will display certain behaviors that can serve as warning signs.

In addition to alcohol as an adjunct to acquaintance rape or date rape, the use of additional drugs such as Rohypnol (roofies), ketamine hydrochloride (Special K), and gamma-hydroxybutyrate (GHB) (see Chapter 7) are playing a greater role in date rapes reported on or near college campuses. Because of the inconspicuous nature of these drugs, they are easily incorporated into drinks without intended victims knowing it. The effects of these drugs are disinhibition, increasing confusion (including the inability to give sexual consent), relaxation of voluntary muscles, and eventual unconsciousness.[13] Despite the publicity garnered by these illicit drugs, the number one date-rape drug on American college campuses is alcohol, where "approximately 50–70 percent of all sexual assaults involve alcohol."[14] The amnesic effect of these drugs reduces the ability of victims to supply information important in the apprehension of date rapists.

Psychologists believe that aside from the physical harm of date rape, a greater amount of emotional damage may occur. Such damage stems from the concept of broken trust. Date rape survivors feel particularly violated because the perpetrator was not a stranger; it was someone they initially trusted, at least to some degree. Once that trust has been broken, developing new relationships with other people becomes much more difficult for the date rape survivor.

Nearly all survivors of date rape seem to suffer from *posttraumatic stress disorder*. They can have anxiety, sleeplessness, eating disorders, and nightmares. Guilt concerning their own behavior, self-esteem, and judgment of other people can be overwhelming, and the individual may require professional counseling. Indeed, all students should be aware of the risk of date rape.

Sexual Harassment   *Sexual harassment* consists of unwanted attention of a sexual nature that creates embarrassment or stress. Examples of sexual harassment include unwanted physical contact, excessive pressure for dates, sexually explicit humor, sexual innuendos or remarks, offers of job advancement based on sexual favors, and

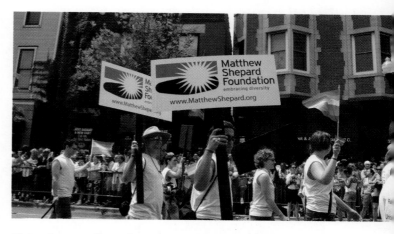

Hate crimes are directed at a person or group solely because of a characteristic such as race, religion, or sexual orientation. Celebrating tolerance and diversity and promoting inclusion can help combat the bigotry that contributes to hate crimes.

overt sexual assault. Unlike more overt forms of sexual victimization, sexual harassment may be applied in a subtle manner and can, in some cases, go unnoticed by coworkers and fellow students. Nevertheless, sexual harassment produces stress that cannot be resolved until the harasser is identified and forced to stop. Both men and women can be victims of sexual harassment.

Sexual harassment can occur in many settings, including employment and academic settings. On the college campus, harassment may be primarily in terms of the offer of sex for grades. If this happens to you, think carefully about the situation and document the specific times, events, and places where the harassment took place. Consult your college's policy concerning harassment. Next, you should report these events to the appropriate administrative officer (perhaps the affirmative action officer, dean of academic affairs, or dean of students). You may also want to discuss the situation with a staff member of the university counseling center.

If harassment occurs in the work environment, the victim should document the occurrences and report them to the appropriate management or personnel official. Reporting procedures will vary from setting to setting. Sexual harassment is a form of illegal sex discrimination and violates Title VII of the Civil Rights Act of 1964.

In 1986 the U.S. Supreme Court ruled that the creation of a "hostile environment" in a work setting was sufficient evidence to support the claim of sexual harassment. This action served as an impetus for thousands of women to step forward with sexual harassment allegations. Additionally, some men are also filing sexual harassment lawsuits against female supervisors.

Bias and Hate Crimes   One sad aspect of any society is how some segments of the majority treat certain

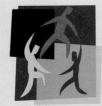

Learning from Our Diversity

Violence Against People with Disabilities

No one is totally free from the risk of senseless violence—children, adults, or college students. No single group, however, is a more tragic target of violence than people with disabilities. Despite the protective efforts of laws such as the Fair Housing Amendments Act, the Americans with Disabilities Act, and the Rehabilitation Act, people with disabilities remain an easily victimized segment of the population.

Because of the high level of vulnerability that disabled persons face, national advocacy groups, such as All Walks of Life, are working to assist the disabled, their caregivers, and the general population in reducing the risk of violence to this group. However, much can also be accomplished on an individual basis. If you are an able-bodied college student, you can probably implement the following suggestions on your campus:

- Encourage your peers who have disabilities to remain vigilant by staying tuned in to their environment. Remind them that simply because they appear to have a disability does not guarantee that they will be protected from harm.
- Support your friends with disabilities in overcoming the challenges imposed by their limitations, particularly when they are in unfamiliar environments or experiencing unusual situations.

- Suggest that your peers with disabilities carry or wear a personal alarm device. Such devices, also frequently carried by able-bodied students, can be purchased in bookstores or sporting goods stores.
- Remind your friends who are disabled to inform others about their schedule plans, for example, when they will be away from school and when they are likely to return.
- Encourage people with disabilities to seek the assistance of an escort (security personnel) when leaving a campus building or a shopping mall to enter a large parking area.
- Be an advocate for your friends with disabilities. For example, if residence hall room doors do not have peepholes at wheelchair height, find out if the doors can be modified.

One additional approach remains controversial. That is the teaching of self-defense techniques to people with disabilities. Groups that advocate instruction to the disabled in the martial arts, such as judo, remind us that "doing nothing will produce nothing." Others contend that a limited ability to use a martial art leads to a false sense of confidence that encourages a disregard for other forms of protection. They further argue that if persons with disabilities try to counter aggression with ineffectively delivered martial arts techniques, they may anger their attacker and actually increase the aggression against themselves.

---

people in the minority. Nowhere is this more violently pronounced than in **bias and hate crimes.** These crimes, which account for just 3 percent of all violent crimes, are defined as crimes that occur "when offenders choose a victim because of some characteristic—for example, race, ethnicity, or religion—and provide evidence that the hate prompted them to commit the crime."[15] During the period from July 2000 through December 2003, about 191,000 hate crimes occurred annually. More than half (55.4 percent) of these incidents were motivated by race, another 30.7 percent were motivated by the victims' association with persons with certain characteristics such as multiracial marriage, 28.7 percent by ethnicity, 18.0 percent by sexual orientation, 12.9 percent by religion, and 11.2 percent by disability (see the box "Violence Against People with Disabilities").[15] Victims of hate crimes are often verbally abused, their property is damaged or destroyed, and too frequently they are physically attacked. Two recent hate-motivated killings shocked the nation. One case involved the beating death of Matthew Shepard, a gay college student who was taken from a Wyoming bar, driven to a rural area, tied to a fence post, and savagely beaten to death. Aaron McKinney, one of the two men accused in the killings, based his defense on "gay panic," contending that he was traumatized by a

homosexual advance as a young child. A second case that shocked the nation was that of James Byrd, Jr., a 49-year-old African American man who was accosted by two white men as he walked along a rural roadway in Texas. After being beaten, spray-painted black, and chained to the rear of a pickup, Byrd was then dragged behind the truck for an extended distance. The trauma Byrd experienced was so severe that he was decapitated and his torso dismembered.

Typically, the offenders in bias or hate crimes are fringe elements of a larger society who believe that the mere presence of someone with a racial, ethnic, sexual orientation, or religious difference is inherently bad for the community, state, or country. Examples of groups commonly known to commit bias and hate crimes in the United States are skinheads, the Ku Klux Klan, and other white supremacist groups. Increasingly, state and federal laws have been enacted to make bias and hate crimes serious offenses.

With a small but growing presence of neo-Nazi groups in Europe and clear evidence that ethnic cleansing took place in Kosovo, Bosnia, Serbia, Croatia, Rwanda, Iraq, Darfur, and the former Soviet Union, bias and hate crimes are a worldwide problem. The recent push on college campuses to promote multicultural education and the celebration of diversity may help today's generation of college graduates understand the importance of tolerance and inclusion and avoid bigotry and exclusion.

Family Violence

Unfortunately, some victims of interpersonal violence are family members. During much of America's relatively brief history, many families were multigenerational, with mothers, fathers, children, and grandparents living together as a family. By the 1950s this arrangement became unusual; the more common family arrangement was mothers and fathers living together with their children. Today, families are more varied and, in some cases, more complex. Many married couples do not have children, and there are also many "blended families" with children from previous and current marriages all living together. In 2007, 50 million children in the United States were living with married parents, and 2.2 million children lived with two unmarried parents. Of the 73.7 million children younger than 18, 67.8 percent lived with married parents, 2.9 percent lived with two unmarried parents, 25.8 percent lived with one parent, and 3.5 percent lived with no parent.[16] For our discussion, we'll use the U.S. Census Bureau's definition of a family: "a group of two or more people who reside together and who are related by birth, marriage, or adoption."

Another way contemporary families differ from families in the past is that today many more women work outside of the home. Since 1950, the labor force participation rate of women has nearly doubled, so that today more than half of all women work. In 2007, women made up 46 percent of the American workforce.[17] Although it is stressful for working spouses to juggle work and domestic responsibilities, and many children are left to take care of themselves after school, the increased income does reduce financial stress at home. Furthermore, female spouses bringing home paychecks may not feel as powerless as those who stay at home all day. Thus, the higher percentage of women in the workforce may be one reason the level of family violence has been declining.

Family violence is the use of physical force by one family member against another, with the intent to hurt, injure, or cause harm. The spectrum of family violence includes intimate partner violence, maltreatment of children, sibling violence, and violence directed at elder family members. One in every six homicides is the result of family violence.

Intimate Partner Violence   **Intimate partner violence** is rape, physical assault, or stalking perpetrated by current and former dates, spouses, and cohabiting partners ("cohabiting" meaning living together at least some of the time as a couple).[11] Most of the victims are women, and a significant percentage of these women are spouses or former spouses of the assailant. Intimate partner violence

can include murder, rape, other sexual assault, robbery, aggravated assault, and simple assault. Violent acts that constitute abuse range from a slap on the face to murder.

According to the Bureau of Justice Statistics, injuries from intimate partner violence have declined in recent years. The number of fatal injuries among intimate partners has declined from 2,944 in 1976 to 1,510 in 2005. Interestingly, almost all of this decline has been in the numbers of male victims. Nonfatal injuries among intimate partners have also declined, from 5.8 per 1,000 in 1993 to 2.3 per 1,000 in 2005.[18] The reasons for the decline in intimate partner violence include the high incarceration rates of violent offenders, better social services for families at risk, and lower levels of unemployment.

The most vulnerable female victims are African American and Hispanic, live in large cities, are young and unmarried, and are from lower socioeconomic groups. However, these trends do not mean that only women from these classifications are vulnerable to violent behavior. Men and women across all economic, racial, and age categories are potential victims.

One of the real difficulties related to intimate violence is the vast underreporting of this crime to law enforcement authorities. The U.S. Department of Justice estimates that about half of the victims of intimate violence do not report the crime to police. Too many victims view their violent situations as private or personal matters and not actual crimes. Despite painful injuries, many victims view the offenses against them as minor. Even psychological abuse, the least frequently reported form of intimate violence, can lead not only to feelings of loss of control and emotional dysfunction, but also to a wide array of physical health problems. Victims of psychological abuse are twice as likely as others to report chronic pain, spastic colon, irritable bowel syndrome, infections, and migraine headaches.[19]

Of course, it is easy to criticize the victims of intimate violence for not reporting the crimes committed against them, but this may be unfair. Why do women stay in these relationships? Many women who are injured

---

Key Terms

bias and hate crimes Criminal acts directed at a person or group solely because of a specific characteristic, such as race, religion, sexual orientation, ethnic background, disability, or other difference.

family violence The use of physical force by one family member against another, with the intent to injure or otherwise cause harm.

intimate partner violence Violence committed against a person by a current or former spouse, date, or cohabiting partner.

may fear being killed if they report the crime. Women may also fear for the safety of their children. Women who receive economic support may fear being left with no financial resources.

However, help is available for victims of intimate abuse. Most communities have family support or intimate violence hot lines that abused people can call for help. Communities are establishing shelters where abused women and their children can seek safety while their cases are being handled by the police or court officials. If you are being abused or know of someone who is the victim of intimate violence, do not hesitate to use the services of these local hot lines or shelters. Also, check the resources listed in the Health Reference Guide at the back of this text.

 TALKING POINTS A close friend confides that her boyfriend sometimes "gets rough" with her. She's afraid to talk to him about it because she thinks that will make things worse. What immediate steps would you tell her to take?

Maltreatment of Children Like many cases of intimate partner violence, child maltreatment tends to be a silent crime. It is estimated that nearly 1 million children are victims of child abuse and neglect each year.[20] Some children are victims of repeated crimes, and since many victims do not report these crimes, the actual incidence of child abuse is difficult to determine.

Child maltreatment includes child abuse and child neglect. Children are abused in various ways. Physical abuse reflects physical injury, such as bruises, burns, abrasions, cuts, and fractures of the bones and skull. Sexual abuse includes acts that lead to sexual gratification of the abuser. Examples include fondling, touching, and various acts involved in rape, sodomy, and incest. Psychological abuse is another form of child abuse. Certainly, children are scarred by family members and others who routinely damage their psychological development. However, this form of abuse is especially difficult to identify and measure.

Child neglect is failure to provide a child with adequate clothing, food, shelter, and medical attention. The incidence of child neglect is approximately three times the incidence of physical abuse and about seven times the incidence of child sexual abuse. Child maltreatment deaths are more often associated with child neglect than with any type of abuse.[20] Educational neglect, such as failure to see that a child attends school regularly, is one of the most common types of child neglect. Each form of maltreatment can have devastating short- and long-term consequences for the child.

Research studies in the various areas of child maltreatment reveal some interesting trends. Abused children are much more likely than are nonabused children to grow up to be child abusers. Abused children are more likely to suffer from poor educational performance, increased health problems, and low levels of overall achievement. Abused and neglected children are significantly more likely than are nonabused children to become involved in adult crime and violent criminal behavior.

It is beyond the scope of this book to discuss in detail how to reduce child abuse. However, the violence directed against children can likely be lessened through a combination of early identification measures and violence prevention programs. Teachers, friends, relatives, social workers, counselors, psychologists, police, and the court system must not hesitate to intervene early in cases of suspected child abuse. In fact, every adult is responsible for reporting suspected child abuse and neglect. To do so, persons should call their local police department or Child Protective Services (within the Department of Public Welfare) and request assistance in filing a report. So long as the report is filed in good conscience (without malice), there will be no negative ramifications for the person filing. The later the intervention, the more likely that the abuse will have worsened. When an individual has abused once, he or she is likely to do it again.

Violence prevention programs can help parents and caregivers learn how to resolve conflicts, improve communication, cope with anger, improve parenting skills, and challenge the view of violence presented in movies and television. These programs may help to stop violence before it begins to damage the lives of young children. The box "Twelve Alternatives to Lashing Out at Your Child" provides helpful guidelines for parents.

Maltreatment of Elders Among the 37 million adults 65 years of age and older, between 1 and 2 million have been injured, exploited, or otherwise mistreated.[21, 22] Particularly vulnerable are women and those of advanced age. More than 65 percent of elder abuse victims were female, and nearly half of the victims were 80 years of age or older. The most common relationships of the perpetrators to the victims were adult-child (32.6 percent) and other family member (21.5 percent).[23]

Many older adults are hit, kicked, attacked with knives, or denied food and medical care; others are robbed of their Social Security checks and automobiles. These crimes probably reflect a combination of factors, particularly the stress of caring for failing older people by middle-aged children who also face the additional demands of dependent children and careers. In many cases, the middle-aged children were themselves abused,

---

Key Terms

child maltreatment The act or failure to act by a parent or caretaker that results in abuse or neglect of a child or that places the child in imminent risk of serious harm.

Twelve Alternatives to Lashing Out at Your Child

- The next time everyday pressures build up to the point where you feel like lashing out—STOP! Try any of these simple alternatives. You'll feel better . . . and so will your child.

- Take a deep breath . . . and another. Then remember you are the adult.

- Close your eyes and imagine you're hearing what your child is about to hear.

- Press your lips together and count to 10 . . . or better yet, to 20.

- Put *your child* in a time-out chair (remember this rule: one time-out minute for each year of age).

- Put *yourself* in a time-out chair. Think about why you are angry: is it your child, or is your child simply a convenient target for your anger?

- Phone a friend.

- If someone can watch the children, go outside and take a walk.

- Take a hot bath or splash cold water on your face.

- Hug a pillow.

- Turn on some music. Maybe even sing along.

- Pick up a pencil and write down as many helpful words as you can think of. Save the list.

- Call for prevention information: 1-800-CHILDREN

Source: Prevent Child Abuse America. www.preventchildabuse.org. Used with permission.

---

or there may be a chemical dependence problem. The alternative, institutionalization, is so expensive that it is often not an option for either the abused or the abuser.

Although protective services are available, abuse of older adults is frequently unseen and unreported. In many cases, the older adults themselves are afraid to report their children's behavior because of the fear of embarrassment that they were not good parents to their children. Regardless of the cause, however, abuse of older adults must be reported to the appropriate protective service so that intervention can occur.

Violence in Our Communities

When family members go to school, attend college, or engage in other community activities, we do not expect them to be injured by the intentional acts of another.

School Violence   Usually, students are safe at school, but occasional, highly publicized fatal school shootings,

like the ones at Columbine High School and Red Lake Indian Reservation, cause parents to ask how safe their children are at school. The National Center for Educational Statistics collects data to determine the frequency, seriousness, and incidence of violence in elementary and high schools. During the 2005–2006 school year, 86 percent of public schools reported one or more violent incidents, serious violent incidents, thefts of items valued at $10 or greater, or other crimes occurring at their school. This amounted to 22 million crimes, a rate of 46 crimes per 1,000 enrolled students. Additionally, 24 percent of public schools reported that bullying was a daily or weekly problem. In 2005, 43 percent of 9th- to 12th-grade students reported they had been in a fight anywhere, and 14 percent said they had been in a fight on school property during the previous 12 months. Also, 19 percent reported that they had carried a weapon in the past 30 days, and 6 percent reported they had carried a weapon in the past 30 days on school property.[24, 25] Nonetheless, the fact that 1 in 20 high school children carried a weapon to school within the past 30 days is frightening.

Weapon carrying is related to another form of interpersonal violence at school—bullying. Bullying includes making fun of another person; spreading rumors about a person; threatening to harm another person; pushing, shoving, tripping, or spitting on a person; pressuring someone to do something he or she does not want to do; excluding someone; or destroying someone's property. In 2005, 28 percent of 12- to 18-year-olds reported that they were bullied at school within the past six months.[24] One natural response to being bullied might be to carry a weapon to school.

In spite of these statistics, the odds of a student suffering a school-associated violent death are less than one in a million. From July 1, 2005, through June 30, 2006, only 14 homicides and 3 suicides of school-aged youth occurred at school. This translates into 1 homicide or suicide of a school-aged youth at school per 3.2 million students enrolled during the 2005–2006 school year.[24] So, while violence at schools has captured the headlines, schools are really a relatively safe place for children to be. Most of the violent crimes committed by juveniles on school days occur after school.[26]

Violence at College   A recent report has summarized violent victimization of college students. Perhaps the most important finding was that college campuses are a relatively safe place to be. College students (ages 18–24 years) experience less violence than do nonstudents in the same age group. Violence rates have declined for both groups since 1995, when rates were 88 per 1,000 for college students and 102 per 1,000 for nonstudents. The 2002 rates are 41 and 56, respectively.[27]

During the period 1995–2002, simple assault (assault without a weapon) accounted for 63 percent of the violent

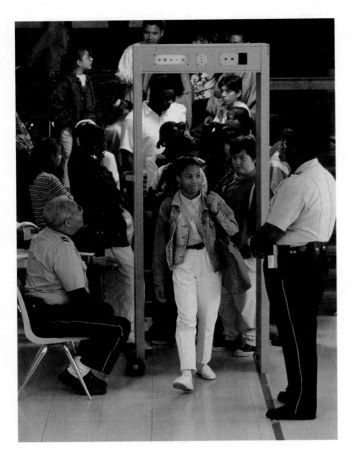

Although young people are safer at school than outside of school, some types of school violence—including fights, threats, vandalism, and weapons carrying—are relatively common. Some schools have instituted strategies such as video surveillance and metal detectors to help reduce the risk of school violence.

victimizations, whereas rape/sexual assault accounted for 6 percent. Males were about twice as likely to be victims of violence as women were. About 93 percent of the crimes occurred off campus and 72 percent occurred at night.[27]

One factor that increases the risk of interpersonal violence on American college campuses is the consumption of alcohol and other drugs. More than 40 percent of victims of violent crimes in college settings perceived their offenders to be using drugs or alcohol. The percentage was even higher for aggravated and simple assault.[27] It should be noted that this is higher than the level of drug use perceived by victims in all settings.[27, 28] To reduce your risk of becoming a victim of interpersonal violence, consider reducing your alcohol intake, pay attention to the alcohol consumption of those around you, and stay away from places where others are drinking heavily.

Campus Safety   Although many of the topics in this chapter are quite unsettling, students and faculty must continue to lead normal lives in the campus environment despite potential threats to our health. The first step in

being able to function adequately is knowing about these potential threats. You have read about these threats in this section on intentional injuries; now you must think about how this information applies to your campus situation.

The campus environment is not immune to many of the social ills that plague our society. At one time the university campus was thought to be a safe haven from the real world. Now there is plenty of evidence to indicate that significant intentional and unintentional injuries can happen to anyone at any time on the college campus.

For this reason, you must make it a habit to think constructively about protecting your safety. In addition to the personal safety tips presented earlier in this section, remember to use the safety assistance resources available on your campus. One of these might be your use of university-approved escort services, especially in the evenings as you move from one campus location to another. Another resource is the campus security department (campus police). Typically, campus police have a 24-hour emergency phone number. If you think you need help, do not hesitate to call this number. Campus security departments frequently offer short seminars on safety topics to student organizations or residence hall groups. Your counseling center on campus might also offer programs on rape prevention and personal protection.

If you are motivated to make your campus environment safer, you might wish to contact Security on Campus, an organization that specifically focuses on campus security (www.securityoncampus.org.). The mission of this organization is to promote on-campus safety for students. We encourage you to become active in making your campus a safer place to live.

Youth and Gang Violence   In the last 30 years, gangs and gang activities have been increasingly responsible for escalating violence and criminal activity. Before that time, gangs used fists, tire irons, and occasionally, cheap handguns ("Saturday night specials") as tools of enforcement. Now, gang members do not hesitate to use more lethal semiautomatic weapons.

The gang problem is most persistent in cities of greater than 50,000 population, where 90 percent of law enforcement agents reported experiencing youth gang activity during 2002–2006.[29] These are areas where many socially alienated, economically disadvantaged young people live. Convinced that society has no significant role for them, gang members can receive support from an association of peers that has well-defined lines of authority. Rituals and membership initiation rites are important in gang socialization. Gangs often control territories within a city. Frequently, gangs are involved in criminal activities, the most common of which are illicit drug trafficking and robberies. In the late 1990s, gang-related murders and drive-by shootings contributed to the high death rate among young people and especially inner-city youth. In 1999 the rate of gang-related murders of young persons reached, on average, 24 deaths every two days—the equivalent of a classroom of dead young persons (below the age of 20) every other day.

Attempting to control gang and youth violence is particularly expensive for communities. When you consider that for every gang-related homicide, there are about 100 nonfatal gang-related intentional injuries, it becomes obvious that gang violence is an expensive health care proposition. Furthermore, gang and youth violence takes an enormous financial and human toll on law enforcement, the judicial system, and corrections departments.

Fortunately, the recent decline in murders and other serious crimes also applies to gang-related crimes. Once again, some observers credit more aggressive police tactics for the decline. Some of the tactics being used to meet this problem are the aggressive "quality of life" policing in some cities and President Clinton's Community Oriented Policing Services (COPS) program to hire new police officers and put them on foot patrols, so they become acquainted with residents. Others believe that the drop in crime should be attributed to factors such as a stronger economy and the fading of the crack market. In Boston, a campaign aimed at youth gangs offered summer jobs to gang members, combined with threats of federal prison sentences for gun violence. This program has significantly reduced firearm-related fatalities among Boston youth.

Regardless, reducing gang and youth violence will be a continuing challenge for the nation in the twenty-first century.

Factors That Contribute to Intentional Injuries

The use and abuse of alcohol and other psychoactive drugs, as discussed in Chapters 7 and 8, are contributing factors to interpersonal violence and the toll of intentional injuries in our society. In 2005, 5 percent of homicides, 10 percent of other violent crimes, and 30 percent of property crimes were drug related.[30] A psychological manifestation of alcohol intoxication is the lowering of inhibitions, and for some this results in a loss of behavior control resulting in acts of interpersonal violence. A drunk or drugged person is more likely than a sober person to become either a victim or a perpetrator of violence. In 2004, 49 percent of state and federal inmates imprisoned for violent crimes reported having used drugs in the month before their offense, and roughly 25 percent reported use at the time of their crime.[31]

Another factor that contributes to the prevalence and deadliness of interpersonal violence is the availability of firearms. Firearms are present in more than half of American homes. In 2002, firearms were the second leading cause of death, after automobiles, accounting for 18.8 percent of all injury deaths. That year, guns were

involved in two-thirds of all homicides in the United States.[32] The ratio of fatalities to nonfatalities for firearm injuries compared to that ratio for all injuries, reveals the lethality of gun violence. For each injury death, there are 9 hospitalizations and 189 more people treated and released. But for firearm injuries, for each injury death, only 1.2 people are hospitalized and only 1 person is treated and released.[33] Firearm deaths are a leading cause of deaths of teenage and young adult men, ages 15 to 24 years. In 2005 there were 4,499 deaths attributed to homicide and legal intervention in this population, a death rate of 10.7 deaths per 100,000.[2] Evidence of the availability of guns is clear from the Youth Risk Behavior Survey conducted by the Centers for Disease Control and Prevention. In 2007, nearly 9 percent of male high school students had carried a gun to school on 1 or more of the past 30 days.[34] Colleges and universities are not immune to gun violence. A recent study found that 4.3 percent of college students had a working firearm at college. Of these students, nearly half stated that they had the gun for protection.[35]

See the box "Violence in the Media: Does It Affect Behavior in the Real World?" for more information on factors contributing to intentional injuries.

The proliferation of firearm use has prompted serious discussions about the enactment of gun control laws. For years, gun control activists have been in direct battle with the National Rifle Association (NRA) and its congressional supporters. Gun control activists want fewer guns manufactured and greater controls over the sale and possession of handguns. Gun supporters believe that such controls are not necessary and that people (the criminals)—not simply the guns—are responsible for gun deaths. This debate will certainly continue.

Identity Theft

In today's cashless, wired society, we make several transactions each day in which personal information is transferred: We write checks, pay bills online, use credit and debit cards at restaurants and for purchases, and withdraw cash from ATMs; we might be asked to provide a Social Security number when we write a check, or give our phone number or address when we shop at a particular store. Each of these transactions provides an opportunity for thieves to obtain your personal information and use it fraudulently.

Identity theft has been on the rise since the early 1990s. In 2005, 6.4 million households (5.5 percent of all

---

Key Terms

identity theft A crime involving the fraudulent use of a person's name, Social Security number, credit line, or other personal, financial, or identifying information.

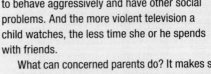
households in the United States), discovered that at least one member had experienced identity theft. The most common type of identity theft was unauthorized use of an existing credit card; the next most prevalent type of theft involved another existing account, such as a bank account. More than one million victims discovered identity theft involving misuse of personal information. Households with incomes of $75,000 or higher were at higher risk for identity theft, as were households located in the West. Households headed by persons 65 and older and rural households were at lower risk.[36]

Here are some of the common ways ID theft occurs. Identity thieves (1) rummage through trash looking for bills and other papers bearing your personal information ("dumpster diving"), (2) steal credit or debit card numbers using a special storage device when processing your card ("skimming"), (3) pretend to be a financial institution or other business and try to get you to reveal personal information ("phishing"), (4) divert your mail by submitting a change of address form for you, or (5) simply steal your wallet, purse, or mail, such as preapproved credit offers, new checks, or other papers. They might also steal your information from your employer by bribing a dishonest employee who has access to it.[37]

Thieves use falsely obtained names, addresses, and Social Security numbers to open credit card accounts and bank accounts, purchase cell phone services, and secure

loans to buy automobiles and other big ticket items. They might even avoid paying taxes by working under false Social Security numbers, or use your identity for other purposes—if they are arrested, for example. Identity thefts can drain a person's bank account and ruin her credit rating before she knows she's become a victim. Often the crime is not discovered until a person wants to make a major purchase—such as a house or a car that requires a credit check.

The Federal Trade Commission suggests a three-prong attack against identity theft, which it labels "Deter-Detect-Defend."[37]

Deter thieves by safeguarding your information:

- Shred financial documents with personal information before you throw them out.

- Protect your Social Security number by not giving it out unless absolutely necessary. Don't carry it in your wallet or write it on your checks; if a business requests it, ask to use another identifier.

- Don't give out personal information unless you know who you are dealing with.

- Never click on links sent in unsolicited e-mails. Use up-to-date firewalls and antispyware and antivirus software to protect your home computer. Refer back to the material on spamming and phishing in Chapter 3 for additional information about e-mail safety.

- Don't use an obvious password like your birthdate, your mother's maiden name, or the last four digits of your Social Security number.

Detect suspicious activity:

- Be aware if bills do not arrive as expected, you receive unexpected credit cards or account statements, you are denied credit for no apparent reason, or you receive calls or letters about purchases you did not make.
- Inspect your credit report. The law requires the major consumer reporting companies (Equifax, Experian, and TransUnion) to give you a free copy of your credit report annually.
- Inspect your financial accounts and billing statements regularly for charges you did not make.

Defend against identity theft as soon as you suspect it:

- Place a "fraud alert" on your credit reports; this tells creditors to follow certain procedures before they open new accounts in your name or make changes to your existing accounts.
- Close any accounts that have been tampered with or established fraudulently. Call the security or fraud departments of each relevant company and follow up in writing. Keep copies of documents and records of your conversations about the theft.
- File a police report and report the theft to the Federal Trade Commission at http://ftc.gov/idtheft.[37]

Terrorism

Although definitions vary, the United Nations defines **terrorism** as any act "intended to cause death or serious bodily harm to civilians or noncombatants with the purpose of intimidating a population or compelling a government or an international organization to do or abstain from doing any act."[38] Over the past 30 years the world has witnessed dozens of acts of terrorism in countries such as Germany, Spain, Indonesia, Kenya, London, Northern Ireland, Japan, and Russia. The United States has not been immune from terrorist acts. To list a few: the World Trade Center bombing in 1993, the Oklahoma City bombing in 1995, the Olympic Park bombing in Atlanta in 1996, and the attacks on the World Trade Center and Pentagon in 2001.

By their very nature, terrorist acts are difficult to prevent. However, it is less likely that your health will be affected by a terrorist act than by your everyday health behavior. As an educated person, you should become knowledgeable about world events and support federal, state, and local security efforts. If you travel abroad, keep in mind that American-style restaurants and night clubs might be more attractive targets for anti-American terrorist acts than locally owned or natively owned establishments.

Unintentional Injuries

The vast majority of injuries that occur each year are **unintentional injuries,** injuries that occur without anyone intending harm. Nearly half of all these injuries occur in or around the home.[1] Nearly twice as many injuries occur in the home as occur outside, and falls are the leading cause of medically consulted injuries in the home. The next most common locations for injuries are recreation areas, and streets and highways.[1] Even though we spend a lot of time at schools and places of work, these venues are relatively safe.

Unintentional injuries account for about two-thirds of all injury deaths annually in the United States. More fatal injuries occur on streets and highways than anywhere else. Of the 117,809 unintentional injury deaths reported in 2005, 37 percent were caused by motor vehicle crashes, 20 percent by unintentional poisonings, 17 percent by falls, and 5 percent by unintentional suffocation. Other causes were drowning, exposure to smoke, fire, and flames, and the accidental discharge of firearms.[2] In 2006, injuries cost an estimated $652 billion, including $330 billion in lost wages and productivity, $116 billion in medical expenses, $135 billion in insurance administration costs, and $42 billion in motor vehicle damage and other costs.[39]

Motor Vehicle Injuries and Safety

Motor vehicle crashes are the leading cause of injury deaths in the United States and, for the 16- to 24-year age group (a majority of those reading this textbook), motor vehicle crashes are the leading cause of *all* deaths. In 2007, 41,059 people were killed and an estimated 2.5 million more were injured in motor vehicle crashes on U.S. streets and highways. The 2006 rates of involvement in fatal crashes are highest for drivers in the 16- to 20-year and the 21- to 24-year age groups; the rates of involvement for male drivers are twice as high as those for female drivers at every age (Figure 19-1). Weekends

---

Key Terms

terrorism Any actions intended to harm or kill civilians in order to intimidate a populace or force a government to take some action.

unintentional injuries Injuries that have occurred without anyone's intending that harm be done.

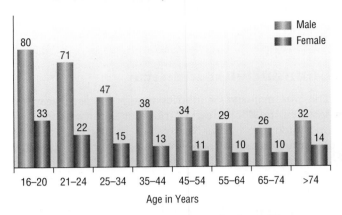

Driver Involvement Rate per 100,000 Licensed Drivers

Male
Female

Figure 19-1 Fatal Motor Vehicle Crashes by Gender and Age
Males are more likely than females to be involved in fatal motor vehicle crashes; rates are highest among young drivers. What could be done to reduce the number of driving fatalities involving young males?

Source: National Highway Traffic Safety Administration. *Traffic Safety Facts 2006.* Washington, DC: U.S. Department of Transportation.

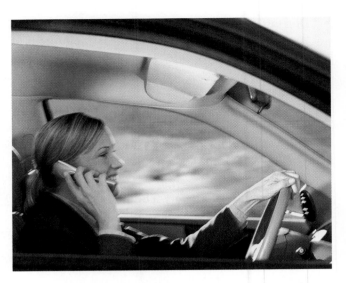

Anything that distracts a driver—talking on a phone, reading a map or notes, eating and drinking, or adjusting vehicle controls—can decrease concentration and slow reaction time. Driver distraction is a key contributing factor in many crashes.

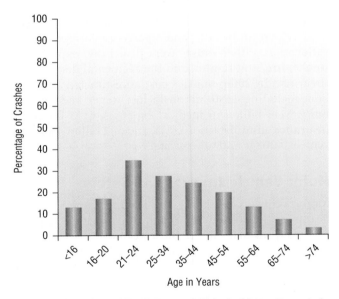

Figure 19-2 Alcohol and Fatal Motor Vehicle Crashes Percent of drivers and motorcycle riders with blood alcohol concentration of 0.08 or higher involved in fatal crashes.

Source: National Highway Traffic Safety Administration. *Traffic Safety Facts 2007.* Washington, DC: U.S. Department of Transportation.

and nights are more dangerous driving times. The most dangerous hours are from midnight to 3 a.m. on Saturdays and Sundays.[40]

As with intentional injuries, alcohol intoxication is often a contributing factor to the number and seriousness of unintentional injuries. This is especially true for motor vehicle crashes. Alcohol involvement increases the likelihood that a crash will occur and that it will result in a fatality. Thirty-two percent of all fatalities in crashes involved an alcohol-impaired driver or motorcycle rider with a blood alcohol concentration (BAC) of 0.08 gram per deciliter or higher. Twenty-two percent of all drivers in fatal crashes had BACs of 0.08 or higher. This figure rises to 35 percent for the 21–24-year age group (Figure 19-2). The percentage of male drivers who died in crashes with a BAC of 0.08 or higher (25 percent) was nearly twice that of female drivers (13 percent).[40]

Motor vehicle crashes also cause disabling injuries. With nearly 2 million such injuries each year, all college students should be concerned about avoiding motor vehicle crashes. With this thought in mind, we offer some important safety tips for motor vehicle operators:

• Make certain that you are familiar with the traffic laws in your state.

• Do not operate an automobile or motorcycle unless it is in good mechanical order. Regularly inspect your brakes, lights, and exhaust system.

• Do not exceed the speed limit. Observe all traffic signs.

• Always wear safety belts, even on short trips. Require your passengers to buckle up. Always keep small children in child restraints.

• Do not drive if you have been drinking alcohol. Give your car keys to a sober, trusted friend.

• Avoid horseplay and other distractions inside a car.

• Be certain that you can hear the traffic outside your car. Keep the car's music system at a reasonable decibel level. (See the box "Cell Phone Safety" for more information.)

• Give pedestrians the right-of-way.

Cell Phone Safety

While Driving

Cell phones that fit easily into a pocket or purse are being used in every place imaginable, including restaurants, theaters, subways, parks, golf courses, and, of course, in cars. And it's in cars that the use of cellular phones is most controversial. A variety of studies and reports indicate a four- to nine-fold increase in the potential for car crashes associated with the driver's use of a cell phone. In July 2001, the state of New York passed the country's first *statewide* ban on the use of handheld cellular phones while driving. Violators of this ban are subject to a $100 fine for the first offense. Since then, at least 25 other states have passed laws regulating cell phone use while operating a motor vehicle.

Research suggests the use of a cell phone decreases driver concentration and delays driver reaction time. The use of mounted, hands-free phones may improve safety, although the safety benefit has been controversial. Experts in traffic safety are careful to point out that there are too many other factors associated with driving to make it fair to blame behind-the-wheel phone use for all or most accidents. These complicating factors include adverse weather conditions, the structural integrity of the cars, the age and health of the drivers, radio, CD, or cigarette use, and interactions between drivers and passengers. The influence of other drivers on the road must also be considered.

States are examining the correlation between use of cell phones while driving and crashes where driver distraction is a causal factor. Generally, state laws are based on issues specific to each state. For example, several states have identified an emerging highway safety trend of cell phone use by novice drivers and have thus restricted use. In some states, localities restrict cell phone use through local ordinances or policies. Other states prohibit localities from implementing such ordinances. These are known as "preemption laws." Highlights of current state cell phone restrictions include the following:

- No state completely bans all types of cell phone use.
- Seventeen states and the District of Columbia ban all cell phone use by novice drivers and by school bus drivers when passengers are present.
- Seven states and the District of Columbia ban text messaging by all drivers.
- Nine states prohibit text messaging by novice drivers.
- Six states legally restrict school bus drivers from texting while driving.
- Eight states have laws that prohibit local jurisdictions from enacting restrictions.

Through better data and studies, states will be better able to identify and guide policy makers on this issue.

If you must use your cell phone in a car, consider these commonsense rules: Get off the main road to a safe parking area to make your call, especially if the call is an important one or one that might upset you. If you must talk while driving, opt for a hands-free phone. Dial when your car is stopped. Keep calls very brief. Don't try to dial or talk in heavy traffic. Keep your eyes on the road. (Or, let a passenger make the call!)

While Walking

Although talking or texting on your cell phone, iPhone, or BlackBerry device while driving can have deadly consequences, texting while walking is also hazardous. All too frequently, people texting while walking have walked into stationary or moving objects, sometimes with injurious consequences. Scraped chins, noses, and foreheads, and broken glasses are among the most common injuries seen almost daily in some emergency departments. Protect yourself from these embarrassing and perhaps costly injuries by refraining from texting while walking.

Source: Governor's Highway Safety Association. Cell Phone Restrictions—State and Local Jurisdictions, 2007. www.ghsa.org/html/stateinfo/laws/cellphone_laws.html; Searcey D, Generation Text: Emailing on the Go Sends Some Users into Harm's Way. *The Wall Street Journal,* July 25, 2008, page 1.

InfoLinks
www.ghsa.org/html/stateinfo/laws/cellphone_laws.html

- Drive defensively at all times. Do not challenge other drivers. Refrain from drag racing.
- Look carefully before changing lanes.
- Be especially careful at intersections and railroad crossings.
- Carry a well-maintained first aid kit that includes flares or other signal devices.
- Drive even more carefully during bad weather.
- Do not drive when you have not had enough sleep.
- Do not ride with a driver who has been drinking.

In spite of the best efforts that people make to prevent motor vehicle crashes, when they occur there is, of course, not only damage to property but also the very real possibility of injury and even death. Remember, poor decisions also affect family members and friends, who pay an emotional price when they experience the loss of companionship when people for whom they care a great deal have been in serious motor vehicle crashes. The effects of motor vehicle–related injuries and injury deaths are also felt in the workplace where they result in economic losses of employers and employees alike.

Motorcycle Safety Some emergency-room physicians call motorcycles "murder-cycles" because of their experience with motorcycle crash victims. The statistics support this grim view. With the death rate for motor-cycles at 40 per 100 million vehicle miles of travel compared to a death rate for cars of 1.5, motorcycles are nearly 27 times more deadly.[40] Therefore, our first recommendation is to not operate or ride on the back of a motorcycle.

If you choose to ride a motorcycle, you can reduce your risk of injury or death by following these suggestions:

- Most important of all, wear a helmet. A variety of studies have supported the effectiveness of helmets in preventing head injuries. Warriors and athletes have worn helmets for centuries to protect themselves from head injuries. Modern examples include construction workers, football players, race car drivers, and military aircraft pilots.

- Wear boots, gloves, and heavy clothing to protect your skin from serious injury when you slide on pavement in a crash.

- Get proper training, such as the Motorcycle Safety Foundation course offered in some states.

- Your risk increases in wet weather. Consider whether a ride in the rain is necessary.

- Do not ride after taking medication that can affect your alertness or performance.

- Never ride after drinking alcohol or taking drugs. About half of motorcyclists killed in accidents had alcohol in their blood.

- Ride defensively. Remember that many drivers do not see you or may not give you the right-of-way you deserve.

For all the reasons discussed in conjunction with automobile accidents, motorcycle accidents can influence the well-being of a wide array of people. However, because of the very high probability of serious injury and death associated with these accidents, the distress suffered by family, friends, witnesses, and coworkers may be even more extensive.

Residential Injuries and Safety

Although more injury deaths occur on our highways and streets, more injuries of all types occur at home. Approximately 1 person in 10 is injured each year at home. It is not that our homes (residence halls, apartments, houses) are particularly dangerous; it is simply that we spend more time at home than anywhere else. Injuries that occur where we live include poisonings, falls, burns, and suffocations.

Poisonings   The leading cause of unintentional injury deaths in homes is poisonings.[41] A few of these are attributable to alcohol, pesticides, or carbon monoxide; but most, by far, are caused by prescription drugs or illegal drugs, particularly prescription narcotics and cocaine. The rate of unintentional poisoning deaths increased 62 percent from 1999 to 2004. The largest increases were among 15- to 24-year-olds (113.3 percent), females (103 percent), and Whites (75.8 percent). Unlike some earlier epidemics of drug abuse, the greatest increase in unintentional poisoning rates has occurred not in East Coast or West Coast cities, but in the Midwest (85.5 percent) and the South (113.3 percent).[41] It is estimated that poisoning accounts for 47 percent of all home unintentional injury deaths.[39]

Prevention of poisoning by prescription drugs requires an understanding of the potency of these agents, particularly the opioid analgesics such as oxycodone. These, and similar drugs, depress respiration to the point where there is insufficient oxygen in the body to sustain a heartbeat. To reduce your risk of a drug overdose, adhere to the following precautions:

- Always read all information provided with your prescription.

- Always precisely follow the directions for taking prescription medications.

- Never exceed the prescribed dosage.

- Never try to obtain prescriptions for the same illness from different physicians.

- Never mix prescription drugs or prescription drugs and supplements (see the box "Safety and Health Care Decisions").

- Never drink alcohol while taking prescription drugs.

- Never take someone else's drugs or give your drugs to someone else.

- Always keep prescription medications in their original container.

- Keep the poison control center telephone number handy.

Other Residential Injuries   The second leading cause of injury deaths in the home is falls. Falls primarily affect the very young and very old, who may be more seriously injured and who may be slower to recover from nonfatal falls. Making sure that flooring is in good repair and that stairways are well lighted and equipped with handrails can reduce the risk of falls.

Exposure to heat, smoke, and flames is another leading cause of residential deaths. Winter is the season when most home fires occur. Make sure that all electrical appliances and heating and cooling systems are in safe working order and that flammable materials are stored safely. Installation of smoke detectors and fire extinguishers can reduce the risk of injuries resulting from a fire. Prepare a fire escape plan.

Safety and Health Care Decisions

In today's complex world of health care, four generalizations regarding the interfacing of traditional allopathic health care and complementary health care can be made. First, as adults age, they are increasingly likely to be under the care of several health care providers, in addition to their primary care physician. In fact, many middle-aged and older adults may be seeing three or more specialists, such as cardiologists, rheumatologists, and endocrinologists, in addition to their family physician or internist. As a result, these individuals may be taking multiple prescription medications simultaneously. Second, over 40 percent of adults report that they are using complementary care, including taking a vast array of dietary supplements. Third, less than 20 percent of adults mention the use of such complementary health care to their physicians, and an even smaller percentage of physicians question patients about their use of complementary health care. Fourth, despite its $50 million budget and newly designated independent status, the National Center for Alternative and Complementary Medicine has yet to carefully evaluate the effectiveness and safety of all the many forms

of health care and the vast array of dietary supplements available in the marketplace.

When these factors are combined, the potential for unanticipated and dangerous drug interactions exists. It is, therefore, imperative that patients proactively inform their physicians about the type and extent of complementary health care they are using. It is equally important that physicians ask their patients about any alternative forms of care being received and any dietary supplements being taken. When this information is not taken into consideration in the patient's plan of care, the complementary care itself may become a negative factor. Therefore, until a great deal more is understood about complementary medical care procedures and the nature of prescription medication–dietary supplement interactions, the use of complementary care should be limited to preventive and palliative measures. In addition, such care should be discontinued during periods of treatment with prescription medications and chemotherapeutic agents or prior to undergoing surgery.

Suffocation affects mostly young children, who can suffocate on a toy, a plastic bag, or other object left within their reach.

Assaults by strangers who enter homes are rare. Nonetheless, there are some precautions you can take:

- Use initials for first names on mailboxes and in phone books.
- Install a peephole and deadbolt locks on doors.
- If possible, avoid living in first-floor apartments. Change locks when moving to a new place.
- Put locks on all windows.
- Require repair people or delivery people to show valid identification.
- Do not use an elevator if it is occupied by someone who makes you feel uneasy.
- Be cautious around garages, laundry rooms, and driveways (especially at night). Use lighting for prevention of assault.
- Be certain that elders have a good understanding of the medications they may be taking. Know the side effects.
- Encourage elders to seek assistance for home repairs.
- Make certain that all door locks, lights, and safety equipment are in good working order.

For young children who are mostly at home and elders whose dependence on homes is often an issue of restricted mobility and a sense of insecurity, homes should be dependably safe environments. Implementing the suggestions made in this section can help make a home safer.

Another dangerous object found in many homes is a firearm. While only 2 to 3 percent of all firearm deaths are classified as unintentional, this represents 700 to 800 tragic and avoidable deaths. Following are some steps you can take to protect yourself and others in your home:

- Consider every gun to be a loaded gun, even if someone tells you it is not loaded.
- Never point a gun at an unintended target.
- Keep your finger off the trigger until you are ready to shoot.
- When moving with a handgun, keep the barrel pointed down.
- Store your gun and ammunition safely in separate locked containers. Use a trigger lock on your gun when not in use.
- Never play with guns at parties. Never handle a gun when intoxicated.
- Make certain that your gun is in good mechanical order.
- Take target practice only at approved ranges.
- Load and unload your gun carefully.
- If you are a novice, enroll in a gun safety course. Your local police, sheriff, or fire department may offer such a course.
- Educate children about gun safety and the potential dangers of gun use. Children must never believe that a gun is a toy.
- Make certain that you follow the gun possession laws in your state. Special permits may be required to carry a handgun.

TALKING POINTS You do not have a firearm in your home, but you're not sure whether your neighbors do, and your child enjoys playing at their house. How might you go about asking your neighbors if they have a gun in their home?

Recreational Injuries and Safety

The thrills we get from risk taking are an essential part of our recreational endeavors. But a significant number of injuries occur in recreational settings. For example, bicycle riding accounted for more than 480,000 emergency department visits in 2006. Only basketball injuries accounted for more sport injury visits to emergency departments.[39] Some injuries occur because we fail to consider important recreational safety information. Do some of the following recommendations apply to you?

- Seek appropriate instruction for your intended activity. Few skill activities are as easy as they look.

- Make certain that your equipment is in excellent working order.

- Involve yourself gradually in an activity before attempting more complicated, dangerous skills.

- Enroll in an American Red Cross first aid course to enable you to cope with unexpected injuries.

- Remember that alcohol use greatly increases the likelihood that people will get hurt.

- Protect your eyes from injury by wearing the recommended eye ware.

- Learn to swim. Most drowning victims are people who never intended to be in the water.

- Obey the laws related to your recreational pursuits. Many laws are directly related to the safety of the participants.

- Be aware of weather conditions. Many outdoor activities turn to tragedy with sudden shifts in the weather. Always prepare yourself for the worst possible weather.

Bicycle Safety With a little common sense and a few precautions, bicycling can be a very safe and enjoyable aerobic activity. Remember these key points:

- Wear a helmet. More than any other precaution, wearing a helmet is paramount and can save your life.

- When cycling at night or when visibility is poor, wear brightly colored reflective clothing.

- Use hand signals so drivers around you know what you plan to do.

- Obey traffic signals just like any other vehicle on the road. You have a right to bicycle on the road, but you also have the same responsibilities as other vehicles. Don't run stop signs or red lights!

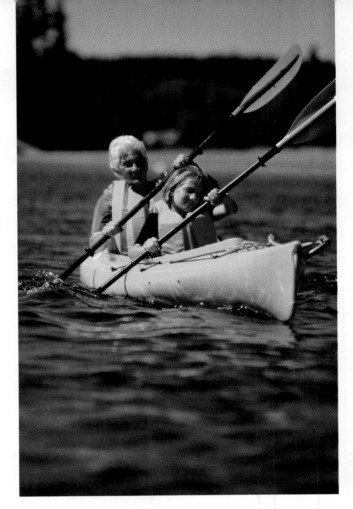

Wearing proper safety gear is an essential safety measure for recreational activities.

- Brake carefully, and use both hand brakes at the same time. Using only the front brake can send you over the handlebars, and using only the back brake can cause a skid. On long downhills or in wet weather, gently tap the brakes to retain control. Be especially careful in wet weather, when wet brake pads are not very helpful.

Boating Safety Most boating deaths result from drowning, when the victim was not wearing a personal flotation device (PFD). Of the 685 boaters who drowned in 2007, most could have been saved if they had been wearing a PFD, according to the U.S. Coast Guard. Two-thirds of the victims in fatal boating accidents drowned and 90 percent of those were not wearing life jackets.[42]

The other major cause of boating accidents and fatalities is "operator error," including (1) inattention, not looking in the direction in which one is moving, (2) carelessness, going out in bad weather or water conditions or while intoxicated, and (3) speeding. In particular, intoxication is a factor in more than half of all boating accidents. Too many casual boaters assume that rules of boating safety do not apply to them. Every boater should learn how to handle high winds, storms, whitecaps, rough waters, and heavy boat traffic. Most boat dealers can give you information about PFDs, "rules of the road," and Coast Guard safety regulations.

Even some experienced boaters tend to go too fast. Some modern watercraft tend to climb out of the water at higher speeds, and less hull in the water means less stability. With less stability, the boat tends to rock from side to side, and this rocking is a warning that you are about to lose control.

Taking Charge of Your Health

- Use the Personal Assessment at the end of this chapter to determine how well you manage your safety at home, in your car, and in your community.
- Assess your behaviors against the recommendations found in the box "Don't Be a Victim of Violent Crime" on page 498.
- Review your attitudes and health behaviors as they relate to people with disabilities, people of the opposite sex, and people

of a different race, ethnicity, religion, or sexual orientation by referring again to the section "Bias and Hate Crimes."
- Find out about the security services available on your campus, and take advantage of them. Post a 24-hour help phone number in your room and on your cell phone.
- Minimize your risk for identity theft by taking the steps outlined in the section "Identity Theft."

- Consider implementing the driving and cell phone safety tips mentioned in the box "Cell Phone Safety."
- If there is a firearm in your place of residence, review and consider firearm safety suggestions on page 513.
- Check recreational safety suggestions on page 514.

SUMMARY

- Each year in the United States, interpersonal violence results in 20,000 deaths and another 2 million nonfatal injuries.
- Rape, other sexual assault, and sexual harassment are forms of sexual victimization in which the victims are often traumatized physically and psychologically.
- Bias and hate crimes are crimes directed at persons or groups solely because of a specific characteristic, such as race, religion, sexual orientation, ethnic background, or disability.
- Family violence includes intimate partner violence, maltreatment of children, and maltreatment of elders.
- Violence in our communities affects our schools and colleges as well as other institutions.

- You can take steps to protect yourself from acts of violence while on campus or at home.
- Alcohol consumption and the availability of firearms are two important factors that contribute to the prevalence and deadliness of interpersonal violence in America.
- Unintentional injuries injure and kill more people than injuries resulting from interpersonal violence.
- Adolescents and young adults have a greater chance of dying in a motor vehicle crash than any other way.
- The leading causes of injury deaths in residential settings are unintentional poisonings, falls, fires, suffocation, and unintentional firearm injuries.
- Bicyclists and motorcyclists can reduce their risk of a head injury by wearing a helmet.

REVIEW QUESTIONS

1. Explain the difference between intentional and unintentional injuries. Give three examples of each.
2. List some myths associated with rape. What are some ways to prevent rapes?
3. Define sexual harassment. Identify some acts that could be considered sexual harassment.
4. What are bias and hate crimes? Who are the perpetrators? Who are the victims?
5. How has the family structure changed over the past several generations? Why are some families under more stress today? Who are the potential victims of family violence?
6. What steps can you take to reduce your risk of becoming a victim of an intentional injury? How do the consumption

of alcohol and the availability of firearms contribute to interpersonal violence in America?
7. What steps can you take to deter identity theft? How would you be able to detect identity theft? What should you do if you suspect your personal information has been stolen?
8. Where do most unintentional injuries occur? Where do most unintentional injury deaths occur?
9. How can you reduce your risk of dying in a fatal motor vehicle crash?
10. List at least eight strategies to make your home safer.

ANSWERS TO THE "WHAT DO YOU KNOW?" QUIZ

1. True   2. True   3. False   4. True   5. False   6. True   7. True

Visit the Online Learning Center (**www.mhhe.com/payne11e**), where you will find tools to help you improve your grade including practice quizzes, key terms flashcards, audio chapter summaries for your MP3 player, and many other study aids.

SOURCE NOTES

1. Adams PF, Barnes PM, Vickerie JL. Summary Health Statistics for the U.S. Population: National Health Interview Survey, 2007. *Vital and Health Statistics,* 10(238). Hyattsville, MD: National Center for Health Statistics, Centers for Disease Control and Prevention, U.S Department of Health and Human Services. November 2008.

2. Kung HC, Hoyert DLM, Xu J, Murphy SL. Deaths: Final Data for 2005. *National Vital Statistics Reports,* 56(10), 1–124. National Center for Health Statistics. Centers for Disease Control and Prevention, U.S Department of Health and Human Services. April 24, 2008.

3. Centers for Disease Control and Prevention, National Center for Injury Prevention and Control, WISQARS (Web-based Injury Surveillance Query and Reporting System). Available at www.cdc.gov/ncipc/wisqars/. Accessed January 7, 2009.

4. Rand M, Catalano SM. National Crime Victimization Survey: Criminal Victimization, 2006. U.S. Department of Justice, Office of Justice Programs, *Bureau of Justice Statistics: Bulletin.* NCJ 219413, December 2007.

5. Pitts SR, Niska RW, Xu J, Burt CW. National Hospital Ambulatory Medical Care Survey: 2006 Emergency Department Summary. *National Health Statistics Reports,* Number 7. Hyattsville, MD: National Center for Health Statistics, 2008.

6. Fox JA. *Homicide Trends in the U.S.* Department of Justice, Office of Justice Programs, Bureau of Justice Statistics, 2006. Available at www.ojp.usdoj.gov/bjs/homicide/tables/totalstab.htm. Accessed January 7, 2009.

7. Blumstein A, Rivara FP, Rosenfeld R. The Rise and Decline of Homicide—and Why. *Annual Review of Public Health,* 21, 505–541, 2000.

8. Bonczar TP. Prevalence of Imprisonment in the U.S. Population, 1974–2001. U.S. Department of Justice, Office of Justice Programs, Bureau of Justice Statistics, *Bureau of Justice Statistics: Special Report,* NCJ 197976, 2003. Available at http://www.ojp.usdoj.gov/bjs/pub/pdf/piusp01.pdf. Accessed January 7, 2009.

9. West HC, Sabol, WJ. Prisoners in 2007. *Bureau of Justice Statistics Bulletin,* NCJ 224280, U.S. Department of Justice, Office of Justice Statistics, 2008. Available at http://www.ojp.usdoj.gov/bjs/pub/pdf/p07.pdf. Accessed January 7, 2009.

10. Catalano, SM. National Crime Victimization Survey: Criminal Victimization, 2005. U.S. Department of Justice, Office of Justice Programs, *Bureau of Justice Statistics: Bulletin.* NCJ 214644, September 2006.

11. Tjaden P, Thoennes N. *Extent, Nature, and Consequences of Intimate Partner Violence: Findings from the National Violence Against Women Survey.* NCJ 181867. Washington, DC: National Institute of Justice, 2000.

12. Fisher BS, Cullen FT, Turner MG. *The Sexual Victimization of College Women.* U.S. Department of Justice, Bureau of Justice Statistics, NCJ 182369. Washington, DC, 2001.

13. Schwartz RH, Milteer R, LeBeau MA. Drug-Facilitated Sexual Assault ("Date Rape"). *Southern Medicine,* 93(6), 558–561, 2000.

14. American College Health Association. *Shifting the Paradigm: Primary Prevention of Sexual Violence.* Baltimore, MD: Author, 2008.

15. Harlow, CW. Hate Crimes Reported by Victims and Police. *Bureau of Justice Special Report, National Criminal Victimization Survey and Uniform Crime Reporting.* U.S. Department of Justice, Office of Justice Programs, NCJ 209911, 2005.

16. U.S. Census Bureau News. 50 Million Children Lived with Married Parents in 2007. Washington, DC: U.S. Census Bureau. Available at http://www.census.gov/Press-Release/www/releases/archives/marital_status_living_arrangements/012437.html. Accessed January 9, 2009.

17. U.S. Department of Labor, Bureau of Labor Statistics. 2008. Women in the Labor Force: A Databook. Report 1011. Available at http://www.bls.gov/cps/wlf-databook-2008.pdf. Accessed January 9, 2009.

18. Catalano S. Intimate Partner Violence in the United States. Bureau of Justice Statistics, U.S. Department of Justice. Available at http://www.ojp.usdoj.gov/bjs/intimate/ipv.htm. Accessed January 9, 2009.

19. Coker AI, et al. Physical Health Consequences of Physical and Psychological Intimate Partner Violence. *Archives of Family Medicine,* 9(5), 451–457, 2000.

20. U.S. Department of Health and Human Services, Administration for Children and Families, Administration on Children, Youth and Families, Children's Bureau. *Child Maltreatment 2004.* Available at http://www.acf.hhs.gov/programs/cb/pubs/cm06/cm06.pdf. Accessed January 9. 2009.

21. U.S. Census Bureau, *Population Estimates.* Available at www.census.gov/popest/estimates.php. Accessed January 9, 2009.

22. National Research Council, *Elder Mistreatment: Abuse, Neglect, and Exploitation in an Aging America,* Washington, DC: National Academies Press, 2003.

23. National Committee for the Prevention of Elder Abuse and the National Adult Protective Services Administration. 2006. The 2004 Survey of State Adult Protective Services: Abuse of Adults 60 Years of Age and Older. Available at http://www.ncea.aoa.gov/NCEAroot/Main_Site/pdf/2-14-06%20FINAL%2060+REPORT.pdf. Accessed January 9, 2009.

24. United States Department of Education, National Center for Education Statistics (2007). Indicators of School Crime and Safety: 2007. NCES 2008-021. Available at http://nces.ed.gov/pubs2008/2008021a.pdf. Accessed January 9, 2009.

25. Centers for Disease Control and Prevention. Youth Risk Behavior Surveillance—United States, 2007. *Morbidity and Mortality Weekly Report,* 57(SS-04), 1–135, 2008. Available at http://nces.ed.gov/pubs2008/2008021a.pdf. Accessed January 9, 2009.

26. Bilchik S. Violence after School. *1999 National Report Series, Juvenile Justice Bulletin,* Washington, DC: U.S. Department of Justice, Office of Justice Programs, Office of Juvenile Justice and Delinquency Prevention. NCJ 178992, November 1999.

27. Baum K, Klaus P. Violent Victimization of College Students, 1995–2002. U.S. Department of Justice, Office of Justice Programs, *Bureau of Justice Statistics Special Report: National Crime Victimization Survey* NCJ 206836, January 2005. Available at www.ojp.usdoj.gov/bjs/pub/pdf/vvcs02.pdf. Accessed January 9, 2009.

28. Bureau of Justice Statistics. 2008. *Criminal Victimization in the United States, 2006, Statistical Tables.* Table 32. Percent Distribution of Victimizations by Perceived Drug or Alcohol Use by Offender. NCJ 223436. Available at http://www.ojp.usdoj.gov/bjs/pub/pdf/cvus0602.pdf. Accessed January 9, 2009.

29. Egley A Jr., O'Donnell CE. Highlights of the 2006 National Youth Gang Survey. *OJJDP Fact Sheet.* July 2008 #05. U.S. Department of Justice, Office of Justice Programs, Office of Juvenile Justice and Delinquency Prevention. Available at http://www.ncjrs.gov/pdffiles1/ojjdp/fs200805.pdf. Accessed January 9, 2009.

30. Dorsey TL, Zawitz MW, Middleton P. *Drugs and Crime Facts.* U.S. Department of Justice, Office of Justice Programs, Bureau of Justice Statistics, NCJ 165148. Available at www.ojp.usdoj.gov/bjs/pub/pdf/dcf.pdf. Accessed February 3, 2007.

31. Mumola CJ, Karberg JC. Drug Use and Dependence, State and Federal Prisoners, 2004. U.S. Department of Justice, Office of Justice Programs, *Bureau of Justice Statistics: Special Report,* NCH 213530, 2006. Available at www.ojp.usdoj.gov/bjs/pub/pdf/dudsfp04.pdf. Accessed February 3, 2007.

32. Miniño AM, Anderson RN. Deaths: Injuries, 2002. *National Vital Statistics Reports,* 54(10), 1–128, 2006.

33. Centers for Disease Control and Prevention. 2001. Surveillance of Fatal and Nonfatal Firearm-Related Injuries—United States, 1993–1998. *Morbidity and Mortality Weekly Report,* 50(SS-2), 1–34. Available at http://www.cdc.gov/mmwr/PDF/ss/ss5002.pdf. Accessed January 15, 2009.

34. Centers for Disease Control and Prevention. 2008. Youth Risk Behavior Surveillance—United States, 2007. *Morbidity and Mortality Weekly Report,* 57(SS-4), 1–44. Available at http://www.cdc.gov/mmwr/PDF/ss/ss5705.pdf. Accessed January 15, 2009.

35. Miller M, Hemenway D, Wechsler H. Guns and Gun Threats at College. *Journal of American College Health,* 51(2), 57–65, 2002.

36. Baum K. 2007. Identity Theft, 2005. U.S. Department of Justice, Office of Justice Programs, *Bureau of Justice Statistics: Special Report,* NCH 219411, 2007.

37. Federal Trade Commission. Deter•Detect•Defend Avoid ID Theft: Fighting Back Against Identity Theft. Available at www.ftc.gov/idtheft. Accessed January 15, 2009.

38. Annan K. [In the second part of the report titled] Larger Freedom. A commentary issued by the United Nations at the Security Council Meeting. March 17, 2005. Available at www.un.org/unifeed/script.asp?scriptId=73. Accessed February 17, 2007.

39. National Safety Council. *Injury Facts® 2008 Edition.* Itasca, IL: Author, 2008.

40. U.S. Department of Transportation, National Highway Traffic Safety Administration. *Traffic Safety Facts 2007 (Early Edition): A Compilation of Motor Vehicle Crash Data from the Fatality Analysis Reporting System and the General Estimates System.* Washington, DC: US Department of Transportation, DOT HS 811 002. Available at http://www-nrd.nhtsa.dot.gov/Pubs/TSF2007EE.PDF. 2008. Accessed January 16, 2009.

41. Centers for Disease Control and Prevention. Unintentional Poisoning Deaths—United States, 1999–2004. *Morbidity and Mortality Weekly Report,* 56(5), 93–96.

42. U.S. Department of Homeland Security, U.S. Coast Guard, Office of Auxiliary and Boating Safety. *Recreational Boating Statistics 2007.* COMDTPUB P16754.21. Available at http://www.uscgboating.org/statistics/Boating_Statistics_2007.pdf. Accessed January 16, 2009.

Personal Assessment

How well do you protect your safety?

This quiz will help you measure how well you manage your personal safety. For each item, circle the number that reflects the frequency with which you do the safety activity. Then, add up your individual scores and check the interpretation at the end.

3 I regularly do this
2 I sometimes do this
1 I rarely do this

1. I am aware of my surroundings and do not get lost.
   3   2   1
2. I avoid locations in which my personal safety would be compromised.
   3   2   1
3. I intentionally vary my daily routine (such as walking patterns to and from class, parking places, and jogging or biking routes) so that my whereabouts are not always predictable.
   3   2   1
4. I walk across campus at night with other people.
   3   2   1
5. I am careful about disclosing personal information (address, phone number, Social Security number, my daily schedule, etc.) to people I do not know.
   3   2   1
6. I carefully monitor my alcohol intake at parties.
   3   2   1
7. I watch carefully for dangerous weather conditions and know how to respond if necessary.
   3   2   1
8. I do not keep a loaded gun in my home.
   3   2   1
9. I never drive a car, truck, or motorcycle after drinking alcohol.
   3   2   1
10. I never ride in a car, truck, or on a motorcycle with a driver who has been drinking alcohol.
    3   2   1
11. I never talk on my cell phone while I am driving.
    3   2   1
12. I never text message while I am driving.
    3   2   1
13. I use my car seat belt.
    3   2   1

14. I drive my car safely and defensively.
    3   2   1
15. I keep my car in good mechanical order.
    3   2   1
16. I keep my car doors locked.
    3   2   1
17. I have a plan of action if my car should break down while I am driving it.
    3   2   1
18. I keep emergency information numbers near my phone.
    3   2   1
19. I keep my first aid skills up to date.
    3   2   1
20. I use deadbolt locks on the doors of my home.
    3   2   1
21. I use the safety locks on the windows at home.
    3   2   1
22. I check the batteries used in my home smoke detector.
    3   2   1
23. I have installed a carbon monoxide detector in my home.
    3   2   1
24. I use adequate lighting in areas around my home and garage.
    3   2   1
25. I have the electrical, heating, and cooling equipment in my home inspected regularly for safety and efficiency.
    3   2   1
26. I use appropriate safety equipment, such as flotation devices, helmets, and elbow pads, in my recreational activities.
    3   2   1
27. I can swim well enough to save myself in most situations.
    3   2   1
28. I use suggestions for personal safety each day.
    3   2   1
29. I have an emergency contact number listed on my cell phone under "ICE."
    3   2   1

TOTAL POINTS _____

Personal Assessment—*continued*

Interpretation

Your total may mean that:

78–87 points   You appear to carefully protect your personal safety.

71–77 points   You adequately protect many aspects of your personal safety.

64–70 points   You should consider improving some of your safety-related behaviors.

Below 64 points   You must consider improving some of your safety-related behaviors.

TO CARRY THIS FURTHER . . .

Although no one can be completely safe from personal injury or possible random violence, there are ways to minimize the risks to your safety. Refer to the text and this assessment to provide you with useful suggestions to enhance your personal safety. Which safety tips will you use today?

20 The Environment and Your Health

chapter

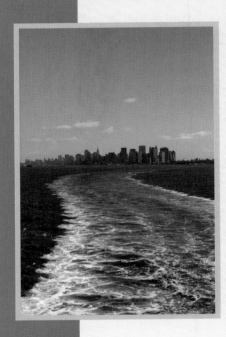

What Do You Know About Environmental Health?

1. The vast majority of your exposure to potentially harmful pollutants occurs in the home and workplace. True or False?

2. Electromagnetic radiation from electrical power lines, microwave ovens, and cell phones has been shown to cause cancer. True or False?

3. If you live in an old house, you and your family are at greater risk for lead poisoning, which can reduce intelligence and increase behavior problems in young children. True or False?

4. The government has tested all chemicals used in household and personal hygiene products to ensure that they do not cause adverse health effects in people. True or False?

5. If you suffer from asthma or other lung diseases, it would be good for your health to move to Los Angeles. True or False?

6. Tap water from a municipal water supplier can contain measurable amounts of potentially harmful pollutants. True or False?

7. Warming of Earth's climate associated with increasing carbon dioxide in the atmosphere from burning fossil fuels can have negative impacts on your health. True or False?

Check your answers at the end of the chapter.

Many college-age students are aware of how human activities damage the health of the environment, but how many know of the risks that their environment poses to their own health? You likely have heard that global warming associated with burning of fossil fuels to power our modern society is causing melting of polar ice caps that endangers the polar bear. You may be aware that over-hunting and habitat destruction associated with logging, farming, urban development, and pollution destroys or degrades natural habitats and puts many species at risk of extinction. But do you know what potentially harmful substances or organisms are in the air you breathe, the water you drink, and the food you eat? Do you know which products you purchase and bring into your home can increase your risk of developing cancer or having a child with birth defects? Are you aware of the materials and appliances in your home that emit noxious or dangerous fumes? Do you know how to maintain your home to minimize your exposure to disease- or allergy-producing organisms? Have you ever felt sad, angry, or hopeless when you read or hear

Figure 20-1 Environmental Problems and Solutions This model shows spatial scales of environmental health risks and appropriate personal responses to environmental problems.

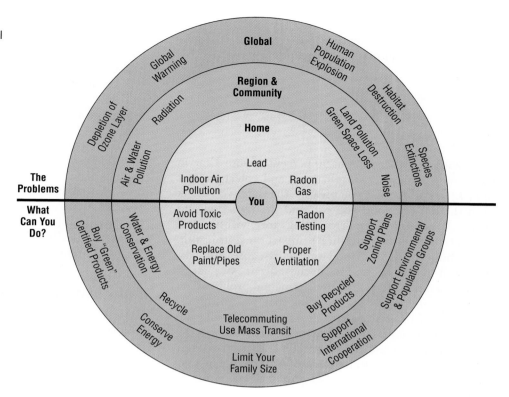

about the loss of a species or a beautiful natural habitat but didn't know what you could do about it? The main focus of this chapter is to make you aware of those components of your environment that may adversely affect your personal health and to provide you with suggestions for how you can manage these environmental factors.

Your **environment** includes a range of conditions that can influence your health, such as the availability of resources (oxygen, water, food) and environmental characteristics, such as temperature, humidity, toxins, allergens, pathogens, noise, and radiation. Conditions in your environment operate across a wide range of spatial scales, from the air immediately surrounding your body to the global earth, air, and ocean system. Your physical health is influenced primarily by your *personal environment,* which comprises conditions immediately around your body, in the home, neighborhood, and workplace. However, this personal environment is influenced by conditions in the larger *community* and *regional environment,* including such conditions as air pollution and water pollution. These local and regional conditions are influenced by conditions of the *global environment,* such as climate and solar radiation.

Your health can be influenced by changes in environmental conditions at the home/workplace, community/region, or global levels. Excessive noise in the workplace or neighborhood can significantly affect your sense of well-being and your ability to work effectively. High ozone levels in the air of your community can limit your ability to enjoy outdoors activities and

cause or exacerbate asthma. Environmental conditions in a particular community and region can enhance or limit opportunities for various types of employment, and so affect occupational health. Few people ever visit a tropical rain forest, wilderness area, or whale sanctuary, but many feel their emotional and spiritual well-being is diminished when they hear these remote places are threatened or destroyed.

The goal of this chapter is to help you identify aspects of your environment that can significantly affect various dimensions of your health, and to suggest ways that you can exert some level of personal control over these environmental influences. The range of options for personal action to improve your environment includes altering personal behaviors and buying habits, becoming involved in the political process related to environmental issues, and supporting various nongovernmental organizations that work to address major environmental problems. Different specific environmental conditions and personal responses will be important at the various spatial scales of your environment (home/workplace, community/region, and global). Figure 20-1 displays a

Key Terms

environment The physical conditions (temperature, humidity, light, presence of substances) and other living organisms that exist around your body.

range of environmental problems that exist at various spatial scales of your environment and a range of personal responses that might be appropriate at each level.

The Personal Environment: Home, Neighborhood, Workplace

On average you spend about 90 percent of your time in your home, workplace, local stores, and entertainment venues.[1] The indoor air you breathe, the water you drink from the tap, the food you eat, and the radiation and noise in your immediate surroundings are environmental factors that have the most direct impact on your health. Some indoor environmental problems cause immediate health effects, such as headaches, dizziness, nausea, or allergic reactions. Other environmental problems act in subtle, cumulative ways, causing major health problems such as cancer or neurological damage that may not become apparent until permanent damage is done.

Of all the different environmental influences on your health, you have the greatest control over factors in your personal environment. You are responsible for maintaining appliances so that they do not produce excessive air pollution. You control the ventilation in your home, allowing you to vent pollutants outside. You select the foods you eat. You choose which products you purchase and can avoid products that contain toxic chemicals. You can eliminate tobacco smoke from your home and workspace. You can identify sources of health risk in the workplace and notify those responsible for environmental safety.

In this section, you will learn to identify important environmental health risks in your personal environment, learn the effects of these environmental factors on your health, and see what you can do to minimize associated risks of health problems. Table 20.1 identifies notable pollutants in the personal environment, and Table 20.2 outlines how to minimize your exposure to these pollutants.

Indoor Air Quality

Indoor air quality within buildings can be influenced by a wide range of factors, including ventilation, humidity, gases given off by building construction materials, furniture and flooring materials, and combustion by-products from stoves and furnaces. When there is a problem with one or more of these factors, people in the

Table 20.1 Pollutants in the Personal Environment

Pollutant	Sources	Health Effects
Carbon monoxide	Poorly functioning furnace, space heater, hot water heater, or gas stove; gasoline/diesel engine exhaust	*At 70–50 ppm:* headache, dizziness, mental confusion, nausea *Above 150 ppm:* death
Volatile organic compounds (VOCs)	Oil paints and paint stripper, cleaning solvents, wood preservatives, aerosol sprays, cleaners, disinfectants, stored fuels, automotive fluids	*Immediate effects:* irritation to eyes, nose, throat; nausea *Long-term effects:* damage to liver, kidney, central nervous system; some VOCs are carcinogenic
Formaldehyde	Home insulation foam, carpet adhesives, plywood, paneling, particleboard, fiberboard, furniture made from these	Irritation to eyes, nose, throat, lungs; long-term exposure may cause lung cancer
Asbestos	Building materials such as floor tiles, noise-dampening tiles, fireproofing	Inhaled asbestos fibers can cause lung damage, emphysema, and lung cancer
Lead	Pre-1980 house paint, plumbing solder, dust from nearby highways	Damages nervous system, kidneys, and blood; in children, causes lower IQ and delayed physical and mental development
Biological pollutants (including *E. coli*)	Disease-causing viruses and bacteria in air or water, dust mites, plant pollen, mold, pet dander, rodent and cockroach feces	Colds and flu; allergic reactions that include itchy eyes, runny nose, sneezing, headache, skin rashes; may induce asthma; waterborne organisms may cause nausea, diarrhea, and fever
Radon	Naturally occurring radioactive substances in soil around the home	Major cause of lung cancer
Mercury and PCBs	Contaminated wild-caught fish and game	Damages nervous system; causes birth defects and cancer
Nitrate	Agricultural fertilizer contamination of groundwater wells	Interferes with oxygen transport by blood; damages reproductive system; may cause several cancers
Vinyl chloride	Pre-1977 PVC pipe in plumbing	Causes cancer
Pesticides	Contamination of water supplies and food	Damages nervous system; interferes with reproductive development; carcinogenic
Phthalates and bisphenol A	Soft plastics in food containers, shampoos, soaps, cosmetics, paints, adhesives, wallpaper, carpet	Interferes with reproductive development; causes cancer and birth defects

Table 20.2 Managing Pollutants in the Personal Environment

Pollutant	How to Minimize Exposure
Carbon monoxide	Proper maintenance of appliances that burn natural gas. Proper use and ventilation of fuel-burning space heaters, cooking grills, fireplaces. Avoid breathing exhaust fumes from autos or power boats. Install a carbon monoxide detector in your home.
Volatile organic compounds (VOCs)	Minimize use of products that emit these substances (e.g., use latex paint instead of oil paint) or use them only in well-ventilated area. Never mix household chemicals (might react to produce VOCs). Do not store VOC-emitting products in your home; dispose of excess product properly.
Formaldehyde	Use only "low-emission" formaldehyde-containing products (carpet, paneling, adhesives). Adequate ventilation of personal environment spaces.
Asbestos	Never disturb intact asbestos-containing materials. Hire qualified contractors to remove asbestos from your home; NEVER do this yourself.
Lead	Do not disturb intact lead-containing paint. Hire qualified contractors to remove old lead-containing paint in your home; use a respirator if you do this yourself.
Biological pollutants	Use exhaust fans or dehumidifiers to maintain relative humidity of your home at 30–50% to minimize growth of mold. Remove all water-damaged carpet and drywall to prevent mold. Regularly clean/vacuum home and eliminate cockroaches and rodents to minimize exposure to allergens. Have tap water tested for *E. coli* and install chlorination or filtration system if present.
Radon	Test home for presence of radon. If test is positive, install a radon reduction system in home.
Mercury and PCBs	Be aware of advisories related to contamination of game, fish, and shellfish in your region. Follow recommended limits for consumption, especially if you are pregnant.
Nitrate	If your water source is a well and you live in an agricultural area, have your water tested. If nitrate is present, drink bottled water or install a reverse osmosis water system in your home.
Vinyl chloride	If your house was built before 1977 and has PVC pipes for the water supply, replace these pipes.
Pesticides	Test your well water or get water quality report from water company. Drink bottled water or install reverse osmosis system if pesticides found in tap water. Eat organically produced food.
Phthalates and BPA	Reduce use of personal hygiene products and cosmetics that list the words "phthalate" in the ingredients. Avoid food and drink containers made of soft plastic; use water bottles made of glass, metal, or plastic labeled as BPA-free. Eliminate all exposure to these if you are pregnant. Do not give soft plastic toys or plastic bottles to your small children unless these items are labeled as phthalate- and BPA-free.

affected building can experience a wide range of symptoms, from headaches and itchy eyes to unconsciousness and death. This section covers some of the most important health risks associated with indoor air quality.

Carbon monoxide is a highly toxic gas that is colorless, odorless and tasteless, and so is not detectable by the unaided senses. Health effects of carbon monoxide vary from mild discomfort to death.[1, 2] Persons who suffer from heart disease may feel chest pain at low concentrations. Regular exposure to low levels in the home or workplace can cause flu-like symptoms that rapidly disappear after you leave the location where you are exposed.

Volatile Organic Compounds
Volatile organic compounds (VOCs) are gases emitted to indoor air from a wide range of household products. These gases often have a "chemical" smell (e.g., gasoline, paint stripper). *Formaldehyde* is a specific VOC that is emitted by many building products (plywood, particleboard, fiberboard, urea foam insulation, and building/carpet adhesives).[2] This indoor air pollutant was the main reason why victims of Hurricane Katrina had to be relocated out of

---

Key Terms

indoor air quality Characteristics of air within homes, workplaces, and public buildings, including the presence and amount of oxygen, water vapor, and a wide range of substances that can have adverse effects on your health.

carbon monoxide A gaseous by-product of the incomplete combustion of natural gas, kerosene, heating oil, wood, coal, gasoline, and tobacco.

volatile organic compounds (VOCs) A wide variety of chemicals that contain carbon and readily evaporate into the air.

---

travel trailer housing provided by FEMA. In hundreds of these travel trailers, indoor air concentrations of form-aldehyde were 4 to 50 times greater than normal levels in homes and well above levels known to cause adverse health effects.[3] People living in these trailers complained of a range of symptoms, including irritated eyes, head-aches, and dizziness. The health effects of volatile organic compounds vary depending on which specific substance is involved, ranging from irritation to eyes and the respi-ratory system to organ damage to cancer. You can con-trol your exposure to toxic volatile organic compounds through your choices of which products you bring into your home and by using VOC-emitting products only in well-ventilated areas.

Tobacco Smoke   Secondhand tobacco smoke is an in-door air pollutant widely recognized as a major health risk, especially for children. For example, this pollutant can increase the risk for acute asthma attacks that require hospital emergency care. Some evidence indicates that regular exposure to tobacco smoke increases the risk of developing asthma in the first place.[4] Exposure to tobacco smoke in the home is also associated with increased risk of sudden infant death syndrome (SIDS), childhood bronchitis, pneumonia and ear infections, cardiovascular disease, and cancer. The health effects of indoor tobacco smoke are covered in more detail in Chapter 9.

Asbestos   Asbestos is a building material that was widely used for its insulation, fire retardant, and noise-dampening properties. When the serious health risks associated with exposure to asbestos fibers became known, governmental agencies banned several asbestos products, and manufacturers voluntarily limited other uses of asbestos. Today, asbestos is most commonly found in older buildings, including homes, schools, and factories. Health effects of asbestos exposure most com-monly occur only after many years of exposure, usually in the workplace.[5] Currently, your greatest risk of expo-sure to asbestos occurs when insulation, floor tiles, and other asbestos-containing substances deteriorate or are damaged during building renovation. These activities release the asbestos fibers to the air, from which they are inhaled into the lungs. However, intact and undisturbed, asbestos-containing products are relatively safe. [5]

Lead   Lead is a toxic metal that was widely used in house paint, as a gasoline additive, and in plumbing solder for metal pipes. As the health consequences of lead toxicity became known, most of these uses of lead were banned. However, lead is a stable substance that remains in the environment today.[6] Lead exposure most commonly occurs in older homes built before 1970 that contain lead-based wall paint. In late 1991, more than 10 years after lead-based paint was banned, the secretary of the U.S. Department of Health and Human Services called

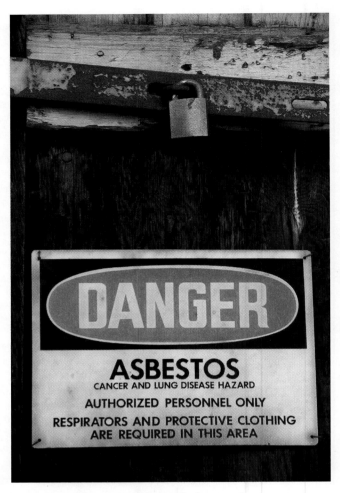

Exposure to asbestos can damage the lungs and cause cancer. Asbestos-containing materials, if damaged and causing the release of asbestos fibers, should be removed by professionals using proper safety gear and precautions.

lead "the number one environmental threat to the health of children in the United States."[7] Exposure to lead from old paint occurs when the paint breaks down into paint flakes and dust, which are then inhaled or swallowed. This risk is especially high for young children, who often put their hands into their mouth.

Lead has serious health effects when ingested or inhaled, especially for children. Blood lead levels as low as 10 micrograms per deciliter in children can delay devel-opment, lower IQ, reduce attention span, and increase behavioral problems. Lead is not readily excreted by the body and will tend to accumulate over time. There are drugs that help the body to excrete lead, but they have adverse side effects and are used only to treat acute lead toxicity.[7]

Biological Pollutants   There are many sources of bio-logical air pollutants within your personal environ-ment. Disease-causing viruses and bacteria are put into the air when infected people or animals sneeze or cough (common cold, flu, measles). Contaminated central air handling systems can be breeding grounds for mold, mildew, and bacteria and can then distribute these contaminants throughout the home. Some people have allergic reactions to spores from mold that grows on moist surfaces inside buildings. Some research indicates that exposure to indoor mold can more than double your risk of developing adult-onset asthma.[4] Pollen from plants around the home or workplace can cause allergic reactions (hay fever) in many people. Household pets, rats, mice, and cockroaches are sources of saliva, urine, feces, and skin dander that can also stimulate strong allergic reactions.[8] The best way for you to minimize biological pollutants is to keep a clean, dry home free of mold and sources of allergens.

Radon **Radon** is an invisible, odorless, tasteless gas that seeps into buildings from the soil surrounding their foundation. It can be detected only using radon detectors. Uranium, the source of radon, can be found in most parts of the world, and this element is present in rocks and soil in parts of all 50 states of the United States. Once radon is produced by decay of uranium, this gas moves through the ground to the air above. Some radon gas may dissolve into groundwater. It is estimated that indoor radon levels sufficient to increase risk of lung cancer occur in 7 percent of homes in the United States, and radon is the second leading cause of lung cancer.[9, 10] You can view state-by-state maps of radon risk zones at the U.S. Environmental Protection Agency's radon website (e.g., to view a map for Indiana, go to the URL http://www.epa.gov/radon/zonemap/indiana.htm). The key to minimizing the health risk of radon is to have your home tested. Inexpensive "do-it-yourself" test kits are available in hardware stores. You can also purchase test kits from the National Safety Council's Radon Hotline (800-767-7236). After the kit is exposed to the air in your home for a specified time period, it is mailed to a laboratory for analysis. If unsafe levels of radon are detected in your home, you should work with a certified contractor to install a radon venting system below and around the house foundation. If you plan to build a new home in a region where high radon levels are common, you should tell your contractor to install radon-resistant features during construction, reducing costs as much as 400 percent.[9]

Nonionizing Radiation Common sources of **nonionizing radiation** in the personal environment are sunlight, electrical devices, electric power transmission lines, and cell phones. This part of the electromagnetic spectrum includes ultraviolet and infrared radiation (in sunlight) and radio frequency radiation (from electronic devices). Most documented health effects of nonionizing radiation are associated with heating tissues or sunburn.

Some have proposed that certain forms of nonionizing radiation may have more serious health effects. A few small studies have documented DNA damage in brain cells of rats exposed to high levels of radiofrequency radiation (RFR) similar to that emitted by early mobile phones. However, other animal studies did not find similar effects. A large-scale study of 420,000 people in Denmark who have been using cell phones for more than 10 years found that they were no more likely to have cancer in the brain, ear, salivary glands, or eye (tissues close to where the cell phone is placed when in use) than people who did not use cell phones.[11] However, a smaller study in Sweden found that people with malignant brain tumors were more likely to have been heavy users of cell phones (analog or digital) or cordless home phones over long periods than were randomly chosen people without cancer.[12] Cell phones are a relatively new technology, and the authors of the Swedish study note that cancers caused by RFR may take many years to develop. Hence, there has not yet been sufficient time to study effects of long-term exposure to RFR. As people use cell phones more, beginning at an ever-younger age, some suggest that it may be prudent to reduce exposure to RFR from these devices.[13] This can be easily done by using a headset attachment to the cell phone to move the cell phone transmitter away from the brain. Advances in cell phone technology are also reducing the amount of RFR emitted by newer cell phones.

Another common source of nonionizing radiation in the human environment is electricity flowing through wires and electronic devices, and electricity transmission lines. A few studies have suggested that exposure to nonionizing radiation around electric devices such as microwave ovens, televisions, tanning lamps, and electric blankets, and electricity transmission lines may slightly increase risk for some cancers.[14, 15, 16] However, attempts to replicate and confirm these small studies have failed, and the vast majority of studies have failed to find any

---

Key Terms

asbestos A class of minerals that have a fibrous crystal structure; a known carcinogen when inhaled.

biological air pollutants Living organisms or substances produced by living organisms that cause disease or allergic reactions, including bacteria, molds, mildew, viruses, dust mites, plant pollen, and animal dander, urine, or feces.

radon A naturally occurring radioactive gas that is emitted during the decay of uranium in soil, rock, and water.

nonionizing radiation Forms of electromagnetic radiation that cannot break chemical bonds but may excite electrons or heat biological materials.

increased risk of adverse health effects associated with household electronics or living near power lines.[13, 17]

Drinking Water

Sources of Drinking Water The safety of drinking water in your home is affected by environmental factors both in the home or neighborhood and in the larger community. The water supply for rural homes is often a well that draws from groundwater and can be much affected by environmental conditions around the home and neighborhood. In urban areas, a municipal water supply system draws from rivers or lakes and then treats the water to make it safe to drink. The community/regional environment plays the dominant role in determining the safety of water from municipal suppliers. However, municipal water can be contaminated by the personal environment as it passes through pipes in the home. Environmental health issues relating to drinking water as influenced by conditions in your home and neighborhood will be covered here. Issues related to municipal water supply are presented later in this chapter.

Approximately 23 million people in the United States obtain their drinking water from groundwater (i.e., from private wells), streams, or cisterns that collect rain water.[18] These households are responsible for ensuring the safety of their own drinking water. Private drinking water supplies that rely on surface waters, or wells that tap shallow groundwater layers, are at risk of contamination by pathogens from home septic systems, contaminants from leaking underground fuel storage tanks, improper disposal of various household chemicals (cleaners, automotive fluids), and agricultural chemicals (fertilizer, pesticides) applied to surrounding farm fields. *Nitrate* from agricultural fertilizer that leaches into shallow groundwater supplies poses a particularly widespread health risk in rural areas. The U.S. Geological Survey estimates that 10 to 20 percent of groundwater sources of drinking water may have levels of nitrate contamination that pose risks to human health.[19] Rural wells

---

> ### Key Terms
>
> **fecal coliform bacteria** A category of bacteria that live within the intestines of warm-blooded animals; the presence of these bacteria is used as an indicator that water has been contaminated by feces.
>
> **endocrine-disrupting chemicals** A large class of substances that can interact with the system of glands, hormones, and tissues that regulate many physiological processes in humans, including growth, development from fetus to adult, regulation of metabolic rate and blood sugar, function of reproductive systems, and development of the brain and nervous system.

---

contaminated by nitrate may also have high levels of other agricultural chemicals. See the section "Endocrine Disrupters" for information on the health effects of pesticides and herbicides.

Leaching of substances from pipes in the plumbing of older homes is another potential source of contamination to drinking water in the home.[20] Metallic pipes can release toxic metals such as lead and copper into the water. Polyvinyl chloride (PVC) pipes manufactured before 1977 may release toxic vinyl chloride into the water. Vinyl chloride is a known human carcinogen. Leaching of toxic substances from pipes into tap water is greatest in pipes with less than a 2-inch diameter when water temperature is high and the water is stagnant in the pipes for more than 24 hours.[20] To reduce your exposure to these contaminants from household plumbing, let the tap run for a couple of minutes before taking water to drink, especially first thing in the morning or if you have been away from home for a long time. In some cases, it may be advisable to replace the old plumbing, but this can be very expensive.

Private water supplies should be tested annually for nitrate and **fecal coliform bacteria.** If you suspect there may be a problem with radon or pesticide contamination, you may need to test your water even more frequently.[18] Testing will generally require that you send samples of your water to a laboratory that tests water quality. You can get a listing of local certified laboratories from your local or state public health department. Some local health departments test private water for free. A private laboratory will charge $10 to $20 to perform a nitrate and bacteria test. Testing for pesticides or organic chemicals may cost from several hundred to several thousand dollars. The results will indicate the concentrations of contaminants and indicate whether each contaminant exceeds a drinking water quality standard.

If your drinking water contains contaminants that exceed safety standards, you should retest the water supply immediately and contact your public health department for assistance. High bacteria concentrations can sometimes be easily controlled by disinfecting a well. Water filters may also remove some contaminants. However, other problems may require a new source of water, such as a deeper well. Alternatively, you may need to rely on bottled water until a new water source can be obtained.[18] You can obtain technical assistance with residential drinking water supply problems from the organization Farm*A*Syst / Home*A*Syst (see the websites http://www.uwex.edu/farmasyst or http://www.uwex.edu/homeasyst). See the box "Reducing Your Contribution to Water Pollution" for steps you can take to help keep your drinking water safe on page 533.

Endocrine Disrupters

Endocrine-disrupting chemicals include a number of infamously dangerous pollutants (dioxin, PCBs, DDT), a large number of pesticides, herbicides, antiseptics, and chemicals used in the manufacture of plastics (phthalates, bisphenol A or BPA) and Teflon (perfluorooctanoic acid, PFOA). These chemicals enter the home and work environment as contaminants of air, food, and water in household plastics, nonstick cookware, and in a range of personal products such as cosmetics, hair spray, perfumes, soap, and shampoo. Many of these substances are not readily eliminated from the body and tend to accumulate; large proportions of the human population in the United States have measurable amounts of these substances in their bodies.[21]

Agricultural pesticides and herbicides that act as endocrine disrupters include some of the most widely used chemicals in our food production system (e.g., the herbicide Atrazine). Your exposure to these chemicals can occur via pesticide residues on fruit and vegetables or contamination of well water (in locations with large areas of farmland). These chemicals have been linked to testicular and breast cancer, reduced sperm production in men, and nervous disorders in children.[22]

Phthalates are a class of endocrine disrupters that has become a recent source of concern after analyses of urine from a random sample of people in the United States indicated that virtually the entire population has measurable quantities of one or more of these chemicals in their bodies.[21] This is likely because of the almost ubiquitous use of phthalates in soft plastics used for food packaging, toys, and many personal hygiene products. Phthalates are released from plastics to air, water, and food and are readily absorbed across the skin and via the lungs and digestive tract. Phthalates disrupt the action of the sex hormones estrogen and testosterone, affecting both reproductive development of fetuses and children and reproductive function of adults.[23] Disruption of hormonal balance at critical stages in the development of a fetus or child can have long-lasting effects.[24] Some have suggested that increases in occurrence of breast and testicular cancer, and decreases in human sperm quality, in recent decades may be linked to exposure to endocrine-disrupting chemicals such as phthalates.[25] As these health risks associated with phthalates have become better documented, major retail stores (e.g., WalMart, Toys R Us, and Target) have required their suppliers to reduce or eliminate these chemicals from the plastics used for children's toys.

Bisphenol A (BPA) is a component of polycarbonate plastic containers used for food and drink and epoxy resins used to line food and drink cans. This substance can leach from the container wall into the food or drink within, which is then consumed. A recent report documented that 93 percent of the U.S. population has measurable amounts of BPA in their body fluids, with the highest levels measured in children and women.[26] The health effects of BPA are currently a source of controversy. The U.S. Food and Drug Administration released a report in April 2008 stating that current evidence indicates BPA is safe at current levels of exposure.[27] However, a paper later published in a prestigious medical journal indicated that current BPA exposure may increase risk of developing type 2 diabetes and heart and liver disease.[28] There is ongoing research to assess the health effects of BPA.

It can be difficult for you to avoid exposure to endocrine-disrupting chemicals when the health effects of many chemicals widely used in consumer products are not yet well known. Both phthalates and BPA have been widely used for decades. Initial studies indicated these substances were not toxic to humans, and so they were deemed safe. Widespread use in various products has resulted in most of the U.S. population having some amounts of these substances in their bodies. Later research has shown that these chemicals may have subtle adverse health effects that develop only after long-term exposure. There are many such chemicals in the various modern consumer products that you bring into your personal environment. These chemicals provide a wide range of benefits. But with the benefits, you may also incur risks. The best way to protect yourself is to be aware of health-related news and to act when new information identifies risks that you can reduce or eliminate from your life.

Noise

Noise can be defined as any undesirable sound. What constitutes "undesirable sound" will vary from one person to the next, but it often involves loud sounds that occur at irregular intervals and cannot be controlled by the listener.[29] In the personal environment of the home, neighborhood, and workplace, noise may include overly loud music, barking dogs, motorcycles and cars with broken muffler systems, loud machinery, appliances and power tools, airplanes flying overhead, and train whistles.

Health Effects of Noise The health effects of environmental noise depend on the intensity, frequency, and nature of the noise. Excessively loud noise can cause physical damage to sensory tissues in your ears, resulting in partial or total hearing loss that can be temporary or permanent. This physical damage will depend on both the intensity (as measured in decibels) and the duration of exposure to the loud noise. A common source of long-term exposure to loud sound that causes hearing loss in many young people is amplified music. Occasional loud rock music at 110 to 120 db may cause only temporary damage. However, daily exposure to such sound levels will cause permanent hearing loss. Jacking up the volume of your iPod or car stereo may be fun today, but is it worth a lifetime of incessant ringing in your ears and diminished hearing later in life? Ironically, damage caused by excessively loud sounds robs you of one of your most important senses, the ability to hear the unamplified human voice.

Even noise at lower levels can cause adverse health effects. The American Speech-Language-Hearing Association reports that low-level noise can elevate blood pressure, reduce sleep, cause fatigue, and disturb digestion. These physical effects of low-level noise can diminish emotional, intellectual, social, and occupational health. Effects reported by the World Health Organization include increased frustration and anxiety, impaired ability to concentrate, reduced productivity and ability to learn, and increased absenteeism and accidents. These effects of noise can increase your feeling of stress and cause you to exhibit anger and aggression that are out of proportion to the immediate source of your irritation.[29] This antisocial behavior may have negative consequences in your personal relationships and occupational health.

The Community and Regional Environment

The community and regional environment is made up of the outdoor air you breathe, local rivers and lakes that provide water and recreation opportunities, surrounding lands (urban, industrial, suburban, rural, agricultural, natural communities), and all the people and other species that live in these areas. A wide range of human activities can degrade this community environment in ways that affect personal health. Air, water, and land pollution include many substances that have significant negative effects on physical health. Loss of natural areas and other recreational and aesthetic "green space" to roads, cities, and industrial development can adversely affect your perceived quality of life, with negative effects on emotional and spiritual health. Degraded environmental conditions in many communities discourage new economic development and may limit occupational health.

While you can exert some influence on the environmental conditions in your community, the influence of any one individual is usually small. Your control over how the community environment affects your personal health is often limited to controlling your exposure to

---

Key Terms

air pollution Substances in the atmosphere that can have adverse effects on human health, crop productivity, and natural communities.

polycyclic aromatic hydrocarbons (PAHs) Air pollutants from fossil fuel combustion.

---

known health risks, such as contaminated water and land or outdoor air pollution. You can also choose to reduce your own contributions to community/regional air, water, and land pollution through conservation of energy and water and recycling solid waste.

Because one person cannot have a significant impact on community environmental problems, many people join organizations that work to improve the environment and quality of life in their community. By working with others of like mind in the political process and in environmental organizations, you become "part of the solution" to major environmental problems that can affect your health and that of your family. For many people, getting involved in solving local environmental problems can provide significant benefits to emotional and spiritual health.

In this section you will learn about aspects of the community and regional environment that can affect your health, and what you can do to exert some level of personal control over these environmental influences.

Air Pollution

Air pollution includes substances that naturally occur in the air (pollen, microbes, dust, sea salt, volcanic ash) and substances produced by human activities (engine exhaust, ozone, various volatile organic compounds, and acid rain). In this section on community and regional environmental influences on health, we focus on those components of air pollution that are produced within a specific region and that have substantial health effects within that community or region.

Sources of Air Pollutants The primary sources of human-caused air pollutants are various kinds of internal combustion engines associated with electric power plants, industry, and transportation (trucks, automobiles, and farm/construction equipment). Oil refineries and chemical production factories also contribute to air pollution in some communities. Electric power stations, industrial facilities, and chemical factories are classified as *point sources* that produce large amounts of pollution from a single location (see the box "Race, Economic Status, and Exposure to Pollution"). Automobiles, trucks, heavy construction/farm equipment, gas stations, lawn mowers, and charcoal grills are *nonpoint sources* of air pollutants. Individually, nonpoint sources produce relatively small amounts of pollution but, when added together, account for a large proportion of community air pollution.

Health Effects of Air Pollutants Air pollutants that are directly produced by internal combustion engines include *carbon monoxide, nitrogen dioxide, sulfur dioxide, polycyclic aromatic hydrocarbons,* and *particulate matter.* Carbon monoxide is a toxic gas that impairs respiration,

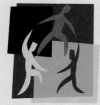

Learning from Our Diversity

Race, Economic Status, and Exposure to Pollution

When it is impossible to prevent all pollution, it is important to know if the risk of adverse health effects due to exposure is fairly distributed across the population. The "environmental justice" movement studies whether people of color and people who are economically or politically disadvantaged are disproportionately exposed to environmental hazards and more likely to suffer associated injury or disease than the general population. This movement gained prominence after a report found that new hazardous waste dumps were being disproportionately located in communities with high proportions of racial minorities and low-income families.* In the years since, researchers have studied this issue in various regions of the United States. Many, but not all, studies have found evidence that environmental hazards are more likely to be in or near areas with a high percentage of minority and low-income population.

Two hypotheses have been proposed for this association between race, class, and pollution: (1) *Industrial siting decisions:* pollution producers prefer to locate their facilities in areas that have cheap real estate and/or where the community is less able to resist (poor and uneducated); and (2) *move-in decisions:* hazardous pollution sources reduce the value of surrounding housing and land, attracting low-income renters and homeowners who tend to be disproportionately of racial and ethnic minorities.† While there is evidence for both phenomena, siting decisions appear to be the primary factor.

Issues of environmental justice are not restricted to industrial pollution and hazardous waste dumps. In recent years, the siting of large confined-animal feeding operations (CAFOs) has stirred much controversy in rural areas of the United States. These mainly corporate-affiliated facilities generate millions of gallons of animal waste that is stored in sewage lagoons. Sewage lagoons can emit large amounts of hydrogen sulfide (rotten egg smell) and ammonia into the atmosphere. These very unpleasant-smelling air pollutants result in adverse physical health effects, diminished quality of life, and reduced land value in the area around the CAFO.‡ Studies in the southeastern United States

have provided evidence that new hog CAFOs were being preferentially sited in areas with high proportions of African American and low-income families.§

Studies of the impact of increased exposure to air pollutants in low-income and minority-dominated communities have documented increased risk of cancer and respiratory distress and decreased academic performance of students in schools located in these communities.** This latter effect acts to strengthen the cycle of poverty, as lowered academic performance by children in poor neighborhoods contributes to reduced future opportunities for economic advancement.

These and other studies have motivated a social and political environmental justice movement that helps disadvantaged communities resist attempts to build new pollutant sources near their neighborhoods. Governmental recognition of the environmental justice issue has resulted in new laws and regulations for land-use planning and permits that require builders of new pollutant sources to specifically address issues of disproportionate pollution exposure of minority and low-income populations. If we all benefit from the products made by industries that produce pollutants, fairness requires that we also share equally the health costs of associated pollutants. If we all share equally the costs and benefits of industry, perhaps there will be greater motivation to develop less-polluting technologies.

*United Church of Christ. *A National Report on the Racial and Socio-Economic Characteristics of Communities with Hazardous Waste Sites.* 1987. UCC Committee for Racial Justice, New York.
†Pastor M, et al. Which Came First? Toxic Facilities, Minority Move-in, and Environmental Justice. *Journal of Urban Affairs,* 23 (1), 1–21. 2001.
‡Donham K, et al. Community Health and Socioeconomic Issues Surrounding Concentrated Animal Feeding Operations. *Environmental Health Perspectives,* 115, 317–320. 2006.
§Wing S, et al. Environmental Justice in North Carolina's Hog Industry. *Environmental Health Perspectives,* 108, 225–231. 2000.
**Pastor M, et al. Reading, Writing, and Toxics: Children's Health, Academic Performance, and Environmental Justice in Los Angeles. *Environment and Planning C: Government and Policy,* 22, 271–290. 2004.

as described under indoor air quality in the previous section. Nitrogen and sulfur oxides interact with water vapor in the air to form small particulates (diameter $<2.5\ \mu m$) that are inhaled into the deepest parts of the lungs. These substances can damage lung tissues, reduce lung capacity, cause coughing and chronic bronchitis, and make worse such ailments as hypersensitivity to allergens, asthma, emphysema, and heart disease. The U.S. Environmental Protection Agency estimates that over 70 million people in the United States live in counties where levels of small-particulate air pollutants exceed human health standards for at least some part of the year.[30] It has been estimated that small-particulate air pollution causes as many as 50,000 to 100,000 premature deaths in the United States per year.[31]

Polycyclic aromatic hydrocarbons (PAHs) have been shown to be carcinogenic to both test animals and humans. Several new studies indicate that PAHs can cross the placenta and have adverse health effects on a developing human fetus.[32, 33] Increased maternal exposure to PAHs was associated with lower birth weight, smaller head circumference, and reduced birth length of newborn children.[32] A study of mothers and newborns living in large cities in the United States, Poland, and China documented a significant association between maternal exposure to PAHs and PAH-linked DNA damage in newborns that is associated with increased risk of cancer.[33] This type of DNA damage was detected in 42 percent and 61 percent of two groups of newborns in New York City (where PAH exposure was lowest), 71 percent

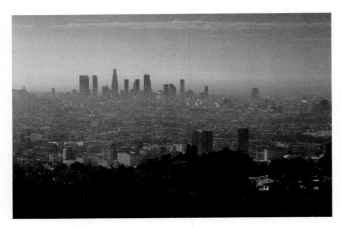

Tropospheric ozone is a key component of smog, which is especially common in certain parts of the United States.

of newborns in Krakow, Poland, and 80 percent of newborns in Tongliang, China (where PAH exposure was highest).

Tropospheric ozone is produced when hydrocarbons, nitrogen oxides, and other small-particulate matter chemically interact in the presence of sunlight. The result is a brownish haze over affected cities, often called *smog*.

Ozone levels are particularly high in locations with warm, sunny climates (southern California) and where natural vegetation produces volatile organic compounds that contribute to the photochemical process that produces ozone (eastern United States). The U.S. Environmental Protection Agency estimates that over 110 million people in the United States live in counties where ozone levels exceed human health standards for at least some part of the year.[30] Most of these people live in southern California and near the East Coast between Virginia and southern Maine (see Figure 20-2).

Key Terms

tropospheric ozone Ozone comprises three oxygen atoms that are bound into a single molecule; tropospheric ozone refers to this substance as it occurs in the lower layer of the atmosphere, close to the ground.

air toxics A class of 177 toxic air pollutants identified by the U.S. Environmental Protection Agency as known or suspected causes of cancer or other serious health effects, such as reduced fertility, birth defects, or adverse environmental effects.

biological water pollutants Disease-causing organisms that are found in water.

toxic pollutants Substances known to cause cancer or other serious health effects.

Inhalation of ozone can cause lung damage that reduces lung capacity. This is a particular health risk to individuals who suffer from asthma, emphysema, or heart disease. On days when ozone concentrations are highest, local hospital emergency room visits associated with respiratory distress increase from 10 to 20 percent.[31] If you suffer from asthma or a chronic cardiovascular disease, you may want to think carefully before living in any of the noncompliance areas shown in Figure 20-2. There is also some evidence that childhood exposure to ozone can actually cause children to become asthmatic.[34, 35]

Air toxics are a diverse collection of hazardous air pollutants produced by electric power plants, industrial sources, and internal combustion engines that constitute an environmental health risk to people. Some of these substances are carcinogenic, some can cause birth defects, and others cause damage to lungs, nervous system, liver, and other organ systems. The most recent inventory of air toxics included data for 177 different pollutants and risk assessments for 133 substances for which health effects data were available.[36] This report estimated that air toxics in the United States will result in increased likelihood of developing cancer for between 1 and 25 individuals per million people in the population. This is a national average risk based on a lifetime of exposure to air pollution levels as they were in 1999. Individuals who live in urban areas would have a risk of 25 per million people, and those living near major highways or certain industrial areas would have a risk of over 50 per million people. As a result of the Clean Air Act of 1970, all air pollution has been steadily declining. Although the number of automotive sources of air pollution has been increasing, better technology and higher fuel efficiency standards are expected to reduce air toxics from this source.

Taking Action on Air Pollution Unfortunately, the degree to which you can control your own exposure to regional air pollution and the associated health risks is limited. In many larger urban areas, where air pollution levels are highest, weather reports in newspapers and on television often include information about air pollution. This information is often conveyed in color-coded alerts. A "yellow" air pollution alert means people who suffer from respiratory or cardiac diseases, or hypersensitivity to allergens, should stay indoors. An "orange" air pollution alert indicates that everyone should limit their outdoor activities to the minimum possible.

You can also help to lower regional air pollution levels by reducing your own contributions to this problem, such as

- Car pool, use mass transit, or telecommute (work at home via a computer network) to reduce air pollution from automobile exhaust.

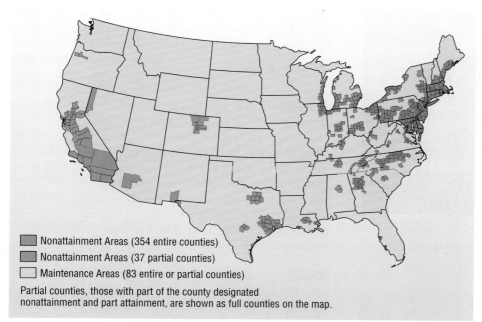

Figure 20-2 Exposure to Unhealthy Air
This map shows counties classified by the EPA as in "nonattainment" of ozone standards in the year 2007, meaning levels of ozone in the county exceeded the limit set by the EPA.
Source: U.S. Environmental Protection Agency.

Nonattainment Areas (354 entire counties)
Nonattainment Areas (37 partial counties)
Maintenance Areas (83 entire or partial counties)
Partial counties, those with part of the county designated nonattainment and part attainment, are shown as full counties on the map.

- Fill your gas tank, mow your lawn, and use your grill during cooler evening hours to reduce your contribution to tropospheric ozone.
- Conserve electricity to reduce emissions from electric power plants.

In areas of the United States where air pollution is especially problematic, local laws may require that you do some of these things on days when conditions result in a "pollution emergency."

Water Pollution

We humans have had a very "schizophrenic" relationship with our rivers and lakes. Water is an essential resource for all living things on our planet, including humans and the plants and animals we use for food. We also value our rivers and lakes for the recreational opportunities and aesthetic benefits they provide. Yet for decades we used these water bodies as convenient dumps for our sewage and industrial wastes.

The problem of water pollution came to national attention on a day in 1968 when children playing with matches set on fire chemical pollutants that covered the Cuyahoga River in Ohio. The subsequent public outcry resulted in major national legislation, including the Clean Water Act of 1972 and the Safe Drinking Water Act of 1974. Since then, substantial progress has been made in reducing water pollution and ensuring safe drinking water supplies. However, the job of cleaning up rivers and lakes in the United States is not complete, and people who come into close contact with contaminated waters or fish from these areas are still at risk for a variety of health problems.

Sources of Water Pollution   Water pollutants in surface waters come from obvious point sources (sewer overflows, confined livestock feedlot operations, sometimes called "factory farms") and from nonpoint sources such as water runoff from urban streets and agricultural areas that carries various chemicals and animal waste into local rivers. In some areas, water drainage from mines carries toxic metals into nearby streams. Some of the most troublesome water pollutants in the United States today are described here.

Biological water pollutants from untreated sewage and drainage from leaking home septic systems include various species of disease-causing viruses, bacteria, and protozoa found in rivers and lakes. The largest sources of biological water pollutants in United States surface waters today are overflows from urban combined septic and storm sewers during heavy rainfall and animal wastes that are carried by runoff of rainfall from agricultural areas. Although much has already been done to eliminate biological contamination from municipal sewer systems, billions of dollars are still required to dig up old combined sewer systems and replace them with separate systems for sewage and storm water runoff. As large animal "factory farms" have become more common in rural America, government agencies have established regulations for the proper handling of the huge amounts of animal sewage they generate. Even so, violations of regulations and occasional accidents result in contamination of local surface waters with animal waste.

A wide variety of **toxic pollutants** can be found in surface and groundwater sources of drinking water. These substances include naturally occurring toxic elements (such as arsenic and mercury) produced by

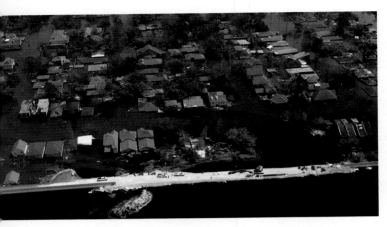

Agricultural runoff and the flow of untreated sewage into rivers during urban flooding are key sources of biological water pollutants.

breakdown of minerals in certain kinds of rock. Various industrial and agricultural human activities produce a wide range of toxic chemicals that find their way into U.S. surface waters, including metals, solvents, plastics, and PCBs (polychlorinated biphenyls). Some toxic substances, including arsenic and mercury, have both natural and human-caused sources. While the dumping of toxic substances into surface waters is now illegal, some of these toxins are very stable and can be found in large quantities in the sediments of rivers and lakes that were polluted before 1972. Cleaning up these toxic sediments can be very costly. A recent decision to dredge and dispose of PCB-contaminated sediments in the Hudson River near Albany, New York, will cost hundreds of millions of dollars.

Agricultural pesticides can be significant toxic water pollutants in parts of the United States where large areas of land are used for crop production. These chemicals include insecticides, fungicides, and herbicides to kill organisms that consume or compete with crop plants. Rainfall can carry these chemicals from croplands into local streams and rivers.

Health Effects of Water Pollution The organisms present in biological pollution cause diseases that are at best uncomfortable (diarrhea) and at worst potentially lethal (dysentery, hepatitis, typhoid fever, and cholera). In the late 1800s, diseases associated with drinking water contaminated by biological pollution were the third leading cause of death in the United States.[37] When surface water polluted with these organisms is used for crop irrigation of fruit and vegetables, these foods can become contaminated and cause disease or death (as seen in recent foodborne *E. coli* outbreaks).

Health effects of agricultural chemicals and other toxic substances depend on the specific chemical.[37]

Taken as a group, these substances have been linked to adverse effects on the blood, liver, spleen, kidney, adrenal gland, thyroid gland, reproductive system (fertility), and cardiovascular system. Some are known or suspected human *carcinogens* (substances that cause cancer), *mutagens* (substances that cause cell mutations), or *teratogens* (substances that cause birth defects). Obvious health effects that occur immediately after exposure to high concentrations of these substances include nausea, fatigue, headache, skin and eye irritation, or tremors. The risks for these immediate adverse health effects are greatest for workers who come in direct contact with the concentrated chemicals. More insidious are health effects such as cancer and birth defects that develop slowly, imperceptibly, after long-term exposure to low concentrations of these chemicals in the environment.

Taking Action on Water Pollution At present, your personal risk of exposure to biological water pollution in the United States is relatively small. Public health departments monitor local surface waters for the presence of fecal coliform bacteria in every U.S. county. While they may or may not cause illness or disease, the presence of fecal coliform organisms is an indicator that water has been contaminated by sewage. All municipal drinking water systems and many private households in the United States treat their water to kill pathogenic organisms. By the end of the twentieth century, deaths due to water pathogens in the drinking water supply were very rare in the United States.[37] It is also important to wash fresh vegetables before eating them, just in case they have been contaminated by polluted irrigation water.

The best way for you to minimize physical health risks posed by waterborne biological or toxic contaminants is to be well informed. Read the annual water quality report from your municipal water supplier that lists the amounts of biological contaminants, agricultural pesticides, and toxic substances detected in its water. If your supplier does not provide a report, you can access the supplier's annual report to the U.S. Environmental Protection Agency at www.epa.gov/safewater/dwinfo.htm. These reports list mean and range (minimum and maximum) concentrations for all regulated contaminants for all samples analyzed in a year. Look at the maximum value to determine if your water system occasionally fails to adequately remove any regulated contaminants. If your water supplier fails to meet health standards, consider drinking bottled, boiled, or filtered water until the supplier fixes the problems. Reverse osmosis water filters can be installed under a household sink and will remove most contaminants from drinking water at a cost of pennies per gallon.

You can also be exposed to toxic water pollutants by eating contaminated fish. Some toxic substances, such as mercury and PCBs, accumulate in high levels in the bodies of shellfish and fish that live in contaminated water. This problem can occur even in remote, apparently pristine areas if there are natural sources of toxic substances such as mercury. People who regularly consume fish from contaminated waters may be at high risk of adverse health effects. To reduce health risks associated with consuming fish, you should be aware of health advisories issued by the public health department or state agencies responsible for fish and game. These advisories are often stated in terms of limits on how much fish may be safely consumed in a specified time period. Pregnant women should be especially careful about consuming shellfish or fish; mercury and PCBs can cause birth defects in the fetus they carry. See Chapter 5 for more information.

You can also be exposed to waterborne pollutants as a result of recreational activities, such as swimming, boating, and backpacking. You can limit your personal risk of exposure to health risks from contaminated water by being aware of "Don't swim" warnings for your local rivers and lakes, usually issued by the public health department. If you are backpacking in an apparently pristine wilderness area, never assume that crystal-clear water in the mountain stream is safe to drink. Backpackers should always filter, boil, or chemically treat drinking water to kill pathogens that may be present even in such remote water sources. See the box "Reducing Your Contribution to Water Pollution" for actions you can take to reduce water pollution in your community.

Land Pollution

We do not physically consume land or soil the way we do air and water, but pollution of land can still result in serious adverse health effects. Disposal of toxic wastes often involves burying them in the ground. When done with proper safeguards, this disposal method can isolate these dangerous materials so they can do no harm to humans or natural systems. If done improperly, these toxic pollutants leach into groundwater or are carried into surface waters by the runoff of rain, where they cause serious ecological problems and pose significant human health risks.

Sources and Components of Solid Waste

Most land pollution today is associated with the disposal of **solid waste.** *Municipal solid waste* consists of everyday items such as product packaging, grass clippings, furniture, clothing, bottles, food scraps, newspapers, appliances, paint, and batteries. Other solid waste produced by business and industry includes waste tires, concrete, asphalt, bricks, lumber, and shingles from demolished buildings, and *sewage sludge* (solids remaining after wastewater treatment). In 2007 the U.S. population produced 254 million tons of solid waste, or about 4.6 pounds of waste per person per day (or 1,680 pounds per person per year).[38]

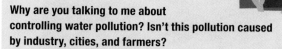

Changing for the Better

Reducing Your Contribution to Water Pollution

Why are you talking to me about controlling water pollution? Isn't this pollution caused by industry, cities, and farmers?

There are a number of actions you can take to reduce your personal contributions to community and regional water pollution, including:

1. Conserve water in the home to reduce the amount that must be processed by the wastewater treatment system.
2. Regularly check that the sewer or septic system on your property is functioning properly.
3. Minimize your use of lawn chemicals, and apply them in a manner that limits runoff into surface waters.
4. Never dispose of any household toxic chemicals (pesticides, solvents, oil-based paint, or automotive fluids) by dumping them down a sink drain, toilet, or storm sewer. These substances can adversely affect wastewater treatment plants.
5. Bring your toxic household chemicals and spent batteries to community-sponsored toxic waste collection centers that will arrange for proper disposal of these toxic substances.
6. To reduce biological contamination of water in remote wilderness areas, backpackers should defecate into a small hole located at least 100 feet from the nearest river or lake. Avoid defecating anywhere on the floodplain of a river; find a spot above the high water mark.

Disposal of Solid Waste

Municipal sanitation departments and private disposal companies are very efficient at removing these wastes from our homes and businesses and putting them someplace where we don't see them. These waste disposal locations include sanitary landfills (wastes are compacted and buried under soil), ocean dumping in garbage barges (with trash sometimes escaping to wash up on beaches), and incinerators (where solid wastes are burned).

As we run out of places to dump our solid waste, some have proposed that we burn it in large incinerators. However, many concerns have been raised about incinerators because they can release toxic substances into the atmosphere. Furthermore, the ash from these incinerators contains concentrated toxic chemicals in forms that can easily leach into ground and surface waters.

Key Terms

solid waste Pollutants that are in solid form, including nonhazardous household trash, industrial wastes, mining wastes, and sewage sludge from wastewater treatment plants.

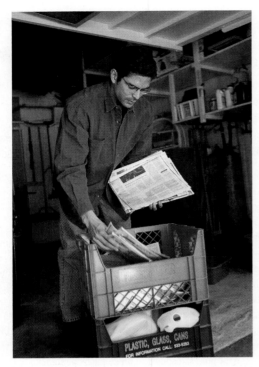
Recycling can reduce land pollution and consumption of natural resources.

Taking Action on Land Pollution   Most of the potential health effects of land pollution have already been described in this chapter under the topics of air and water pollution. Most human exposure to pollutants that are deposited on land occurs when those toxic substances end up in the air or water. You can limit your risk of these health effects by being aware of where solid wastes are disposed, both at the present time and in the past. You should be particularly aware of proximity to a local landfill or waste disposal site if your water source is a private well that draws from groundwater that might be contaminated.

You can reduce your personal contribution to the solid waste problem of your community by following the Three R's:

- *Reduce* waste by consuming less, accepting less packing on the products you buy, and composting yard

waste or using a lawn mower with a mulching blade to eliminate grass clippings and leaves.

- *Reuse* bottles, zipper-closure storage bags, cloth shopping bags, and cloth diapers to reduce solid waste.

- *Recycle* newspapers, magazines, aluminum and steel cans, glass bottles, and many plastic containers instead of disposing of them in the trash.

You can also buy products made of recycled materials, such as recycled paper and plastic "wood" products, to support the market for recycled waste. Electronic equipment poses special waste and recycling challenges; see the box "The High-Tech Revolution and E-Waste."

Loss of Green Space

Loss of **green space** represents another kind of land pollution that can affect your quality of life and health. In many parts of the United States, green space is being converted to housing developments, shopping malls, industrial sites, and highways. Hundreds of large, brightly lit signs along the highways pollute the visual environment. Wildlife species disappear from your community and surroundings as their habitats are destroyed.

While development of green space for human uses may provide job opportunities and be beneficial for your occupational health, the "urban sprawl" nature of much of this development can adversely impact your physical, emotional, and spiritual health. Recent studies have shown that urban development that increases commute times to work or school is associated with decreased physical activity and increased prevalence of obesity and high blood pressure.[39] Increased time spent in a car commuting to work often comes at the expense of time spent in physical activities. The replacement of green space with urban sprawl can also adversely affect your emotional health and quality of life when you no longer see wild animals in your backyard or you feel that your community is becoming ugly.

Some communities have created land-use (zoning) plans that allow for economic development while protecting recreational and aesthetic values in their communities. These zoning plans can be controversial, as they try to balance the rights of private property owners with the welfare of the entire community. You can contribute toward protecting environmental quality in your community by supporting land-use planning and enforceable zoning laws that protect green space while allowing for responsible economic development.

Ionizing Radiation

Sources and Effects of Radiation   *Radiation* is a general term that refers to various forms of energy that are emitted by atoms and molecules when they undergo

---

Key Terms

green space Areas of land that are dominated by domesticated or natural vegetation, including rural farmland, city lawns and parks, and nature preserves.

ionizing radiation Electromagnetic radiation that is capable of breaking chemical bonds, such as X-rays and gamma rays.

The High-Tech Revolution and E-Waste

The high-tech revolution has produced mountains of obsolete electronic equipment that contains large amounts of toxic substances. Hundreds of millions of old computers, containing millions of pounds of lead, cadmium, chromium, and mercury, need to go somewhere. These toxic metals cause a wide range of severe health effects if they end up in the air, drinking water, or food supply.*[†] Only 6 percent of obsolete computers disposed of after 1998 were recycled. The remainder was deposited in landfills across the country. It is estimated that 70 percent of heavy metals such as lead and mercury going into U.S. landfills today comes from electronic waste. Several states, including California and Massachusetts, have banned disposal of computer monitors in landfills.*

While recycling computers is seen as the ideal solution to the problem of waste disposal, it is estimated that in 2007 only 18 percent of discarded TVs and computer products were recycled; only 10 percent of cell phones were recycled. In 2005, 61 percent of TVs and computer monitors collected for recycling were exported to other countries for recycling.[†] Most of these were exported to poor Asian countries where low-paid workers extract useful metals but with minimal or no protection from the toxic materials in the electronics. Materials that cannot be recycled are dumped into rivers or burned in open-air pits, exposing workers and surrounding communities to toxic substances. The practice of shipping toxic computer waste to underdeveloped countries is now banned by an international treaty, but the United States is the only developed nation that has not ratified this treaty. The "free market" justification for the practice of shipping toxic computer waste to underdeveloped countries is that this practice provides jobs and helps poor people. But some question the morality of giving poor people the choice between poverty and poisons.*

Given that the use of computers and electronics will only increase in the future, we must develop environmentally responsible computer recycling systems. Some computer manufacturers are already initiating computer take-back programs. In 2002, Rep. Mike Thompson introduced The Computer Hazardous-Waste Infrastructure Program (CHIP) Act that would require the Environmental Protection Agency to help set up computer recycling across the United States. As of 2008, the U.S. Congress has passed no legislation that specifically addresses e-waste disposal. Currently, the EPA regulates e-waste disposal under general hazardous waste disposal regulations that have so many loopholes, a recent U.S. Government Accountability Office report called for a major overhaul of these regulations.[‡]

The other, and perhaps most important, approach to the computer waste problem is to develop electronic equipment that is less toxic and more easily recycled. This will require development of and investment in new technologies. In our free market system, this will happen only when electronics manufacturers share the cost of dealing with e-waste.

*Puckett J., and others. *Exporting Harm: The High-Tech Trashing of Asia.* 2002. http://www.ban.org/E-waste/technotrashfinalcomp.pdf
[†]U.S. Environmental Protection Agency. *eCycling—Frequent Questions.* 2008. http://www.epa.gov/osw/conserve/materials/ecycling/faq.htm#recycled
[‡]U.S. Government Accountability Office. 2008. Electronic Waste: E.P.A. Needs to Better Control Harmful U.S. Exports Through Stronger Enforcement and More Comprehensive Management. GAO-08-1044. 67p.

---

change, including radio waves, infrared waves, visible light, ultraviolet waves, X-rays, and gamma rays. Each kind of radiation has different effects on biological materials and health. **Ionizing radiation** causes damage to biological structures such as DNA that can result in serious adverse health effects. Ionizing radiation is produced by nuclear reactions, and sources include medical X-rays, naturally occurring radioactive minerals such as uranium and radon, various radioactive materials used by industry, nuclear reactors and their waste products, and nuclear bomb explosions.

The health effects of exposure to X-rays and gamma radiation depend on many factors, including the duration, type, and dose of radiation and your individual sensitivity. Heavy exposure to these forms of radiation can occur if you are near a nuclear bomb blast or downwind of a major nuclear reactor accident. In such cases, exposure can cause *radiation sickness,* including intense fatigue, nausea, weight loss, hair loss, fever, bleeding from the mouth, and compromised immune system, usually resulting in death.

Exposure to lower levels of nuclear radiation can cause damage to eyes, skin, and reproductive organs and may result in birth defects in children. Since September 11, 2001, government officials have warned about the possibility of terrorists using "*dirty bombs,*" whereby conventional explosives are combined with radioactive materials. The resulting dispersion of radioactive matter by the conventional bomb blast and wind would contaminate land well beyond the area affected by the blast.

The Challenge of Nuclear Waste Disposal In the coming years, huge amounts of radioactive waste must be permanently stored where it cannot escape into our environment. Nuclear reactors that generate 20 percent of the U.S. electricity supply have been accumulating highly radioactive wastes on-site. The U.S. government plans to store these wastes permanently in underground salt caves below Yucca Mountain, Nevada. A major health concern raised about the U.S. nuclear waste disposal program is the need to transport large quantities of highly radioactive waste by truck or train across the United States. However, the current situation is not safe either. Hundreds of tons of high-level radioactive waste are dispersed across the country in shallow, water-filled temporary holding tanks adjacent to nuclear power plants.

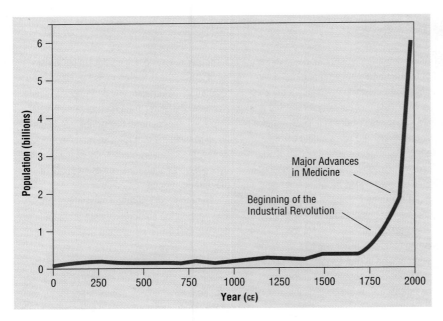

Figure 20-3 Growth of the Earth's Human Population
Source: U.S. Census Bureau, www.census.gov/ipc/www/worldhis.html.

The Global Environment

The global environment is made up of the atmosphere, oceans, continental land masses, and all the living organisms that exist on Earth. Interactions among these components of the global environment influence the characteristics of solar radiation at the ground level, climate (temperature, precipitation, seasonal variation), production of food plants and animals, availability of freshwater, energy requirements for heating and cooling of human habitations, the geographic distribution of diseases, the composition of natural communities (deserts, tundra, rain forest), and the survival and extinction of species.

Some of the characteristics of the global environment have obvious and direct effects on human physical health, such as the presence of disease-causing organisms or solar UV radiation that can increase the risk of skin cancer. Other effects of the global environment on personal health are less well documented, such as the adverse effects on emotional or spiritual health associated with the extinction of species or destruction of beautiful natural communities. Many scientists warn that the global environment is being degraded by the combined forces of ever more powerful technology being used by a rapidly increasing global human population. In this section we briefly describe major concerns regarding the global environment and how these might affect personal health. We end this section and the chapter with some thoughts about how you can take some degree of personal control over these global environmental problems and their influence on your health.

Human Population Explosion

Many scientists warn that the human population is increasing at a rate that cannot be sustained by the resources of the Earth (see Figure 20-3). There are currently over 6 billion people in the global human population, and this is projected to increase to over 10 billion in the next 50 years. Every year, the world's population grows by about 78 million people, with 97 percent born in the poorest countries.[40]

Effects of Human Population Growth The effects of the human population explosion on personal health depend on who you are and where you live. Many of the poorer nations of Asia, Africa, and South America will not be able to feed their people; starvation and associated diseases will be major health problems for these populations. Growing populations in dry regions are exceeding their freshwater supply, and hundreds of millions of people must drink from contaminated water sources. Every year, 5 million children die from waterborne diarrhea diseases associated with unsanitary drinking water.[40] By 2025, 2.5 billion people may live in regions where available freshwater is insufficient to meet their needs.

In many extremely poor countries, hungry people will destroy most or all of the remaining natural communities (tropical rain forests, African savanna) in vain efforts to grow food on lands that are not suited for agriculture. Overcultivation of farmlands to meet the demand for food has already degraded the fertility of a land area equivalent to that of the United States and

Canada combined.[40] Hungry people who live on oceanic islands often destroy their coral reefs trying to make a living by using dynamite or cyanide to catch fish. In Africa hungry people hunt wild game for food, putting more and more species at risk of extinction.

Competition among nations for limited supplies of water and oil is often a root cause of political tensions, terrorism, and war. Political upheaval in the Middle East, recent terrorist attacks on U.S. targets, and the war in Iraq can be partially explained by competition for scarce resources (water, land, and oil). The genocide that killed hundreds of thousands in Rwanda in 1994–1995 has been traced to inequitable distribution of land and associated hunger in some parts of that country.[41] Many fear that such social instability and strife will be the inevitable result of competition for scarce resources, associated with excessive human population growth and overconsumption of limited resources.

Reducing Human Population Growth

The solutions to the human population growth problem are simple in theory, but often complex in their implementation. Basic population ecology theory states that the rate of population growth can be reduced if (1) women have fewer children over their lifetime and (2) if they delay the birth of their first child. A somewhat counterintuitive pattern is that population growth rate slows when infant survival rate is increased by better health care. It has been documented in many countries that women choose to have fewer children if they are confident that their children will survive.[40]

Simply providing education opportunities to girls can have major and long-lasting effects that act to reduce population growth. Girls who become educated delay having their first child; educated women have half the pregnancies of their uneducated sisters.[40] Educated women are more likely to be employed outside the home. This has two effects: working women are too busy to care for large numbers of children, and women with an independent income have greater status and influence in deciding how many children they will have. Of course, universal access to birth control information and affordable contraception are also needed to allow women to have only as many children as they desire.

While this combination of commonsense actions can drastically reduce future human population growth, these proactive initiatives are often held hostage to political and cultural controversies. The sad result is that human populations may ultimately be controlled by increased death rates associated with starvation, disease, and war rather than reduced birth rates. For more information on issues related to population growth, visit the websites listed in the box "Organizations Related to Environmental and Population Control Concerns" on page 542.

Global Climate Change

Greenhouse Gases A wide range of human activities add **greenhouse gases** to the atmosphere that trap heat and cause a net gain of energy and increase in temperature in the Earth system. This increase in global temperature is called the "greenhouse effect" or "global warming." Greenhouse gases include water vapor, carbon dioxide, methane, chlorofluorocarbons, ozone, and nitrous oxides. Human-caused sources of greenhouse gases include carbon dioxide from both industrial and agricultural activities, including the burning of coal, oil, and natural gas, conversion of natural communities (grasslands, forests, and wetlands) to human uses, methane emissions from leaking natural gas pipelines, large herds of cattle, flooded rice fields, tropospheric ozone (described earlier in this chapter), chlorofluorocarbons from air-conditioner fluids, and nitrous oxide from agricultural fertilizer use. The average concentration of carbon dioxide in the atmosphere has increased 35 percent since the 1700s and currently exceeds the range of natural variation over the past 650,000 years. This increase is mostly due to burning of fossil fuels, and the rate of fossil fuel burning continues to increase. Atmospheric concentrations of the other greenhouse gases (methane and nitrous oxides) have also increased substantially during this period.[42]

There is growing evidence that increases in atmospheric greenhouse gases are associated with changes in global climate. Chemical analyses of gas bubbles in glacial ice core samples from the polar ice caps indicate that atmospheric carbon dioxide and methane concentrations have been closely related to changes in global temperature through several cycles of ice ages and warm periods during the past 420,000 years; when carbon dioxide and methane concentrations increased, so did atmospheric temperature.[42] The current increase in greenhouse gases is also associated with increasing global temperature. According to the websites for the National Oceanic and Atmospheric Administration (NOAA) and the World Meteorological Association, the year 2006 was the warmest ever recorded in the United States and the sixth warmest year for the entire Earth; the nine years from

> **Key Terms**
>
> **greenhouse gases** A category of gases in the atmosphere that allow solar radiation to pass through the atmosphere to the Earth but then trap the heat that is radiated from the Earth back toward space; greenhouse gases include water vapor, carbon dioxide, methane, nitrous oxide, and tropospheric ozone.

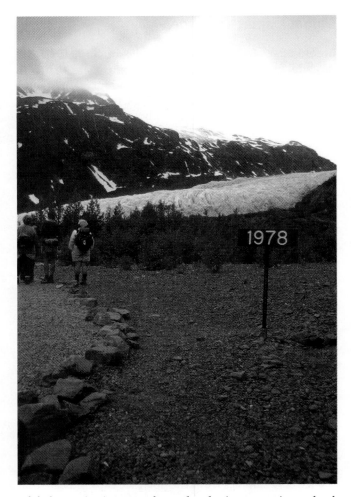

Global warming is expected to melt polar ice caps, raise sea level, and flood coastal areas. One result of recent warming is melting glaciers. The sign in this photo shows how far this Alaskan glacier has retreated since 1978.

1998 to 2006 were among the 25 warmest years in the United States since 1895. The rate of increase in temperature has been accelerating since the mid-1970s.

Most scientists around the world believe that the changes in global climate described previously are the first evidence of global climate change related to human activities. However, a vocal minority of scientists still question the relative contributions of humans versus natural processes, and whether or not this warming trend is a short-term phenomenon or the beginning of a long-term trend (see the box "Hype Versus Useful Information").

Effects of Climate Change Because climate is such a fundamental characteristic of the environment, global warming is expected to have diverse and widespread effects, including melting of the polar ice caps that raises sea level and floods coastal areas (including major coastal cities) and increased frequency and severity of

hurricanes and other destructive weather events. Effects of climate change on human health include increased heat stress, loss of life in storms and floods, expansion of the ranges of disease-carrying insects (such as mosquitoes) from subtropical regions into temperate regions (such as the United States), increased abundance of waterborne pathogens, decreased air and water quality, and decreased food availability associated with severe weather and water shortages. In 2003 a highly unusual heat wave in western Europe killed 35,000 people. While it is unknown if this event was linked to global warming, it proved the potential for severe climate events to have major impacts, even in economically developed countries. In less developed countries, millions of people have died from drought-related famine and severe storms (hurricanes and typhoons).

Taking Action on Climate Change Your ability as an individual to take personal responsibility for addressing the global warming problem is limited, but all good things must start with individuals willing to do the right thing. Ways you can reduce your personal contribution to global warming include:

- Conserve electricity at home by purchasing the most efficient appliances and heating/cooling systems, using compact fluorescent or LED lighting, and turning off computers, TVs, and lights when not in use. Compact fluorescent lighting consumes only 10 percent of the electricity compared with incandescent or halogen lighting.

- Insulate and weatherproof your home, and set your thermostat to lower temperatures in winter and higher temperatures in summer to reduce energy use for heating and cooling.

- Drive the most fuel-efficient vehicle that meets your needs, use mass transit if available, or telecommute for work if possible.

- Reduce, reuse, and recycle to reduce demand and production for consumer products.

- Use alternative energy sources (solar, wind, geothermal) as they become available at prices you can afford.

- Support governmental action to encourage development of alternative energy sources and discourage emissions of greenhouse gases. This is most effectively done through organized actions of groups dedicated to these causes and through active participation in the political process.

 TALKING POINTS How can you encourage your children to develop sound habits regarding their environment and their personal health? What changes can you make in your own habits to serve as a better example for them?

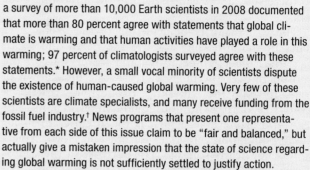

Hype Versus Useful Information

"The media" is one of the most powerful forces in American society and has influence across much of the Earth's human population. In the past 20 years, the media has experienced two very divergent trends: consolidation of "mainstream media" (newspapers, magazines, radio, and television) by a small number of large multinational corporations and fragmentation of media as more people create and view media via the Internet. Mainstream media controlled by for-profit corporations often filters news for its entertainment value. What is deemed sufficiently entertaining is hyped and repeated; uninteresting information is simply ignored. The explosion of Internet-based media has produced legions of bloggers and websites that present opinion and special-interest perspectives with little or no objectivity or error-checking. It is left to the consumer of Internet media to determine the credibility of the various sources of information.

The "entertainment filter" of mainstream media producers may not interact well with issues of environmental health. Many environmental problems are complex and affect human health in subtle ways over long periods. For example, the U.S. population is being exposed to hundreds, if not thousands, of chemicals that have not been tested for human toxicity. They are found in our air, water, and food supply. They are found in our bodily fluids and hair. Some have been shown to cause cancer and birth defects in laboratory animals. The U.S. Environmental Protection Agency estimates that air pollution in major U.S. cities contributes to thousands of deaths from respiratory and cardiovascular disease each year. In the last 20 to 30 years, cancer rates in the U.S. population have increased substantially, while fertility of men as measured by sperm counts has been declining by 1 to 3 percent per year. When was the last time you heard about these issues on the evening news or read about them in a newspaper or magazine? By way of comparison, many people know that the polar bear is endangered by global warming and melting of the polar ice cap. Although Al Gore demonstrated in *An Inconvenient Truth* that it is possible to communicate complex environmental issues in an entertaining manner, mainstream media producers seem to lack the motivation to do this with other complex issues.

When the mainstream media does cover an environmental health story, it is often presented as a debate to make it more interesting.

All too often, these debates give the misperception that an environmental health issue is unresolved, leading to inaction. For example, a survey of more than 10,000 Earth scientists in 2008 documented that more than 80 percent agree with statements that global climate is warming and that human activities have played a role in this warming; 97 percent of climatologists surveyed agree with these statements.* However, a small vocal minority of scientists dispute the existence of human-caused global warming. Very few of these scientists are climate specialists, and many receive funding from the fossil fuel industry.† News programs that present one representative from each side of this issue claim to be "fair and balanced," but actually give a mistaken impression that the state of science regarding global warming is not sufficiently settled to justify action.

On the positive side, it has never been easier to obtain information about environmental health issues on the Internet. Detailed reports can be downloaded from websites of the U.S. Environmental Protection Agency and the Centers for Disease Control. You can read articles in scientific journals and browse websites that present a diversity of information and opinions. However, when you "Google" an environmental health issue, you will need to exercise judgment about what you believe. Advocacy groups and industrial groups all have their own web presence where they promote their perspectives. The mainstream news media has self-correcting mechanisms; inaccurate statements are often exposed and the mistakes made public. Similar mechanisms have not been developed for the Internet. See the "Building Media Literacy Skills" box in Chapter 1 for suggestions about how to be a discerning user of information on the Web. These skills will help you identify important issues and questions and give you a better basis on which to make informed decisions for yourself.

*Doran P., and M. Zimmerman. 2009. Survey: Scientists Agree Human-Induced Warming Is Real. *Eos, Transactions, American Geophysical Union,* 20(3).
†Union of Concerned Scientists. 2007. Smoke, Mirrors, and Hot Air: How ExxonMobile Uses Big Tobacco's Tactics to Manufacture Uncertainty on Climate Science. http://www.ucsusa.org/assets/documents/global_warming/exxon_report.pdf

Stratospheric Ozone Depletion

The *stratospheric ozone layer* is a concentration of ozone molecules located about 10 to 25 miles above the Earth's surface. This "ozone layer" contains about 90 percent of the planet's ozone. Stratospheric ozone is a naturally occurring gas formed by the interaction of atmospheric oxygen and components of solar radiation. Unlike tropospheric (low-elevation) ozone, which has many adverse health and ecological effects, the stratospheric ozone layer has the beneficial health effect of protecting living organisms on the Earth's surface from harmful solar ultraviolet (UV) radiation.

Causes of Ozone Depletion   It has been well documented that chemical reactions between stratospheric ozone and certain human-made air pollutants can significantly reduce the ozone layer, causing increased UV radiation at the Earth's surface. The chemicals that cause ozone depletion include chlorofluorocarbons (CFCs, used as coolants in many air-conditioning and refrigeration systems, in insulating foams, and as solvents), halons (used in fire suppression systems), and methyl bromide (used in pesticides). When these substances are released to the atmosphere and rise to the stratosphere, they release either chlorine or bromine molecules. One chlorine molecule can destroy 100,000 ozone molecules, and these substances can remain in the atmosphere for years.[43]

The vast majority of depletion of the ozone layer occurs in the atmosphere above the north and south poles; the colder temperatures and ice crystals in the atmosphere over the poles increases the breakdown of ozone. In 2006 the Antarctic "ozone hole" reached a record size of 10.6 million square miles. Thankfully, the Arctic ozone hole, which is much closer to major human population centers in Europe and North America, was not nearly so large. The decrease in the stratospheric ozone layer has been associated with as much as a 50 percent increase in UV radiation at the ground level in Antarctica.[43] The ozone layer above the United States has decreased by only 5 to 10 percent.

Effects of Ozone Layer Depletion and Increased UV Radiation

For people, overexposure to UV rays can lead to skin cancer, cataracts (clouding of the lens of the eye), and weakened immune systems. Increased UV can also lead to reduced crop yield and reduced plant production in natural communities. The latter can result in less food for all the other species in the communities and disruption of the ocean's food chain.

Taking Action on Ozone Depletion

In response to the well-documented links between certain air pollutants and depletion of the ozone layer, and links between UV radiation and adverse health and ecological effects, the world community has worked to eliminate the use of ozone-depleting chemicals. For example, a complete ban on the production of halons and CFCs went into effect in the mid-1990s. As the amounts of ozone-depleting chemicals in the atmosphere decrease, the ozone layer is projected to recover to natural levels by the year 2050.[43] However, there remain thousands of tons of CFCs in older refrigeration and air-conditioning systems, including those in older automobiles. You can contribute to reducing ozone-depleting chemicals in the atmosphere by always having your refrigerator and air-conditioning systems serviced by licensed technicians who have the equipment to capture and properly dispose of old CFC chemicals.

To limit your risk of skin cancer and other UV-related health problems that can be exacerbated by ozone layer depletion, you should limit your exposure to direct sunlight, and when you are outside you should wear sunscreen on exposed skin. You should also wear sunglasses that are rated as eliminating over 95 percent of UV radiation. When traveling to parts of North America, Europe,

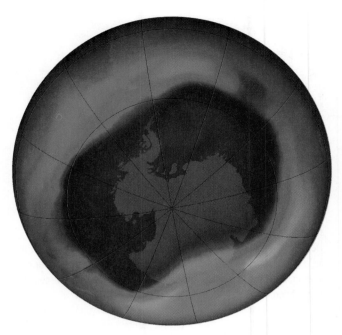

The "ozone hole" over Antarctica in 2006 was the largest to date. The depleted ozone layer in the atmosphere is expected to recover, but the process is slow and will likely take until about 2050.

South Africa, South America, and Australia that are close to the polar ozone holes, you should be aware of UV index information presented by the popular media. During months when the polar ozone holes are larger, you may want to further restrict your exposure to direct sunlight.

 TALKING POINTS Your sister is a sun worshipper who loves the look of a deep, dark tan. How might you persuade her to protect her skin from the rays of the sun?

Loss of Natural Habitats and Species Extinctions

Causes of Habitat Destruction and Species Extinctions

On every continent, an exploding human population armed with ever more powerful technology is altering or completely taking over the habitats of other species that share our planet. Over 20 percent of the total land surface of Earth has been converted entirely for human uses, and as much as 40 to 50 percent has been degraded by human activities.[44] Humans currently use 50 percent of the Earth's freshwater runoff, mostly for agricultural irrigation. Dams for electric power generation have impacted 94 percent of the rivers in the world.[45]

Human impact on the biosphere is not limited to the land. Humans consume 25 to 35 percent of the energy flow in coastal ocean waters.[44] As of 2003, 29 percent of all ocean fish populations exploited for human consumption had collapsed due to overharvesting. If current trends continue, all populations of ocean fish currently used for human food production will collapse by the year 2050.[46] Worldwide, 30 percent of all coral reefs have been destroyed by human activities. Coastal water pollution has been linked to increased frequency of fish kills and massive "dead zones" where nothing else can live.[45]

The cumulative effects of all these human-caused changes to the Earth's land and oceans have increased the species extinction rate by 100 to 1,000 times over rates estimated for the period before human domination. The primary causes of these extinctions are habitat loss due to human activities and overharvesting of species by humans.[45]

Personal Health Effects of Habitat Destruction and Species Extinctions

The effects on personal health associated with worldwide loss of natural communities and species extinctions are highly variable from person to person. Pharmaceutical companies have found many substances produced by species in various natural communities to be useful sources of drugs to treat human illnesses. As the richness of species on Earth is depleted by extinction, we lose a wealth of genetic material that could be of great importance to human health. The degradation and loss of natural ecosystems also undermines the systems that function to make Earth a livable planet, contributing to such problems as global climate change, freshwater shortages, and increased frequency of destructive flooding.

Some have proposed that human evolution predisposes us to be most happy when we are surrounded by natural beauty; this is called the *biophilia hypothesis*.[47] Many have written about the human psychological benefits from natural communities. John Muir, a famous early U.S. environmentalist, wrote:

> Climb the mountains and get their good tidings.
> Nature's peace will flow into you as sunshine flows into trees.
> The winds will blow their own freshness into you, and the storms their energy, while cares drop off like autumn leaves.

Wallace Stegner wrote a passage that appears in the Wilderness Act passed by the U.S. Congress in 1964 to protect areas of intact U.S. ecosystems for the enjoyment of future generations:

> We simply need that wild country available to us, even if we never do more than drive to its edge and look in. For it can be a means of reassuring ourselves of our sanity as creatures, a part of the geography of hope.

Both Muir and Stegner refer to the psychological benefits that humans derive simply from the knowledge that natural communities and wildlife species still exist somewhere on our planet. Try to imagine how you would feel about a world completely dominated and degraded by a massive human population; no great herds of caribou, zebra, and wildebeest moving like a tide across the landscape; no wolves, lions, tigers, or elephants to excite the imagination; no monarch butterflies sipping nectar in your backyard on their migration from Maine to Mexico; no dolphins and orcas playing in the ocean waves; no humpback whales singing in the depths; no coral reef wonderlands; no great, ancient trees stretching out of sight toward a clear blue sky; no expansive grasslands rippling in the breeze as far as the eye can see; the sky and waters tainted with pollution; the climate itself hostile to human civilization. The effects of such a dark and dismal world on the human psyche seem unimaginable. The thought of forever losing the natural wonders of our planet could have profoundly adverse effects on our emotional, psychological, and spiritual well-being. For many, the thought of such a dark future can cause anger, frustration, depression, hopelessness, and despair.[48]

Taking Action on Habitat Destruction and Species Extinction

How can you or any one person exert any degree of personal control over such a great and complex threat to your physical, emotional, and spiritual health? Start with the little things. Conserve energy, recycle and reuse, limit your consumption of resources to what you need, and join with others to support organizations that are working to solve these big problems (see the listing in the box "Organizations Related to Environmental and Population Control Concerns"). If you want to make a bigger personal commitment to solving global environmental problems, you could limit your own family size to at most two children. For a list of many more ways to reduce your personal impact on the Earth, go to the website www.earthshare.org/green-tips.html.

Another way you can reduce the negative environmental effects of your personal consumption of natural resources is to "buy green" when you can. In recent years, environmental organizations have begun certification programs so that the consumer can identify which products are produced by "Earth-friendly" means (for more information, see www.newdream.org/buy). Examples of such products include sustainably harvested timber, shade-grown coffee, and organic food and cotton (see the box "Is Organic Food Good for the Environment?"). These products are often more expensive, because they are produced by methods that lack the efficiency of environmentally destructive production systems. When you "buy green," you support Earth-friendly producers and reduce economic pressure to destroy natural communities. Many "buy-green" organizations also work to improve economic conditions in villages where their producers live. These efforts improve educational opportunities and health care, resulting in reduced birth rates,

Organizations Related to Environmental and Population Control Concerns

Population Issues

The following organizations provide material and informational support to women and men worldwide who seek to protect their reproductive health and to control their family size.

United Nations Population Fund: www.unfpa.org

International Planned Parenthood Federation: www.ippf.org

The Population Institute: Provides information on the social and environmental consequences of rapid population growth, and advocacy for governmental support of voluntary family planning programs: www.populationinstitute.org

Environmental Political Advocacy Groups

The private environmental organizations listed use the political and legal system to promote responsible use of the Earth's ecosystems and resources and to provide information to the public about a full range of environmental issues. Some also employ scientists, policy analysts, and lawyers in support of lobbying and litigation in support of environmental protection.

Sierra Club: www.sierraclub.org

Wilderness Society: www.wilderness.org

National Wildlife Federation: www.nwf.org

Natural Resources Defense Council: www.nrdc.org

Environmental Defense: www.environmentaldefense.org

The League of Conservation Voters: A political action organization that provides information to voters on the voting records of politicians regarding environmental issues. This organization also campaigns to elect candidates who support environmentally responsible policies: www.lcv.org

Conservation of Natural Communities and Endangered Species

The Nature Conservancy: Uses private donations to purchase, protect, and manage important natural communities and habitats in the United States and throughout the world (117 million acres worldwide, as of 2007). www.nature.org

World Wildlife Fund: Privately funded organization that works to protect endangered species and threatened habitats around the world and to reduce pollution and climate change: www.panda.org

Sources of Environmental Information

World Resources Institute: A privately funded "think tank" that compiles environmental and economic data from around the world and publishes environmental policy analyses to promote a worldwide transition to an ecologically sustainable, socially just society: www.worldwatch.org

U.S. Environmental Protection Agency: The agency within the U.S. federal government responsible for monitoring environmental quality and enforcing environmental laws and regulations. This agency provides a wide range of environmental information to the public: www.epa.gov

Considering Complementary Care

Is Organic Food Good for the Environment?

Certified "organic" food in the U.S. is produced under guidelines set out by the Organic Foods Production Act. The guidelines in this law stipulate materials and practices that enhance the balance of natural systems and that integrate parts of the farming system into an ecological whole.

The primary goal of organic agriculture is to optimize the health and productivity of interdependent communities of soil life, plants, animals, and people. Organic farms that produce grain, fruits, and vegetables may not use synthetic pesticides or fertilizers. Meat producers must feed their livestock only organically produced feedstuffs. In addition, many organic meat producers forego the use of growth hormones and antibiotics that stimulate livestock growth rates. Although organic foods have not been shown to be any more nutritious than nonorganic food, organic foods have fewer chemical residues that may adversely impact human health.* A recent study documented that when elementary school children were switched from a conventional diet to an organic food diet, pesticide residues in their urine dropped to nondetectable levels. As soon as the children were returned to a conventional diet, the concentration of pesticide residues in their urine increased again.† Hence, people who are concerned about the health effects of pesticides, antibiotics, and hormone residues in their food might consider switching to certified organic foods.

This description of organic food suggests that organic farming practices are also good for the environment. Organic farming puts far less pollution into local water and air, and fewer chemicals into the food supply. Local farmers can often make greater profits through direct sales of organic produce to local cooperatives or other consumer-supported agriculture organizations. This may help preserve local green space against encroachment by suburban developers. Hence, organic farming can certainly be good for the local community environment. It is unclear whether a wholesale shift to organic farming methods would be able to supply enough food to feed a growing global human population without bringing more areas (including natural areas, parks, and preserves) under cultivation.‡ However, there is also uncertainty about whether intensive, chemical-dependent agricultural systems that degrade soil and are dependent on fossil fuels are sustainable in the long term.

*Cable News Network Interactive. 1998. In-Depth: Organic Food. http://www.cnn.com/HEALTH/indepth.food/organic/index.html
†Lu C et al. Organic diets significantly lower children's dietary exposure to organo-phosphorous pesticides. *Environmental Health Perspectives,* 114(2), 260–263, 2006.
‡Center for Global Food Issues. 2002. Growing More Food per Acre Leaves More Land for Nature. http://www.highyieldconservation.org

slowing the human population growth that is the root cause for many environmental problems.

The combined actions of 6 billion people making personal choices will determine the future of the Earth's environment and thus the future of humankind. The solutions to the great environmental problems looming in the future begin with you, today. Your positive actions and faith in fellow humans to do the right thing will not only benefit the future, but also enhance your emotional well-being in the present.

Taking Charge of Your Health

- All environmental problems and their associated health risks begin with personal choices regarding resource consumption, waste disposal, and electing leaders who set policies and regulations. When you make your choices, consider the environmental consequences and act in ways that promote a healthy environment for all people and other living things on Earth.

- Be aware of environmental hazards in the air, water, and materials in your personal environment and work to minimize or eliminate these hazards.

- Reduce your own consumption of natural resources, and dispose of wastes responsibly.

- Be aware of government policies regarding natural resource exploitation, pollution, and habitat destruction.

- Vote for leaders who are more concerned with the quality of the environment of all people and other species than they are for economic special interests.

- When that small voice inside you says, "Forget it, there is nothing I can do," don't listen! That voice is leading you toward a life of cynicism and despair. For your own psychological, emotional, and spiritual well-being, have faith that the actions of individuals can accumulate to bring about world change.*

*For more information, see Ellison K. A Question of Faith. *Frontiers in Ecology and the Environment,* 1(1), 56, 2003.

SUMMARY

- Environmental influences on personal health operate over a wide range of spatial scales, from the personal spaces of your home and workplace, to the common spaces of your community and region, to the global environment that supports all life on Earth.
- You can exert the greatest degree of control over your exposure to pollutants within the personal environment of your home and workplace. You can identify environmental health risks in your personal environment, and then eliminate or reduce these risks by changing your buying habits and eliminating pollutant sources.
- Air pollution in major urban areas can cause serious adverse health effects, especially for people who suffer from respiratory or cardiac disease.
- Much progress has been made in reducing community water pollution, but water and fish in many rivers and lakes still contain chemicals and pathogens that can adversely affect your health.
- Loss of green space in your community and regional environment, associated with urban sprawl and unregulated land development, can diminish your perceived quality of life, and reduce opportunities for exercise, which is important for maintaining good physical health.

- While you have limited personal control over the environment of your community and region, you can still work to enhance your environment by joining others of like mind in groups that advocate environmental protection through the democratic political process.
- At the current rate of human population growth, most scientists of the world warn of increased starvation and disease, decreased standards of living, and increased conflict over progressively decreasing supplies of natural resources.
- Pollutants produced by humans are responsible for changes in the atmosphere that are altering climate patterns and allowing harmful solar radiation to reach the surface of the Earth.
- Changes in the global environment have potential to increase risks to human health and to significantly harm many other species and natural communities.
- While individuals can do little to address global environmental problems, the solutions all start with individual choices about family size, resource consumption, and political candidates. The best path to a livable future for humankind is to do your part and have faith that others will do theirs.

REVIEW QUESTIONS

1. Identify the sources and the potential health effects of the following common indoor air pollutants: carbon monoxide, volatile organic compounds, and biological pollutants such as mold, mildew, pollen, and pet dander. Describe actions you could take to minimize health risks from these pollutants.

2. What health risks are associated with lead and asbestos? What actions can you take to minimize these risks?

3. Tropospheric ozone and small-particulate matter are community and regional air pollutants that have been linked to serious health risks. For each of these substances, describe the main human sources, the effect(s) on human physical health, and what actions you could take to minimize your own risk of adverse health effects from these air pollutants.

4. What are "air toxics" and where do you think you are most likely to be exposed to these substances? What do you think you could do to minimize your personal health risk from air toxics?

5. What are some pollutants that might be in drinking water from a tap in your home? What are the main sources of these pollutants? What can you do to minimize the risk to your personal health from water pollutants?

6. What is "green space," and why is it important to your personal health? What personal actions could you take to protect green space in your community or region?

7. What policies should the U.S. foreign aid agencies implement in poor underdeveloped countries to help them reduce their population growth rate? Explain how these policies would work toward this goal.

8. Global warming and stratospheric ozone depletion are large-scale changes in the global environment with uncertain, but potentially significant, health consequences. For each of these global changes, describe the cause(s) of environmental change, the potential health effects, and what might be done to minimize these effects.

9. Loss of natural habitats and species extinctions are major ecological problems, but do these phenomena represent any risk to *your* personal health? Your answer should reflect your own perceptions and should provide some explanation for your assessment.

10. A well-known environmentalist slogan is "Think globally, but act locally." Based on what you've learned in this chapter, describe how you think this slogan applies to your personal actions in response to environmental health risks.

ANSWERS TO THE "WHAT DO YOU KNOW?" QUIZ

1. True   2. False   3. True   4. False   5. False   6. True   7. True

Visit the Online Learning Center (**www.mhhe.com/payne11e**), where you will find tools to help you improve your grade including practice quizzes, key terms flashcards, audio chapter summaries for your MP3 player, and many other study aids.

SOURCE NOTES

1. U.S. Environmental Protection Agency. *Healthy Buildings, Healthy People: A Vision for the 21st Century*, 2003. http://www.epa.gov/iaq/hbhp/index.html

2. U.S. Environmental Protection Agency. *The Inside Story: A Guide to Indoor Air Quality*, 1995. http://www.epa.gov/iaq/pubs/insidest.html

3. U.S. Centers for Disease Control. *Final Report on Formaldehyde Levels in FEMA-Supplied Travel Trailers, Park Models and Mobile Homes*, 2008. Available at http://www.cdc.gov/nceh/ehhe/trailerstudy

4. Thorn J et al. Adult-Onset Asthma Linked to Mold and Tobacco Smoke Exposure. *Allergy*, 56, 287–292, 2001.

5. U.S. Environmental Protection Agency. *Sources of Indoors Air Pollution: Asbestos*, 2003. http://www.epa.gov/iaq/asbestos.html

6. U.S. Environmental Protection Agency. *Sources of Indoor Air Pollution: Lead (Pb)*, 2003. www.epa.gov/iaq/lead.html

7. U.S. Department of Health and Human Services, Public Health Service, Agency for Toxic Substances and Disease Registry. *Case Studies in Environmental Medicine: Lead Toxicity*, 1995. www.atsdr.cdc.gov/HEC/CSEM/lead.

8. U.S. Environmental Protection Agency. *Sources of Indoors Air Pollution: Biological Pollutants*, 2003. http://www.epa.gov/iaq/biologic.html

9. National Safety Council. *Radon*, 2002. http://www.nsc.org/ehc/radon.htm

10. National Academy of Science. *The Health Effects of Exposure to Radon (BEIR VI)*.1999. National Academy Press. http://books.nap.edu/books/0309056454/html/

11. Schüz J et al. Cellular Telephone Use and Cancer: Update of a Nationwide Danish Cohort. *Journal of the National Cancer Institute*, 98(23), 1707–1713, 2006.

12. Hardell L et al. Pooled Analysis of Two Case-Control Studies on Use of Cellular and Cordless Telephones and the Risk for Malignant Brain Tumors Diagnosed in 1997–2003. *International Archives of Occupational and Environmental Health*, 79(8), 630–639, 2006.

13. Ahlbom A et al. Epidemiology of Health Effects of Radiofrequency Exposure. *Environmental Health Perspectives*, 112(17), 2004.

14. UK Childhood Cancer Study Investigators. Childhood Cancer and Residential Proximity to Power Lines. *British Journal of Cancer*, 83, 1573–1580, 2000.

15. Savitz DA, Loomis DP. Magnetic Field Exposure in Relation to Leukemia and Brain Cancer Mortality Among Electric Utility Workers. *American Journal of Epidemiology*, 141(2), 123–128, 1995.

16. Greenland S, Sheppard AR, et al. A Pooled Analysis of Magnetic Fields, Wirecodes, and Childhood Leukemia. *Epidemiology*, 11, 624–634, 2000.

17. U.S. Food and Drug Administration. 2008. Center for Devices and Radiological Health. http://www.fda.gov/cdrh/wireless/research.html

18. U.S. Environmental Protection Agency. Water on Tap: What You Need to Know, 2003. http://www.epa.gov/safewater/

19. U.S. Environmental Protection Agency. *Factsheet on: Nitrate / Nitrite*, 2002. http://www.epa.gov/safewater/dwh/t-ioc/nitrates.html

20. U.S. Environmental Protection Agency. *Permeation and Leaching*, 2002. http://www.epa.gov/ogwdw/disinfection/tcr/pdfs/whitepaper_tcr_permeation-leaching.pdf

21. U.S. Centers for Disease Control and Prevention. *Third National Report on Human Exposure to Environmental Chemicals*. 2005. http://www.cdc.gov/exposurereport/report.htm

22. Gray LE, Ostby J. Effects of Pesticides and Toxic Substances on Behavioral and Morphological Reproductive Development: Endocrine Versus No-Endocrine Mechanisms. *Toxicology and Industrial Health*, 14, 159–184, 1998.

23. U.S. Environmental Protection Agency. *Endocrine Disrupting Chemicals Risk Management Research*, http://www.epa.gov/ord/NRMRL/EDC

24. Adibi J, et al. Pre-Natal Exposures to Phthalates Among Women in New York City and Krakow, Poland. *Environmental Health Perspectives*, 111(14), 1719–1722, 2003.

25. Landrigan P, Garg A, Droller D. Assessing the Effects of Endocrine Disruptors in the National Children's Study. *Environmental Health Perspectives*, 111(13), 1678–1682, 2003.

26. U.S. Centers for Disease Control and Prevention. *National Report on Human Exposure to Environmental Chemicals: Spotlight on Bisphenol A*, 2008. http://www.cdc.gov/exposurereport/pdf/factsheet_bisphenol.pdf

27. U.S. Food and Drug Administration. *Bisphenol A*, 2009. http://www.fda.gov/oc/opacom/hottopics/bpa.html

28. Lang IA et al. Association of Urinary Bisphenol A Concentration with Medical Disorders and Laboratory Anomalies in Adults. *Journal of the American Medical Association*, 300(11), 1303–1310, 2008.

29. Bell P. Noise, Pollution, and Psychopathology. In Ghadirian A, Lehmann H (Eds.), *Environment and Psychopathology*. New York: Springer, 1993.

30. U.S. Environmental Protection Agency. *Report on the Environment*, 2008. http://www.epa.gov/indicators

31. Dockery D, Pope C III. Acute Respiratory Effects of Particulate Air Pollution. *Annual Review of Public Health*, 15, 107–132, 1994.

32. Perera F et al. Effects of Transplacental Exposure to Environmental Pollutants on Birth Outcomes in a Multiethnic Population. *Environmental Health Perspectives*, 111(2), 201–205, 2003.

33. Perera F et al. DNA Damage from Polycyclic Aromatic Hydrocarbons Measured by Benzo[a] Pyrene-DNA Adducts in Mothers and Newborns from Northern Manhattan, the World Trade Center Area, Poland, and China. *Cancer, Epidemiology Biomarkers & Prevention*, 14, 709–714, 2005.

34. National Institute of Environmental Health Sciences. *Asthma*, 2008. http://www.niehs.nih.gov/health/topics/conditions/asthma/index.cfm

35. McConnell R, et al. Asthma in Exercising Children Exposed to Ozone. *Lancet*, 359, 386–391, 2002.

36. U.S. Environmental Protection Agency. *The National Air Toxics Assessment*, 2008. http://www.epa.gov/ttn/atw/natamain/index.html

37. U.S. Environmental Protection Agency. Drinking Water and Your Health, What You Need to Know, List of Drinking Water Contaminants & MCLs, 2003. http://www.epa.gov/safewater/mcl.html#1

38. U.S. Environmental Protection Agency. *Non-Hazardous Waste—Municipal Solid Waste*, 2008. http://www.epa.gov/osw/basic-solid.htm

39. Ewing R, et al. Relationship Between Urban Sprawl and Physical Activity, Obesity and Morbidity. *American Journal of Health Promotion*, 18(1), 47–57, 2003.

40. The Population Institute. http://www.populationinstitute.org/

41. Gasana J. Remember Rwanda? *World Watch*, 15(5), 24–33, 2002.

42. Intergovernmental Panel on Climate Change. *IPCC Fourth Assessment Report: Working Group 1 Report, The Physical Science Basis*, 2007. http://www.ipcc.ch/ipccreports/ar4-wg1.htm

43. U.S. Environmental Protection Agency. *The Science of Ozone Depletion*, 2003. http://www.epa.gov/docs/ozone/science/index.html

44. Vitousek P et al. Human Domination of Earth's Ecosystems. *Science*, 277, 494–499, 1997.

45. World Resources Institute. 2003. http://www.wri.org

46. Worm B et al. Impacts of Biodiversity Loss on Ocean Ecosystem Services. *Science*, 314, 787–790, 2006.

47. Wilson E. *Biophilia: The Human Bond with Other Species.* Cambridge, MA: Harvard University Press, 1984.

48. Gardner GT, Stern PC. *Environmental Problems and Human Behavior.* Needham Heights, MA: Allyn & Bacon, 1996.

Personal Assessment

Are you an environmentalist?

When asked, many people will say that they are an "environmentalist," including political leaders who are widely criticized for decisions perceived by others to be environmentally destructive. So what is an "environmentalist"? One definition of environmentalism is that it is an ideology that values and reveres Nature, and works to protect and preserve natural systems for both ethical reasons and because humankind depends on these systems for life. However, beyond this general statement environmentalists encompass a wide diversity of beliefs and practices. For some, their environmental beliefs are a form of religion, others function mainly in the political process, and some operate like terrorist groups who use violence to fight human economic development on behalf of Earth.* The wide diversity of beliefs and practices encompassed under "environmentalism" creates a situation whereby almost anyone could claim to be an environmentalist. Perhaps more useful criteria for determining if you are an environmentalist would be (1) your awareness of how various human activities create environmental health hazards or degrade natural systems; (2) your willingness to consider your own role in creating environmental problems; and (3) your willingness to act in ways that reduce your personal risk from environmental hazards and your contribution to the causes of these hazards. These three criteria define a hierarchy of commitment to environmental protection. First you have to know a problem exists. Then you have to recognize your own part in creating that problem. The last, and most difficult, step is that you must be willing to reduce or eliminate your contribution to environmental problems. Your answers to the following questions will help you think about where you really stand on protecting the environment for yourself, your community, and all the rest of life on Earth.

Awareness of Environmental Problems

1. Have you ever read the water quality assessment provided by the supplier of your drinking water?
2. If your drinking water is from a well, do you know about potential sources of contamination (landfills or other waste disposal sites, large agricultural areas, confined feedlot livestock operations) in your watershed?
3. If your drinking water supply is from a well, do you know if your water contains potentially harmful contaminants?
4. Do you know whether or not your community wastewater treatment system occasionally dumps raw sewage into the local river during high rainfall events?
5. If you use a gas furnace or kerosene space heater, do you know whether or not these appliances are functioning properly so as to maximize energy efficiency and minimize risks from indoor air pollution?
6. Have you ever made a note of air pollution alerts or information about high ultraviolet radiation published in a local newspaper or presented on a local TV news program?
7. Have you ever searched for information on air, water, and land pollution in your community?
8. When you eat fish, are you aware of health advisories regarding contaminants in fish (for example, mercury, PCBs) and recommendations that you limit the amount of the fish you consume?
9. When you purchase products, do you look at packaging materials for warnings that the product contains toxic chemicals?
10. When you listen to loud music, do you think about potential long-term damage to your hearing and the nuisance noise you create for your neighbors?
11. Do you know if your community (city, county, state) has a land-use management (zoning) plan?
12. When you see new economic developments (malls, superstores, warehouses, suburban housing developments) being constructed, do you wonder if a wildlife habitat is being destroyed?
13. Do you know the proposed human causes of global warming and the potential consequences of this change in climate?
14. Do you know the causes and potential health effects of depletion of the stratospheric ozone layer?
15. Do you know the link between the wood you buy at a store like Menard's, Lowe's, and Home Depot and species extinctions?

Willingness to Consider Your Personal Environmental Impact

16. When you think about having a family of your own, do you worry about contributing to a rapidly growing human population that is responsible for widespread environmental degradation?
17. When you think about purchasing a vehicle, do you consider fuel efficiency more important than "image" sold by advertisers?
18. When you consider purchasing any product, do you consider the resources used, and pollution created, to produce that product?
19. When you purchase an electric appliance or a gas-powered device, do you consider energy efficiency?
20. When planning to build a new home, do you consider how your choices regarding location and amount of

land could contribute to loss of green space and natural habitat?

21. When you use or dispose of household, yard, and automotive chemicals and fluids, do you consider that you may be contributing to local water pollution?

22. When you hear about global warming, do you recognize that your own use of electricity and gas-powered vehicles contributes to this problem?

23. Did you know that if you vent your home or automotive air-conditioning system coolant while performing do-it-yourself maintenance, you are contributing to the depletion of the stratospheric ozone layer?

24. When you purchase lumber, do you wonder if the wood you are buying was harvested using environmentally sound practices or if critical wildlife habitats or wilderness was destroyed to produce the lumber?

25. Do you consider how your vote in public elections can affect government policies that impact the environment?

Willingness to Alter Your Lifestyle to Protect Yourself and the Environment

26. Would you limit the number of your own children to one or two so as to reduce your contribution to the problem of global human population explosion?

27. When you purchase a vehicle, is energy efficiency your main concern?

28. Would you use mass transit to travel from home to work, if it were available, to reduce your contribution to local air pollution and the need for paving more land to expand highways?

29. When you buy a home, would you seek to minimize the distance from work and schools to reduce gas consumption, minimize air pollution, and reduce demand for construction of new roads?

30. When you buy a home, would you look for a smaller, energy-efficient home to minimize your contribution to natural resource exploitation and pollution associated with energy consumption?

31. When you buy lighting, do you buy energy-efficient lights (compact fluorescent and LED lightbulbs) that are initially more expensive, but more efficient and less expensive over the long term?

32. When furnishing your home, would you seek out water-efficient toilets, faucets, and shower heads that conserve freshwater and reduce demands on waste water treatment systems?

33. Do you set the thermostat in your home to cooler temperatures in winter and warmer temperatures in summer to conserve energy?

34. Would you invest money and effort to better insulate your home so as to reduce energy needed for heating and cooling?

35. When buying food, would you be willing to pay more for organically grown foods that were produced without the use of pesticides and fertilizers that pollute the surrounding environment?

36. Would you buy locally grown foods to support farmers (and their green spaces) in your community and reduce energy spent on long-distance transport?

37. When purchasing wood products, would you buy more expensive wood that is certified to have been harvested using environmentally sound practices?

38. Would you be willing to have something less than the perfect lawn to avoid using fertilizers and pesticides that contaminate local waterways?

39. Would you limit your personal consumption of material goods to mainly those things you need, so as to reduce exploitation of natural resources?

40. When you dispose of household chemicals, automotive fluids, and spent batteries, do you make the extra effort to be sure they do not end up polluting the environment, like taking them to a toxic waste collection site?

41. Do you make the effort to recycle paper, glass, plastic, and metals?

42. When you make purchases, do you look for products made from recycled materials (for example, post-consumer recycled paper, "plastic wood," fleece clothing made from recycled plastic)?

43. Do you limit the noise that you produce (loud music, loud car or motorcycle engines, barking dogs) to reduce noise pollution in your neighborhood?

44. Do you contribute financial support to environmental groups that promote conservation and protection of natural resources through the legal and political systems?

45. When you consider candidates for public office, do you vote for the candidates who have strong records or position statements for environmental protection?

Interpretation

If the majority of your answers to questions 1 to 15 are yes, you are likely "environmentally aware." That is, you pay attention to news stories about environmental issues or have taken an environmental science course.

If most of your answers to questions 16 to 25 are yes, you are "environmentally conscious." That is, you are not only aware of the problems, but beginning to think about how these problems are related to your own lifestyle.

If the majority of your answers to questions 26 to 45 are yes, you are likely "environmentally active." That is, you are personally involved in efforts to address environmental problems through your own lifestyle choices and through the political process.

*Wikipedia (The Free Encyclopedia). www.wikipedia.org/wiki/environmentalism.

part seven

Completing Life's Journey

This last part comprises a single chapter on a topic that inevitably affects each of us: dying and death. Traditional-age students may think that death will not touch their lives until they grow older. Yet many young people must face the reality of death much sooner, when a loved one is lost to an accident, a disease, suicide, or some other tragedy.

1. **Physical Dimension**
   Unless we die suddenly at a young age, most of us will enjoy years of good physical health before we begin a period of gradual decline. Eventually, we may experience an extended period of failing health before dying of a chronic condition, such as heart disease. However, many people today experience their highest level of physical health late in life. An adequate activity level, weight management, smoking cessation, and moderation of alcohol use can increase the likelihood that an older adult will be able to enjoy good physical health well into his or her later years.

2. **Psychological Dimension**
   The process of dying and death can be emotionally draining for both the dying person and his or her loved ones. The death of a spouse, close friend, or child, especially when it is unexpected, can be emotionally taxing. The grieving person may feel anger, sadness, regret, and a range of other complex emotions. Indeed, coping with death can be a great challenge to the emotional stability of even the healthiest person.

3. **Social Dimension**
   The dying process and the event of a loved one's death offer opportunities for reaching out to others. In fact, many people who have had these experiences report that having a social support system was essential to maintaining their emotional balance during the ordeal. The families of people who are dying must also deal effectively with health care professionals, funeral directors, and estate executors.

4. **Intellectual Dimension**
   Complex decisions about treatment options must be made. Loved ones may be left to sort out the finances of a family member who has died. These difficult situations require an ability to analyze many variables in order to make sound choices.

5. **Spiritual Dimension**
   Those who have a strong religious faith may find comfort in their beliefs, while others may find that their faith is shaken by the experience. Those who are not religious may look for other ways to find meaning in the event.

6. **Occupational Dimension**
   The dying process often unfolds slowly. A person who is terminally ill may have to continue working for months or even years before he or she becomes so ill that work is no longer possible. Such an illness can make work difficult. However, some people find that their job provides a welcome diversion as well as a social support network.

Accepting Dying and Death

What Do You Know About Dying and Death?

1. Signing a donor card or the organ-donor option on your driver's license ensures that your organs will be donated when you die. True or False?

2. Death is defined as a state when one's heartbeat can no longer be detected and breathing has ceased. True or False?

3. There are only two states in the United States where physician-assisted suicide is legal. True or False?

4. It is advisable to bring children to funerals to help them better understand and accept death. True or False?

5. Hospice care is provided primarily in the patient's home. True or False?

6. The average cost for a funeral service is around $6,500. True or False?

7. Only 25 percent of people choose cremation for disposal of their bodies. True or False?

Check your answers at the end of the chapter.

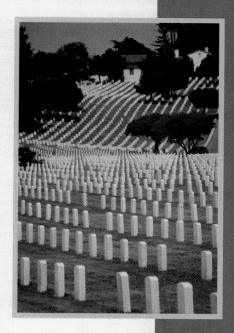

The Experience of Dying

The primary goal of this chapter is to help people realize that accepting the reality of death can motivate us to live a more enjoyable, healthy, productive, and contributive life. Each day in our lives becomes even more meaningful when we have fully accepted the reality that someday we will die. We can then live each day to its fullest.

Our personal awareness of death can give us a framework from which to appreciate and conduct our lives. It helps us to prioritize our activities so that we can accomplish our goals (in our work, our relationships with others, and our recreation) before we die. Quite simply, death can help us to appreciate living.

Dying in Today's Society

Since the 1920s, the way people experience death in this society has changed. Formerly, most people died in their own homes, surrounded by family and friends. Young children frequently lived in the same home with their aging grandparents and saw them grow older and eventually die. Death was seen as a natural extension of life. Children grew up with a keen sense of what death meant, both to the dying person and to the grieving survivors.

Times have indeed changed. Today about 80 percent of people die in hospitals, nursing homes, and assisted living facilities, rather than in their own homes. The extended family is seldom at the bedside of the dying person.[1] Sometimes, frantic efforts are made to keep a dying person alive. Although medical technology has improved our lives, some people believe that it has reduced our ability to die with dignity. Some are convinced that our way of dying has become more artificial and less natural than it used to be. The trend toward hospice care may be a positive response to this high-tech manner of dying.

Many families are forced to deal with death unexpectedly when a loved one dies in an accident or by violence. The emotions they feel are somewhat different from the ones normally evoked when a friend or relative dies of a disease or failing health in old age.

As the baby boomers age over the next 30 years, the number of people age 85 and older will more than double, to 9 million. This means that the topic of death and dying will become increasingly common and relevant for us all as we cope with the loss of our parents, grandparents, friends, and other family members.

Definitions of Death

Death was once easy to define. People were considered dead when a heartbeat could no longer be detected and when breathing ceased. Now, with the technological advances in medicine, especially emergency medicine, some patients who give every indication of being dead can be resuscitated. Critically ill people, even those in comas, can now be kept alive for years with many of their bodily functions maintained by medical devices, including feeding tubes and respirators.

Thus death can be a very challenging concept to define.[2] Many professional associations and ad hoc interdisciplinary committees have struggled with this problem and have developed criteria by which to establish death. The Uniform Determination of Death Act of 1981 is adhered to by most states in defining death. It states, "An individual who has sustained either (1) irreversible cessation of circulatory and respiratory functions, or (2) irreversible cessation of all functions of the entire brain, including the brain stem, is dead."[3]

Clinical determinants of death measure bodily functions. Often judged by a physician, who can then sign a legal document called a *medical death certificate,* these clinical criteria include the following:

1. Lack of heartbeat and breathing.
2. Lack of central nervous system function, including all reflex activity and environmental responsiveness. This can often be confirmed by an *electroen-*

cephalograph reading. If no brain wave activity is recorded after an initial measurement and a second measurement after 24 hours, the person is said to have undergone *brain death.*

3. The presence of *rigor mortis,* indicating that body tissues and organs are no longer functioning at the cellular level. This is sometimes called *cellular death.*

The legal determinants used by government officials are established by state law. A person is not legally dead until a physician, *coroner,* or health department officer has signed a death certificate. However, some argue that death should be defined as occurring when there is an irreparable lack of consciousness or loss of the structures that support thinking even if the brain stem is still functioning. This would allow faster harvesting of donor organs, such as hearts for transplant patients.

Psychological States of Dying

People who have a terminal illness undergo a process of self-adjustment (see the box "Challenging Death"). The stages in this process have helped form the basis for the modern movement of death education. Knowing these stages may help you understand how people adjust to other important losses in their lives.

Perhaps the most widely recognized name in the area of death education is Dr. Elisabeth Kübler-Ross. As a psychiatrist working closely with terminally ill patients at the University of Chicago's Billings Hospital, Kübler-Ross could observe the emotional reactions of dying people. In her classic book *On Death and Dying,* Kübler-Ross summarized the psychological stages that dying people often experience.[4]

- *Denial.* This is the stage of disbelief. Patients refuse to believe that they actually will die. Denial can serve as a temporary defense mechanism and can allow patients the time to accept their prognosis on their own terms.

- *Anger.* A common emotional reaction after denial is anger. Patients can feel as if they have been cheated. By expressing anger, patients can vent some of their fears, jealousies, anxieties, and frustrations. Patients often direct their anger at relatives, physicians and nurses, religious figures, and healthy people.

- *Bargaining.* Terminally ill people follow the anger stage with a bargaining stage. In an effort to avoid their inevitable death, they attempt to strike bargains—often with God or a church leader. Some people undergo religious conversions. The goal is to buy time by promising to repent for past sins, to restructure and rededicate their lives, or to make a large financial contribution to a religious cause.

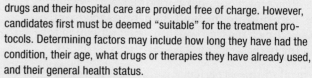
- *Depression.* When patients realize that, at best, bargaining can only postpone their fate, they may begin an unpredictable period of depression. In a sense, terminally ill people are grieving for their own anticipated death. They may become quite withdrawn and refuse to visit with close relatives and friends. Prolonged periods of silence or crying are normal components of this stage and should not be discouraged.

- *Acceptance.* During the acceptance stage, patients fully realize that they will die. Acceptance ensures a relative sense of peace for most dying people. Anger, resentment, and depression are usually gone. Kübler-Ross describes this stage as one without much feeling. Patients feel neither happy nor sad. Many are calm and introspective and prefer to be left either alone or with a few close relatives or friends.

The psychological stages of dying include two more important points. Just as each person's life is totally unique, so is each person's death. Unfolding deaths vary as much as do unfolding lives. Some people move through Kübler-Ross's stages of dying very predictably, but others do not. It is not uncommon for some dying people to avoid one or more of these stages entirely or to revisit a stage more than once.

The second important point about Kübler-Ross's stages of dying is that the family members or friends of dying people often pass through similar stages as they observe their loved ones dying. When informed that a close friend or relative is dying, many people also experience varying degrees of denial, anger, bargaining, depression, and acceptance. Because of this, as caring people we need to recognize that the emotional needs of the living must be fulfilled in ways that do not differ appreciably from those of the dying.[5]

 TALKING POINTS Have you lost a family member, friend, or pet? If so, how did you cope with this loss? What stages of grief did you experience?

Near-Death Experiences

Death ends our physical existence. Perhaps this is the ultimate connection between death and our physical dimension of health. Many people believe that, in a positive sense, death brings a sense of relief and comfort—two qualities one may need most when one is dying. The classic work of Raymond Moody,[6] who examined reports of people who had near-death experiences, suggests that we may have less to fear about dying than we have generally thought.

In a comprehensive study of more than 100 people who had near-death experiences, Kenneth Ring reported that these people shared a core experience.[7] This experience was composed of some or all of the following stages:

1. Realization of the person's death
2. An out-of-body experience in which the dying person floats above his or her body and witnesses the activities that are occurring

3. Movement into a blue tunnel
4. Encountering loved ones who have died
5. A shaft of intense light that generally leads upward or lies in the distance
6. A sense of well-being and peace
7. Reviewing one's life
8. Reaching a boundary or border
9. Returning to the body, sometimes reluctantly
10. Feeling a sense of warmth when returning to the body

Central to this experience is the need to decide whether to move toward death or to return to the body that has been temporarily vacated.

Experts do not agree whether near-death experiences are truly associated with death or more closely associated with the depersonalization that some people experience during particularly frightening situations. In a scientific sense, near-death experiences are impossible to prove. However, there has also been research suggesting that oxygen deprivation may cause these near-death experiences. Science can neither verify nor deny the existence of out-of-body experiences.[1]

Regardless, for those who have had near-death experiences, simply knowing that death might not be such an unpleasant experience appears to be comforting. Most seem to have formed a more positive orientation toward living.[1]

Interacting with Dying People

Facing the impending death of a friend, relative, or loved one is a difficult experience. If you have yet to go through this situation, be assured that, as you grow older, your opportunities will increase. This is part of the reality of living.

Most counselors, physicians, nurses, and ministers who spend time with terminally ill people suggest that you display honesty, respect, and compassion when interacting with dying people. Just the thought of talking with a dying person may make you feel uncomfortable, especially if you have not had this experience before. Sometimes, to make ourselves feel less anxious or depressed, we may tend to deny that the person we are with is dying. Our words and nonverbal behavior reveal that we prefer not to face the truth. Our words become stilted as we gloss over the facts and merely attempt to cheer up both our dying friend and ourselves. This behavior is rarely beneficial or supportive—for either party.

Often people say they don't know how to behave or what to say when with a person who is dying. It is helpful to be as genuine and emotionally supportive as possible. Sometimes people try to avoid talking about death or the severity of the person's illness, but this is not being honest or genuine. It can be comforting for terminally ill patients to be able to talk openly about what is happening

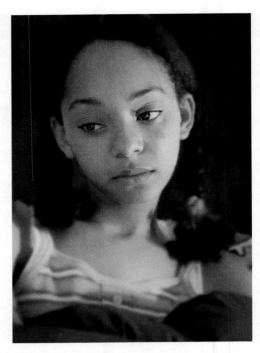

Talking honestly, answering questions, and providing support can help a child cope with loss.

to them, to be able to express any thoughts or feelings and talk about funeral arrangements. It can be stressful to pretend that the situation is not as serious as it is, and the dying person may be trying to put on a "brave face" for everyone else and take care of others and make them feel comfortable. Talking about daily events, reading the newspaper or a book, holding hands, giving a back massage, and providing music to listen to are other helpful ways of interacting with dying people.

Talking with Children About Death

Because most children are curious about everything, we should not be surprised that they are also fascinated about death. From very young ages, children are exposed to death through mass media, adult conversations ("Aunt Emily died today," "Uncle George is very ill"), and their discoveries (a dead squirrel on the road, a crushed bug, the death of a pet). The way children learn about death greatly affects their ability to recognize and accept their own mortality and to cope with the deaths of others.

Psychologists encourage parents and older friends to avoid shielding children from or misleading children about the reality of death. Young children need to realize that death is not temporary and is not like sleeping. Parents should make certain they understand children's questions about death before they give an answer. Most children want simple, direct answers to their questions, not long, detailed dissertations, which often confuse the issues. For example, when a 4-year-old asks her father, "Why is Tommy's dog dead?" an appropriate answer might be, "Because he got very, very sick and his heart stopped beating." Getting involved in a long discussion about "doggy heaven" or the causes of specific canine diseases may not be necessary or appropriate.

When a child suffers the loss of a near relative, informing the child is a painful task. Adults are usually present when a near relative dies, but children in Western societies are unlikely to be present at the time of death. In the death of a parent, the surviving parent usually must tell the child. The surviving parent sometimes tells the child the news much later, and often in a misleading way.

Two crucial pieces of information that help children to cope with death are knowing that the person will never come back and that the body has been buried or burned to ashes.[8] It is for these reasons that it is recommended that children be brought to funerals, so that they can better understand and accept death. Children's fantasies about death and burial can be more frightening to them than reality, especially if they are not told the truth about death. For example, a common tendency is to tell young children that the deceased has "gone to sleep." Since children tend to take things literally, they may develop a fear of going to sleep themselves, since they now associate sleeping with dying. Seeing the dead body at the funeral can dispel these myths.

People often hide their feelings of loss in an effort to be strong and protect children from emotional pain. However, it is good role modeling for children to see how adults mourn and grieve the loss of a loved one and that mourning assists with normalizing this part of the life cycle.

By telling children about the death of a loved one, using language that is age-appropriate, straightforward, and honest, you can help them to begin to learn that death is not something to be feared but something to be accepted. Sharing feelings, answering questions truthfully without too much detail, and giving him or her sympathy and support to cope with losses is the best gift you can give to a grieving child.

End-of-Life Options and Decisions

Many decisions related to dying and death can be anticipated and discussed with family members. Areas to consider include the type of care you'd like at the end of your life and whether you plan to donate organs.

Hospice Care for the Terminally Ill

The thought of dying in a hospital ward, with institutional furniture, medical equipment, and strict visiting hours, is not the way most people envision spending their list days of life. Perhaps this thought alone has helped encourage the concept of **hospice care.** Hospice care is an alternative approach to dying for terminally ill patients and their families. The goal of hospice care is to maximize the quality of life of dying people and their family members. Popularized in England during the 1960s, the hospice helps people die comfortably and with dignity by using one or more of the following strategies:

- *Pain control.* Dying people usually are not treated for their terminal disease; they are given appropriate drugs to keep them free from pain, alert, and in control of their faculties. Drug dependence is of little concern, and patients can receive pain medication when they feel they need it.

- *Family involvement.* Family members and friends are trained and encouraged to interact with the dying person and with each other. Family members often care for the dying person at home. If the hospice arrangement includes a hospice ward in a hospital or a separate building (also called a hospice), the family members have no restrictions on visitation.

- *Multidisciplinary approach.* The hospice concept promotes a team approach.[9] Specially trained physicians, nurses, social workers, counselors, and volunteers work with the patient and family to fulfill important needs. The needs of the family receive nearly the same priority as those of the patient.

- *Patient decisions.* Contrary to most hospital approaches, hospice programs encourage patients to make their own decisions. The patient decides when to eat, sleep, go for a walk, and just be alone. By maintaining a personal schedule, the patient is more apt to feel in control of his or her life, even as that life is slipping away.

Another way the hospice differs from the hospital approach is in the care given to the survivors. Even after the death of the patient, the family receives a significant amount of follow-up counseling. Helping families with their grief is an important role of the hospice team.

The number of hospices in the United States has climbed quickly to more than 4,100. According to the National Hospice and Palliative Care Organization, hospices served at least 1.4 million patients in 2007.[10] People seem to be convinced that the hospice system does work effectively. Part of this approval may be the cost factor. The cost of caring for a dying person in a hospice is usually

---

Key Terms

hospice care (hos pis) An approach to caring for terminally ill patients that maximizes the quality of life and allows death with dignity.

less than the cost of full (inpatient) services provided by a hospital. Although insurance companies are delighted to see the lower cost of hospice care, many are still uncertain how to define hospice care. Thus not all insurance companies are fully reimbursing patients for their hospice care. Before you discuss the possibility of hospice care for members of your family, you may want to consider the extent of hospice coverage in your health insurance policy.

Euthanasia and Physician-Assisted Suicide

There are two types of euthanasia: **indirect (passive) euthanasia** and **direct (active) euthanasia.**

Indirect Euthanasia Indirect or passive euthanasia is when people are allowed to die without being subjected to life-sustaining efforts such as being placed on life support. Examples of indirect euthanasia include physicians' orders of "do not resuscitate" (DNR) and "comfort measures only" (CMO).

Indirect euthanasia is increasingly occurring in a number of hospitals, nursing homes, and medical centers. Physicians who withhold lifesaving techniques or drug therapy treatments or who disconnect life-support systems from terminally ill patients are practicing indirect euthanasia. Although some people still consider this form of euthanasia a type of murder, indirect euthanasia seems to be gaining legal and public acceptance for people with certain terminal illnesses—near-death cancer patients, brain-dead accident victims, and hopelessly ill newborn babies.

Direct Euthanasia Direct or active euthanasia is when people are intentionally put to death. It is usually performed through the administration of large amounts of depressant drugs, which eventually causes all central nervous system functioning to stop. Although direct euthanasia is commonly practiced on house pets and laboratory animals, it is illegal for humans in the United States, Canada, and other developed countries. There have been accusations that medical personnel performed euthanasia on hospital patients who could not be given adequate treatment during Hurricane Katrina. There are documented cases of patients receiving seemingly lethal doses of morphine—some argue it was a palliative measure to alleviate pain, while others cry "murder." However, in 1992, the Netherlands became the first country to enact legislation that permits euthanasia under strict guidelines. Belgium and Switzerland have enacted similar laws.

Physician-Assisted Suicide In recent years, physician-assisted suicide has been the focus of some important news stories. In July 1997, the U.S. Supreme Court unanimously ruled that dying people have no fundamental constitutional right to physician-assisted suicide. In effect, this ruling left the decision to individual states to permit or prohibit physician-assisted suicide.

More than 30 states have enacted laws prohibiting assisted suicide, and many other states have essentially prohibited it through common law.[11] Two states allow physician-assisted suicide. Oregon passed a law in 1994 that legalized assisted suicide, referred to as the Death with Dignity Act. In November 2008, Washington followed suit by passing the Washington Initiative 1000 allowing physician-assisted suicides. This allows doctors to prescribe fatal doses of barbiturates and other drugs to adults of sound mind who have less than 6 months to live. It requires the patient to be at least 18 years of age and of sound mind, make two oral and one written request for the medication with 15 days between the first request and the final one, consult with two physicians, and notify pharmacists and state health authorities before proceeding with physician-assisted suicide. A fatal drug is prescribed, and the patient may ingest it orally at his or her discretion, with or without the doctor present. It remains illegal for physicians to administer lethal injections. To date, there have been over 200 legal physician-assisted suicides in Oregon.

Even though physician-assisted suicide is legal in the state of Oregon, many physicians are unwilling to prescribe the lethal medication. Being confined to their bed or home, living a long way from a large urban area, experiencing difficulty finding a willing physician, dying before completing the requirements of the law, and encountering opposition from family and friends are some of the reasons why greater numbers of terminally ill patients are not obtaining medication to end their lives.

Another news story concerned the April 1999 Michigan conviction of Dr. Jack Kevorkian, a retired pathologist who has aided in the suicides of over 100 people. Kevorkian was convicted of second-degree murder and delivery of a controlled substance in the assisted suicide of Thomas Youk, a 52-year-old patient with Lou Gehrig's disease. This suicide had been televised on the CBS show *60 Minutes*. Kevorkian was sentenced to 10 to 25 years in prison and was paroled in 2007, contingent on his promise that he would not assist in any more suicides.[12]

Interestingly, most physicians will not inform patients if they are terminally ill. A recent study showed that only one-third of doctors reported that they routinely tell their patients that they are dying. This lack of information can make it difficult for the dying person, family, and friends to make decisions and prepare for this event.

 TALKING POINTS Would you want to know that you were dying if your doctor knew you were terminally ill? How would this information change the way you spent the rest of your life and the decisions you would make?

Figure 21-1 (Sample Living Will)

New York Living Will — Page 1 of 2

INSTRUCTIONS

This Living Will has been prepared to conform to the law in the State of New York, as set forth in the case In re Westchester County Medical Center, 72 N.Y.2d 517 (1988). In that case the Court established the need for "clear and convincing" evidence of a patient's wishes and stated that the "ideal situation is one in which the patient's wishes were expressed in some form of writing, perhaps a 'living will.'"

PRINT YOUR NAME

I, _____, being of sound mind, make this statement as a directive to be followed if I become permanently unable to participate in decisions regarding my medical care. These instructions reflect my firm and settled commitment to decline medical treatment under the circumstances indicated below:

I direct my attending physician to withhold or withdraw treatment that merely prolongs my dying, if I should be in an **incurable or irreversible mental or physical condition with no reasonable expectation of recovery,** including but not limited to: (a) a **terminal condition;** (b) a **permanently unconscious condition;** or (c) a **minimally conscious condition in which I am permanently unable to make decisions or express my wishes.**

I direct that my treatment be limited to measures to keep me comfortable and to relieve pain, including any pain that might occur by withholding or withdrawing treatment.

CROSS OUT ANY STATEMENTS THAT DO NOT REFLECT YOUR WISHES

While I understand that I am not legally required to be specific about future treatments **if I am in the condition(s) described above I feel especially strongly about the following forms of treatment:**

[ ] I do not want cardiac resuscitation.
[ ] I do not want mechanical respiration.
[ ] I do not want artificial nutrition and hydration.
[ ] I do not want antibiotics.

However, **I do want** maximum pain relief, even if it may hasten my death.

@2005 National Hospice and Palliative Care Organization 2006 Revised

New York Living Will - Page 2 of 2

ADD PERSONAL INSTRUCTIONS (IF ANY)

Other directions:

SIGN AND DATE THE DOCUMENT AND PRINT YOUR ADDRESS

These directions express my legal right to refuse treatment, under the law of New York. I intend my instructions to be carried out, unless I have rescinded them in a new writing or by clearly indicating that I have changed my mind.

Signed _____ Date _____

Address _____

WITNESSING PROCEDURE

I declare that the person who signed this document appeared to execute the living will willingly and free from duress. He or she signed (or asked another to sign for him or her) this document in my presence.

YOUR WITNESSES MUST SIGN AND PRINT THEIR ADDRESS

Witness 1 _____

Address _____

Witness 2 _____

Address _____

@ 2005 National Hospice and Palliative Care Organization 2006 Revised

Courtesy of Caring Connections
1700 Diagonal Road, Suite 625, Alexandria, VA 22314
www.caringinfo.org, 800/658-8898

Figure 21-1 Sample Living Will   Living wills and other advance directives must conform to specific state laws. To obtain a copy of the living will for your state, visit the website for the National Hospice and Palliative Care Organization (www.caringinfo.org).

Source: Copyright © 2007 National and Palliative Care Organization. All rights reserved. Reproduction and distribution by an organization or organized group without the written permission of the National Hospice and Palliative Care Organization is expressly forbidden.

Advance Health Care Directives

Because some physicians and families have difficulty supporting indirect euthanasia, many people are starting to use legal documents called *advance health care directives.*[13] One of these health care directives is the **living will** (Figure 21-1). This is a document that confirms a dying person's desire to be allowed to die peacefully and with a measure of dignity if a time should arise when little hope exists for recovery from a terminal illness or severe injury. All 50 states and the District of Columbia have living will statutes. The living will requires that physicians or family members carry out a person's wishes to die naturally, without receiving life-sustaining treatments.[13] About one-third of U.S. citizens have signed living wills. The Terri Schiavo case has drawn increased attention to health care advance directives, because she neither had a living will nor did she designate a health care agent; see the box "The Controversy Surrounding the Death of Terri Schiavo" for more information.

A second important document that can assist terminally ill or incapacitated patients is the **durable power of attorney for health care.** This legal document authorizes another person (sometimes called a *health care*

Key Terms

indirect (passive) euthanasia Allowing people to die without the use of life-sustaining procedures.

direct (active) euthanasia Intentionally causing death.

living will A legal document that requires physicians or family members to carry out a person's wishes to die naturally, without receiving life-sustaining treatments.

durable power of attorney for health care A legal document that designates who will make health care decisions for people unable to do so.

The Controversy Surrounding the Death of Terri Schiavo

Terri Schiavo's death became a legal battle, media event, religious debate, and was even brought into the political spotlight. She was 26 years old when she had heart failure because of a chemical imbalance that may have been caused by an eating disorder, bulimia nervosa. This left her severely brain damaged for 15 years. While she was in hospice care in a vegetative state, her husband and her parents were in a legal battle over whether to remove the feeding tube that was keeping her alive. If she had had a living will, this would have helped to make her wishes more clear, but it may not have precluded the legal debate. Advance directives such as living wills and durable powers of attorney for health care are legal documents that communicate the person's wishes about being kept alive with life support should they become incapacitated.

Both Terri Schiavo's husband and her parents claimed to know her end-of-life wishes, but none of them was named as her health care agent or proxy, giving a specific person the legal right to make this determination. Michael, her husband, stated that she had made casual comments about not wanting

to be on life support if she were ever incapacitated. She had further stated to him that she didn't ever want to be a burden to him or her family. Her parents countered by saying that she was a devout Roman Catholic who believed in the sanctity of life.

The tug-of-war that ensued between her family members, as well as the publicity surrounding her dying wishes, spurred thousands of people to consider completing living wills. In fact, the Aging with Dignity organization estimated that requests for advance directives increased 10-fold because of the Schiavo case. They further reported that they have distributed over 1 million copies of living wills since this case, and orders for more living wills continue to flood in at a rate of 200 an hour.

Bitter legal battles continued for 12 years between these families. The case was brought to the U.S. Supreme court six times and refused each time. The judges stated that any action on their part would be improper. There was a great deal of public outcry, with some referring to her death as "judicial homicide."

Terri Schiavo remained in hospice care for 5 years before she died. Because she hadn't preplanned her funeral, there was continued

acrimony and disagreement concerning the disposition of her body. Her husband stated that Terri had expressed her wish to be cremated, but her parents asserted that because of her Roman Catholic faith, she would not have wanted cremation and would have wanted to be buried. Michael Schiavo had her cremated and her ashes buried at an undisclosed location so that her parents, her brother, and the media wouldn't create a disturbance.

This young woman's death brought to the forefront many important issues that we all must face regarding death and dying. Should your family keep you alive with life support and, if so, for how long? Who should make these decisions? Do we have a legal right to die? Should the courts decide our fate? Having a living will, health care agent, hospice care, and preplanned funeral arrangements could clarify your wishes and possibly preclude a court battle.

Sources: Life and Death Tug of War: The Whole Terri Schiavo Story. *World Net Daily,* March 24, 2005; Terri Schiavo Dies in Florida Hospice. *Fox News,* March 31, 2005; Terri Schiavo Has Died. *CNN.com,* March 31, 2005; Terri Schiavo Dies, but Battle Continues. *U.S. News,* March 31, 2005.

---

agent or proxy) to make specific health care decisions about treatment and care under specified circumstances, such as when patients are in vegetative states and cannot communicate their medical wishes. This document helps tell hospitals and physicians which person will help make the critical medical decisions. You can complete both a living will and a durable power of attorney for health care document.

Organ Donation

For some, the decision to donate body tissue and organs is rewarding and comforting. Organ donors understand that their sacrifice can help give life or improve the quality of life for another person. In this sense, their death can mean life for others.

Certain states permit people to state on their driver's license that they wish to donate their organs. There is a new, more convenient way to register for organ donation through a nonprofit organization called Donate Life America at www.donatelife.net. Thirty-one states have agreed to have this online registration option as of 2008. However, family consent (by next of kin) is also

required at the time of death for organ or tissue donation to proceed. Recently, hospitals have been required by federal law to inform the family of a deceased person about organ donation at the time of death. Thus, those who wish to donate organs at the time of death should discuss these wishes with their family as soon as possible so that family members will support the donation after the individual has died.

The issue of major organ donation today is the shortage of donors—the need for organs is much greater than our current supply.[14] Other critical issues, including interagency cooperation and screening procedures for donated organs, have largely been resolved (see the box "Organ Donation: Fact or Fiction?"). The scarcity of suitable organs is a life-threatening issue for over 100,000 persons on waiting lists for transplant organs (Table 21.1). There is also an increase in the types of transplants that can be conducted. For example, the first face transplant in the United States was performed in 2008, the fourth such transplant performed worldwide since 2005. Demand for organs has risen considerably since 1990, but the number of donors has remained fairly stable. Currently, 77 people receive organ transplants each day; another 110 people

Building Media Literacy Skills

Organ Donation: Fact or Fiction?

From people not really being dead when their organs are harvested, to medical personnel not doing all that they can to save people's lives in order to obtain more organ donors, there are many myths surrounding organ donation. Perhaps this is one of the biggest reasons the need for donated organs far surpasses the number of available organs. Here are some common myths and facts about organ donation.

Myth To be an organ donor, I just have to sign an organ donor card or indicate my preference on my driver's license.

Reality By signing a donor card, you indicate your wish to be a donor. However, at the time of death, your next-of-kin will still be asked to sign a consent form for donation. If you wish to be an organ donor, it is important to tell you family about this decision so that your wishes will be honored at the time of death. It is estimated that about 35 percent of potential donors never become donors because family members refuse to give consent.

Myth Donating organs will cost my family money.

Reality Your family pays for your medical care and funeral costs, but not for organ donation. Costs related to donation are paid by the recipient, usually through insurance, Medicare, or Medicaid.

Myth Being an organ donor can only help one other person.

Reality Each organ and tissue donor saves or improves the lives of as many as 50 people.

Myth I won't be able to have an open-casket funeral.

Reality Donation does not interfere with having an open casket service. Surgical techniques are used to retrieve organs and tissues, and all incisions are closed.

Myth I have to be 18 years old or older to donate.

Reality All individuals can indicate their intent to donate, although persons younger than 18 years of age must have a parent's or guardian's consent. Newborns as well as senior citizens have been organ donors.

Myth I have to have had no previous medical conditions in order to be an organ donor.

Reality False. Transplant professionals will evaluate the condition of your organs at the time of your death and determine if your organs are suitable for donation. You should consider yourself a potential organ and tissue donor, indicate your intent to donate on your driver's license, donor card, or state donor registry, and discuss your decision with family members.

Myth If I sign a donor card, it will affect the quality of medical care I receive at the hospital.

Reality No! The medical team trying to save your life is separate from the transplant team. Every effort is made to save your life before donation is considered.

Myth It would be against my religion's beliefs.

Reality Virtually all religious denominations approve of organ and tissue donation as representing the highest humanitarian ideals and the ultimate charitable act.

Myth The need for organs is the same across all ethnicities.

Reality Minorities overall have a particularly high need for organ transplants because some diseases of the kidney, heart, lung, pancreas, and liver are found more frequently in racial and ethnic minority populations than in the general population. For example, African Americans, Asians and Pacific Islanders, and Hispanics are three times more likely than Whites to suffer from end-stage renal (kidney) disease, often as the result of high blood pressure and other conditions that can damage the kidneys. In addition, similar blood type is essential in matching donors to recipients. Because certain blood types are more common in ethnic minority populations, increasing the number of minority donors can increase the frequency of minority transplants.

It is hoped that knowing the real facts will ease people's minds about the process and enable them to make well-informed choices about organ donation and perhaps save another person's life.

Sources: Adapted from U.S. Department of Health and Human Services Health Resources and Services Administration. Find Answers: Organ Donation and Transplantation. http://answers.hrsa.gov/ November 3, 2009. Congressional Kidney Caucus. 25 Facts about Organ Donation and Transplantation. http://www.house.gov/mcdermott/kidneycaucus/25facts.html February, 2002.

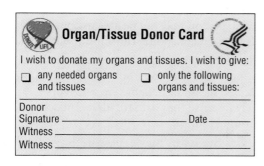

You can request a free national donor card like the one shown above at www.organdonor.gov. You can also contact the United Network for Organ Sharing (UNOS) at 1-888-894-6361 or www.unso.org.

join a waiting list every day—one person every 13 minutes. In 2008 nearly 7,000 people—19 per day—died waiting for an organ transplant.[15]

Because it can take 10 years before transplant patients receive an organ donation, a novel way has been developed to link donors with those in need via the Internet. In 2004, Dr. Jeremiah Lowney started MatchingDonors.com to shorten this wait time. People seeking kidney donors pay $49 a week, or $595 for unlimited usage, to find potential donors; however, 70 percent of the site's members have had this fee waived because of lack of ability to afford these costs. Some worry this is an unregulated system and so there may be potential for fraud

The Grieving Process

The grieving process consists of four phases, each of which varies in length and form in each individual. These phases are composed of the following:

1. *Internalization of the deceased person's image.* By forming an idealized mental picture of the dead person, the grieving person is freed from dealing too quickly with the reality of the death.

2. *Intellectualization of the death.* Mental processing of the death and the events leading up to its occurrence move the grieving person to a clear understanding that death has occurred.

3. *Emotional reconciliation.* During this third and often delayed phase, the grieving person allows conflicting feelings and thoughts to be expressed and eventually reconciled with the reality of the death.

4. *Behavioral reconciliation.* Finally, the grieving person can comfortably return to a life in which the death has been fully reconciled. The survivor reestablishes old routines and adopts new patterns of living where necessary. The grieving person has largely recovered.

The friends of a grieving person sometimes make the mistake of encouraging a return to normal behavior too quickly. When friends urge the grieving person to return to work right away, make new friends, or become involved in time-consuming projects, they may be preventing necessary grieving. It is not easy or desirable to forget about the fact that a spouse, friend, or child has recently died.

Table 21.1 Sample Patient Waiting List for Organ Transplant from the United Network for Organ Sharing (UNOS)

Type of Transplant	Patients Waiting for Transplant
Kidney transplant	79,487
Liver transplant	15,871
Pancreas transplant	1,523
Intestine transplant	215
Heart transplant	2,787
Heart-lung transplant	86
Lung transplant	1,952
	*Total Patients: 101,769

*Some patients are waiting for more than one organ, therefore the total number of patients is less than the sum of patients waiting for each organ.

Note: UNOS policies allow patients to be listed with more than one transplant center (multiple-listing), thus the number of registrations is greater than the actual number of patients. Waiting lists are updated weekly at www.unos.org/data. April 24, 2009. For more information, see the U.S. Department of Health and Human Services Organ Procurement & Transplantation Network (OPTN) at www.unos.org.

or selling organs. The site had more than 5,800 donors registered in 2009.

Grief and Coping

The emotional feelings that people experience after the death of a friend or relative are collectively called *grief.* *Mourning* is the process of experiencing these emotional feelings in a culturally defined manner. (See the box "The Grieving Process" for more information.)

Grief and the Resolution of Grief

The expression of grief is seen as a valuable process that gradually permits people to accept the loss of the deceased. Expressing grief, then, is a sign of good health.

Although people experience grief in remarkably different ways, most people have some of the following sensations and emotions:

- *Physical discomfort.* Shortly after the death of a loved one, grieving people display a similar pattern of physical discomfort. This discomfort is characterized by "sensations of somatic distress occurring in waves lasting from 20 minutes to an hour at a time, a feeling of tightness in the throat, choking with shortness of breath, need for sighing, and an empty feeling in the abdomen, lack of muscular power, and an intense subjective distress described as a tension or mental pain. The person soon learns that these waves of discomfort can be precipitated by visits, by mentioning the deceased, and by receiving sympathy."[16]

- *Sense of numbness.* Grieving people may feel as if they are numb or in a state of shock. They may deny the death of their loved one.

- *Feelings of detachment from others.* Grieving people see other people as being distant from them, perhaps because the others cannot feel the loss. A person in grief can feel very lonely. This is a common response.

- *Preoccupation with the image of the deceased.* The grieving person may not be able to complete daily tasks without constantly thinking about the deceased.

- *Guilt.* The survivor may be overwhelmed with guilt. Thoughts may center on how the deceased was neglected or ignored. Sensitive survivors feel guilt merely because they are still alive. Indeed, guilt is a common emotion.

- *Hostility.* Survivors may express feelings of loss and remorse through hostility, which they direct at other family members, physicians, lawyers, and others. Sometimes survivors may feel anger at the deceased person, perhaps at the suddenness of the death, at

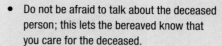
leaving the survivor to deal with problems, or at abandoning the survivor. Such a feeling may cause the survivor to feel guilty and ashamed. Survivors should know that such hostility can be a normal part of grieving.

- *Disruption in daily schedule.* Grieving people often find it difficult to complete daily routines. They can suffer from an anxious type of depression. Seemingly easy tasks take a great deal of effort. Starting new activities and relationships can be difficult. Social interaction skills can be temporarily lost.

- *Delayed grief.* In some people, the typical pattern of grief can be delayed for weeks, months, and even years.

The grief process continues until the bereaved person can establish new relationships, feel comfortable with others, and look back on the life of the deceased person with positive feelings (see the box "Helping the Bereaved"). Although the duration of the grief resolution process varies with the emotional attachments one has to a deceased person, the grieving process usually lasts for 18 months. One should seek professional help when grieving is characterized by unresolved guilt, extreme hostility, physical illness, significant depression, and a lack of other meaningful relationships. Trained counselors, physicians, and hospice workers can all play significant roles in helping people through the stages of grief.

Coping with Death from Specific Causes

Coping with Death from a Terminal Illness   Watching a family member or friend slowly die can bring mixed emotions, from being glad to have that person with you as long as possible to wishing that the person would not have to suffer. It can be painful to see the person you know gradually slip away. In addition, he or she may become someone who seems more like a stranger to you and may not even recognize you or acknowledge your presence. Some people say that they are thankful for the time they have with this person and to be able to say good-bye. However, others may feel a false sense of hopefulness that the person is beating the illness only to feel shocked and devastated when the illness begins to progress at a faster rate. The research does suggest that we cope better with loss when we are expecting it, when we have time to prepare and take whatever action we feel necessary in response to it. In this way, a protracted illness can facilitate the ability to cope that people who experience loss through accidental death, natural disaster, suicide, or murder do not have.

Coping with Death from Accident, Natural Disaster, Terrorism, or War   Deaths that occur from natural disasters or accidental deaths bring some unique challenges. Accidental death is the number-one cause of death for 15- to 34-year-olds, and so college students may encounter this more often than terminal illnesses. Though any type of trauma or crisis is more difficult to deal with when it is unexpected, accidental death seems particularly devastating in that you are unprepared and shocked by the news. Often people have more trouble accepting this type of death because it is so unexpected that it seems unreal.

Death from natural disasters are typically uncommon and unlikely and so are even more difficult to comprehend and accept. We tend to cope better with events we

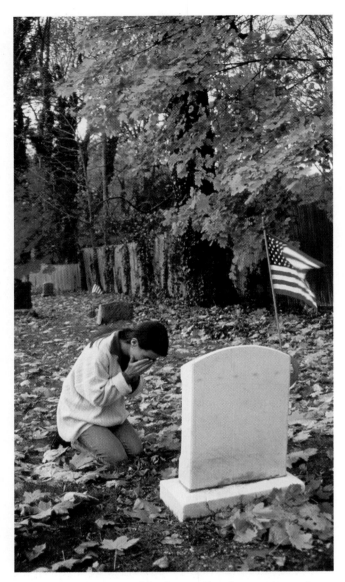

The cause and manner of death can affect the experience of grief. The death of a young soldier in war can be difficult to accept and can lead to a mix of emotions—pride, anger, and profound loss.

can understand and explain. Yet this may be impossible to do with accidental deaths such as from a car accident or from incidents without a clear cause of death. Part of finding an explanation can also involve blaming someone: "I should have known he was too tired to drive." People can feel more vulnerable and fearful after accidents and disasters and become more hesitant in their day-to-day living. Things that you may not have questioned begin to seem potentially dangerous, such as going swimming after a friend has drowned or driving after a car accident.

Death associated with terrorism is something that Americans have not had to face, as other countries have, until 9/11. Since that time, Americans have felt less safe on their own soil and traveling abroad. People have changed their lifestyles in terms of the trips they take, having a survival kit at home, stockpiling food and water, and encountering stringent security. Organizations, hospitals, and government agencies are developing responses to bioterrorism and other types of terrorist attacks.

Those who say good-bye to a soldier going off to combat may dread that the soldier will die in the war. Even though we know this is a possibility, such a death is very difficult to accept, especially when the soldier is young, as many are. Those who have lost a loved one to war might have mixed emotions—pride at the person's courage, heroics, and sacrifice, and anger at the enemy or the government. When a soldier goes missing in action, loved ones lack closure and may remain hopeful that he or she will be found alive and well. When people die in a war thousands of miles away, their deaths can seem unreal because of the distance and the different worlds people and their loved ones have been living in.

Coping with Death by Suicide People react similarly to suicides as they do to accidental death, because both means of death are sudden and unexpected. Making sense of these types of death is difficult, and coping with a completed suicide brings the added burden of understanding the reason and motivation behind the death. If you hold religious beliefs that tell you committing suicide is a sin, this can lead to additional misunderstanding and anger. As with death by murder, this type of death is a crime, and so there are legal as well as religious and moral implications in accepting a person's decision to take his or her own life.

Family members frequently say they feel ashamed and embarrassed by the suicide because of these connotations. They worry that others will see them and their family as crazy. All these concerns usually mean that coping with death by suicide can be a longer process than coping with other types of death. It is helpful for people to understand the events that led up to and contributed to a person's choosing to take his or her life.

Chapter 2 discussed the warning signs and factors that contribute to suicide. Often people blame themselves for not seeing the warning signs or not acting on those they did see. There can also be a sense of feeling unimportant or unloved by this person because you tell yourself "If she really cared about me, she would have fought to stay with me and not left me." Survivors of suicide often feel abandoned and rejected. If your relationship with this person was distant, if you hadn't talked to him or her for a while or you had recently had an argument, you may feel guilty and blame yourself, saying "If only I had been nicer or called her more often, this might not have happened."

Coping with Death by Murder Shock, anger, guilt, confusion, and vulnerability are some of the emotions people commonly experience when they cope with a murder. You don't expect murder to happen—certainly not to someone you know. It can be difficult to comprehend the taking of someone's life, which makes it even more difficult to accept such a loss. You may blame yourself for not protecting the victim in some way or not doing something to prevent it from happening. If the suspect hasn't been identified or apprehended, you may feel angry at the police for not doing more or feel frightened that you live in a world that seems suddenly very unsafe and frightening. If the murderer has been apprehended, it can take years before the trial is over, making it hard to have a sense of closure.

Coping with the Death of a Child

Adults face not only the death of their parents and friends but perhaps also the death of a child. Whether because of sudden infant death syndrome (SIDS), chronic illness, accident, or suicide, adults are sometimes forced to grieve the loss of someone who was "too young to die."

Parents and children are bound by physical and emotional ties like no other relationship. When the tragic death of a young child severs that bond, the pain and anguish the parents feel can be too much to bear. The death of a child can be the most devastating loss parents can experience, and many say that they feel part of them died with their child.

Miscarriage Most pregnancies progress to full term and result in the birth of a healthy child. However, researchers now believe that about one-third of pregnancies end in miscarriage. Since accurate home-pregnancy tests were developed, many women began learning early in the first trimester that they are pregnant. Thus, rather than mistaking the miscarriage for a late heavy menstrual period, more women now know that their pregnancy has ended. Most then go through a grieving process.

In addition, other couples may learn of complications that lead them to choose an elective abortion, or the baby may die during birth or during infancy. Though most people know that such things can happen, many believe that such tragedies happen only to others. When they face the death or potential loss of a child, parents often find their beliefs shaken and their faith tested.

Miscarriage can be especially difficult for the mother. She may think that something she did (or did not do) caused the miscarriage. The exact cause of a miscarriage may never be determined, and the woman needs to be reassured that she did not cause any abnormalities in the fetus.

A miscarriage can be painful and stressful for the woman. Physical symptoms may not occur when the baby dies but may be delayed for some time. Mild or moderate depression, sleeping difficulties, recurring images of the miscarriage, loss of appetite, and abdominal discomfort and cramping may occur weeks or months after a miscarriage. Not surprisingly, fathers can also experience similar symptoms of loss and depression after a miscarriage.

Supportive comments acknowledging how painful their loss is can be helpful to the parents. If an unhealthy fetus is miscarried or aborted, sometimes people try to rationalize the loss for the parents by saying it was "nature's way" of preventing the birth of an imperfect child. Such comments are not only insensitive, but they also imply that the parents should be grateful that they lost the baby. Even seemingly innocent comments can cause pain in the wrong context.

Losing an Infant or Young Child Even after a baby is delivered, there are health risks. Sometimes newborn babies die. The support of family and friends is especially important when a couple is trying to recover from the death of a child. Friends and coworkers can help by acknowledging the death of the child and offering support. Often people will not mention the baby because they think that the parents will become upset, but not talking about the baby can cause greater pain for the parents. Calling to offer support or showing up in person can also help.

Parents often want to hold on to the memory of the child. Such feelings are normal and do not mean that the parents are clinging to their grief in an unhealthy way. Remembering the child can give a sense of meaning to parents' lives. Parents often do something constructive to help them remember their baby and accept this loss. Putting together a scrapbook, donating the baby's clothes and toys to charity, writing memoirs, or setting up a place for remembrance can help the family keep memories of the baby.

Eventually, the grief will lose its intensity. It may flare up again around "anniversaries" (the baby's birthday, the date of the baby's death), but gradually things will become bearable. The family will be forever changed by the experience. The death of a child can change the parents' value system, and their spiritual beliefs may be challenged as well.

Sometimes parents become more protective and focused on their remaining children, creating a new set of problems. It is also not uncommon for parents to take their anger over their loss out on each other, sometimes resulting in so much distance, resentment, and bitterness that they eventually divorce.[9] So, how people come to terms with the loss of their child is important to the continued health and healing of the family unit.

Grieving for a Dead Child Coping with the death of a child is particularly difficult because it seems so unnatural and wrong for a child to precede his or her parents in death. Experts agree that grieving adults, particularly the parents, should express their grief fully and proceed cautiously to return to normal routines. They can avoid many pitfalls. Adults who are grieving for dead children should do the following:

- *Avoid trying to cope with grief by using alcohol or drugs.*
- *Make no important life changes.* Moving to a different home, relocating, or changing jobs usually doesn't help parents deal any better with the grief they are experiencing.
- *Share their feelings with others.* Grieving adults should share their feelings, particularly with other adults who have experienced a similar loss. Group support is available in many communities.
- *Avoid trying to erase the death.* Giving away clothing and possessions that belonged to the child cannot erase the adult's memories of the child.
- *Give themselves the time and space to grieve.* On the anniversary of the child's death or on the child's birthday, family members should give themselves special time just for grieving.
- *Don't attempt to replace the child.* Do not quickly have another child or use the deceased child's name for another child.

For most adults, grief over the death of a child will require an extended time. Eventually, however, life can return to normal.

Coping with the Death of a Parent, Spouse, or Sibling

In some ways, coping with the death of a parent, spouse, or sibling is similar to coping with the death of a child. In each case, survivors must live with the significant loss of a family member. Each death produces some degree of emotional trauma for each survivor, followed by a period of grief. Gradually, the force of the grieving process lessens as the survivors put the death into a perspective that they can live with. Despite the similarities, there are some differences involving the death of a parent, spouse, or sibling.

Death of a Parent   The death of a parent can be especially difficult because parents have formed a foundation in most people's lives. In a sense, parents have always "been there." There is a sense of a loss of security that a parent provided for his or her children. A "safety net" for the children disappears. Perhaps for the first time, adult children genuinely see themselves as getting older. When a parent dies, the children realize they have become the new matriarchs and patriarchs, the leaders of their families.

When a parent dies, adult children are reminded of their own mortality.[3] It is not unusual for this realization to push adult children into serious reflection about their own lives. They may, for the first time, evaluate their lives to determine whether the dreams they had as young adults have materialized. This evaluation can be a positive experience for midlife adults, if it encourages them to refocus on the real priorities in their lives.

Some may consider the death of a mother to be more traumatic than the death of a father.[3] Perhaps this is because the mother traditionally has had the role of the primary nurturing caregiver in a family. From the mother's nine months of pregnancy through a child's adult life, the maternal role produces a special bond between a mother and her child. Perhaps another reason why a mother's death is especially traumatic is the fact that men tend to die at younger ages than women do. Thus, a mother's death typically follows a father's death and leaves the adult child with the emptiness of "feeling orphaned."

Death of a Spouse   There is great variability in the way a person adapts to the death of a spouse depending on the length of the marriage (or relationship), the age of the person at death, the children from that marriage, financial resources, the vitality of the relationship, the manner in which the spouse died, and the health status of the widow or widower.

Some couples become so interconnected that the death of one leaves the survivor feeling utterly alone and not whole. A spouse's death might also create a single-parent family, thereby making day-to-day activities quite challenging for the survivor. Some couples may need to assume roles and responsibilities that are unfamiliar and difficult for them, such as handling finances and doing home repairs (see the box "Aftercare").

The death of a spouse can also result in the loss of a primary source of one's social interactions.[3] It is important for the remaining spouse to maintain a network of family and friends for social support and interaction. This social support will be crucial in determining how well the survivor will adjust to his or her new situation. Fortunately, there are support groups for recently widowed persons. These can be found in local communities through churches or social support agencies. Support groups also exist on the Internet for those who wish to seek an online form of support.

Death of a Sibling   The death of a brother or a sister can be very difficult for the surviving sibling(s). It is common for children to feel great guilt for outliving their sibling. They may wonder why the death happened to the sibling rather than them. They may start to question their own mortality and feel more vulnerable to death themselves. Survivors may feel overwhelmed with guilt and believe that they, in some strange way, caused the death. For example, the surviving child who frequently had wished "that his brother was dead" (a common sibling rivalry wish) may believe that his wish caused the car accident that killed his brother.

Aftercare: Attending to the Spiritual Needs of Grieving Families and Friends

Several years ago, funeral homes wanted the public to feel they were not just focusing on the deceased but providing comprehensive service to the mourners. This sparked the concept of "aftercare," which refers to providing services to the family and friends of the deceased through the difficult times following the funeral. Funeral homes now offer counseling such as group meetings of widows or widowers where they can talk to one another about the difficulties they are having, especially during the holidays and special events of remembrance. Funeral homes also coordinate special services in the cemetery or chapel during holidays such as Memorial Day or Mother's Day where everyone is invited and different ministers are invited to speak.

Some funeral homes offer seminars for the survivors on topics such as financial planning, cooking, auto and home repair, and parenting. Children are also provided supportive play therapy groups to give them a place to express their feelings of loss. Some advertise that they help with processing life insurance benefits, Social Security, and pension claims for a deceased's family. They also act as a community referral and resource agency to assist other life transitions especially during the first year after the death. Thus, the roles of funeral director and funeral home are expanding beyond helping to put the deceased to rest to also helping the survivors to live happy, fulfilling lives.

The manner in which parents communicate and respond to the situation can help the surviving child come to terms with the sibling death. Parents need to keep the lines of communication open, listen to the child's concerns, avoid becoming overly protective of the child, and avoid attempting to re-create in the living child certain qualities of the deceased child.[3] Children must be allowed to express their feelings. Talking with mental health experts in the field of grief and bereavement can be especially helpful to children. Individual counseling sessions and group sessions are available in most communities.

Rituals of Death

Our society has established many rituals associated with death that help the survivors accept the reality of death, ease the pain associated with the grief process, and provide a safe disposal of the body. Our rituals give us the chance to formalize our good-byes to a person and to receive emotional support and strength from family members and friends (see the box "Cultural Differences in Death Rituals" on page 565). In recent years, more of our rituals seem to be celebrating the life of the deceased. In doing this, our rituals also reaffirm the value of our own lives.

Most of our funeral rituals take place in funeral homes, churches, and cemeteries. Funeral homes (or mortuaries) are business establishments that provide a variety of services to the families and friends of the deceased. The services are carried out by funeral directors, who are licensed by the state in which they operate. Most funeral directors are responsible for preparing the bodies for viewing, filing death certificates, preparing obituary notices, establishing calling hours, assisting in the preparation and details of the funeral, selecting a casket, transporting mourners to and from the cemetery, and counseling the family. Although licensing procedures vary from state to state, most new funeral directors

must complete one year of college, one year of mortuary school, and one year of internship with a funeral home before taking a state licensing examination.

Full Funeral Services

An ethical funeral director will attempt to follow the wishes of the deceased's family and provide only the services requested by the family. Most families want traditional, **full funeral services.** Three significant components of the full funeral services are as follows.

Embalming *Embalming* is the process of using formaldehyde-based fluids to replace the blood components. Embalming helps preserve the body and return it to a natural look. Embalming permits friends and family members to view the body without being subjected to the odors associated with tissue decomposition. Embalming is often an optional procedure, except when death results from specific communicable diseases or when body disposition (disposal) is delayed.

Calling Hours Sometimes called a *wake* or *visiting hours,* this is an established time when friends and family members can gather in a room to share their emotions and common experiences about the deceased. Generally in the same room, the body will be in a casket, with the lid open or closed. Open caskets help some people to confirm that death truly did occur. Some families prefer not to have any calling hours.

> **Key Terms**
>
> **full funeral services** All the professional services provided by funeral directors.

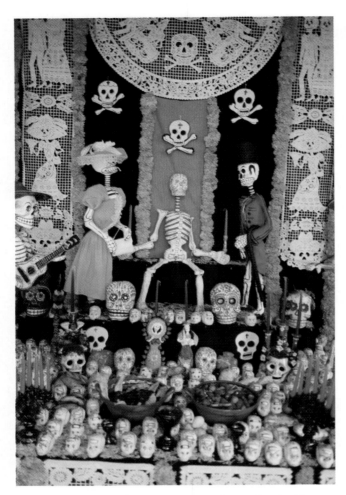

There are cultural differences in the rituals associated with death. Day of the Dead, which originated in Mexico, is a celebration of the dead and the continuation of life, characterized by both sadness and joy. Graves may be decorated with orange marigolds, the deceased's favorite foods, sugared skulls, and figurines of skeletons.

Funeral Service   *Funeral services* vary according to religious preference and the emotional needs of the survivors. Although some services are held in a church, most funeral services today take place in a funeral home, where a special room might serve as a chapel. Some services are held at the graveside. Families may also choose to have a simple memorial service within a few days after the funeral. Completing the Personal Assessment at the end of this chapter will help you think about what kind of funeral arrangements, if any, you would prefer for yourself.

Memorial Service

Some families prefer to have a **memorial service** in addition to (or instead of) the full funeral services. The memorial service is usually a celebration of the life of

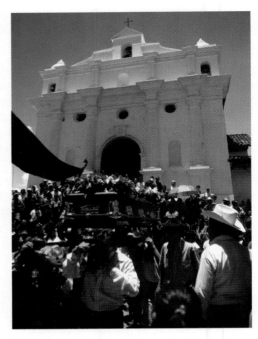

Guatemalan funerals, such as this one, have their own cultural rituals.

the deceased person. This service may have elements of a religious service, with eulogies spoken by friends and relatives of the dead person. Frequently, the public is invited to attend a memorial service. A memorial service typically takes place weeks or months after a person's death, and may follow an earlier, private funeral service. Thus, the body of the deceased person is rarely present at a memorial service.

Disposition of the Body

Ground Burial   We dispose of bodies in one of four ways. Ground burial is the most common method. About 70 percent of all bodies undergo ground burial. The casket is almost always placed in a metal or concrete *vault* before being buried. The vault serves to further protect the body (a need only of the survivors) and to prevent collapse of ground because of the decaying of caskets. Most cemeteries require the use of a vault.

Entombment   A second type of disposition is *entombment*. Entombment refers to nonground burial, most often in structures called **mausoleums.** A mausoleum contains a series of shelves where caskets or urns of cremated remains can be sealed in vaultlike spaces called **niches.** Entombment also can take place in the floors, walls, or basements of buildings, especially in large, old churches. For example, the bodies of many famous British religious, cultural, and government leaders are entombed in the **crypts** of Westminster Abbey in London.

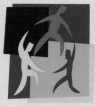

Learning from Our Diversity

Cultural Differences in Death Rituals

Death rituals vary considerably among ethnic and religious groups. Even within the broad categories of ethnic, racial, or religious distinction, differences exist in how groups of people dispose of their deceased. For example, funeral rituals may differ between Orthodox Jews and Conservative Jews. Furthermore, groups of people living in the United States may not be able to follow the traditional funeral rituals of their home countries because they lack the necessary resources and community support. However, some general cultural differences in funeral rituals can be seen in the following examples.

According to Purnell and Paulanka, funeral rituals by the Amish are carried out in the deceased person's home. The church community takes care of the arrangements for visitors, relieving the grieving family of these tasks. In some Amish communities, a wakelike "sitting up" takes place in which family members are supported by friends throughout the night. The funeral itself is simple, with burial in an unadorned wooden coffin, often made by the local Amish carpenter. Children are encouraged to see death as a transition to a better life. Although the Amish clearly feel the pain of their loss, they often may not express this grief openly.

Muslim death rituals are based on their belief that death is the result of God's will. Death is foreordained. For Muslims (and for members of many other religious groups), life in this world is seen as a preparation for eternal life. At death, the deceased's bed is turned to face the Holy City of Mecca, and verses of hope and acceptance are read from the Qur'an. The dead body is washed three times by a Muslim of the same sex as the deceased and then it is wrapped in white material and buried as soon as possible, usually in a brick or cement-lined grave facing Mecca. Prayers are offered for the dead at the cemetery, at the mosque, or at the home. Unless the deceased is a husband or close relative, women usually do not attend the burial. Cremation is not practiced among Muslims.

In Judaism, death is seen as part of the life cycle. Traditional Jews believe in an afterlife in which a person's soul continues to flourish. In this afterlife, people are judged by their actions in life. People who have lived righteous lives are likely to be rewarded in the next world. Judaism does not have a form of last rites; any Jew may ask for God's forgiveness.

At traditional Jewish funerals, the body is rarely embalmed, unless there are unusual circumstances causing burial to be delayed. Burial routinely takes place within a short time after death. Cosmetic restoration is used minimally, if at all. The body is wrapped in a shroud and placed in an unadorned wooden casket. Traditionally, flowers are not displayed at the funeral or at the cemetery. The funeral service is directed at honoring the deceased, while praising God and encouraging people to reaffirm their faith. Traditionally, a 7-day period of immediate mourning (*shiva*) takes place after the burial. After this period there are established mourning periods. For example, mourning for a relative typically lasts 30 days; for a parent, 1 year.

Source: LD Purnell and BJ Paulanka, *Transcultural Healthcare* (Philadelphia: F.A. Davis, 1998).

Cremation   *Cremation* is a third type of body disposition. In the United States, 30 percent of all bodies are cremated.[17] This practice is increasing. Generally, both the body and casket (or cardboard cremation box) are incinerated so that only the bone ash from the body remains. The body of an average adult produces about 5 to 7 pounds of bone ash. These ashes then are placed in containers called *urns,* and then buried, entombed, or scattered, if permitted by state law. The itemized crematory fee ($600–$1,000) is much less than the fee for ground burial. Some families choose to cremate after having full funeral services.[18]

Anatomical Donation   A fourth method of body disposition is *anatomical donation.* Separate organs (such as corneal tissue, kidneys, or the heart) can be donated to a medical school, research facility, or organ donor network. Some people choose to donate their entire body to medical science. Often this is done through prior arrangements with medical schools. Bodies still require embalming. After they are studied, the remains are often cremated and returned to the family, if requested. Just as with an organ donation, those who wish to donate their bodies should discuss their wishes with family members beforehand so that their wishes can be carried out at the time of death.

Costs

The full funeral services (also referred to as death-care services) offered by a funeral home cost upward of $6,000, with other expenses added to this price. Casket prices

---

Key Terms

memorial service A broad term for a ceremony that honors the life of a person who has died.

mausoleum (moz oh **lee** um**)** An above-ground structure, which frequently resembles a small stone house, into which caskets can be placed for disposition.

niche A recessed area in a mausoleum where a casket can be placed.

crypts Burial locations generally in the walls, floors, or basements of churches.

---

vary significantly, with the average cost between $1,500 and $2,500. Costs can vary tremendously depending on the type of casket, funeral services, and arrangements. Some people are opting to have plastic surgery as part of the funeral preparations, which would certainly increase the cost of death-care services. When all the expenses associated with a typical funeral are totaled, the average cost is approximately $6,500.[19]

Regardless of the rituals you select for the handling of your body (or the body of someone in your care), you may want to make prearrangements. You can ease your survivors' burden by putting your wishes in writing. *Funeral prearrangements* relieve the survivors of many of the details that must be handled at the time of your death and can better ensure that your wishes will be carried out. You can gather much of the information for your obituary notice and your wishes for the disposition of your body. You can make prearrangements with a funeral director, family member, or attorney. Many individuals also prepay the costs of their funeral. By making arrangements before the need arises, you can have peace of mind. Currently, about 30 to 40 percent of funerals are preplanned and prepaid. However, there may be some risk involved with prepaying funeral arrangements, such as if the funeral home goes out of business or sells the business to another owner who doesn't honor these arrangements, or if items are not available or included at the time of the funeral service.

Personal Preparation for Death

We hope that this chapter helps you to develop a new framework about death and form your own personal perspective on death and dying. Remember that the ultimate goal of death education is a positive one—to help you best use and enjoy your life. Becoming aware of the reality of your own mortality is a step in the right direction. Reading about the process of dying, grief resolution, and the rituals surrounding death can also help you accept that someday you too will die.

You can prepare for the reality of your own death in some additional ways. Preparing a will, purchasing a life insurance policy, making funeral prearrangements, preparing a living will, and considering an anatomical or organ donation are measures that help you to prepare for your death. At the appropriate time, you might also wish to talk with family and friends about your death. You may discover that an upbeat, positive discussion about death can help relieve some of your apprehensions and those of others around you.

Another suggestion to help you emotionally prepare for your death is to prepare your *obituary notice* or **eulogy.** Include all the things you would like to have said about you and your life. Now compare your obituary notice and eulogy with the current direction your life seems to be taking. Are you doing the kinds of activities for which you want to be known? If so, great! If not, perhaps you will want to consider why your current direction does not reflect how you would like to be remembered. How do you want to restructure your life to better fit your life's goals, meaning, and purpose?

Another suggestion to help make you aware of your eventual death is to write your own **epitaph,** an inscription on a grave marker or monument. Before doing this, you might want to visit a cemetery. Reading the epitaphs of others may help you develop yours.

To assist you in expanding and accepting your awareness of your own mortality, consider answering the following questions: (1) If I had only one day to live, how would I spend it? (2) What one accomplishment would I like to achieve before I die? (3) After I am dead, what two or three things will people miss most about me? By answering these questions and accomplishing a few of the tasks suggested in this section, you will have a good start on accepting your own death and understanding the value of life itself.

Key Terms

eulogy A composition or speech that praises someone; often delivered at a funeral or memorial service.

epitaph An inscription on a grave marker or monument.

Taking Charge of Your Health

- Start considering how you might plan for your funeral by completing the Personal Assessment at the end of this chapter.
- Consider completing a living will and designating a health care agent or proxy. Discuss your wishes with your family and friends.

- Consider completing an organ donor card, purchase life insurance, and/or prepare a will.
- If you don't already know, ask your family about their end-of-life wishes.
- Write your own eulogy, epitaph, or obituary.

- If you have experienced a loss, where would you place yourself in the psychological stages of grief? If appropriate, explore with a trusted friend, family member, spiritual leader, or counselor how you can move closer to a sense of acceptance of this loss.

SUMMARY

- Death is determined primarily by clinical and legal factors.
- Euthanasia can be performed through either direct or indirect measures.
- Currently, physician-assisted suicide is legal in only two states, Oregon and Washington.
- The most current advance health care directives are the living will and the durable power of attorney for health care.
- Denial, anger, bargaining, depression, and acceptance are the five classic psychological stages that dying people commonly experience, according to Kübler-Ross.
- When a parent dies, a child needs support and the truth, especially two crucial pieces of information: that the dead parent will never return and that the body has been buried in the ground or cremated.
- Death in our society is associated with many rituals to help survivors cope with the loss of a loved one and to ensure proper disposal of the body.
- The shortage of organ donations is the biggest problem facing people who need a transplant to save their lives.
- Hospice care is an alternative end-of-life health care option for terminally ill patients and their families.
- We dispose of bodies in four ways: ground burial, entombment, cremation, and anatomical donation.

REVIEW QUESTIONS

1. Identify and explain the clinical and legal determinants of death, and identify who establishes each of them.
2. Explain the difference between direct and indirect euthanasia.
3. What is physician-assisted suicide, and in what states is it legal?
4. How does a living will differ from a durable power of attorney as a health care document? Why are these advance health care directives becoming increasingly popular?
5. Identify and explain the five psychological stages that dying people tend to experience. Explain each stage.
6. Identify and explain the four strategies that form the basis of hospice care. What are the advantages of hospice care for the patient and the family?
7. Define the term *grief*. Identify and explain the sensations and emotions most people have when they experience grief. When does the grieving process end?
8. What purposes do the rituals of death serve? What are the significant components of the full funeral service?
9. What are the four ways in which bodies are disposed?
10. Define these terms: *mausoleum, niche, crypt, vault, urn, eulogy, obituary,* and *epitaph.*

ANSWERS TO THE "WHAT DO YOU KNOW?" QUIZ

1. False   2. False   3. True   4. True   5. True   6. True   7. False

Visit the Online Learning Center (**www.mhhe.com/payne11e**), where you will find tools to help you improve your grade including practice quizzes, key terms flashcards, audio chapter summaries for your MP3 player, and many other study aids.

SOURCE NOTES

1. Leming MR, Dickinson GE. *Understanding Dying, Death and Bereavement* (5th ed.). New York: Harcourt, 2001.
2. Kastenbaum RJ. *Death, Society, and Human Experience* (6th ed.). Boston: Allyn & Bacon, 1998.
3. DeSpelder L, Strickland A. *The Last Dance: Encountering Death and Dying* (7th ed.). New York: McGraw-Hill, 2005.
4. Kübler-Ross E. *On Death and Dying* (reprint ed.). New York: Collier Books, 1997.
5. Kübler-Ross E. *To Live Until We Say Goodbye* (reprint ed.). Upper Saddle River, NJ: Prentice Hall, 1997.
6. Moody RA. *The Last Laugh: A New Philosophy of Near Death Experiences, Apparitions, and the Paranormal.* Charlottsville, VA: Hampton Roads, 1999.
7. Ring K. *Life at Death: A Scientific Investigation of the Near-Death Experience.* New York: Coward, McCann and Geoghegan, 1980.
8. Bendiksen R, Fulton R (Eds.). *Death and Identity* (3rd ed.). Philadelphia: Charles Press, 1994.
9. Staudacher, C. *Beyond Grief.* Oakland, CA: New Harbinger, 1987.
10. National Hospice and Palliative Care Organization. *Facts and Figures on Hospice Care in America,* 2008, www.nhpco.org, November 2008.
11. www.pbs.org/wgbh/pages/frontline/kevorkian/law, "The Law on Assisted Suicide," December 16, 1999.
12. Doctor of Death to Be Paroled Soon, *The Star Press,* December 14, 2006.
13. Partnership for Caring. *Facts about Advance Directives,* www.partnershipforcaring.org, October 10, 2000.
14. Organ Donors' Lives on the Line, *St. Louis Post,* May 22, 2005.
15. United Network for Organ Sharing. *The Critical Organ Shortage,* www.unos.org, April 24, 2009.
16. Lindemann E. Symptomology and Management of Acute Grief. In Fulton et al. (Eds.), *Death and Dying: Challenge and Change.* Boston: Addison-Wesley, 1978.
17. New Creations Personalize Cremation, *USA Today,* October 20, 2006.
18. Bowman J (Licensed Funeral Director). Personal correspondence, September 25, 2001.
19. Plan Funeral Now to Make Sure You Have the Final Word. *USA Today,* July 28, 2006.

Personal Assessment

Planning Your Funeral

In line with this chapter's positive theme of the value of personal death awareness, here is a funeral service assessment that we frequently give to our health classes. This inventory can help you assess your reactions and thoughts about the funeral arrangements you would prefer for yourself.

After answering each of the following questions, you might wish to discuss your responses with a friend or close relative.

1. Have you ever considered how you would like your body to be handled after your death?

   _____ Yes   _____ No

2. Have you already made funeral arrangements for yourself?

   _____ Yes   _____ No

3. Have you considered a specific funeral home or mortuary to handle your arrangements?

   _____ Yes   _____ No

4. If you were to die today, which of the following would you prefer?

   _____ Embalming   _____ Ground burial
   _____ Cremation   _____ Entombment
   _____ Donation to medical science

5. If you prefer to be cremated, what do you want done with your ashes?

   _____ Buried   _____ Entombed
   _____ Scattered
   _____ Other; please specify _____

6. If your funeral plans involve a casket, which of the following do you prefer?

   _____ Plywood (cloth covered)
   _____ Hardwood (oak, cherry, mahogany, maple, etc.)
   _____ Steel (sealer or nonsealer type)
   _____ Stainless steel
   _____ Copper or bronze
   _____ Other; please specify _____

7. How important is a funeral service for you?

   _____ Very important
   _____ Somewhat important
   _____ Somewhat unimportant
   _____ Very unimportant
   _____ No opinion

8. What kind of funeral service do you want for yourself?

   _____ No service at all
   _____ Visitation (calling hours) the day before the funeral service; funeral held at church or funeral home
   _____ Graveside service only (no visitation)
   _____ Memorial service (after body disposition)
   _____ Other; please specify

9. How many people do you want to attend your funeral service or memorial service?

   _____ I do not want a funeral or memorial service
   _____ 1–10 people
   _____ 11–25 people
   _____ 26–50 people
   _____ Over 50 people
   _____ I do not care how many people attend

10. What format would you prefer at your funeral service or memorial service? Select any of the following that you like:

	Yes	No
Religious music	_____	_____
Nonreligious music	_____	_____
Clergy present	_____	_____
Flower arrangements	_____	_____
Family member eulogy	_____	_____
Eulogy by friend(s)	_____	_____
Open casket	_____	_____
Religious format	_____	_____
Other; please specify _____		

11. Using today's prices, how much do you expect to pay for your total funeral arrangements, including cemetery expenses (if applicable)?

   _____ Less than $4,500
   _____ Between $4,501 and $6,000
   _____ Between $6,001 and $7,500
   _____ Between $7,501 and $9,000
   _____ Between $9,001 and $13,000
   _____ Above $13,000

TO CARRY THIS FURTHER . . .

Which items had you not thought about before? Were you surprised at the arrangements you selected? Will you share your responses with anyone else? If so, whom?

First Aid

Accidents are the leading cause of death for people ages 1 to 37. Injuries sustained in accidents can often be tragic. They are grim reminders of our need to learn first aid skills and to practice preventive safety habits.

First aid knowledge and skills allow you to help people who are in need of immediate emergency care. They also can help you save yourself if you should become injured. We recommend that our students enroll in American Red Cross first aid and safety courses, which are available in local communities or through colleges or universities. In this appendix, we briefly present some information about common first aid emergencies. (Please note that our information is *not* a substitute for comprehensive American Red Cross first aid instruction.)

First Aid

- Keep a list of important phone numbers near your phone (your doctor, ambulance service, hospital, poison control center, police and fire departments).
- In case of serious injury or illness, call the appropriate emergency service immediately for help (if uncertain, call "911" or "0").

Common First Aid Emergencies

Specific Problem	What to Do
Asphyxiation Victim stops breathing and skin, lips, tongue, and fingernail beds turn bluish or gray.	Tip head back with one hand on forehead and other lifting the lower jaw near the chin. Look, listen, and feel for breathing. If the victim is not breathing, place your mouth over victim's mouth, pinch the nose, get a tight seal, and give 2 slow breaths. Do a pulse check. If no pulse is detected, CPR must be administered. (Note: Some states require CPR training for those who administer CPR.) If there is a pulse but no breathing, give breaths once every 5 seconds for an adult, once every 3 seconds for a child, once every 3 seconds for infants (do not exaggerate head tilt for babies). Recheck pulse and breathing every 2 minutes.
Bleeding Victim bleeding severely can quickly go into shock and die within 1 or 2 minutes.	Use universal precautions. With the palm of your hand, apply firm, direct pressure to the wound with a clean dressing or pad. Elevate the body part if possible. Do not remove blood-soaked dressings; use additional layers, continue to apply pressure, and elevate the site.
Choking Accidental ingestion or inhalation of food or other objects causes suffocation that can quickly lead to death. There are over 3,000 deaths annually, mostly of infants, small children, and the elderly.	The procedure of giving 5 back blows followed by 5 abdominal thrusts is easy to learn; however, the correct technique must be learned from a qualified instructor. The procedure varies somewhat for infants, children, adults, pregnant women, and obese people.
Hyperventilation A situation in which a person breathes too rapidly; often the result of fear or anxiety; may cause confusion, shortness of breath, dizziness, or fainting. Intentional hyperventilation before an underwater swim is especially dangerous, since it may cause a swimmer to pass out in the water and drown.	Have the person relax and rest for a few minutes. Provide reassurance and a calming influence. Having the victim take a few breaths from a paper bag (not plastic) may be helpful. Do not permit swimmers to practice hyperventilation before attempting to swim.

appendix

Common First Aid Emergencies *continued*

Specific Problem	What to Do
Bee Stings Not especially dangerous except for people who have developed an allergic hypersensitivity to a particular venom. Those who are not hypersensitive will experience swelling, redness, and pain. Hypersensitive people may develop extreme swelling, chest constriction, breathing difficulties, hives, and shock signs.	For nonsensitive people: Scrape stinger from skin and apply cold compresses or over-the-counter topical preparation for insect bites. For sensitive people: Get professional help immediately. Scrape the stinger from skin; position the person so that the stung body part is below the level of the heart; help administer prescribed medication (if available); apply cold compresses.
Poisoning Often poisoning can be prevented with adequate safety awareness. Children are frequent victims.	Call the poison control center immediately; follow the instructions provided. Keep syrup of ipecac on hand.
Shock A life-threatening depression of circulation, respiration, and temperature control; recognizable by a victim's cool, clammy, pale skin; weak and rapid pulse; shallow breathing; weakness; nausea; or *unconsciousness.*	Keep the victim calm; loosen tight clothing. Help the victim to a comfortable, reclining position with legs elevated 8–12 inches (*if there are head, neck, back, or internal injuries, do not move the person at all;* if breathing is difficult, help the person to sit or semi-recline). Prevent loss of body heat; cover if necessary. Do not give food or fluids. Seek further emergency assistance.
Burns Burns can cause severe tissue damage and lead to serious infection and shock.	Minor burns: immerse in cold water 10–15 minutes; dry; apply antibiotic agent and loose sterile dressing; do not apply butter or grease to burns. Major burns: cover affected area with sterile or clean dressings; do not try to clean the burn area or break blisters. Seek medical attention. Chemical burns: flood the area with running water.
Broken Bones Fractures are a common result of car accidents, falls, and recreational accidents.	Do not move the victim unless absolutely necessary to prevent further injury. Immobilize the affected area. Give care for shock while waiting for further emergency assistance.

Source: American Red Cross. *First Aid: Responding to Emergencies* (4th ed.). Staywell Publishers, 2006.

570   **Appendix**   First Aid

Epilepsy: Recognition and First Aid

Seizure Type	What It Looks Like	Often Mistaken for	What to Do	What Not to Do
Convulsive				
Generalized tonic-clonic (also called grand mal)	Sudden cry, fall, rigidity, followed by muscle jerks, frothy saliva on lips, shallow breathing or temporarily suspended breathing, bluish skin, possible loss of bladder or bowel control, usually last 2–5 minutes; normal breathing then starts again; there may be some confusion and/or fatigue, followed by return to full consciousness	Heart attack Stroke Unknown but life-threatening emergency	Protect from nearby hazards Loosen ties or shirt collars Place folded jacket under head Turn on side to keep airway clear; reassure when consciousness returns Look for medical identification *after* seizure subsides or protective steps have been taken If single seizure lasted less than 5 minutes, ask if hospital evaluation wanted If multiple seizures, or if one seizure lasts longer than 5 minutes, seek medical attention	Don't put any hard implement in the mouth Don't try to hold tongue; it can't be swallowed Don't try to give liquids during or just after seizure Don't use artificial respiration unless breathing is absent after muscle jerks subside Don't restrain
Nonconvulsive				
	This category includes many different forms of seizures, ranging from temporary unawareness (petit mal) to brief, sudden, massive muscle jerks (myoclonic seizures)	Daydreaming, acting out, clumsiness, poor coordination, intoxication, random activity, mental illness, and many others	Usually no first aid necessary other than to provide reassurance and emotional support If behavior during seizure places person in potentially hazardous situation (e.g., traffic, machinery), gently guide person away from hazard Medical evaluation is recommended	Do not shout at, restrain, or grab a person having a nonconvulsive seizure (unless danger threatens); do not expect verbal instructions to be obeyed

A

abortion Induced premature termination of a pregnancy.

absorption The passage of nutrients or alcohol through the walls of the stomach or intestinal tract into the bloodstream.

abuse Any use of a drug in a way that is detrimental to health or well-being.

acceptable macronutrient distribution range (AMDR) The range of intakes for energy sources associated with adequate nutrient intake and reduced risk of chronic disease.

acquired immunity (AI) A form of immunity resulting from exposure to foreign protein (most often wild, weakened, or killed pathogenic organisms).

acupuncture Insertion of fine needles into the body to alter electroenergy fields and treat disease.

acute Having a sudden onset and a prompt resolution.

acute alcohol intoxication A potentially fatal elevation of BAC, often resulting from heavy, rapid consumption of alcohol.

acute rhinitis The common cold; the sudden onset of nasal inflammation.

adaptive thermogenesis The physiological response of the body to adjust its metabolic rate to the presence of food.

addiction Compulsive, uncontrollable dependence on a substance, habit, or practice to such a degree that cessation causes severe emotional or physiological reactions.

additive effect The combined (but not exaggerated) effect produced by the concurrent use of two or more drugs.

adipose tissue Tissue made up of fibrous strands around which specialized cells designed to store liquefied fat are arranged.

aerobic energy production The body's primary means of energy production, used when the respiratory and circulatory systems can process and transport sufficient oxygen to muscle cells to convert fuel to energy.

agent The causal pathogen of a particular disease.

agoraphobia A fear of being in situations from which there is no escape or in which help would be unavailable should an emergency arise; often associated with panic disorder.

air pollution Substances found in the atmosphere that can have adverse effects on human health, crop productivity, and natural communities.

air toxics A class of 188 toxic air pollutants identified by the U.S. Environmental Protection Agency as known or suspected causes of cancer or other serious health effects, such as reduced fertility, birth defects, or adverse environmental effects.

alarm stage The first stage of the stress response, involving physiological, involuntary changes that are controlled by the hormonal and nervous system; the fight or flight response is activated in this stage.

alcohol abuse Patterns of alcohol use that create problems for the drinker's school and job performance, other responsibilities, and interpersonal relationships. Individuals persist in drinking even though they are having legal problems and know that their drinking is causing them problems. Also called *problem drinking*.

alcohol dependence Tolerance, withdrawal, and a pattern of compulsive use of alcohol. A primary, chronic disease with genetic, psychosocial, and environmental factors affecting its development. Also called *alcoholism*.

allopathy (ah **lop** ah thee) A system of medical practice in which specific remedies (often pharmaceutical agents) are used to produce effects different from those produced by a disease or injury.

alveoli (al **vee** oh lie) Thin, saclike terminal ends of the airways; the site at which gases are exchanged between the blood and the lungs.

Alzheimer's disease Adult-onset form of dementia resulting from loss of acetylcholine production within specific areas of the brain.

amenorrhea The absence of menstruation.

amino acids The building blocks of protein; can be manufactured by the body or obtained from dietary sources.

anabolic steroids (ann uh **bol** ick) Drugs that function like testosterone to produce increases in muscle mass, strength, endurance, and aggressiveness.

anaerobic energy production The body's alternative means of energy production, used when the available oxygen is insufficient for aerobic energy production. Anaerobic energy production is a much less efficient use of stored energy.

anal intercourse A sexual act in which the erect penis is inserted into the rectum of a partner.

androgyny (an **droj** en ee) The blending of both masculine and feminine qualities.

andropause Significant decrease in androgenic hormone production in aging men; also called male menopause.

angina pectoris (an **jie** nuh **peck** tor is) Chest pain that results from impaired blood supply to the heart muscle.

anorexia nervosa An eating disorder in which the individual weighs less than 85 percent of the expected weight for his or her age, gender, and height; has an intense fear of gaining weight; and, in females, ceases to menstruate for at least three consecutive months. People with anorexia perceive themselves as overweight, even though they are underweight.

antagonistic effect The effect produced when one drug reduces or offsets the effects of a second drug.

antibodies Chemical compounds produced by the body's immune system to destroy antigens and their toxins.

antioxidants Substances that may prevent cancer by interacting with and stabilizing unstable molecules known as free radicals.

artificially acquired immunity (AAI) A type of acquired immunity resulting from the body's response to pathogens introduced into the body through immunizations.

asbestos A class of minerals that have a fibrous crystal structure; a known carcinogen when inhaled.

asphyxiation Death resulting from lack of oxygen to the brain.

atherosclerosis The buildup of plaque on the inner wall of arteries.

attention deficit hyperactivity disorder (ADHD) An above-normal rate of physical movement; often accompanied by an inability to concentrate on a specified task.

autoimmune disorders Disorders caused by the immune system's failure to recognize the body as "self"; thus the body mounts an attack against its own cells and tissues.

axon The portion of a neuron that conducts electrical impulses to the dendrites of adjacent neurons; neurons typically have one axon.

B

ballistic stretching A "bouncing" form of stretching in which a muscle group is lengthened repetitively to produce multiple, quick, forceful stretches.

basal metabolic rate (BMR) The amount of energy, expressed in calories, that the body requires to maintain basic functions.

basic needs Deficiency needs that are viewed as essential and fundamental, including physiological needs, safety and security, belonging and love, and esteem needs.

behavior therapy A behavior modification therapy based on the learning principles of reinforcement therapy, stimulus-response, and conditioning responses to change behavior.

benign Noncancerous; localized nonmalignant tumors contained within a fibrous membrane.

beta blockers Drugs that reduce the workload of the heart, which results in angina pectoris.

beta endorphins Mood-enhancing, pain-reducing, opiatelike chemicals produced within the smoker's body in response to the presence of nicotine.

bias and hate crimes Criminal acts directed at a person or group solely because of a specific characteristic, such as race, religion, ethnic background, sexual orientation, or other difference.

bigorexia An obsession with getting bigger and more muscular, and thinking that your body is never muscular enough.

binge drinking Five or more drinks on the same occasion (at the same time or within the span of a couple of hours) on at least 1 day in the last 2-week period.

binge eating disorder An eating disorder formerly referred to as compulsive overeating disorder; binge eaters use food to cope in the same way that bulimics do and also feel out of control, but do not engage in compensatory purging behavior.

biological air pollutants Living organisms or substances produced by living organisms that cause disease or allergic reactions, including bacteria, molds, mildew, viruses, dust mites, plant pollen, and animal dander, urine, or feces.

biological water pollutants Disease-causing organisms that are found in water.

biopsychological model A model that addresses how biological, psychological, and social factors interact and affect psychological health.

bipolar disorder A mood disorder characterized by alternating episodes of depression and mania.

birth control All of the methods and procedures that can prevent the birth of a child.

blackout An inability to remember events that occur during a period of alcohol use, including things that a person said or did during that time.

blastocyst Early stage of the developing life form that embeds itself into the endometrial lining of the uterus.

blood alcohol concentration (BAC) The percentage of alcohol in a measured quantity of blood; BAC can be determined directly, through the analysis of a blood sample, or indirectly, through the analysis of exhaled air.

body dysmorphic disorder (BDD) A secret preoccupation with an imagined or slight flaw in one's appearance.

body image One's subjective perception of how one's body appears to oneself and others.

body mass index (BMI) A mathematical calculation based on weight and height; used to determine desirable body weight.

bolus theory A theory of nicotine addiction based on the body's response to the bolus (ball) of nicotine delivered to the brain with each inhalation of cigarette smoke.

bonding Important initial recognition established between the newborn and those adults on whom the newborn will depend.

bradycardia Slowness of the heartbeat, as evidenced by a resting pulse rate of less than 60 beats per minute.

brand name Specific patented name assigned to a drug by its manufacturer.

bulimia nervosa An eating disorder in which individuals engage in episodes of binging, consuming unusually large amounts of food and feeling out of control, and then engaging in some compensatory purging behavior to eliminate the food.

c

calcium channel blockers Drugs that prevent arterial spasms; used in the control of blood pressure and the long-term management of angina pectoris.

calendar method A form of periodic abstinence in which the variable lengths of a woman's menstrual cycle are used to calculate her fertile period.

caliper A device used to measure the thickness of a skinfold from which percentage of body fat can be calculated.

caloric balance Caloric intake and caloric expenditure are equal and body weight remains constant.

calories Units of heat (energy); specifically, 1 calorie is the amount of energy needed to raise the temperature of 1 gram of water by 1 degree C. In common usage,

on food labels, and in this book, the term *calorie* is used to refer to a larger energy unit, *kilocalorie* (1,000 calories).

carbohydrates The body's primary source of energy for all body functioning; chemical compounds including sugar, starches, and dietary fibers.

carbon monoxide A gaseous byproduct of the incomplete combustion of natural gas, kerosene, heating oil, wood, coal, gasoline, and tobacco; a compound that can "inactivate" red blood cells.

carcinogens Environmental agents, including chemical compounds within cigarette smoke, that stimulate the development of cancerous changes within cells.

cardiac arrest Immediate death resulting from a sudden change in the rhythm of the heart causing loss of heart function.

cardiac muscle Specialized muscle tissue that forms the middle (muscular) layer of the heart wall.

cardiorespiratory endurance The ability of the heart, lungs, and blood vessels to process and transport oxygen required by muscle cells so that they can contract over a period of time. Cardiorespiratory endurance is produced by exercise that requires continuous, repetitive movements.

cardiovascular Pertaining to the heart (*cardio*) and blood vessels (*vascular*).

catabolizing The metabolic process of breaking down tissue for the purpose of converting it to energy.

cell-mediated immunity Immunity provided principally by the immune system's T cells, both working alone and in combination with highly specialized B cells; also called *T cell–mediated immunity*.

cellulite Tissue composed of fat cells intertwined around strands of fibrous connective tissue.

cerebrovascular occlusions (ser **ee** bro **vas** kyou lar) Blockages to arteries supplying blood to the cerebral cortex of the brain; cause of the most common type of stroke.

cesarean delivery (si **zare** ee an) Surgical removal of a fetus through the abdominal wall.

chemical name Name used to describe the molecular structure of a drug.

chemoprevention Cancer prevention using food, dietary supplements, or medications thought to bolster the immune system or reduce the damage caused by carcinogens.

child maltreatment The act or failure to act by a parent or caregiver that results in abuse or neglect of a child or that places the child in imminent risk of serious harm.

chiropractic Manipulation of the vertebral column to relieve malalignments and cure illness.

chlamydia The most prevalent sexually transmitted disease; caused by a nongono-coccal bacterium.

cholesterol A primary form of fat found in the blood; lipid material manufactured within the body, as well as derived from dietary sources.

chronic Develops slowly and persists for an extended period of time.

chronic bronchitis Persistent inflammation and infection of the smaller airways within the lungs.

chronic fatigue syndrome (CFS) An illness that causes severe exhaustion, fatigue, aches, and depression; mostly affects women in their 40s and 50s.

chronic stress Remaining at a high level of physiological arousal for an extended period of time; it can also occur when an individual is not able to immediately react to a real or a perceived threat.

cilia (**sill** ee uh) Small, hairlike structures that extend from cells that line the air passages.

circadian rhythms The internal, biological clock that helps coordinate physiological processes with the 24-hour light/dark cycle.

clinical depression A psychological disorder in which individuals experience a lack of motivation, decreased energy level, fatigue, social withdrawal, sleep disturbance, disturbance in appetite, diminished sex drive, feelings of worthlessness, and despair.

club drug One of a variety of psychoactive drugs typically used at raves, bars, and dance clubs.

cognitive-behavioral therapy An action-oriented form of therapy that assumes that maladaptive, or faulty, thinking patterns cause maladaptive behavior and negative emotions; treatment focuses on changing an individual's thoughts or cognitive patterns in order to change his or her behavior and emotional state.

cohabitation Sharing of a residence by two unrelated, unmarried people; living together.

coitus (**co** ih tus) Penile-vaginal intercourse.

cold turkey Immediate, total discontinuation of use of a drug; associated withdrawal discomfort.

colonoscopy (co lun **os** ko py) Examination of the entire length of the colon, using a flexible fiberoptic scope to inspect the structure's inner lining.

compliance Willingness to follow the directions provided by another person.

computerized axial tomography (CT) scan An X-ray procedure designed to illustrate structures within the body that would not normally be seen through conventional X-ray procedures.

condom A shield designed to cover the erect penis and retain semen upon ejaculation; "rubber."

congestive heart failure Inability of the heart to pump out all the blood that returns to it; can lead to dangerous fluid accumulations in veins, lungs, and kidneys.

consumer fraud Marketing of unreliable and ineffective services, products, or information under the guise of curing disease or improving health; quackery.

contraception Any method or procedure that prevents fertilization.

contraceptive patch Contraceptive skin patch containing estrogen and progestin; replaced each week for a three-week period.

contraceptive ring Thin, polymer contraceptive device containing estrogen and progestin; placed deep within the vagina for a three-week period.

contraceptive sponge A small, pillow-shaped contraceptive device that contains a spermicide; placed deep in the vagina to cover the cervical opening.

contraindications Factors that make the use of a drug inappropriate or dangerous for a particular person.

coronary arteries Vessels that supply oxygenated blood to heart muscle tissues.

coronary artery bypass surgery A surgical procedure designed to improve blood flow to the heart by providing alternate routes for blood to take around points of blockage.

corpus luteum (kore pus **loo** tee um) The cellular remnant of the graafian follicle after the release of an ovum.

cross-tolerance Transfer of tolerance from one drug to another within the same general category.

cruciferous vegetables (crew **sif** er us) Vegetables, such as broccoli, whose plants have flowers with four leaves in the pattern of a cross.

crypts Burial locations generally in the walls, floors, or basements of churches.

crystal methamphetamine A dangerous form of methamphetamine that quickly produces intense physical and psychological exhilaration when smoked.

cunnilingus (cun uh **ling** gus) Oral stimulation of the vulva or clitoris.

curette A metal scraping instrument that resembles a spoon, with a cup-shaped cutting surface on its end.

current use At least one drink in the past 30 days.

cyanosis Blue coloration of the lips, skin, and nail beds caused by inadequate oxygenation of the blood.

D

degenerative A slow but progressive deterioration of the body's structure or function.

dehydration Abnormal depletion of fluids from the body; severe dehydration can be fatal.

delirium tremens (DTs) Uncontrollable shaking, combined with irrational hallucinations, caused by abstinence from alcohol following habitual alcohol use.

dementia The loss of cognitive abilities, including memory and reason.

dendrite The portion of a neuron that receives electrical stimuli from adjacent neurons; neurons typically have several such branches or extensions.

dependence A general term that refers to the need to continue using a drug for psychological or physical reasons or both.

depressants A category of drugs that sedate the user by slowing central nervous system function; they produce tolerance and strong psychological and physical addiction in users.

designated driver A person who abstains from or carefully limits alcohol consumption to be able to safely transport other people who have been drinking.

desirable weight The weight range deemed appropriate for people, taking into consideration gender, age, and frame size.

diaphragm A soft rubber cup designed to cover the cervix.

diastolic pressure (**dye** uh stol ick) Blood pressure against blood vessel walls when the heart relaxes.

Dietary Reference Intakes (DRIs) Measures that refer to three types of reference values: Estimated Average Requirement, Recommended Dietary Allowance, and Tolerable Upper Intake Level.

dilation The gradual expansion of an opening or passageway, such as the cervix.

dilation and evacuation (D&E) Second-trimester abortion procedure that requires greater dilation, suction, and curettage than first-trimester vacuum aspiration procedures.

dilation and suction curettage (D&C) (kyoo re **taage**) A surgical procedure in which the cervical canal is dilated to allow the uterine wall to be scraped; vacuum aspiration.

direct (active) euthanasia Intentionally causing death.

dissonance (**dis** son ince) A feeling of uncertainty that occurs when a person believes two equally attractive but opposite ideas.

distillation The process of heating an alcohol solution and collecting its vapors into a more concentrated solution.

distress Stress that diminishes the quality of life; commonly associated with disease, illness, and maladaptation.

dose-response curve The size of the effect of a drug on the body related to the amount of the drug administered.

drink 12 ounces of beer, 5 ounces of wine, or 1.5 ounces of liquor.

drug Any substance, natural or artificial, other than food, that by its chemical or physical nature alters structure or function in the living organism.

durable power of attorney for health care A legal document that designates who will make health care decisions for people unable to do so.

duration The length of exercise time of each training session; for aerobic fitness, 20 to 60 minutes is recommended.

dynamic therapy An intensive therapy based on the belief that effective treatment must focus on the psychological forces underlying the individual's problems.

dysmenorrhea Abdominal pain caused by muscular cramping during the menstrual cycle.

E

ectopic pregnancy A pregnancy in which the fertilized ovum implants at a site other than the uterus, typically in a fallopian tube.

electrical impedance A method used to measure the percentage of body fat using a harmless electrical current.

embolism A potentially fatal condition in which a circulating blood clot lodges in a smaller vessel.

embryo Developmental stage from the end of the second week after conception until the end of the eighth week.

emergency contraception Contraceptive measures used to prevent pregnancy within five days after unprotected intercourse; also called *postcoital* or *morning-after* contraception.

emotional intelligence The ability to understand others and act wisely in human relations and measure how well one knows one's emotions, manages one's emotions, motivates oneself, recognizes emotions in others, and handles relationships.

empowerment The nurturing of an individual's or group's ability to be responsible for their own health and well-being.

endocrine-disrupting chemicals A large class of substances that can interact with the system of glands, hormones, and tissues that regulate many physiological processes in humans, including growth, development from fetus to adult, regulation of metabolic rate and blood sugar, function of reproductive systems, and development of the brain and nervous system.

enriched Foods that have been resupplied with some of the nutritional elements (B vitamins and iron) removed during processing.

enucleated egg An ovum with the nucleus removed.

environment The physical conditions (temperature, humidity, light, presence of substances) and other living organisms that exist around your body.

environmental tobacco smoke Tobacco smoke, regardless of source, that stays within a common source of air.

enzymes Organic substances that control the rate of physiological reactions but are not altered in the process.

epidemic A highly significant increase in the number of cases of an infectious illness in a given time period in a given geographical area.

epitaph An inscription on a grave marker or monument.

erection The engorgement of erectile tissue with blood; characteristic of the penis, clitoris, nipples, labia minora, and scrotum.

erotic dreams Dreams whose contents elicit a sexual response.

estimated average requirement (EAR) The intake value that is estimated to meet the requirement in 50 percent of an age- and gender-specific group.

eulogy A composition or speech that praises someone; often delivered at a funeral or memorial service.

eustress Stress that enhances the quality of life.

excitement stage Initial arousal stage of the sexual response pattern.

exercise A subcategory of physical activity; it is planned, structured, repetitive, and purposive in the sense that an improvement or maintenance of physical fitness is an objective (Casperson et al., 1985).

exhaustion stage The point at which the physical and psychological resources used to deal with stress have been depleted.

exocrine glands Glands whose secretions are released through tubes or ducts, such as sweat glands.

F

false labor Conditions that resemble the start of true labor; may include irregular uterine contractions, pressure, and discomfort in the lower abdomen.

family violence The use of physical force by one family member against another, with the intent to injure or otherwise cause harm.

fat density The percentage of a food's total calories that are derived from fat; above 30 percent reflects higher fat density.

FDA Schedule 1 A list of drugs that have a high potential for abuse but no medical use.

fecal coliform bacteria A category of bacteria that live within the intestines of warm-blooded animals; the presence of these bacteria is used as an indicator that water has been contaminated by feces.

fellatio (feh **lay** she oh) Oral stimulation of the penis.

fermentation A chemical process whereby plant products are converted into alcohol by the action of yeast cells on carbohydrate materials.

fertility The ability to reproduce.

fetal alcohol syndrome (FAS) Characteristic birth defects noted in the children of some women who consume alcohol during their pregnancies.

fetus Developmental stage from the beginning of the ninth week after conception until birth.

fiber The plant material that cannot be digested; found in cereal, fruits, and vegetables.

fight or flight response The physiological reaction to a stressor that prepares the body for confrontation or avoidance.

fistula A fissure, break, or hole in the wall of an organ.

flaccid (fla sid) Nonerect; the state of erectile tissue when vasocongestion is not occurring.

flexibility The ability of joints to function through an intended range of motion.

follicle-stimulating hormone (FSH) A gonadotropic hormone required for initial development of ova (in the female) and sperm (in the male).

food allergy A reaction in which the immune system attacks an otherwise harmless food or ingredient; allergic reactions can range from mildly unpleasant to life-threatening.

food intolerance An adverse reaction to a specific food that does not involve the immune system; usually caused by an enzyme deficiency.

foreplay Activities, often involving touching and caressing, that prepare individuals for sexual intercourse.

formaldehyde A chemical widely used in glues, adhesives, paints, and numerous household products; also a by-product of combustion. Readily evaporates at room temperature; a major indoor pollutant.

frequency The number of exercise sessions per week; for aerobic fitness, 3–5 days are recommended.

full funeral services All the professional services provided by funeral directors.

functional foods Foods capable of contributing to the improvement/prevention of specific health problems.

G

Gail Score A numerical expression of the risk of developing invasive breast cancer, based on several variables such as age of first menstrual period, age at first live birth, results of previous biopsies, family history of breast cancer, and others. A score of 1.66% reflects a high level of risk.

gait Pattern of walking.

gaseous phase The portion of tobacco smoke containing carbon monoxide and many other physiologically active gaseous compounds.

gateway drug An easily obtainable legal or illegal drug that represents a user's first experience with a mind-altering drug; this drug can serve as the "gateway" to the use of other drugs.

gender General term reflecting a biological basis of sexuality; the male gender or the female gender.

gender adoption The long process of learning the behavior that is traditional for one's gender.

gender identification Achievement of a personally satisfying interpretation of one's masculinity or femininity.

gender identity Recognition of one's gender.

gender preference Emotional and intellectual acceptance of one's own gender.

general adaptation syndrome (GAS) Sequenced physiological responses to the presence of a stressor, involving the alarm, resistance, and exhaustion stages of the stress response.

generalized anxiety disorder (GAD) An anxiety disorder that involves experiencing intense and nonspecific anxiety for at least six months, in which the intensity and frequency of worry is excessive and out of proportion to the situation.

gene replacement therapy An experimental therapy in which a healthy human gene is incorporated into a harmless virus to be delivered to cells that have an abnormal version of the gene.

generic name Common or nonproprietary name of a drug.

green space Areas of land that are dominated by domesticated or natural vegetation, including rural farmland, city lawns and parks, and nature preserves.

greenhouse gases A category of gases in the atmosphere that allow solar radiation to pass through the atmosphere to the Earth, but then trap the heat that is radiated from the Earth back toward space; greenhouse gases include water vapor, carbon dioxide, methane, nitrous oxide, and tropospheric ozone.

H

hallucinogens Psychoactive drugs capable of producing hallucinations (distortions of reality).

health A reflection of one's ability to use the *intrinsic* and *extrinsic* resources related to each dimension of our holistic makeup to participate fully in the activities that contribute to growth and development,

with the goal of feeling a sense of well-being as one evaluates one's progress through life.

health claims Statements authorized by the FDA as having scientific proof of claims that a food, nutrient, or dietary supplement has an effect on a health-related condition.

health promotion A movement in which knowledge, practices, and values are transmitted to people for use in lengthening their lives, reducing the incidence of illness, and feeling better.

herbalism An ancient form of healing in which herbal preparations are used to treat illness and disease.

high-density lipoprotein (HDL) The type of lipoprotein that transports cholesterol from the bloodstream to the liver, where it is eventually removed from the body; high levels of HDL are related to a reduction in heart disease.

high-risk health behavior A behavioral pattern, such as smoking, associated with a high risk of developing a chronic illness.

high sensitivity C-reactive protein (hsCRP) A chemical compound found in the blood that is associated with inflammation; high levels are related to increased risk of coronary heart disease.

holistic health A view of health in terms of its physical, emotional, social, intellectual, spiritual, and occupational makeup.

homeopathy (hoe mee **op** ah the) The use of minute doses of herbs, minerals, or other substances to stimulate healing.

homicide The intentional taking of one person's life by another person.

homocysteine An amino acid found in the bloodstream; high levels of homocysteine are thought to be related to an increased risk of coronary heart disease.

hormone replacement therapy (HRT) Medically administered hormones to replace hormones lost as the result of menopause; also called postmenopausal hormone therapy (PHT).

hospice care (**hos** pis) An approach to caring for terminally ill patients that maximizes the quality of life and allows death with dignity.

host negligence A legal term that reflects the failure of a host to provide reasonable care and safety for people visiting the host's residence or business.

hot flashes Unpleasant, temporary feelings of warmth experienced by women during and after menopause, caused by blood vessel dilation.

human cloning The replication of a human being.

humanistic therapy A treatment approach based on the belief that people, left to their own devices, will naturally grow in positive and constructive ways.

human papillomavirus (HPV) Sexually transmitted viruses, some of which are capable of causing precancerous changes in the cervix; causative agent for genital warts.

humoral immunity Immunity responsible for the production of critically important immune system elements known as *antibodies;* also called *B cell–mediated immunity.*

hydrostatic weighing Weighing the body while it is submerged in water.

hypercellular obesity A form of obesity that results from having an abnormally high number of fat cells.

hyperglycemia The condition of having an abnormally high blood glucose level.

hypertonic saline solution A salt solution with a concentration higher than that found in human fluids.

hypertrophic obesity A form of obesity in which there is a normal number of fat cells, but the individual fat cells are enlarged.

hypervitaminosis Excessive accumulation of vitamins within the body; associated with the fat-soluble vitamins.

hypoglycemia The condition of having an abnormally low blood glucose level.

hypothyroidism A condition in which the thyroid gland produces an insufficient amount of the hormone thyroxin.

hypoxia Oxygenation deprivation at the cellular level.

I

identity theft A crime involving the fraudulent use of a person's name, Social Security number, credit line, or other personal, financial, or identifying information.

immune system The system of cellular chemical elements that protects the body from invading pathogens, abnormal cells, and foreign proteins.

indirect (passive) euthanasia Allowing people to die without the use of life-sustaining procedures.

indoor air quality Characteristics of air within homes, workplaces, and public buildings, including the presence and

amount of oxygen, water vapor, and a wide range of substances that can have adverse effects on your health.

infatuation A relatively temporary, intensely romantic attraction to another person.

inhalants Psychoactive drugs that enter the body through inhalation.

inhibitions Inner controls that prevent a person from engaging in certain types of behavior.

insulin A hormone produced by the islet cells of the pancreas that is necessary for the normal utilization of glucose.

intensity The level of effort put into an activity; for aerobic fitness, 40 to 85 percent of heart rate range is recommended.

intentional injuries Injuries that are purposefully inflicted either by the victim or by another person.

interstitial cell stimulating hormone (ICSH) (in ter **stish ul**) A gonadotropic hormone of the male required for the production of testosterone.

intervention An organized process that involves encouraging a chemically addicted individual to enter into drug treatment; usually coordinated by family and friends along with a mental health professional.

intimacy Any close, mutual, verbal, or nonverbal behavior within a relationship.

intimate partner violence Violence committed against a person by a current or former spouse, date, or cohabiting partner.

intoxication Dysfunctional and disruptive changes in physiological and psychological functioning, mood, and cognitive processes, resulting from the consumption of a psychoactive substance.

intrapsychic stressors Our internal worries, self-criticisms, and negative self-talk.

intrauterine device (IUD) A small, plastic, medicated or unmedicated contraceptive device that prevents pregnancy when inserted in the uterus.

in vitro Outside the living body, in an artificial environment.

ionizing radiation Electromagnetic radiation that is capable of breaking chemical bonds, such as X-rays and gamma rays.

isokinetic exercises (eye so kin **et** ick) Muscular strength training exercises in which machines are used to provide variable resistances throughout the full range of motion at a fixed speed.

isometric exercises (eye so **met** rick) Muscular strength training exercises in which

the resistance is so great that the object cannot be moved.

isotonic resistance exercises Muscular strength training exercises in which traditional barbells and dumbbells are used.

L

learned helplessness A theory of motivation explaining how individuals can learn to feel powerless, trapped, and defeated.

learned optimism An attribution style regarding permanence, pervasiveness, and personalization; how people explain both positive and negative events in their lives, accounting for success and failure.

living will A legal document that requires physicians or family members to carry out a person's wishes to die naturally, without receiving life-sustaining treatments.

low-density lipoprotein (LDL) The type of lipoprotein that transports the largest amount of cholesterol in the bloodstream; high levels of LDL are related to heart disease.

lumpectomy A surgical treatment for breast cancer in which a minimal amount of breast tissue is removed; when appropriate, this procedure is an alternative to mastectomy, in which the entire breast and underlying tissue are removed.

luteinizing hormone (LH) (**loo** ten eye zing) A gonadotropic hormone of the female required for fullest development and release of ova; ovulating hormone.

Lyme disease A bacterial infection transmitted by deer ticks.

M

magnetic resonance imaging (MRI) scan An imaging procedure that uses a powerful magnet to generate an image of body tissue.

mainstream smoke Smoke inhaled and then exhaled by a smoker.

mania An extremely excitable state characterized by excessive energy, racing thoughts, impulsive and/or reckless behavior, irritability, and being prone to distraction.

manual vacuum aspiration (MVA) An abortion procedure performed in the earliest weeks after a pregnancy is established.

masturbation Self-stimulation of the genitals.

mausoleum (moz oh **lee** um) An above-ground structure, which frequently resembles a small stone house, into which caskets can be placed for disposition.

medical abortion An abortion caused by the use of prescribed drugs.

memorial service A broad term for a ceremony that honors the life of a person who has died.

menopause The decline and eventual cessation of hormone production by the female reproductive system.

metabolism The chemical process by which substances are broken down or synthesized in a living organism to provide energy for life.

metaneeds Secondary concerns, such as spirituality, creativity, curiosity, beauty, philosophy, and justice, that can be addressed only after the basic needs are met.

metastasis (muh **tas** ta sis) The spread of cancerous cells from their site of origin to other areas of the body.

minipills Low-dose progesterone (progestin) oral contraceptives.

misuse The inappropriate use of legal drugs intended to be medications.

modeling The process of adopting the behavioral patterns of a person one admires or has bonds with.

monogamous (mo **nog** a mus) Paired relationship with one partner.

mononucleosis ("mono") A viral infection characterized by weakness, fatigue, swollen glands, sore throat, and low-grade fever.

morbidity Pertaining to illness and disease.

mortality Pertaining to death.

mucus Clear, sticky material produced by specialized cells within the mucous membranes of the body; mucus traps much of the suspended particulate matter within tobacco smoke.

multifactorial Requiring the interplay of many factors; refers to the cause of a disease or condition.

multiorgasmic capacity The potential to have several orgasms within a single period of sexual arousal.

murmur An atypical heart sound that suggests a backflow of blood into a chamber of the heart from which it has just left.

muscular endurance The aspect of muscular fitness that deals with the ability of a muscle or muscle group to repeatedly contract over a long period of time.

muscular fitness The ability of skeletal muscles to perform contractions; includes muscular strength and muscular endurance.

muscular strength The component of muscular fitness that deals with the ability to contract skeletal muscles to a maximal level; the maximal force that a muscle can exert.

mutual monogamy A pattern of dating in which a person is involved exclusively with one partner.

myocardial infarction Heart attack; the death of heart muscle as a result of a blockage in one or more of the coronary arteries.

N

narcolepsy A sleep-related disorder in which a person has a recurrent, overwhelming, and uncontrollable desire to sleep, often at inappropriate times.

narcotics Opiates; psychoactive drugs derived from the Oriental poppy plant. Narcotics relieve pain and induce sleep.

naturally acquired immunity (NAI) A type of acquired immunity resulting from the body's response to naturally occurring pathogens.

nature The innate factors that genetically determine personality traits.

naturopathy (na chur **op** ah thee) A system of treatment that avoids drugs and surgery and emphasizes the use of natural agents, such as sunshine, to correct underlying imbalances.

negative caloric balance Caloric intake is less than caloric expenditure, resulting in weight loss.

neuron A nerve cell.

neurotransmitters Chemical messengers that transfer electrical impulses across the synapses between nerve cells.

niche A recessed area in a mausoleum where a casket can be placed.

nicotine A physiologically active, dependence-producing drug found in tobacco.

nocturnal emission Ejaculation that occurs during sleep; "wet dream."

nomogram A graphic means of finding an unknown value.

nonionizing radiation Electromagnetic radiation that cannot break chemical bonds, but may excite electrons (ultraviolet radiation) or heat biological materials.

nontraditional-age students An administrative term used by colleges and universities for students who, for whatever reason,

are pursuing undergraduate work at an age other than that associated with traditional college years (18–24).

norepinephrine (nor epp in **eff** rin) An adrenaline-like neurotransmitter produced within the nervous system.

nurture The effect that the environment, people, and external factors have on personality.

nutrient-dense foods Foods that provide substantial amounts of vitamins and minerals and comparatively few calories.

nutrients Elements in foods that are required for the growth, repair, and regulation of body processes.

O

obesity A condition in which a person's body weight is 20 percent or more above desirable weight as determined by standard height/weight charts.

obsessive-compulsive disorder An anxiety disorder characterized by obsessions (intrusive thoughts, images, or impulses causing a great deal of distress) and compulsions (repetitive behaviors aimed at reducing anxiety or stress that is associated with the obsessive thoughts).

oncogenes Faulty regulatory genes that are believed to activate the development of cancer.

oral contraceptive pill A pill taken orally, composed of synthetic female hormones that prevent ovulation or implantation; "the pill."

orgasmic platform Expanded outer third of the vagina, which grips the penis during sexual intercourse.

orgasmic stage Third stage of the sexual response pattern; the stage during which neuromuscular tension is released.

osteoarthritis Arthritis that develops with age; largely caused by weight bearing and deterioration of the joints.

osteopathy (os tee **op** ah thee) A system of medical practice in which allopathic principles are combined with specific attention to postural mechanics of the body.

osteoporosis Decrease in bone mass that leads to increased incidence of fractures, primarily in postmenopausal women.

outercourse Sexual activity that does not involve intercourse.

overload principle The principle whereby a person increases the resistance load to levels above which he or she is normally accustomed to; this principle also applies to other types of fitness training.

overweight A condition in which a person's excess fat accumulation results in a body weight that exceeds desirable weight by 1–19 percent.

ovolactovegetarian diet (oh voe **lack** toe veg a **ter** ee in) A diet that excludes all meat but does allow the consumption of eggs and dairy products.

ovulation The release of a mature egg from the ovary.

oxidation The process that removes alcohol from the bloodstream.

P

pandemic An epidemic that has crossed national boundaries, thus achieving regional or international status (HIV/AIDS, avian flu, and novel H1N1 are pandemics).

panic disorder An anxiety disorder characterized by panic attacks, in which individuals experience severe physical symptoms. These episodes can seemingly occur "out of the blue" or because of some trigger, and can last for a few minutes or for hours.

Pap test A cancer screening procedure in which cells are removed from the cervix and examined for precancerous changes.

particulate phase The portion of tobacco smoke composed of small suspended particles.

passively acquired immunity (PAI) A temporary immunity achieved by providing extrinsic antibodies to a person exposed to a particular pathogen.

pathogen A disease-causing agent.

pelvic inflammatory disease (PID) An acute or chronic infection of the peritoneum, or lining of the abdominopelvic cavity, and fallopian tubes; associated with a variety of symptoms or none at all and a potential cause of sterility.

percutaneous coronary intervention (PCI) Any of a group of procedures used to treat patients suffering from an obstruction in an artery; typically involves inserting a slender balloon-tipped tube into an artery of the heart.

perfectionism A tendency to expect perfection in everything one does, with little tolerance for mistakes.

perineum In the female, the region between the vulva and the anus.

periodic abstinence Birth control methods that rely on a couple's avoidance of

intercourse during the ovulatory phase of a woman's menstrual cycle; also called *fertility awareness* or *natural family planning*.

periodontal disease Destruction of soft tissue and bone that surround the teeth.

peripheral artery disease (PAD) Atherosclerotic blockages that occur in arteries that supply blood to the legs and arms.

peritonitis (pare it ton **eye** tis) Inflammation of the peritoneum, or lining of the abdominopelvic cavity.

permanence The first dimension of an individual's attribution style, related to whether certain events are perceived as temporary or long lasting.

personality A specific set of consistent patterns of behavior and traits that helps to identify and characterize an individual; personality comprises thoughts, feelings, behaviors, motivation, instinct, and temperament.

personalization The final dimension of attribution style, related to whether an individual takes things personally or is more balanced in accepting responsibility for positive and negative events.

pervasiveness The second dimension of an individual's attribution style, related to whether events are perceived as specific or general.

pesco-vegetarian diet A vegetarian diet that includes fish, dairy products, and eggs along with plant foods.

phenylpropanolamine (PPA) (**fen** ill **pro** pa **nol** ah **meen**) The active chemical compound found in some over-the-counter diet products and associated with increased risk of stroke.

physical activity Any bodily movement produced by skeletal muscles that results in energy expenditure (Casperson et al., 1985).

physical fitness A set of attributes that people have or achieve that relates to the ability to perform physical activity (Casperson et al., 1985).

phytochemicals Physiologically active components of foods that are believed to deactivate carcinogens and to function as antioxidants.

placebo pills (pla **see** bo) Pills that contain no active ingredients.

placenta The structure through which nutrients, metabolic wastes, and drugs (including alcohol) pass from the bloodstream of the mother into the bloodstream of the developing fetus.

plateau stage Second stage of the sexual response pattern; a leveling off of arousal immediately before orgasm.

platelet adhesiveness The tendency of platelets to clump together, thus enhancing the speed at which the blood clots.

platonic Close association between two people that does not include a sexual relationship.

polycyclic aromatic hydrocarbons (PAHs) Air pollutants from fossil fuel combustion.

positive caloric balance Caloric intake greater than caloric expenditure, resulting in weight gain.

postmenopausal hormone therapy (PHT) Medically administered hormones to replace hormones lost as the result of menopause; also called hormone replacement therapy (HRT).

postpartum The period after the birth of a baby during which the uterus returns to its prepregnancy size.

postpartum depression A form of depression that affects women in the weeks and months following childbirth.

posttraumatic stress disorder An anxiety disorder that sometimes develops following exposure to an extreme stressor involving threat of death or serious injury. Symptoms include recurrent and distressing thoughts or nightmares about the event, emotional numbness, feelings of detachment, sleep disturbance, hypervigilance, and irritability.

potentiated effect A phenomenon whereby the use of one drug intensifies the effect of a second drug.

preventive or prospective medicine Physician-centered medical care in which areas of risk for chronic illnesses are identified so that they might be lowered.

primary care health providers Health care providers who generally see patients on a routine basis, particularly for preventive health care.

primary prevention Measures intended to deter first-time drug use.

probiotics Living bacteria ("good bugs") that help prevent disease and strengthen the immune system.

problem drinking An alcohol use pattern in which a drinker's behavior creates personal difficulties or difficulties for other people.

process addictions Addictions in which people compulsively engage in behaviors such as gambling, shopping, gaming, or sexual activity to such an extreme degree that these addictions can cause serious financial, emotional, social, and health problems similar to those caused by drug and alcohol addictions.

Prochaska's Transtheoretical Model of Health Behavior Change Six predictable stages—precontemplation, contemplation, preparation, action, maintenance, and termination—people go through in establishing new habits and patterns of behavior.

procrastination A tendency to put off completing tasks until some later time, sometimes resulting in increased stress.

procreation Reproduction.

prophylactic mastectomy Surgical removal of the breasts to prevent breast cancer in women who are at high risk of developing the disease.

prophylactic oophorectomy Surgical removal of the ovaries to prevent ovarian cancer in women at high risk of developing the disease.

prostate-specific antigen (PSA) test A blood test used to identify prostate-specific antigen, an early indicator that the immune system has recognized and mounted a defense against prostate cancer.

proteins Compounds composed of chains of amino acids; primary components of muscle and connective tissue.

proto-oncogenes (pro toe **on** co genes) Normal regulatory genes that may become oncogenes.

psychiatrist A medical doctor with specialized training in the diagnosis and treatment of psychological disorders through the use of biological and medical interventions.

psychoactive drug Any substance capable of altering feelings, moods, or perceptions.

psychological dependence Craving a drug for emotional reasons and to maintain a sense of well-being; also called *habituation*.

psychological health A broadly based concept pertaining to cognitive functioning in conjunction with the way people express their emotions, cope with stress, adversity, and success, and adapt to changes in themselves and their environment.

psychologist A doctoral-level practitioner with specialized training in the diagnosis and treatment of psychological disorders through the use of psychotherapy.

psychosocial sexuality Masculine and feminine aspects of sexuality.

pulmonary emphysema An irreversible disease process in which the alveoli are destroyed.

purging Using vomiting, laxatives, diuretics, enemas, or other medications, or means such as excessive exercise or fasting to eliminate food.

Q

quack A person who earns money by purposely marketing inaccurate health information, unreliable health care, or ineffective health products.

quackery The practice of disseminating or supplying inaccurate health information, unreliable health care, or ineffective health products for the purposes of defrauding another person.

R

radon A naturally occurring radioactive gas that is emitted during the decay of uranium in soil, rock, and water.

recessive inheritance pattern The inheritance of traits whose expression requires that they be carried by both biological parents.

Recommended Dietary Allowance (RDA) The dietary intake level sufficient to meet the nutrient requirements of nearly all individuals in an age- and gender-specific group.

refractory phase That portion of the male's resolution stage during which sexual arousal cannot occur.

regulatory genes Genes that control cell specialization replication, DNA repair, and tumor suppression.

resistance stage The second stage of the stress response, during which the body attempts to reestablish its equilibrium, or internal balance.

resolution stage Fourth stage of the sexual response pattern; the return of the body to a preexcitement state.

retinal hemorrhage Uncontrolled bleeding from arteries within the eye's retina.

rheumatic heart disease Chronic damage to the heart (especially the heart valves) resulting from a streptococcal infection within the heart; a complication of rheumatic fever.

risk factor A biomedical index such as serum cholesterol level or a behavioral pattern such as smoking associated with a chronic illness.

S

salt sensitive Term used to describe people whose bodies overreact to the presence of sodium by retaining fluid, thus increasing blood pressure.

sarcopenia A reduction in the size of muscle fibers, related to the aging process.

satiety (suh **tie** uh tee) The feeling of no longer being hungry; a diminished desire to eat.

saturated fats Fats that promote cholesterol formation; they are in solid form at room temperature; primarily animal fats.

schizophrenia One of the most severe mental disorders, characterized by profound distortions in one's thought processes, emotions, perceptions, and behavior. Symptoms may include hallucinations, delusions, disorganized thinking, and/or maintaining a rigid posture and not moving for hours.

sclerotic changes (skluh **rot** ick) Thickening or hardening of tissues.

seasonal affective disorder (SAD) A type of depression that develops in relation to the changes in the seasons.

secondary prevention Measures aimed at early detection, intervention, and treatment of drug abuse before severe physical, psychological, emotional, or social consequences can occur.

secondary virginity The discontinuation of sexual intercourse after initial exploration.

self-actualization The highest level of psychological health, at which one reaches his or her highest potential and values truth, beauty, goodness, faith, love, humor, and ingenuity.

self-antigens The cells and tissues that stimulate the immune system's autoimmune response.

self-care movement The trend toward individuals taking increased responsibility for prevention or management of certain health conditions.

self-concept An individual's internal picture of himself or herself; the way one sees oneself.

self-esteem An individual's sense of pride, self-respect, value, and worth.

self-fulfilling prophecy The tendency to inadvertently make something more likely to happen as a result of one's own expectations and attitudes.

semen A secretion containing sperm and nutrients discharged from the urethra at ejaculation.

semivegetarian diet Also called "flexitarian," a diet that significantly reduces but does not eliminate meat consumption and allows consumption of dairy products and eggs.

serial monogamy A pattern of dating in which a person is involved in a series of exclusive relationships, one after the other.

set point A genetically programmed range of body weight, beyond which a person finds it difficult to gain or lose additional weight.

sex chromosomes The X and Y chromosomes that determine sex; chromosomes other than the autosomes.

sex flush The reddish skin response that results from increasing sexual arousal.

sexual fantasies Fantasies with sexual themes; sexual daydreams or imaginary events.

sexually transmitted diseases (STDs) Infectious diseases that are spread primarily through intimate sexual contact.

shingles Painful fluid-filled skin eruptions along underlying sensory nerve pathways—caused by reactivation of once-sequestered herpes zoster (chicken pox) viruses.

shock The profound collapse of many vital body functions; evident during acute alcohol intoxication and other serious health emergencies.

sidestream smoke Smoke that comes from the burning end of a cigarette, pipe, or cigar.

sigmoidoscopy Examination of the sigmoid colon (lowest section of the large intestine), using a short, flexible fiberoptic scope.

skinfold measurement A measurement to determine the thickness of the fat layer that lies immediately beneath the skin; used to calculate body composition.

sleep apnea A condition in which abnormalities in the structure of the airways lead to periods of greatly restricted air flow during sleep, resulting in reduced levels of blood oxygen and placing greater strain on the heart to maintain adequate tissue oxygenation.

smegma Cellular discharge that can accumulate beneath the clitoral hood or the foreskin of an uncircumcised penis.

social phobia A phobia characterized by feelings of extreme dread and embarrassment in situations in which public speaking or social interaction is involved.

social worker A professional with a master's degree in social work. Social workers provide both mental health and social services to the community and are the largest group of professionals to provide psychological services.

solid waste Pollutants that are in solid form, including nonhazardous household trash, industrial wastes, mining wastes, and sewage sludge from wastewater treatment plants.

solution-focused therapy A goal-oriented approach that helps clients change by looking for solutions rather than dwelling on problems.

specific phobia An excessive and unreasonable fear about a particular situation or object that causes anxiety and distress and interferes with a person's functioning.

spermatogenesis (sper mat oh **jen** uh sis) The process of sperm production.

spermicides Chemicals capable of killing sperm.

spontaneous abortion Any cessation of pregnancy resulting from natural causes; also called a *miscarriage.*

stalking Repeated visual or physical proximity, nonconsensual communication, or threats that would cause fear in a reasonable person.

static stretching The slow lengthening of a muscle group to an extended stretch; followed by a holding of the extended position for 15 to 60 seconds.

stem cells Premature (pluripotent) cells that have the potential to turn into any kind of body cell.

stent A device inserted inside a coronary artery during a percutaneous coronary intervention (PCI) to prevent the artery from narrowing at this site.

sterilization Generally permanent birth control techniques that surgically disrupt the normal passage of ova or sperm.

stimulants Psychoactive drugs that stimulate the function of the central nervous system.

stress The physiological and psychological state of disruption caused by the presence of an unanticipated, disruptive, or stimulating event.

stressors Factors or events, real or imagined, that elicit a state of stress.

stress response The physiological and psychological responses to positive or negative events that are disruptive, unexpected, or stimulating.

synapse (**sinn** aps) The location at which an electrical impulse from one neuron is transmitted to an adjacent neuron; also referred to as a *synaptic junction.*

synergistic effect A heightened, exaggerated effect produced by the concurrent use of two or more drugs.

synesthesia A sensation of combining of the senses, such as perceiving color by hearing or perceiving taste by touching it.

systemic (sis **tem** ic) Distributed or occurring throughout the entire body system.

systolic pressure (sis **tol** ick) The blood pressure against blood vessel walls when the heart contracts.

T

tachycardia Excessively rapid heartbeat, as evidenced by a resting pulse rate of greater than 100 beats per minute.

tar A chemically rich, syrupy, blackish-brown material obtained from the particulate matter within cigarette smoke when nicotine and water are removed.

target heart rate (THR) The number of times per minute the heart must contract to produce a cardiorespiratory training effect.

teratogenic agent Any substance that is capable of causing birth defects.

terrorism Any actions intended to harm or kill civilians in order to intimidate a populace or force a government to take some action.

tertiary prevention Treatment and rehabilitation of drug-dependent people to limit physical, psychological, emotional, and social deterioration or prevent death.

test anxiety A form of performance anxiety that generates extreme feelings of distress in exam situations.

therapeutic cloning The use of certain human replication techniques to reproduce body tissues and organs.

thermic effect of food (TEF) The amount of energy our bodies require for the digestion, absorption, and transportation of food.

thorax The chest; the portion of the torso above the diaphragm and within the rib cage.

threshold dose The smallest amount of a drug to have an observable effect on the body.

titration (tie **tray** shun) The particular level of a drug within the body; adjusting the level of nicotine by adjusting the rate of smoking.

tolerable upper intake level (UL) The maximum level of daily nutrient intake that is unlikely to pose risks of adverse health effects for almost all of the individuals in the group for whom it is designed.

tolerance An acquired reaction to a drug in which the continued intake of the same dose has diminished effects.

toxic pollutants Substances known to cause cancer or other serious health effects.

toxic shock syndrome (TSS) A potentially fatal condition caused by the proliferation of certain bacteria in the vagina whose toxins enter the general blood circulation.

trace elements Minerals whose presence in the body occurs in very small amounts; micronutrient elements.

traditional-age students College students between the ages of 18 and 24.

transcervical balloon tuboplasty The use of inflatable balloon catheters to open blocked fallopian tubes; a procedure used for some women with fertility problems.

trans-fatty acid An altered form of an unsaturated fat molecule in which the hydrogen atoms on each side of the double bond(s) are on opposite sides. Also called *trans fat*.

transgendered Refers to persons whose appearance and behaviors do not conform to society's traditional gender role expectations.

transient ischemic attack (TIA) (**tran** see ent iss **key** mick) Strokelike symptoms caused by the temporary spasm of cerebral blood vessels.

transsexualism A sexual variation in which a person rejects his or her biological sexuality.

transvestism Atypical behavior in which a person derives sexual pleasure from dressing in the clothes of the opposite gender.

trimester A three-month period; human pregnancies encompass three trimesters.

tropospheric ozone Ozone is composed of three oxygen atoms that are bound into a single molecule. Tropospheric ozone refers to this substance as it occurs in the lower layer of the atmosphere, close to the ground.

tumor Mass of cells; may be cancerous (malignant) or noncancerous (benign).

type A personality A personality type that tends to be competitive, ambitious, and impatient; often associated with heart attacks and other stress-related conditions.

type B personality A personality type that tends to be more relaxed and patient.

U

underweight A condition in which the body is below the desirable weight.

unintentional injuries Injuries that have occurred without anyone's intending that harm be done.

urethra (yoo **ree** thra) The passageway through which urine leaves the urinary bladder.

V

vasectomy A surgical procedure in which the vasa deferens are cut to prevent the passage of sperm from the testicles; the most common form of male sterilization.

vegan vegetarian diet (**vee** gun *or* **vay** gun) A vegetarian diet that excludes the consumption of all animal products, including eggs and dairy products.

virulent (**veer** yuh lent) Capable of causing disease.

vitamins Organic compounds that facilitate the action of enzymes.

volatile organic compounds (VOCs) A wide variety of chemicals that contain carbon and readily evaporate into the air.

W

wellness A process intended to aid individuals in unlocking their full potential through the development of an overall wellness lifestyle.

Wernicke-Korsakoff syndrome A syndrome that results from vitamin B_1 deficiency, often as the result of alcoholism. Symptoms include impaired short-term memory, psychosis, impaired coordination, and abnormal eye movements.

withdrawal (coitus interruptus) (**co** ih tus in ter **rup** tus) A contraceptive practice in which the erect penis is removed from the vagina before ejaculation.

withdrawal illness An uncomfortable, perhaps toxic response of the body as it attempts to maintain homeostasis in the absence of a drug; also called *abstinence syndrome*.

X

xenotransplant A transplant of tissue from an animal, such as a pig, to a human recipient.

Y

Yerkes-Dodson Law A bell-shaped curve demonstrating that there is an optimal level of stress for peak performance; this law states that too little or too much stress is not helpful, whereas a moderate level of stress is positive and beneficial.

young adult years The segment of the life cycle from ages 18 to 24; a transitional period between adolescence and adulthood.

Z

zero-tolerance laws Laws that severely restrict the right to operate motor vehicles for underage drinkers who have been convicted of driving under the influence of alcohol or any other drug.

zygote A fertilized ovum.

Chapter 1

Page 1, 3: © BananaStock/JupiterImages; **6:** © Colin Paterson/Getty Images; **10:** U.S. Air Force photo by Tech. Sgt. Mark Borosch; **13:** © The McGraw-Hill Companies, Inc./Gary He, photographer; **16:** © Brand X Pictures/PunchStock; **17:** © Comstock/JupiterImages.

Chapter 2

Page 32: © Javier Pierini/Getty Images; **38:** Royalty-Free/Corbis; **40:** © BananaStock/JupiterImages; **49:** © The McGraw-Hill Companies, Inc./Gary He, photographer; **54:** © Comstock/JupiterImages.

Chapter 3

Page 60: © Image Source/JupiterImages; **65:** © The McGraw-Hill Companies, Inc./Gary He, photographer; **70:** © The McGraw-Hill Companies, Inc./Andrew Resek, photographer; **78:** © JupiterImages; **79:** © Royalty-Free/Corbis.

Chapter 4

Page 88: © Thinkstock Images/JupiterImages; **93:** © The McGraw-Hill Companies, Inc./Gary He, photographer; **96 all:** Courtesy of Leonard Kaminsky; **100:** © The McGraw-Hill Companies, Inc./Andrew Resek, photographer; **104:** © The McGraw-Hill Companies, Inc./Lars A. Niki, photographer; **112, 113 all:** Courtesy Stewart Halperin.

Chapter 5

Page 114: © Royalty-Free/Corbis; **118:** © The McGraw-Hill Companies, Inc./Andrew Resek, photographer; **129:** © Royalty-Free/Corbis; **131:** © RubberBall Production/Getty Images; **135:** © Mitch Hrdlicka/Getty Images; **146:** © UpperCut Images/Getty Images.

Chapter 6

Page 151: © Royalty-Free/Corbis; **154:** © The McGraw-Hill Companies, Inc./John Flournoy, photographer; **157:** Photo courtesy of Life Measurement, Inc., Concord, CA; **162:** © The McGraw-Hill Companies, Inc./Lars A. Niki, photographer; **165 left:** © The McGraw-Hill Companies, Inc./John Flournoy, photographer; **165 right:** © Royalty-Free/Corbis; **172:** © The McGraw-Hill Companies, Inc./Jill Braaten, photographer; **176:** BananaStock/PunchStock.

Chapter 7

Page 186: © Royalty-Free/Corbis; **187:** © The McGraw-Hill Companies, Inc./Gary He, photographer; **190 top and bottom:** © The McGraw-Hill Companies, Inc./Gary He, photographer; **190 middle:** © Royalty-Free/Corbis; **193:** © BananaStock/PunchStock; **200:** © U.S. Drug Enforcement Administration; **204:** © BananaStock/PunchStock.

Chapter 8

Page 212: © Imagestate Media (John Foxx)/Imagestate; **213:** © Royalty-Free/Corbis; **217:** © The McGraw-Hill Companies, Inc./Jill Braaten, photographer; **223:** Courtesy Mothers Against Drunk Driving; **227:** © D. Falconer/PhotoLink/Getty Images.

Chapter 9

Page 236: © PhotoAlto/JupiterImages; **241:** © The McGraw-Hill Companies, Inc./Gary He, photographer; **244:** © BananaStock/PunchStock; **252 both:** Courtesy of Wayne Jackson; **253:** © The McGraw-Hill Companies, Inc./Christopher Kerrigan, photographer; **254:** © 1998 Copyright IMS Communications Ltd./Capstone Design. All Rights Reserved; **255:** © National Cancer Institute; **256:** © Sarah Hill; **259:** © Royalty-Free/Corbis; **264:** © Stockbyte/JupiterImages.

Chapter 10

Page 270: © Stockdisc/PunchStock; **275:** © BananaStock/PunchStock; **281 top:** © Keith Brofsky/Getty Images; **281 bottom:** © The McGraw-Hill Companies, Inc./Rick Brady, photographer.

Chapter 11

Page 294: Photo provided by Ball Memorial Hospital, Muncie, IN; **303 both:** © The Skin Cancer Foundation, www.skincancer.org; **305:** © Kerry-Edwards 2004, Inc./Sharon Farmer, photographer; **318 left:** © Pablo Martinez Monsivais/AFP/Getty Images; **318 right:** © National Cancer Institute/Bill Branson, photographer.

Chapter 12

Page 325: © Stockdisc/PunchStock; **329, 331, 332:** © Custom Medical Stock Photo; **345:** © Rufus F. Folkks/Corbis.

Chapter 13

Page 351: © Steve Allen/Getty Images; **363:** © PhotoAlto; **370:** © The McGraw-Hill Companies, Inc./Christopher Kerrigan, photographer; **375:** © F. Schussler/PhotoLink/Getty Images; **377:** © Steven J. Nussenblatt/Custom Medical Stock Photo; **379:** © Custom Medical Stock Photo.

Chapter 14

Page 387: © BananaStock; **391 left:** © Thinkstock/JupiterImages; **394 right:** © Brand X Pictures/JupiterImages.

Chapter 15

Page 404: © Brand X Pictures/Punchstock; **411:** © The McGraw-Hill Companies, Inc./Christopher Kerrigan, photographer; **412, 417:** © Ryan McVay/Getty Images; **419:** © Bucinna Studio/Getty Images; **420:** © Thinkstock.

Chapter 16

Page 425, 433, 435: © The McGraw-Hill Companies, Inc./Kristan Price, photographer; **436:** Courtesy Stewart Halperin; **439:** Courtesy Organon USA; **440:** © The McGraw-Hill Companies, Inc./Christopher Kerrigan, photographer.

Chapter 17

Page 447: © Liquidlibrary/JupiterImages; **449:** © E. Dygas/Getty Images; **451, 453:** © Science Photo Library/Photo Researchers; **454:** © Brand X Pictures/JupiterImages; **459:** © BananaStock/PunchStock; **462:** © The McGraw-Hill Companies, Inc./Jill Braaten, photographer.

Chapter 18

Page 467: © Image Source/JupiterImages; **469:** © Keith Brofsky/Getty Images; **476:** © Creatas/PunchStock; **480:** © The McGraw-Hill Companies, Inc./Jill Braaten, photographer; **484:** © Kent Kundson/PhotoLink/Getty Images.

Chapter 19

Page 497: © Fancy Photography/Veer; **501:** © The McGraw-Hill Companies, Inc./Jill Braaten, photographer; **506:** © Don Tremain/Getty Images; **510:** © Adam Gault/Getty Images; **514:** © Keith Thomas/Brand X Pictures/JupiterImages.

Chapter 20

Page 520: © Image 100/Corbis; **524:** © Alex L. Fradkin/Getty Images; **530:** © Kent Knudson/PhotoLink/Getty Images; **532:** © Jocelyn Augustino/FEMA; **534:** © Royalty-Free/Corbis; **538:** © Dr. Parvinder Sethi.

Chapter 21

Page 549, 552, 560: © Royalty-Free/Corbis; **564 left:** © D. Normark/PhotoLink/Getty Images; **564 right:** © Melba Photo Agency/PunchStock.

A

AA. *See* Alcoholics Anonymous
AAI. *See* artificially acquired immunity
abdominal isolation devices, 97
abdominal strength, 113
abdominoplasty, 173–174
Abdul, Paula, 178
abortion, 442–444
   pill, 440
   spontaneous, 452
   vacuum aspiration, 442–443
absorption, 213, 214
abstinence, 429–430
   periodic, 428*t*, 430, 431, 431*f*
abuse, 190–191
academic stressors, 69–71
acceptance stage, of dying, 551
accidental death, 223
accidents
   boating, 514
   from drunk driving, 222
   grief and coping with death from, 559–560
   vehicle, 509–510, 510*f*
acculturation, obesity and, 163
acetaminophen, 216, 365
Achilles tendinitis, 110*t*
acid-base balance, 120
acme stage, of infection, 355
ACNM. *See* American College of Nurse-Midwives
ACOAs. *See* adult children of alcoholics
Acomplia, 264
acquired immunity (AI), 356, 356*f*, 357
acquired immunodeficiency syndrome (AIDS). *See* HIV/AIDS
ACSM. *See* American College of Sports Medicine
ACTH. *See* adrenocorticotropic hormone theory
action stage, of Prochaska's Transtheoretical Model of Health Behavior Change, 14
active immunity, 357
activities of daily living (ADLs), 92
activity requirements, 159
acupuncture, 229–230, *476*, 476
acute alcohol intoxication, 214, 215
acute (severe) community-acquired pneumonia, 365
acute conditions, 326, 327
acute rhinitis, 361
acute stage, of infection, 355
AD. *See* Alzheimer's disease
ADA. *See* Americans with Disabilities Act (1990)
adaptive thermogenesis, 162
ADD. *See* attention deficit disorder
Adderall, 196, 197, 198
addictions, 190–191
   compulsion in, 187
   exposure in, 187
   Internet, 46
   loss of control in, 187
   nicotine, 242–243
   process, 186–187, 188
addictive behavior, 187–188
   codependence, 188
addictive effect, 203
adenocarcinoma, 298, 299*f*
adipose tissue, 158–159
ADLs. *See* activities of daily living
adolescents
   bisexuality of, 411
   gonorrhea in, 378
   HBV in, 370
   with HIV/AIDS, 371*t*

   menstruation and, 396
   smoking and, 245
   vitamin D for, 121
adoption, 461–462
   gender, 389, 390–391
adrenocorticotropic hormone theory (ACTH), 61, 64*f*, 242
adult children of alcoholics (ACOAs), 225
Adult Immunization Schedule, 359
adult stem cells, 358
adults
   CFS in, 366
   immunization recommendations for, 360*f*
   living with AIDS, 375*f*
   obesity in US, 151
   sexual partners of, 376*f*
advance health care directives, 555–556
advanced practice nurses (APNs), 480
advertising, 72. *See also* media literacy
   alcohol, 228, 229
   smoke and susceptibility to, 245
   as sources of health information, 468
   tobacco marketing, 238–240
AED. *See* automated external defibrillator
aerobic energy production, 90–91
aerobics
   anaerobic v., 90
   low-impact, 104–105
AFDC. *See* Aid to Families with Dependent Children
African Americans
   alcohol advertising and, 228
   alcohol and, 217
   cancer among, 300*t*
   color vision deficiency in, 329–330, 347
   CVD and, 273, 275
   family violence of, 503
   health insurance of, 483
   with HIV/AIDS, 371, 371*t*
   lactose intolerance in, 142
   marijuana use of, 201
   nicotine addictions of, 242
   obesity of, 151, 163
   Parkinson's disease in, 343
   physician office visits of, 8
   poverty of, 163
   sickle cell trait/disease in, 328–329, 457
   smoking cessation of, 262
   smoking patterns of, 237*t*, 253, 254
   stress coping of, 62
   substance abuse of, 194
   suicide and, 48
   uterine cancer in, 315
   victimization rate of, 500
age
   as CVD risk factor, 273
   obesity and, 158
Agency for Healthcare Research and Quality, 475
agent, 352, 353
aging. *See also* menopause
   accepting changes of, 5–6
   AD, 343, 345, 346–347, 348
   alcohol and, 217, 219
   arthritis, 142, 152, 346, 377
   caregiving, 6, 343, 482
   CVD, 275, 280
   developmental tasks, 4, 5–6
   exercise and, 101–102, 199
   health care costs, 485–486
   health concerns of, 100–101
   health screening, 280

index